Lecture Notes in Computer Science 7917

Commenced Publication in 1973
Founding and Former Series Editors:
Gerhard Goos, Juris Hartmanis, and Jan van Leeuwen

James C. Gee   Sarang Joshi
Kilian M. Pohl   William M. Wells
Lilla Zöllei (Eds.)

Information Processing in Medical Imaging

23rd International Conference, IPMI 2013
Asilomar, CA, USA, June 28–July 3, 2013
Proceedings

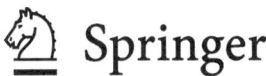 Springer

Volume Editors

James C. Gee
Kilian M. Pohl
University of Pennsylvania, Department of Radiology, Philadelphia, PA, USA
E-mail: gee@mail.med.upenn.edu; pohl.kilian@gmail.com

Sarang Joshi
University of Utah, Department of Bioengineering, Salt Lake City, UT, USA
E-mail: sjoshi@sci.utah.edu

William M. Wells
Harvard Medical School and Brigham and Women's Hospital
Department of Radiology, Boston, MA, USA
E-mail: sw@bwh.harvard.edu

Lilla Zöllei
Harvard Medical School and Massachussetts General Hospital
A.A. Martinos Center for Biomedical Imaging, Charlestown, MA, USA
E-mail: lzollei@nmr.mgh.harvard.edu

ISSN 0302-9743   e-ISSN 1611-3349
ISBN 978-3-642-38867-5   e-ISBN 978-3-642-38868-2
DOI 10.1007/978-3-642-38868-2
Springer Heidelberg Dordrecht London New York

Library of Congress Control Number: 2013939662

CR Subject Classification (1998): I.4, I.5, I.2.5-6, G.3, J.3, I.3

LNCS Sublibrary: SL 6 – Image Processing, Computer Vision, Pattern Recognition,
and Graphics

Typesetting: Camera-ready by author, data conversion by Scientific Publishing Services, Chennai, India

Printed on acid-free paper

Springer is part of Springer Science+Business Media (www.springer.com)

Preface

The 23rd International Conference on Information Processing in Medical Imaging (IPMI) was held June 28–July 3, 2013, at the Asilomar Conference Grounds near Pacific Grove, California, USA. The conference was the latest in a series of biennial scientific meetings, the last being held in July of 2011 at the Kloster Irsee in Bavaria, Germany, during which new developments in the acquisition, analysis, and use of medical images were presented. IPMI is one of the longest running conferences devoted to these topics in medical imaging. The first IPMI conference was held in 1969, when a group of young scientists working in nuclear medicine gathered to discuss the current problems in their field. Since that time the conference has expanded into other medical imaging acquisition modalities, including ultrasound, optics, magnetic resonance, and x-ray imaging techniques. IPMI is now widely recognized as one of the most exciting and influential meetings in medical imaging, with a unique emphasis on active participation from all attendees and a strong commitment to vigorous discussion and open debate.

A wide variety of topics are covered at IPMI meetings, all within a single-track format. This year 199 full-length manuscripts were submitted to the conference. Of these, 26 papers were selected for oral presentation and 38 were accepted as posters. Submissions were carefully reviewed by at least three members of the Scientific Review Committee, who evaluated the novelty, methodological development, and scientific rigor of each manuscript. The Paper Selection Committee, along with the Co-chairs, took on the difficult task of creating a meeting program. Using the rankings and detailed comments of the reviewers of each manuscript, and adding to that their own judgment of the merits of each manuscript, they designed the meeting program represented in this volume. The many high-quality manuscripts submitted for consideration made the selection process extremely difficult, and many excellent papers did not make it into the final program. This is an unfortunate inevitability of the high selectivity for which IPMI is known.

A key goal of IPMI is to encourage active participation of the most talented and promising young investigators in the field in an environment that also fosters in-depth interactions with senior researchers. To achieve this goal, all IPMI participants were involved in small study groups where they prepared for the upcoming conference presentations. After reading their assigned papers, graduate students, post-docs, and young faculty members discussed their understanding of related work in the field with senior investigators and together formulated both clarifying and probing questions for the oral presenters. The study groups thus led off the discussion of each paper, ensuring a lively and vigorous dialog. Further emphasis on the young researcher was made through the competition for the prestigious Erbsmann award. The Francois Erbsmann Prize is awarded for the best contribution by a young scientist who is the first author of a paper and a first-time IPMI oral presenter. This year 23 of the 26 oral presenters were eligible for the Erbsmann Prize.

IPMI 2013 featured a keynote talk about the current frontiers of neuroimaging by Dr. Bruce Rosen, M.D., Ph.D., Professor in Radiology at Harvard Medical School and Director of the Athinoula A. Martinos Center for Biomedical Imaging. Dr. Rosen is the recipient of numerous awards in recognition of his contributions to the field of functional MRI, including, most recently, the 2011 Outstanding Researcher award from the Radiological Society of North America (RSNA), and the Rigshospitalet's International KFJ Prize from the University of Copenhagen/Rigshospitalet. Dr. Rosen is a Fellow and Gold Medal winner for his contributions to the field of Functional MRI from the International Society for Magnetic Resonance in Medicine, a Fellow of the American Institute for Medical and Biological Engineering, and a member of the Institute of Medicine of the National Academies.

The IPMI 2013 conference featured the traditions that past IPMI attendees have come to expect as part of the unique character of the meeting. Most importantly, each oral presentation was allowed unlimited time for discussion to give the audience the opportunity to resolve all questions regarding the methods and results. IPMI discussions can go on for hours, involving virtually every attendee in the room! Session Chairs play a key role at IPMI as they strive to ensure that these extended discussions are productive and continuing to add to the group's understanding of the nature and significance of each presentation's original contribution.

IPMI is traditionally held in a small and sometimes remote location. This year's venue, the Asilomar State Beach and Conference Grounds, is a breathtaking 107 acres of ecologically diverse beachfront land that is situated within the quaint and scenic town of Pacific Grove, CA, USA.

Attendees were housed in rustic accommodations and enjoyed communal meals in a common dining hall, as well as late-night conversations at the reception, conference banquet, bonfire events, and nearby watering holes. On Tuesday afternoon, the traditional IPMI soccer match was held, pitting the American team against "the rest of the world." As you may have heard, at the last IPMI, the American team ended a prolonged losing streak, which significantly ups the ante on this long-running rivalry. At the time of this writing the outcome of the latest match is uncertain.

These proceedings contain the IPMI 2013 papers in the order they were presented at the meeting. We hope that this volume serves as a valuable source of information for the participants, as well as a reminder of the great conference experience that we had. For those who were not able to attend the conference, we hope that these proceedings provide you with an excellent summary of the latest research contributions to the medical imaging field. We look forward to the next IPMI conference, which is currently planned for 2015 on the Isle of Skye, Scotland, UK. More information will be posted on www.ipmi-conference.org as it becomes available.

July 2013   William M. Wells
                                                                                      Sarang Joshi
                                                                                      Kilian M. Pohl

Acknowledgments

The organization of the 23rd IPMI conference was only possible through the efforts and contributions of several organizations and many individuals. First of all, the IPMI 2013 Co-chairs would like to thank the members of the Scientific Review Committee for providing so many high-quality reviews within a very limited time frame; because of these reviews, we were able to make a fair selection of the best papers for the final program. We also express our gratitude to the Paper Selection Committee members, who each read many papers and their reviews and traveled to Salt Lake City for a marathon organizational meeting that resulted in an outstanding final program. We also thank previous IPMI organizers, particularly James Duncan, Jerry Prince,Horst Hahn, Stephen Pizer, and Gábor Székely, for sharing their experiences and insights with us.

We thank Trey Campbell at Brigham and Women's Hospital for his invaluable assistance in the preparation of our R13 proposal to the NIH. For expert help with our IPMI website, we are grateful to Bilwaj Gaonkar. We thank as well Jeffrey Duda and Benjamin Kandel for their essential help in preparing this proceedings volume. Thanks also to Microsoft Corporation for assistance with their excellent CMT conference management system, which we used for the automation of submissions and review of manuscripts. We also thank Jerry Prince for providing the template for this front matter.

Finally, we are grateful to the following organizations for their generous financial support:

IBM Research
Scientific Computing and Imaging Institute (SCI), University of Utah
National Institute of Biomedical Imaging and Bioengineering (NIBIB) [1]

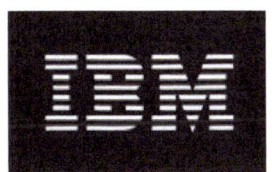  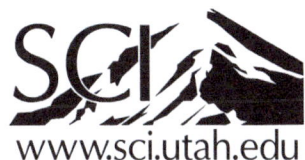

---
[1] Funding for this conference was made possible (in part) by 1R13EB 017075-01 from the National Institute of Biomedical Imaging and Bioengineering. The views expressed in written conference materials or publications and by speakers and moderators do not necessarily reflect the official policies of the Department of Health and Human Services; nor does mention of trade names, commercial practices, or organizations imply endorsement by the U.S. Government.

Francois Erbsmann Prizewinners

1987 (Utrecht, the Netherlands): **John M. Gauch**, University of North Carolina, Chapel Hill, NC, USA.
J.M. Gauch, W.R. Oliver, S.M. Pizer: Multiresolution shape descriptions and their applications in medical imaging.

1989 (Berkeley, CA, USA): **Arthur F. Gmitro**, University of Arizona, Tucson, AZ, USA.
A.F. Gmitro, V. Tresp, V. Chen, Y. Snell, G.R. Gindi: Video-rate reconstruction of CT and MR images.

1991 (Wye, Kent, UK): **H. Isil Bozma**, Yale University, New Haven, CT, USA.
H.I. Bozma, J.S. Duncan: Model-based recognition of multiple deformable objects using a game-theoretic framework.

1993 (Flagstaff, AZ, USA): **Jeffrey A. Fessler**, University of Michigan, Ann Arbor, MI, USA.
J.A. Fessler: Tomographic reconstruction using information-weighted spline smoothing.

1995 (Brest, France): **Maurits K. Konings**, University Hospital, Utrecht, The Netherlands.
M.K. Konings, W.P.T.M. Mali, M.A. Viergever: Design of a robust strategy to measure intravascular electrical impedance.

1997 (Poultney, VT, USA): **David Atkinson**, Guys Hospital, London, UK.
D. Atkinson, D.L.G. Hill, P.N.R. Stoyle, P.E. Summers, S.F. Keevil: An autofocus algorithm for the automatic correction of motion artifacts in MR images.

1999 (Visegrad, Hungary): **Liana M. Lorigo**, Massachusetts Institute of Technology, Cambridge, MA, USA.
L.M. Lorigo, O. Faugeras, W.E.L. Grimson, R. Keriven, R. Kikinis, C.-F. Westin: Co-dimension 2 geodesic active contours for MRA segmentation.

2001 (Davis, CA, USA): **Viktor K. Jirsa**, Florida Atlantic University, FL, USA.
V.K. Jirsa, K.J. Jantzen, A. Fuchs, J.A. Scott Kelso: Neural field dynamics on the folded three-dimensional cortical sheet and its forward EEG and MEG.

2003 (Ambleside, UK): **Guillaume Marrelec**, INSERM, France.
G. Marrelec, P. Ciuciu, M. Pélégrini-Issac, H. Benali: Estimation of the hemodyamic response function in event-related functional MRI: Directed acyclic graphs for a general Bayesian inference framework.

2005 (Glenwood Springs, Colorado, USA) **Duygu Tosun**, Johns Hopkins University, Baltimore, USA.
D. Tosun, J.L. Prince: Cortical surface alignment using geometry driven multi-spectral optical flow.

2007 (Kerkrade, The Netherlands) **Ben Glocker**, Technische Universität München, Garching, Germany.
B. Glocker, N. Komodakis, N. Paragios, G. Tziritas, N. Navab: Inter- and intra-modal deformable registration: Continuous deformations meet efficient optimal linear programming.

2009 (Williamsburg, Virginia, USA): **Maxime Descoteaux**, NeuroSpin, IFR 49 CEA Saclay, France.
M. Descoteaux, R. Deriche, D. Le Bihan, J.-F. Mangin, C. Poupon: Diffusion propagator imaging: Using Laplace's equation and multiple shell acquisitions to reconstruct the diffusion propagator.

2011 (Kloster Irsee, Germany): **Hubert Fonteijn**, University College London, UK.
H. Fonteijn, M. Clarkson, M. Modat, J. Barnes, M. Lehmann, S. Ourselin, N. Fox, D. Alexander: An event-based disease progression model and its application to familial Alzheimer's disease.

Organization

Conference Chairs

William M. Wells	Harvard Medical School, USA
Sarang Joshi	University of Utah, USA
Kilian M. Pohl	University of Pennsylvania, USA

Organizing Committee

James C. Gee	University of Pennsylvania, USA
Tina Kapur	Harvard Medical School, USA
Lilla Zöllei	Harvard Medical School, USA

Paper Selection Committee

Daniel Alexander	University College London, UK
James Duncan	Yale University, USA
Xavier Pennec	INRIA Sophia Antipolis, France
Lilla Zöllei	Harvard Medical School, USA

Scientific Committee

Stephen Alyward	Kitware Inc., USA
Amir Amini	University of Louisville, USA
Jeffrey Anderson	University of Utah, USA
John Ashburner	University College London, UK
Brian Avants	University of Pennsylvania, USA
Suyash Awate	University of Utah, USA
Christian Barillot	Institut de Recherche en Informatique et Systèmes Aléatoires / Centre National de la Recherche Scientifique, France
Pierre-Louis Bazin	Max Planck Institute for Human Cognitive and Brain Sciences, Germany
Faisal Beg	Simon Fraser University, Canada
Sylvain Bouix	Harvard Medical School, USA
Djamal Boukerroui	Heudiasyc, France
Michael Brady	University of Oxford, UK
M. Jorge Cardoso	University College London, UK
Owen Carmichael	University of California, Davis, USA
Gary Christensen	University of Iowa, USA
Albert Chung	The Hong Kong University of Science and Technology, Hong Kong

Ela Claridge	The University of Birmingham, UK
Louis Collins	McGill University, Canada
Tim Cootes	Manchester University, UK
Antonio Criminisi	Microsoft Research, USA
Christos Davatzikos	University of Pennsylvania, USA
Benoit Dawant	Vanderbilt University, USA
Marleen de Bruijne	Erasmus MC - University Medical Center Rotterdam, The Netherlands
Rachid Deriche	INRIA Sophia Antipolis, France
Stanely Durrleman	University of Utah, USA
Aaron Fenster	Robarts Research Institute, Western University, Canada
Thomas Fletcher	University of Utah, USA
Alejandro Frangi	University of Sheffield, UK
James Gee	University of Pennsylvania, USA
Guido Gerig	University of Utah, USA
Ben Glocker	Microsoft Research, UK
Polina Golland	Massachusetts Institute of Technology, USA
Michael Goris	Stanford University School of Medicine, USA
Matthias Guenther	Fraunhofer MEVIS, Germany
Horst Hahn	Fraunhofer MEVIS, Germany
Justin Haldar	University of Southern California, USA
Jo Hajnal	Imperial College London, UK
Ghassan Hamarneh	Simon Fraser University, Canada
Joel Hass	University of California, Davis, USA
Joachim Hornegger	University of Erlangen, Germany
Ivana Isgum	University Medical Center Utrecht, The Netherlands
Anand Joshi	University of Southern California, USA
Nico Karssemeijer	Radboud University Nijmegen Medical Centre, The Netherlands
Boklye Kim	University of Michigan, USA
Ender Konukoglu	Harvard Medical School, USA
Frithjof Kruggel	University of California, Irvine, USA
Jan Kybic	Czech Technical University, Czech Republic
Tobias Lasser	Technical University of Munich, Germany
Richard Leahy	University of Southern California, USA
Boudewijn Lelieveldt	Leiden University Medical Center, The Netherlands
Alex Leow	University of Illinois at Chicago, USA
Frederik Maes	Katholieke Universiteit Leuven, Belgium
Stephen Marsland	Massey University, New Zeland
Dimitri Metaxas	Rutgers University, USA
Charles Meyer	University of Michigan, USA
Bernard Ng	INRIA Saclay, France
Mads Nielsen	University of Copenhagen, Denmark

Wiro Niessen	Erasmus MC - University Medical Center Rotterdam, The Netherlands
Marc Niethammer	University of North Carolina at Chapel Hill, USA
Alison Noble	University of Oxford, UK
Lauren O'Donnell	Harvard Medical School, USA
Sebastien Ourselin	University College London, UK
Xenophon Papademetris	Yale University, USA
Nikos Paragios	Ecole Centrale de Paris, France
Franjo Pernus	University of Ljubljana, Slovenia
Dzung Pham	Johns Hopkins University, USA
Stephen Pizer	University of North Carolina at Chapel Hill, USA
Marcel Prastawa	University of Utah, USA
Jerry Prince	Johns Hopkins University, USA
Jinyi Qi	University of California, Davis, USA
Anand Rangarajan	University of Florida, USA
Joseph Reinhardt	University of Iowa, USA
Torsten Rohlfing	SRI International, USA
Karl Rohr	University of Heidelberg, IPMB, and DKFZ Heidelberg, Germany
Daniel Rueckert	Imperial College London, UK
Mert Sabuncu	Harvard Medical School, USA
Julia Schnabel	University of Oxford, UK
Christof Seiler	Stanford University, USA
Dinggang Shen	University of North Carolina at Chapel Hill, USA
Pengcheng Shi	Rochester Institute of Technology, USA
Kaleem Siddiqi	McGill University, Canada
Ivor Simpson	University College London, UK
Lawrence Staib	Yale University, USA
Colin Studholme	University of Washington, USA
Martin Styner	University of North Carolina at Chapel Hill, USA
Gábor Székely	ETH Zurich, Switzerland
Chris Taylor	University of Manchester, UK
Jean-Philippe Thiran	Ecole Polytechnique Federale de Lausanne (EPFL), France
Bertrand Thirion	INRIA Saclay, France
Matthew Toews	Harvard Medical School, USA
Alain Trouvé	Ecole Normale Supérieure, France
Zhuowen Tu	University of California, Los Angeles, USA
Carole Twining	University of Manchester, UK
Koen Van Leemput	Harvard Medical School, USA

Baba Vemuri	University of Florida, USA
Simon Warfield	Harvard Medical School, USA
Demian Wassermann	Harvard Medical School, USA
Carl-Fredrik Westin	Harvard Medical School, USA
Ross Whittaker	University of Utah, USA
Laurent Younes	Johns Hopkins University, USA
Paul Yushkevich	University of Pennsylvania, USA
Darko Zikic	Microsoft Research, USA

IPMI 2013 Board

Harrison H. Barrett
Christian Barillot
Aaron B. Brill
Gary E. Christensen
Alan C.F. Colchester
James S. Duncan
Michael L. Goris
Nico Karssemeijer
Richard M. Leahy
Stephen M. Pizer
Jerry L. Prince
Gábor Székely
Chris Taylor
Andrew Todd-Pokropek
William M. Wells

Table of Contents

Dynamic Imaging

Poster Session I

Cortical Surface Registration I

Diffusion MRI

Functional Imaging

Torso Image Analysis

Cortical Surface Registration II

Poster Session II

Tract Analysis

Statistical Analysis II

Matched Signal Detection on Graphs: Theory and Application to Brain Network Classification

Chenhui Hu[1,2], Lin Cheng[3], Jorge Sepulcre[1],
Georges El Fakhri[1], Yue M. Lu[2], and Quanzheng Li[1]

[1]Center for Advanced Medical Imaging Science, NMMI, Radiology,
Massachusetts General Hospital, Boston, MA 02114
{sepulcre@nmr.,elfakhri@pet.,Li.Quanzheng@}mgh.harvard.edu
[2]School of Engineering and Applied Sciences,
Harvard University, Cambridge, MA 02138
{hu4,yuelu}@seas.harvard.edu
[3]Department of Engineering, Trinity College, Hartford, CT 06106
lin.cheng@trincoll.edu

Abstract. We develop a matched signal detection (MSD) theory for signals with an intrinsic structure described by a weighted graph. Hypothesis tests are formulated under different signal models. In the simplest scenario, we assume that the signal is deterministic with noise in a subspace spanned by a subset of eigenvectors of the graph Laplacian. The conventional matched subspace detection can be easily extended to this case. Furthermore, we study signals with certain level of smoothness. The test turns out to be a weighted energy detector, when the noise variance is negligible. More generally, we presume that the signal follows a prior distribution, which could be learnt from training data. The test statistic is then the difference of signal variations on associated graph structures, if an Ising model is adopted. Effectiveness of the MSD on graph is evaluated both by simulation and real data. We apply it to the network classification problem of Alzheimer's disease (AD) particularly. The preliminary results demonstrate that our approach is able to exploit the sub-manifold structure of the data, and therefore achieve a better performance than the traditional principle component analysis (PCA).

Keywords: Matched subspace detection, graph-structured data, graph Laplacian, brain networks, classification, Alzheimer's disease.

1 Introduction

Matched subspace detection is a classic tool that determines whether a multidimensional signal lies in a given linear subspace or not [1]. It has achieved a great success in applications such as radar, hyperspectral imaging and medical imaging [2]. The subspace is either governed by the physical system that generates the signal, or could be inferred from training data. Subspace learning

J.C. Gee et al. (Eds.): IPMI 2013, LNCS 7917, pp. 1–12, 2013.

or dimensionality reduction is a central issue in machine learning. One popular method is principal component analysis (PCA), which projects the original data to a linear subspace spanned by the leading eigenvectors of the data matrix. A common assumption of PCA is that the data are generated from a linear subspace. In fact, many real data are sampled from a nonlinear low-dimensional *sub-manifold*, which is embedded in a high-dimensional ambient space [3]. Examples include images, gene data, social network records, and sensor network measurements. These types of data may be better modeled as signals supported on graph structures,[1] instead of conventional signals in Euclidean spaces. In this setting, the signal subspace can be effectively learnt by graph spectral methods, *e.g.*, Isomap, Locality Linear Embedding (LLE), Laplacian eigenmaps [4,5].

Motivated by the requirement of classifying graph-structured data in many emerging problems, we are interested in developing a similar detection framework for graph-signals in this paper. Specifically, we formulate hypothesis tests to decide which graph structure a signal is more likely to embed in. Instead of building combinatorial tests on graph [6,7], we exploit the matched subspace detection technique to make our setup generic to handle a variety of situations. Intuitively, the tests are dependent on the relation between the signal and the graphs, *i.e.*, the signal models. To this end, we first assume that the signal lies in a subspace spanned by a subset of eigenvectors of the graph Laplacian matrix. The classic matched subspace detection can be applied directly. Then, we consider signals that are *smooth* on graph, as specified by a bounded variation metric. The maximum likelihood estimator (MLE) of the true signal is derived by solving a constrained optimization problem. When the noise variance is negligible, we find the test becomes a weighted energy detector. More generally, we presume the signal is randomly drawn from a prior distribution. It ends up with comparing the signal variations on the hypothetic graphs, if an Ising model is adopted.

We apply the proposed detection theory to brain network classification for AD. As one of the most common forms of dementia, AD is believed to be a brain network disease, and is characterized by progressive impairment of memory and other cognitive capacity, which eventually causes death. It affects nearly 36 million people in the world with an expected number 65.7 million by 2030 [8]. While conventional clinical diagnosis might be inaccurate, Positron Emission Tomography (PET) imaging of brain amyloid using Pittsburgh Compound-B (PIB) tracer provides sensitive and consistent biomarkers in the early stage of the disease [9]. We carry out leave-one-out tests on 30 AD patients and 40 normal control (NC) subjects. Experimental results show that when using the MSD on graph, the probabilities of false alarm and miss are 2/40 and 0/30, respectively. In contrast, the associated probabilities are 6/40 and 5/30, if a linear PCA is used; or 5/40 and 3/30, if we use support vector machine (SVM). This preliminary result indicates the MSD on graph provides an effective way for AD network classification, probably due to the effectiveness of exploiting the sub-manifold structure of the data.

---

[1] For short, we will also refer to them as graph-signals.

2   Signal Models

Since we aim to classify graph-structured data, such as neuroimaging data, it is necessary to introduce the statistical signal models on graph before presenting the hypothesis testing models. A brain network can be represented by a *weighted graph* $\mathcal{G}(\mathcal{V}, \mathcal{E}, W)$ with vertex set $\mathcal{V}(|\mathcal{V}| = N)$ and edge set $\mathcal{E}$. For such graph, the similarity or associativity between vertex i and j is given by $W_{ij} \geq 0$. Besides, we introduce a diagonal degree matrix D with $D_{ii} = \sum_{j=1}^{N} W_{ij}$. Then, the *Laplacian matrix* of the graph is defined as $L \overset{\text{def}}{=} D - W$. Note that L is symmetric, we can decompose it into $L = F\Lambda F^T$, where Λ is diagonal with $\Lambda_{ii} = \lambda_i$ being the i-th smallest eigenvalue of L and the columns of F, f_is, are the associated eigenvectors. By nature, the eigenvalues of L satisfy: $0 = \lambda_1 \leq \lambda_2 \cdots \leq \lambda_N$.

Let $\mathcal{H}$ be a Hilbert space on $\mathcal{V}$. A signal x on graph $\mathcal{G}$ is a $N \times 1$ vector in $\mathcal{H}$, with each entry being a real value assigned to a vertex (see Fig. 1 for an example). Since F is orthogonal, the projection of x onto its column space is

$$\widehat{x} = F^T x. \tag{1}$$

Accordingly, we have $x = F\widehat{x}$. We refer to $\widehat{x}$ as the *graph Fourier transform* (GFT) of x and x the inverse GFT of $\widehat{x}$ [10,11], based on the fundamental connection between (1) and the classical discrete Fourier transform (DFT): the eigenvectors of the Laplacian matrice form a DFT basis, for any circulant graph.

To facilitate the proposed hypothesis tests (whether a signal is embedded in a given graph structure), prior information could be applied. It could simply be additional constraints. Alternatively, we can assume that the signal follows a prior distribution, which could be learnt from the training data. Next, we illustrate the signals with both types of prior information in this section.

2.1   Finite Support Graph-Signals

In many applications, the GFT component of the signal is more likely to be close to zero as the corresponding eigenvalue becomes large. This is largely due to the *smoothness* of the signal on graph, since a higher eigenvalue reflects a stronger variation of the eigenvector [12,13]. Analogous to the traditional signal, we call the f_is frequency components for GFT. Generally, we can define signals that are only supported on selected frequency components, namely the *finite support signals*, as specified by $\{x \mid \widehat{x}_{i \notin I_S} = 0, I_S \subset \{1, \cdots, N\}\}$. Usually, the supporting eigenvectors in I_S are chosen on the basis of the amplitudes of the GFT components. By introducing a binary diagonal matrix S with $S_{ii} = 1$ only if $\widehat{x}_i \neq 0$, we can write $x = FS\widehat{x}$.

2.2   Constrained Graph-Signals

To improve the robustness of a hypothesis test, prior information is usually applied. One common prior is to add regularization to the GFT coefficients in the form of a penalty function $C(\cdot)$, which imposes a reward or penalty when

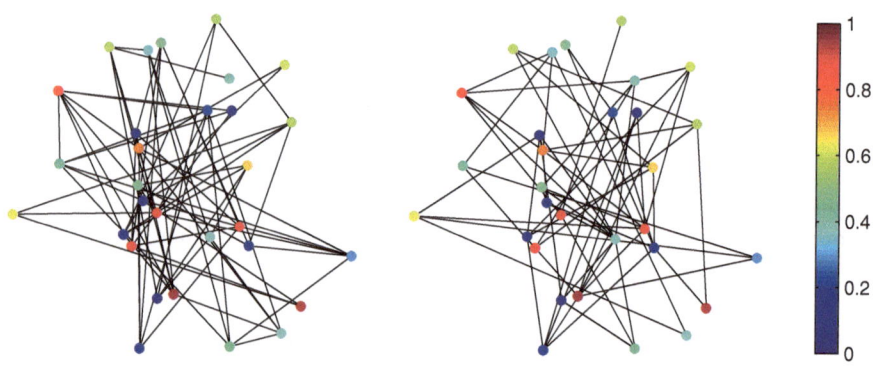

Fig. 1. A same graph-signal displayed on two graph structures. Both graphs have 30 vertices but different connections, each of which has a unit weight. The values of the signal on the vertices are encoded in the color of the dots.

the signal is in a certain shape. Due to the uncertainty caused by the noise, the hypothesis tests involve the estimation of maximum likelihood (ML) with unknown parameters. Under the constraint, we maximize the following penalized ML instead of ML:

$$\arg\max_{\theta} LL(\widehat{x}, \theta_{\setminus \widehat{x}}) - \gamma \cdot C(\widehat{x}), \qquad (2)$$

where $LL(\cdot)$ is the log-likelihood function, $\gamma > 0$ is a trade-off factor, and $\theta = \{\widehat{x}, \theta_{\setminus \widehat{x}}\}$ denotes the set of all unknown but *deterministic* parameters. In Section 3.2, we replace the corresponding parameter with its penalized MLE and obtain a general likelihood ratio (GLR) test.

2.3   Probabilistic Graph-Signals

Perviously, we treat the signal as deterministic but unknown due to noise. From a Bayesian perspective, we can also assume that the signal is randomly generated from a prior distribution.

The distribution could be expressed in the graph domain. In [15,16], the authors proposed a so-called *Ising model* as follows

$$\mathbb{P}(x) \propto \exp(-x^T L x). \qquad (3)$$

The exponent term in the above equation is the variation of x on the graph for that $x^T L x = \sum_{i,j} W_{ij}(x_i - x_j)^2$ [12]. PIB-PET images for a certain subject group may obey this model, since the correlated brain regions should yield similar measurements. In the GFT domain, we consider a multivariate Gaussian distribution of the GFT coefficients. We will define a probabilistic MSD on graph in Section 3.3 based on above probabilistic graph-signals.

3   Decision Models

Let $y \in \mathbb{R}^N$ be an observed signal defined on a potential graph. There are two hypotheses $H_j, j = 0, 1$, representing that y is embedded in either graph $\mathcal{G}_0$ or $\mathcal{G}_1$, with the associated Laplacian matrix L_0 or L_1, respectively. The graphs are defined on the same set of vertices. Fig. 1 shows a same graph-signal on two different hypothetic graphs, where every edge has a unit weight. Our goal is to formulate a hypothesis test to decide which graph fits the signal more accurately. We refer to the procedure as *matched signal detection* (MSD) on graph.

We first presume that y is a contaminated version of a signal x with additive Gaussian noise, since the observed signal may not fit the learnt model completely. Namely, we express $y = x + n$, with $n \sim \mathcal{N}(\mathbf{0}, \Phi)$. Without loss of generality, we assume $\Phi = \xi^2 I$. Followed from (1), we have

$$y = F\widehat{x} + n. \tag{4}$$

Because the observation y is random, the most general form of the likelihood ratio (LR) test would be

$$\frac{l(\theta_1; y)}{l(\theta_0; y)} = \frac{\mathbb{P}(y|H_1)}{\mathbb{P}(y|H_0)} \underset{H_0}{\overset{H_1}{\gtrless}} \frac{\pi_0}{\pi_1} = \eta, \tag{5}$$

where $l(\cdot)$ indicates the likelihood function, θ_j and π_j are the set of parameters and prior probability under H_j, respectively. By default, we choose equal priors, *i.e.*, $\eta = 1$. In accordance with the signal models in last section, we present more concrete versions of (5) in terms of different types of MSD on graph.

3.1   Simple MSD on Graph

The basic form of MSD on graph follows immediately from the conventional matched subspace detection, if the subspace is spanned by a subset of the eigenvectors of the Laplacian matrix under each hypothesis. Suppose the eigendecomposition of L_j possesses the form $L_j = F_j \Lambda_j F_j^T$, from the orthogonality of F_j, we could obtain the test statistic

$$T_1(y) = \frac{\|(I - S)F_0 y\|_2^2}{\|(I - S)F_1 y\|_2^2}, \tag{6}$$

where S is the indicative matrix of the GFT support defined in Section 2.1.

3.2   CMSD on Graph

We adopt CMSD as a shorthand for the constrained MSD problem, when the graph-signal model with constraint in Section 2.2 is taken into account. By multiplying F^T to both sides of (4), we obtain

$$\widehat{y} = \widehat{x} + \widehat{n}, \tag{7}$$

where $\widehat{\ }$ denotes the GFT of the corresponding parameter. Since F is orthonormal, $\widehat{n}$ is still a white Gaussian noise of the same distribution as n.

The constraint function may be selected in various ways. For instance, if we prefer a sparse $\widehat{x}$ as that in [17], we can let $C(\widehat{x}) = \|\widehat{x}\|_1$. Here we introduce the following quadratic penalty function

$$C(\widehat{x}) = \sum_{i \in I_S} \alpha_i \widehat{x}_i^2, \tag{8}$$

with α_i being a non-negative weight. We might assign a larger penalty weight on the GFT coefficient which is less informative. For the CMSD with above quadratic constraint, we have the following theorem

Theorem 1. *Given the cost function (8) under two hypotheses and denote by $\widehat{y}_{i,j}$ the i-th entry of $F_j^T y$, the GLRT statistic can be expressed as*

$$T_2(y) = \frac{\sum_{i \in I_S} \alpha_i \widehat{y}_{i,0}^2}{\sum_{i \in I_S} \alpha_i \widehat{y}_{i,1}^2}, \tag{9}$$

if the noise variances are unknown but significantly small.

Proof. See Appendix A.

We then present a specific form of CMSD by imposing a smoothness constraint to the graph-signals measured on the graph structure. This kind of constraint is common and is particularly suitable for neuroimaging data, since brain imaging data generated from similar physiological mechanisms would vary smoothly along a certain sub-manifold structure. To measure the degree of smoothness, for $s > 0$, we define the following metric on graph for

$$V_{\mathcal{G},s}(x) = \frac{x^T L^s x}{x^T x}. \tag{10}$$

Lemma 1. *(1) $x^T L^s x = \sum_i \lambda_i^s \widehat{x}_i^2$; (2) $V_{\mathcal{G},1}(f_i) = \lambda_i$,*

The proof is omitted due to limitation of space. Lemma 1 indicates the smoothness measurement is a special case of the constraint in (8). From the lemma, we observe that the signal will have a large variation when its GFT components are concentrated on high frequency components, *i.e.*, f_i with large λ_i.

We consider the smoothness constraint as a *bounded variation* of the signal. Namely, we assume $V_{\mathcal{G},s}(x) < r$ holds for $0 < r < \lambda_N$. In particular, when $s = 1$, we obtain that $\sum_{i=1}^N \lambda_i \widehat{x}_i^2 < r \sum_{i=1}^N \widehat{x}_i^2$, *i.e.*, $\sum_{i=1}^N (\lambda_i - r)\widehat{x}_i^2 < 0$. Under this constraint and by the KKT condition, we have

$$\frac{\partial}{\partial \widehat{x}} \left\{ N \log \xi + \frac{1}{2\xi^2} \|\widehat{x} - \widehat{y}\|_2^2 + \gamma \|R\widehat{x}\|_2^2 \right\} = 0, \tag{11}$$

$$\gamma \left(\sum_{i=1}^N (\lambda_i - r)\widehat{x}_i^2 \right) = 0, \quad \gamma \geq 0. \tag{12}$$

Notice that R is a diagonal matrix with $R_{ii} = (\lambda_i - r)^{1/2}$ and γ is a dual variable. Following the proof of Theorem 1, we get $\hat{x}_i = \frac{\hat{y}_i}{1+\gamma\xi^2(\lambda_i - r)}$ from (11). Replacing $\hat{x}_i$ in (12) with this, we can write

$$\sum_{i<\tau} \frac{(r - \lambda_i)\hat{y}_i^2}{(1 + \gamma\xi^2(\lambda_i - r))^2} = \sum_{i>\tau} \frac{(\lambda_i - r)\hat{y}_i^2}{(1 + \gamma\xi^2(\lambda_i - r))^2}, \tag{13}$$

where $\tau = \max\{i | \lambda_i < r\} + \frac{1}{2}$. If we assume that the noise variance ξ can be estimated from the average residual energy of the projection as

$$\xi = \sqrt{\frac{\sum_{i=N'+1}^{N} \hat{y}_i^2}{N - N'}}, \tag{14}$$

with $N' < N$ being an integer threshold, then from (13) we can solve out the dual parameter γ. After that, the MLE of $\hat{x}$ can be readily obtained. Plugging it to the likelihood expression in (5), we will reach the GLRT.

3.3   PMSD on Graph

A more general MSD is to consider random graph-signals, which gives rise to the probabilistic MSD (PMSD) on graph. We assume that the p.d.f. of $\hat{x}$ is $g_j(\hat{x})$ under H_j. By independence of the noise on the signal, the LR is

$$LR = \frac{\int g_1(\hat{y} - t)h_1(t)dt}{\int g_0(\hat{y} - t)h_0(t)dt}, \tag{15}$$

where $h_j(\cdot)$ denotes the p.d.f. of the white Gaussian noise under H_j.

If the GFT coefficients of the true signal follow a Gaussian distribution $\mathcal{N}(\mathbf{0}, \Sigma_j)$, the test statistic would be $\hat{y}^T (\Phi_0^{-1} - \Phi_1^{-1})\hat{y}$, where $\Phi_j = \Sigma_j + \xi_j^2 I$. In particular, if we apply the Ising model (3) to the true signal, we will have $g_j(\hat{x}) \propto e^{-(F_j\hat{x})^T L_j (F_j\hat{x})} = e^{-\hat{x}^T \Lambda_j \hat{x}}$. It turns out that $\hat{y}$ is distributed as $\mathcal{N}(\mathbf{0}, \Lambda_j^\dagger + \xi_j^2 I)$, by viewing g_j as a degenerated Gaussian distribution. Here $\Lambda_j^\dagger$ is the pseudoinverse of Λ. When the noise variances are known, the LRT statistic reduces to

$$T_3(y) = \sum_i \beta_{i,0}\hat{y}_{i,0}^2 - \sum_i \beta_{i,1}\hat{y}_{i,1}^2, \tag{16}$$

with $\beta_{1,j} = \xi_j^{-2}$ and $\beta_{i,j} = (\lambda_{i,j}^{-1} + \xi_j^2)^{-1}$, for $i \geq 2$. In a special noise-free case, the statistic in (16) becomes $y^T(L_0 - L_1)y$, which is simply a measure of the difference of the signal variations on the two graph structures.

4   Experimental Validation

4.1   Numerical Simulation

In this section, we evaluate the MSD on a pair of small-world networks. It has been reported that human brain networks have a small-world topology that supports both segregated and distributed information processing with a minimized

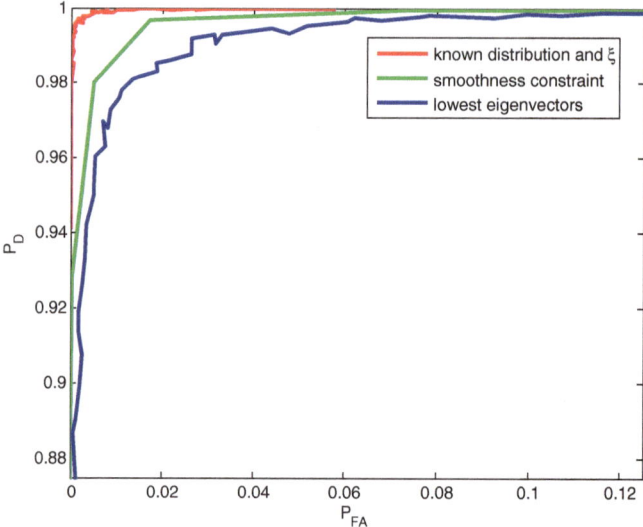

Fig. 2. ROC curves for hypothesis tests upon small-world networks of 40 vertices with vertex degree and rewiring probability being $(12, 0.05)$ and $(20, 0.5)$, respectively

cost [18]. The alternation of the graph structures is often caused by certain diseases. Previously, people used graph metrics, like degree distribution, average shortest path length, clustering coefficient, *etc.*, to classify different networks. Here we fulfill the task upon two networks characterized by the Watts-Strogatz model [19], using the MSD schemes developed in Section 3.

The networks are constructed from random rewiring of a circulant graph with 40 vertices. The number of edges of each vertex and the rewiring probability are $(12, 0.05)$ under H_0, and $(20, 0.5)$ under H_1, respectively. We assume that the GFT coefficients of the signals are distributed as $\mathcal{N}(\mathbf{0}, \Sigma)$ with Σ being diagonal and $\Sigma_{ii} = \exp(-i/10)$ for both hypotheses. The standard deviation of the noise $\xi = 0.1$. In the first case, we presume that the signal distribution and noise level are known. As shown in Fig. 2, we can apply the PMSD to get an almost perfect ROC curve in red. In the second case, we impose a smoothness constraint specified by an upper bound equal to λ_{20} on the signal variation (10) in each graph. At last, we implement the simple MSD via picking up the first 20 eigenvectors. The green and the blue lines display the associated ROC curves for them. We find that the CMSD can outperform the simple MSD and is slightly inferior to the optimal case. Notice that the areas under the ROC curves are all close to 1, verifying the effectiveness of the proposed approaches.

4.2   AD Network Classification

We then apply the proposed MSD to the classification of PIB-PET images and compare it with PCA in this section. The data set consists of 30 AD patients and 40 Normal Control (NC). Part of the data has been studied in [20] as well. Among the normal subjects, 20 are labeled as PIB positive and the rest as PIB negative based on the beta-amyloid binding level. Each image has a dimension of $20 \times 24 \times 18$ with $8mm \times 8mm \times 8mm$ voxels, downsampled from $2mm \times 2mm \times 2mm$ voxels for computational efficiency. In the pre-processing of the data, we first mask out the area out of the brain. Next, we apply Automated Anatomical Labeling (AAL) [21] to map the effective voxels to 116 volumes-of-interest (VOIs). The data is then averaged within each VOI for further analysis.

As an initial step, we build a similarity graph over 42 regions among all the VOIs that are regarded to be potentially related to AD. Table 1 in [22] lists the names of the VOIs spread over the frontal, parietal, occipital, and temporal lobes. For an arbitrary group, let $\{R_1, \cdots, R_p\}$ be the p selected VOIs and suppose we have m samples. The observation in the i-th region of subject j is denoted by x_{ij}. We construct a weighted graph over the p brain volumes, by assigning a positive weight W_{ij} to the edge between R_i and R_j as follows

$$W_{ij} = \exp\left(-\frac{\|x_i - x_j\|^2}{\rho^2}\right), \tag{17}$$

where $x_i = (x_{i1}, \cdots, x_{im})^T$, $x_j = (x_{j1}, \cdots, x_{jm})^T$, and $\rho > 0$ is a scaling factor (here we set $\rho = 1$). The kernel function in (17) is known as a heat kernel [3]. After building graphs for both groups, we project a newly observed signal to the sets of eigenvectors of the graph Laplacian matrices. The decision is made through comparing the test statistic (6) against one. We present the major steps of our data processing in Fig. 3.

We perform leave-one-out tests to evaluate the proposed MSD on graphs. Fig. 4 demonstrates the projection errors, *i.e.*, the numerator and denominator in (6), when the true signal belongs to NC and AD, respectively. Here we merely choose the first 4 eigenvectors as the supporting set. The error rates in Fig. 4(a) and 4(b) are 2/40 and 0/30, compared with the rates 6/40 and 5/30 when we use linear PCA, namely we form a matrix by aligning the existing data and use the principle left eigenvectors of the data matrix to carry out the matched subspace detection. We've also carried out the classification by SVM [23], which gives the probabilities of false alarm and miss 5/40 and 3/30. It shows the advantage of the MSD on graph over the traditional method and indicates that the data could have an intrinsic sub-manifold structure. We also observe that there are less differences of projection errors in NC than in AD. This might be due to the following reasons: (1) The PIB binding levels of NC subjects are about 20% lower than those of the AD subjects on average; (2) We reduce the dimension of the raw data by mapping it to a few VOIs, indicating some information may not be retained; (3) We use a simple strategy to construct the weighted graphs which could be improved via more sophisticated schemes (*e.g.*, [24]). This observation also implies that if we slightly increase the threshold of our hypothesis test, we can achieve 100% detection rate. In addition, we find that the two miss-classified subjects (Number 29 and 31) in Fig. 4(a) are both PIB positive, which may indicate that they are more likely to develop AD.

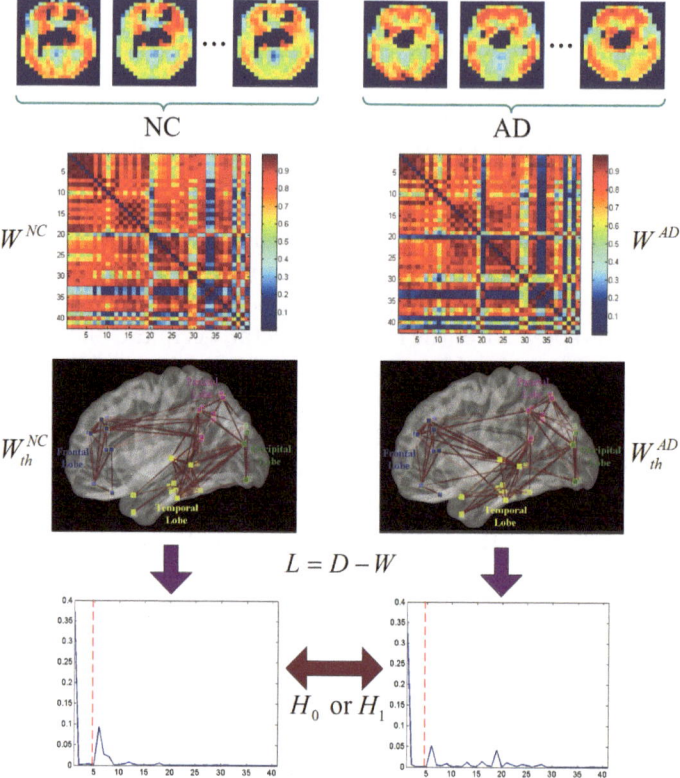

Fig. 3. Main steps (from the top to the bottom) of the MSD implementation for AD network classification. W^{NC}, W^{AD} are the weighted graphs constructed from the imaging data listed in the first row; while W_{th}^{NC}, W_{th}^{AD} are their corresponding thresholded versions with 135 edges. The last row illustrates the projection energy distributions of a signal on the two sets of eigenvectors of the graph Laplacians.

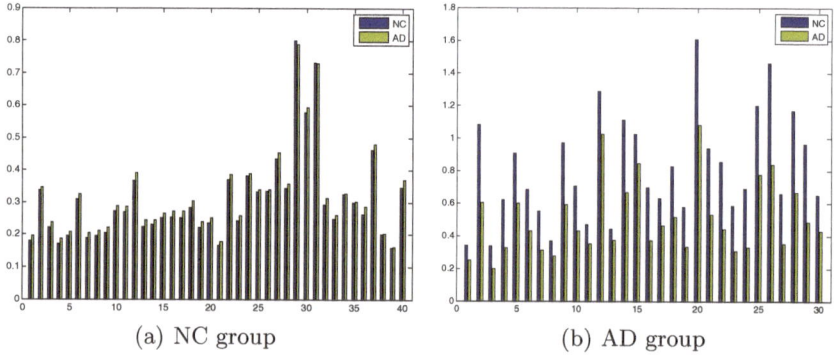

(a) NC group   (b) AD group

Fig. 4. Projection errors in the leave-one-out tests when the true data is from either NC or AD group. Note that the x-axis is the index of subjects.

5   Conclusion

In this paper, we formulate the MSD for graph-structure data under different signal models. We consider the signals that are either smooth on the graph or randomly generated from a known prior distribution. In the first setting, GLRT can be obtained by solving a constrained optimization problem. Specially, when the noise variance is negligible, it results in a weighted energy detector. In the second case, the test statistic is the difference of the signal variations on the graphs, if an Ising model is employed. We test the effectiveness of the MSD on simulated and real data by applying it to AD network classification. Compared with the linear PCA, our method demonstrates a better performance due to its ability of exploiting the sub-manifold structure of the neuroimaging data.

Appendix A: Proof of Theorem 1

Define a diagonal matrix R as such $R_{ii} = \alpha_i^{1/2}$ for $i \in I_S$, and $R_{ii} = 0$ elsewhere, then the penalty function can be written as $C(\hat{x}) = \|R\hat{x}\|_2^2$. We need to estimate the set of parameters $\theta = \{\hat{x}, \xi\}$ from the following

$$\arg\min_{\hat{x},\xi} N \log \xi + \frac{1}{2\xi^2}\|\hat{x} - \hat{y}\|_2^2 + \gamma\|R\hat{x}\|_2^2, \tag{18}$$

when the noise variance is unknown. Denote by $Q(\hat{x}, \xi)$ the objective function in the above equation and set $\frac{\partial Q}{\partial \hat{x}} = 0$, we obtain $(\hat{x} - \hat{y})/\xi^2 + \gamma R^2 \hat{x} = 0$, i.e., $\hat{x} = (I + \xi^2 \gamma R^2)^{-1}\hat{y}$. Similarly, let $\frac{\partial Q}{\partial \xi} = 0$, we have $\xi^2 = \|\hat{x} - \hat{y}\|_2^2 = \|(I + \xi^2 \gamma R^2)^{-1}\hat{y} - \hat{y}\|_2^2$. If $\xi \ll \frac{1}{\gamma \max_i\{\alpha_i\}}$, we can proceed with the approximation $\xi^2 = \|\xi^2 \gamma R^2 \hat{y}\|_2^2$, indicating that $\xi = \gamma^{-1}\|R\hat{y}\|_2$. Plugging it into (5) leads to the constrained test here.

References

1. Scharf, L.L., Friedlander, B.: Matched Subspace Detectors. IEEE Trans. on Signal Proc. 42, 2146–2157 (1994)
2. Li, Z., Li, Q., Yu, X., Conti, P.S., Leahy, R.M.: Lesion Detection in Dynamic FDG-PEG Using Matched Subspace Detection. IEEE Trans. on Medical Imaging 28, 230–240 (2009)
3. Belkin, M., Niyogi, P.: Using Manifold Structure for Partially Labeled Classification. In: Advances in Neural Information Processing Systems, vol. 15, pp. 929–936 (2002)
4. Saul, L.K., Weinberger, K.Q., Ham, J.H., Sha, F., Lee, D.D.: Spectral Methods for Dimensionality Reduction. In: Chapelle, O., Schoelkopf, B., Zien, A. (eds.) Semisupervised Learning, pp. 293–308. MIT Press, Cambridge (2006)
5. Cai, D., He, X., Han, J.: Spectral regression: A Unified Approach for Sparse Subspace Learning. In: 7th IEEE Int. Conf. on Data Mining, pp. 73–82 (2007)
6. Addario-Berry, L., Broutin, N., Devroye, L., Lugosi, G.: On Combinatorial Testing Problems. The Annals of Statistics 38, 3063–3092 (2010)

7. Arias-Castro, E., Candes, E.J., Durand, A.: Detection of an Anomalous Cluster in a Network. The Annals of Statistics 39, 278–304 (2011)
8. Brookmeyer, R., Johnson, E., Ziegler-Graham, K., Arrighi, H.M.: Forecasting the Global Burden of Alzheimers Disease. Alzheimer's and Dementia 3, 186–191 (2007)
9. Mintun, M.A., Larossa, G.N., Sheline, Y.I., Dence, C.S., Lee, S.Y., Mach, R.H., Klunk, W.E., Mathis, C.A., DeKosky, S.T., Morris, J.C.: [11C] PIB in a Non-demented Population Potential Antecedent Marker of Alzheimer Disease. Neurology 67, 446–452 (2006)
10. Zhu, X., Rabbat, M.: Approximating Signals Supported on Graphs. In: IEEE Int. Conf. on Acoustics, Speech and Signal Processing, pp. 3921–3924 (2012)
11. Shuman, D.I., Ricaud, B., Vandergheynst, P.: A Windowed Graph Fourier Transform. In: IEEE Statistical Signal Processing Workshop (SSP), pp. 133–136 (2012)
12. Bougleux, S., Elmoataz, A., Melkemi, M.: Discrete Regularization on Weighted Graphs for Image and Mesh Filtering. In: Sgallari, F., Murli, A., Paragios, N. (eds.) SSVM 2007. LNCS, vol. 4485, pp. 128–139. Springer, Heidelberg (2007)
13. Spielman, D.A.: Spectral Graph Theory and Its Applications. In: 48th Annual IEEE Symposium on Foundations of Computer Science, pp. 29–38 (2007)
14. Tipping, E.M., Bishop, C.M.: Probabilistic Principal Component Analysis. Jour. of the Royal Stat. Soci.: Series B (Stat. Meth.) 61, 611–622 (1999)
15. Sharpnack, J., Singh, A.: Identifying Graph-Structured Activation Patterns in Networks. In: Proc. of Neural. Info. Proc. Sys. (2010)
16. Grimmett, G.: Probability on Graphs: Random Processes on Graphs and Lattices, vol. 1. Cambridge University Press (2010)
17. Paredes, J.L., Wang, Z., Arce, G.R., Sadler, B.M.: Compressive Matched Subspace Detection. In: Proc. 17th European Signal Processing Conf., pp. 120–124 (2009)
18. Bassett, D.S., Bullmore, E.: Small-World Brain Networks. The Neuroscientist 12, 512–523 (2006)
19. Watts, D.J., Strogatz, S.H.: Collective Dynamics of "Small-World" Networks. Nature 2, 393–440 (1998)
20. Buckner, R.L., Sepulcre, J., Talukdar, T., Krienen, F.M., Liu, H., Hedden, T., Andrews-Hanna, J.R., Sperling, R.A., Johnson, K.A.: Cortical Hubs Revealed by Intrinsic Functional Connectivity: Mapping, Assessment of Stability, and Relation to Alzheimer's Disease. The Journal of Neuroscience 29, 1860–1873 (2009)
21. Tzourio-Mazoyer, N., Landeau, B., Papathanassiou, D., Crivello, F., Etard, O., Delcroix, N., Mazoyer, B., Joliot, M.: Automated Anatomical Labeling of Activations in SPM Using a Macroscopic Anatomical Parcellation of the MNI MRI Single-Subject Brain. Neuroimage 15, 273–289 (2002)
22. Huang, S., Li, J., Sun, L., Liu, J., Wu, T., Chen, K., Fleisher, A., Reiman, E., Ye, J.: Learning Brain Connectivity of Alzheimer's Disease from Neuroimaging Data. In: Advances in Neural Information Processing Systems, vol. 22, pp. 808–816 (2009)
23. Cristianini, N., Shawe-Taylor, J.: An Introduction to Support Vector Machines and Other Kernel-Based Learning Methods. Cambridge University Press (2000)
24. Hu, C., Cheng, L., Sepulcre, J., Fakhri, G.E., Lu, Y.M., Li, Q.: A Graph Theoretical Regression Model for Brain Connectivity Learning of Alzheimer's Disease. In: Int. Symp. on Biomedical Imaging (2013, to appear)

Exploring High-Order Functional Interactions via Structurally-Weighted LASSO Models

Dajiang Zhu[1], Xiang Li[1], Xi Jiang[1], Hanbo Chen[1],
Dinggang Shen[2], and Tianming Liu[1]

[1] Cortical Architecture Imaging and Discovery Lab, Department of Computer Science,
University of Georgia, Athens, GA, USA
[2] Department of Radiology,
University of North Carolina at Chapel Hill, Chapel Hill, NC, USA

Abstract. A major objective of brain science research is to model and quantify functional interaction patterns among neural networks, in the sense that meaningful interaction patterns reflect the working mechanisms of neural systems and represent their relationships with the external world. Most current research approaches in the neuroimaging field, however, focus on pair-wise functional/effective connectivity and are thus unable to handle high-order, network-scale functional interactions. In this paper, we propose a novel structurally-weighted LASSO (SW-LASSO) regression model to represent the functional interaction among multiple regions of interests (ROIs) based on resting state fMRI (rsfMRI) data. In particular, the structural connectivity constraints derived from diffusion tenor imaging (DTI) data are used to guide the selection of the weights, thus adaptively adjusting the penalty levels of different coefficients which correspond to different ROIs. The robustness and accuracy of our models are evaluated and demonstrated via a series of carefully designed experiments. In an application example, the generated regression graphs show different assortative mixing patterns between Mild Cognitive Impairment (MCI) patients and normal controls (NC). Our results indicate that the proposed model has promising potential to enable the construction of high-order functional networks and their applications in clinical datasets.

Keywords: High-order functional interaction, LASSO.

1   Introduction

One of the major research objectives of brain science is to model and quantify the functional interaction patterns among neural networks at different spatial and temporal scales, in that meaningful interaction patterns reflect the working mechanisms of neural systems and represent their relationships with the external world. However, inferring robust and meaningful interaction patterns from high-dimensional neuroimaging datasets impose significant challenges from computational perspectives. For instance, so far, many previous studies have been focused on the *pairwise* functional connectivity analyses of networks of brain regions [1-3] based on resting state fMRI (rsfMRI) data. Though these pairwise functional connectivity

J.C. Gee et al. (Eds.): IPMI 2013, LNCS 7917, pp. 13–24, 2013.

analyses could provide useful information regarding neural systems, their descriptive power is limited. The major reason is that higher-order functional interactions among brain nodes cannot be captured in pair-wise connectivity analysis. The characterizing difference between functional interaction and connectivity, from a computational perspective, is that functional interaction models the relationship among multiple (n>=3) brain regions, while functional connectivity considers the temporal relationship between only two regions. Fig. 1 shows an example of functional pair-wise connectivities (Fig.1a) and high-order interactions (Fig.1b) proposed in this paper. In Fig.1, red and green bubbles represent the target Region of Interest (ROI) and other ROIs we want to study, respectively. With pair-wise analysis, each time we may only examine the functional relationship between the target ROI with one single ROI and obtain a single correlation, no matter what the overall interactions are like within the network. Through our proposed higher-order regression model in this work, however, all other ROIs (green bubbles in Fig.1b) will be considered simultaneously and those ROIs which have genuine functional interactions with the target ROI would stand out (deep pink bubbles).

Intuitively, there are two major advantages of studying higher-order interactions using our methods instead of pair-wise connectivity analysis. First, the latter only focuses on the relationship between two regions. Using Fig. 1a as an example, it can be seen that a pair-wise functional connectivity analysis, e.g., Pearson correlation, will have to examine the correlation between one ROI (red) and other ROIs separately, limiting the information that can be extracted. By using our proposed method (Fig. 1b), though, all ROIs could be simultaneously characterized and those have genuine functional interactions with the target ROI can be identified. Second, our method makes it possible to consider "directionality" when studying functional interactions. Traditional pair-wise functional correlation methods have been limited because of no directional information is available, which is critically important to brain network analysis. In comparison, high-order regression model could compensate to some extent such that the direction of regression will provide an informative reference for further inferring of genuine functional interaction directions among the brain network.

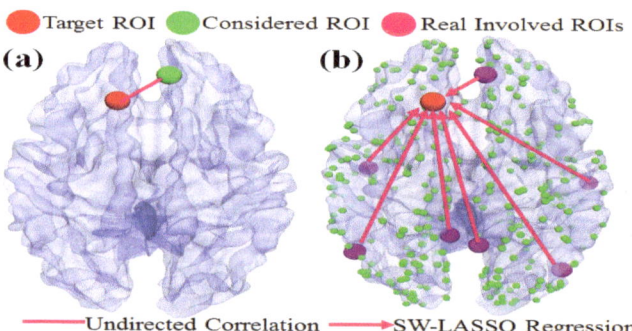

Fig. 1. Illustration of pair-wise functional connectivity (a) and high-order interaction (b). Green bubbles represent the candidate ROIs we considered and the deep pink ones are those really involved in our SW-LASSO regression procedure. Undirected line in (a) refers to traditional correlation; Arrows in (b) indicate the direction of the regression.

In the literature, there have been several existing methods which attempted to deal with the functional interactions among multiple ROIs such as Independent Component Analysis (ICA) [4], Granger Causality Mapping (GCM) [5-6], dynamic causal modeling (DCM) [7], multivariate autoregressive model (MAR) [8], structural equation modeling (SEM) [9], joint MAR-SEM model [10], and Bayesian graphical models [11-12]. Compared with those published approaches [4-12], our method is novel in the following aspects. First, we used the method in [13] to define 358 cortical ROIs at the connectome scale which encode the most consistent structural connectivities of the human brain. In comparison with the traditional ways for defining ROIs such as those relying on Brodmann brain atlas and image registration methods, these 358 ROIs will offer substantially finer granularity, much better functional homogeneity, much more accurate functional localization, and automatically-established cross-subjects correspondences [13]. In comparison with those methods that are intrinsically limited to brain networks of small sizes [7, 11, 12], our methods can deal with large-scale (e.g., hundreds of) brain ROIs. Second, we propose a novel structurally-weighted LASSO (SW-LASSO) regression model and use it to represent the functional interactions based on rsfMRI data. The LASSO properties ensure that the truly involved ROIs will be effectively selected and structural connectivity constraint will guide the regression process. The neuroscience basis of using structural connectivity information as the weight to constrain the regression process is that if two brain regions have strong structural connections, they tend to have strong functional dependence between each other [14-17]. Our experimental results indicate that the regressed coefficients are relatively robust and reproducible (Section 3.1, 3.2). Moreover, the functional interactions based on the regression result have shown promising potential to enable constructing high-order brain functional networks and studying their dynamic changes (Section 3.3).

2   Methods

The main steps in our proposed framework are outlined in Fig.2. First, by maximizing the consistency of structural connectivity profiles [13], we predicted the 358 cortical ROIs in the new datasets. Then the structural connectivity patterns among the ROIs were derived from DTI data and used as prior knowledge in our SW-LASSO regression model, along with the rsfMRI BOLD signals. At last, the learned coefficients matrix were normalized and reorganized as series of directed graphs according to their temporal order for further analysis.

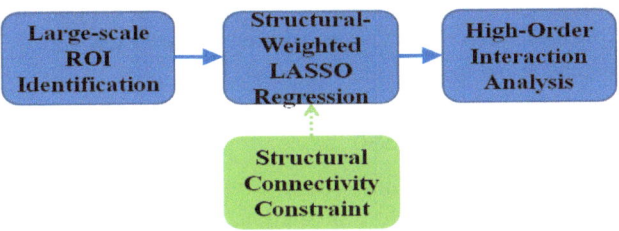

Fig. 2. The flowchart of our proposed computational framework

2.1   Dataset Acquisition

We used two independent multimodal DTI/rsfMRI datasets to develop, evaluate and apply the proposed computational framework in Fig.2.

Dataset 1: Sixteen participants (8 Mild Cognitive Impairment (MCI) patients and 8 normal controls (NC)) were recruited to participate in this study. FMRI and DTI scans were acquired on a GE 3T Signa scanner using an 8-channel head coil. Acquisition parameters were as follows: rsfMRI: 64x64 matrix, 4mm slice thickness, 256x256 FOV, TR=5s, TE=25ms, flip angle = 90°; DTI: 128×128 matrix, 2mm slice thickness, 256mm FOV, 60 slices, TR=17000ms, TE= min-full, 30 optimized gradient directions, b-value=1000. All scans were aligned to the AC-PC line beforehand.

Dataset 2: Twenty participants (10 MCI patients and 10 NC) were recruited and scanned in a 3.0 Tesla scanner (GE Signa EXCITE, GE Healthcare). For rsfMRI, 34 slices were acquired in the same plane (as the low resolution T1-weighted images) using a SENSE inverse-spiral pulse sequence with echo time (TE) = 32 ms, repetition time (TR) = 2 s, FOV = 25.6 cm2, matrix = 64 × 64 × 34, 3.8 mm^3. For DTI, 25 direction diffusion-weighted whole-brain volumes were acquired axially parallel to the AC-PC line using diffusion weighting values, b = 0 and 1000 s/mm^2, flip angle = 90°, TR = 17 s and TE = 78 ms. The imaging matrix was 256 x 256 with a rectangular FOV of 256 x 256 mm^2 and 72 slices with a slice thickness of 2.0 mm.

Preprocessing steps of these two DTI/rsfMRI datasets are similar to those in [13].

2.2   Cortical ROI Identification

Recently, we developed and validated an effective data-driven strategy that discovered 358 consistent cortical ROIs with correspondence in over 240 brains [13]. Each identified ROI was optimized to possess maximal group-wise consistency of DTI-derived fiber shape patterns. In this work, the 358 cortical ROIs are predicted in each of the subjects in section 2.1 and are then used as the network nodes for rsfMRI signal extraction and functional interaction modeling.

It should be noted here that the 358 cortical ROIs are originally constructed on healthy brains. Even though some previous works suggested that structural atrophy can be seen in MCI patients [18], no reports indicate the large scale alternations of structural connectivity exist in MCI patients so far. Therefore we adopted the prediction procedure in [13] and transferred the 358 ROIs to the two MCI datasets described in section 2.1. Briefly, the prediction is similar to the cortical ROI optimization process [13]: the consistency of the structural profiles between the new brain and the ROI models will be maximized as showed in Eq. (1).

$$E\ (S_M, S_N) = \sum |D_{MN}| \qquad (1)$$

where S_M represent the cortical ROI models, S_N is the new brain that needs to be predicted, D_{MN} is defined as the DTI-derived fiber shape distance [13]. The details of the algorithm can be found in [13].

2.3   LASSO and Weighted LASSO

The LASSO [19] is one of the most commonly used high-dimensional regression models for variable selection, feature prediction, and sparse learning. The LASSO estimates are defined as:

$$\hat{\beta}(\text{LASSO}) = \arg\min \|y - \sum_{i=1}^{n} x_i \beta_i\|^2 + \lambda \sum_{i=1}^{n} |\beta_i| \qquad (2)$$

The second term in Eq. (2) is known as the "ℓ_1 penalty" which makes the LASSO continuously shrink the coefficients toward zero as λ increases. If λ is large enough, some coefficients will be exactly zero and thus the feature selection is achieved automatically. But the LASSO shrinkage produces biased estimates for those large coefficients, and hence it could be suboptimal considering the estimation risk [20]. Many improved LASSO methods have been proposed in the literature including the adaptive LASSO [20], which tends to assign each covariate different penalty parameters to avoid having larger coefficients penalized more heavily than small coefficients. However, we still face two problems in practice: variable selection is highly unstable and some preferred features are not selected. To alleviate this, we propose to adjust the regression procedure using external or domain constraints.

In this paper, we introduce a novel weighted LASSO model that uses structural connectivity information derived from DTI tractography data as the constraint to construct the weight. The major difference between our method and the adaptive LASSO [20] is that the latter uses ℓ_2 initial estimation to adjust and reweight ℓ_1 penalty in an iterative algorithm, while our method will decide the weight directly according to the structural brain connectivity analysis based on DTI data. The neuroscience basis of our method is that axonal fiber connections are the structural substrates of functional interactions, and a variety of neuroscience research studies have reported this strong correlation [1, 14-16, 21]. That is, stronger structural connections among ROIs indicate higher functional interactions, and this principle can be used as the biologically meaningful guidance in the search of functional interaction patterns during LASSO regression. Another advantage of introducing the structural connectivity constraint is the consideration of computational complexity: the regression space grows exponentially as the number of ROIs increases [11, 12]. By using meaningful structural information, one can efficiently and effectively reducing the search space, which is grounded on sound neuroscience principle [1, 14-16, 21]. Therefore, in comparison with previous models [4-12], the major methodological advantage of our SW-LASSO model is that it achieves high-order functional interaction modeling while being computationally treatable in dealing with large-scale brain networks.

2.4   Construction of Weights Using Structural Connectivity Constraint

After we predicted the 358 cortical ROIs, we came up with the structural connectivity matrix based on the number of fibers connecting one ROI to the others. As shown in Fig.3a, the line colors encode the number of fibers between any pair of ROIs (green bubbles). Fig. 3b shows the structural connectivity matrix constructed based on Fig.3a. Then, for each ROI, we calculated the percentages of the fibers connecting to the other ROIs: $f_{i,j}$ represents the ratio of the number of fibers connecting the i-*th* and j-*th* ROI over the total number of fibers connecting to the i-*th* ROI. Thus, we have $\sum_{j=1}^{n} f_{i,j} = 1$, $i \neq j$ and here n=358. In our weighted LASSO regression model, a lower weight value represents a smaller penalty to the corresponding variable, making it more likely to be included in the selected regression model. So we define the weight as:

$$w_{i,j} = 1 - f_{i,j}/\text{p}, \quad \text{p}>1 \qquad (3)$$

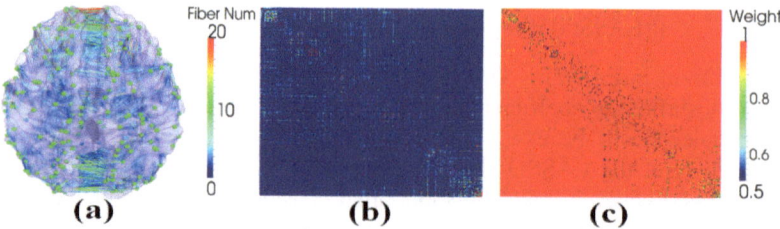

Fig. 3. Illustration of constructing weight constraint. (a) Structural connectivity patterns among 358 cortical ROIs. The color of lines encodes the number of fibers between any pair of ROIs. (b) The corresponding structural connectivity matrix of (a). (c) The generated weight matrix based on Eq. (3) when p equals 2.

Fig. 3 (c) shows the corresponding weight matrix (p=2), and we can see that stronger structural connectivity will have a lower weight value. Another issue that needs to be noted is that the weight matrix is not symmetric, since $f_{i,j}$ and $f_{j,i}$ are not necessarily equal.

2.5   SW_LASSO Regression

In this section, we will formally define the structural weighted LASSO (SW-LASSO) regression model used in this paper. Suppose we have response y_r and k regressors $X_r:\{x_1, x_2, ..., x_k\}$ (k=357). For both responses and regressors, we have N (N=10000) (N=10000) sample values. $y_r(j)$ and $x_i(j)$ represent the j-th sample value of response and the i-th regressor x_i respectively, i=1, 2, ..., k and j=1,2, ..., N. Then, we perform weighted ℓ_1 constrained regression of y_r on X_r:

$$\hat{\beta}_{Lasso}=\arg \min\{\sum_{j=1}^{N}(y_r(j) - \sum_{i=1}^{k} \beta_i\, x_i(j))^2\}+\lambda\sum_{i=1}^{k}(1 - f_{r,i}/p)|\beta_i| \qquad (4)$$

Eq. (4) is similar in concept to the adaptive LASSO [20], but the major difference is that the weight term comes from the DTI-derived structural connectivity, instead of learning from the dataset.

Since we are trying to infer every ROI by the other ROIs, we must make sure that the number of samples is large enough, compared with the 357 regressors. In this paper, we proposed a novel combined spatial-temporal sampling strategy as illustrated in Fig.4: 1) we divide the rsfMRI BOLD signals into a series of time windows and each time window contains ten time points (represented as T1 to T10 in Fig.4). The SW-LASSO regression process will be executed for each time window separately; 2) at each time point, we have 1000 groups of regressor samples and in each group the 357 samples (green dots) will be randomly selected from the neighborhood (27 neighbors) of the original ROI (red dots) in the volumetric image space. Hence, we totally achieve ten thousand samples for each round of regression.

In comparison with traditional pair-wise functional connectivity analysis that only considers the temporal correlation of two ROIs [1-3], here, we considered that one ROI is functionally interacting with multiple ROIs in the network, and thus its time series can be regressed by other rsfMRI time series via the optimally weighted linear

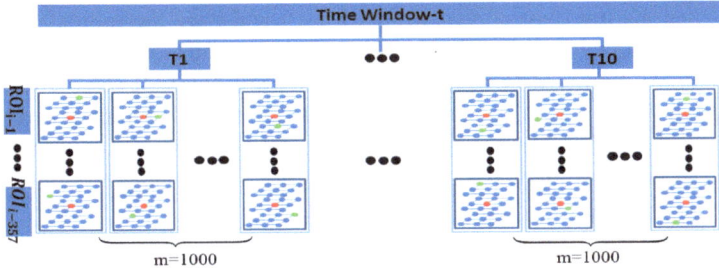

Fig. 4. Combined spatial-temporal sampling. As an example, one time window is showed here. Each time window contains ten time points, which are from T1 to T10 (temporal sampling). At each time point, we have 1000 groups of regressor samples and in each group the 357 samples will be randomly selected from the neighborhood of the original ROI in the volumetric image space. The red and green dots represent the original ROI and the real sampling locations, respectively.

regression model in Eq. (4). Since the structural connectivity mapping already demonstrated that one ROI could be structurally connected to multiple other ROIs (Figs. 3a-3b), it is reasonable to assume that one ROI may functionally interact with multiple ROIs. During the regression, we fixed p=2 as an experimentally determined value while λ was determined by fivefold cross-validation. It is evident that Eq. (4) is essentially a ℓ_1 penalization problem which can be solved very efficiently [20]. In this this work, we adopted the LARS algorithm [22] to computationally solve Eq. (4) based on the widely used SPAMS sparse learning package [23].

3   Experimental Results

This result section includes three parts as follows. Sections 3.1 and 3.2 focus on the evaluation of reproducibility and regression accuracy of the proposed SW-LASSO model. Section 3.3 provides an assortativity analysis based on the learned coefficient matrix which displayed interesting difference between MCI subjects and normal controls.

3.1   Reproducibility of SW-LASSO

In section 2.5, we adopted a novel combined spatial-temporal strategy to achieve enough regression samples. Here, we evaluate the effect of sampling to the final regression result. We randomly picked one subject and repeated the sampling process for three times. The SW-LASSO regression procedure was applied to each round of sampling separately, and the result was shown in Fig. 5(a): four ROIs are displayed on the top two rows of the figure and the regression results are consistent through visual inspection. To quantitatively measure the robustness of proposed sampling method, we define the measure of consistence (MOC) as follows:

$$\text{MOC} = \sum_{i,j} \frac{M_{1ij} - M_{2ij}}{M_1 + M_2} \tag{5}$$

where M_1 and M_2 are two regression matrices; i and j are the indices of row and column. We calculated the MOC between any two rounds and the result is shown in Fig. 5(b). We can clearly see that the MOCs are below 0.1 for all 358 ROIs and most of them are in the range from 0.06 to 0.08, which is very small considering the information loss during the regression process. Notably, we achieved similar experimental results in Fig.5 for other subjects, suggesting the robustness and reproducibility of the SW-LASSO model.

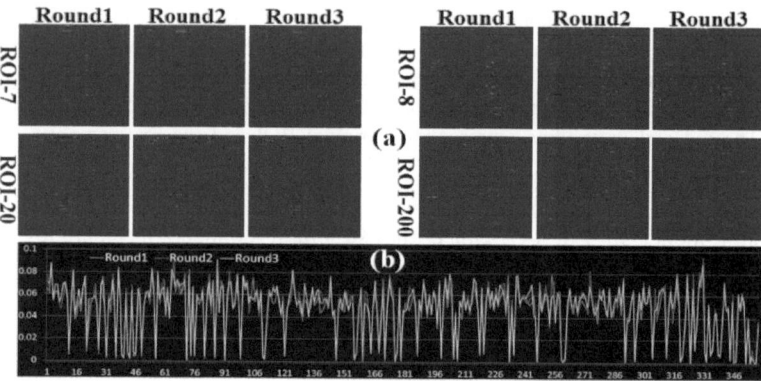

Fig. 5. Reproducibility of combined spatial-temporal sampling. The regression results of four ROIs in three independent sampling rounds are shown in (a). (b) shows the MOC (vertical axis) of all 358 ROIs (horizontal axis).

3.2   Accuracy of SW-LASSO

To measure how well the proposed structurally-weighted LASSO regression model fits the rsfMRI signals, or how well each of the cortical ROI's rsfMRI signal can be predicted by other 357 ROIs' rsfMRI signals, we employed the coefficient of determination (COD) [24] as a quantitative metric, and the results are shown in Fig. 6. From the figure, we can see that the fMRI BOLD signals of most cortical ROIs can be explained or represented by the other ROIs with more than 60%. Considering the low SNR of fMRI signals, the average COD value is 70%, which is quite satisfactory. This result suggests that the SW-LASSO can reasonably model high-order functional interactions among brain ROIs. One possible reason that might lead to the fact that

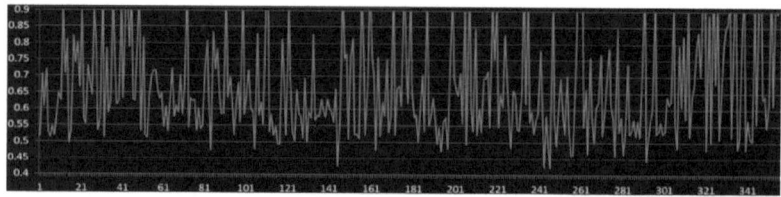

Fig. 6. Evaluation of accuracy for 358 cortical ROIs. COD values are shown in the vertical direction and the horizontal axis shows the cortical ROI index.

around 30% fMRI signals are unpredictable is that some interacting functional regions are still not covered by the current 358 cortical ROIs. Once denser cortical ROIs are included in the future, the average COD value by the SW-LASSO could be improved.

3.3   Assortative Analysis

Because the learned coefficients cannot be directly compared across different subjects, we need to normalize them before further analysis. Thus, we reorganized the data according to the temporal order, and for each time window we had a 358*358 matrix as shown in Fig.7. Actually, this matrix describes the overall regression dependency within a specific small time period. By doing this, we acquired a series of directed graphs automatically, each of which encodes the high-order interactions among 358 cortical ROIs.

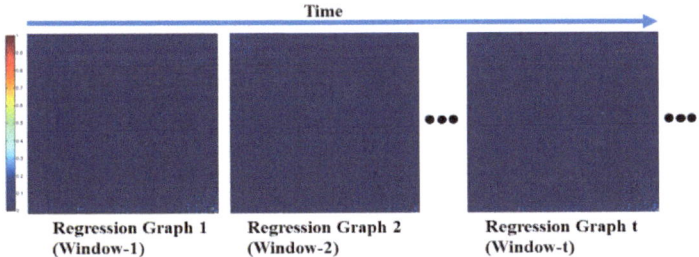

Fig. 7. Generated regression graphs along with the temporal order. Each regression graph is a 358*358 matrix which encodes the high-order functional interactions among the 358 cortical ROIs.

In this paper, we adopted the assortative [25] analysis on the generated graphs of two independent MCI datasets. Nodes in a network might show preference of connecting to other nodes that either have the similar (assortative mixing) or opposite properties (disassortative mixing), and in most cases the properties refer to the degree of the node. The type of mixing can be determined by assortativity coefficient which is defined as below:

$$R = \tfrac{1}{2} \Sigma_{jk} jk(e_{jk} - q_j q_k) \tag{6}$$

where j, k represent the degree of two ends of edge and q, e_{jk} are the distribution of remaining degree and joint probability distribution of the remaining degrees of the two nodes, respectively. Put simply, the assortativity coefficient reflects the Pearson correlation between the degrees of pairs of linked nodes. R ranges from -1 to 1, which correspond to complete disassortative and perfect assortative.

We calculated the assortativity coefficient for both MCI datasets and found a very interesting result, as shown in Fig.8. Specifically, the regression graphs of normal controls showed obvious disassortative mixing. MCI patients, however, tend to display assortative mixing. Remarkably, this observation is reproducible in two independent multimodal MCI datasets, as shown in Figs.8a and 8b. This suggests that in healthy brains, the active regions which often functionally interact with many other regions tend to communicate with those regions with little interactions. On the contrary, in MCI patients, the active regions tend to interact with other active regions as well. Notably, this result has supporting evidence from the literature report [26] on the default mode network (DMN): the DMN ROIs in Alzheimer's disease subjects tend to functionally interact with more other DMN ROIs than healthy controls. That is, Alzheimer's disease might initially involve DMN regions, which results in Alzheimer's patients demonstrating higher-functional activity in the DMN than healthy controls.

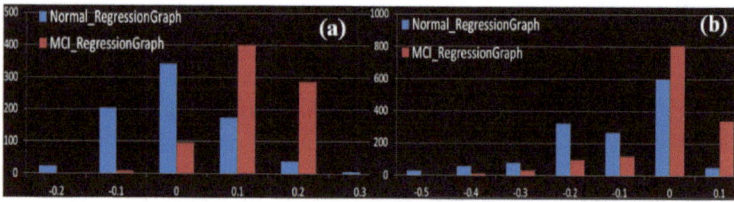

Fig. 8. (a) and (b) display the results of assortative mixing analysis on two separate MCI datasets. Horizontal axis shows the assortativity coefficient and the vertical axis represents the number of regression graphs.

4   Discussion and Conclusion

In this paper, we proposed a novel SW-LASSO regression model to represent the higher-order functional interactions among large-scale cortical ROIs in brain networks. Our major methodological contribution is that by introducing meaningful structural connectivity constraint, we can effectively examine the functional dependences of ROIs within the large-scale brain network. Since the search space grows exponentially with the increment of the number of brain ROIs we are considering, using the structural connectivity constraint to prune the ROI candidates is an efficient and effective strategy, considering the close relationship between the brain's structural connection and function. Therefore, the SW-LASSO model achieves a desirable trade-off between modeling high-order functional interaction and being computationally efficient in dealing with large-scale brain networks. Our experimental evaluation results have demonstrated the reasonably good robustness and accuracy of the proposed SW-LASSO model in characterizing high-order functional interactions. Importantly, the application of the SW-LASSO regression model in two separate MCI datasets revealed interesting findings, lending further support to the effectiveness and usefulness of the proposed methods.

Notably, the SW-LASSO regression model also has limitations, partly due to several key challenges in modeling high-order functional interactions. First, as pointed out in the literature [11], a major challenge in modeling multivariate functional interactions stems from the astronomical size of the possible space of alternative graph models. If represented as a graph, the number of possible directed interaction graph structures relating N brain regions or regions of interest (ROIs) is $4^{((N-1)*N)/2}$. However, the current SW-LASSO regression model in Eq.(4) only considers a small portion of possible alternative graph structures. In the future, more types of graph structures such as the chain-dependency structures [27] should be considered. Second, the current SW-LASSO regression model cannot deal with the temporal dynamics of functional interactions. Essentially, there is growing evidence from the literature [28-29] indicating that functional connectivities/interactions are under dynamic state changes at different time scales, even in resting state. It is still largely unknown how frequently high-order functional interactions within brain networks temporally transit and what the underlying principles are. In the future, the SW-LASSO regression model should be extended to account for temporal dynamics, in order to investigate those dynamic phenomena and principles.

References

[1] Honey, C.J., Sporns, O., Cammoun, L., Gigandet, X., Thiran, J.P., Meuli, R., Hagmann, P.: Predicting human resting-state functional connectivity from structural connectivity. PNAS 106(6), 2035–2040 (2009)

[2] Fox, M.D., Raichle, M.E.: Spontaneous fluctuations in brain activity observed with functional magnetic resonance imaging. Nat. Rev. Neurosci. 8, 700–711 (2007)

[3] Bullmore, E., Sporns, O.: Complex brain networks: graph theoretical analysis of structural and functional systems. Nat. Rev. Neurosci. 186(10) (2009)

[4] Calhoun, V.D., Adali, T., Pearlson, G.D., Pekar, J.J.: A method for making group inferences from functional MRI data using independent component analysis. Hum. Brain Mapping 14(3), 140–151 (2001)

[5] Roebroeck, A., Formisano, E., Goebel, R.: Mapping directed influence over the brain using Granger Causality and fMRI. NeuroImage 25, 230–242 (2005)

[6] Deshpande, G., Santhanam, P., Hu, X.: Instantaneous and causal connectivity in resting state brain networks derived from functional MRI data. NeuroImage 54(2), 1043–1052 (2011)

[7] Friston, K.J., Harrison, L., Penny, W.: Dynamic causal modelling. NeuroImage 19(3), 1273–1302 (2003)

[8] Harrison, L., Penny, W.D., Friston, K.: Multivariate autoregressive modeling of fMRI time series. NeuroImage 19, 1477–1491 (2003)

[9] Protzner, A.B., McIntosh, A.R.: Testing effective connectivity changes with structural equation modeling: what does a bad model tell us? Hum. Brain. Mapp. 27, 935–947 (2006)

[10] Kim, J., Zhu, W., Chang, L., Bentler, P.M., Ernst, T.: Unified Structural Equation Modeling Approach for the Analysis of Multisubject, Multivariate Functional MRI Data. Human Brain Mapping 28, 85–93 (2007)

[11] Ramsey, J., Hanson, S., Hanson, C., Halchenko, Y., Poldrack, R., Glymour, C.: Six problems for causal inference from fMRI. NeuroImage 49(2), 1545–1558 (2010)

[12] Ramsey, J.D., Hanson, S.J., Glymour, C.: Multi-subject search correctly identifies causal connections and most causal directions in the DCM models of the Smith et al. simulation study. NeuroImage 58(3), 838–848 (2011)

[13] Zhu, D., Li, K., Guo, L., Jiang, X., Zhang, T., Zhang, D., Chen, H., Deng, F., Faraco, C., Jin, C., Wee, C., Yuan, Y., Lv, P., Yin, Y., Hu, X., Duan, L., Hu, X., Han, J., Wang, L., Shen, D., Miller, L.S., Li, L., Liu, T.: DICCCOL: Dense Individualized and Common Connectivity-based Cortical Landmarks. Cerebral Cortex 23(4), 786–800 (2012)

[14] Li, K., Guo, L., Faraco, C., Zhu, D., Deng, F., Zhang, T., Jiang, X., Zhang, D., Chen, H., Hu, X., Miller, L.S., Liu, T.: Individualized ROI Optimization via Maximization of Group-wise Consistency of Structural and Functional Profiles. In: NIPS (2010)

[15] Zhu, D., Zhang, D., Faraco, C., Li, K., Deng, F., Chen, H., Jiang, X., Guo, L., Miller, L.S., Liu, T.: Discovering Dense and Consistent Landmarks in the Brain. In: Székely, G., Hahn, H.K. (eds.) IPMI 2011. LNCS, vol. 6801, pp. 97–110. Springer, Heidelberg (2011)

[16] Zhu, D., Li, K., Faraco, C., Deng, F., Zhang, D., Jiang, X., Chen, H., Guo, L., Miller, L.S., Liu, T.: Optimization of Functional Brain ROIs via Maximization of Consistency of Structural Connectivity Profiles. NeuroImage 59, 1382–1393 (2011)

[17] Honey, C.J., Sporns, O., Cammoun, L., Gigandet, X., Thiran, J.P., Meuli, R., Hagmann, P.: Predicting human resting-state functional connectivity from structural connectivity. PNAS 106(6), 2035–2040 (2009)

[18] Karas, G., Sluimer, J., Goekoop, R., Flier, W., Rombouts, S.A.R.B., Vrenken, H., Scheltens, P., Fox, N., Barkhof, F.: Amnestic mild cognitive impairment: structural MR imaging findings predictive of conversion to Alzheimer disease. AJNR 29(5), 944–949 (2008)

[19] Tibshirani, R.: Regression shrinkage and selection via the LASSO. Journal of the Royal Statistical Society 58, 267–288 (1996)

[20] Zou, H.: The adaptive lasso and its oracle properties. J. Amer. Statist. Assoc. 101(476), 1418–1429 (2006)

[21] Passingham, R.E., Stephan, K.E., Kötter, R.: The anatomical basis of functional localization in the cortex. Nat. Rev. Neurosci. 3(8), 606–616 (2002)

[22] Efron, B., Hastie, T., Johnstone, I., Tibshirani, R.: Least Angle Regression. The Annals of Statistics 32, 407–499 (2004)

[23] http://www.di.ens.fr/willow/SPAMS/

[24] Dougherty, E.R., Kim, S., Chen, Y.D.: Coefficient of determination in nonlinear signal processing. Signal Process. 80(10), 2219–2235 (2000)

[25] Newman, M.E.J.: Assortative Mixing in Networks. Physical Review Letters 89 (2002)

[26] Bero, A.W., Yan, P., Roh, J.H., Cirrito, J.R., Stewart, F.R., Raichle, M.E., Lee, J.M., Holtzman, D.M.: Neuronal activity regulates the regional vulnerability to amyloid-beta deposition. Nature Neuroscience 14, 750–756 (2011)

[27] Neapolitan, R.E.: Learning Bayesian Networks. Prentice Hall (2004)

[28] Chang, C., Gary, G.H.: Time - frequency dynamics of resting-state brain connectivity measured with fMRI. NeuroImage 50(1), 81–98 (2010)

[29] Majeed, W., Magnuson, M., Hasenkamp, W., Schwarb, H., Schumacher, E.H., Barsalou, L., Keilholz, S.D.: Spatiotemporal dynamics of low frequency BOLD fluctuations in rats and humans. NeuroImage 54, 1140–1150 (2011)

Feature-Based Alignment
of Volumetric Multi-modal Images

Matthew Toews[1], Lilla Zöllei[2], and William M. Wells[1]

[1] Brigham and Women's Hospital, Harvard Medical School
{mt,sw}@bwh.harvard.edu
[2] A.A. Martinos Center, Massachussetts General Hospital, Harvard Medical School
lzollei@nmr.mgh.harvard.edu

Abstract. This paper proposes a method for aligning image volumes acquired from different imaging modalities (e.g. MR, CT) based on 3D scale-invariant image features. A novel method for encoding invariant feature geometry and appearance is developed, based on the assumption of locally linear intensity relationships, providing a solution to poor repeatability of feature detection in different image modalities. The encoding method is incorporated into a probabilistic feature-based model for multi-modal image alignment. The model parameters are estimated via a group-wise alignment algorithm, that iteratively alternates between estimating a feature-based model from feature data, then realigning feature data to the model, converging to a stable alignment solution with few pre-processing or pre-alignment requirements. The resulting model can be used to align multi-modal image data with the benefits of invariant feature correspondence: globally optimal solutions, high efficiency and low memory usage. The method is tested on the difficult RIRE data set of CT, T1, T2, PD and MP-RAGE brain images of subjects exhibiting significant inter-subject variability due to pathology.

1 Introduction

Multiple medical imaging modalities, e.g. MR and CT images of the brain, are useful in highlighting complementary aspects of anatomy, however, they must first be aligned within a common spatial reference frame or atlas. A straight forward approach is to align all images to a single reference image or template via standard image registration methods, however, alignment and subsequent image analysis may be biased by the choice of template [1]. Group-wise alignment aims to reduce bias by jointly aligning image data. While a significant body of literature has addressed group-wise alignment of mono-modal image data [2–5], the more difficult context of multi-modal data is rarely addressed [6, 7].

Pair-wise image alignment is challenging due to factors such as pathology, resection, variable image cropping, multi-modal appearance changes and inter-subject variability. In the general case, it may be difficult to justify assumptions of smooth, one-to-one correspondence between images adopted by many registration techniques. Practical algorithms must be robust to poor initial misalignment, for example due to DICOM error [8]. Group-wise alignment poses several

J.C. Gee et al. (Eds.): IPMI 2013, LNCS 7917, pp. 25–36, 2013.
© Springer-Verlag Berlin Heidelberg 2013

additional challenges. Typical iterative algorithms compute multiple image-to-image or model-to-image alignment solutions for each image, and thus memory and computational requirements are generally linear and super-linear in the number of images, respectively. In the context of multi-modal data, a mechanism is required in order to address inter-modality intensity differences, e.g. simultaneously learning models of tissue classes [6] or the joint intensity relationship between modalities [7].

We propose a new group-wise alignment method to address these challenges. Rather than attempting to model a potentially complex global intensity relationship, we propose learning a collection of locally linear intensity relationships throughout the image. To do this effectively, we adopt a model based on local scale-invariant image features [9, 10], similar to approaches used with mono-modal 2D images [5, 11] and in full 3D volumes [12]. Local scale-invariant features can be repeatably extracted in the presence of global variations in image geometry and intensity, and encoded for computing global correspondence between images despite a high degree of occluded or missing image content. Recent efficient 3D scale-invariant feature encodings [12] are particularly useful for group-wise alignment, since once extracted, the memory and computational requirements of multiple, iterative alignment phases are significantly reduced in comparison to intensity-based methods.

This paper extends the feature-based alignment technique [12], and makes two primary technical contributions. A novel scale-invariant feature encoding is presented for computing inter-modality image correspondences, based on locally inverted intensity profiles, that significantly increases the number of correspondences possible between different image modalities. Similar ideas have been presented in the context of 2D image data [13], however, these do not generalize to volumetric data due to 3D orientation. A novel probabilistic model is then developed, incorporating this encoding into a feature-based model. A fully automatic algorithm iterates between model learning and model-to-image alignment, converging efficiently to a group-wise alignment solution with no pre-processing or pre-alignment. Previous approaches to multi-modal, group-wise alignment have assumed minor deformations around pre-aligned images of healthy subjects [6] or an individual subject [7].

Experiments demonstrate group-wise alignment on the challenging Retrospective Image Registration Evaluation (RIRE) multi-modal brain image data [14], where all subjects exhibit a high degree abnormal variability due to pathology. The inverted intensity encoding is crucial in achieving fully automatic and efficient group-wise alignment solutions. The model resulting from group-wise alignment can be used subsequently for globally optimal alignment of new multi-modal images of the same domain.

2 Invariant Feature Extraction

A scale-invariant feature in 3D is defined geometrically by a scaled local coordinate system S within image I. Let $S = \{X, \sigma, \Theta\}$, where $X = \{x, y, z\}$

is a 3-parameter location specifying the origin, σ is a 1-parameter scale and $\Theta = \{\hat{\theta}_1, \hat{\theta}_2, \hat{\theta}_3\}$ is a set of three orthonormal unit vectors $\hat{\theta}_1, \hat{\theta}_2, \hat{\theta}_3$ specifying the orientations of the coordinate axes. Invariant feature extraction begins by identifying a set of location/scale pairs $\{(X_i, \sigma_i)\}$ in an image. This is done by detecting spherical image regions centered on location X_i with radius proportional to scale σ_i that locally maximize a function $f(X, \sigma)$ of image saliency. For example, SIFT feature extraction identifies local extrema of the difference-of-Gaussian (DoG) function [9]:

$$\{(X_i, \sigma_i)\} = \text{local} \operatorname*{argmax}_{X, \sigma} |f(X, \kappa\sigma) - f(X, \sigma)|, \tag{1}$$

where $f(X, \sigma)$ is the convolution of the image I with a Gaussian kernel of variance σ^2 and κ is a multiplicative scale sampling rate. DoG detection generalizes trivially from 2D to higher dimensions and can be efficiently implemented using Gaussian scale-space pyramids [9, 15]. Following detection, each region is assigned an orientation Θ, and an image patch centered on X_i and proportional in size to σ_i is cropped from the image, reoriented and rescaled after which image intensity is encoded. We adopt the 3D orientation assignment and intensity encoding methods described in [12]. Briefly, orientation is assigned based on dominant image gradient orientations ∇I computed within regions $\{(X_i, \sigma_i)\}$. Let $H(\nabla I)$ be a spherical 3D histogram generated from image gradient samples ∇I within region (X, σ). Orthonormal unit vectors $\Theta = \{\hat{\theta}_1, \hat{\theta}_2, \hat{\theta}_3\}$ are determined as follows:

$$\hat{\theta}_1 = \operatorname*{argmax}_{\hat{\theta}} \{H(\nabla I)\},$$

$$\hat{\theta}_2 = \operatorname*{argmax}_{\hat{\theta}} \left\{H(\hat{\theta}_1 \times (\nabla I \times \hat{\theta}_1))\right\}, \qquad \hat{\theta}_3 = \hat{\theta}_1 \times \hat{\theta}_2. \tag{2}$$

With geometry S_i identified, region (X, σ) is cropped from the image, scaled and reoriented according to σ and Θ to a canonical image patch of fixed size, after which intensity is encoded. An efficient 3D version of the gradient orientation histogram (HoG) descriptor [9] is adopted as in [12], where spatial location and gradient orientation are quantized uniformly into eight spatial locations and eight 3D orientations, resulting in a compact $8 \times 8 = 64$-element vector.

A challenge in invariant feature matching is to reliably identify and characterize instances of the same anatomical structure in images acquired from different modalities, e.g. CT and MR. Regions identified in Equation (1) are essentially image blobs approximating center-surround patterns reminiscent of mammalian visual receptive fields [16]. Given that relationship between intensities arising from the same tissues in different modalities is generally non-linear and multimodal in nature [17], patterns in different image modalities arising from the same underlying anatomical structure will generally vary to the extent they cannot be extracted.

It has been noted, however, that multi-modal image registration can be achieved by assuming a locally linear intensity relationship, with either positive or negative correlation [18]. Generalizing this observation, we propose that the same holds true for distinctive image patterns localized in scale and space. Our reasoning is as follows: distinctive patterns present in different images arise from the interface between different tissue classes in the image. Although multiple tissue classes may be present within a local window, in many instances the image content may be dominated by a small number of intensity classes, e.g. white and grey matter, in which case the intensity relationship may be approximated as locally linear.

In can be shown that the set of image regions $\{(X_i, \sigma_i)\}$ identified via Equation (1) remains constant across linear intensity variations, either positive or negative. Negative linear variations, or intensity inversions, however, cause an inversion of the image gradient, which has a major affect on feature orientation Θ and intensity encoding. Thus in order to correctly normalize and compare features across intensity inversion, primary and secondary coordinate axes must be inverted in order to correctly align spatial locations, which is equivalent to a rotation of π about axis $\hat{\theta}_3$, see Figure 1 b). The same inversion must be performed on the spatial locations and orientation bins of the associated orientation GoH encoding, see Figure 1 c). Note that the tertiary coordinate axis remains unchanged as the cross product does not change with the negation of vectors $\hat{\theta}_3$.

Note that different image modalities may generally exhibit local intensity mappings other than linear relationships. In such cases, features cannot be extracted and matched, and alternative methods are necessary. Considering both positive and negative correlations significantly increases the number of possible correspondences. To illustrate the usefulness of inverted features, for the T2-MP-RAGE pair in Figure 1, only 2 correct correspondences are identified via nearest neighbor descriptor matching of conventional features (a), however, 22 additional correspondences are identified throughout the brain when inverted feature correspondences are considered (b).

3   Feature-Based Group-Wise Alignment

The feature-based alignment (FBA) method [12] is limited to a single image modality and requires pre-aligned training images. This section extends the FBA model to multiple image modalities, and presents a novel group-wise alignment algorithm that can achieve alignment without assuming pre-alignment.

Let S_{ij} represent the geometry of the jth feature extracted in the ith image, and let I_{ij} represent its associated intensity encoding. Let $\bar{IS} = \{(I_{ij}, S_{ij})\}$ represent a vector of feature appearance/geometry pairs extracted in N images. Let $\bar{T} = \{T_i\}$ be a set of unknown coordinate transforms, where T_i maps locations image i to a common reference or atlas space. In the context of this paper, T_i is a global 7-parameter similarity transform, about which further deformations are described independently in the neighborhood of local features. $\bar{T}$ is modeled here as a random variable characterized by the posterior $p(\bar{T}|\bar{IS})$. Group-wise alignment aims to identify the transform set $\bar{T}_{MAP}$ maximizing the posterior probability, which can be expressed using Bayes' theorem as follows:

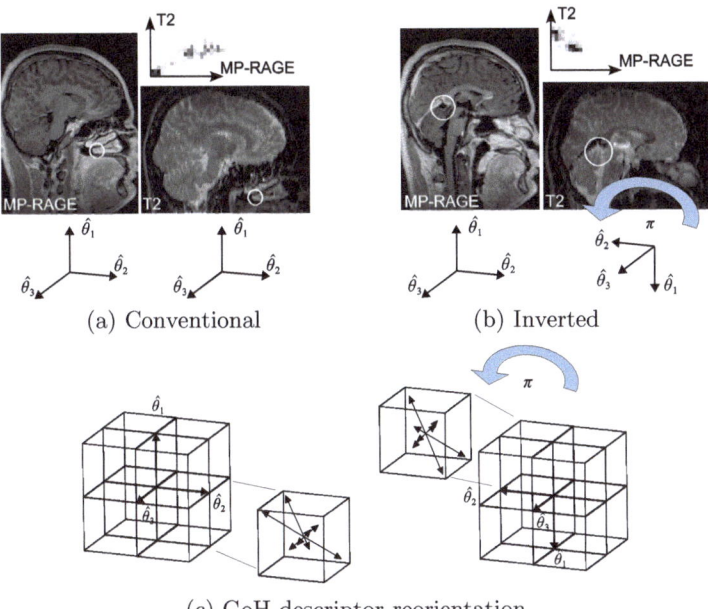

(a) Conventional   (b) Inverted

(c) GoH descriptor reorientation

Fig. 1. (a) and (b) illustrate scale-invariant feature correspondences automatically computed between MP-RAGE and T2 modalities. White circles illustrate feature locations and scales, graphs above the images illustrate the local joint intensity relationship associated with features. Intensities associated with tissues within the brain (b) generally exhibit an intensity inversion between these modalities, this is not the case for structures external to the brain such as bone and air-filled sinuses (a). (c) illustrates reorientation of the GoH intensity encoding in the case of intensity inversion. From left to right, a rotation of π about $\hat{\theta}_3$ is applied both to the 8 spatial location bins (boxes) and to the 8 orientation bins which they each contain (arrows).

$$\bar{T}_{MAP} = \underset{\bar{T}}{\mathrm{argmax}} \left\{ p(\bar{T}|\bar{IS}) \right\} \propto \underset{\bar{T}}{\mathrm{argmax}} \left\{ p(\bar{IS}|\bar{T})p(\bar{T}) \right\}. \qquad (3)$$

In Equation (3), $p(\bar{IS}|\bar{T})$ is the probability of image feature set $\bar{IS}$ conditional on transform set $\bar{T}$, $p(\bar{T})$ is the prior probability of transform set $\bar{T}$. The prior probability can be expressed as $p(\bar{T}) = \prod_i p(T_i)$, under the assumption that transforms for different images T_i and T_j, $i \neq j$ are independent. Factor $p(\bar{IS}|\bar{T})$ can be expressed as:

$$p(\bar{IS}|\bar{T}) = \prod_{i,j} p(I_{ij}, S_{ij}|\bar{T}) = \prod_{i,j} p(I_{ij}, S_{ij}|T_i), \qquad (4)$$

where the two equalities in Equation (4) follow from two modeling assumptions. The first is the assumption of conditionally independent features (I_{ij}, S_{ij}) given transform set $\bar{T}$. Intuitively, this states that the appearance and geometry (I_{ij}, S_{ij}) of one image feature provide no information regarding the appearance and geometry of another feature, provided image-wise mappings $\bar{T}$ are known. The second equality results from the assumption of conditional independence of features I_{ij}, S_{ij} and all transforms $T_j, i \neq j$ given transform T_i.

Alignment is driven by distinctive local image features, for instance scale-invariant features arising from tissue patterns in the brain. In a single image modality, such features can be characterized by their geometry, e.g. location, scale and orientation, and by their appearance, e.g. intensity encoding. In the case of multiple modalities, structures are also characterized by distinct modes of appearance, for example conventional and inverted intensities as in the previous section. Features may be incorporated as a latent random variable and marginalized out in determining $\bar{T}_{MAP}$. As in [12], we consider a discrete random variable of feature identity $F = \{f_{k,l}\}$, where $f_{k,l}$ indicates a specific anatomical structure $k \in \{1, \ldots, K\}$ and binary local appearance mode $l \in \{0,1\}$ (e.g. conventional or inverted). Marginalization is expressed as a sum over discrete model feature instances $f_{k,l}$:

$$p(I_{ij}, S_{ij}|T_i) = \sum_{k,l} p(S_{ij}, I_{ij}, f_{k,l}|T_i) = \sum_{k,l} p(S_{ij}, I_{ij}|f_{k,l}, T_i)p(f_{k,l}). \quad (5)$$

The right-hand side of Equation (5) results from Bayes' theorem and the assumption of independence between F and T_i, i.e. $p(f_{k,l}|T_i) = p(f_{k,l})$. Intuitively, this independence assumption indicates that transform T_i provides no additional information regarding the probability of model feature $f_{k,l}$. Factor $p(f_{k,l})$ is the discrete probability of model feature $f_{k,l}$ and $p(S_{ij}, I_{ij}|f_{k,l}, T_i)$ represents the probability of feature geometry and appearance (S_{ij}, I_{ij}) conditional on latent model feature $f_{k,l}$ and transform T_i. This factor can be further expressed as:

$$p(S_{ij}, I_{ij}|f_{k,l}, T_i) = p(I_{ij}|S_{ij}, f_{k,l}, T_i)p(S_{ij}|f_{k,l}, T_i) = p(I_{ij}|f_{k,l})p(S_{ij}|f_{k,l}, T_i), \quad (6)$$

assuming conditional independence of feature intensity encoding I_{ij} and feature geometry and transform (S_{ij}, T_i) given specific model feature $f_{k,l}$. Factor $p(I_{ij}|f_{k,l})$ is a conditional density over feature intensity encoding I_{ij} given model feature $f_{k,l}$, taken to be a Gaussian density over conditionally independent descriptor elements. Factor $p(S_{ij}|f_{k,l}, T_i)$ is a conditional density over feature geometry given model feature $f_{k,l}$ and transform T_i, which can be factored into conditional distributions over feature location, scale and orientation:

$$p(S_{ij}|f_{k,l}, T_i) = p(X_{ij}|f_{k,l}, T_i)p(\sigma_{ij}|f_{k,l}, T_i)p(\Theta_{ij}|f_{k,l}, T_i). \quad (7)$$

In Equation (7), factor $p(X_{ij}|\sigma_{ij}, f_{k,l}, T_i)$ is a density over extracted feature location X_{ij}, conditioned on model feature $f_{k,l}$ and transform T_i, here taken to be an isotropic Gaussian density with variance proportional to σ_{ij}. $p(\sigma_{ij}|f_{k,l}, T_i)$ is a density over extracted feature scale, conditioned on $(f_{k,l}, T_i)$, here taken to be a Gaussian density in $\log \sigma$. $p(\Theta_j|f_{k,l}, T)$ is a von Mises density [19] over independent angular deviations of coordinate axes, here approximated as an isotropic Gaussian density over Θ for simplicity under a small angle assumption. The final expression for the posterior probability of $\bar{T}$ becomes $p(\bar{T}|\bar{I}\bar{S}) \propto$

$$\prod_i p(T_i) \prod_j \sum_{k,l} p(f_{k,l}) p(I_{ij}|f_{k,l}) p(X_{ij}|f_{k,l}, T_i) p(\sigma_{ij}|f_{k,l}, T_i) p(\Theta_{ij}|f_{k,l}, T_i). \quad (8)$$

3.1   Group-Wise Alignment

The goal of group-wise alignment is to estimate transform vector $\bar{T}$ from feature data $\bar{IS}$ extracted in a set of images. If the model feature set F and the parameters of its associated probability factors are known, then the posterior in Equation (8) can be maximized directly by independently maximizing transforms T_i associated with individual images. They are unknown, however, and determining $\bar{T}$ and F is thus a circular problem. We propose an iterative solution which alternates between estimating $\bar{T}$ and F, in an attempt to converge to reasonable estimates of both. The algorithm consists of 1) initialization, 2) model estimation 3) image alignment and 4) feature updating, where steps 2-4 repeated iteratively until estimates of $\bar{T}$ converge. Note that alignment is based solely on scale-invariant features extracted once in each image.

1) **Initialization** involves setting individual transforms T_i to approximately correct alignment solutions according to location, orientation and scale. The primary requirement is that a subset of initializations to be approximately correct, the group-wise alignment is robust to a significant degree of error and a high number of completely incorrect transforms. This is performed here by choosing one image as an initial reference frame, then aligning all images to this model via a 3D Hough transform [20]. Due to inter-subject and inter-modality differences, many images may not initially align correctly, however, only a small subset is required to bootstrap model estimation.

2) **Model Estimation** aims to identify a set of model feature set $F = \{f_{k,l}\}$ and associated factors in Equation (8) from features extracted in training images. Equation (8) takes the form of a mixture model with K components, defined by conditional densities over model feature appearance and geometry $p(I_{ij}|f_{k,l}) p(S_{ij}|f_{k,l}, T_i)$ and mixing proportions $p(f_{k,l})$. The model parameters could thus potentially be estimated via methods such as expectation maximization [21] or Dirichlet process modeling [22], however, there are several challenges that make this difficult. First, the number of mixture components K is unknown and potentially large. Moreover, the current set of transforms $\bar{T}^t$ may be noisy and contain a high number of incorrect, outlier transforms T_i. A robust clustering process similar to the mean shift algorithm [23] is used to identify clusters of features that are similar in terms of their geometry and appearance as in [12]. Each cluster represents a single model feature $f_{k,l}$, and feature instances in a cluster are used to estimate parameters for associated probability factors, i.e. Gaussian means, variances and mixing proportions. Note that for the purpose of estimation, all model features are assumed to bear conventional appearance $l = 0$. Intensity-inversion $l = 1$ is incorporated later in alignment.

3) Alignment proceeds by maximizing $p(\bar{T}|\bar{I}S)$ via marginalization, as in Equation (8). With known model feature set F, this proceeds by maximizing each individual transform T_i independently:

$$T_{iMAP} = \underset{T_i}{\mathrm{argmax}} \left\{ p(T_i|\bar{I}S) \right\}. \tag{9}$$

Maximization proceeds by determining candidate model-to-image correspondences between features in image i and learned intensity distributions $p(I_{i,j}|f_{k,l})$. A candidate correspondence exists between model feature $f_{k,l}$ and image feature descriptor $I_{i,j}$ if $I_{k,l}$ and $I_{i,j}$ are nearest neighbors (NN) according to the Euclidean metric, where $I_{k,l}$ represents the mean of density $p(I_{i,j}|f_{k,l})$. Candidate correspondences are used to identify model-to-image similarity transform candidates T_i for evaluation under $p(T_i|I)$ in manner similar to the Hough transform [20]. Note that T_{iMAP} is globally optimal in the space of similarity transforms. This procedure can be carried out efficiently via approximate nearest neighbor techniques [24], and by considering only a subset of the most frequently occurring model features, as identified by $p(f_{k,l})$ in learning. Although a single image feature can potentially be attributed to multiple model features, appearance descriptors representing distinctive image patterns lie in sparse, high dimensional space, where it can be assumed that there is at most one significantly probable model correspondence.

Two types of alignment are considered here, conventional and multi-modal. Conventional alignment considers only appearance mode $l = 0$, whereas multi-modal alignment marginalizes over both conventional and inverted features $l = 0, 1$ under the assumption that $p(f_{k,l=0}) = p(f_{k,l=1})$. Multi-modal alignment has the capacity to identify correspondences despite local intensity inversions, however, it runs a higher probability of identifying incorrect correspondences and requires a higher search time. Experiments contrast conventional vs. multi-modal alignment.

4) Feature Update with $\bar{T}^t$ estimated, the geometry of each image feature $S_{i,j}$ is updated according to T_{iMAP}^t for subsequent iterations. Feature intensity encodings are invariant under similarity transforms and need not be updated.

4   Experiments

Experiments use the high-resolution RIRE data set [14], consisting of brain images of nine subjects and five modalities: CT, T1, T2, PD and MP-RAGE, for a total of 39 images (not all modalities are available for all subjects). Groupwise alignment of this data set is challenging for several reasons: all subjects exhibit significant anatomical abnormalities due to large brain tumors, there are no healthy or normal subjects. Images are acquired with a high degree of anisotropy which varies between modalities and subjects, with (X,Y,Z) voxels sizes of approximately (0.86,0.86,3.00) for T1,T2,PD, (0.98,1.37,0.98) for MP-RAGE and (0.45,0.45,3.00) for CT.

While several authors report multi-modal group-wise registration for recovering small deformations about known ground truth for a single subject [7, 25] or healthy subjects [6], we are not aware of literature addressing the more challenging context of inter-subject, multi-modal alignment involving significant abnormality and no pre-alignment. The only image preprocessing applied here is to resample images as isotropic, with voxels sizes 0.86mm for T1,T2,PD, 0.98mm for MP-RAGE and 0.45mm for CT. Knowledge of the image modality, the voxel size, image orientation or translation is not required or used.

Feature extraction requires approximately 25 seconds per volume of size $256 \times 256 \times 200$. Features arising from degenerate structures that cannot be reliably localized in 3D such as surfaces are identified and discarded via an analysis of the local structure tensor as in [26]. Model learning makes use of approximately 83K features, requiring 8.3MB of memory, note original image data in isotropic floating point format require 1700MB. Individual learning and fitting phases require approximately 25 and 10 seconds each on a 2.4GHz processor. The total running time here is ≈ 22 minutes, note that mono-modal group-wise registration algorithms require ≈ 19 hours for comparable amounts of data [3, 4].

Group-wise alignment converges in 7 iterations for both conventional and multi-modal alignment as shown in the upper left graph of Figure 2, when set $\bar{T}$ no longer changes with further iterations. The lower left graph of Figure 2 shows the relative numbers of conventional and inverted model-to-subject correspondences as a function of t for multi-modal alignment. In early iterations, a relatively large percentage of correspondences (e.g. 15% at $t = 1$) result from inverted matches, as relatively few model features exist due to initial misalignment. Inverted matches make up increasingly smaller portions of correspondences (e.g. 3%, $t = 7$), as improved alignment results in a larger set of model features. After convergence, a model with a stable latent feature set F has been learned, reflecting features present in the alignment/training image. This model can be used with either conventional alignment in order to efficiently align additional images of modalities present in training, or with multi-modal alignment to align images of new modalities unseen in training.

Recall that each mapping T_i represents a coarse global transform between images, about which individual image-to-model feature correspondences reflect refined, localized deformations. While T_i do not represent highly accurate transforms, images resampled according to T_i can be used to visually assess general success/failure of alignment. Multi-modal alignment successfully aligns all subjects, whereas conventional alignment produces three failure cases with clearly incorrect alignment solutions, see Figure 3. All failures arise from CT images, which have low image contrast in the brain and produce fewer features than other modalities. Precise quantification of alignment error could be performed on a feature-by-feature basis by contrasting the discrepancy of image-to-model correspondence with human labelers as in [11], we leave this for future work. The vast majority of correspondences in successful alignment solutions appear qualitatively correct, typical examples are shown in Figure 1.

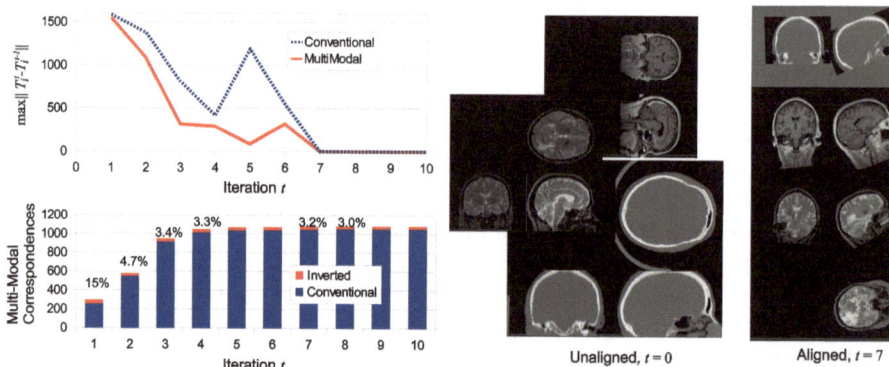

Fig. 2. The upper left graph illustrates transform set $\bar{T}$ change vs. iteration t, where change is measured by the maximum Frobenius norm affine transform matrix difference $max\|T_i^t - T_i^{t-1}\|$. Learning converges after 7 iterations, after which $\bar{T}$ does not change. The lower left graph shows the relative numbers of conventional and inverted correspondences over iteration t, where the percentages reflect the proportion of inverted correspondences. Image sets to the right show images before alignment $t = 0$ and resampled after convergence according to T_i at $t = 7$. Note the slightly elevated orientation in aligned images; since alignment here is fully automatic, the final geometry of group-wise alignment is determined by the data.

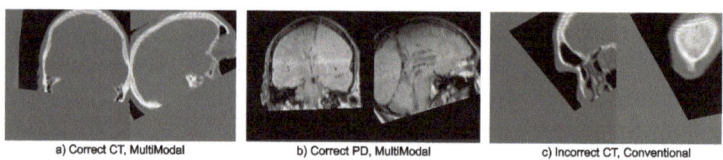

Fig. 3. a) and b) show typical instances of correct multi-modal alignment solutions, c) shows one of three clearly incorrect conventional alignment solutions

5   Discussion

This paper investigates a new method for addressing group-wise alignment of difficult, multi-modal image data. Inverted scale-invariant feature correspondences are proposed, which address multi-modality in the form of locally inverted joint intensity relationships. For several combinations of brain modalities, e.g. MP-RAGE and T2, this results in a significant increase in the number of image correspondences identified in comparison to conventional correspondence which assumes a positive linear joint intensity relationship.

Inverted correspondences form the basis for a novel feature-based model and group-wise alignment algorithm, which is shown to be effective in the case of a difficult, multi-modal brain image data set. Experiments demonstrate that considering multi-modality in the form of locally inverted intensity mappings leads to successful group-wise alignment, where conventional feature-based alignment fails. Although allowing for a wider range of intensity mappings potentially permits a higher number of incorrect correspondences and alignment solutions, these are unlikely to occur in practice due to smoothness of natural images.

Once a feature-based model of multi-modal intensity patterns has been learned for a set of modalities, it serves as prior knowledge for efficient and robust alignment of images of the same modalities considering strictly positive intensity correlations. This is analogous to theoretical findings in dense image registration, where the use of multi-modal vs. mono-modal similarity measures can be explained in terms of the informativness of the Bayesian prior [27].

A significant practical contribution of this paper is a system that is able to achieve group-wise alignment of difficult, multi-modal image data. The code used in this paper for feature extraction and inversion is available to the research community [1], which will facilitate the use of scale-invariant feature technology in medical image analysis. We have evaluated our group-wise alignment method several difficult contexts, including infant brain MR exhibiting intensity contrast changes and multi-subject truncated body CT scans, and results are promising.

Acknowledgements. Support was received from NIH grants P41-EB-015902, P41-RR-013218, R00 HD061485-03, P41-EB-015898 and P41-RR-019703.

References

1. Joshi, S., David, B., Jomier, M., Gerig, G.: Unbiased diffeomorphic atlas construction for computational anatomy. NeuroImage LVI(23), 151–160 (2004)
2. Twining, C.J., Cootes, T., Marsland, S., Petrovic, V., Schestowitz, R., Taylor, C.J.: A unified information-theoretic approach to groupwise non-rigid registration and model building. In: Christensen, G.E., Sonka, M. (eds.) IPMI 2005. LNCS, vol. 3565, pp. 1–14. Springer, Heidelberg (2005)
3. Learned-Miller, E.: Data driven image models through continuous joint alignment. IEEE TPAMI 28(2), 236–250 (2005)
4. Wu, G., Wang, Q., Jia, H., Shen, D.: Feature-based groupwise registration by hierarchical anatomical correspondence detection. Human Brain Mapping 33(2), 253–271 (2012)
5. Zhang, P., Cootes, T.F.: Automatic construction of parts+geometry models for initializing groupwise registration. IEEE TMI 31(2), 341–358 (2012)
6. Lorenzen, P., Prastawa, M., Davis, B., Gerig, G., Bullitt, E., Joshi, S.: Multi-modal image set registration and atlas formation. MIA 10(3), 440 (2006)
7. Spiclin, Z., Likar, B., Pernus, F.: Groupwise registration of multimodal images by an efficient joint entropy minimization scheme. IEEE TIP 21(5), 2546–2558 (2012)
8. Guld, M.O., Kohnen, M., Keysers, D., Schubert, H., Wein, B., Bredno, J., Lehmann, T.M.: Quality of dicom header information for image categorization. In: Int. Symposium on Medical Imaging, vol. 4685, pp. 280–287. SPIE (2002)
9. Lowe, D.G.: Distinctive image features from scale-invariant keypoints. IJCV 60(2), 91–110 (2004)

---

[1] `www.spl.harvard.edu/publications/item/view/2335`

10. Mikolajczyk, K., Schmid, C.: A performance evaluation of local descriptors. IEEE TPAMI 27(10), 1615–1630 (2005)
11. Toews, M., Arbel, T.: A statistical parts-based appearance model of anatomical variability. IEEE TMI 26(4), 497–508 (2007)
12. Toews, M., Wells III, W.: Efficient and robust model-to-image alignment using 3d scale-invariant features. Medical Image Analysis 17(3), 271–282 (2013)
13. Chen, J., Tian, J.: Real-time multi-modal rigid registration based on a novel symmetric-sift descriptor. Progress in Natural Science 19(5), 643–651 (2009)
14. West, J., Fitzpatrick, J., Wang, M., Dawant, B., Maurer Jr., C., Kessler, R., Maciunas, R., Barillot, C., Lemoine, D., Collignon, A., et al.: Comparison and evaluation of retrospective intermodality brain image registration techniques. Journal of Computer Assisted Tomography 21(4), 554–568 (1997)
15. Burt, P.J., Adelson, E.H.: The laplacian pyramid as a compact image code. IEEE Transactions on Communications 31(4) (1983)
16. Hubel, D.H., Wiesel, T.N.: Receptive fields, binocular interaction and functional architecture in the cat's visual cortex. Journal of Physiology 160 (1962)
17. Roche, A., Malandain, G., Pennec, X., Ayache, N.: The correlation ratio as a new similarity measure for multimodal image registration. In: Wells, W.M., Colchester, A.C.F., Delp, S.L. (eds.) MICCAI 1998. LNCS, vol. 1496, pp. 1115–1124. Springer, Heidelberg (1998)
18. Andronache, A., von Siebenthal, M., Szekely, G., Cattin, P.: Non-rigid registration of multi-modal images using both mutual information and cross-correlation. MIA 12, 3–15 (2008)
19. Evans, Hastings, Peacock: Statistical Distributions, 2nd edn. John Wiley and Sons (1993)
20. Ballard, D.: Generalizing the hough transform to detect arbitrary shapes. Pattern Recognition 13(2), 111–122 (1981)
21. Duda, R.O., Hart, P.E., Stork, D.G.: Pattern classification, 2nd edn. Wiley (2001)
22. Rasmussen, C.E.: The infinite gaussian mixture model. In: Neural Information Processing Systems, pp. 554–560 (2001)
23. Comaniciu, D., Meer, P.: Mean shift: A robust approach toward feature space analysis. IEEE TPAMI 24(5), 603–619 (2002)
24. Beis, J.S., Lowe, D.G.: Shape indexing using approximate nearest-neighbour search in high-dimensional spaces. In: CVPR, pp. 1000–1006 (1997)
25. Wachinger, C., Navab, N.: Structural image representation for image registration. In: MMBIA, pp. 23–30 (2010)
26. Rohr, K.: On 3D differential operators for detecting point landmarks. Image and Vision Computing 15(3), 219–233 (1997)
27. Zöllei, L., Jenkinson, M., Timoner, S., Wells, W.M.: A marginalized MAP approach and EM optimization for pair-wise registration. In: Karssemeijer, N., Lelieveldt, B. (eds.) IPMI 2007. LNCS, vol. 4584, pp. 662–674. Springer, Heidelberg (2007)

Bayesian Estimation of Regularization and Atlas Building in Diffeomorphic Image Registration

Miaomiao Zhang, Nikhil Singh, and P. Thomas Fletcher

Scientific Computing and Imaging Institute, University of Utah, Salt Lake City, UT

Abstract. This paper presents a generative Bayesian model for diffeomorphic image registration and atlas building. We develop an atlas estimation procedure that simultaneously estimates the parameters controlling the smoothness of the diffeomorphic transformations. To achieve this, we introduce a Monte Carlo Expectation Maximization algorithm, where the expectation step is approximated via Hamiltonian Monte Carlo sampling on the manifold of diffeomorphisms. An added benefit of this stochastic approach is that it can successfully solve difficult registration problems involving large deformations, where direct geodesic optimization fails. Using synthetic data generated from the forward model with known parameters, we demonstrate the ability of our model to successfully recover the atlas and regularization parameters. We also demonstrate the effectiveness of the proposed method in the atlas estimation problem for 3D brain images.

1 Introduction

Deformable image registration is often formulated as a maximum a posteriori (MAP) optimization problem, in which an image match likelihood term is regularized by a prior that encourages smooth deformations. In the diffeomorphic image registration setting, the log prior is in the form of the geodesic energy arising from a metric on an infinite-dimensional manifold of diffeomorphisms. In this framework, the level of smoothness is typically controlled by parameters describing the metric on the tangent space of the diffeomorphism group, as well as the noise variance in the image match term. However, despite the probabilistic motivation for the diffeomorphic registration problem, these model parameters are not estimated in current practice, but rather specified in an ad hoc manner. Part of the reason for this is that the estimation problem is inherently difficult, due to the fact that the log posterior of the metric parameters does not have a closed form and is computationally problematic to solve using direct optimization.

Further issues arise in the MAP formulation of diffeomorphic atlas building, where a template image, or atlas, is estimated along with the diffeomorphic registrations between the template and each input image. Current approaches [9,18] optimize over both the template image and the diffeomorphic transformations. However, in the MAP formulation the diffeomorphisms should be treated as hidden random variables and not parameters to be estimated. The current practice

J.C. Gee et al. (Eds.): IPMI 2013, LNCS 7917, pp. 37–48, 2013.

of optimizing over the diffeomorphisms is a mode approximation of the posterior distribution. Allassonnière et al. [1] shows that the common mode approximation scheme performs poorly under image noise, even for a simple 1D template estimation problem where the transformations are discrete shifts. As we show in this paper, the mode approximation in the diffeomorphism setting has similar difficulties when atlas estimation is combined with estimation of the metric and noise variance.

In this paper we propose a truly probabilistic formulation of the diffeomorphic atlas building problem. We develop an algorithm that can for the first time estimate the parameters controlling the smoothness of the diffeomorphisms and the image noise variance. This estimation procedure is a Monte Carlo Expectation Maximization (MCEM) algorithm, where the expectation step integrates over the posterior distribution of the diffeomorphic image transformations. We sample from this distribution using a novel Hamiltonian Monte Carlo (HMC) method on the space of the diffeomorphisms. Because we have a generative Bayesian model, we generate a synthetic data set from known parameters by sampling from the forward model, and then we show that our MCEM estimation procedure is able to recover those parameters. We also demonstrate that, unlike our MCEM algorithm, the mode approximation algorithm is unable to jointly estimate the atlas and the correct parameters. Finally, we show an example of an atlas and smoothness parameters estimated from real 3D brain images.

2 Related Work

Several works have proposed probabilistic motivations of the "groupwise" image registration problem, both in the small deformation [5,21] and diffeomorphic [9,17,18] setting. In these approaches a set of input images are registered to a template, which is simultaneously estimated in an alternating optimization strategy. Allassonniére et al. [1] were the first to point out that atlas estimation via this alternating optimization scheme is not completely faithful to the probabilistic interpretation. They go on to propose a fully generative probability model for an image atlas and population. Later, Allassonniére et al. [2] developed a stochastic approximative expectation maximization (SAEM) algorithm to estimate the atlas and registration parameters. This estimation was done by appropriately marginalizing over the posterior distribution for the image deformations using a Monte Carlo sampling procedure.

Another related area of research involves Bayesian models of the segmentation problem. Van Leemput [10] developed a Bayesian model of the image segmentation problem that includes an atlas image and a generative deformation and image intensity model. He introduced a sampling procedure for image deformations also based on HMC, although his registration is based on a small deformation model and ours is in the diffeomorphic setting. Iglesias et al. [8] later extended this work to include uncertainty in the registration parameters, by introducing hyperpriors on the parameters and integrating over their posterior. Risholm et al. [13,14] also formulated a Bayesian model for elastic image registration and provided an MCMC method for sampling deformations, with the goal of quantifying uncertainty in the image registrations. Simpson et al. [15] furthermore inferred the level of regularization in non-rigid registration by a hierarchical Bayesian model.

Our work is the first in the diffeomorphic setting to bring MCMC sampling and correct parameter estimation via marginalization of the image transformations. Ma et al. [11] introduced a Bayesian formulation of the diffeomorphic image atlas problem, but also estimated the atlas using a mode approximation to alternate between atlas and registration optimizations. They do not estimate the registration parameters. There has been some work on stochastic flows of diffeomorphisms [6], which are Brownian motions, i.e., small perturbations integrated along a time-dependent flow. This differs from the prior distribution in our work, which is on the tangent space of initial velocity fields, rather than on the entire time-dependent flow. Our formulation leads to random geodesics in the space of diffeomorphisms, and makes possible an efficient sampling procedure for MCMC sampling.

3   A Bayesian Model for Diffeomorphic Atlas Building

We define a generative probabilistic model for atlas building in the setting of large deformation diffeomorphic metric mappings (LDDMM) [4], which we begin by reviewing. In this framework, the registration between two images, $I_0, I_1 \in L^2(\Omega, \mathbb{R})$, is the minimizer of the energy,

$$E(v, I_0, I_1) = \int_0^1 (Lv_t, v_t)\, dt + \frac{1}{2\sigma^2}\|I_0 \circ \phi_1^{-1} - I_1\|^2. \tag{1}$$

Here $v \in L^2([0,1], V)$ is a time-varying velocity field in a reproducing kernel Hilbert space, V, equipped with a metric, $L : V \to V^*$, a positive-definite, self-adjoint, differential operator, mapping to the dual space, V^*. The notation (m, v) denotes the pairing of a momentum vector $m \in V^*$ with a tangent vector $v \in V$. The deformation ϕ is defined as the integral flow of v, that is, $(d/dt)\phi(t, x) = v(t, \phi(t, x))$. We use subscripts for the time variable, i.e., $v_t(x) = v(t, x)$, and $\phi_t(x) = \phi(t, x)$. When the energy above is minimized over all initial velocities, it yields a squared distance metric between the two input images, i.e.,

$$d(I_0, I_1)^2 = \min_{v \in V} E(v, I_0, I_1).$$

Using this distance metric between images, the atlas estimation problem can be formulated as a least-squares estimation problem, or in other words, a Fréchet mean. Given input images $I_1, \ldots, I_N$, the diffeomorphic atlas building problem is to find a template image $\hat{I}$ and initial velocities v^k that minimize the sum-of-squared distances function, i.e.,

$$\hat{I} = \arg\min_I \frac{1}{N} \sum_{k=1}^N d(I, I_k)^2. \tag{2}$$

Because the distance function between images is itself a minimization problem, the atlas estimation is typically done by alternating between the minimization in (1) to find the optimal v^k and the minimization in (2) to update the atlas $\hat{I}$. However, in a probabilistic interpretation of the energy (1) as a negative log posterior, the initial velocities v^k should be regarded as latent random variables. The maximization step is only a mode approximation to this posterior.

For a continuous domain $\Omega \subset \mathbb{R}^n$, direct interpretation of (1) as a negative log posterior is problematic, as the image match term would be akin to isotropic Gaussian noise in the infinite-dimensional Hilbert space $L^2(\Omega, \mathbb{R})$. This is not a well-defined probability distribution as it has infinite measure. More appropriately, we can instead consider our input images, I_k, and our atlas image, I, to be measured on a discretized grid, $\Omega \subset \mathbb{Z}^n$. That is, images are elements of the finite-dimensional Euclidean space $l^2(\Omega, \mathbb{R})$. We will also consider velocity fields v^k and the resulting diffeomorphisms ϕ^k to be defined on the discrete grid, Ω. Now our noise model is i.i.d. Gaussian noise at each image voxel, with likelihood given by

$$p(I_k \,|\, v^k, I) = \frac{1}{(2\pi)^{M/2}\sigma^M} \exp\left(-\frac{\|I \circ (\phi^k)^{-1} - I_k\|^2}{2\sigma^2}\right), \qquad (3)$$

where M is the number of voxels, σ^2 is the noise variance, and the norm inside the exponent is the Euclidean norm of $l^2(\Omega, \mathbb{R})$.

The negative log prior on the v^k is a discretized version of the squared Hilbert space norm above. Now consider L to be a discrete, self-adjoint, positive-definite differential operator on the domain Ω. The prior on each v^k is given by a multivariate Gaussian,

$$p(v^k) = \frac{1}{(2\pi)^{\frac{M}{2}}|L^{-1}|^{\frac{1}{2}}} \exp\left(-\frac{(Lv^k, v^k)}{2}\right), \qquad (4)$$

where d is the dimension of v^k, and $|L|$ is the determinant of L. In this work, we use a metric of the form $L = -\alpha\Delta + \beta$, where Δ is the discrete Laplacian, and α and β are positive numbers. In the sequel, we consider $\theta = (\alpha, \sigma, I)$ to be parameters that we wish to estimate. We fix β to a small number to ensure that the L operator is nonsingular. Putting together the likelihood (3) and prior (4), we arrive at the log joint posterior for the diffeomorphisms, via initial velocities, v^k, as

$$\log \prod_{k=1}^{N} p\left(v^k \,|\, I_k; \theta\right) \propto \frac{N}{2} \log|L| - \frac{1}{2} \sum_{k=1}^{N} (Lv^k, v^k)$$
$$- \frac{MN}{2} \log \sigma - \frac{1}{2\sigma^2} \sum_{k=1}^{N} \|I \circ (\phi^k)^{-1} - I_k\|^2. \qquad (5)$$

4   Estimation of Model Parameters

We now present an algorithm for estimating the parameters, θ, of the probabilistic image atlas model specified in the previous section. These parameters include the image atlas, I, the smoothness level, or metric parameter, α, and the standard deviation of the image noise, σ. We treat the v^k, i.e., the initial velocities of the image diffeomorphisms, as latent random variables with log posterior given by (5). This requires integration over the latent variables, which is intractable in closed form. We thus develop a Hamiltonian Monte Carlo procedure for sampling v^k from the posterior and use this in a Monte Carlo Expectation Maximization algorithm to estimate θ. It consists of two main steps:

1. **E-step.** We draw a sample of size S from the posterior distribution (5) using HMC with the current estimate of the parameters, $\theta^{(i)}$. Let v^{kj}, $j = 1, \ldots, S$, denote the jth point in this sample for the kth velocity field. The sample mean is taken to approximate the Q function,

$$Q(\theta \mid \theta^{(i)}) = E_{v^k \mid I_k; \theta^{(i)}} \left[\sum_{k=1}^{N} \log p \left(v^k \mid I_k; \theta \right) \right]$$

$$\approx \frac{1}{S} \sum_{j=1}^{S} \sum_{k=1}^{N} \log p \left(v^{kj} \mid I_k; \theta \right). \tag{6}$$

2. **M-step.** Update the parameters by maximizing $Q(\theta \mid \theta^{(i)})$. The maximization is closed form in I and σ, and a one-dimensional gradient ascent in α.

4.1 Background on Geodesic Shooting of Diffeomorphisms

Before presenting our MCEM estimation algorithm, we provide a brief background on the computations we will use for geodesic shooting and gradients for diffeomorphic image matching. Details of these methods are found in [19,20,16].

Deformation Momenta: The tangent space at identity, $V = T_{\mathrm{Id}}\mathrm{Diff}(\Omega)$, consists of all vector fields with finite Sobolev norm. Let $V^* = T_{\mathrm{Id}}^*\mathrm{Diff}(\Omega)$ denote its dual space. The velocity, $v \in V$, maps to its dual deformation momenta, $m \in V^*$, via the operator L such that $m = Lv$. The operator $K : V^* \to V$ denotes the inverse of L, so that $v = Km$. Note that constraining ϕ to be a geodesic with initial momentum $m_0 = m(0)$ implies that ϕ, m and I all evolve in a way entirely determined by the metric L, and that the deformation is determined entirely by the initial momenta, m_0.

EPDiff for Geodesic Evolution: Given the initial velocity, $v_0 \in V$, or equivalently, the initial momentum, $m_0 \in V^*$, the geodesic path $\phi(t)$ is constructed via integration of the following EPDiff equation [3,12]:

$$\frac{\partial m}{\partial t} = -\mathrm{ad}_v^* m = -(Dv)^T m - Dm\, v - m\,\mathrm{div}(v), \tag{7}$$

where D denotes the Jacobian matrix, and the operator ad^* is the dual of the negative Lie bracket of vector fields,

$$\mathrm{ad}_v w = -[v, w] = Dvw - Dwv.$$

The deformed image $I(t) = I_0 \circ \phi^{-1}(t)$ evolves via the equation

$$\frac{\partial I}{\partial t} = -v \cdot \nabla I.$$

Image Matching Gradient: In our HMC sampling procedure, we will need to compute gradients, with respect to initial momenta, of the diffeomorphic image matching problem in (1), for matching the atlas I to an input image I_k.

Following the optimal control theory approach in [19], we add Lagrange multipliers to constrain the diffeomorphism $\phi^k(t)$ to be a geodesic path. This is done by introducing time-dependent adjoint variables, $\hat{m}, \hat{I}$ and $\hat{v}$, and writing the augmented energy,

$$\tilde{E}(m_0) = E(Km_0, I, I_k) + \int_0^1 \langle \hat{m}, \dot{m} + \mathrm{ad}_v^* m \rangle dt + \int_0^1 \langle \hat{I}, \dot{I} + \nabla I \cdot v \rangle dt + \int_0^1 \langle \hat{v}, m - Lv \rangle dt,$$

where E is the diffeomorphic image matching energy from (1), and the other terms correspond to Lagrange multipliers enforcing: a) the geodesic constraint, which comes from the EPDiff equation (7), b) the image transport equation, $\dot{I} = -\nabla I \cdot v$, and c) the constraint that $m = Lv$, respectively.

The optimality conditions for m, I, v are given by the following time-dependent system of ODEs, termed the *adjoint equations*:

$$-\dot{\hat{m}} + \mathrm{ad}_v \hat{m} + \hat{v} = 0, \qquad -\dot{\hat{I}} - \nabla \cdot (\hat{I}v) = 0, \qquad -\mathrm{ad}_{\hat{m}}^* m + \hat{I} \nabla I - L\hat{v} = 0,$$

subject to initial conditions

$$\hat{m}(1) = 0, \qquad \hat{I}(1) = \frac{1}{\sigma^2}(I(1) - I_k).$$

Finally, after integrating these adjoint equations backwards in time to $t = 0$, the gradient of $\tilde{E}$ with respect to the initial momenta is

$$\nabla_{m_0} \tilde{E} = Km_0 - \hat{m}_0. \tag{8}$$

4.2   Hamiltonian Monte Carlo (HMC) Sampling

Hamiltonian Monte Carlo [7] is a powerful MCMC sampling methodology that is applicable to a wide array of continuous probability distributions. It utilizes Hamiltonian dynamics as a Markov transition probability and efficiently explores the space of a target distribution. The integration through state space results in more efficient, global moves, while it also uses gradient information of the log probability density to sample from higher probability regions. In this section, we derive a HMC sampling method to draw a random sample from the posterior distribution of our latent variables, v^k, the initial velocities defining the diffeomorphic image transformations from the atlas to the data.

To sample from a pdf $f(x)$ using HMC, one first sets up a Hamiltonian $H(x,\mu) = U(x) + V(\mu)$, consisting of a "potential energy", $U(x) = -\log f(x)$, and a "kinetic energy", $V(\mu) = -\log g(\mu)$. Here $g(\mu)$ is some proposal distribution (typically isotropic Gaussian) on an auxiliary momentum variable, μ. An initial random momentum μ is drawn from the density $g(\mu)$. Starting from the current point x and initial random momentum μ, the Hamiltonian system is integrated forward in time to produce a candidate point, $\tilde{x}$, along with the corresponding forward-integrated momentum, $\tilde{\mu}$. The candidate point $\tilde{x}$ is accepted as a new point in the sample with probability

$$P(\text{accept}) = \min(1,\ \exp(-U(\tilde{x}) - V(\tilde{\mu}) + U(x) + V(\mu)).$$

This acceptance-rejection method is guaranteed to converge to the desired density $f(x)$ under fairly general regularity assumptions on f and g.

In our model, to sample v^k from the posterior in (5), we equivalently sample m^k from the dual momenta, using $v^k = Km^k$, so we define our potential energy as $U(m^k) = -\log p(m^k|I_k;\theta)$. We use the prior distribution on the dual momenta as our proposal density, in other words, we use $p(K\mu)$ defined as in (4), taking care to include the appropriate change-of-variables. This gives the kinetic energy, $V(\mu) = (\mu, K\mu)$. This gives us the following Hamiltonian system to integrate in the HMC:

$$\frac{dm^k}{dt} = \frac{\partial H}{\partial \mu} = K\mu,$$

$$\frac{d\mu}{dt} = -\frac{\partial H}{\partial m^k} = -\nabla_{m^k}\tilde{E},$$

where the last term comes from the gradient defined in (8). As is standard practice in HMC, we use a "leap-frog" integration scheme, which better conserves the Hamiltonian and results in high acceptance rates.

4.3 The Maximization Step

We now derive the M-step for updating the parameters $\theta = (\alpha, \sigma, I)$ by maximizing the HMC approximation of the Q function, which is given in (6). This turns out to be a closed-form update for the noise variance σ^2 and the atlas I, and a simple one-dimensional gradient ascent for α.

From (5) and (6), it is easy to derive the closed-form update for σ as

$$\sigma^2 = \frac{1}{MNS} \sum_{j=1}^{S}\sum_{k=1}^{N} \|I_0 \circ (\phi^{kj})^{-1} - I^k\|^2. \tag{9}$$

For updating the atlas image I, we set the derivative of the Q function approximation which with respect to I to zero. The solution for I gives a closed-form update,

$$I = \frac{\sum_{j=1}^{S}\sum_{k=1}^{N} I^k \circ \phi^{kj}|D\phi^{kj}|}{\sum_{j=1}^{S}\sum_{k=1}^{N} |D\phi^{kj}|}.$$

The gradient ascent over α requires that we take the derivative of the metric $L = -\alpha\Delta + \beta I$, with respect to α. We do this in the Fourier domain, where the discrete Laplacian is a diagonal operator. For a 3D grid, the coefficients A_{xyz} of the discrete Laplacian at coordinate (x, y, z) in the Fourier domain is

$$A_{xyz} = -2\left(\cos\frac{2\pi x}{W-1} + \cos\frac{2\pi y}{H-1} + \cos\frac{2\pi z}{D-1}\right) + 6,$$

where W, H, D are the dimension of each direction. Hence, the determinant of the operator L is

$$|L| = \prod_{x,y,z} A_{xyz}\alpha + \beta.$$

The gradient of the HMC approximated Q function, with respect to α, is

$$\nabla_\alpha Q(\theta\,|\,\theta^{(i)}) \approx \frac{1}{2}\sum_{j=1}^{S}\sum_{k=1}^{N}\left[\sum_{x,y,z}\frac{A_{xyz}}{A_{xyz}\alpha+\beta} - \langle -\Delta v^{kj}, v^{kj}\rangle\right].$$

5   Results

We demonstrate the effectiveness of our proposed model and MCEM estimation routine using both 2D synthetic data and real 3D MRI brain data. Because we have a generative model, we can forward simulate a random sample of images from a distribution with known parameters $\theta = (\alpha, \sigma, I)$. Then, in the next subsection, we test if we can recover those parameters using our MCEM algorithm. Figure 1 illustrates this process. We simulated a 2D synthetic dataset starting from a atlas image, I, of a binary circle with resolution 100×100. We then generated 20 smooth initial velocity fields from the prior distribution, $p(v^k)$, defined in (4), setting $\alpha = 0.025$ and $\beta = 0.001$. Deformed circle images were constructed by shooting the initial velocities by the EPDiff equations and transforming the atlas by the resulting diffeomorphisms, ϕ^k. Finally, we added i.i.d. Gaussian noise according to our likelihood model (3). We used a standard deviation of $\sigma = 0.05$, which corresponds to an SNR of 20 (which is more noise than typical structural MRI).

Parameter Estimation on Synthetic Data. In our estimation procedure, we initialized α with 0.002 for noise free, and 0.01 for noise corrupted images. The step size of 0.005 for leap-frog integration is used in HMC with 10 units of time discretization in integration of EPDiff equations.

Figure 2 compares the true atlas and estimated atlases in the clean and noisy case. Figure 3 shows the convergence graph for α and σ estimation. It shows that our method recovers the model parameters fairly well. However, the iterative mode approximation algorithm does not recover the α parameter as nicely as our method. In the noisy case, the mode approximation algorithm estimates α as 0.0152, which is far from the ground truth value of 0.025. This is compared with our estimation of 0.026. In addition, in the noise free example, the mode approximation algorithm blows up due to the σ dropping close to 0, thus making the image match term numerically too high and the geodesic shooting unstable.

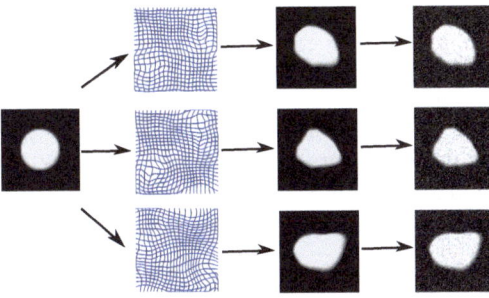

Fig. 1. Simulating synthetic 2D data from the generative diffeomorphism model. From left to right: the ground truth template image, random diffeomorphisms from the prior model, deformed images, and final noise corrupted images.

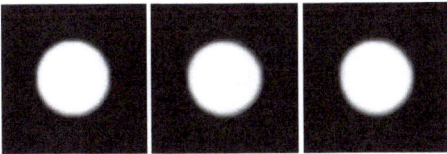

Fig. 2. Atlas estimation results. Left: ground-truth template. Center: estimated template from noise free dataset. Right: estimated template from noise corrupted dataset.

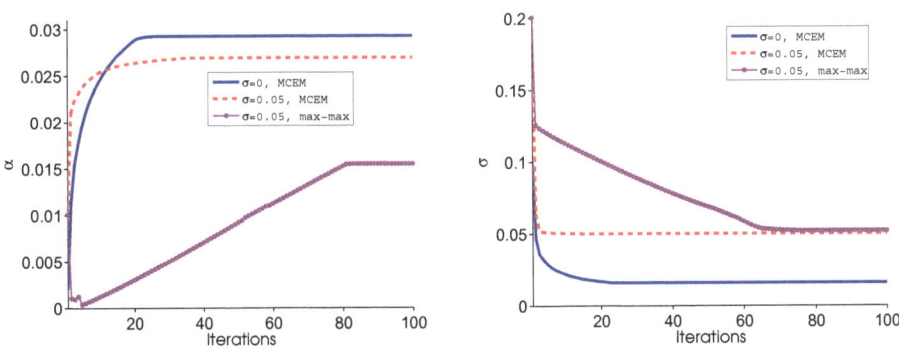

Fig. 3. Estimation of α, σ. Left: α estimation. Right: σ estimation. In our MCEM method, final estimated α and σ for noise free data are 0.028, 0.01, and for noise data are 0.026, 0.0501. Compared with max-max method, for the noise data, estimated α and σ are 0.0152, 0.052.

Atlas Building on 3D Brain Images. To demonstrate the effectiveness of our method on the real data, we apply our MCEM atlas estimation algorithm to a set of brain MRI from ten healthy subjects. The MRI have resolution

$108 \times 128 \times 108$ and are skull-stripped, intensity normalized, and co-registered with rigid transforms. We set the initial $\alpha = 0.01$, $\beta = 0.001$ with 15 time-steps.

The left side of Figure 4 shows coronal and axial slices from the 3D MRI used as input. The right side shows the initialization (greyscale average of the input images), followed by the final atlas estimated by our method. The final atlas estimate correctly aligns the anatomy of the input images, producing a sharper average image. The algorithm also jointly estimated the smoothness parameter to be $\alpha = 0.028$ and the image noise standard deviation to be $\sigma = 0.031$.

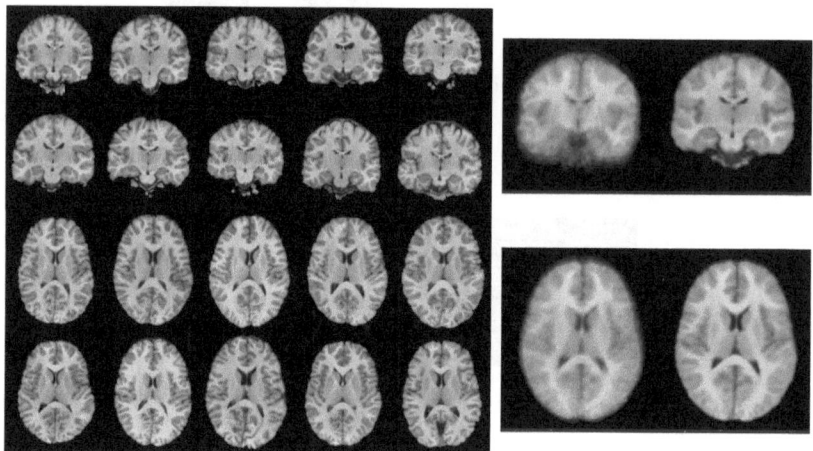

Fig. 4. Left: coronal and axial slices from the input 3D MRIs. Middle: initial greyscale average of the input images. Right: final atlas estimated by our MCEM estimation procedure.

Image Matching Accuracy. Finally, we demonstrate that another benefit of our HMC sampling methodology is improved performance in the standard image registration problem under large deformation shooting. Rather than use a direct gradient descent to solve the image registration problem, we instead can find the posterior mean of the model (5), where for image matching we fix the "atlas", I, as the source image and have just one target image, I_1. The stochastic behavior in the sampling helps to get out of local minima, where the direct gradient descent can get stuck. We compared our proposed method with direct gradient descent image registration by geodesic shooting from [19]. We used the authors' uTIlzReg package for geodesic shooting, which is available freely online. For the comparison, we registered the image pair shown in the first two panels of Figure 5, which requires a large deformation. The source and target images are 50×50. We used $\alpha = 0.02, \beta = 0.001$ for smoothing kernel, and $h = 40$ time-steps between $t = 0$ and $t = 1$. Note that we only want to compare the image matching here, so we fix the α and σ parameters.

Figure 5 demonstrates the results of the direct geodesic shooting registration with our HMC posterior mean. It shows that the geodesic shooting method gets

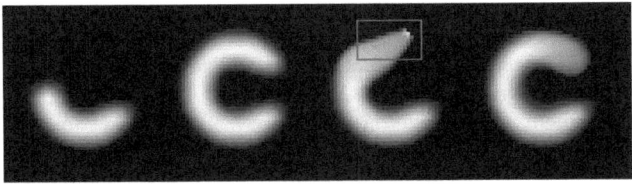

Fig. 5. The first two images from left to right are the source and target image respectively. Third is the matched image obtained by geodesic shooting method using [19]. Last image is the matched image from our MCEM method.

stuck in a local minima and cannot make it to the target image even with a large number of time-steps ($h = 60$) in the time discretization (we tried several time discretizations up to 60, and none worked). Though our method did not match perfectly in the tip of the "C", it still recovers the full shape while retaining a diffeomorphic transformation.

6   Conclusion

We presented a novel generative model of the diffeomorphic atlas estimation problem. Our method is the first to jointly estimate the regularity parameter, noise variance, and image atlas. It faithfully treats the diffeomorphic transformations from the atlas to the input images as unobserved random variables. We introduced a MCMC sampling scheme to integrate over these transformations. While we chose a particular parameterized form for the metric operator L, other metrics are also possible in our framework. This work opens up the possibility of extensions for rigorous probabilistic modeling of shape variability through diffeomorphisms.

Acknowledgements. This work was supported by NIH Grant R01 MH084795, NIH Grant 5R01EB007688, and NSF CAREER Grant 1054057.

References

1. Allassonnière, S., Amit, Y., Trouvé, A.: Toward a coherent statistical framework for dense deformable template estimation. Journal of the Royal Statistical Society, Series B 69, 3–29 (2007)
2. Allassonnière, S., Kuhn, E.: Stochastic algorithm for parameter estimation for dense deformable template mixture model. In: ESAIM-PS, vol. 14, pp. 382–408 (2010)
3. Arnol'd, V.I.: Sur la géométrie différentielle des groupes de Lie de dimension infinie et ses applications à l'hydrodynamique des fluides parfaits. Ann. Inst. Fourier 16, 319–361 (1966)
4. Beg, M.F., Miller, M.I., Trouvé, A., Younes, L.: Computing large deformation metric mappings via geodesic flows of diffeomorphisms. International Journal of Computer Vision 61(2), 139–157 (2005)

5. Bhatia, K., Hajnal, J., Puri, B., Edwards, A., Rueckert, D.: Consistent groupwise non-rigid registration for atlas construction. In: ISBI (2004)
6. Budhiraja, A., Dupuis, P., Maroulas, V.: Large deviations for stochastic flows of diffeomorphisms. Bernoulli 16, 234–257 (2010)
7. Duane, S., Kennedy, A., Pendleton, B., Roweth, D.: Hybrid Monte Carlo. Physics Letters B, 216–222 (1987)
8. Iglesias, J.E., Sabuncu, M.R., Van Leemput, K., The Alzheimer's Disease Neuroimaging Initiative: Incorporating parameter uncertainty in Bayesian segmentation models: Application to hippocampal subfield volumetry. In: Ayache, N., Delingette, H., Golland, P., Mori, K. (eds.) MICCAI 2012, Part III. LNCS, vol. 7512, pp. 50–57. Springer, Heidelberg (2012)
9. Joshi, S., Davis, B., Jomier, M., Gerig, G.: Unbiased diffeomorphic atlas construction for computational anatomy. NeuroImage 23(suppl. 1), 151–160 (2004)
10. Van Leemput, K.: Encoding probabilistic brain atlases using Bayesian inference. IEEE Transactions on Medical Imaging 28, 822–837 (2009)
11. Ma, J., Miller, M.I., Trouvé, A., Younes, L.: Bayesian template estimation in computational anatomy. NeuroImage 42, 252–261 (2008)
12. Miller, M.I., Trouvé, A., Younes, L.: Geodesic shooting for computational anatomy. Journal of Mathematical Imaging and Vision 24(2), 209–228 (2006)
13. Risholm, P., Pieper, S., Samset, E., Wells III, W.M.: Summarizing and visualizing uncertainty in non-rigid registration. In: Jiang, T., Navab, N., Pluim, J.P.W., Viergever, M.A. (eds.) MICCAI 2010, Part II. LNCS, vol. 6362, pp. 554–561. Springer, Heidelberg (2010)
14. Risholm, P., Samset, E., Wells III, W.: Bayesian estimation of deformation and elastic parameters in non-rigid registration. In: Fischer, B., Dawant, B.M., Lorenz, C. (eds.) WBIR 2010. LNCS, vol. 6204, pp. 104–115. Springer, Heidelberg (2010)
15. Simpson, I.J.A., Schnabel, J.A., Groves, A.R., Andersson, J.L.R., Woolrich, M.W.: Probabilistic inference of regularisation in non-rigid registration. NeuroImage 59, 2438–2451 (2012)
16. Singh, N., Hinkle, J., Joshi, S., Thomas Fletcher, P.: A vector momenta formulation of diffeomorphisms for improved geodesic regression and atlas construction. In: International Symposium on Biomedial Imaging (ISBI) (April 2013)
17. Twining, C.J., Cootes, T., Marsland, S., Petrovic, V., Schestowitz, R., Taylor, C.J.: A unified information-theoretic approach to groupwise non-rigid registration and model building. In: Christensen, G.E., Sonka, M. (eds.) IPMI 2005. LNCS, vol. 3565, pp. 1–14. Springer, Heidelberg (2005)
18. Vialard, F.-X., Risser, L., Holm, D., Rueckert, D.: Diffeomorphic atlas estimation using Kärcher mean and geodesic shooting on volumetric images. In: MIUA (2011)
19. Vialard, F.-X., Risser, L., Rueckert, D., Cotter, C.J.: Diffeomorphic 3d image registration via geodesic shooting using an efficient adjoint calculation. International Journal of Computer Vision, 229–241 (2012)
20. Younes, L., Arrate, F., Miller, M.I.: Evolutions equations in computational anatomy. NeuroImage 45(1S1), 40–50 (2009)
21. Zöllei, L., Jenkinson, M., Timoner, S., Wells, W.M.: A marginalized MAP approach and EM optimization for pair-wise registration. In: Karssemeijer, N., Lelieveldt, B. (eds.) IPMI 2007. LNCS, vol. 4584, pp. 662–674. Springer, Heidelberg (2007)

Gradient Competition Anisotropy for Centerline Extraction and Segmentation of Spinal Cords

Max W.K. Law[1,2,*], Gregory J. Garvin[2,4], Sudhakar Tummala[2],
KengYeow Tay[2,3], Andrew E. Leung[2,3], and Shuo Li[1,2]

[1]GE Healthcare, Canada
[2] University of Western Ontario, London, Canada
[3] London Health Sciences Centre, London, Canada
[4] St. Joseph's Health Care London, London, Canada
max.w.k.law@gmail.com

Abstract. Centerline extraction and segmentation of the spinal cord
– an intensity varying and elliptical curvilinear structure under strong
neighboring disturbance are extremely challenging. This study proposes
the gradient competition anisotropy technique to perform spinal cord
centerline extraction and segmentation. The contribution of the proposed
method is threefold – 1) The gradient competition descriptor compares
the image gradient obtained at different detection scales to suppress
neighboring disturbance. It reliably recognizes the curvilinearity and orientations of elliptical curvilinear objects. 2) The orientation coherence
anisotropy analyzes the detection responses offered by the gradient competition descriptor. It enforces structure orientation consistency to sustain strong disturbance introduced by high contrast neighboring objects
to perform centerline extraction. 3) The intensity coherence segmentation quantifies the intensity difference between the centerline and the
voxels in the vicinity of the centerline. It effectively removes the object
intensity variation along the structure to accurately delineate the target
structure. They constitute the gradient competition anisotropy method
which can robustly and accurately detect the centerline and boundary of
the spinal cord. It is validated and compared using 25 clinical datasets.
It is demonstrated that the proposed method well suits the applications
of spinal cord centerline extraction and segmentation.

1 Introduction

Centerline and boundary detection of the spinal cord in T1-weighted (T1-) and
T2-weighted (T2-) magnetic resonance (MR) images are beneficial to the diagnosis of spinal cord compression, myelopathy, spinal cord atrophy and multiple
sclerosis. In T1- and T2-MR images, a spinal cord is a grey elliptical curvilinear object surrounded by different tissues, including dark bone cortex/spinal
cavity/cartilaginous tissues, dark to grey ligaments and nerve roots, grey bone
marrow and dark grey to bright cerebro-spinal fluid (CSF). The intensity of the

---

* Corresponding author.

J.C. Gee et al. (Eds.): IPMI 2013, LNCS 7917, pp. 49–61, 2013.
© Springer-Verlag Berlin Heidelberg 2013

spinal cord and the surrounding tissues can noticeably change because of the reduced amount of white matter of the spinal cord towards the inferior direction, fluid motion artifacts, partial volume effects and bias fields. Considering the strong disturbance introduced by adjacent tissues (Figs. 1a-f) and the inconsistent intensity of the spinal cord, the detection of the spinal cord centerline and boundary are extremely challenging tasks.

Prior curvilinear structure detection approaches [1–9] mainly focus on detection of circular tubular objects. They scarcely discuss the analysis of elliptical curvilinear structures surrounded by high contrast neighboring objects. Owing to the lack of a suitable curvilinear structure descriptor, previous spinal cord detection approaches rely on extensive user inputs, training data and prior assumption of the spinal cord. Koh *et. al.* [10] segmented the surrounding structures of a spinal cord to include the spinal cord in the segmentation result. An atlas-based non-rigid registration algorithm was proposed for voxel-wise classification for spinal cord segmentation [11]. McIntosh and Harmarneh [12] designed a set of criteria including structure surface smoothness, structure cross section circularity and intensity consistency, along with user guided centerline extraction to segment the spinal cord. Horsfield *et. al.* [13] formulated an active surface model for spinal cord segmentation which requires manually supplied spinal cord centerlines. Coulon *et. al.* [14] presented a gradient based active surface model which merely refines manually segmented spinal cord surfaces.

This paper proposes the gradient competition anisotropy to detect elliptical curvilinear structure under strong neighboring disturbance. The proposed method possesses three components - 1) the gradient competition descriptor sustains neighboring disturbance to detect elliptical curvilinear objects; 2) the orientation coherence anisotropy reliably extracts structure centerlines even if high contrast neighboring objects present; 3) the intensity coherence segmentation well handles the intensity inconsistency along the structure.

The gradient competition descriptor captures the structure orientation and curvilinearity. The curvilinearity and orientation, along with the orientation coherence constitute a Riemannian metric for orientation coherence anisotropy centerline extraction. Based on minimizing the intensity difference between the centerline and the voxels in the vicinity of the centerline, the spinal cord is delineated by the intensity coherence segmentation. Distinct from the aforementioned existing spinal cord detection approaches, the proposed method is general to the

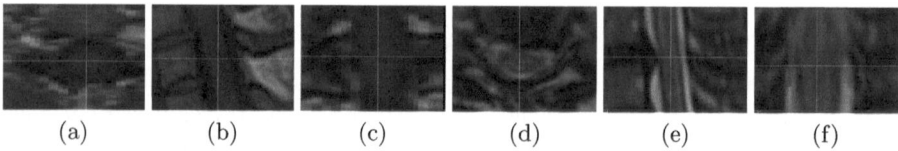

(a)	(b)	(c)	(d)	(e)	(f)

Fig. 1. Local image patches of two volumetric cervical spinal scan. (a-c) T1-MR image, the crosses belong to a manually selected center of the spinal cord; (d-f) T2-MR image, the crosses belong to a manually selected center of the spinal cord. (a,d) Axial planes; (b, e) Sagittal planes; (c, f) Coronal planes.

detection of different curvilinear structures. It also handles both T1- and T2-MR images. It is validated and compared using 10 T1- and 15 T2-MR images in the experiment. It is shown that the proposed method well suits the tasks of elliptical curvilinear structure detection under strong neighboring disturbance, so as the spinal cord centerline extraction and segmentation.

2   Methodology

2.1   Gradient Competition Descriptor

The anisotropic descriptor is developed based on aggregating image gradients at a spherical surface δS_r,

$$f(\boldsymbol{x}; r, \hat{\rho}) = \frac{1}{4\pi r^2} \int_{\delta S_r} \left((\hat{\rho}\hat{\rho}^T) \nabla I(\boldsymbol{x} + r\hat{n}) \right) \cdot \hat{n} dA, \qquad (1)$$

where r is the radius of the spherical surface, $\hat{\rho}$ is an arbitrary detection direction, $\hat{n}$ and dA are the outward normal and infinitesimal area of the spherical surface respectively. Derivatives are evaluated by convolving images with the first derivatives of Gaussian having a unit voxel-length scale factor. The term $\hat{\rho}\hat{\rho}^T \nabla I$ reports the gradient along $\hat{\rho}$. This descriptor reports positive (negative) responses when δS_r touches an ascending (descending) edge [6, 2].

Inside a curvilinear structure, the optimal detection direction which produces the strongest response lies on the structure cross-sectional plane. If $\hat{\rho}$ is parallel to the curvilinear structure orientation, the response is minimal. Given the optimal detection direction, the above measure reaches its maximum at the curvilinear object centerline when r is the semi-width of the object, i.e. the contact area between δS_r and the curvilinear object boundary is maximized. The optimal detection direction is obtained according to,

$$\hat{a}_{1,r} = \arg\max_{\hat{\rho}} |f(\boldsymbol{x}; r, \hat{\rho})|.^1 \qquad (2)$$

The response $f(\cdot; q, \hat{a}_{1,q})$ is competed with the strongest responses reported in a smaller detection scale to penalize oversize detection scales,

$$\lambda_{1,r} = \max(f(\cdot; r, \hat{a}_{1,r}), 0) - \max_{u \in \{l, 2l, \ldots, r\}} |f(\cdot; u, \hat{a}_{1,r})|, \qquad (3)$$

where l is the minimum voxel length. The above equation assumes that the target curvilinear object is darker than its surrounding (spinal cords in T2-MR images). Detection of bright structure (spinal cords in T1-MR images) is achieved by conducting the analysis on the inverted image. On spinal cord detection, the above gradient competition suppresses the disturbance introduced by

---

[1] The optimization of Equations 2 and 5 are achieved by performing eigendecomposition on a 3-by-3 symmetric tensor $(4\pi r^2)^{-1} \int_{S_r} \mathbf{H} dV$ and a 2-by-2 symmetric tensor $(4\pi r^2)^{-1} \int_{S_r} [\frac{\partial}{\partial \hat{b}_1} \frac{\partial}{\partial \hat{b}_2}][\frac{\partial}{\partial \hat{b}_1} \frac{\partial}{\partial \hat{b}_2}]^T (I) dV$ respectively, where $\mathbf{H}$ is the image Hessian, $\hat{b}_1 \times \hat{b}_2 = \hat{b}_1 \times \hat{a}_{1,r_1} = \hat{b}_2 \times \hat{a}_{1,r_1} = 0$ and V is the infinitesimal volume.

neighboring structures, such as CSF, ligaments and bone cortex when extracting responses inside the spinal cord. The optimal detection scale is,

$$r_1 = \arg \max_{r \in \{Z_0, Z_0+l, \ldots Z_1\}} \lambda_{1,r}, \tag{4}$$

where Z_0 and Z_1 are the minimum and maximum possible semi-widths of the spinal cord respectively[2]. To conform with the elliptical curvilinear object, a different detection scale is obtained in the orthogonal space of $\hat{a}_{1,r_1}$ [15],

$$\hat{a}_{2,r} = \arg \max_{\hat{\rho}, \forall \hat{\rho} \perp \hat{a}_{1,r_1}} |f(\cdot; r, \hat{\rho})|,^1 \tag{5}$$

$$\lambda_{2,r} = \max(f(\cdot; r, \hat{a}_{2,r}), 0) - \max_{u \in \{l, 2l, \ldots, r\}} |f(\cdot; u, \hat{a}_{2,r})|, \quad r_2 = \arg \max_{r \in \{Z_0, Z_0+l, \ldots Z_1\}} \lambda_{2,r}. \tag{6}$$

A curvilinear structure orientation field is retrieved as $\hat{v} = \hat{a}_{1,r_1} \times \hat{a}_{2,r_2}$. The object curvilinearity is defined as the sum of the intensity changes cross the boundaries, subtracted by the local intensity fluctuation along the structure,

$$\gamma = \lambda_{1,r_1} + \lambda_{2,r_2} - \max_{r \in [l, 2l, \ldots Z_1]} |f(\cdot; r, \hat{v})|. \tag{7}$$

2.2   Orientation Coherence Anisotropy

The gradient competition descriptor offers a scalar curvilinearity response γ and an orientation field $\hat{v}$. The spinal cord centerline has both large curvilinearity and low orientation discrepancy. An anisotropic speed functional is constructed to capture the spinal cord centerline,

$$\arg \max_{\mathcal{P} \in \mathbf{P}_{\boldsymbol{p}_0, \boldsymbol{p}_1}} \int_{\mathcal{P}} (\gamma(\mathcal{P}(p)) |\hat{v}(\mathcal{P}(p)) \cdot \mathcal{P}'(p)|) \, dp, \tag{8}$$

where p is the length parameterization of the path $\mathcal{P}$, $\mathbf{P}_{\boldsymbol{p}_0, \boldsymbol{p}_1}$ is a family of paths which connect the points $\boldsymbol{p}_0$ and $\boldsymbol{p}_1$. $\boldsymbol{p}_0$ and $\boldsymbol{p}_1$ are the manually supplied end points of the spinal cord. Equation 8 finds the fastest pathway to travel from $\boldsymbol{p}_0$ to $\boldsymbol{p}_1$ to extract the spinal cord centerline.

However, the structure orientation field can be adversely affected by noise or ambiguous object boundaries. Computation of the optimal path can be deteriorated by the inaccurately estimated structure orientation, leading to an incorrect path which follows the large curvilinearity responses induced by adjacent high contrast objects . This is overcome by considering the orientation coherence between the path and the structure orientation in a local region,

$$\arg \max_{\mathcal{P} \in \mathbf{P}_{\boldsymbol{p}_0, \boldsymbol{p}_1}} \int_{\mathcal{P}} J_{\text{Speed}}(p, \mathcal{P}, \mathcal{P}') dp, \text{ where}$$

$$J_{\text{Speed}}(p, \mathcal{P}, \mathcal{P}') = \gamma(\mathcal{P}(p)) \left(\int g_\sigma(\boldsymbol{y}) \left(\hat{v}(\mathcal{P}(p) + \boldsymbol{y}) \cdot \mathcal{P}'(p) \right)^2 dV \right)^{\frac{1}{2}}. \tag{9}$$

---

[2] Z_0 and Z_1 are $1.5mm$ and $20mm$ in this study.

where g_σ is a Gaussian function with a scale factor σ, dV is the infinitesimal volume. Given σ is defined according to the minimum width of the detection target[3], the structure orientation at the spinal cord centerline is coherent within the effective Gaussian window, i.e. $\left(\int g_\sigma(\boldsymbol{y})(\hat{v}(\mathcal{P}(p)+\boldsymbol{y})\cdot\mathcal{P}'(p))^2 dV\right)^{\frac{1}{2}} \approx |\hat{v}(\mathcal{P}(p))\cdot\mathcal{P}'(p)|$ and Equation 9 resembles Equation 8. When the object orientation becomes ambiguous, the locally random orientation field lowers the preference of the optimal path orientation. It is distinct to Equation 8 which always forces the path to follow the orientation field. Thus, the optimal path extraction is more robust against less accurate orientation fields caused by noise or ambiguous object boundaries. Equation 9 is reformulated in a tensorial form to compute the corresponding optimal path, $J_{\text{Speed}}(p,\mathcal{P},\mathcal{P}')$ becomes,

$$\left(\gamma^2(\mathcal{P}(p))(\int g_\sigma(\boldsymbol{y})(\mathcal{P}'(p))^T\left(\hat{v}(\mathcal{P}(p)+\boldsymbol{y})\hat{v}^T(\mathcal{P}(p)+\boldsymbol{y})\right)\mathcal{P}'(p)dV)\right)^{\frac{1}{2}}$$
$$=\sqrt{(\mathcal{P}'(p))^T\left(\int\gamma^2(\mathcal{P}(p))g_\sigma(\boldsymbol{y})\hat{v}(\mathcal{P}(p)+\boldsymbol{y})\hat{v}^T(\mathcal{P}(p)+\boldsymbol{y})dV\right)\mathcal{P}'(p)}. \quad (10)$$

Let $\mathbf{M}$ denote the resultant tensors of integrating the orientation field outer product in Equation 10. The computation of $\mathbf{M}$ is independent to the path $\mathcal{P}$,

$$\mathbf{M}(\boldsymbol{x}) = \gamma^2(\boldsymbol{x})\left(\int g_\sigma(\boldsymbol{y})\hat{v}(\boldsymbol{x}+\boldsymbol{y})\hat{v}^T(\boldsymbol{x}+\boldsymbol{y})dV\right). \quad (11)$$

$\mathbf{M}$ can be regarded as a tensor defining an anisotropic local speed. It embodies the curvilinearity and orientation field provided by the gradient competition descriptor. A minimum time of arrival function $\mathcal{T}(\boldsymbol{x})$ is defined as,

$$\mathcal{T}(\boldsymbol{x}) = \min_{\mathcal{P}\in\mathbf{P}_{p_0,\boldsymbol{x}}}\int_\mathcal{P} J(p,\mathcal{P},\mathcal{P}')dp, J(p,\mathcal{P},\mathcal{P}') = \sqrt{\mathcal{P}'(p)^T\mathbf{N}^{-1}(\mathcal{P}(p))\mathcal{P}'(p)}, \quad (12)$$

where $\mathcal{T}(\boldsymbol{p}_0) = 0$, $\mathbf{N} = \mathbf{M} + \epsilon\mathbf{I}$, ϵ is a small constant (10^{-4} in this paper) to avoid singularity and $\mathbf{I}$ is an identity matrix. The optimal path is acquired using gradient descent according to $\mathcal{L}' \propto \mathbf{N}\nabla\mathcal{T}$. The first variation of $\mathcal{T}$ is,

$$\delta\mathcal{T} = \frac{\partial J}{\partial\mathcal{P}'}\delta\mathcal{P} + \int_{p0}^x\left(\frac{\partial J}{\partial\mathcal{P}} - \frac{d}{ds}\frac{\partial J}{\partial\mathcal{P}'}\right)dp. \quad (13)$$

The second term on the right hand side of the above equation vanishes according to the Euler condition, i.e.

$$\nabla\mathcal{T} = \frac{\partial\mathcal{T}}{\partial\mathcal{P}} = \frac{\partial J}{\partial\mathcal{P}'} = \frac{\mathbf{N}^{-1}\mathcal{P}'}{\sqrt{\mathcal{P}'^T\mathbf{N}^{-1}\mathcal{P}'}}. \quad (14)$$

It can be expressed in a form of Eikonal equation,

$$\nabla\mathcal{T}^T\mathbf{N}\nabla\mathcal{T} = \frac{\mathcal{P}'^T(\mathbf{N}^{-1})^T\mathbf{N}\mathbf{N}^{-1}\mathcal{P}'}{\mathcal{P}'^T\mathbf{N}^{-1}\mathcal{P}'} = 1. \quad (15)$$

The Eikonal equation is solved by the anisotropic fast marching algorithm [16].

---

[3] The full width of half maximum of the Gaussian function is decided according to the minimum width of the spinal cord, i.e. $\sigma = 0.5(2\ln 2)^{-0.5}Z_0$.

The optimal path of Equation 12 is acquired based on the minimal Riemannian arc-length governed by the tensorial metric $\mathbf{M}^{-1}$. When the local orientation is coherent, $\mathbf{M}$ is a stick tensor, giving a γ^2 and null speed along the structure orientation and structure cross-sectional plane respectively. Such a tensor yields an infinite anisotropy, leading to a strong preference to align the optimal path along the structure orientation. If the orientation is locally random, $\mathbf{M}$ becomes a ball-tensor, possessing unit anisotropy and a $\frac{1}{3}\gamma^2$ isotropic speed. The reduced speed $\frac{1}{3}\gamma^2$ leads to a more conservative path search, while the tensor has a minimal anisotropy, implying a less restrictive path orientation preference. As such, the tensor anisotropy is governed by the local orientation field coherence. It effectively avoids the optimal path from following a random orientation field and producing incorrect centerline extraction.

2.3 Intensity Coherence Segmentation

Let $\boldsymbol{y_x}$ denotes a centerline position which is closest to the voxel $\boldsymbol{x}$. An intensity difference function is formulated,

$$\mathcal{E} = |I(\boldsymbol{x}) - I(\boldsymbol{y_x})|. \tag{16}$$

The spinal cord is segmented by partitioning the vicinity of the centerline into two regions. The desired region is the one connecting to the centerline with the consideration of intensity coherence (i.e. minimizing the intensity difference),

$$\tilde{\alpha}, \tilde{\beta} = \underset{\substack{\alpha \in [0,1], \\ \beta \in \{0,1\}}}{\arg\min} \int_{\Omega_{\mathcal{L},Z_1}} \underbrace{\alpha\mathcal{E} + (1-\alpha)|\mathcal{E} - \mu|}_{\text{Image term}} + \underbrace{\kappa|\nabla\alpha|}_{\text{Smoothness}} + \underbrace{\beta C_{\mathcal{L}}(\alpha) + (1-\beta)\bar{C}_{\mathcal{L}}(\alpha)}_{\text{Connectivity constraint}} dV,$$

$$\mu = \int_{\Omega_{\mathcal{L},Z_1}} (1-\alpha)\mathcal{E}dV \left(\int_{\Omega_{\mathcal{L},Z_1}} (1-\alpha)dV \right)^{-1}, \tag{17}$$

where κ is the smoothness strength which is $0.1 \max(\mathcal{E})$ in our experiment, $\Omega_{\mathcal{L},Z_1}$ is the region within the distance Z_1 to $\mathcal{L}$, C is ∞ inside the regions $\{\alpha > 0.5\}$ isolated from $\mathcal{L}$ and 0 otherwise, $\bar{C}$ is the inverse of C and the final spinal cord segmentation is $\{\tilde{\alpha} > 0.5\} \cap \{\tilde{\beta} = 1\}$. The minimization of the above functional with respect to α is solved iteratively based on the convex relaxed Potts model [17]. The minimization with respect to β is achieved by assigning $\tilde{\beta} = 1$ when $C(\tilde{\alpha}) = 0$. The intensity difference offsets the intensity fluctuation along the structure. Therefore, minimizing the intensity difference well segments a structure along which the intensity is significantly varying.

3   Experiment

The experiments employ one numerical tensor field (Fig. 2a), three numerical volumes (Fig. 3a-c), 10 clinical T1-MR and 15 clinical T2-MR images captured from

25 subjects concerning the cervical and upper thoracic spines[4]. Various components of the proposed method, including the gradient competition descriptor, orientation coherence anisotropy centerline extraction and intensity coherence segmentation are examined. They are compared against five existing approaches using different criteria - the gradient competition descriptor is compared with the multiscale Vesselness measure (Vesselness) [1] and Optimally Oriented Flux approach (OOF) [6] based on curvilinear object orientation estimation accuracy[5]; the orientation coherence anisotropy centerline extract is studied along with the vesselness measure [1] incorporated in the fast marching method [18] (Vesselness-FM) [6] and a state-of-the-art 4D fast marching method (4D-Anisotropy) [4] based on centerline extraction accuracy; and intensity coherence segmentation and the multiphase convex relaxed optimization [19] of Chan-Vese functional (Convex-CV)[7] [20] are examined using spinal cord segmentation accuracy.

The first experiment (Fig. 2a) mimics a tensor field computed according to the outer product of the orientation fields of two adjacent tubes. The red region represents the target tube for centerline extraction while the green region corresponds to a high contrast tube (green tensors have a 50% larger trace than the red counterparts) attached to the target. The vertical red tensors mimic the erroneously detected object orientation, which is perpendicular to the target tube. Assigning this stick tensor field to $\hat{v}\hat{v}^T$ in Equation 11 with $\sigma = 0$, i.e. orientation coherence is unconsidered, the resultant optimal path is attracted by the green tensors and leaves the target object, giving an incorrect centerline extraction. Fig. 2b shows the tensor field $\mathbf{M}$ obtained by using the tensor field in Fig. 2a for $\hat{v}\hat{v}^T$ and $\sigma = 1$ voxel-length in Equation 11. The erroneously oriented tensors in Fig. 2a become elliptical tensors in Fig. 2b. Employing the orientation coherence allows the optimal path to pass through these tensors with lower orientation preference and reports a correct extraction.

---

[4] The scans were acquired by Siemens Avanto 1.5T MRI at St. Joseph's Hospital, London, Canada, using the following protocol: voxelsize $3.3 \times 0.5729 \times 0.5729 mm^3$ (T1-MR), $0.4375 \times 0.4375 \times 1 mm^3$ (T2-MR); slice dimension 640×640; $T_R = 2500, T_E = 29$ (T1-MR), $T_R = 1500, T_E = 150$ (T2-MR); flip angle $150°$. The University of Western Ontario Research Ethics Board for Health Sciences Research Involving Human Subjects approved the use of the clinical data with the requirement for informed consent being waived.

[5] The structure orientations of Vesselness and OOF are the eigenvectors of the minimal magnitude eigenvalues of the Hessian matrices and OOF tensors at the selected scales.

[6] The fast marching method finds the optimal path which connects p_0 and p_1 to minimize the sum of the inverted vesselness response along the path.

[7] Each spinal image is partitioned into three regions, which correspond to the bright, grey and dark structures, $\arg\min_{(\alpha_1,\alpha_2,\alpha_3)} \sum_{n=\{1,2,3\}} \int \alpha_n (I - \mu_n)^2 + \alpha_n H_n + \kappa|\nabla\alpha_n|dV, \mu_n = \int \alpha_n I dV (\int \alpha_n dV)^{-1}$ and $\mu_1 < \mu_2 < \mu_3$, $\sum_{n=\{1,2,3\}} \alpha_n = 1$. The voxels where $\mathcal{L}$ traverses are employed as the hard constraint, i.e. H_1 and H_3 are zero except $H_1(\mathcal{L}) = H_3(\mathcal{L}) = \infty$, and H_2 is always zero. Connectivity analysis is performed on the resultant region $\{\{\alpha_2 > \alpha_1\} \cap \{\alpha_2 > \alpha_3\}\}$. The final segmentation is the connected component which encloses $\mathcal{L}$.

Table 1. The acute angular error (radian) of the structure orientation estimated at the ground truth structure centerline

	Major radius	8	6	4
Structure	Proposed method	0.1019 ± 0.0923	0.0774 ± 0.0337	0.0802 ± 0.0309
Orientation	Vesselness	0.2485 ± 0.1725	0.2281 ± 0.1272	0.1852 ± 0.1104
	OOF	0.3178 ± 0.2045	0.1928 ± 0.1336	0.1167 ± 0.0968
Major axis	Proposed method	0.1222 ± 0.1341	0.1210 ± 0.0864	Not Available
Minor axis	Proposed method	0.0525 ± 0.0364	0.1055 ± 0.0932	Not Available

Table 2. Quantitative centerline extraction comparison. An extraction is regarded as successful if the entire extracted centerline stays within the ground truth spinal cord. "Success rate" is the successful proportion of cases among all cases.

	T1 Images		T2 Images	
	Average distance	Success rate	Average distance	Success rate
Proposed method	$1.1853 \pm 0.7831 mm$	100%	$0.7895 \pm 0.4536 mm$	100%
Proposed method without curvilinearity	$1.9543 \pm 1.0565 mm$	100%	$1.4213 \pm 0.8108 mm$	100%
Vesselness-FM	$3.9686 \pm 2.8130 mm$	20%	$1.9087 \pm 1.3180 mm$	73.33%
4D-Anisotropy	$4.5478 \pm 3.3011 mm$	0%	$1.4456 \pm 1.1852 mm$	100%

Table 3. Quantitative segmentation results (Mean±Standard Deviation)

T1 Images	DSC	Signed distance	Absolute distance
Proposed method	0.8156 ± 0.0786	$-0.1650 \pm 0.5863 mm$	$0.9645 \pm 0.4156 mm$
Proposed method (Ellipsoid)	0.7057 ± 0.1439	$-0.7079 \pm 0.9854 mm$	$1.2788 \pm 0.6675 mm$
Multiphase CV-Functional	0.7132 ± 0.1733	$-0.4087 \pm 0.9018 mm$	$1.0087 \pm 0.5854 mm$
T2 Images	DSC	Signed distance	Absolute distance
Proposed method	0.8905 ± 0.0299	$-0.2521 \pm 0.3663 mm$	$0.4812 \pm 0.2567 mm$
Proposed method (Ellipsoid)	0.7214 ± 0.1987	$-0.6915 \pm 0.5978 mm$	$1.1795 \pm 0.7109 mm$
Multiphase CV-Functional	0.8201 ± 0.1535	$0.4520 \pm 0.9705 mm$	$0.9087 \pm 0.7018 mm$

The second test employs the numerical volumes which consist of nested elliptical and circular curvilinear objects. The target elliptical curvilinear structure is enclosed by another one, and is also adjacent to nested circular curvilinear objects. These neighboring structures exhibit a higher boundary contrast than the target structure (Fig. 3a). Table 1 details the accuracy of estimating different directions of the elliptical object. The proposed method outperforms existing approaches in terms of the structure orientation estimation. Mathematically, Vesselness and OOF merely select one object scale at each position. This is insufficient to capture the elliptical object which has two scales at each centerline position. In contrast, λ_1 and λ_2 of the proposed method correspond to two detection scales. The proposed method has larger performance advantages over existing approaches when the eccentricity of the elliptical structure soars. Without eccentricity (Table 1, major radius=4), the proposed method still yields a better result because of the gradient competition descriptor (Equations 3 and 6). The competition suppresses the detection responses obtained using oversize scales and effectively removes the neighboring disturbance during detection. On the contrary, OOF doesn't have the gradient competition and Vesselness relies on the second derivatives of Gaussian which involves large regions around the target during detection. Their detection performance is unsatisfactory when

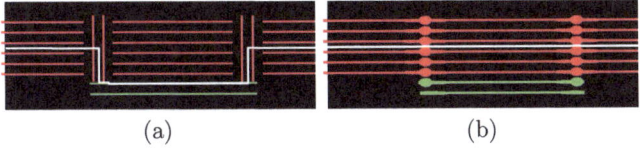

(a)   (b)

Fig. 2. The white curves are the optimal paths extracted from the corresponding tensor fields, which are shown as the red or green lines and ellipses. p_0 and p_1 are at the center points at the left-most and right-most slices. For better illustration, the tensors with very small traces are not shown.

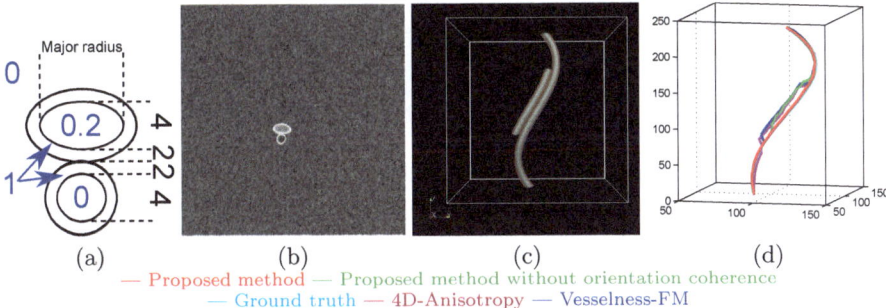

(a)   (b)   (c)   (d)
— Proposed method — Proposed method without orientation coherence
— Ground truth — 4D-Anisotropy — Vesselness-FM

Fig. 3. (a) The description of three numerical volumes, major radius $= 4, 6, 8$. The blue and black numbers indicate the intensity of different image regions and the dimensions of different structures respectively. The image is corrupted by additive Gaussian noise with magnitude 0.2. (b-d) Major radius $= 8$, (b) the middle axial slice of the volume; (c) the x-z view of the isosurfaces of the curvilinear objects with isovalues 0.4 (green) and 0.9 (orange); (d) the centerline extraction results.

strong neighboring disturbance exists even if the target is circular. Finally, Table 1 also evidences the accurate minor and major axes estimated by the gradient competition descriptor of the proposed method.

We further investigate the impact of the neighboring disturbance during centerline extraction. It is noted that the circular tube has a higher boundary contrast than the target object (1 versus 0.8, Fig. 3a). It thus produces larger responses that undesirably attract the optimal paths of Vesselness-FM and 4D-Anisotropy to pass through the circular tube (Fig. 3d). Without employing the orientation coherence (i.e. $\sigma = 0$ for Equations 9-11), the proposed method also fails to keep the optimal path inside the target structure. Analogous results are obtained from the clinical data (Fig. 4). They resemble the discovery in the previous experiment using the numerical tensor field.

Based on the clinical data, the quantitative centerline extraction result is shown in Table 2. The proposed method shows an outstanding performance as compared to other approaches. The low success rates of Vesselness-FM and 4D-Anisotropy hint that these two methods are sensitive to the high contrast tissues adjacent to the spinal cord. In addition, the proposed method is tested

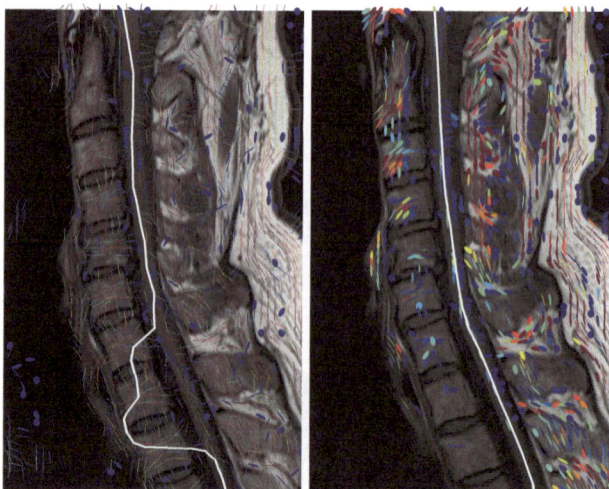

Fig. 4. The extracted centerline based on Equation 10 without (left), and with (right) local orientation coherence. The white curves are the extracted optimal paths. The color lines and ellipses represent the stick tensor $\hat{v}\hat{v}^T$ (left) and the tensor $\mathbf{M}$ (right). Their orientation and eccentricity correspond to the directions and anisotropy of these tensors. The tensors are colored according to the largest eigenvalues, pure blue and red are the minimum and maximum value in the image volume respectively. For better illustration, isotropic tensors and tensors having very small traces are not shown.

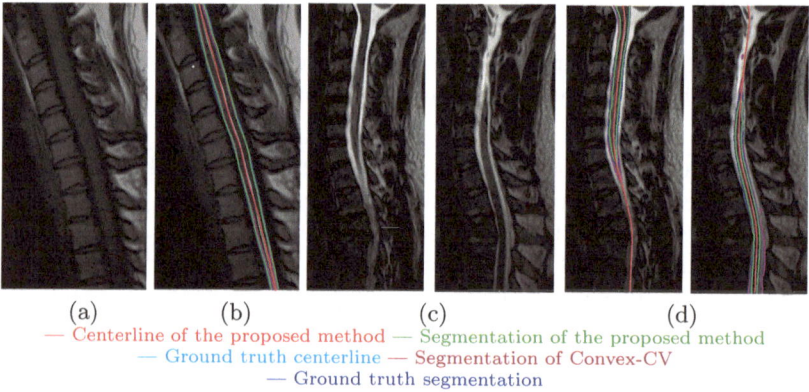

| (a) | (b) | (c) | (d) |

— Centerline of the proposed method — Segmentation of the proposed method
— Ground truth centerline — Segmentation of Convex-CV
— Ground truth segmentation

Fig. 5. Sagittal slices and corresponding segmentation results of 2 clinical cases. (a, b) The mid-sagittal slice of a T1 case. (c, d) Two sagittal slices of a T2 case.

with the curvilinearity measure removed, i.e. γ is removed from Equation 11. Nonetheless, the optimal path follows the spinal cord and offers a 100% success rate, despite the less accurate extraction. This mirrors that the orientation coherence anisotropy offers the robustness against neighboring disturbance, while the curvilinearity helps providing an accurate extraction.

The spinal cord segmentation results are shown in Table 3^8. The proposed method is more accurate than Convex-CV. It is noted that the voxel intensity at $\mathbf{p}_0$ are on average 32.28% and 60.72% higher than that at $\mathbf{p}_1$ in our T1- and T2-MR images respectively. Such significant intensity changes along the spinal cord boosts the Chan-Vese functional and deteriorates the segmentation. In the proposed method, the discrepancy is offset by measuring the intensity difference between reference voxels to the closest centerline positions (Equation 16). The envelop of the ellipsoids constructed according to $\mathcal{L}, r_1, r_2, \hat{a}_{1,r_1}$ and $\hat{a}_{2,r_2}$ is also compared to the ground truth spinal cord. It illustrates that the gradient competition descriptor satisfactorily estimates the local ellipsoids that well approximate the spinal cord. Fig. 5 visualizes the segmentation results obtained by the proposed method and Convex-CV. The largely overlapping curves between the proposed method and the ground truth confirms the promising segmentation accuracy of the proposed method.

4   Perspective and Conclusion

This study proposes the gradient competition anisotropy for spinal cord centerline extraction and segmentation in T1- and T2-MR images. In the proposed method, the gradient competition descriptor provides an accurate elliptical curvilinear structure detection which is robust against neighboring disturbance. The curvilinearity and orientation field are used to formulate the tensorial orientation coherence anisotropy metric. Despite the high contrast neighboring objects which produce large curvilinearity, the metric encourages the optimal path traversing the target object, and accurately extracts the spinal cord centerlines. The centerline based intensity coherence segmentation model eliminates intensity discrepancy along the structure to perform accurate segmentation.

In the comparison against existing approaches, the proposed method is noticeably more accurate in terms of structure orientation estimation, centerline extraction and structure segmentation. The proposed method merely requires the minimum and maximum scales of the detection target. It is therefore general to handle different elliptical curvilinear objects under strong neighboring disturbance. From this perspective, our experiment compares the proposed method against closely related general curvilinear structure detection methods, including the widely utilized vesselness measure [1], the improved variant of flux measure [6] and the state-of-the-art 4D fast marching algorithm [4]. Applying the proposed method to other curvilinear structure detection applications, such as coronary artery and carotid artery detection will be one of the future directions

---

[8] DSC (Dice Similarity Coefficient) is computed as $\frac{2|A \cap M|}{|A|+|M|}$ where A and M are the segmented regions of different methods and ground truth respectively. The distance between the segmented regions and ground truth is computed as, at each point on the segmented surface, the Euclidean distance between that point to the closest one on the ground truth. Four samples are drawn for each voxel-length. In the signed distance calculation, negative and positive numbers represent under-segmentation and over-segmentation respectively.

of this research. Finally, the spinal cord segmentation allows retrieval of clinically relevant information, such as the spinal cord cross-sectional area, spinal cord volume and intensity profiles. Studying the segmentation performance of the proposed method, and extracting disease-specific statistics from the segmented regions based on a large dataset comprising categorized abnormal spines is the current research direction.

Acknowledgement. This work was supported by GE Healthcare and Mitacs through the Mitacs-Elevate fellowship granted to the first author of this paper.

References

1. Frangi, A.F., Niessen, W.J., Vincken, K.L., Viergever, M.A.: Multiscale vessel enhancement filtering. In: Wells, W.M., Colchester, A.C.F., Delp, S.L. (eds.) MICCAI 1998. LNCS, vol. 1496, pp. 130–137. Springer, Heidelberg (1998)
2. Law, M.W.K., Chung, A.C.S.: An oriented flux symmetry based active contour model for three dimensional vessel segmentation. In: Daniilidis, K., Maragos, P., Paragios, N. (eds.) ECCV 2010, Part III. LNCS, vol. 6313, pp. 720–734. Springer, Heidelberg (2010)
3. Olabarriaga, S.D., Breeuwer, M., Niessen, W.J.: Minimum cost path algorithm for coronary artery central axis tracking in CT images. In: Ellis, R.E., Peters, T.M. (eds.) MICCAI 2003. LNCS, vol. 2879, pp. 687–694. Springer, Heidelberg (2003)
4. Benmansour, F., Cohen, L.: Tubular structure segmentation based on minimal path method and anisotropic enhancement. IJCV 92(2), 192–210 (2011)
5. Bouix, S., Siddiqi, K., Tannenbaum, A.: Flux driven automatic centerline extraction. MedIA 9(3), 209–221 (2005)
6. Law, M.W.K., Chung, A.C.S.: Three dimensional curvilinear structure detection using optimally oriented flux. In: Forsyth, D., Torr, P., Zisserman, A. (eds.) ECCV 2008, Part IV. LNCS, vol. 5305, pp. 368–382. Springer, Heidelberg (2008)
7. Law, M.W.K., Chung, A.C.S.: Efficient implementation for spherical flux computation and its application to vascular segmentation. TIP 18(3), 596–612 (2009)
8. Wörz, S., Rohr, K.: Segmentation and quantification of human vessels using a 3-D cylindrical intensity model. TMI 16(8), 1994–2004 (2007)
9. Law, M.W.K., Chung, A.C.S.: A deformable surface model for vascular segmentation. In: Yang, G.-Z., Hawkes, D., Rueckert, D., Noble, A., Taylor, C. (eds.) MICCAI 2009, Part II. LNCS, vol. 5762, pp. 59–67. Springer, Heidelberg (2009)
10. Koh, J., Kim, T., Chaudhary, V., Dhillon, G.: Automatic segmentation of the spinal cord and the dural sac in lumbar MR images using gradient vector flow field. In: IEEE EMBS, pp. 3117–3120 (2010)
11. Chen, M., Carass, A., Cuzzocreo, J., Bazin, P.L., Reich, D., Prince, J.L.: Topology preserving automatic segmentation of the spinal cord in magnetic resonance images. In: IEEE ISBI. From Nano to Macro., pp. 1737–1740 (2011)
12. McIntosh, C., Hamarneh, G.: Spinal crawlers: Deformable organisms for spinal cord segmentation and analysis. In: Larsen, R., Nielsen, M., Sporring, J. (eds.) MICCAI 2006. LNCS, vol. 4190, pp. 808–815. Springer, Heidelberg (2006)
13. Horsfield, M., Sala, S., Neema, M., Absinta, M., Bakshi, A., Sormani, M., Rocca, M., Bakshi, R., Filippi, M.: Rapid semi-automatic segmentation of the spinal cord from magnetic resonance images: Application in multiple sclerosis. NeuroImage 50(2), 446–455 (2010)

14. Coulon, O., Hickman, S., Parker, G., Barker, G., Miller, D., Arridge, S.: Quantification of spinal cord atrophy from magnetic resonance images via a b-spline active surface model. MRM 47(6), 1176–1185 (2002)
15. Law, M.W.K., Tay, K., Leung, A., Garvin, G.J., Li, S.: Dilated divergence based scale-space representation for curve analysis. In: Fitzgibbon, A., Lazebnik, S., Perona, P., Sato, Y., Schmid, C. (eds.) ECCV 2012, Part II. LNCS, vol. 7573, pp. 557–571. Springer, Heidelberg (2012)
16. Mirebeau, J.M.: Anisotropic fast-marching on cartesian grids using lattice basis reduction (2012) (Preprint)
17. Chan, T., Esedoglu, S., Nikolova, M.: Algorithms for finding global minimizers of image segmentation and denoising models. SIAM J. App. Math. 66(5), 1632–1648 (2006)
18. Hassouna, M., Farag, A.: Multistencils fast marching methods: A highly accurate solution to the eikonal equation on cartesian domains. PAMI 29(9), 1563–1574 (2007)
19. Bae, E., Yuan, J., Tai, X.C.: Global minimization for continuous multiphase partitioning problems using a dual approach. IJCV 92(1), 112–129 (2011)
20. Chan, T., Vese, L.: Active contours without edges. TIP 10(2), 266–277 (2001)

Automated Segmentation of the Cerebellar Lobules Using Boundary Specific Classification and Evolution

John A. Bogovic[1], Pierre-Louis Bazin[2], Sarah H. Ying[3], and Jerry L. Prince[1]

[1] Department of Electrical and Computer Engineering, Johns Hopkins University, Baltimore, MD, USA
[2] Department of Neurophysics, Max Plank Institute for Human Cognitive and Brain Sciences, Leipzig, Germany
[3] Departments of Radiology, Neurology and Opthamology, Johns Hopkins School of Medicine, Baltimore, MD, USA

Abstract. The cerebellum is instrumental in coordinating many vital functions ranging from speech and balance to eye movement. The effect of cerebellar pathology on these functions is frequently examined using volumetric studies that depend on consistent and accurate delineation, however, no existing automated methods adequately delineate the cerebellar lobules. In this work, we describe a method we call the Automatic Classification of Cerebellar Lobules Algorithm using Implicit Multi-boundary evolution (ACCLAIM). A multiple object geometric deformable model (MGDM) enables each boundary surface of each individual lobule to be evolved under different level set speeds. An important innovation described in this work is that the speed for each lobule boundary is derived from a classifier trained specifically to identify that boundary. We compared our method to segmentations obtained using the atlas-based and multi-atlas fusion techniques, and demonstrate ACCLAIM's superior performance.

1 Introduction

The human cerebellum is a remarkably complex structure that coordinates numerous vital functions of the human body. It is involved in tasks such as eye-movement, speech, balance, fine motor control, motor learning, and cognition [12,16]. As in the cerebrum, cerebellar functions tend to be localized to particular regions. As well, cerebellar diseases and degeneration often target specific regions of the cerebellum and are associated with specific patterns of symptoms [23]. The cerebellum has been shown to be affected in diseases ranging from attention-deficit and hyperactivity disorder [14] to chronic alcoholism [17]. Continued research into the nature of these patterns will require accurate estimates of the sizes and shapes of the constituent sub-regions of the cerebellum. Furthermore, more detailed and anatomically meaningful sub-regions will provide the best insight into the particular workings of the cerebellum.

J.C. Gee et al. (Eds.): IPMI 2013, LNCS 7917, pp. 62–73, 2013.

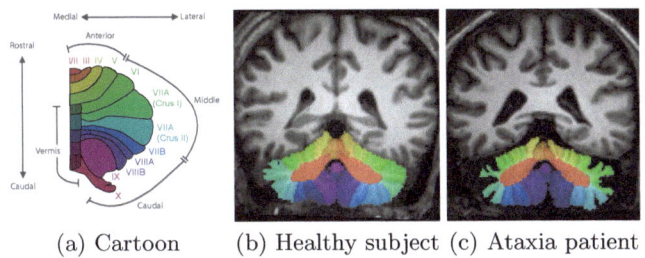

(a) Cartoon   (b) Healthy subject (c) Ataxia patient

Fig. 1. Figures showing (a) a cartoon of the cerebellar vermis and lobules (one hemisphere), and (b) and (c) MR images of the cerebellum labeled by an expert human rater

The cerebellar cortex consists of a thin sheet of highly convoluted gray matter wrapped around a central mass of white matter called the corpus medullare (CM). Fissures divide the gray matter into small branches called lobules, numbered from I to X. The most prominent fissures define the boundaries of the lobes of the cerebellum. Lobules I–V form the anterior lobe, VI–VII are the middle lobules, and VIII–X are the caudal lobules. Fig. 1 shows a cartoon representation of the cerebellar lobules, and magnetic resonance images of a control subject and patient annotated with cerebellar lobule labels. Notice the significant gray matter atrophy in the patient.

Despite the importance of the cerebellar lobules, progress has been slow in developing automated segmentation methods. While several manual and automatic methods [15] exist, the level of human interaction and expertise limits the potential scope of studies. Current automatic segmentation methods for the cerebellar lobules rely on registration with an atlas, for example the SUIT atlas of Diedrichsen et al. [10]. The multi-atlas segmentation framework improves upon single-atlas methods in that they better incorporate inter-subject variability and take advantage of "statistical fusion" techniques [20]. However, neither of these approaches produces adequate segmentation results of the cerebellar lobules. Furthermore, neither of these methods controls the topology of the resulting segmentation; an important capability if subsequent analyses require point correspondences between subjects.

In this work, we describe an Automatic Classification of Cerebellar Lobules Algorithm using Implicit Multi-boundary evolution (ACCLAIM). Given a magnetic resonance (MR) image, ACCLAIM produces a topologically correct and accurate lobule parcellation despite variability due to cerebellar atrophy. The multiple-object geometric deformable model (MGDM) framework [5] is used to find a locally optimal segmentation relative to a topologically correct initialization. MGDM's capability in enabling the specification of speeds on object *boundaries* rather than on the objects themselves was key in obtaining desired behavior during evolution.

ACCLAIM applies speed functions derived from a novel boundary classification method to evolve the boundaries between lobule labels. This involves training a classifier to detect individual boundary surfaces between objects. Boundary detection is similar to edge detection, the difference being that while *edges* are low-level image features without semantic meaning, *boundaries* are a high-level concept relative to specific objects. For example, while an edge exists at locations between low and high intensity, a boundary exists at the interface between two specific anatomical regions (e.g., different cerebellar lobules, in our case). This aspect of our work shares a philosophy with the work of [19] in the use of low-level, discriminative image features with high-level semantic concepts. Bogovic et al. [5] included a preliminary demonstration of automatic cerebellum parcellation using MGDM but resulted in a coarser parcellation and did not include boundary classification speeds or quantitative validation.

ACCLAIM yields a 28 label parcellation of the cerebellum. We group some regions to form a 24 label parcellation to enable direct comparison with SUIT. We validated ACCLAIM using both control subjects and patients with a spinocerebellar ataxia (SCA) type 6: a genetic disease that can cause severe cerebellar atrophy, see Fig. 1. Direct comparisons with atlas and multi-atlas based approaches demonstrate ACCLAIM's superior performance.

2   Methods

2.1   Subject Cohort, Image Acquisition, and Preprocessing

A cohort of 15 subjects (9 females) is used for training and validation, with ages ranging from 30 to 71 years. Nine of the subjects have been diagnosed with cerebellar ataxia. The input image to ACCLAIM is a magnetization-prepared rapid gradient echo (MPRAGE) acquired using a 3.0T MR scanner (Intera, Phillips Medical Systems, Netherlands). The parameters of the MPRAGE are: 132 slices, axial orientation, 1.1mm slice thickness, 8° flip angle, TE = 3.9ms, TR = 8.43ms, FOV 21.2 × 21.2 cm, matrix 256 × 256 (resolution: 0.828125 × 0.828125 × 1.1mm). A human expert rater manually labeled the cerebellar lobules from these images, the results of which we use as ground-truth for training and validation of our method.

ACCLAIM starts by resampling the acquired MR volume to $0.8 \times 0.8 \times 0.8$mm voxels using windowed sinc interpolation and then corrects for intensity inhomogeneity using N3 [18]. The intensities are then linearly scaled to the range $[0, 1]$ with all intensities at or above the 99.99^{th} percentile mapped to unity. SPECTRE [7] is used to mask the brain (cerebrum and cerebellum) and TOADS [4] is used to obtain a mask around the cerebellum and a soft classification of its tissues as gray or white matter.

2.2   Topology and Statistical Atlas

We briefly describe the construction and use of the statistical and topology atlases in ACCLAIM. First, a group-wise registration was performed using all subjects in the cohort using the symmetric image normalization (SyN) algorithm [1]. The ground truth labels were transformed to the group mean, and the probability for each object was computed. We determined the most likely object at each point and resampled that label map to a coarse resolution ($2 \times 2 \times 2$mm) in order to ensure that the features of each object will be sufficiently "thick" [2] after being registered to the image to be segmented. Next, we ensured that each object had spherical topology and enforced that all lobule labels are connected to the corpus medullare, and that lobules are connected to the adjacent lobules in the rostral and caudal directions (see Fig. 1(a)). ACCLAIM rigidly registers the topology atlas to the novel subject as an initial segmentation, and uses the registered probabilistic atlas as a prior during parcellation.

The groupwise registration also yields a mean average appearance of the cerebellum which we register to a masked MPRAGE of a novel subject's cerebellum, also using the SyN algorithm. We ran SyN using cross correlation as the similarity measure, and set the maximum number of iterations at the coarse, medium, and fine levels to 40, 30, and 20, respectively. This coregisters our probabilistic atlas with the subject.

2.3 Multiple-Object Geometric Deformable Model (MGDM)

MGDM is a multiple-object extension to the geometric deformable model framework for active contours [5]. It uses a decomposition of the signed distance functions (SDFs) of all objects that enables efficient evolution of all objects while preventing overlaps or gaps from forming. It also allows speeds to be specified on boundaries between objects as well as on the objects themselves.

The MGDM decomposition of object level sets (ϕ_i), begins by computing a series of "neighbor functions" by:

$$\begin{aligned} \forall x, \; L_0(x) &= i & \text{iff } \phi_i(x) < 0 \\ L_k(x) &= \arg \min_{j \neq L_n(x)} \phi_j(x) & \forall \, k > 0, \, 0 \leq n < k \end{aligned} \tag{1}$$

These functions can be interpreted as the the current segmentation (L_0) and the set of closest neighboring objects L_k at a point x. These can be used to define a series of distance functions as follows:

$$\begin{aligned} \forall x, \quad \varphi_0(x) &= \phi_{L_1}(x) \\ \varphi_k(x) &= \phi_{L_{k+1}}(x) - \phi_{L_k}(x) \; k > 0 \end{aligned} \tag{2}$$

The first of these φ_0 give the distance to the nearest boundary (i.e., to the closest neighbor). The φ_k functions indicate how much further the $k+1$-th neighbor is from x than the k-th neighbor. An important advantage of this decomposition is the fact that only the first few of these functions are required in order to perform the geometric deformable model computations. This is because at any given voxel, storing the first K distance functions allows the SDF for the nearest $K+1$ neighboring objects to be exactly reconstructed.

One can think of this decomposition as representing *boundaries* rather than objects. This enables MGDM to evolve the boundary surfaces between objects rather than the objects themselves. We denote boundaries as unordered pairs of labels, where (i, j) or (j, i) denote the boundary between objects i and j. We also associate every point x with the boundary it is closest to, and can so build a set of points $\mathcal{B}_{i,j}$ associated with boundary (i, j):

$$\mathcal{B}_{i,j} = \{x : [L_0(x) = i \cap L_1(x) = j] \cup [L_0(x) = j \cup L_1(x) = i]\} . \tag{3}$$

In other words, the closest boundary is between the current object at x (L_0) and the nearest neighboring object (L_1). This allows MGDM to evolve the distance function at x under speeds defined for the nearest boundary rather than for the object to which x belongs.

As a result, the evolution of the kth MGDM distance function φ_k is defined by the evolution equation

$$\frac{\partial \varphi_k(x)}{\partial t} = f_{L_k, L_{k+1}}(x) |\nabla \widehat{\phi}_{L_k}(x)| , \tag{4}$$

where $f_{L_k, L_{k+1}}(x)$ gives the speed for the (L_k, L_{k+1}) boundary at x and $\widehat{\phi}_{L_k}$ is the estimate of the distance function for object L_k reconstructed from the set of MGDM distance functions. Furthermore, if $L_n = i$ and $L_m = j$, and $m > n$, then the distance to the (i, j) boundary can be computed using:

$$\psi_{i,j}(x) = \sum_{k=n}^{m-1} \varphi_k(x). \tag{5}$$

This capability of MGDM is used in the following section, where we learn a classifier for each boundary. In particular, this enables us to select voxels near the boundary both during training and when detecting a boundary for a novel subject, and in applying appropriate level set speeds according to the nearest boundary.

2.4   Boundary Detection and Evolution

The use of image intensity statistics within objects has been an important technique in the level set literature for finding object boundaries [9,13]. In the cerebellum, however, image intensity is not sufficient to distinguish the cerebellar lobules from one another because they all share similar intensities. Instead, many classical segmentation approaches use the magnitude of the image gradient, $|\nabla I(x)|$ as an indicator of a boundary location [8,22], and develop a level set speed of the form:

$$f(x) = -\mathbf{v}(x) \cdot \nabla \phi(x),$$
$$\text{where } f(x) = 0 \Rightarrow |\nabla I(x)| > \epsilon \tag{6}$$

where $\mathbf{v}(x)$ describes a vector field, most often obtained as the gradient of a stopping or potential function [8], or using gradient vector flow (GVF) [22]. The field is designed such that the speed zero only where an edge is detected. We adopt a similar framework in this work, as a vector is computed at each spatial location x to determine the level set speed.

Rather than detecting edges, we learn the appearance of the (i, j) boundary by training a classifier that discriminates between on-boundary $(c_{i,j} = 1)$ and off-boundary $(c_{i,j} = 0)$ image locations for all boundaries. Specifically, we estimate

$$p = p_x(c_{i,j}|I) \tag{7}$$

where $p_x(c_{i,j}|I)$ denotes the conditional probability that x is on boundary (i, j) given the image intensities I. While machine learning techniques have been used in the past for edge detection, to our knowledge this work is the first to use unique classifiers for each boundary surface. The semantic meaning of these boundaries and the MGDM representation make this approach possible. Our level set speed for the (i, j) boundary is given by the GVF field of the conditional probabilty map, obtained by finding the $\mathbf{v}_{i,j}$ that minimizes:

$$E = \int_x \mu ||\mathbf{v}_{i,j}||^2 + ||\nabla p||^2 ||\mathbf{v}_{i,j} - \nabla p||^2. \tag{8}$$

The final resulting vector field speed is:

$$f_{i,j}^b(x) = -\mathbf{v}_{i,j}(x) \cdot \nabla \widehat{\phi}_i(x). \tag{9}$$

Note from Eqs. 3 and 4 that $f_{i,j}^b(x)$ only affects the evolution of the distance function φ_0 where x is nearest to the (i, j) boundary (i.e., $x \in \mathcal{B}_{i,j}$). Next, we simplify the conditional probability $p_x(c_{i,j}|I) \approx p_x(c_{i,j}|\mathbf{u}(x))$ where the vector $\mathbf{u}(x)$ is a set of features computed at x.

The cerebellar lobules are separated by *fissures* containing cerebral spinal fluid (CSF), which appear as lines or planes of lower intensity. These fissures can be thinner or wider depending on the particular subject, level of atrophy, and particular fissure. Therefore, we compute these features at a variety of scales as in [21]. We found that the eigenvalues of the image Hessian provide a good trade-off between the number of features and the classification performance. As a result, the feature vector at voxel x is:

$$\mathbf{u}(x) = [\lambda_1^\sigma(x)\ \lambda_2^\sigma(x)\ \lambda_3^\sigma(x)]_{\sigma \in \{0.5, 1.0, 2.0, 3.0\}} \tag{10}$$

where λ_n^σ is the nth eigenvalue of the Hessian matrix at x at the σ scale. Since each scale yields three eigenvalues, a total of 12 features are used by the classifier.

In this work we used random forests [6] to perform classification and estimate $p_x(c_{i,j}|\mathbf{u}(x))$. Random forests consist of a set of bootstrap aggregated decision trees and have been shown to achieve robust and accurate classification while avoiding overfitting. We trained an ensemble of 20 decision trees, with each decision node considering a random subset of $\log_2(M) + 1$ of the M total input features (4 of the 12 in our case) as described in [6]. Novel observations are classified by every decision tree in the ensemble. The probability that the observation belongs to a particular class can be computed as:

$$p_x(c_{i,j}|\mathbf{u}(x)) = \frac{1}{N} \sum_i^N h_i(\mathbf{u}(x)), \tag{11}$$

where $h_i(\mathbf{u}(x)) \in \{0,1\}$ gives the prediction of the ith decision tree. We used the implementation found in the open-source Weka machine learning software [11].

We next create a set of training data $\mathcal{T}$ from the training subjects $\mathcal{S}$. Each observation in the training data for the (i, j) boundary consists of an ordered pair $(\mathbf{u}(x), c_{i,j}(x))$. At this stage, a decision remains as to which voxels should be included in the training data for a given boundary. One straightforward choice would be to include all voxels, but this could result in voxels being classified as "on-boundary" for multiple boundaries, as well as needlessly increasing computational burden. Rather, we include voxels x within a small window ($\Delta = 4$mm) around a given boundary in the training data for that boundary, with "on-edge" observations being those within a distance $\delta = 1$mm of the boundary. As a result, the training data can be expressed as

$$\mathcal{T} = \begin{cases} (\mathbf{u}^s(x), 0) : \delta < \psi^s_{i,j}(x) \le \Delta, s \in \mathcal{S} \} \cup \\ \{(\mathbf{u}^s(x), 1) : \psi^s_{i,j}(x) \le \delta, s \in \mathcal{S} \} \end{cases} \tag{12}$$

where $\psi^s_{i,j}(x)$ indicates the distance to the boundary (i, j) at point x for subject s as computed by Eq. 5. We used these data to train the ensemble of decision trees h_i. Next, we describe how ACCLAIM uses these during the segmentation of a novel subject.

In order to take advantage of the ensemble of classifiers, we must compute the vector field defining the level set speeds for all boundaries. First, the conditional probabilities are estimated by:

$$p_x(c_{i,j}|\mathbf{u}(x)) = \begin{cases} \dfrac{1}{N} \displaystyle\sum_i^N h_i(\mathbf{u}(x)), & \widehat{\psi}_{i,j}(x) \le \Delta \\ 0, & \widehat{\psi}_{i,j}(x) > \Delta \end{cases} \tag{13}$$

where $\widehat{\psi}_{i,j}(x)$ is the distance to the (i, j) boundary estimated from ACCLAIM's current segmentation. This estimate is needed only to determine the window in which computations will be performed, and to avoid false positives far from the expected boundary location. An example of a prediction made by our trained random forest classifier $p_x(c_{i,j}|\mathbf{u}(x))$ is shown in Fig. 2(b). We can observe that voxels for two distinct regions have high probabilities of being on the boundary. We would like to ensure that the anatomical feature that is detected belongs to a single fissure and not to two or more fissures. We applied the fast marching topology correction method of [3] to obtain a corrected probability map $\widehat{p}_x(c_{i,j}|\mathbf{u}(x))$ (shown in Fig. 2(c)), in order to remove extraneous portions of the detected region.

Finally, the GVF field is computed from the topology corrected probability map by minimizing Eq. 8. A maximum of 20 iterations were allowed with $\mu = 0.3$. Fig. 2(d) visualizes the resulting field.

2.5   Boundary Evolution Speed Functions

ACCLAIM uses level set speeds based on the probabilistic atlas, image intensity, tissue classification, and the boundary classification field. We evolve each

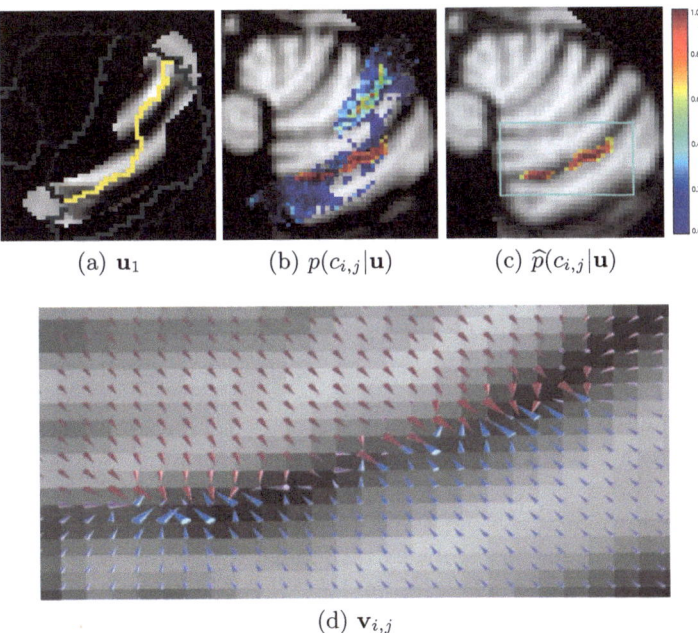

(a) $\mathbf{u}_1$ (b) $p(c_{i,j}|\mathbf{u})$ (c) $\widehat{p}(c_{i,j}|\mathbf{u})$

(d) $\mathbf{v}_{i,j}$

Fig. 2. A trained classifier is given image features, one of which is shown in (a). The yellow pixels show the current estimate of the boundary to be evolved, while gray pixels show other nearby boundaries. The classifier produces a probability map shown in (b) indicating how likely it is that a given voxel lies on the boundary between two lobules. The topology of this probability map is corrected, the result of which is given in (c). Finally a GVF field is computed from the topologically correct probabilities as shown in (d). The arrows of the GVF are scaled by the square root of their magnitude and colored according to their y component: blues and reds indicate positive and negative y components, respectively.

boundary using different weights of the speeds, and give two examples here (omitting others for space considerations). First, a tissue boundary between lobules and CSF or WM uses the speed

$$f_{i,j}(x) = (0.1)\kappa - (2.5)\left[(I(x) - \mu_j)^2 - (I(x) - \mu_i)^2\right] - (0.3)\left[l_j(x) - l_i(x)\right]$$
$$-(1.0)\left[r_{CSF}(x) - r_{GM}(x)\right]$$
$$(14)$$

where $i \in \{\text{Lobule I} - \text{VIII}\} \cap j \in \{\text{Background/CSF}\}$. Second, a lobule-to-lobule boundary uses the speed

$$f_{i',j'}(x) = (0.3)\kappa - (0.4)\left[l_{j'}(x) - l_{i'}(x)\right] - (1.6)\left[\mathbf{v}_{i',j'}(x) \cdot \nabla\phi_{i'}(x)\right] \qquad (15)$$

where $i' \in \{\text{Lobule}; \text{I} - \text{VIII}\} \cap j' \in \{\text{Lobule I} - \text{VIII}\}$. In these examples, κ denotes the mean curvature of the boundary, $l_i(x)$ denotes the probability of finding object i at x from the probabilistic atlas, μ_i denotes the mean intensity in object i, and $r_{tissue}(x)$ denotes the membership function of a tissue class.

3   Results

We ran ACCLAIM using each subject in the cohort and compared the results to an expert's segmentation. The results shown here use all subjects for training, with subject-wise leave-one-out validation planned. We expect cross-validation experiments to produce similar results to those shown because the training procedure for random forests bootstraps the training data. Evaluation was performed at three levels of hierarchy: whole cerebellum, lobe-level (I-V, VI-VII, VIII-X), and lobule-level. We examined the overlap between the true and automatically obtained labels using the Dice similarity coefficient (DSC), and the accuracy of the volumes produced using the intraclass correlation coefficient (ICC). Figure 3 shows a boxplot of the DSC between the expert's and automatic labels for the three level of hierarchy. As is to be expected, the overlap is lower for smaller labels. We observe that ACCLAIM performs best for the whole cerebellum, the cerebellar lobe labels (in the gray shading), and most of the lobule labels. ACCLAIM's improvement over the competing methods is perhaps most marked for the small lobules V and X. From Table 1, we see that ACCLAIM produces better or comparable ICCs for most lobules with mean ICC across all lobules of 0.62, 0.31, and 0.71 for SUIT, multi-atlas, and ACCLAIM, respectively.

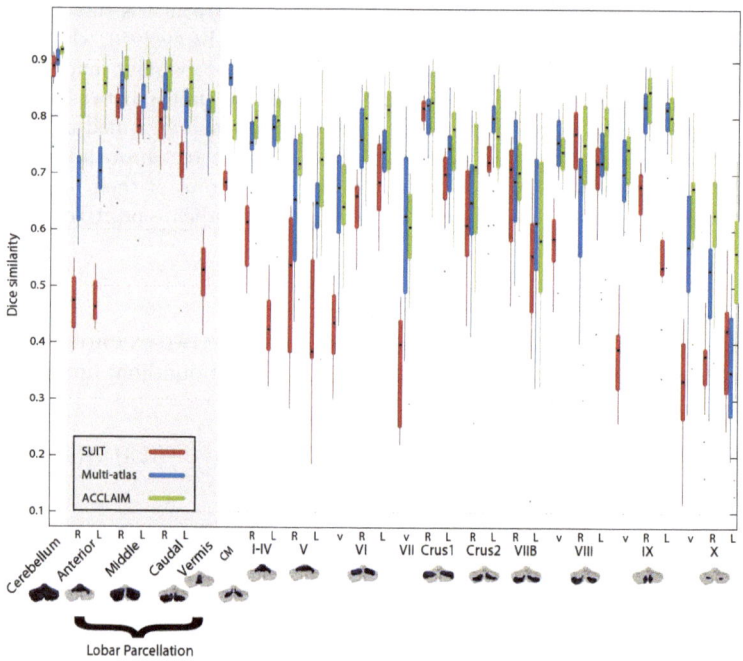

Fig. 3. Box plots Dice similarity coefficients

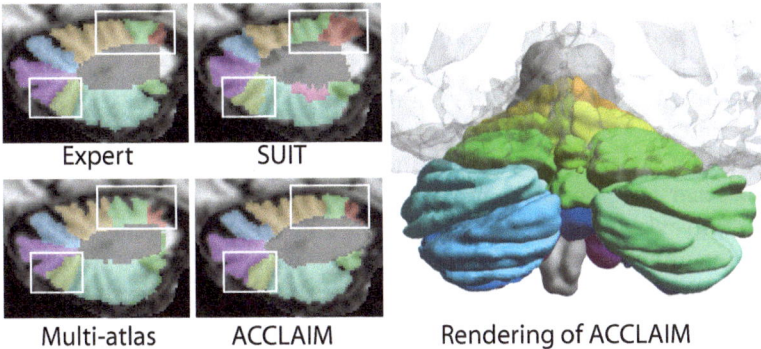

Expert   SUIT

Multi-atlas   ACCLAIM   Rendering of ACCLAIM

Fig. 4. Examples of cerebellar lobule segmenations using the SUIT, multi-atlas, and ACCLAIM methods. Shown also is a rendering of a cerebellar lobule segmentation produced by ACCLAIM, (with a transparent cerebrum for reference).

Table 1. Inter-rater intraclass correlation coefficients computed relative to the expert human rater. Bold values indicate the method with the highest estimated ICC for a particular label. Values in parentheses give the 95% confidence interval.

	Absolute ICC		
Region	SUIT	Multi-atlas	ACCLAIM
I-IVL	0.7473 (0.41 , 0.91)	0.4100 (-0.11 , 0.78)	**0.7865** (0.45 , 0.92)
I-IVR	0.5683 (-0.01 , 0.85)	0.4427 (-0.10 , 0.79)	**0.7561** (0.43 , 0.91)
VL	0.5595 (0.07 , 0.83)	0.4525 (-0.08 , 0.78)	**0.6584** (0.08 , 0.88)
VR	**0.7707** (0.30 , 0.92)	0.4734 (-0.07 , 0.80)	0.7017 (0.33 , 0.89)
VIv	**0.7648** (0.04 , 0.93)	0.3595 (-0.12 , 0.74)	0.7613 (0.43 , 0.91)
VIL	0.6144 (-0.09 , 0.89)	0.6281 (0.20 , 0.86)	**0.7895** (0.49 , 0.92)
VIR	**0.8884** (0.70 , 0.96)	0.5985 (0.13 , 0.85)	0.8349 (0.59 , 0.94)
VIIv	0.3602 (-0.12 , 0.74)	0.3222 (-0.11 , 0.71)	**0.6736** (0.29 , 0.88)
VIIACrus1L	0.6851 (-0.04 , 0.91)	0.3718 (-0.11 , 0.75)	**0.8371** (0.59 , 0.94)
VIIACrus1R	0.8369 (0.58 , 0.94)	0.3705 (-0.08 , 0.72)	**0.8667** (0.65 , 0.94)
VIIACrus2L	0.5519 (-0.08 , 0.85)	0.2086 (-0.23 , 0.62)	**0.7027** (0.31 , 0.89)
VIIACrus2R	0.7829 (0.48 , 0.92)	0.1728 (-0.10 , 0.54)	**0.8709** (0.50 , 0.96)
VIIBL	**0.8014** (0.50 , 0.93)	0.2968 (-0.19 , 0.68)	0.7663 (0.45 , 0.91)
VIIBR	**0.4279** (-0.07 , 0.76)	0.1431 (-0.13 , 0.50)	0.3346 (-0.20 , 0.71)
VIIIv	0.5068 (0.04 , 0.80)	0.1792 (-0.12 , 0.55)	**0.6504** (0.21 , 0.87)
VIIIL	0.6222 (0.14 , 0.86)	0.2632 (-0.13 , 0.64)	**0.8464** (0.61 , 0.95)
VIIIL	0.6849 (0.29 , 0.88)	0.4651 (-0.02 , 0.78)	**0.9401** (0.83 , 0.98)
IXv	0.2349 (-0.08 , 0.63)	0.4248 (-0.04 , 0.75)	**0.5759** (0.09 , 0.84)
IXL	0.7674 (0.15 , 0.93)	0.3584 (-0.10 , 0.72)	**0.8093** (0.52 , 0.93)
IXR	**0.8400** (0.60 , 0.94)	0.2629 (-0.12 , 0.64)	0.8390 (0.59 , 0.94)
Xv	**0.7920** (0.47 , 0.93)	-0.0491 (-0.16 , 0.20)	0.1733 (-0.37 , 0.62)
XL	0.2610 (-0.07 , 0.67)	-0.0033 (-0.04 , 0.09)	**0.4667** (0.00 , 0.78)
XR	0.1353 (-0.06 , 0.48)	-0.0218 (-0.05 , 0.09)	**0.7068** (0.10 , 0.91)
Mean (Sd)	0.6176 (0.2112)	0.3100 (0.1815)	0.7108 (0.1802)

4   Discussion and Conclusion

In this work, we presented ACCLAIM, a segmentation algorithm for the cerebellar lobules that takes advantage of the MGDM level set decomposition and evolution, boundary-specific speeds, and topology preservation. Tissue memberships, image intensity (based) speeds, and our novel boundary classification speed were used to evolve the boundaries of the cerebellar lobules.

Our novel boundary classification technique enabled us to locate the fissures between pairs of lobules and to design forces that enable MGDM to evolve them to the desired position. A key benefit of our approach is its use of a unique classifier for every boundary in the image, rather than attempting to learn a single classifier that performs well over the entire image. Our approach might still be improved by including a priori known information about boundaries for a particular application. In the case of the cerebellar lobules, for example, a segmentation of the cerebellar white matter branches could be helpful in constraining the regions in which the algorithm should expect a boundary, and could improve initial "window" estimates.

We compared ACCLAIM to a single-atlas method using the SUIT template, and a multi-atlas method using diffeomorphic registration and robust label fusion. Of the three methods tested, ACCLAIM performed best overall, both in terms of the volumes of the labels estimated and the labels' overlap with those produced by an expert rater. The results in Table 1 suggest that ACCLAIM produces a segmentation with better agreement of lobule volumes than the competing methods. The lobar parcellation shown in the grayed area of Fig. 3 may be the most useful regions to consider when performing automated labeling because their relatively large size and the presence of intensity cues enables them to be reliably labeled. They are also likely to provide sufficient detail for most functional/anatomical studies since the cerebellar lobes differentiate several important functions [12].

In conclusion, ACCLAIM achieves superior segmentations of the cerebellar lobules across a range of control subjects and patients. The label configuration is topologically correct, and can therefore enables subjects to be mapped to a canonical representation and used in sophisticated analyses of shape. When compared to other state-of-the-art automatic methods, our method produces labels with a higher degree of agreement with an expert human rater both in terms of both volume and spatial overlap.

Acknowledgements. This work was supported in part by NIH/NINDS grant 1R01NS056307 and NIH/NIDA grant 1K25DA025356. We are grateful to Annie Du for her manual delineations of the cerebellar lobules and to Aaron Carass for his numerous helpful comments on the experiments.

References

1. Avants, B.B., Epstein, C.L., Grossman, M., Gee, J.C.: Symmetric diffeomorphic image registration with cross-correlation: Evaluating automated labeling of elderly and neurodegenerative brain. MIA 12(1), 26–41 (2008)
2. Bazin, P.-L., Ellingsen, L.M., Pham, D.L.: Digital homeomorphisms in deformable registration. In: Karssemeijer, N., Lelieveldt, B. (eds.) IPMI 2007. LNCS, vol. 4584, pp. 211–222. Springer, Heidelberg (2007)
3. Bazin, P.L., Pham, D.L.: Topology Correction of Segmented Medical Images using a Fast Marching Algorithm. CMPB 88(2), 182–190 (2007)

4. Bazin, P.L., Pham, D.L.: Topology-preserving tissue classification of magnetic resonance brain images. IEEE TMI 26(4), 487–496 (2007)
5. Bogovic, J.A., Prince, J.L., Bazin, P.-L.: A Multiple Object Geometric Deformable Model for Image Segmentation. CVIU 117(2), 145–157 (2013)
6. Breiman, L.: Random Forests. Machine Learning 45, 5–32 (2001)
7. Carass, A., Cuzzocreo, J., Wheeler, M.B., Bazin, P.L., Resnick, S.M., Prince, J.L.: Simple paradigm for extra-cerebral tissue removal: algorithm and analysis. NeuroImage 56(4), 1982–1992 (2011)
8. Caselles, V., Kimmel, R., Sapiro, G.: Geodesic Active Contours. Intl. J. Comp. Vision 22(1), 61–79 (1997)
9. Chan, T.F., Vese, L.A.: Active contours without edges. IEEE TIP 10(2), 266–277 (2001)
10. Diedrichsen, J., Balsters, J.H., Flavell, J., Cussans, E., Ramnani, N.: A probabilistic MR atlas of the human cerebellum. NeuroImage 46(1), 39–46 (2009)
11. Hall, M., Frank, E., Holmes, G., Pfahringer, B., Reutemann, P., Witten, I.H.: The WEKA Data Mining Software: An Update. SIGKDD Explorations 11(1) (2009)
12. Ito, M.: The cerebellum and neural control. Raven, New York (1984)
13. Kim, J., Fisher, J.W., Yezzi, A., Cetin, M., Willsky, A.S.: A nonparametric statistical method for image segmentation using information theory and curve evolution. IEEE TIP 14(10), 1486–1502 (2005)
14. Mostofsky, S.H., Reiss, A.L., Lockhart, P., Denckla, M.B.: Evaluation of cerebellar size in attention-deficit hyperactivity disorder. J. Child Neurol. 13(9), 434–439 (1998)
15. Pierson, R., Corson, P.W., Sears, L.L., Alicata, D., Magnotta, V., O'Leary, D., Andreasen, N.C.: Manual and semiautomated measurement of cerebellar subregions on MR images. NeuroImage 17(1), 61–76 (2002)
16. Schmahmann, J.D.: An emerging concept. The cerebellar contribution to higher function. Arch. Neurol. 48, 1178–1187 (1991)
17. Seitz, D., Widmann, U., Seeger, U., Nägele, T., Klose, U., Mann, K., Grodd, W.: Localized proton magnetic resonance spectroscopy of the cerebellum in detoxifying alcoholics. Alcoholism, Clinical and Experimental Research 23(1), 158–163 (1999)
18. Sled, J.G., Zijdenbos, A.P., Evans, A.C.: A nonparametric method for automatic correction of intensity nonuniformity in MRI data. IEEE Transactions on Medical Imaging 17(1), 87–97 (1998)
19. Tu, Z., Chen, X., Yuille, A.L., Zhu, S.C.: Image Parsing: Unifying Segmentation, Detection, and Recognition. IJCV 63(2), 113–140 (2005)
20. Warfield, S.K., Zou, K.H., Wells, W.M.: Simultaneous truth and performance level estimation (STAPLE): An algorithm for the validation of image segmentation. IEEE TMI 23(7), 903–921 (2004)
21. Witkin, A.: Scale-space filtering. In: Proc. Int. Joint Conf. Artificial Intelligence, Karlsruhe, West Germany, pp. 1019–1021 (1983)
22. Xu, C., Prince, J.L.: Snakes, shapes, and gradient vector flow. IEEE Trans. Imag. Proc. 7(3), 359–369 (1998)
23. Ying, S.H., Choi, S.I., Perlman, S.L., Baloh, R.W., Zee, D.S., Toga, A.W.: Pontine and cerebellar atrophy correlate with clinical disability in SCA2. Neurology 66(3), 424–426 (2006)

Tree-Space Statistics and Approximations for Large-Scale Analysis of Anatomical Trees

Aasa Feragen[1,2], Megan Owen[3], Jens Petersen[1], Mathilde M.W. Wille[4],
Laura H. Thomsen[4], Asger Dirksen[4], and Marleen de Bruijne[1,5]

[1] Department of Computer Science, University of Copenhagen, Denmark
[2] Max Planck Institute for Intelligent Systems and Max Planck Institute
for Developmental Biology, Tübingen, Germany
[3] David R. Cheriton School of Computer Science, University of Waterloo, Canada
[4] Lungemedicinsk Afdeling, Gentofte Hospital, Denmark
[5] Erasmus MC - University Medical Center Rotterdam, The Netherlands
{aasa,phup,marleen}@diku.dk
http://www.image.diku.dk/aasa

Abstract. Statistical analysis of anatomical trees is hard to perform due
to differences in the topological structure of the trees. In this paper we
define statistical properties of leaf-labeled anatomical trees with geometric edge attributes by considering the anatomical trees as points in the
geometric space of leaf-labeled trees. This tree-space is a geodesic metric
space where any two trees are connected by a unique shortest path, which
corresponds to a tree deformation. However, tree-space is not a manifold,
and the usual strategy of performing statistical analysis in a tangent
space and projecting onto tree-space is not available. Using tree-space
and its shortest paths, a variety of statistical properties, such as mean,
principal component, hypothesis testing and linear discriminant analysis
can be defined. For some of these properties it is still an open problem
how to compute them; others (like the mean) can be computed, but efficient alternatives are helpful in speeding up algorithms that use means
iteratively, like hypothesis testing. In this paper, we take advantage of a
very large dataset ($N = 8016$) to obtain computable approximations, under the assumption that the data trees parametrize the relevant parts of
tree-space well. Using the developed approximate statistics, we illustrate
how the structure and geometry of airway trees vary across a population
and show that airway trees with Chronic Obstructive Pulmonary Disease come from a different distribution in tree-space than healthy ones.
Software is available from http://image.diku.dk/aasa/software.php.

1 Introduction

Anatomical trees, such as vessels, airways or dendrites, are transportation networks that play an important role in the development of diseases. In order to
better understand disease and its interaction with the anatomical tree geometry and structure, one needs to be able to perform statistical analysis of sets of
anatomical trees, including both the topological structure of the trees and the

J.C. Gee et al. (Eds.): IPMI 2013, LNCS 7917, pp. 74–85, 2013.
© Springer-Verlag Berlin Heidelberg 2013

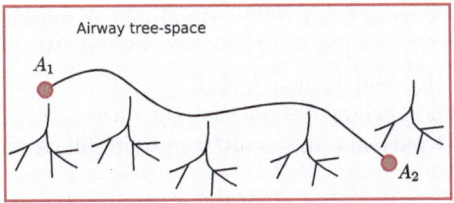
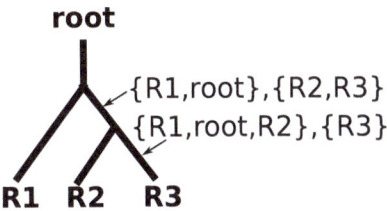

Fig. 1. Left: Tree-space is path connected space,i.e., any two trees can be joined by a path in tree-space. Moving along such a path corresponds to a deformation of trees. **Right:** Tree edges are defined by partitions of the leaf label set.

shape of the branches. In particular, detection of disease or disease phenotype based on anatomical tree structure and geometry could improve computer-aided tools for diagnosis and prognosis of disease. However, since anatomical trees have different topological structures, it is not obvious how they should be compared. In particular, two trees can have different topologies but be geometrically and functionally similar, like the trees along the tree-space path in Fig. 1.

Background and Related Work. There are several tree-space constructions that treat trees as a continuous family of objects where tree topology changes as part of a continuous deformation of the tree [4, 9]. However, the geometry of these tree-spaces does not allow for an easy transfer of standard statistical properties. For instance, tree-spaces have corners and branching points, and so manifold statistics do not apply. For this reason, most statistical measurements are still not available for tree-structured data, although the statistical analysis of tree- and graph-structured data is increasingly studied in mathematical and applied statistics [10,13,23]. Recent results include the existence, uniqueness and computation of Fréchet means [2, 7, 16, 21] and first results on principal components analysis [17]; however, how principal components should be defined and computed remains an open problem. Most available tools have so far only been used to analyze small datasets [7]. *Tree kernels* [8] form an alternative method for analyzing tree-structured data, which gives access to machine learning algorithms for e.g., classification or regression. However, tree kernels do not operate in a true space of trees, and cannot produce tree-valued solutions, such as an average tree, or the variation along a principal component or between classes.

Our Contributions. We choose a set of statistics that in different ways are useful in understanding dataset and class variation, although at present we do not know how to compute them all exactly: *principal components (PCA), two-sample hypothesis testing, linear discriminant analysis*. Hypothesis tests can already be computed to a high precision using available algorithms for means [16], whereas the others cannot. Using automatic airway branch labeling [10] on a database of airway trees, we obtain a large set of leaf-labeled airway trees. Treating the large dataset as a discretization of the relevant parts of tree-space, we define approximations of the listed statistics, which can be computed for large datasets in very limited time. Using the developed methods, we perform a large-scale study on a real dataset consisting of 8016 airway trees from 1692 individuals, of which 842 are diagnosed with Chronic Obstructive Pulmonary Disease (COPD). With our newly developed tools, we can quantify and visualize statistical properties of the airway population such as means and variance, show that the airway tree-shape differs significantly between COPD patients and healthy individuals, and visualize this difference.

Organization. The paper is organized as follows: In Sec. 2 we briefly introduce the tree-space used in this paper. In Sec. 3 we review known methods for computing mean trees, and then define and compute or approximate geodesic PCA, hypothesis tests for means and variances, and geodesic linear discriminant analysis. A detailed description of the airway dataset is given in Sec. 4, and the presented methods and results are discussed in detail in Sec. 5.

2   Tree-Space

The tree-space $\mathcal{T}$ used here is a straight-forward generalization of the space of phylogenetic trees originally defined in [4], where scalar edge length attributes have been generalized to multi-dimensional edge shape vectors in $(\mathbb{R}^3)^d$, consisting of d equidistantly sampled points along the edge (in this paper $d = 5$, giving an edge shape space $\mathbb{R}^{15}$). The space $\mathcal{T}$ is *path connected*, i.e., any two trees can be joined by a path in tree-space, corresponding to a tree deformation, see Fig. 1. Any two trees in tree-space have a unique *shortest* path joining them [4], whose length defines a distance between the two trees, giving a metric d on $\mathcal{T}$.

Each point in $\mathcal{T}$ is a leaf-labeled tree with root r and 20 leaves labeled by the 20 airway segmental branch labels $\mathcal{L} = \{L1, ..., L10, R1, ..., R10\}$. Each edge in the tree is combinatorially represented as a partition of $\mathcal{L} \cup \{r\}$ into the leaves descending from the edge, and the remaining leaves (including r), see Fig. 1. If S is the set of possible partitions of $\mathcal{L} \cup \{r\}$, then each tree uniquely corresponds to a vector in $(\mathbb{R}^{15})^S$, where each consecutive set of 15 coordinates corresponding to a possible edge (identified with a partition of $\mathcal{L} \cup \{r\}$). If the edge associated with that partition appears in the tree, then those 15 coordinates will be its branch vector; otherwise they are all 0. Certain edges can never appear in a tree together (e.g., an edge that splits $\{R1, R2\}$ off from the rest of the tree and an edge that splits $\{R1, R3\}$ off), so not all vectors are possible trees. *Tree-space* $\mathcal{T}$ is precisely those vectors in $(\mathbb{R}^{15})^S$ that correspond to trees; thus, $\mathcal{T}$ is a proper subset of Euclidean space. The shortest-path distance between two trees is the length of the shortest path between them which stays within $\mathcal{T}$, measured in the ambient Euclidean space. There is no analytic formula for this distance, but it can be computed recursively in polynomial time [18].

Figure 3 shows portions of the spaces of leaf-labeled trees with 3 and 4 leaves and edge length attributes. Tree-space is not a manifold, because it has a branching structure and corners: it can be decomposed into *orthants* where tree structure is constant, and where the orthants are glued together along subspaces containing contracted versions of the orthant trees, see Fig. 2. This geometric structure complicates statistical analysis. First, while the concept of "direction"

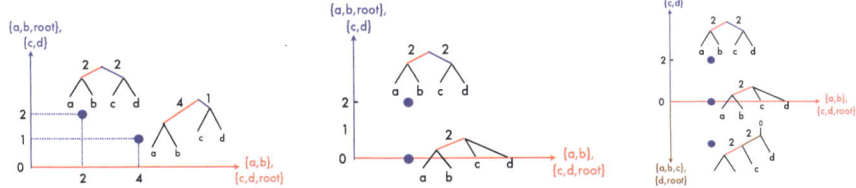

Fig. 2. Tree-space is a union of *orthants*, where each orthant is the non-negative part of a Euclidean space, corresponding to a specific leaf-labeled tree topology. **Left:** Within orthants the leaf-labeled tree topology is constant. **Middle:** In trees at the boundary of an orthant, at least one edge is contracted and described by a zero vector. **Right:** Orthant boundaries correspond to intermediate tree topologies. For simplicity, tree-space is illustrated using trees with edge length attributes rather than 3D shape. The same behavior carries over to edges with shape-vector attributes.

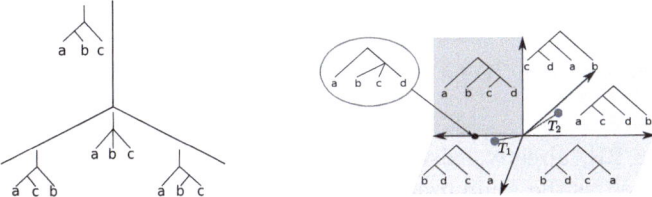

Fig. 3. Portions of tree-space $\mathcal{T}$ for trees with 3 and 4 leaves. At orthant boundaries, a large number of orthants may meet, creating *self-intersections* or *corners*.

makes sense locally within an orthant, where the space locally looks Euclidean, it does not make sense on a global level. In linear spaces, directions are defined by lines, and on manifolds, lines and directions are defined by geodesics and their tangent vectors. In tree-space, whenever a geodesic curve hits a corner or a branching point, there will be multiple geodesic extensions of the curve beyond the corner or branching point. This makes the extension of notions like PCA difficult, as we will return to below. A second difficulty occurs with optimization problems – iterative procedures like gradient descent become computationally intractable when they step close to the orthant boundaries, which can have many neighboring orthants in which the gradient has to be evaluated. In the worst case, if an iterative algorithm goes near the zero tree, the number of gradients that need to be evaluated is exponential in the number of leaves.

While the understanding of tree-space geometry is important, it is not a contribution of this paper, and we refer to [4, 16, 18] for a detailed description.

3   Tree-Space Statistics: Theory and Results

We will formulate statistical properties as solutions to optimization problems in the tree-space $\mathcal{T}$ [4]. Whereas optimization in tree-space is a very hard problem, we make the assumption that our finite dataset $\mathcal{X} \subset \mathcal{T}$ is large enough to give a good approximate parametrization of the regions of tree-space in which our solutions will be found. More precisely, given the optimization problem

$$S = \mathrm{argmin}_{x \in \mathcal{T}} f(x),$$

where $f \colon \mathcal{T} \to \mathbb{R}$ is an objective function whose minimizer is a statistic that we would like to compute, we shall instead solve the optimization problem

$$S = \mathrm{argmin}_{x \in \mathcal{X}} f(x),$$

where we only consider solutions that are themselves part of the dataset $\mathcal{X}$. The resulting statistics are called *set statistics*.

We define a set of tree-space statistics covering the most basic types of data analysis, along with computable approximations. We demonstrate the usefulness of our algorithms by analyzing a set of 8016 airway trees extracted from repeated CT scans of 1692 subjects. For a detailed description of the dataset, see Sec. 4.

3.1   The Mean Airway Tree

Given a subset $X = \{x_i\}_{i=1}^N \subset \mathcal{X}$, an iterative optimization scheme, *Sturm's algorithm* [2, 16, 21], already exists for computing the *Fréchet mean* of X in tree-space, defined as the minimizer

$$\mu = \mathrm{argmin}_{x \in \mathcal{T}} \sum_{i=1}^N d^2(x, x_i).$$

Sometimes a faster approximation may be useful, and we define the set mean:

$$\mu = \mathrm{argmin}_{x \in \mathcal{X}} \sum_{i=1}^N d^2(x, x_i)$$

Experiments. We compute set and Sturm means for our entire dataset $X = \mathcal{X}$ with $\sharp \mathcal{X} = 8016$. Plotting the Sturm mean and set mean together (Fig. 4) supports our basic hypothesis (*set statistics are good approximations*) since the set mean is visually a close approximation to the Sturm mean.

3.2   Analysis of Variance: Tree-Space PCA

Principal component analysis (PCA) is a basic tool for dimensionality reduction and analysis of variance in Euclidean spaces. In Euclidean and manifold PCA, the first principal component is often defined as the line, or more generally the geodesic curve γ, that minimizes the squared projection error [11, 12]:

$$PC1 = \mathrm{argmin}_\gamma \sum_{i=1}^N d^2(x_i, \mathrm{pr}_\gamma(x_i)), \tag{1}$$

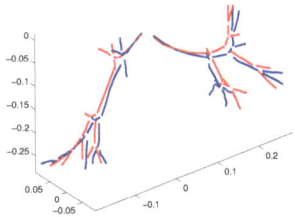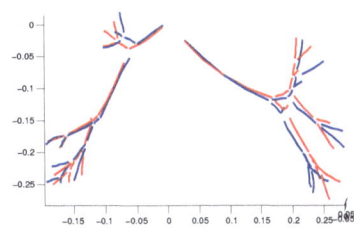

Fig. 4. Left and middle: The similarity of Sturm's Fréchet mean [16] (blue) to the approximate set mean (red) for 8016 airway trees supports the hypothesis that the dataset approximates the relevant parts of tree-space well near the population center

where projection[1] is defined as $\mathrm{pr}_\gamma(x_i) = \mathrm{argmin}_{x \in \gamma} d(x, x_i)$, which is computed in tree-space using a golden ratio search along the geodesic, as done by Nye [17].

On manifolds the best-fit geodesic line is found by optimizing over all geodesic lines passing through the Fréchet mean, parameterized by their tangent directions. However, since the concept of direction is not well defined in tree-space, this approach does not carry over. Nye [17] computes a version of the first principal component by requiring it to pass through the *majority consensus tree* (a summary tree used in phylogenetics [3]), and considering only a subset of geodesics that have unique extensions beyond corners. Even this is computationally infeasible, and MCMC simulation methods are used to find the geodesic.

We choose to find the first principal component for $X = \{x_i\}_{i=1}^N \subset \mathcal{X}$ by optimizing over geodesic segments connecting pairs of trees, parametrized by the endpoint trees:

$$PC1 = \mathrm{argmin}_{x,x' \in \mathcal{T}} \sum_{i=1}^N d^2(x_i, \mathrm{pr}_{\gamma_{x,x'}}(x_i)), \qquad (2)$$

where $\gamma_{x,x'}$ is the (unique) geodesic joining x to x'. However, since tree-space optimization is hard, finding the optimal line segment is also an open problem.

Proposition 3. *PC1 exists, but is not unique.*

Proof. Let $\bar{B}(\bar{0}, r) = \{x \in \mathcal{T} | d(x, \bar{0}) \le r\}$ be the smallest closed ball about the tree-space origin which contains all data points. It is enough to optimize over geodesics whose endpoints lie in the compact ball $\bar{B}(\bar{0}, r)$, and a minimizer of (2) exists by compactness. The minimizing solution can be extended to a longer geodesic segment which is also a PC1; thus, the PC1 is not unique. ☐

Even though PC1 is not unique, it will usually contain a unique minimal segment containing all projected data points. In order to achieve a computable solution, we randomly sample endpoint pairs from our dataset and select the optimal geodesic segment, see Algorithm 1.

---

[1] The projection of a point onto a geodesic is unique in any $CAT(0)$ space ($\mathcal{T}$ is $CAT(0)$ [4]), as follows directly from the $CAT(0)$ property. This is also noted in [17].

Algorithm 1. Computing set PCA in tree-space

1: **Input:** Dataset $\mathcal{X} \subset \mathcal{T}$, subset $X = \{x_i\}_{i=1}^N \subset \mathcal{X}$ for which PC1 is computed; number M of random endpoint samples.
2: $m = 1$
3: **while** $m \leq M$ **do**
4:     Select random $x, x' \in \mathcal{X}$; endpoints$(m) = (x, x')$;
5:     Compute geodesic $\gamma_{x,x'}$.
6:     Compute projected dataset $\mathrm{pr}_{\gamma_{x,x'}}(X)$.
7:     score$(m) = \sum_{i=1}^N d^2(x_i, \mathrm{pr}_{\gamma_{x,x}}(x_i))$.
8:     $m = m + 1$
9: **end while**
10: $(x_0, x_0') = $ endpoints$(\mathrm{argmin}_m\{\mathrm{score}(m)\})$; $PC1 = \gamma_{x_0,x_0'}$.

Note that in $\mathbb{R}^d$, PCA serves many purposes: visualization of variance along PCs, dataset visualization (like multidimensional scaling), and dimensionality reduction. Our version of tree-space PC1 primarily serves the first purpose.

Experiments. Fig. 5 show $PC1$ computed from $X = \mathcal{X}$ consisting of 8016 airway trees belonging to 1692 subjects ($M = 18286$). Note that along PC1 the shape changes both in terms of vertical scale and angle of the lungs, which is consistent with deformation due to differences in inspiration level. In addition, there are topological changes arising from topological variance in the data.

3.3   Hypothesis Testing in Tree-Space

We define one hypothesis test for the sample means and two for sample variance.

Hypothesis Test for the Mean. Let $A = \{a_i\}_{i=1}^{N_1}$ and $B = \{b_j\}_{j=1}^{N_2}$ be two samples from tree-space. To test for difference in means we use the univariate approach of Terriberry et al [22], with test statistic $T(A, B) = d(\hat{\mu}_A, \hat{\mu}_B)$, where $\hat{\mu}_A, \hat{\mu}_B$ are the Sturm or set means from Sec. 3.1. Under the null hypothesis the samples A and B are drawn from the same distribution on $\mathcal{T}$, and randomly permuting the elements of A and B should not affect the value of T.

Form the two-class data set $X = A \cup B \subset \mathcal{X}$ and consider partitions of X into datasets of size N_1 and N_2. Due to the size of X we cannot check all possible permutations, but compute the test statistics $T_m = d(\hat{\mu}_{A_m}, \hat{\mu}_{B_m})$, $m = 1, \ldots, M$, for M random partitions $X = A_m \cup B_m$, with $|A_m| = N_1$ and $|B_m| = N_2$. Comparing the T_m to the original statistic value $T_0 = d(\hat{\mu}_A, \hat{\mu}_B)$ we obtain a p-value approximating the probability of observing T_0 under the null hypothesis:

$$p = \frac{1 + \sum_{T_m \geq T_0, m \in \{1,\ldots,M\}} 1}{M + 1},$$

where the additional 1 is added to avoid $p = 0$, which is impossible in the limit where all permutations are tested [14].

Hypothesis Test for the Variance. Again, let A and B be two tree-space samples. Testing the equality of the variances σ_A and σ_B is formulated as a permutation test based on tree-space distances and means, using the test statistics

$$S_1(A, B) = \| \tfrac{1}{N_1} \sum_{i=1}^{N_1} d(x_i, \hat{\mu}_A)^2 - \tfrac{1}{N_2} \sum_{j=1}^{N_2} d(y_i, \hat{\mu}_B)^2 \|,$$
$$S_2(A, B) = \| \tfrac{1}{N_1^2} \sum_{i=1}^{N_1} \sum_{j=1}^{N_1} d(x_i, x_j)^2 - \tfrac{1}{N_2^2} \sum_{i=1}^{N_2} \sum_{j=1}^{N_2} d(y_i, y_j)^2 \|,$$

where S_1 tests variance about the mean, and S_2 tests the dataset spread.

Experiments. The defined test statistics were applied to samples from COPD patients and healthy subjects ($\sharp Z = 1692$, 842 with COPD and 850 healthy), one scan from each subject. There were 732 women and 960 men. The pairs of classes females/males and COPD/healthy were shown to come from tree-space distributions with different means and variances (Table 1). The tests used three different mean computations: The set mean optimized over the set $X = A \cup B$ with one airway tree per subject ($\sharp X = 1692$); the set mean optimized over the set $\mathcal{X}$ of all available airway trees ($\sharp \mathcal{X} = 8016$) and the Sturm mean. Only the latter two detected significant differences for means (5% significance level). Note that the set $\mathcal{X}$ of 8016 airway trees was only used as a tree-space discretization, while the samples $X = A \cup B$ were the same in all tests.

Table 1. Computed p-values for class separation for tests on mean (T) and variance (S_1 and S_2). Recall that S_2 does not use the mean value. The $p = 1$ appears because the two set means coincide in this case.

Test statistic	Gender class separation			COPD class separation		
	Set mean ($N = 1692$) $m = 10\,000$	Set mean ($N = 8016$) $m = 10\,000$	Sturm mean $m = 1\,000$	Set mean ($N = 1692$) $m = 10\,000$	Set mean ($N = 8016$) $m = 10\,000$	Sturm mean $m = 1\,000$
T	0.12	0.0011	0.00099	0.49	1.0	0.00099
S_1	0.0034	0.045	0.00099	0.00099	0.000099	0.00099
S_2		0.0084			0.000099	

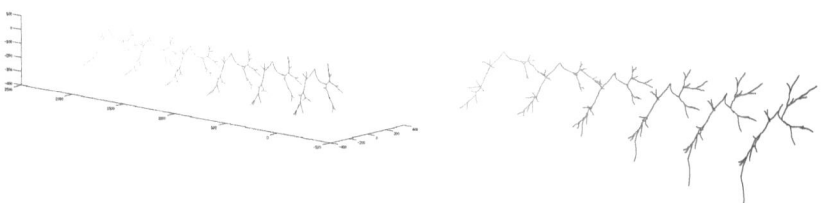

Fig. 5. Left: Trees sampled along PC1. Note the changing tree topology. **Right:** The LDA geodesic segment γ_{LDA} shows trees with long branches in the COPD cluster, most likely due to missed branches in the segmentation.

3.4   Classification: Linear Discriminant Analysis in Tree-Space

A basic classification method in Euclidean space $\mathbb{R}^d$ is *Fisher's linear discriminant analysis (LDA)* [1,5], which searches for a linear codimension 1 classification boundary. The classification boundary is determined by any line which is orthogonal to it, up to a translation along the line, and by visualizing the data objects found along such a perpendicular line one can visualize how between-class variation affects the data objects. Whereas the concept of a linear classification boundary is not well-defined in tree-space, we can use our well-defined geodesic lines and projections onto them to formulate a version of tree-space LDA. One of the advantages of working in tree-space as opposed to analyzing trees using tree kernels is that every point in tree-space corresponds to a tree. Thus, with a version of Fisher's LDA in tree-space, the change in the geometric trees between the extremes of the classes can be visualized.

In Euclidean space $\mathbb{R}^d$, optimizing over LDA classification boundaries is equivalent to optimizing over lines $L \in \mathcal{L}$ orthogonal to the classification boundary, where $\mathcal{L}$ is the set of all lines in $\mathbb{R}^d$. The translation of the classification boundary is equivalent to a classification threshold for projected datapoints onto the line. When $N > d$ for dataset size N, given a training set $X = A \cup B$ consisting of two classes A and B, the optimal LDA line is defined as maximizing the distance between projected class means, normalized by projected class scatter $\hat{s}^2(\mathrm{pr}_l(A)) = \sum_{x \in A}(\mathrm{pr}_l(x) - \mu_{\mathrm{pr}_l(A)})^2$, etc. [5]:

$$L = \mathrm{argmax}_{l \in \mathcal{L}} \frac{d^2\left(\hat{\mu}(\mathrm{pr}_l(A)), \hat{\mu}(\mathrm{pr}_l(B))\right)}{\hat{s}^2(\mathrm{pr}_l(A)) + \hat{s}^2(\mathrm{pr}_l(B))}. \tag{4}$$

We define a version of tree-space LDA analogous to (4):

$$\mathrm{argmax}_{x,x' \in \mathcal{T}} \frac{d^2(\hat{\mu}(\mathrm{pr}_{\gamma_{x,x'}}(A)), \hat{\mu}(\mathrm{pr}_{\gamma_{x,x'}}(B))}{\hat{s}^2(\mathrm{pr}_{\gamma_{x,x'}}(A)) + \hat{s}^2(\mathrm{pr}_{\gamma_{x,x'}}(B))}, \tag{5}$$

which we approximate, as with PCA, by only considering geodesic segments that pass between elements of a dataset $\mathcal{X}$ (often bigger than the training set X):

$$\gamma_{LDA} = \mathrm{argmax}_{x,x' \in \mathcal{X}} \frac{d^2(\hat{\mu}(\mathrm{pr}_{\gamma_{x,x'}}(A)), \hat{\mu}(\mathrm{pr}_{\gamma_{x,x'}}(B))}{\hat{s}^2(\mathrm{pr}_{\gamma_{x,x'}}(A)) + \hat{s}^2(\mathrm{pr}_{\gamma_{x,x'}}(B))}. \tag{6}$$

Projected means and scatters on the geodesic segment can be reformulated as computing means and scatters on the real line, which is fast. Searching over all possible point pairs is not feasible, so as with PCA, we only use a set of randomly selected pairs of geodesic endpoints from the dataset. Given the LDA geodesic segment γ_{LDA}, we classify new points x_0 by assigning the class whose projected class mean is closer to the projection $\mathrm{pr}_{\gamma_{LDA}}(x_0)$. Note, however, that more refined methods for classification on the 1-dimensional geodesic line segment can easily be incorporated.

Algorithm 2. Computing set LDA in tree-space

1: **Input:** Classes A, B; number M of geodesic endpoint permutations.
2: $m = 1$
3: **while** $m \leq M$ **do**
4:    Select random $x, x' \in \mathcal{X}$, endpoints$(m) = (x, x')$
5:    Compute geodesic $\gamma_{x,x'}$
6:    Compute projected samples $\mathrm{pr}_{\gamma_{x,x'}}(A)$, $\mathrm{pr}_{\gamma_{x,x'}}(B)$
7:    Compute projected sample means $\hat{\mu}(\mathrm{pr}_{\gamma_{x,x'}}(A))$, $\hat{\mu}(\mathrm{pr}_{\gamma_{x,x'}}(B))$ and scatters $\hat{s}(\mathrm{pr}_{\gamma_{x,x'}}(A))$ and $\hat{s}(\mathrm{pr}_{\gamma_{x,x'}}(B))$
8:    score$(m) = \frac{d^2(\hat{\mu}(\mathrm{pr}_{\gamma_{x,x'}}(A)), \hat{\mu}(\mathrm{pr}_{\gamma_{x,x'}}(B)))}{\hat{s}^2(\mathrm{pr}_{\gamma_{x,x'}}(A)) + \hat{s}^2(\mathrm{pr}_{\gamma_{x,x'}}(B))}$
9:    $m = m + 1$
10: **end while**
11: $(x_0, x_0') = $ endpoints$(\mathrm{argmin}_m\{$score$(m)\})$; $\gamma_{LDA} = \gamma_{x_0,x_0'}$

Note: In the Euclidean setting, when $d > N$, there will exist a line in $\mathbb{R}^d$, called *the maximal data piling direction* (MDP) [1], such that the classes A and B project onto two separate, single points. The MDP direction will coincide with the line L defined by (4) (as opposed to Fisher's LDA [1]), since this line gives zero denominators in (4). For $N \geq d$, LDA = MDP [1]. Thus, our version of LDA is really a generalization of MDP, and a generalization of LDA when $N > d$.

Experiments. We apply LDA by dividing the set of 1692 airway trees (one from each of 1692 subjects, 842 with COPD) into a training set (846, 421 with COPD) and a test set (846 individuals, 421 with COPD). Note that the dimension of tree-space is $d = 585$, so we have $d < N$. The LDA algorithm was ran with $M = 11829$, and a classification accuracy of 55.3% was obtained. Since LDA does not just give a binary classification, but in fact a whole geodesic segment, it is also useful for visualizing the differences between classes. The LDA geodesic segment γ_{LDA} is shown in Fig. 5.

4   Data

The developed techniques were applied to the analysis of the shape of airway trees classified by gender and COPD diagnosis. The airway trees were segmented [20] from 8016 CT-scans of 1692 subjects from a national lung cancer screening trial. Centerlines were extracted from the interior surface using the front propagation method of [15]. As the resulting centerlines are disconnected at bifurcation points, the end points were connected using a shortest path search within an inverted distance map of the interior surface. All images of the same subject were registered and the resulting deformation fields were used to remove centerline errors, such as spurious branches, following the approach of [19]. Based on the centerline shape, 20 segmental leaf labels ($R1 - R10, L1 - L10$) were automatically assigned to each airway tree using a geodesic labeling scheme [10], and branches below the segment level were discarded, producing a set of leaf-labeled airway trees with a fixed leaf label set. Airways for which not all leaf labels could be assigned were left out. For classification and hypothesis testing experiments, a set of 1692 trees were selected, one from each subject, of which 842 were diagnosed with COPD and 732 were women.

5 Discussion and Conclusion

We have defined a series of new tree-space statistics along with computable approximations of them. The main advantage of our approach is the ability to perform large-scale statistical analysis of real-world datasets and learn about connections between illness and anatomical tree geometry and structure in new ways. We show that the distribution of airway tree-shape is different in patients with COPD compared to healthy individuals. We provide a visual demonstration of mean tree-shape and tree-shape variability along the principal component. We perform LDA both for classification and visualization of the classification mechanism, and visualize the variation along the LDA component, which is consistent with increased difficulty of segmentation in COPD patients. There are no exact algorithms for computing some of our defined statistics, such as PCA or LDA, but the approximations give a rough estimate of the expected behavior of the optimal solutions. This may help in further developing how tree-space statistics should ideally be defined.

There are several disadvantages to our approach. Set statistics require a large dataset, which is not always available, and even when such a dataset is available it does not always give a good discretization of tree-space. Furthermore, due to the computational complexity of computing distances between large, unordered trees [6], we work with airway trees which have been labeled and cut off at the segmental level, reducing trees with $100 - 500$ branches to trees with ~ 40 branches, most likely discarding relevant information.

These disadvantages have potential solutions, which will be topics of future work. Small sample sizes can be helped using sampling methods in tree-space, e.g. similar to those used by Nye [17], ideally initialized by the original data set. Methods should be developed to take advantage of larger parts of the tree, either by developing heuristics for computing distances between unordered trees, or by using alternative distance measures.

In Summary: We propose a set of tree statistics along with computable approximations and show that they work on a real medical dataset. Software will be made available online upon publication of the paper.

Acknowledgements. This research was supported by the Danish Council for Independent Research | Technology and Production Sciences; the Lundbeck Foundation; AstraZeneca; The Danish Council for Strategic Research; Netherlands Organisation for Scientific Research. M.O. was supported by a Fields-Ontario Postdoctoral Fellowship. The authors wish to thank Steve Marron and Tom Nye for insightful discussions.

References

1. Ahn, J., Marron, J.S.: The maximal data piling direction for discrimination. Biometrika 97(1), 254–259 (2010)

2. Bacak, M.: A novel algorithm for computing the Fréchet mean in Hadamard spaces (2012) (Preprint), http://arxiv.org/abs/1210.2145
3. Barthélémy, J.P.: The median procedure for n-trees. J. Class. 3, 329–334 (1986)
4. Billera, L.J., Holmes, S.P., Vogtmann, K.: Geometry of the space of phylogenetic trees. Adv. in Appl. Math. 27(4), 733–767 (2001)
5. Duda, R.O., Hart, P.E., Stork, D.G.: Pattern Classification, 2nd edn. Wiley (2001)
6. Feragen, A.: Complexity of computing distances between geometric trees. In: Gimel'farb, G., Hancock, E., Imiya, A., Kuijper, A., Kudo, M., Omachi, S., Windeatt, T., Yamada, K. (eds.) SSPR & SPR 2012. LNCS, vol. 7626, pp. 89–97. Springer, Heidelberg (2012)
7. Feragen, A., Hauberg, S., Nielsen, M., Lauze, F.: Means in spaces of tree-like shapes. In: ICCV (2011)
8. Feragen, A., Petersen, J., Grimm, D., Dirksen, A., Pedersen, J.H., Borgwardt, K., de Bruijne, M.: Geometric tree kernels: Classification of COPD from airway tree geometry. In: Gee, J.C., Joshi, S., Pohl, K.M., Wells, W.M., Zöllei, L. (eds.) IPMI 2013. LNCS, vol. 7917, pp. 171–183. Springer, Heidelberg (2013)
9. Feragen, A., Lo, P., de Bruijne, M., Nielsen, M., Lauze, F.: Towards a theory of statistical tree-shape analysis. IEEE TPAMI (in press, 2013)
10. Feragen, A., Petersen, J., Owen, M., Lo, P., Thomsen, L.H., Wille, M.M.W., Dirksen, A., de Bruijne, M.: A hierarchical scheme for geodesic anatomical labeling of airway trees. In: Ayache, N., Delingette, H., Golland, P., Mori, K. (eds.) MICCAI 2012, Part III. LNCS, vol. 7512, pp. 147–155. Springer, Heidelberg (2012)
11. Fletcher, P.T., Lu, C., Pizer, S.M., Joshi, S.: Principal geodesic analysis for the study of nonlinear statistics of shape. TMI 23, 995–1005 (2004)
12. Huckemann, S., Hotz, T., Munk, A.: Intrinsic shape analysis: geodesic PCA for Riemannian manifolds modulo isometric Lie group actions. Statist. Sinica 20(1), 1–58 (2010)
13. Jain, B.J., Obermayer, K.: Structure spaces. JMLR 10, 2667–2714 (2009)
14. Knijnenburg, T.A., Wessels, L.F.A., Reinders, M.J.T., Shmulevich, I.: Fewer permutations, more accurate p-values. Bioinformatics 25(12), i161–i168 (2009)
15. Lo, P., van Ginneken, B., Reinhardt, J.M., de Bruijne, M.: Extraction of Airways from CT (EXACT'09). In: 2. Int. WS. Pulm. Im. Anal., pp. 175–189 (2009)
16. Miller, E., Owen, M., Provan, J.S.: Averaging metric phylogenetic trees (2012) (Preprint), http://arxiv.org/abs/1211.7046
17. Nye, T.M.W.: Principal components analysis in the space of phylogenetic trees. Ann. Statist. 39(5), 2716–2739 (2011)
18. Owen, M., Provan, J.S.: A fast algorithm for computing geodesic distances in tree space. ACM/IEEE Trans. Comp. Biol. Bioinf. 8, 2–13 (2011)
19. Petersen, J., Gorbunova, V., Nielsen, M., Dirksen, A., Lo, P., de Bruijne, M.: Longitudinal analysis of airways using registration. In: 4. Int. WS. Pulm. Im. Anal. (2011)
20. Petersen, J., Nielsen, M., Lo, P., Saghir, Z., Dirksen, A., de Bruijne, M.: Optimal graph based segmentation using flow lines with application to airway wall segmentation. In: Székely, G., Hahn, H.K. (eds.) IPMI 2011. LNCS, vol. 6801, pp. 49–60. Springer, Heidelberg (2011)
21. Sturm, K.-T.: Probability measures on metric spaces of nonpositive curvature. Contemp. Math., vol. 338, pp. 357–390 (2003)
22. Terriberry, T.B., Joshi, S.C., Gerig, G.: Hypothesis testing with nonlinear shape models. In: Christensen, G.E., Sonka, M. (eds.) IPMI 2005. LNCS, vol. 3565, pp. 15–26. Springer, Heidelberg (2005)
23. Wang, H., Marron, J.S.: Object oriented data analysis: sets of trees. Ann. Statist. 35(5), 1849–1873 (2007)

Predicting Cognitive Data from Medical Images Using Sparse Linear Regression

Benjamin M. Kandel[1,4], David A. Wolk[2], James C. Gee[3,4], and Brian Avants[3,4]

[1] Department of Bioengineering, University of Pennsylvania
[2] Department of Neurology and Penn Memory Center, University of Pennsylvania
[3] Department of Radiology, University of Pennsylvania
[4] Penn Image Computing and Science Laboratory (PICSL)

Abstract. We present a new framework for predicting cognitive or other continuous-variable data from medical images. Current methods of probing the connection between medical images and other clinical data typically use voxel-based mass univariate approaches. These approaches do not take into account the multivariate, network-based interactions between the various areas of the brain and do not give readily interpretable metrics that describe how strongly cognitive function is related to neuroanatomical structure. On the other hand, high-dimensional machine learning techniques do not typically provide a direct method for discovering which parts of the brain are used for making predictions. We present a framework, based on recent work in sparse linear regression, that addresses both drawbacks of mass univariate approaches, while preserving the direct spatial interpretability that they provide. In addition, we present a novel optimization algorithm that adapts the conjugate gradient method for sparse regression on medical imaging data. This algorithm produces coefficients that are more interpretable than existing sparse regression techniques.

1 Introduction

The advent of large population databases that seek to establish imaging-based biomarkers has spurred a need for generalizable prediction models in imaging. To serve this need, we seek to develop new statistical standards wherein models are trained on input data, the parameters of the model are fixed, and the model is then evaluated on unseen test datasets. This system of analysis both provides a validation of its accuracy in terms of the units of the dependent variable, as opposed to p-values, and also mimics the realistic restrictions of translational applications.

Despite this need, the large majority of medical imaging research uses traditional voxel-based morphometry (VBM) [1] which employs mass univariate testing. VBM generates statistical maps that display the correlation coefficient between a given voxel and an outcome or variable of interest and gives no indication of how these models will generalize. In contrast to VBM, several recent

J.C. Gee et al. (Eds.): IPMI 2013, LNCS 7917, pp. 86–97, 2013.
© Springer-Verlag Berlin Heidelberg 2013

approaches [22] may be used to combine voxels across the brain to *explicitly optimize prediction*, rather than to test for an association or correlation. The distinction is important, as the *p*-value is not intended as a goodness-of-fit metric and does not guarantee accurate prediction estimates. Multivariate prediction approaches instead seek the best *combination of* voxels for predicting a given outcome, rather than testing for associations one voxel at a time. This provides a second motivation for multivariate voxel-driven prediction: they implement a network-like model which fits naturally with the neural network basis of cognition.

Toward this end, much effort has recently been invested in developing prediction-based methods of analyzing medical images. Such techniques have included efforts to diagnose Alzheimer's Disease from medical images [8], among many other applications. One drawback that many of these methods share, however, is that they do not directly produce anatomically informative results. This drawback is inherent to the high-dimensional and non-linear nature of the algorithms used to analyze the data [9]. On the other hand, these methods do not have the drawbacks that mass-univariate methods such as VBM have.

We present here a method that combines advantages of traditional linear regression and high-dimensional machine learning approaches to analyzing medical image data. Our method leverages the inherently multivariate nature of imaging information to produce a sparse and anatomical prediction model for a univariate response. We demonstrate how careful use of cross-validation can provide assurance that results obtained from a sample population can be confidently applied to another population. Underlying our method is an adaptation of sparse linear regression. Drawing on recent advances in sparse regression and optimization techniques for sparsity-constrained problems, we show that sparse regression can both produce anatomically meaningful results and also give good prediction accuracy for a variety of psychometric and other clinical data. In addition, by using the framework of linear regression, we maintain the applicability of the mature analytical tools that have been developed for linear regression, including confidence intervals and significance metrics.

In sum, our contributions are: 1) An imaging-specific implementation of penalized regression; 2) Evaluation on a range of distinct response variables; 3) A cross-validation paradigm that completely separates training and testing; 4) A fully specified method of setting parameters; 5) Empirical demonstration that the models produced by our method are more accurate and generalizable than a state-of-the-art algorithm, elastic net; and 6) Establishing contrasting biologically plausible substrates for distinctive cognitive domains and aging.

2 Methods

2.1 Sparse Regression Background

Linear regression finds a linear transformation x that minimizes the error between an observed outcome variable b and the observed data A:

$$\arg\min_{x} \quad \|Ax - b\|_2^2. \tag{2.1}$$

In the context of medical imaging as considered in this work, A is an $n \times p$ matrix of n vectorized images, each with p voxels; x is a $p \times 1$ transformation matrix to be solved for; and b is the known $n \times 1$ response variable, such as a psychometric score. Because A is "fat", i.e. $p \gg n$, it is not invertible and some form of regularization is necessary to solve for x.

Recently, much effort has been invested in finding *sparse* solutions to linear least squares problems, that is, solutions that have only a few non-zero components [6]. In the context of predicting clinical or cognitive data from medical images, sparse solutions include only a few anatomical regions of interest to predict a given outcome [15,17]. Sparsity is crucial for generating clinically and neurobiologically meaningful predictive results for two reasons. First, we can validate a proposed approach by verifying that the anatomical regions associated with a given clinical outcome are consonant with existing neuroanatomical knowledge. Second, by highlighting the effect of a given anatomical region, sparse regression techniques can discover novel brain-behavior associations by selecting specific brain regions that are predictive of a given clinical result.

The most direct way of enforcing sparsity constraints on solutions to linear regression problems of the form 2.1 is to restrict the number of non-zero entries in x using a metric known as the ℓ_0 "norm" which returns the number of non-zero entries in its argument. This modifies Equation 2.1 by restricting the number of non-zero entries in x to be less than a given level of sparsity s, as follows:

$$\arg\min_{x} \quad \|Ax - b\|_2^2, \qquad (2.2)$$
$$\text{subject to} \quad \|x\|_0 \leq s.$$

Solving this problem is known to be NP-hard, so a wide variety of approaches have been proposed to solve the problem [25]. One method for finding a solution to Equation 2.2 that has attracted much attention in recent years is replacing the ℓ_0 penalty with the convex ℓ_1 penalty [22], as the two penalties give identical solutions for many problems[11].

Incorporating feasibility constraints into optimization techniques has been a subject of research for over 50 years, and optimization methods dealing with feasibility constraints are mature and perform well. One of the most widely-used methods for incorporating hard feasibility constraints is known as projected gradient descent [5]. In this method, the solution is constructed by following a gradient descent algorithm, with the modification that if the gradient descent takes the solution out of the feasible set, the projection operator returns the solution to the point in the feasible set that is closest (in Euclidean distance) to the optimal, but infeasible, solution. Mathematically, if x_i is the estimate of the minimum of function $f(x)$ at the i'th iteration, the estimate at iteration $i+1$ is given as

$$x_{i+1} = P_F\left(x_i - \alpha \nabla f\left(x\right)\right), \qquad (2.3)$$

where $P_F\left(\cdot\right)$ is the projection (or "proximal") operator that finds the point within the feasible set F that is closest to the operand and α is the step size.

For ℓ_1 norms, the projection operator is known as a "soft-thresholding" or "shrinkage" operator, and has a simple closed-form expression [10]:

$$\arg\min_v \|u - v\|_2^2 + \gamma\|v\|_1 = S(u, \gamma), \tag{2.4}$$

where the soft-thresholding operator $S(u, \gamma)$ is evaluated entry-wise and is defined as

$$S(u_i, \gamma) = \begin{cases} u_i - \gamma, & u_i > \gamma \\ 0, & -\gamma \geq u_i \leq \gamma \\ u_i + \gamma, & u_i < -\gamma \end{cases}. \tag{2.5}$$

Although the shrinkage operator does not explicitly define a feasible set with a desired amount of sparsity, it is simple to run a search over possible values of γ to obtain the value of γ that will return a solution with the desired amount of sparsity, as in [27]. We denote the operator that finds the appropriate level of γ for achieving sparsity s as $G(u, s)$. Requiring only the desired level of sparsity as an input to the algorithm as opposed to a penalty value avoids the well-documented [12] instability of solutions of ℓ_1-constrained solutions with regard to choice of penalty on the ℓ_1 norm. In addition to the sparsity penalty, we also include in the projection operator an optional minimum cluster size threshold, as is commonly performed in VBM-type analyses. We have found that including a (optional) minimum cluster threshold size generally improves robustness of results (see Figure 1) and, critically, helps prevent overfitting.

The fundamental difference between imaging data and other types of data is that in imaging data, the spatial information contained in the data is important. Because we are interested in obtaining neuroanatomically interpretable solutions, we wish to constrain our sparse solutions to be coherent and smooth, as in [4]. A few scattered non-zero voxels throughout the brain do not give rise to meaningful anatomical conclusions and these voxels will be difficult to locate in new datasets. That is, searching for individual voxels in the brain, as opposed to regions, is likely to give rise to spurious regression curves that cause overfitting on the data. Instead, we aim to recover coherent regions in the brain that are large enough and smooth enough to correspond to anatomically meaningful regions. To achieve anatomical coherence, we add a penalty to the norm of the gradient of the coefficient vector to our objective function:

$$\arg\min_x \quad \frac{1}{2}\|Ax - b\|_2^2 + \frac{\lambda_1}{2}\|x\|_2^2 + \frac{\lambda_2}{2}\|\nabla x\|_2^2, \tag{2.6}$$
$$\text{subject to} \quad \|x\|_1 \leq s.$$

λ_1 is the value of the ridge penalty, commonly used to regularize least-squares solutions to linear equations, and λ_2 is the value of the smoothing penalty applied to the coefficient vector x. Taking the derivative, we get

$$A^{\mathrm{T}}(Ax - b) + \lambda_1 x + \lambda_2 \Delta x, \tag{2.7}$$

which gives us our update step for projected gradient descent (Equation 2.3).

Instead of the classical gradient descent, we used a projected conjugate gradient algorithm. Optimization algorithms of this type have been proposed before [20], but to the best of our knowledge the formulation of the projected conjugate gradient algorithm in this context is novel. Pseudocode for the projected conjugate gradient algorithm we used is given in Algorithm 1. For extracting multiple areas in the brain that contribute independently to the outcome variable of interest, we used a variant of Orthogonal Matching Pursuit [24]. After using Algorithm 1 for determining the solution to the problem $Ax = b$, we subtracted the component of b that is not orthogonal to x_0 ($b_1 = b - Ax_0$), and then used the component of b that is orthogonal to x_0 for the next round of sparse predictions. In this way, we retrieve multiple areas of the brain that contribute to different components of cognitive ability.

Algorithm 1. Algorithm for optimizing sparse regression vector

---

Input: A, b, s, α. ▷ Input data A, predicted data b, sparseness level s, step size α.
$x_0 \leftarrow$ random seed. ▷ Initialize regression vector.
$p_0 \leftarrow A^\mathrm{T}\left(b - Ax\right) - \lambda_1 x - \lambda_2 \Delta x$ ▷ Initialize direction with negative of gradient.
$r_0 \leftarrow p_0$ ▷ Initialize residual.
$k \leftarrow 0$ ▷ Initialize iterator.
while not converged **do**
 $x_{k+1} \leftarrow x_k + \alpha p_k$ ▷ Update solution.
 $\gamma_{\mathrm{opt}} \leftarrow G\left(x_{k+1}, s\right)$ ▷ Find appropriate value of γ for desired sparsity.
 $x_{k+1} \leftarrow S\left(x_{k+1}, \gamma_{\mathrm{opt}}\right)$ ▷ Project solution to entry in sparse feasible set.
 $r_{k+1} \leftarrow A^\mathrm{T}\left(b - Ax_{k+1}\right) - \lambda_1 x_{k+1} + \lambda_2 \Delta x_{k+1}$ ▷ Update residual.
 $\beta \leftarrow \dfrac{r_k^\mathrm{T} r_k}{r_{k-1}^\mathrm{T} r_{k-1}}$
 $p_k \leftarrow r_k + \beta p_{k-1}$ ▷ Update direction.
 $k \leftarrow k + 1$.
end while
Output: x_k.

2.2 Prediction Methodology

One of the motivations for moving from a correlation-based statistical approach to a prediction-based approach is that a prediction-based approach provides falsifiable hypotheses. These can be tested using the model that is an output of the sparse regression algorithm within cross-validation. To provide more rigorous and generalizable results, we use a two-step cross-validation approach. In the first step, we use cross-validation within the training data to tune sparsity and cluster threshold parameters (Figure 1). Using cross-validation in the training data also enables us to average the coefficient vector over several trials, which helps minimize the dependence on initialization of the algorithm. The coefficient vectors returned from each fold are then averaged to return a final result for use on the test data. Thus, the model parameters are selected and fixed via exploration of the training data and applied, with set coefficients, to evaluate prediction accuracy in unseen datasets.

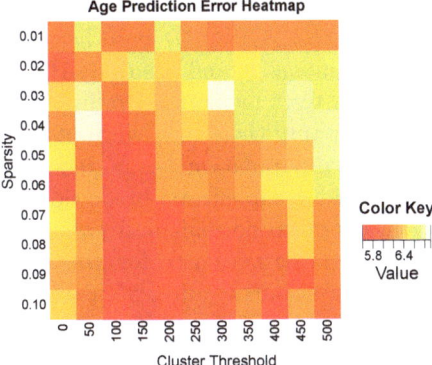

Fig. 1. Heat map of errors for age prediction (lower is better), used to tune parameters. Units are in years. We found that for most tests, a sparsity of 0.04-0.05 and a cluster threshold of 100-250 generally provided the most stable results.

In the second step of cross-validation, stepwise forward regression using the Bayesian Information Criterion (BIC) [21] was used to select the coefficient vectors necessary for constructing an optimal linear model predicting the outcome of interest from the training imaging data. The optimal linear model was then trained on the training data and used to predict the outcome variable in the test data. Two-thirds of the data was used for training, and the other one-third was used for testing.

2.3   Clinical Data

Test data for the study consisted of 216 scans of patients collected in the course of the Penn Memory Center/Alzheimer's Disease Center longitudinal cohort. Subjects were scanned on Siemens Sonata, Espree, Verio, or Trio Tim scanners using an MPRAGE T1 sequence. All scans were resampled to 2x2x2 mm isotropic resolution for analysis. The patient population had a mean age of 71.8 with standard deviation of 8.41. Of the 216 subjects, a definitive diagnosis was available for 191. There were 36 normal controls, 59 mild cognitive impairment (MCI) patients, 71 patients with Alzheimer's Disease, and 25 with a variety of other conditions.

For analysis, we employed a standard pipeline wherein all images were diffeomorphically registered to a common template using ANTs [3] and cortical thickness measurements were computed using DiReCT [7].

2.4   Predictions

To evaluate the accuracy of our sparse linear prediction method for predicting a variable of interest, we began by predicting age because of the unambiguous ground truth measurement and because of the availability of comparison results. Competing methods have reported accuracies of mean absolute errors ranging from 5 to 6.5 years [26,13,2]. In addition to age, we predict a set of cognitive scans that correspond to distinct cognitive and neuroanatomical domans:

The Boston Naming Test, which tests language ability; Consortium to Establish a Registry for Alzheimer's Disease (CERAD) word list memory test ("WordList-Trial1"), which tests working memory; and the CERAD 5-minute delayed recall test ("WordListTotal"), which tests memory encoding and longer-term memory [18]. Age was predicted using only the scans, without any clinical data, as the ages of the control and diseased population was matched. All subjects were used in the age prediction. To avoid group effects, prediction of cognitive scores was done by grouping the patients into normals and patients with dementia. Only subjects with a definitive diagnosis were used for prediction of cognitive scores.

As a comparison to state-of-the-art results, we used the popular "elastic net" model [14], which combines the ℓ_2 ridge penalty with an ℓ_1 "Lasso" penalty on the coefficient vector. We used the implementation in the R `glmnet` package. In a similar manner to our method of parameter tuning on training data, we used the `cv.glmnet` function to find optimal parameters in the training data and the `predict.cv.glmnet` function to predict the outcome variables in the test data. The elastic net optimization algorithm uses a version of Least Angle Regression [12], which is similar to the variant of Orthogonal Matching Pursuit we used to create successive coefficient vectors using our sparse regression algorithm, so we did not generate more than one coefficient vector using elastic net.

A smoothed version of Lasso algorithm, called the "fused Lasso" algorithm [23], has been proposed. We were not able to run the optimization algorithm on problems of the magnitude considered here, as the time necessary for computing the fused Lasso increases significantly with the number of predictors and exponentially with the dimensionality of the problem. We typically deal with tens or hundreds of thousands of predictors and three-dimensional arrays, making the resulting optimization problem infeasible for fused Lasso.

Our algorithm implementation is open-source, and detailed instructions for replicating the results found here, including input data, are available from `https://github.com/bkandel/KandelSparseRegressionIPMI.git`.

3   Results

We used cortical thickness measurements to predict age and three cognitive tests with different neurobiological substrates to demonstrate that our algorithm achieves state-of-the-art prediction results while obtaining anatomically interpretable prediction coefficients. Numerical results for all trials are presented in Table 1. Our results for predicting age compare favorably with the errors of 5-6.5 years reported in the literature. The linear models produced by our method achieved higher significance (lower p-value) and higher correlation with test data than the model from the elastic net in every case. In addition, our models achieved higher generalizability (training / testing error) for every case except WordList1, where the elastic net failed to discover a significant correlation at all.

In addition to achieving greater generalizability, our method produced more interpretable coefficient vectors than the elastic net. For predicting age, our

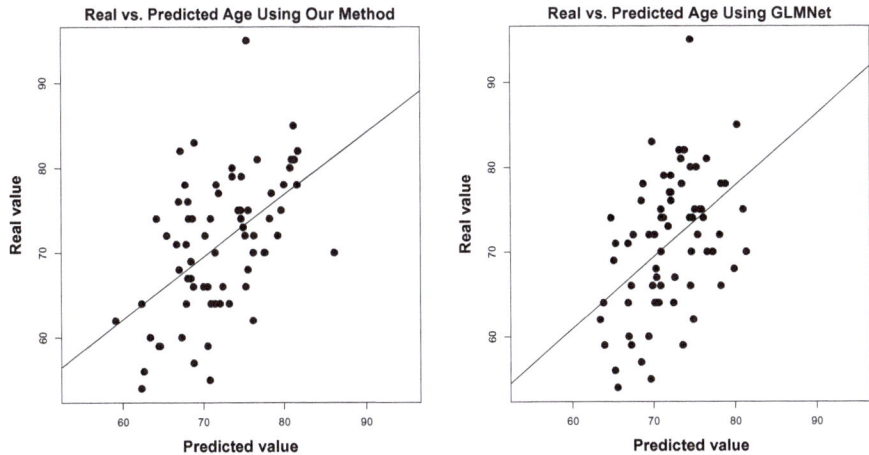

(a) Predictions of age from cortical thickness measurements using our method and the elastic net ("GLMNet"). Quantitative results are in Table 1.

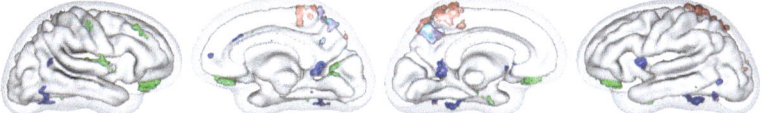

(b) Coefficients retained for predicting age using our method. Precuneal, orbitofrontal, and motor strip cortical areas were returned. Different colors represent coefficient vectors retained in successive runs of the sparse regression algorithm (see Section 2.1).

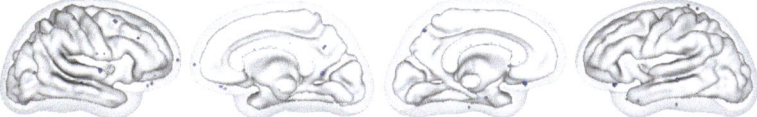

(c) Coefficients retained for predicting age using the elastic net. No clearly discernable anatomical pattern emerged although many of the elastic net voxels may be contained within the voxels selected by our method.

Fig. 2. Age results

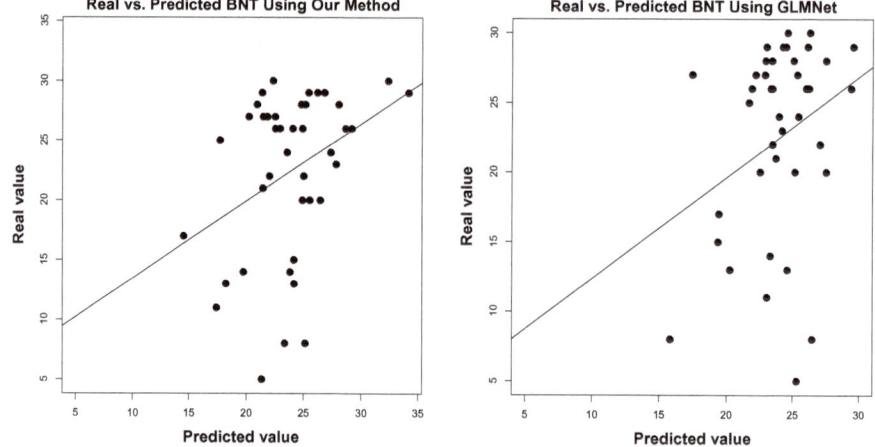

(a) Predictions of Boston Naming Test (BNT) from cortical thickness measurements using our method and the elastic net ("GLMNet"). Quantitative results are in Table 1.

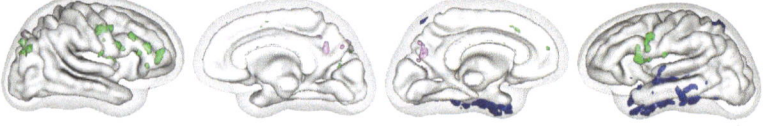

(b) Coefficients retained for predicting BNT using our method. Broca's and Wernicke's areas were retained, as were the lateral and inferior temporal lobe.

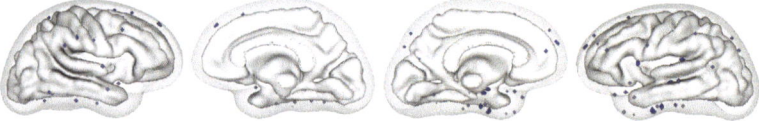

(c) Coefficients retained for predicting BNT using the elastic net. As before, no clearly discernable pattern emerged.

Fig. 3. BNT results.

Table 1. Table of p-value, correlation coefficient ("Co. Coef."), average training and testing errors, and generalizability (Gen.), defined as training error / testing error, for our sparse regression method and the elastic net. Our method produced more significant models with higher correlation in every case.

| | Our method | | | | | Elastic net | | | | |
	p-value	Cor. Coeff.	Train Error	Test Error	Generalizability	p-value	Cor. Coeff.	Train Error	Test Error	Generalizability
Age	3.25e-06	0.521	3.7	5.58	0.663	4.74e-05	0.463	3.12	5.86	0.533
BNT	0.0211	0.359	2.44	5.29	0.46	0.0599	0.296	1.6	5.06	0.316
WordList1	0.000508	0.513	0.813	1.32	0.616	0.331	0.154	1.31	1.59	0.823
WordListTotal	1.44e-06	0.673	1.2	2.01	0.599	0.0015	0.48	0.612	2.47	0.248

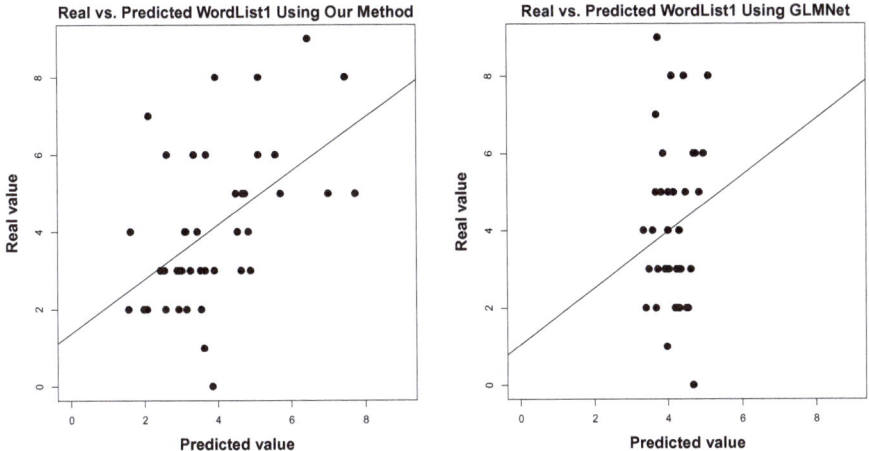

(a) Prediction for the CERAD word list memory test, "WordList1". Quantitative results are in Table 1.

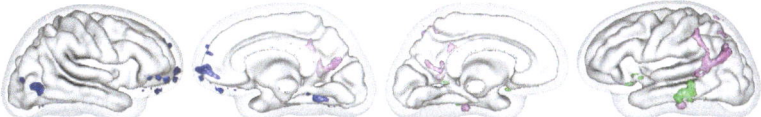

(b) Coefficients retained for predicting "WordList1," the CERAD word list memory test, using our method. Lateral parietal and temporal lobe and lateral frontal lobe were returned.

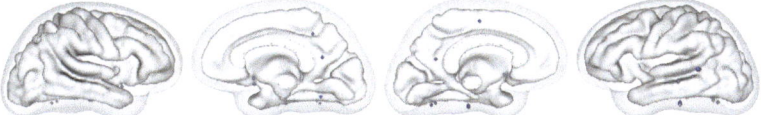

(c) Coefficients retained for predicting "WordList1" using the elastic net.

Fig. 4. WordList1 results

method found that the precuneal, orbitofrontal, and motor strip cortical regions were important (Figure 2). For BNT, we found that Broca's and Wernicke's areas were retained, as were the lateral and inferior temporal lobe (Figure 3). For WordList1, the word list memory CERAD test, we found that lateral parietal and temporal lobe and lateral frontal lobe were returned (Figure 4). WordListTotal, the delayed recall CERAD test, returned left medial temporal lobe and precuneus (figure omitted due to space restrictions). A detailed clinical explanation of these areas is beyond the scope of this brief paper, but the areas found to predict the cognitive tests show dissociation for each test and match well with each test's known neurological substrate. The elastic net found scattered non-zero coefficients, but they did not form a recognizable anatomical pattern for each test and did not dissociate the different cognitive tests.

4   Discussion and Conclusion

We have presented a method that both provides neuroanatomically meaningful information about a population and also uses learning techniques to predict the results of psychometric tests. Our prediction method maintains the direct anatomical interpretability of VBM-type studies, but incorporates a multivariate learning approach that incorporates the networked nature of neurological function. The method has prediction accuracy that is competitive with the state of the art. In addition, the anatomical regions associated with cognitive scores match closely with current understanding of neuroanatomical specificity. These results provide confidence that the method is capable of producing anatomically and neurobiologically meaningful and accurate results.

Acknowledgements. BK was supported by the Department of Defense National Defense Science & Engineering Graduate Fellowship Program. This research was also supported by NIH grants AG17586, AG15116, NS44266, NS53488, DA022807, DA014129, NS045839, P30-AG010124, and the Dana foundation.

References

1. Ashburner, J., Friston, K.J.: Voxel-based morphometry–the methods. NeuroImage 11(6 pt. 1), 805–821 (2000); PMID: 10860804
2. Ashburner, J.: A fast diffeomorphic image registration algorithm. NeuroImage 38(1), 95–113 (2007)
3. Avants, B.B., Epstein, C.L., Grossman, M., Gee, J.C.: Symmetric diffeomorphic image registration with cross-correlation: Evaluating automated labeling of elderly and neurodegenerative brain. Medical Image Analysis 12(1), 26–41 (2008)
4. Batmanghelich, N., Taskar, B., Davatzikos, C.: A general and unifying framework for feature construction, in image-based pattern classification. In: Prince, J.L., Pham, D.L., Myers, K.J. (eds.) IPMI 2009. LNCS, vol. 5636, pp. 423–434. Springer, Heidelberg (2009)
5. Bertsekas, D.: On the goldstein-levitin-polyak gradient projection method. IEEE Transactions on Automatic Control 21(2), 174–184 (1976)
6. Candès, E.J., Romberg, J., Tao, T.: Robust uncertainty principles: Exact signal reconstruction from highly incomplete frequency information. IEEE Transactions on Information Theory 52(2), 489–509 (2006)
7. Das, S.R., Avants, B.B., Grossman, M., Gee, J.C.: Registration based cortical thickness measurement. NeuroImage 45(3), 867–879 (2009); PMID: 19150502

8. Davatzikos, C., Resnick, S.M., Wu, X., Parmpi, P., Clark, C.M.: Individual patient diagnosis of AD and FTD via high-dimensional pattern classification of MRI. NeuroImage 41(4), 1220–1227 (2008)
9. Davatzikos, C.: Why voxel-based morphometric analysis should be used with great caution when characterizing group differences. NeuroImage 23(1), 17–20 (2004)
10. Donoho, D.L.: De-noising by soft-thresholding. IEEE Transactions on Information Theory 41(3), 613–627 (1995)
11. Donoho, D.L.: For most large underdetermined systems of linear equations the minimal l1-norm solution is also the sparsest solution. Communications on Pure and Applied Mathematics 59(6), 797–829 (2006)
12. Efron, B., Hastie, T., Johnstone, I., Tibshirani, R.: Least angle regression. The Annals of Statistics 32(2), 407–499 (2004)
13. Franke, K., Ziegler, G., Klöppel, S., Gaser, C.: Estimating the age of healthy subjects from t1-weighted MRI scans using kernel methods: Exploring the influence of various parameters. NeuroImage 50(3), 883–892 (2010)
14. Friedman, J., Hastie, T., Tibshirani, R.: Regularization paths for generalized linear models via coordinate descent. Journal of Statistical Software 33(1), 1 (2010)
15. Ganesh, G., Burdet, E., Haruno, M., Kawato, M.: Sparse linear regression for reconstructing muscle activity from human cortical fMRI. NeuroImage 42(4), 1463–1472 (2008)
16. Goldstein, A.A.: Convex programming in Hilbert space. Bulletin of the American Mathematical Society 70(5), 709–710 (1964)
17. Lee, H., Lee, D.S., Kang, H., Kim, B.-N., Chung, M.K.: Sparse brain network recovery under compressed sensing. IEEE Transactions on Medical Imaging 30(5), 1154–1165
18. Morris, J.C., Heyman, A., Mohs, R.C., Hughes, J.P., van Belle, G., Fillenbaum, G., Mellits, E.D., Clark, C.: The consortium to establish a registry for Alzheimer's disease (CERAD). Part i. Clinical and neuropsychological assessment of Alzheimer's disease. Neurology 39(9), 1159–1165 (1989); PMID: 2771064
19. Natarajan, B.K.: Sparse approximate solutions to linear systems. SIAM Journal on Computing 24(2), 227–234 (1995)
20. Schwartz, A., Polak, E.: Family of projected descent methods for optimization problems with simple bounds. Journal of Optimization Theory and Applications 92(1), 1–31 (1997)
21. Schwarz, G.: Estimating the dimension of a model. The Annals of Statistics 6(2), 461–464 (1978)
22. Tibshirani, R.: Regression shrinkage and selection via the lasso. Journal of the Royal Statistical Society. Series B (Methodological) 58(1), 267–288 (1996)
23. Tibshirani, R., Saunders, M., Rosset, S., Zhu, J., Knight, K.: Sparsity and smoothness via the fused lasso. Journal of the Royal Statistical Society: Series B (Statistical Methodology) 67(1), 91–108 (2005)
24. Tropp, J.A., Gilbert, A.C.: Signal recovery from random measurements via orthogonal matching pursuit. IEEE Transactions on Information Theory 53(12), 4655–4666 (2007)
25. Tropp, J.A., Wright, S.J.: Computational methods for sparse solution of linear inverse problems. Proceedings of the IEEE 98(6), 948–958 (2010)
26. Wang, B., Pham, T.D.: MRI-based age prediction using hidden markov models. Journal of Neuroscience Methods 199(1), 140–145 (2011)
27. Witten, D.M., Tibshirani, R., Hastie, T.: A penalized matrix decomposition, with applications to sparse principal components and canonical correlation analysis. Biostatistics 10(3), 515–534 (1937); PMID: 19377034

A Multiple Hypothesis Based Method for Particle Tracking and Its Extension for Cell Segmentation*

Liang Liang, Hongying Shen, Panteleimon Rompolas, Valentina Greco,
Pietro De Camilli, and James S. Duncan

Yale University, New Haven, CT 06520, USA
liang.liang@yale.edu

Abstract. In biological studies, it is often required to track thousands
of small particles in microscopic images to analyze underlying mechanisms of cellular and subcellular processes which may lead to better
understanding of some disease processes. In this paper, we present an
automatic particle tracking method and apply it for analyzing an essential subcellular process, namely clathrin mediated endocytosis using
total internal reflection microscopy. Particles are detected by using image
filters and subsequently Gaussian mixture models are fitted to achieve
sub-pixel resolution. A multiple hypothesis based framework is designed
to solve data association problems and handle splitting/merging events.
The tracking method is demonstrated on synthetic data under different
scenarios and applied to real data. We also show that, by equipping with
a cell detection module, the method can be extended straightforwardly
for segmenting cell images taken by two-photon excitation microscopy.

1 Introduction

With the rapid development in fluorescence microscopy, biologists can observe
the dynamics of individual particles and investigate the underlying mechanisms
of cellular processes which may reveal mechanisms of some disease processes.
We are particularly interested in clathrin mediated endocytosis (CME). CME
[1] is an essential cellular process that cells use to take up nutrients, to internal-
ize plasma membrane proteins, and to recycle lipid components on the plasma
membrane. The process consists of several stages [1] as illustrated in Fig. 1:
clathrin coat assembly, clathrin coat maturation, clathrin coated pits (CCPs)
fission into clathrin coated vesicles, and finally vesicles uncoating clathrin. CCP
intensity increases as it grows up, and remains relatively stable when it matures,
and decreases when it releases its coat. CCP motion is a kind of constrained
Brownian motion.

The study of this process has profound implications in neuroscience and vi-
rology. For instance, CME is the major route for synaptic vesicle recycling in
neurons critical for synaptic transmission [1], and dysfunction of the process may
be the symptom of certain disease [1]. It is also one of the pathways through

---

* This work was supported in part by the Keck Foundation.

J.C. Gee et al. (Eds.): IPMI 2013, LNCS 7917, pp. 98–109, 2013.

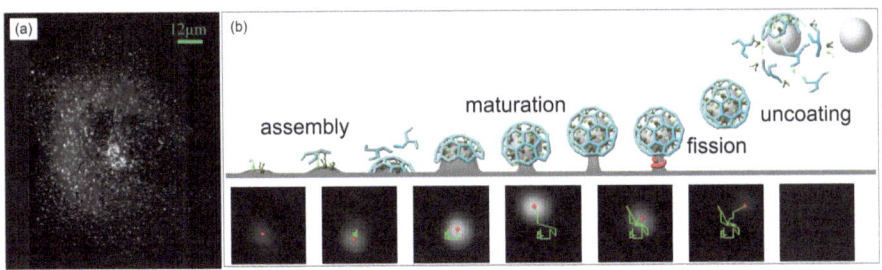

Fig. 1. (a) A Cell image. (b) Different stages of CME, and an image sequence (smoothed) showing a CCP in different stages. Clathrin is fluorescently labeled. The red dots indicate the center positions and the green lines represent the trajectories.

which viruses enter cells [2]. Since typical image datasets from an experiment consist of several thousand image frames, manual processing is almost infeasible. In the literature, there are some particle tracking methods for different biological applications [3,4,5]. For example, in [3], a method is presented to track quantum dots which can rapidly switch between acceleration mode and steady speed mode which are described by multiple motion models. Since the properties of CCPs are different from those particles, those methods are not directly applicable for our application. Due to the importance and complexity of CME, it is worth developing a method for CCP tracking.

Tracking frameworks are also essential for managing multiple trajectories. Most of the particle tracking methods in literature consider tracking as a MAP (maximum a posteriori) problem, and try to solve it in various ways. Some methods use stochastic sampling based frameworks, e.g., particle filter [6] to explore the probability space of the trajectories spatially and temporally when the tracking problem is nonlinear and non-Gaussian. Many other methods are based on the classical multiple hypothesis tracking (MHT) framework [7] and its variants [8,9,4,3]. In the MHT framework, particle tracking can be decomposed to three sub-tasks: particle detection, particle state estimation and prediction, and linking between established trajectories and newly detected particle locations. The known issue of the MHT framework is the solution space will expand exponentially fast, and many methods [10] have been proposed to overcome the issue. The results from MHT based methods are strictly reproducible compared to the stochastic approach, and therefore we choose MHT as the base framework.

The MHT framework has an implicit assumption that the observations of the targets are already given by the detection module, except that it is not known which observation corresponds to which target and vise versa. The assumption can be violated if the observations are imperfect. splitting and merging events occur frequently in our application. For example, some CCPs may temporarily crowd together and then move apart. As a result, there are many suspicious observations obtained by the detection module, each of which may correspond to several particles, and the number of the corresponding real particles and their states are all unknowns. A method in [11] uses k-means based functions to cut the suspicious observations to pieces, and find the best result. That concept is not applicable for our application because the local intensity profile of the crowded particles is a mixture of Gaussian functions, and small spatial segments of the profile are meaningless. Another method in [12] tries to fit more than one Gaussian functions around each suspicious observation. Since the number of the real particles is unknown, and the goodness of fitting will increase as the number of the Gaussian functions increases, the optimal number of Gaussian functions can not be determined.

In this paper, we present an extended version of the classical MHT framework. Since it considers more types of hypotheses, it can handle the splitting/merging events effectively without user intervention, and prevent independent CCP trajectories from linking together. The models used in the paper are based on our previous works [13]. The proposed method is quantitatively evaluated on synthetic image datasets and it is also applied to real data. The method is not limited for CCP analysis only, and we show that by using an ellipse-shaped cell detection module, the method can be used for cell segmentation.

2   Tracking Framework

In this section, we describe the general framework including hypothesis generation and optimization by integer programming. In section 3, we will show how to apply the framework for CCP tracking.

2.1   The Extended MHT Framework

Let $\mathbf{I}_t$ be the image taken at time t (frame index). Let $\mathbf{X}_t$ be the joint state of all targets (i.e., particles) at time t, assembled from each target's state $X_t^{(k)}$. Let $\mathbf{D}_t$ be the observation set, and $D_t^{(j(k,t))}$ be the observation of the target k at time t. The goal is to find the target states $\{\widehat{\mathbf{X}}_t\}_{t=1}^{t_{max}}$ that maximize the posterior probability (MAP) given the dataset $\{\mathbf{I}_t\}_{t=1}^{t_{max}}$, i.e., maximize the energy $\mathbf{E}$:

$$\mathbf{E} = \log p\left(\{\mathbf{X}_t\}_{t=1}^{t_{max}} \,\middle|\, \{\mathbf{I}_t\}_{t=1}^{t_{max}}\right) \tag{1}$$

Here, $\{\mathbf{X}_t\}_{t=1}^{t_{max}} = \{\mathbf{X}_1, ..., \mathbf{X}_{t_{max}}\}$. Since it is difficult to find the optimal solution directly, we try to maximize the lower bound $\widehat{\mathbf{E}}$ of the above energy. Assuming the targets are statistically independent of each other, then we obtain

$$\widehat{\mathbf{E}} = \sum_k \alpha^{(k)} E_P^{(k)} + \sum_t E_{I_t} \tag{2}$$

$$E_P^{(k)} = \log p\left(\{X_t^{(k)}\}_{t=1}^{t_{max}}\right) + \sum_t \log p\left(D_t^{(j(k,t))} \,\middle|\, X_t^{(k)}\right) \tag{3}$$

$$E_{I_t} = \log p\left(\mathbf{I}_t \,\middle|\, \mathbf{D}_t\right) \tag{4}$$

Each target trajectory $\{X_t^{(k)}\}_{t=1}^{t_{max}}$ is a hypothesis and has an indicator $\alpha^{(k)} \in \{0,1\}$. If $\alpha^{(k)} = 1$, the trajectory k is selected as a real trajectory, and if $\alpha^{(k)} = 0$,

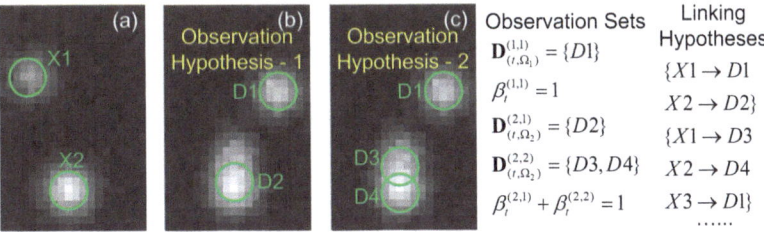

Fig. 2. (a) Two particles in time t-1. (b) Two observations at time t. (c) Three observations at time t.

it is discarded as a false trajectory. By considering different correspondences between the target tags and the observations, multiple trajectory hypotheses can be generated. One to one correspondence is assumed, which is the constraint of the maximization problem.

If we only use the above equations as the framework, then it will just be the classical MHT. We further extend the framework by considering multiple observation hypotheses. In most cases, each image $\mathbf{I}_t$ can be segmented into small regions $\{\Omega_m\}_{m=1}^{m_{max}}$. Each sub-image $\mathbf{I}_{(t,\Omega_m)}$ contains one ore more observations. In each image region, we find many observation sets, and each set of them, $\mathbf{D}_{(t,\Omega_m)}^{(m,n)}$ indexed by n, can describe the sub-image independently. Therefore, we extend the Eq.(4) to

$$E_{I_t} = \sum_m \sum_n \beta_t^{(m,n)} E_{I_t}^{(m,n)} \tag{5}$$

$$E_{I_t}^{(m,n)} = \log p\left(\mathbf{I}_{(t,\Omega_m)} \middle| \mathbf{D}_{(t,\Omega_m)}^{(m,n)}\right) \tag{6}$$

$$\sum_n \beta_t^{(m,n)} = 1, \ and \ \beta_t^{(m,n)} \in \{0,1\} \tag{7}$$

Each observation set $\mathbf{D}_{(t,\Omega_m)}^{(m,n)}$ is a hypothesis and has an indicator $\beta_t^{(m,n)} \in \{0,1\}$. If $\beta_t^{(m,n)} = 1$, the observation set is selected as real observation, and if $\beta_t^{(m,n)} = 0$, then it is false. Each single observation in the set also has an indicator equal to $\beta_t^{(m,n)}$. If there is only one observation in the set, then its indicator is 1. The method for generating observation sets is not defined here, we leave it to be implemented in different applications. By generating multiple observation hypotheses and finding the best hypothesis, the problem caused by splitting/merging can be solved. Fig. 2 shows the observation hypotheses generated in a simple scenario.

2.2 Solving the Optimization Problem

After obtaining the hypotheses of trajectories and observations, the only task left is to find the set of hypotheses as a solution that is feasible and maximizes the energy in Eq.(1). In a feasible solution, there must not exist any observation which is shared by more than one trajectories, and there must not exist any pair of observation sets, each of which explains the same image region. The feasibility definition is used to ensure one to one correspondences. Eq.(2) and its constraints can be rewritten to the matrix forms, given by

$$maximize : \widehat{\mathbf{E}} = E'\boldsymbol{\gamma} \tag{8}$$
$$subject\ to : \mathbf{A}\boldsymbol{\alpha} = \widetilde{\boldsymbol{\beta}} \tag{9}$$
$$\mathbf{B}\boldsymbol{\beta} = 1 \tag{10}$$

After integer programming is applied, the solution is obtained as a binary vector $\boldsymbol{\gamma}$ defined as $\boldsymbol{\gamma} = [\boldsymbol{\alpha}, \boldsymbol{\beta}]'$. $\boldsymbol{\alpha}$ and $\boldsymbol{\beta}$ are two binary vectors assembled from every unknown $\alpha^{(k)}$ and every unknown $\beta_t^{(m,n)}$ respectively. $\widetilde{\boldsymbol{\beta}}$ is a vector assembled from all the observation indicators, and therefore its length equals to the total number of individual observations. We note that some of the observation indicators are known as 1. E is a vector assembled from all the corresponding $E_P^{(k)}$ and $E_{I_t}^{(m,n)}$. $\mathbf{A}$ is a sparse binary matrix. Only if the trajectory k has the observation indexed by l, then $\mathbf{A}(l, k) = 1$. The summation of the indicators of the trajectories that have the same observation (e.g., the one indexed by l) is equal to the indicator of the observation, which is the one-to-one mapping constraint described by Eq.(9). $\mathbf{B}$ is a sparse binary matrix. 1 is a vector and all its elements are equal to 1. Eq.(10) is just the matrix form of Eq.(7).

3   Tracking Clathrin Coated Pits in 2D+t

3.1   State Space Models and Filters

We assume particle dynamics can be modeled using linear state space models [14] with a certain probability distribution at each time. Each model is given as

$$X_t^{(k)} = F_t^{(i)} X_{t-1}^{(k)} + U_t^{(i,k)} + W_t^{(i)} \tag{11}$$
$$D_t^{(j(k,t))} = H X_t^{(k)} + V_t^{(j(k,t))} \tag{12}$$

Here, $F_t^{(k)}$ is the state transition matrix. $U_t^{(i,k)}$ is the external input. $W_t^{(i)}$ is the process noise with covariance matrix $Q_t^{(i)}$. H is a constant observation matrix. $V_t^{(j(k,t))}$ is the observation noise with covariance matrix $R_t^{(j(k,t))}$. Each of these noise sources is assumed to be Gaussian and independent. The model parameters can be estimated from training data.

We define the state of particle k at time t as $X_t^{(k)} = [x_t^{(k)}, y_t^{(k)}, a_t^{(k)}, \dot{a}_t^{(k)}, r_t^{(k)}]'$. $[x_t^{(k)}, y_t^{(k)}]$ is its position. $a_t^{(k)}$ is its intensity, and $\dot{a}_t^{(k)}$ is the rate of intensity change over time. $r_t^{(k)}$ is its relative radius. We use two linear state space models. For particle motion, the first model describes it as free Brownian motion, and the second model describes it as confined motion because each particle is linked to the plasma membrane through its neck and can only move within a restricted region until the fission stage [1]. For intensity variation, both models describe it as a linear process. The matrices are given by

$$F_t^{(1)} = \begin{bmatrix} 1&0&0&0&0 \\ 0&1&0&0&0 \\ 0&0&1&1&0 \\ 0&0&0&1&0 \\ 0&0&0&0&1 \end{bmatrix} , F_t^{(2)} = \begin{bmatrix} 0&0&0&0&0 \\ 0&0&0&0&0 \\ 0&0&1&1&0 \\ 0&0&0&1&0 \\ 0&0&0&0&1 \end{bmatrix} , U_t^{(2,k)} = \begin{bmatrix} \bar{x}_{t-1}^{(k)} \\ \bar{y}_{t-1}^{(k)} \\ 0 \\ 0 \\ 0 \end{bmatrix} , H = \begin{bmatrix} 1&0&0&0&0 \\ 0&1&0&0&0 \\ 0&0&1&0&0 \\ 0&0&0&0&1 \end{bmatrix}$$

$U_t^{(1,k)}$ is a zero vector, and $U_t^{(2,k)}$ is the force that keeps the particle staying near its neck joint which is estimated by the time-average position $[\bar{x}_t^{(k)}, \bar{y}_t^{(k)}]$. $\bar{x}_t^{(k)} = \frac{1}{t-t_1+1} \sum_{\tau=t_1}^{t} x_\tau^{(k)}$, and t_1 is the time the particle appears. Also, let t_2 be the time the particle disappears. Then the particle lifetime is $t_2 - t_1 + 1$.

Since the process is assumed to be Markovian, we obtain

$$p\left(\{X_t^{(k)}\}_{t=1}^{t_{max}}\right) = p\left(X_1^{(k)}\right) \prod_{t=2}^{t_{max}} p\left(X_t^{(k)} | X_{t-1}^{(k)}\right) \tag{13}$$

To deal with appearing/disappearing, we set $X_{t_1-1}^{(k)} = [x_{t_1}^{(k)} + 0.707\Delta, y_{t_1}^{(k)} + 0.707\Delta, 0, \dot{a}_{t_1}^{(k)}, r_{t_1}^{(k)}]'$ and $X_{t_2+1}^{(k)} = [x_{t_2}^{(k)} + 0.707\Delta, y_{t_2}^{(k)} + 0.707\Delta, 0, \dot{a}_{t_2}^{(k)}, r_{t_2}^{(k)}]'$ where Δ is the maximum displacement. We define $p(X_{t_1}^{(k)} | X_{t-1}^{(k)}) = p(X_{t_1}^{(k)} | X_{t_1-1}^{(k)})$ for $t < t_1 - 1$ and $p(X_t^{(k)} | X_{t-1}^{(k)}) = p(X_{t_2+1}^{(k)} | X_{t_2}^{(k)})$ for $t > t_2 + 1$, which means the states are irrelevant before the particle is created and after it disappears.

The computation of $E_P^{(k)}$ is simplified. In the right side of Eq.(3), the second term can be ignored because observation noise level is much smaller than process noise level in our application. The element in Eq.(13) can be approximated as

$$\log p\left(X_t^{(k)} | X_{t-1}^{(k)}\right) \approx - \left\| H\left(X_t^{(k)} - \tilde{X}_t^{(k)}\right) \right\|_{\tilde{Q}_t^{(i^*)}}^2 \tag{14}$$

Here, $\tilde{X}_t^{(k)}$ is the predicted state, and $\tilde{Q}_t^{(i^*)} = H Q_t^{(i^*)} H'$ where i^* is the index of the most probable model at time t. The vector norm is defined as $\|X\|_Q^2 = X'Q^{-1}X$. We insert the H matrix in the norm to ensure that only observable features are used to evaluate the goodness of each trajectory.

For state estimation and prediction, we use the well known IMM filter [14,3]. In addition, the feasible range of the observation of a particle is also calculated, which is realized by using the gating technique [9].

3.2   Initial Detection

The fluorescence intensity in the 2D x-y plane can be well modeled using Gaussian mixtures, which is well studied in literature [5]. Before it is captured by the EMCCD camera, the 2D fluorescence image f_t can be modeled as the sum of Gaussian mixture G_t and background b_t, given by

$$f_t(x, y) = G_t(x, y) + b_t(x, y) \tag{15}$$

The Gaussian mixture G_t has multiple components, i.e., $G_t = \sum_j G_t^{(j)}$. Each component corresponds to a feature/observation vector $D_t^{(j)} = [x_t^{(j)}, y_t^{(j)}, a_t^{(j)}, r_t^{(j)}]$, given by

$$G_t^{(j)}(x, y) = a_t^{(j)} \exp\left[-\frac{(x - x_t^{(j)})^2 + (y - y_t^{(j)})^2}{2(r_t^{(j)})^2}\right] \tag{16}$$

The image $\mathbf{I}_t$ from the EMCCD camera is determined by the fluorescence image f_t and the noise sources [15], which can be approximated as

$$\mathbf{I}_t(x, y) \approx f_t(x, y) + N_t\left(0, \sigma_{(t,x,y)}^2\right) \tag{17}$$

$$\log p\left(\mathbf{I}_t \,|\mathbf{D}_t\right) \approx -\sum_{(x,y)} \frac{(f_t(x, y) - \mathbf{I}_t(x, y))^2}{\sigma_{(t,x,y)}^2} \tag{18}$$

N_t is Gaussian noise with variance $\sigma_{(t,x,y)}^2 = 2\left(G_t(x, y) + b_t(x, y)\right)$ and zero-mean. The approximation is only used for feature estimation not for simulation.

According to the above analysis, we have developed a detection method [16]. Initial positions of the particles are identified in each image by using matched filters. Then, image background is estimated and Gaussian mixture models are fitted to obtain the full observation vectors. By thresholding the filtered images, each image is segmented into regions containing particles.

3.3   Multiple Hypothesis Generation

We use four types of trajectory hypotheses: initiation/appearing, extension, termination, and breaking. Let's assume that trajectories (hypotheses) up to time $t - 1$ and observations at time t have been obtained. The first three can be made straightforwardly. A hypothesis of trajectory breaking is made, if the intensity curve of an established trajectory has more than two local minima. The breaking points are at the local minima. This hypothesis will help to prevent independent trajectories jointing together.

Since the initial detection may not be accurate, multiple observation hypotheses are generated. Let's suppose that trajectories up to time $t - 1$ have been obtained. In the image $\mathbf{I}_t$, each segmented region Ω_m intersects the predicted observation regions of the particles $\{X^{(k_1)}, X^{(k_2)}, ...\}$. Then, for each subset $\{X^{(k_{h_1})}, X^{(k_{h_2})}, ...\}$ of the particles, we can find their observation set $\mathbf{D}_{(t,\Omega_m)}^{(m,n)}$ which maximizes the energy:

$$E_O^{(m,n)} = \log p\left(\mathbf{I}_{(t,\Omega_m)} \,\Big|\, \mathbf{D}_{(t,\Omega_m)}^{(m,n)}\right) - \lambda_a \sum_h \left(a_t^{(k_h)} - \tilde{a}_t^{(k_h)}\right)^2 \tag{19}$$

subject to (for each k_h)

$$\left(x_t^{(k_h)} - \tilde{x}_t^{(k_h)}\right)^2 + \left(y_t^{(k_h)} - \tilde{y}_t^{(k_h)}\right)^2 < \Delta^2 \tag{20}$$

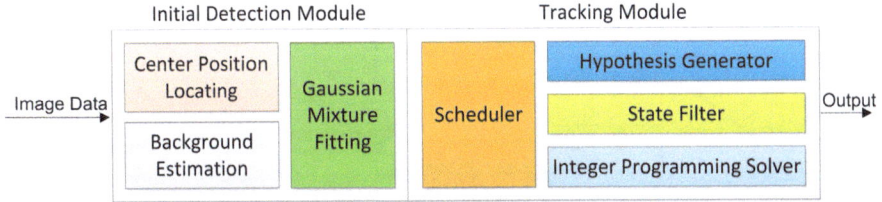

Fig. 3. The diagram of the tracking process

The first term in Eq.(19) is just $E_{I_t}^{(m,n)}$ calculated using Eq.(18) by considering the pixels only in the region. The second term in Eq.(19) ensures that each estimated intensity $a_t^{(k_h)}$ will agree with its predicted value $\widetilde{a}_t^{(k_h)}$ to some degree controlled by λ_a. Eq.(20) ensures that each estimated position $(x_t^{(k_h)}, y_t^{(k_h)})$ is within a circle centered at its predicted position $(\widetilde{x}_t^{(k_h)}, \widetilde{y}_t^{(k_h)})$ with radius $\triangle$.

3.4 The Tracking Process

The tracking process is illustrated in Fig. 3. After the initial detection result is obtained by processing all the images, the tracking module starts. Once it is finished, the order of the image sequence is reversed and the tracking module performs again to provide the final result. As the reader may notice, splitting-hypothesis is not mentioned in section 3.3. However, by tracking in the backward time direction, the problem can be solved, because a splitting event in the forward timeline is equivalent to a merging event in the reversed timeline.

3.5 Evaluation on Synthetic Data

Synthetic datasets are created with different signal to noise ratios (SNRs) and particle densities. A set of CCP trajectories are obtained from real data, and are adjusted by smoothing and rescaling their intensity-time curves. Each simulated trajectory can be generated by randomly sampling from that dataset and randomly putting to image plane. After the clean images are obtained, each image is convolved with point spread function, and then noises are added. Two types of noises are considered in simulation: the Poisson (shot) noise of input photon and the excess noise generated in the EMCCD. The SNR of each dataset is defined as the average SNR of individual particles. By varying the background noise level, the SNR of each dataset can be tuned in a large range. We choose two particle densities: $0.005/\text{pixel}^2$ and $0.008/\text{pixel}^2$ to represent the densities of different regions.

To measure tracking performance, Jaccard similarity is calculated for the tracking result on each dataset, given by

$$J = \frac{TP}{TP + FN + FP} \tag{21}$$

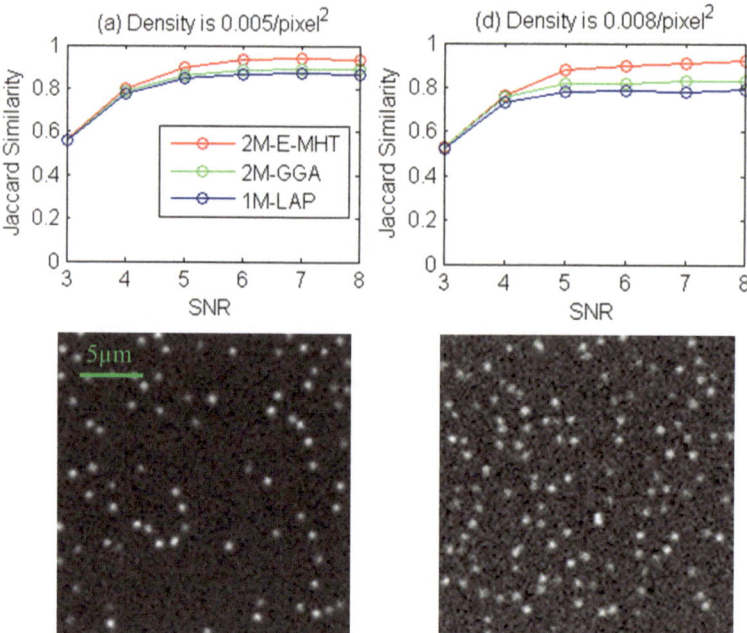

Fig. 4. Top Row: the Jaccard similarity scores of the three methods in different scenarios. Botom Row: Tow synthetic image samples (128x128 pixel, and 1 pixel=180nm): (a) Density=0.005/pixel^2 and SNR=8. (b) Density=0.008/pixel^2 and SNR=5.

True (false) positive TP (FP) is the total number of correct (wrong) associations in the recovered trajectories, and false negative FN is the sum of the lifetimes of the ground truth trajectories minus the true positive. Before the calculations, the best match between the recovered trajectories and the ground truth trajectories is found. The distance threshold is set to be 3 (pixel), which means if the distance between two positions in two trajectories is greater than the threshold, then the two positions do not match to each other, i.e., a wrong association occurs.

To evaluate the proposed method, we may compare it to some particle tracking methods in the literature. However, since different parameters and detection methods are used for different applications, direct comparisons are very difficult and unfair. Instead, we choose two representative methods modified from two general particle tracking methods. The first method uses Brownian motion model and linear assignment programing (LAP), which is based on the method in [4]. We name the first method as 1M-LAP where M means model. The second method uses the two models with IMM filter described in section 3.1 and global greedy assignment (GGA), which is based on the method in [3]. We name the second method as 2M-GGA. Both of the two methods use the same detection module described in section 3.2. We name our proposed method as 2M-E-MHT where E means extended.

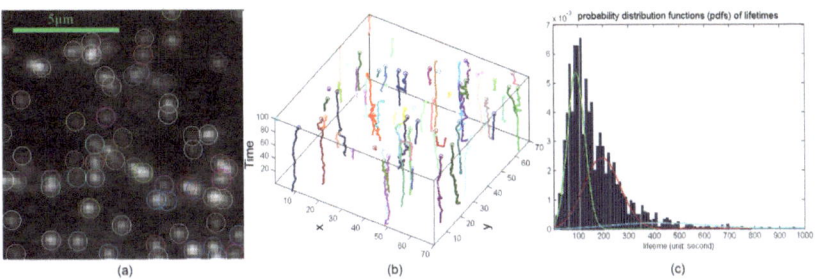

Fig. 5. (a) A sample image with circles indicating detected particles. (b) Sample trajectories over time (vertical axis), uint in x-y plane is pixel. (c) Lifetime distributions.

The performance scores are shown in Fig. 4. The method 1M-LAP has the lowest performance because it uses the least amount of information. By using better models, the method 2M-GGA does better than the method 1M-LAP in some scenarios. By applying the extended MHT framework with the CCP models, the proposed method 2M-E-MHT performs consistently better than the other two methods when SNR is greater than 4.

3.6   Evaluation on Real Data

Wild type mouse fibroblasts were transiently transfected with GFP tagged µ2 subunit of Adaptor Protein 2 complex by electroporation, and were immediately plated at subconfluent densities ontofibronectin-coated 35mm glass bottom culture dishes (MatTek, Ashland, MA, USA) for 24 hours. Images were acquired using a Nikon TiEinverted microscope equipped with 100× oil objective lens (1.49-NA). Excitation light was provided by 488nm diode-pumped solid-state lasers coupled to the TIRF illuminator through an optical fiber. The output from the lasers was controlled by an acousto-optic tunable filter, and fluorescence signal was acquired with an EM-CCD camera (DU-887; Andor).

Examples of detected particles and the trajectories are shown in Fig. 5(a) and (b), respectively. The lifetime histogram is shown in Fig. 5(c). Mixture Gaussian distribution functions are fitted to the normalized histograms, and three populations are indentified. Other analysis can be performed based on tracking result, and details are omitted due to space limit.

4   Extension for Cell Segmentation

The method can be extended for 3D tracking in other applications by extending the detection method to 3D and using relevant state models. Here, we show that the method can be indeed extended for 3D cell segmentation.

Stem cells play a key role in hair regeneration [17], however, the underlying mechanisms still remain unclear. For this research, we have acquired cell images in the epidermis by using two-photon excitation microscopy which can penetrate

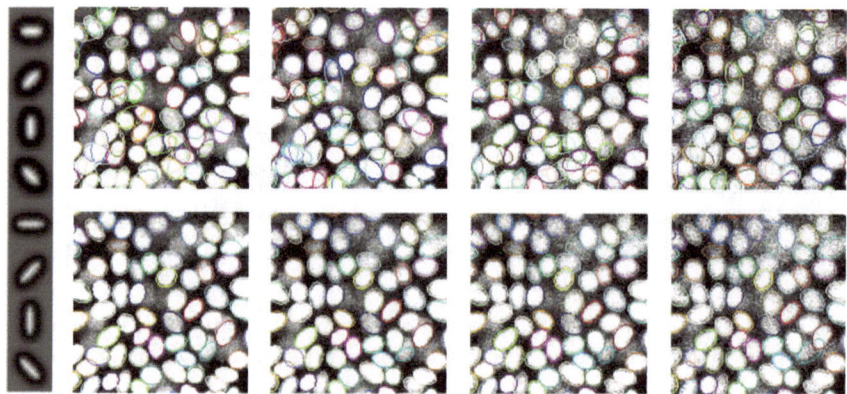

Fig. 6. Leftmost: Samples of the ellipse-shaped filters. Top row: Cell observation hypotheses over 4 successive z-steps. Bottom row: The selected cell observations.

deep tissues. By considering the z-slices as time frames, segmentation in 3D just becomes tracking in 2D+t. Each cell is just a 'big particle'. The strategy of hypothesis generation is similar to that described in section 3.3. For each pixel location on each z-slice image, we apply ellipse-shaped filters with different sizes and orientations as shown in Fig.6, and select the best ellipse that has the highest filter output. Therefore, multiple cell observation hypotheses are generated for each image as shown in Fig.6. To calculate energies related to observation hypotheses, we set λ_a in Eq.(19) as zero, and set $\log p \left(\mathbf{I}_{(t,\Omega_m)} \middle| \mathbf{D}_{(t,\Omega_m)}^{(m,n)} \right)$ to be equal to the sum of the corresponding filter outputs. To link the cell observations in 2D images, the same four types of "trajectory" hypotheses are used, and we only use the second model described in section 3.1. After applying integer programming, the best set of hypotheses are selected as shown in Fig.6.

This method is full automatic and works for crowded cells because of the advantage of the filter based approach, and is relatively easy to be implemented. Since cells can be generally represented by ellipses, the method can serve as an automatic initial segmentation method.

5   Conclusions

We have proposed a tracking method and applied it for clathrin mediated endocytosis analysis, and shown the extension for cell segmentation. The original MHT framework is extended by considering more types of hypotheses, and the related optimization problem is solved using integer programming. For CCP tracking, special strategies are designed for multiple hypothesis generation. The tracking method has been demonstrated on synthetic data and real data. By considering the z-slices as time frames, the method can be extended for 3D cell segmentation. The method is currently being used to investigate the mechanisms of clathrin mediated endocytosis, and we will expect more applications.

References

1. Slepnev, V.I., Camilli, P.D.: Accessory factors in clathrin-dependent synaptic vesicle endocytosis. Nature Reviews Neuroscience 1, 161–172 (2000)
2. Brandenburg, B., Zhuang, X.: Virus trafficking – learning from single-virus tracking. Nature Reviews Microbiology 5, 197–208 (2007)
3. Genovesio, A., Liedl, T., Emiliani, V., Parak, W.J., Coppey-Moisan, M., Olivo-Marin, J.-C.: Multiple particle tracking in 3-d+t microscopy: method and application to the tracking of endocytosed quantum dots. IEEE Transactions on Image Processing 15(5), 1062–1070 (2006)
4. Jaqaman, K., Loerke, D., Mettlen, M., Kuwata, H., Grinstein, S., Schmid, S.L., Danuser, G.: Robust single-particle tracking in live-cell time-lapse sequences. Nature Methods 5, 695–702 (2008)
5. Carter, B.C., Shubeita, G.T., Gross, S.P.: Tracking single-particles: a user-friendly quantitative evaluation. Physical Biology 2(1), 60–72 (2005)
6. Smal, I., Draegestein, K., Galjart, N., Niessen, W.J., Meijering, E.H.W.: Particle filtering for multiple object tracking in dynamic fluorescence microscopy images: Application to microtubule growth analysis. IEEE Transactions on Medical Imaging 27(6), 789–804 (2008)
7. Reid, D.B.: An algorithm for tracking multiple targets. IEEE Transactions on Automatic Control 24, 843–854 (1979)
8. Chenouard, N., Bloch, I., Olivo-Marin, J.-C.: Multiple hypothesis tracking in microscopy images. In: IEEE International Symposium on Biomedical Imaging: From Nano to Macro, pp. 1346–1349 (2009)
9. Feng, L., Xu, Y., Yang, Y., Zheng, X.: Multiple dense particle tracking in fluorescence microscopy images based on multidimensional assignment. Journal of Structural Biology 173, 219–228 (2011)
10. Poore, A.B.: Some assignment problems arising from multiple target tracking. Mathematical and Computer Modelling 43, 1074–1091 (2006)
11. Genovesio, A., Olivo-Marin, J.-C.: Split and merge data association filter for dense multi-target tracking, pp. 677–680 (2004)
12. Thomann, D., Rines, D.R., Sorger, P.K., Danuser, G.: Automatic fluorescent tag detection in 3d with super-resolution: application to the analysis of chromosome movement. Journal of Microscopy 208(1), 49–64 (2002)
13. Liang, L., Shen, H., De Camilli, P., Toomre, D.K., Duncan, J.S.: An expectation maximization based method for subcellular particle tracking using multi-angle TIRF microscopy. In: Fichtinger, G., Martel, A., Peters, T. (eds.) MICCAI 2011, Part I. LNCS, vol. 6891, pp. 629–636. Springer, Heidelberg (2011)
14. Li, X.R., Jilkov, V.P.: Survey of maneuvering target tracking. Part v. Multiple-model methods. IEEE Transactions on Aerospace and Electronic Systems 41(4), 1255–1321 (2005)
15. Robbins, M.S., Hadwen, B.J.: The noise performance of electron multiplying charge-coupled devices. IEEE Transactions on Electron Devices 50(5), 1227–1232 (2003)
16. Liang, L., Xu, Y., Shen, H., Camilli, P.D., Toomre, D., Duncan, J.S.: Automatic detection of subcellular particles in fluorescence microscopy via feature clustering and bayesian analysis. In: IEEE Workshop on Mathematical Methods in Biomedical Image Analysis, pp. 161–166 (2012)
17. Rompolas, P., Deschene, E.R., Zito, G., Gonzalez, D.G., Saotome, I., Haberman, A.M., Greco, V.: Live imaging of stem cell and progeny behaviour in physiological hair-follicle regeneration. Nature (2012)

A Multiple Model Probability Hypothesis Density Tracker for Time-Lapse Cell Microscopy Sequences

Seyed Hamid Rezatofighi[1,2], Stephen Gould[1], Ba-Ngu Vo[3],
Katarina Mele[2], William E. Hughes[4,5], and Richard Hartley[1,6]

[1] College of Engineering & Computer Sci., Australian National University, ACT, AU
[2] Quantitative Imaging Group, CSIRO Math., Informatics & Statistics, NSW, AU
[3] Department of Electrical and Computer Engineering, Curtin University, WA, AU
[4] The Garvan Institute of Medical Research, NSW, AU
[5] Department of Medicine, St. Vincent's Hospital, NSW, AU
[6] National ICT (NICTA), AU
`hamid.rezatofighi@anu.edu.au`

Abstract. Quantitative analysis of the dynamics of tiny cellular and subcellular structures in time-lapse cell microscopy sequences requires the development of a reliable multi-target tracking method capable of tracking numerous similar targets in the presence of high levels of noise, high target density, maneuvering motion patterns and intricate interactions. The linear Gaussian jump Markov system probability hypothesis density (LGJMS-PHD) filter is a recent Bayesian tracking filter that is well-suited for this task. However, the existing recursion equations for this filter do not consider a state-dependent transition probability matrix. As required in many biological applications, we propose a new closed-form recursion that incorporates this assumption and introduce a general framework for particle tracking using the proposed filter. We apply our scheme to multi-target tracking in total internal reflection fluorescence microscopy (TIRFM) sequences and evaluate the performance of our filter against the existing LGJMS-PHD and IMM-JPDA filters.

1 Introduction

Recent developments in time-lapse cell microscopy imaging systems have had a great impact on the analysis of cellular and intracellular dynamics. To help this analysis, automated tracking methods have been extensively used in biological applications in the last decade [1–8]. Despite significant technical advances made in automatically tracking moving objects, particle tracking remains a challenging task due to the complex nature of biological applications. The microscopic sequences are usually populated with visually similar tiny structures having intricate motion patterns and sophisticated interactions with other structures such as spawning (mitosis) and merging. Moreover, the structures may enter, exit, or temporarily disappear from the field of view or be occluded by other cellular objects. In addition in some imaging techniques, e.g. fluorescence microscopy

J.C. Gee et al. (Eds.): IPMI 2013, LNCS 7917, pp. 110–122, 2013.
© Springer-Verlag Berlin Heidelberg 2013

imaging, the sequences are contaminated with high levels of noise which complicates detection. Thus for success in biological applications, particle tracking
methods should be able to track an unknown and time-varying number of similar
structures in the presence of clutter noise and detection uncertainty.

To this end, many tracking approaches have been proposed. Bayesian tracking approaches have become popular for many cell tracking applications in recent years [1–8]. These tracking methods can theoretically deal with the aforementioned difficulties by incorporating prior knowledge of object dynamics and
measurement models. Recently, a new generation of Bayesian filters based on Random Finite Set (RFS) theory has been proposed in the literature [9, 10]. In this
approach, the state of targets and measurements are modeled as random finite
sets. Then, the Bayesian filtering framework is used to recursively estimate and
update the joint posterior density of the targets' states as a random finite set. This
elegant formulation avoids explicit track management and associations between
measurements and targets which makes this approach advantageous compared to
the traditional Bayesian tracking algorithms such as Kalman [1–3] and Particle
[4–6] filters. Mahler [10] recently proposed a computationally tractable RFS filter, the so called Probabilistic Hypothesis Density (PHD). Due to its good performance and significantly low processing time, the filter has been recently used
in various applications such as computer vision [11]. In biological applications, we
know of only two published applications of this filter to cell tracking [7, 8]. In these
papers, the microscopic structures' motion is modeled using single linear Gaussian
dynamics. However, in many biological applications, a single motion model cannot mimic maneuvering dynamics of structures. Thus, these approaches cannot
be extended to other similar applications.

In this paper, we propose a general framework for tracking cellular and subcellular structures using the multiple model approach or the jump Markov system
(JMS) implementation of the PHD filter [12]. To our knowledge, this is the first
application of the multiple model approach of the PHD filer to biological imaging. The main contribution of this paper is a new closed-form for the multiple
model Gaussian mixture PHD (LGJMS-PHD) filter. As required for biological
applications, this new form is more general than the closed-form suggested by
Pasha *et al.* [12]. Moreover, since the identity of trajectories is not considered in
the PHD filter formulation, we propose a scheme for identity propagation in this
filter. To show the efficiency of the proposed framework, we apply it to particle tracking in a specific biological application and compare the tracking results
against the results of the existing LGJMS-PHD filter [12] and the IMM-JPDA
filter [1], which is the most relevant traditional filter for this task.

2 Background

Let $x_{k,1}, ..., x_{k,N_k}$ and $z_{k,1}, ..., z_{k,M_k}$ be the states of all N_k targets and all M_k
measurements at time k, respectively. Over time, some of these targets may
disappear, new targets may appear, and the surviving targets evolve to new

states based on their dynamics. Moreover, due to sensor limitations, only some targets are detected at each time step and many measurements are spurious detections (clutter). We can conveniently describe each time slice by two random finite sets, $X_k = \{x_{k,1}, ..., x_{k,N_k}\}$ and $Z_k = \{z_{k,1}, ..., z_{k,M_k}\}$. In the RFS based Bayesian tracking approach, the goal is to estimate the joint multi-target posterior density of the states at each time step k using the set of all measurements up to this time step. This posterior density, $p(X_k|Z_{1:k})$, can be described by a discrete probability distribution and a joint probability density on the targets' cardinality and state, respectively [9]. The Bayesian filtering framework is used to recursively estimate this combinational posterior density using multi-target transition density $f(X_k|X_{k-1})$ and measurement likelihood $g(Z_k|X_k)$. Although the filter provides an elegant Bayesian formulation of the multi-target filtering problem, it is computationally intractable [9]. To overcome this problem, Mahler [10] proposed to propagate the probability hypothesis density, or posterior intensity, of the targets $v_k(x)$ which is the first statistical moment of the probability density function $p(X_k|Z_{1:k})$. This alleviates the computational burden of the RFS filter while still using the RFS concept. It has been shown that this posterior intensity can be calculated using the following recursive equations,

$$v_{k|k-1}(x) = \int p_{S,k}(\acute{x}) f_{k|k-1}(x|\acute{x}) v_{k-1}(\acute{x}) d\acute{x} + \int \beta_{k|k-1}(x|\acute{x}) v_{k-1}(\acute{x}) d\acute{x} + \gamma_k(x), \quad (1)$$

$$v_k(x) = [1 - p_{D,k}(x)] v_{k|k-1}(x) + \sum_{z \in Z_k} \frac{p_{D,k}(x) g_k(z|x) v_{k|k-1}(x)}{\kappa_k(z) + \int p_{D,k}(x) g_k(z|x) v_{k|k-1}(x) dx}, \quad (2)$$

where $p_{S,k}(\cdot)$ and $p_{D,k}(\cdot)$ are survival and detection probabilities, and $\kappa_k(\cdot)$, $\beta_{k|k-1}(\cdot)$ and $\gamma_k(\cdot)$ denote the clutter, spawn and birth intensities, respectively [10].

3   Our Framework for Particle Tracking

Since the PHD filter recursion accommodates complexities such as the birth and spawn models, data association uncertainty, clutter noise, and detection uncertainty in its formulation, it is a suitable tracker for many the biological applications. However, this recursion involves integrals and does not have a closed-form solution in general. The Sequential Monte Carlo implementation of this filter, so called SMC-PHD (or particle-PHD) filter [9], is a generic solution for propagating the intensity distribution. However, the drawback of this approach is the high computational cost due to the large number of required particles [13]. In the case where the target dynamics and measurement model are both linear and Gaussian, and the birth and spawn terms can be expressed as a mixture of Gaussians, there is a closed-form for this recursion so called Gaussian mixture PHD (GM-PHD) filter which is computationally efficient [13].

We now tailor a framework using this filter for particle tracking in biological applications. To propose a practical tracker for densely populated particles with reasonable processing time, we assume linear Gaussian models. Moreover, we model maneuvering dynamics of the particles with multiple such models. Although, the JMS model for the PHD filter was previously proposed by Pasha *et al.* [12], we introduce a more general closed-form implementation.

The State and Measurement Vectors: Sequences acquired from time-lapse cell microscopy imaging systems usually contain hundreds of cellular structures appearing as similar tiny particles occupying few pixels in the image. Thus, using shape similarity between objects in order to associate the measurements to the tracks may not be helpful. Typically in this approach, the (kinematic) state vector, $\xi \in \mathbb{R}^n$, includes basic features such as position x, velocity $\dot{x}$, acceleration $\ddot{x}$, intensity I, and direction ϕ of particles [1–3, 5–8].

The measurement vector z contains what can be measured from the sequences, e.g., the intensity of each pixel. However, the intensity of each pixel is usually a non-linear function of the state vector [5, 6]. Therefore in this case, SMC-PHD filter which is computationally intensive, is required for the tracking framework. In contrast, a simple detection approach can be usually applied for calculation of an estimated position $\hat{x}$ or an estimated intensity $\hat{I}$ of each particle. Although the detections include many false alarms, the PHD filter can properly deal with this while using the more efficient Gaussian mixture model.

Modeling Maneuvering Behavior of Particles: In many biological applications, the cellular structures exhibit intricate motion patterns and maneuvering dynamics which cannot properly described by a single linear Gaussian motion model. Instead, the motions can appropriately model by several linear dynamic models [1–3, 5]. Therefore, we propose a multiple model approach for simulating the motion model of these structures as follows.

For notational convenience, we remove the time index k in our formulation. However, the random variables and intensity distributions are generally time-indexed variables and distributions. All random variables $(\cdot)_k$ at time k and $(\cdot)_{k-1}$ at time $k-1$ are simply shown by $(\cdot)$ and $(\acute{\cdot})$, respectively.

Assume that the maneuvering dynamics of the structures can be properly modeled by $\mathcal{M}$ linear Gaussian models and measurement likelihood has also a linear Gaussian form for each model $r = \{1, ..., \mathcal{M}\}$ such that $\tilde{f}(\xi|\acute{\xi}, r) = \mathcal{N}\left(\xi; F(r)\acute{\xi}, Q(r)\right)$ and $g(z|\xi, r) = \mathcal{N}(z; H(r)\xi, R(r))$, where $F(r)$, $H(r)$, $Q(r)$ and $R(r)$ are the transition, the measurement, and the process and measurement noise covariance, matrices for model r, respectively.

In some biological applications [1, 14], the transition from a dynamic model to another model depends not only on the current model but also on the state of the structures, i.e., its position or velocity. Thus, a more accurate model includes a state-dependent transition probability $t(r|\acute{r}, \acute{\xi})$. Therefore, the transition density $f(\cdot|\cdot)$ for the augmented state vector $\mathrm{x} = (\xi, r)$ can be written as

$$f(\mathrm{x}|\acute{\mathrm{x}}) = \tilde{f}(\xi|\acute{\xi}, r)t(r|\acute{r}, \acute{\xi}) \tag{3}$$

where $\tilde{f}(\cdot|\cdot)$ is the state transition density for a specific model r. In this approach, it is supposed that $t(r|\acute{r}, \acute{\xi})$ can be expressed by an affine mixture of Gaussians,

$$t(r|\acute{r}, \acute{\xi}) = w_t^{(0)}(r, \acute{r}) + \sum_{j=1}^{J_t(r,\acute{r})} w_t^{(j)}(r, \acute{r}) \mathcal{N}\left(\acute{\xi}; \mu_t^{(j)}(r, \acute{r}), \Sigma_t^{(j)}(r, \acute{r})\right), \qquad (4)$$

where $w_t^{(j)}, J_t(r, \acute{r}), \mu_t^{(j)}(r, \acute{r})$ and $\Sigma_t^{(j)}(r, \acute{r})$ are given model parameters and are tuned based on prior knowledge about the application. Note $0 \leqslant t(r|\acute{r}, \acute{\xi}) \leqslant 1$ and $\sum_r t(r|\acute{r}, \acute{\xi}) = 1, \forall \acute{\xi}, \acute{r}$. The $w_t^{(j)}(\cdot)$ can be negative so that these conditions are met. Instead of having a constant transition probability matrix, the definition $t(\cdot|\cdot)$ as the form of Eq. 4 lets us to adaptively change the transition probability weights $w_t^{(j)}(\cdot)$ based an a set of Gaussian functions of the state $\acute{\xi}$.

Modeling Spawn Term: Similarly, the state of spawned structures may be affected by the state of their parents in these applications [15]. Therefore, the spawned intensity for the augmented state $\mathrm{x} = (\xi, r)$ is given by

$$\beta(\mathrm{x}|\dot{\mathrm{x}}) = \tilde{\beta}(\xi|\acute{\xi}, \acute{r})\pi(r|\acute{r}, \acute{\xi}), \qquad (5)$$

where $\tilde{\beta}(\cdot|\cdot)$ is the spawned intensity of the state ξ for the model r and $\pi(r|\acute{r}, \acute{\xi})$ is the state-dependent spawned transition probability. In this approach, it is assumed that the $\tilde{\beta}(\cdot|\cdot)$ and $\pi(\cdot|\cdot)$ can be represented by a Gaussian mixture and an affine mixture of Gaussians, respectively.

$$\tilde{\beta}(\xi|\acute{\xi}, \acute{r}) = \sum_{j=1}^{J_\beta(\acute{r})} w_\beta^{(j)}(\acute{r}) \mathcal{N}\left(\xi; F_\beta^{(j)}(\acute{r})\acute{\xi} + d_\beta^{(j)}(\acute{r}), Q_\beta^{(j)}(\acute{r})\right), \qquad (6)$$

$$\pi(r|\acute{r}, \acute{\xi}) = w_\pi^{(0)}(r, \acute{r}) + \sum_{l=1}^{J_\pi(r,\acute{r})} w_\pi^{(l)}(r, \acute{r}) \mathcal{N}\left(\acute{\xi}; \mu_\pi^{(l)}(r, \acute{r}), \Sigma_\pi^{(l)}(r, \acute{r})\right), \qquad (7)$$

where $J_\beta(\cdot), w_\beta^{(j)}(\cdot), F_\beta^{(j)}(\cdot), d_\beta^{(j)}(\cdot), Q_\beta^{(j)}(\cdot), J_\pi(\cdot), w_\pi^{(l)}(\cdot), \mu_\pi^{(l)}(\cdot)$ and $\Sigma_\pi^{(l)}(\cdot)$ are given parameters for these models [12] and are set based on a prior knowledge of the spawn phenomena in the application and such that $0 \leqslant \pi(r|\acute{r}, \acute{\xi}) \leqslant 1, \forall \acute{\xi}, \acute{r}$. The interpretation for $\pi(\cdot|\cdot)$ is similar to $t(\cdot|\cdot)$ in Eq. 4.

State-dependent Survival and Detection Probabilities: The probabilities that a target survives, $p_{S,k}(\cdot)$, or is detected by the detection scheme, $p_{D,k}(\cdot)$, may depend on its state. For example, the cellular structures may fuse or may disappear from the field of view around specific locations. Similarly, the probability of detection may vary such that the structures with faint intensity may not be detected as well as other structures [7]. Therefore, state-dependent survival and detection probabilities, $p_{S,k}(\cdot)$ and $p_{D,k}(\cdot)$, can enhance the tracking results. In our framework, we assume that these probabilities can be represented by Gaussian mixture models.

$$p_S(\acute{\xi}, \acute{r}) = w_S^{(0)}(\acute{r}) + \sum_{l=1}^{J_S(\acute{r})} w_S^{(l)}(\acute{r}) \mathcal{N}\left(F(r)\acute{\xi}; \mu_S^{(l)}(\acute{r}), \Sigma_S^{(l)}(\acute{r})\right), \quad 0 \leqslant p_S(\acute{\xi}, \acute{r}) \leqslant 1 \; \forall \acute{\xi}, \acute{r} \quad (8)$$

$$p_D(\xi,r)=w_D^{(0)}(r)+\sum_{l=1}^{J_D(r)}w_D^{(l)}(r)\mathcal{N}\Big(\xi;\mu_D^{(l)}(r),\Sigma_D^{(l)}(r)\Big),\quad 0\leqslant p_D(\xi,r)\leqslant 1\quad\forall\xi,r.\ (9)$$

The parameters of the survival and detection probabilities such as $w_S^{(l)}(\cdot)$, $J_S(\cdot)$, $\mu_S^{(l)}(\cdot)$, $\Sigma_S^{(l)}(\cdot)$, $w_D^{(l)}(\cdot)$, $J_D(\cdot)$, $\mu_D^{(l)}(\cdot)$ and $\Sigma_D^{(l)}(\cdot)$ are set based on the application.

Modeling Birth Term: In most of the previous applications, the locations of spontaneous births are either unknown or uniformly distributed everywhere in the image background [1, 5–7]. However in this filtering framework, a prior on birth locations is required to estimate the birth intensity distribution. To address this, we use a Gaussian term with very high variance, as the birth intensity distribution of the state ξ such that $\tilde{\gamma}(\xi) = w_\gamma \mathcal{N}(\xi;\mu_\gamma,\Sigma_\gamma)$, where w_γ represents the expected number of new born structures. This allows that any detected measurement has the same chance to be detected as new born targets. The birth intensity distribution for the augmented state $\mathrm{x} = (\xi,r)$ is then given by $\gamma(\xi,r) = \tilde{\gamma}(\xi)\pi_\gamma(r)$, where $\pi_\gamma(r)$ is the probability of birth for model r [12].

A Closed-form PHD Recursion: Our model differs from Pasha *et al.* [12] by the introduction of state-dependent models for $t(\cdot|\cdot)$ and $\pi(\cdot|\cdot)$. Therefore, the closed-form for the predicted intensity $v_{k|k-1}(\cdot)$ will be different from [12]. However, the updated intensity $v_k(\cdot)$ are obtained similar to the general closed-form proposed in their paper. In order to show that there is a closed-form for the predicted intensity (Eq. 1) using the above models, two Lemmas are required:

Lemma 1: The product of a Gaussian and a conditional Gaussian has a weighted Gaussian form such that $\mathcal{N}(x;\mu,\Sigma)\mathcal{N}(z;Hx + d,R) = \lambda_b\mathcal{N}(x;\mu_b,\Sigma_b)$, where $\lambda_b = \mathcal{N}(z;H\mu+d,R+H\Sigma H^T)$, $\mu_b = \mu+K(z-d-H\mu)$, and $\Sigma_b = (I-KH)\Sigma$, where $K = \Sigma H^T(H\Sigma H^T + R)^{-1}$.

Lemma 2: The product of two Gaussian distributions is a weighted Gaussian such that $\mathcal{N}(x;\mu_1,\Sigma_1)\mathcal{N}(x;\mu_2,\Sigma_2) = \lambda_c\mathcal{N}(x;\mu_c,\Sigma_c)$, where $\lambda_c = \mathcal{N}(\mu_1;\mu_2,\Sigma_1+\Sigma_2)$, $\Sigma_c = (\Sigma_1^{-1} + \Sigma_2^{-1})^{-1}$ and $\mu_c = \Sigma_c(\Sigma_1^{-1}\mu_1 + \Sigma_2^{-1}\mu_2)$.

According to Eq. 1, the $v_{k|k-1}(\cdot)$ is composed of three terms including intensity distributions due to existing targets $v_f(\cdot)$, spawned targets $v_\beta(\cdot)$ and spontaneous births $v_\gamma(\cdot)$ as $v_{k|k-1}(\mathrm{x}) = v_f(\mathrm{x}) + v_\beta(\mathrm{x}) + v_\gamma(\mathrm{x})$. Supposing that the posterior intensity v_{k-1} at time $k-1$ has a Gaussian mixture form

$$v_{k-1}(\acute{\mathrm{x}}) = v_{k-1}(\acute{\xi},\acute{r}) = \sum_{i=1}^{J(\acute{r})} w^{(i)}(\acute{r})\mathcal{N}\left(\acute{\xi};\mu^{(i)}(\acute{r}),\Sigma^{(i)}(\acute{r})\right),\qquad(10)$$

and by substituting Eqs. 3, 8 and 10 into the first term of Eq. 1 and using Lemmas 1–2, it can be shown that $v_f(\cdot)$ has Gaussian mixture form,

$$v_f(\xi,r) = \sum_{\acute{r}}\sum_{i=1}^{J(\acute{r})}\sum_{l=0}^{J_S(\acute{r})}\sum_{j=0}^{J_t(r,\acute{r})} w_f^{(i,l,j)}(r,\acute{r})\mathcal{N}\left(\xi;\mu_f^{(i,l,j)}(r,\acute{r}),\Sigma_f^{(i,l,j)}(r,\acute{r})\right).\ (11)$$

The equations for $w_f^{(i,l,j)}$, $\mu_f^{(i,l,j)}$ and $\Sigma_f^{(i,l,j)}$ can be easily calculated using the aforementioned lemmas and we omit them here due to space restrictions. Similarly by substituting Eqs. 5 and 10 into the second term of Eq. 1 and using Lemmas 1–2, it can be shown that $v_\beta(\cdot)$ also has a Gaussian mixture form as

$$v_\beta(\xi,r) = \sum_{\acute{r}} \sum_{i=1}^{J(\acute{r})} \sum_{j=1}^{J_\beta(r,\acute{r})} \sum_{l=0}^{J_\pi(r,\acute{r})} w_\beta^{(i,j,l)}(r,\acute{r}) \mathcal{N}\left(\xi; \mu_\beta^{(i,j,l)}(r,\acute{r}), \Sigma_\beta^{(i,j,l)}(r,\acute{r})\right). \quad (12)$$

As above, equations for $w_\beta^{(i,j,l)}$, $\mu_\beta^{(i,j,l)}$ and $\Sigma_\beta^{(i,j,l)}$ can be calculated using the lemmas. Finally, the last term in Eq. 1 is Gaussian term equal to

$$v_\gamma(\mathbf{x}) = \gamma(\xi,r) = w_\gamma \pi_\gamma(r) \mathcal{N}\left(\xi; \mu_\gamma, \Sigma_\gamma\right). \quad (13)$$

Consequently, $v_{k|k-1}(\cdot)$, which is sum of Eqs. 11, 12 and 13, is a Gaussian mixture. The closed-form suggested here for $v_{k|k-1}(\cdot)$ is more general than what is proposed in [12] and is applicable for an enhanced particle tracking in biological applications where the transition probabilities $t(\cdot|\cdot)$ and $\pi(\cdot|\cdot)$, and survival and detections probabilities, $p_S(\cdot|\cdot)$ and $p_D(\cdot|\cdot)$, are state-dependant functions. The proposed scheme, however, is completely general and supports simpler models where some or all of these terms are state-independent.

Tag Propagation Scheme: In the PHD filtering framework, the identity of trajectories is not considered in the filter recursions and thus, the dynamics of an individual target cannot be evaluated. A method for propagating the identity of the tracks in Gaussian mixture probability hypothesis density (GM-PHD) filter is proposed in [16]. However, the method uses a heuristic technique to find the identity of crossing targets that is only applicable for the GM-PHD filter. Here, we propose a better solution for propagating track identities and solving crossing targets. Our solution applies to both GM-PHD and LGJMS-PHD filters. Supposing the identity of each Gaussian term in the posterior intensity v_{k-1} is known, the tags are propagated in our framework as follows.

Prediction step: The Gaussian terms in $v_f(\cdot)$ keep the identities of their parents v_{k-1} as these terms are related to existing targets which move based on their dynamics. For each Gaussian term spawned by an existing term with index i in the spawned term $v_\beta(\cdot)$, a new tag is assigned. For Gaussian terms introduced by the birth model, no tag is assigned in this step.

Update step: The Gaussian terms with existing identities, initially keep their tags after the update step. For each updated Gaussian term introduced by the birth model, a new tag is assigned in this step. This idea is based on the assumption that each generated measurement is either due to the targets or clutter and a single target cannot generate more than one measurement at each time frame.

Next, the state estimation procedure (i.e. thresholding on Gaussian terms) [13] is applied to revise the tags. Noting that an existing target cannot have more than one state at each time frame, if multiple target states are assigned with

Gaussian terms having identical tags, the term with the highest weight keeps its identity and the remaining terms are assigned by a new tag.

A solution for crossing targets: From the PHD recursion, it can be seen that the number of intensity components increases as time progresses. Therefore, this filter is usually followed by a pruning step that eliminates and merges Gaussian terms [12, 13]. This step is applied to decrease computational burden and remove unlikely intensity distributions. However, it leads to identity loss in crossing targets. To avoid this, we simply suggest that merging between intensity terms can be performed only if their tags are identical. More precisely, the merging for the Gaussian terms with the different tags is not allowed in this approach.

4   Experimental Results

We applied the proposed scheme for multi-target tracking in 2-D Total Internal Reflection Fluorescence Microscopy (TIRFM) sequences. TIRFM is an imaging technique that enables the selective excitation of fluorescently tagged proteins within a few hundred nanometers of the plasma membrane of a cell. This selective excitation characteristic of TIRFM has made it an ideal imaging technique for visualizing subcellular structures such as vesicles that are on or close to the plasma membrane [17]. The vesicles are very tiny subcellular structures and are seen in TIRFM sequences as small bright spots moving with different dynamics while appearing or disappearing from the field of view or are occluded by or spawned from other structures. Moreover, due to limitations in TIRFM acquisition process, the sequences are contaminated with a high level of noise [18].

We modeled the state of each vesicle by its position, $x = (x_x, x_y)$, and velocity, $\dot{x} = (\dot{x}_x, \dot{x}_y)$. The measurements $z = (\hat{x}_x, \hat{x}_y)$ were provided by the detection scheme proposed by Rezatofighi *et al.* [18]. Then, we applied our LGJMS-PHD filter using two linear dynamic models including random walk and small acceleration motion model [1, 3, 5]. The transition probability $t(\cdot|\cdot)$ were defined similar to the function suggested in [1]. This function can be easily represented as an affine mixture of Gaussians. Since the vesicles are spawned independently from the state of their parents, a state independent form of the spawned transition probability was used in this application $\pi(r|\acute{r}, \acute{\xi}) = \pi(r|\acute{r})$. Moreover, $p_S(\cdot)$ in this current implementation is independent of the state of targets $p_S(\acute{\xi}, \acute{r}) = p_S(\acute{r})$.

Since the main source of noise in this imaging technique is an intensity dependent noise (Poisson noise) [5], the signal to noise ratio (SNR) in the areas with higher intensity levels is lower. Therefore, the vesicles located in this area have lower detection probability. To improve the probability of detection, we defined it as a Gaussian mixture function of the target positions, x. Since the locations where spontaneous births may occur is unknown in this application, the birth intensity distribution is set as Gaussian distribution centered on the image with very high standard deviation.

Evaluation on Realistic Synthetic Data: Due to complexity of the data, there is no reliable manual ground truth on the TIRFM sequences. To quantitatively evaluate the proposed tracking algorithm, it was first evaluated using

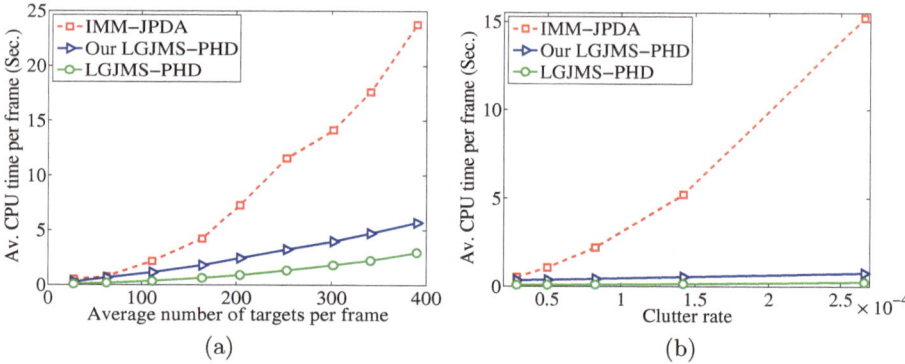

Fig. 1. The average CPU time per frame required for tracking the targets using the IMM-JPDA, the previous LGJMS-PHD and the proposed LGJMS-PHD filters in sequences with (a) different target densities and a constant clutter rate and (b) different clutter rate and a fixed average number of targets.

realistic synthetic sequences generated by the framework proposed in [19]. The sequences simulated using this framework appropriately reflect the difficulties existing in real TIRFM sequences while providing accurate ground truth.

Moreover, we quantitatively compared the results of our LGJMS-PHD filter against the result of the IMM-JPDA filter proposed in [1]. Since this filter is a combination of a multiple model Bayesian filter and a very robust data-association technique, it is the most relevant traditional Bayesian tracking filter for comparison with our framework. In addition, our results are also compared against the result of the previously implemented LGJMS-PHD filter [12] when the $t(\cdot|\cdot)$, $\pi(\cdot|\cdot)$, $p_S(\cdot|\cdot)$ and $p_D(\cdot|\cdot)$ are independent of target state. To maximize the validity of our experiments, we chose identical parameters and models such as the same state vector, clutter rate, measurements and dynamic models, for all filters. For other parameters which are not in common, we attempted to find the values that resulted in the best performance for the competing models.

In the first experiment, we compared the processing time required for these filters to track different numbers of targets in a fixed clutter rate. Here, clutter rate (λ_c) is defined as the average number of false measurements per pixel per frame. In Fig. 1(a), we see the both LGJMS-PHD filters require noticeably lower processing time for tracking large number of targets. However, since our LGJMS-PHD filter propagates more Gaussian terms for each target in each recursion, its processing time is higher than the time required for the original LGJMS-PHD filter. In the second experiment, we evaluated the performance of the tracking filters in different clutter rates but a fixed average number of targets. Fig. 1(b) shows that the processing time for the both LGJMS-PHD filters is significantly less than the IMM-JPDA filter.

To qualitatively assess the performance of these tracking methods, we used a metric based on optimal subpattern assignment (OSPA) [20]. This metric is the sum of two errors: cardinality and location. The cardinality error is related

Table 1. Comparison of the performance of the IMM-JPDA, the previous LGJMS-PHD filter and our LGJMS-PHD filters using OSPA metric [20] (lower value is better)

Method	Location error	Cardinality error	OSPA
IMM-JPDA filter [1]	**3.70**	3.53	7.23
LGJMS-PHD [12]	3.98	2.12	6.10
Our LGJMS-PHD	3.92	**1.80**	**5.72**

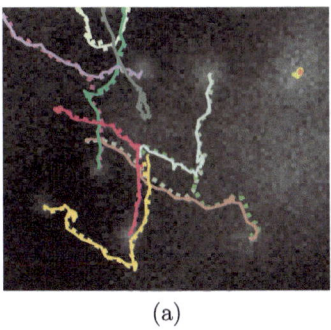
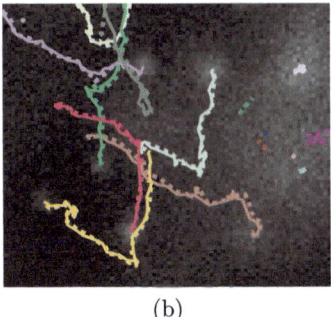

(a)   (b)

Fig. 2. An example where the PHD filter fails to accurately track several crossing targets with maneuvering motions. The ground truth (solid line) and tracking results (dashed line) for (a) our LGJMS-PHD and (b) the IMM-JPDA filters. The results of the PHD and IMM-JPDA filters include some labeling errors and false tracks, respectively.

to missed or false tracks while location error shows track accuracy error and labeling error. In Table 1, the performance of these tracking filters is compared using this metric. To this end, we applied the filters for tracking targets in synthetic sequences including on average 164 targets per frame and clutter rate $\lambda_c = 1.01 \times 10^{-4}$. According to the table, the overall tracking performance for our LGJMS-PHD filter using this metric is better than the other filters. Compared to the previous LGJMS-PHD filter, this is an expected result as we have a better model for the $t(\cdot|\cdot)$ and $p_D(\cdot|\cdot)$.

In comparison with the IMM-JPDA filter, the both PHD filters have slightly higher location error. This is mostly due to labeling error in very hard scenarios such as several crossing targets with maneuvering dynamics. Intuitively, JPDA uses joint probability association of measurements to update the tracks while the PHD filters use the first statistical moment of this joint probability. Thus, the PHD filters can not work as well as the IMM-JPDA filter in these cases (Fig. 2). In addition, the primary weakness of the PHD recursion is a loss of higher order cardinality information which causes noisy tracks specially when the density of targets are very high [21]. Therefore, this also affects track accuracy and increases the location error. In contrast, both PHD filters have the lower cardinality error compared to the IMM-JPDA filter due to less false and missed tracks. This is due to incorporating new born targets and clutter models in their recursions while there is no principled formulation for the IMM-JPDA filter. Fig. 2(b) shows that

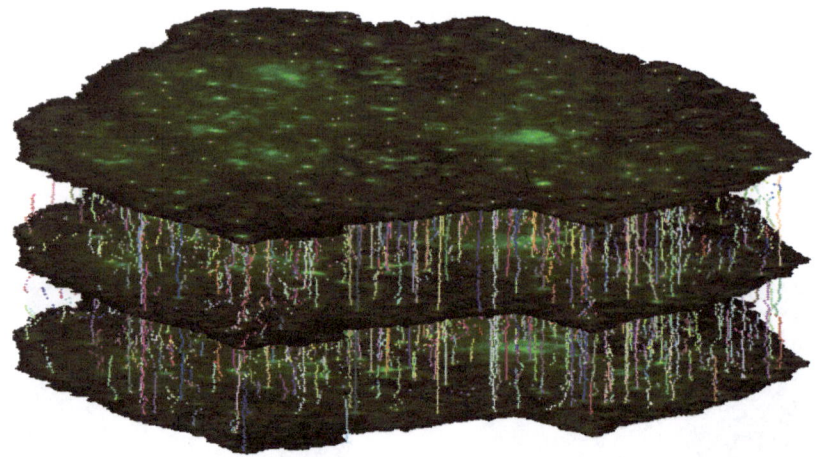

Fig. 3. Tracking result of our LGJMS-PHD filter for 100 real TIRFM sequences

the result of the IMM-JPDA filter includes several false tracks which do not exist in the result of our PHD filter (Fig. 2(a)).

Evaluation on Real Data: The three tracking filters were also tested on real TIRFM sequences. Because manual delineation of trajectories for generating reliable ground truth for our data is an arduous and subjective task, the results of the tracking were visually assessed by an expert. The real sequences include about 300 targets per frame moving through a cell membrane with an effective region size of 200×210 pixels.

In this data, there are particles that are barely visible. To detect and track these particles, the threshold in the detection method should be set low. This increases clutter rate which dramatically increases the processing time and false tracks in the IMM-JPDA filter. In contrast, the proposed LGJMS-PHD filter allows us to track a significantly larger number of faint vesicles while keeping false track rate low with significantly lower processing time compared to the IMM-JPDA filter. However, the tracks resulted from the PHD filters are slightly noisy as previously mentioned. Furthermore, they have more labeling errors in very hard scenarios where there are many crossing targets with different dynamics.

5   Conclusion

In this paper, we proposed a new closed-form recursion for the LGJMS-PHD filter by incorporating state-dependent transition probability functions $t(\cdot|\cdot)$ and $\pi(\cdot|\cdot)$. This new closed-form is more general than what was proposed previously in the literature and therefore, allows more accurate PHD trackers for biological applications. Compared to traditional Bayesian trackers such as IMM-JPDA, the proposed filter has noticeably lower processing time in the cases where there are numerous targets and noisy detections. Therefore, it can be an accurate particle tracker in these applications especially when the number of crossing targets with maneuvering motions is reasonably restricted. In addition, our filter can properly detect and track spawned particles which is not well-principled in other traditional Bayesian filters. The main weakness of the PHD filters, including ours, is that they generate noisy tracks in area with very high target density. To address this problem, we plan to use an improved version of the PHD filter, so called cardinalized PHD (CPHD) filter [21], in our future work.

References

1. Rezatofighi, S.H., Gould, S., Hartley, R., Mele, K., Hughes, W.E.: Application of the IMM-JPDA filter to multiple target tracking in total internal reflection fluorescence microscopy images. In: Ayache, N., Delingette, H., Golland, P., Mori, K. (eds.) MICCAI 2012, Part I. LNCS, vol. 7510, pp. 357–364. Springer, Heidelberg (2012)
2. Yang, L., Qiu, Z., Greenaway, A., Lu, W.: A new framework for particle detection in low-SNR fluorescence live-cell images and its application for improved particle tracking. IEEE Trans. Biomed. Eng. 59(7), 2040–2050 (2012)
3. Feng, L., Xu, Y., Yang, Y., Zheng, X.: Multiple dense particle tracking in fluorescence microscopy images based on multidimensional assignment. J. Struct. Biol. 173(2), 219–228 (2011)
4. Yuan, L., Zheng, Y.F., Zhu, J., Wang, L., Brown, A.: Object tracking with particle filtering in fluorescence microscopy images: Application to the motion of neurofilaments in axons. IEEE Trans. Med. Imag. 31(1), 117–130 (2012)
5. Smal, I., Meijering, E., Draegestein, K., Galjart, N., Grigoriev, I., Akhmanova, A., Van Royen, M., Houtsmuller, A., Niessen, W.: Multiple object tracking in molecular bioimaging by rao-blackwellized marginal particle filtering. Med. Image Anal. 12(6), 764–777 (2008)
6. Smal, I., Draegestein, K., Galjart, N., Niessen, W., Meijering, E.: Particle filtering for multiple object tracking in dynamic fluorescence microscopy images: Application to microtubule growth analysis. IEEE Trans. Med. Imag. 27(6) (2008)
7. Wood, T., Yates, C., Wilkinson, D., Rosser, G.: Simplified multitarget tracking using the PHD filter for microscopic video data. IEEE Trans. Circ. Syst. Vid. 22(5), 702–713 (2012)
8. Juang, R., Levchenko, A., Burlina, P.: Tracking cell motion using GM-PHD. In: Proc. ISBI, pp. 1154–1157 (2009)
9. Vo, B.N., Singh, S., Doucet, A.: Sequential monte carlo methods for multitarget filtering with random finite sets. IEEE Trans. Aerosp. Electron. Syst. 41(4) (2005)
10. Mahler, R.: Multitarget bayes filtering via first-order multitarget moments. IEEE Trans. Aerosp. Electron. Syst. 39(4), 1152–1178 (2003)
11. Maggio, E., Taj, M., Cavallaro, A.: Efficient multitarget visual tracking using random finite sets. IEEE Trans. Circ. Syst. Vid. 18(8), 1016–1027 (2008)
12. Pasha, S., Vo, B.N., Tuan, H., Ma, W.: A gaussian mixture PHD filter for jump markov system models. IEEE Trans. Aerosp. Electron. Syst. 45(3), 919–936 (2009)
13. Vo, B.N., Ma, W.: The gaussian mixture probability hypothesis density filter. IEEE Trans. Signal Process. 54(11), 4091–4104 (2006)
14. Keller, P., Pampaloni, F., Lattanzi, G., Stelzer, E.: Three-dimensional microtubule behavior in xenopus egg extracts reveals four dynamic states and state-dependent elastic properties. Biophys. J. 95(3), 1474–1486 (2008)

15. Cohen, A., Gomes, F., Roysam, B., Cayouette, M.: Computational prediction of neural progenitor cell fates. Nature Methods 7(3), 213–218 (2010)
16. Panta, K., Clark, D., Vo, B.N.: Data association and track management for the gaussian mixture probability hypothesis density filter. IEEE Trans. Aerosp. Electron. Syst. 45(3), 1003–1016 (2009)
17. Burchfield, J., Lopez, J., Mele, K., Vallotton, P., Hughes, W.: Exocytotic vesicle behaviour assessed by total internal reflection fluorescence microscopy. Traffic 11, 429–439 (2010)
18. Rezatofighi, S.H., Hartley, R., Hughes, W.: A new approach for spot detection in total internal reflection fluorescence microscopy. In: Proc. ISBI, pp. 860–863 (2012)
19. Rezatofighi, S.H., Pitkeathly, W., Gould, S., Hartley, R., Mele, K., Hughes, W., Burchfield, J.: A framework for generating realistic synthetic sequences of total internal reflection fluorescence microscopy images. In: Proc. ISBI (2013)
20. Ristic, B., Vo, B.N., Clark, D., Vo, B.T.: A metric for performance evaluation of multi-target tracking algorithms. IEEE Trans. Signal Process. 59(7) (2011)
21. Vo, B.T., Vo, B.N., Cantoni, A.: Analytic implementations of the cardinalized probability hypothesis density filter. IEEE Trans. Signal Process. 55(7) (2007)

Multi-layer Deformation Estimation
for Fluoroscopic Imaging

J. Samuel Preston[1], Caleb Rottman[1], Arvidas Cheryauka[2], Larry Anderton[2],
Ross T. Whitaker[1], and Sarang Joshi[1]

[1] Scientific Computing and Imaging (SCI) Institute, University of Utah
{jsam,crottman,whitaker,sjoshi}@sci.utah.edu
[2] GE Healthcare
{arvi.cheryauka,larry.anderton}@med.ge.com

Abstract. Accurate estimation of motion in fluoroscopic imaging sequences is critical for improved frame interpolation/extrapolation, tracking of surgical instruments, and Digital Subtraction Angiography (DSA). The projection of multiple transparent objects undergoing multiple complicated deformations in 3D onto a single 2D view makes this motion estimation problem quite challenging and ill-suited to existing techniques used in medical image analysis. We propose a novel method for jointly decomposing the observed image into a set of additive layers each associated with its corresponding smooth nonlinear deformation, which together model the non-smooth motion observed in the projection images across several frames. A total variation based regularization penalty is used to incorporate the known structure of the input frames for well posedness of the layer separation problem. We present the use of this model for frame interpolation and artifact reduction in DSA. Results are included from synthetic and real clinical datasets.

1 Introduction

Registration and motion estimation are a mainstay of modern medical image analysis, used for comparison and analysis of structures between patients or across multiple timepoints, motion prediction for treatment planning, and motion compensation for improved reconstruction and denoising, among other applications. Estimating a dense deformation field representing correspondences between image locations is an under-constrained problem, but correspondences modeling image differences due to motion, growth, and inter-subject variability of biological structures has been shown to be well-modeled by smooth deformation fields [12]. Fluoroscopic imaging is an important tool commonly used for diagnosis and interventional procedures. Motion estimation from fluoroscopic imaging is needed for accurate frame interpolation or motion extrapolation. This provides opportunities for lower framerates by reducing the exposure of the patient to ionizing radiation. In addition, Digital Subtraction Angiography (DSA) is a common technique for analyzing the vascular structure for diagnosis as well as interventional procedures [8]. In DSA, a radiographic contrast agent

J.C. Gee et al. (Eds.): IPMI 2013, LNCS 7917, pp. 123–134, 2013.

is injected into a blood vessel, and then a pre-contrast frame (or mask) is subtracted from all the subsequent frames. Ideally, the resulting subtraction would only show the intensity change due to the injected contrast. In practice, normal physiological motion due to breathing and heartbeat as well as other patient motion introduces artifacts in the subtracted images, and so motion estimation between the mask and current frames is needed to suppress these artifacts.

Unlike standard 3D image based deformation estimation problems in which each point in the reference image is assumed to map to a single point in the target image, fluoroscopic imaging techniques generate a projection of a three-dimensional object onto a two-dimensional imaging plane. This results in a motion estimation problem in which smooth motion of the true 3D object projects on to a non-smooth motion in the acquired image, and the intensity of each pixel at one timepoint contributes to the intensity of multiple dispersed locations in another timepoint. A 'true' motion model for this situation would reconstruct the 3D scene and smooth 3D motion field associated with each frame of the imaging sequence. This has been studied in scenes with opaque objects as structure from motion, which is still a difficult and open area of research. As we are primarily interested in estimating realistic deformations and frames as seen from the same viewpoint as the original series, we propose instead to model the motion as a number of additive layers each undergoing a smooth transformation. To achieve our goals, these layers need not represent a segmentation of objects in the scene – they must only separate overlapping objects where contradictory motion violates a smooth-deformation model. The sum of smoothly deforming layers can then accurately describe the motion in the original frames. Our method will jointly estimate these layers and corresponding deformations.

2   Background

While there has been extensive work on layer-based representations of 3D scenes in the computer vision community, the vast majority have assumed opaque objects, segmenting the optical flow field into regions undergoing similar transformations and estimating a set of deformations and unique pixel assignments ([18,19], *etc.*). In cases where transparency or reflections are considered, layer extraction models use only two layers, and even then only in constrained situations such as linear or repetitive motion, or with pairs of images obtained with different compositing functions [13, 16, 17].

Estimation of multiple motions at each point has been studied via the double optical flow constraint proposed in [14] which estimates two motion vectors at each point. Other similar formulations and extensions attempt regularize these fields into consistent motion models or increase the number of motions captured at each point [7, 10, 11, 15]. These formulations do not attempt layer extraction (estimation of the layer intensities) and cannot be used to generate interpolated or motion compensated frames.

In applications to X-ray imaging, Close *et al.* [6] propose an ad hoc hierarchical algorithm for layer extraction in analysis of angiographic stenosis.

This formulation assumes linear transformation of layers, and the sequential layer estimation and removal seems error prone. Chen *et al.* [4] propose a method for two layer extraction with one layer being static and the availability of dual-energy X-rays, which is a far more constrained situation than we wish to model. Auvray *et al.* [1] attempt motion compensation for denoising of fluoroscopic sequences using the three-frame motion constraint of [10]. Although this formulation is derived in terms of translational motion, it is used to solve for nonlinear motion. Also, although multiple motion layers are estimated, only two motions may occur at any point. Further, only motions and regions of influence are modeled, not the actual layer intensities. This greatly constrains the type of prediction or compensation for which this technique can be used.

3   Methods

Focusing on data from fluoroscopic imaging provides both simplifications and complications when compared to working with video sequences with transparency and reflections, a case often studied in the literature. With the exception of objects completely attenuating the imaging signal (a case we will ignore), we can assume that all objects are 'translucent', such that we do not have to consider occlusions. Also, unlike a video sequence in which a panning of the camera to follow a moving object may create one 'layer' whose extent is much larger than the area captured by a single frame, we assume the object being imaged stays mostly within the field of view, with relatively small portions moving in and out of frame. However, unlike much of the work on video analysis, we will not assume that layer motions can be described by a homographies or even low-order polynomial parameterizations. Further, we will not assume a 'dominant' motion between frames, and will therefore avoid a hierarchical motion decomposition.

3.1   Frame Generation Model

We are interested in modeling a time series of fluoroscopic imaging frames as a number of superimposed layers each undergoing a smooth deformation. For a scene with multiple objects, we will model the X-ray intensity at the detector as $\beta \exp(-\sum_i \mu_i d_i)$, where μ_i is the attenuation coefficient, d_i is the thickness of the ith object, and β is a constant representing the maximum transmission value. Assuming a log-transformed image (although in practice clinical data may have some approximation applied), our model subtracts the contribution of each layer from M, a maximum observed image intensity. This produces layers where zero values are be interpreted as the absence of an object.

Assume we are given a series of F frames acquired at evenly spaced time intervals, and that we wish to represent this series with N layers. The frames will be indexed by time, where the first frame occurs at time t_0 and frame F occurs at time t_T, with $T = F - 1$. These input frames will be labeled $I_0(\mathbf{x}) \ldots I_T(\mathbf{x})$. We will model each layer $\{L_n\}_{n=0\ldots N-1}$ as undergoing its own smooth deformation $\phi^n(\mathbf{x},t), t \in [t_0, t_T]$ using the standard large deformation model [3, 5], where $\phi(\mathbf{x},t)$ is defined via the time-varying velocity field $\mathbf{v}^n(\mathbf{x},t)$, $\phi(\mathbf{x},t) = \phi(\mathbf{x},t_0) + \int_{t_0}^t \mathbf{v}(\phi(\mathbf{x},s),s)\,ds$, where $\phi(\mathbf{x},t_0) = \mathbf{x}$. Smoothness of the deformation ϕ is enforced by penalizing $\int_{t_0}^{t_T} \|\mathbf{v}(\mathbf{x},t)\|_V^2 \, dt$, where $\|\mathbf{v}\|_V^2 = <\mathcal{L}\mathbf{v}, \mathbf{v}>_2$ for smooth velocity field $\mathbf{v}$, and $\mathcal{L}$ is a differential operator penalizing non-smoothness. Under reasonable smoothness assumptions the deformation $\phi(\mathbf{x},t)$ is guaranteed to be diffeomorphic, guaranteeing the existence of $\phi^{-1}(\mathbf{x},t)$. Following [3] we will use the notation $\phi_{t,s}(\mathbf{x}) = \phi(\phi^{-1}(\mathbf{x},t_t),t_s)$ for the deformation moving the point $\mathbf{x}$ at time t_t to its location at time t_s. Going forward we will also drop explicit mention of the spatial parameter $\mathbf{x}$ for notational convenience. The model for frame t is then

$$I_t = M - \sum_{n=0}^{N-1} L_t^n + \mathcal{N}(0, \sigma^2), \tag{1}$$

where $L_t^n = L^n \circ \phi_{t,0}^n$ and $\mathcal{N}(0, \sigma^2)$ represents the corruption of the ideal image by additive zero-mean Gaussian noise. Although this is not technically correct for our log-transformed photon count model, we assume the process is sufficiently close to a Gaussian model.

3.2   Layer Gradient Penalty

Our method jointly estimates both the layers and the deformations. Even with the smoothness constraint on the deformations imposed by the large deformation model this is an extremely underconstrained problem. In order to formulate a well posed estimation problem, some assumptions regarding the properties of the layers must be made. We wish to separate overlapping objects in the input frames into different layers in our model. Reducing the number of edges in layer images will help with this goal, as the overlapping of transparent objects introduces an edge which will appear in multiple layers if proper separation has not been achieved. A natural choice would be to impose a total variation penalty on the layer images. Such a penalty encourages sparsity of gradients within an image, and more importantly for our application, encourages sparsity of gradients across the layer images. Even with the 'smooth layers' constraint, the formulation permits ambiguous solutions for even simple motion as shown in Figure 1. This shows a small object moving to the right between two timepoints. Solution (a) is the 'expected' solution, however we see that solution (b) may actually be the optimal solution given the tradeoff between deformation[1] and gradient penalties. In order to improve this situation we note that other information is available which can improve the solution. Consistent motion across

---

[1] A pure translation will not be penalized by our smoothness penalty, however in realistic 2D scenes a pure translation would be uncommon, so for purposes of this example we can associate increased size of deformation with increasing smoothness penalty.

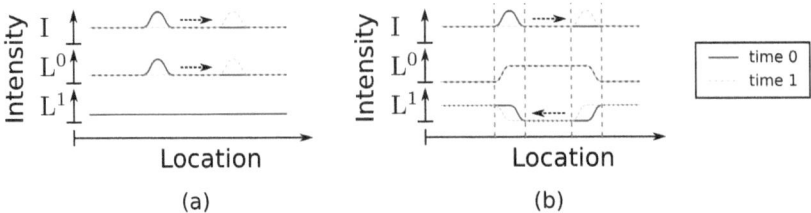

Fig. 1. A 1D example of two possible solutions accounting for the movement of a small object with two layers. Note that a larger deformation is required in case (a), and more edges are required in case (b).

multiple frames can remove ambiguity. We can also use the frame data to improve the layer smoothness penalty. We know that if there is an edge in a frame, that edge should exist in at least one layer. Further, if some location contains no edge in a frame, no edge should exist at that location in any layer at that time. Observe that this is violated in Figure 1 (b). However, as our goal is to separate objects into different layers, we do not want to force every edge into every layer. Consider the following penalty

$$\int_\Omega \|\nabla L^n\|_2 - \nabla L^n \cdot \mathbf{n}_0 \, dx, \tag{2}$$

where $\mathbf{n}_0$ represents the normals of the pseudo-attenuation frame $M - I_0$ taken with a 'cutoff' regularization based on parameter ϵ:

$$\mathbf{n}_0 = \begin{cases} -\frac{\nabla I_0}{\|\nabla I_0\|_2} & \text{if } \|\nabla I_0\|_2 \geq \epsilon, \\ 0 & \text{if } \|\nabla I_0\|_2 < \epsilon. \end{cases} \tag{3}$$

This looks like a standard TV penalty on the layer L^n except where an edge occurs in the frame I_0. Here the penalty is eliminated if the gradient in the layer aligns (in the same direction) with the gradient of the frame, and is doubled if they align in opposite directions. Also note that this value is always nonnegative, as $\nabla L^n \cdot \mathbf{n}_0$ takes its maximum value when $\mathbf{n}_0 = \frac{\nabla L^n}{\|\nabla L^n\|_2}$, resulting in zero penalty. It is also zero if ∇L^n is zero, meaning there is no penalty for a layer *not* representing an edge in I_0. Of course, noise in the frame will cause incorrect estimates of the normals. It will be important for our results to have nonzero normals only where true edges in the frame exist. To ensure this, we will calculate normals from $\bar{I}_0$, a denoised version of frame I_0. As we desire sparse gradients, a standard total variation based denoising method is employed. We note that a penalty very similar to (2) is proposed in [9] for the purposes of denoising, where the normals used are estimates the 'true' normals of the image being denoised, and are approximated by the normals of the TV-denoised image.

The undeformed layers are estimated at time t_0, and therefore equation (2) only makes sense for the normals of frame I_0. We do not wish to bias our solution to the configuration of objects observed at t_0, so we propose a version incorporating all frames

$$\sum_{t=0}^{T} \int_{\Omega} \|\nabla L^n\|_2 - \nabla L^n \cdot \tilde{\mathbf{n}}_t \, d\mathbf{x}, \tag{4}$$

where $\tilde{\mathbf{n}}_t$ represents the normals of the denoised version of $M - I_t$ taken after deforming it to time t_0, once again with cutoff ϵ:

$$\tilde{\mathbf{n}}_t = \begin{cases} -\frac{\nabla(\bar{I}_t \circ \phi_{t,0})}{\|\nabla(\bar{I}_t \circ \phi_{t,0})\|_2} & \text{if } \|\nabla(\bar{I}_t \circ \phi_{t,0})\|_2 \geq \epsilon, \\ 0 & \text{if } \|\nabla(\bar{I}_t \circ \phi_{t,0})\|_2 < \epsilon. \end{cases} \tag{5}$$

As standard numerical solutions of TV denoising do not result in perfectly uniform image regions, the parameter ϵ is chosen to ignore very small gradients, in our case approximately one percent of the input image intensity range.

3.3 Energy Formulation

We will formulate the estimation as an energy minimization problem. Given the current constraints, the energy will have the form

$$E_{\text{total}} = E_{\text{data}} + \lambda_L E_{\text{layer}} + \lambda_{\mathbf{v}} E_{\text{def}}, \tag{6}$$

where E_{data} is the data attachment term, E_{layer} is the layer gradient penalty, and E_{def} enforces the deformation smoothness constraints. The constants λ_L and $\lambda_{\mathbf{v}}$ control the tradeoff between the goals pursued by the different terms. We can now explicitly state the penalty terms. The data term will come directly from the frame generation equation (1)

$$E_{\text{data}} = \sum_{t=0}^{T} \|\hat{I}_t - I_t\|_2^2, \tag{7}$$

where $\hat{I}_t$ is the estimated frame at time t_t; $\hat{I}_t = M - \sum_{n=0}^{N-1} L_t^n$. The layer gradient penalty, as outlined above, is

$$E_{\text{layer}} = \sum_{n=0}^{N-1} \sum_{t=0}^{T} \left\| \|\nabla L^n\|_2 - \nabla L^n \cdot \tilde{\mathbf{n}}_t \right\|_1, \tag{8}$$

and the deformation smoothness, again as discussed above, is

$$E_{\text{def}} = \sum_{n=0}^{N-1} \int_{t_0}^{t_T} \|\mathbf{v}_t^n\|_V^2 \, dt, \tag{9}$$

where $\|\cdot\|_V$ is dependent on our choice of $\mathcal{L}$. In this work we will use $\mathcal{L} = \nabla^2$, the Laplacian operator. Note that we also should normalize for the number of frames, but for brevity we have absorbed this in our constants λ_L and $\lambda_{\mathbf{v}}$. Our problem is then formulated as

$$\underset{\{L^n\}_n, \{\mathbf{v}_t^n\}_{n,t}}{\arg \min} E_{\text{total}}\left(\{I_t\}_t, \{L^n\}_n, \{\mathbf{v}_t^n\}_{n,t}\right). \tag{10}$$

3.4   Residual Layers

Although the smooth deformation of layers described above can adequately describe the motion caused by breathing, heartbeat, and other deformations of 3D anatomy, there are some important cases for fluoroscopic imaging which violate this model. Specifically, the introduction of new objects such as tools during interventional procedures or contrast agents during angiography are not handled by our model. In order to accommodate these cases, additional layers with specific properties meant to model these situations are introduced.

We will look at the case of a radiographic contrast medium introduced into the vascular system to increase the contrast between blood vessels and surrounding tissue, thereby exposing vessel blockages, leaks, and abnormalities . The contrast enters the frame as a large dark object, and spreads rapidly from frame to frame. In order to model the contrast, we introduce a 'residual' layer which accounts for inter-frame changes not well modeled by a deformation. Based on the observed properties of contrast, we model it as a smooth contiguous object. The layer should also be sparse, containing mostly zero values. We therefore estimate a layer at each timepoint which is not subject to deformation, and impose a TV penalty and L^1 penalty on this layer. The model for our estimated frame is then $\hat{I} = M - \sum_{n=0}^{N-1} L_t^n - b_t$, where b_t is the residual layer at t_t, $t \in \{0 \ldots T\}$, and we introduce a new term to the energy minimization

$$E_{\text{res}} = \lambda_{\text{TV}} \sum_{t=0}^{T} \left\| \|\nabla b_t\|_2 \right\|_1 + \lambda_{L^1} \sum_{t=0}^{T} \|b_t\|_1. \tag{11}$$

again accounting for normalization over the number of frames in the constants λ_{TV} and λ_{L^1}.

3.5   Discretization and Solution

Since the time interval between frames is arbitrary in our formulation, we choose unit temporal spacing, $t_0 = 0, t_1 = 1, \ldots, t_T = T$. We expect small deformations between subsequent frames, so our discretization of a time-varying velocity field $\mathbf{v}(\mathbf{x}, t)$ will match the frame times such that there is one piecewise-constant (in time) velocity field $\mathbf{v}_t(\mathbf{x})$ corresponding to each frame I_t, $t \in \{0 \ldots T-1\}$. Euler integration in time will be used for generating ϕ from v, and bilinear interpolation is used for deformation of images and composition of deformations. For reverse-time integration, the small-deformation approximation $v^{-1} = -v$ will be used.

In order to optimize the layer gradient penalty (8), we use a primal-dual strategy based on [20]. This choice is based on properties of the regularized primal variation as $\nabla L_t^n \rightarrow 0$ with $\nabla I_t \neq 0$, which could force some portion of ∇I_t into each layer. Noting that $\|\nabla L^n\|_2 = \nabla L^n \cdot \frac{\nabla L^n}{\|\nabla L^n\|_2}$ and choosing a dual variable $\mathbf{p}^n s.t. \|\mathbf{p}^n\|_2 \leq 1$ approximating $\frac{\nabla L^n}{\|\nabla L^n\|_2}$ for $n \in \{0 \ldots N-1\}$, we rewrite (8) as

$$E_{\text{layer}} = \sum_{n=0}^{N-1} \sum_{t=0}^{T} \left\| \nabla L^n \cdot (\mathbf{p}^n - \tilde{\mathbf{n}}_t) \right\|_1. \tag{12}$$

This transforms the minimization (10) in to a max/min problem. When including a residual layer in our formulation, we also introduce a dual variable $\mathbf{q}_t$ for each residual image b_t in order to solve the total variation penalty. The L^1 penalty is solved using a 'shrinkage'-based [2] L^1 update on b_t.

A multiscale algorithm is used to ensure correct deformations are found even in cases of large movements of small structures such as vessels. At each scale level $\bar{I}_t$ is computed from the appropriately downsampled version of I_t, and $\tilde{\mathbf{n}}_t$ is then calculated from $\bar{I}_t$ via equation (5). The algorithm iteratively updates each $\{L^n\}_n$, $\{\mathbf{p}^n\}_n$, and $\{\mathbf{v}_t^n\}_{n,t}$ (and $\{\mathbf{q}_t\}_t$ and $\{b_t\}_t$ if using residual layers), taking appropriate gradient descent steps on the primal variables, and gradient ascent steps on the dual variables followed by reprojection onto their constraints, repeating until convergence.

4   Results

We first present results on a synthetic dataset meant to approximate a fluoroscopic image sequence of a contrast-enhanced vessel structure (see the first column of Figure 2). This is included to highlight characteristics of solutions this algorithm produces. Results are then presented on the clinical angiography dataset the synthetic data was meant to approximate (see first column of Figure 3). Finally results are presented for the DSA application using the deformation with residual model on a clinical dataset (Figure 5 (a) and (b)). Values for the λ constants were determined experimentally. The synthetic and clinical data frames are 256×256 and 512×512 pixels, respectively. Optimization was run on a NVIDIA Tesla C1060. Each gradient descent iteration on the clinical data at the finest scale level takes approximately 310 ms. Results presented were run for 4000 iterations at each scale level to ensure convergence.

The synthetic data is generated from four layers; a static 'rib', a slowly moving 'diaphragm', and two 'vessel' layers representing a vessel tree undergoing a nonlinear deformation with branches overlapping from the imaged viewpoint. Although the data is generated from four layers, experimental results reveal that three layers are sufficient to capture the independent motion of different structures, and additional layers do not improve the result.

The results in Figure 2 are a representative example of the solutions found by our algorithm. While the results are not correct from a segmentation perspective, in a given region any objects displaying contradictory motion are separated. Note that the diaphragm object has been removed from the upper portion of L^0, allowing the vessel to cross the diaphragm boundary. While we employ a total variation based regularization on the layers in order to help separate objects and estimate coincident motions, we do not typically want the highly denoised results shown in columns (b) and (c). In fact, we see areas at the tips of the vessel structure where fine detail has been obliterated by the de-noising properties of the estimation. If the set of estimated deformations are consistent with the motion of the imaged objects, it is possible to re-estimate only the layer intensities given these fixed deformations. In this case very little regularization

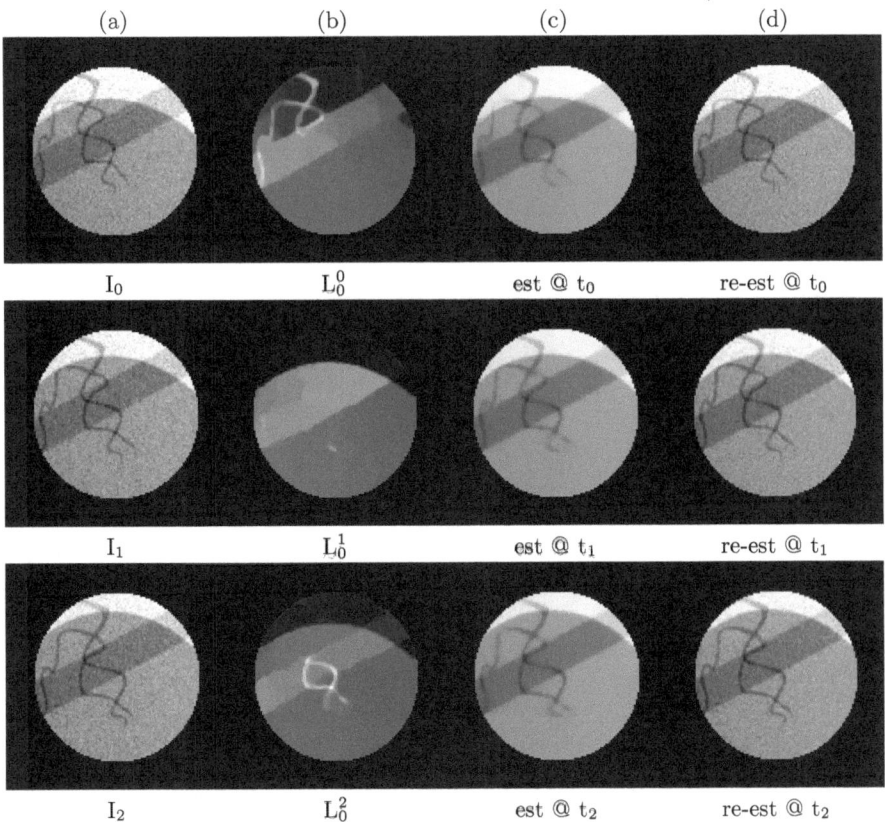

Fig. 2. Results of layer and deformation estimation on synthetic dataset. Column (a) shows the input frames. Column (b) shows each layer at t_0. Column (c) shows the estimated frame at each timepoint. Column (d) show the reconstruction with re-estimated layers.

is necessary in the intensity estimation, and the resulting layers preserve the noise texture and much of the fine detail of the original images, as shown in column (d). By temporal interpolation we can use our layer model to generate intermediate frames, as shown in Row (a) of Figure 4 where the re-estimated layers have been used.

Figure 3 shows results on a clinical angiography dataset. A Three-layer model has again been chosen based on experimental results. Note the separation of the most prominent vessel from the diaphragm. Once again, we show initial denoised layers as well as re-estimated layers. Row (b) of Figure 4 shows an interpolated frame between times t_0 and t_1. Note the crossing of vessels in the upper portion of the image.

Figure 5 shows the results of using a residual layer and two deforming layers to estimate the motion and contrast between two frames of an angiographic

132   J. Samuel Preston et al.

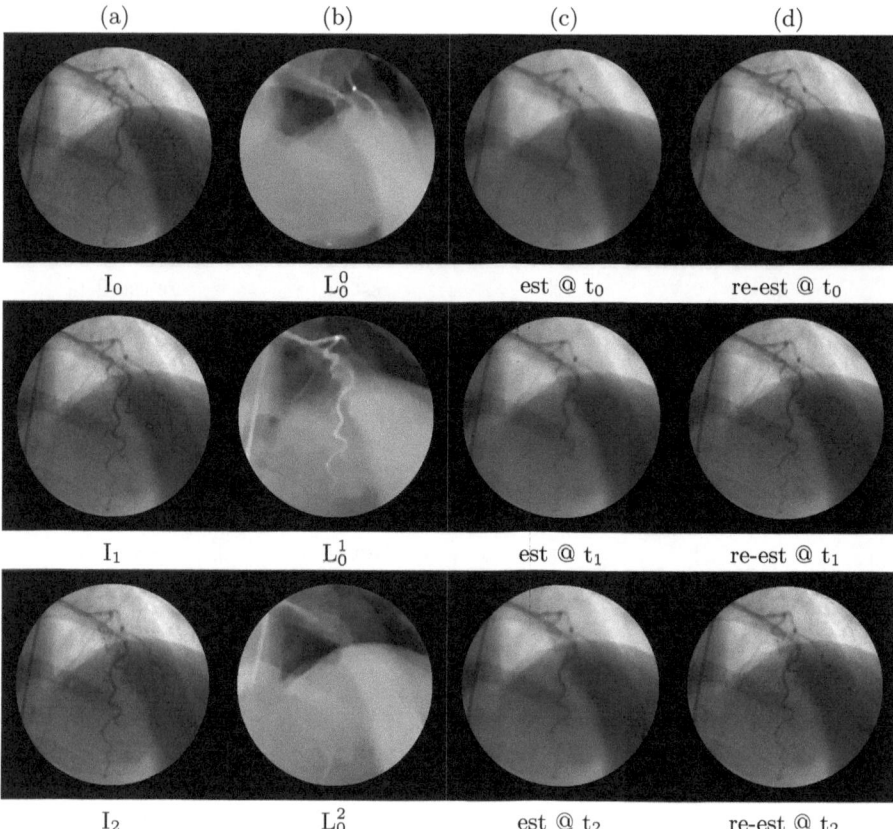

Fig. 3. Results of layer and deformation estimation on clinical dataset. Column (a) shows the input frames. Column (b) shows each layer at t_0. Column (c) shows the estimated frame at each timepoint. Column (d) show the reconstruction with re-estimated layers.

sequence to diagnose stent placement for treatment of an abdominal aortic aneurysm, and compares against static subtraction and elastic registration.

In this paper we proposed a model of dynamic X-ray images that consists of a set of superimposed, smoothly deforming layers, that combine additively to describe the spatio-temporal behavior of projected 3D motion. We also described an estimate procedure and demonstrated the feasibility of this technique for motion modeling in fluoroscopic imaging. We observed that this process should not be considered as a conventional segmentation problem; the estimated layers need not be a segmentation of physical objects in the scene in order to accurately represent the observed sequence. The estimation of such a layered model is inherently difficult. It is under constrained and there are many feasible solutions, even for simple examples. To address this challenge we propose regularizing the problem with a set of both general and application-specific penalties or models. For this we have introduced a novel penalty of gradients in the layers which forces layer edges to align with those in the observations. Also, we have introduced a

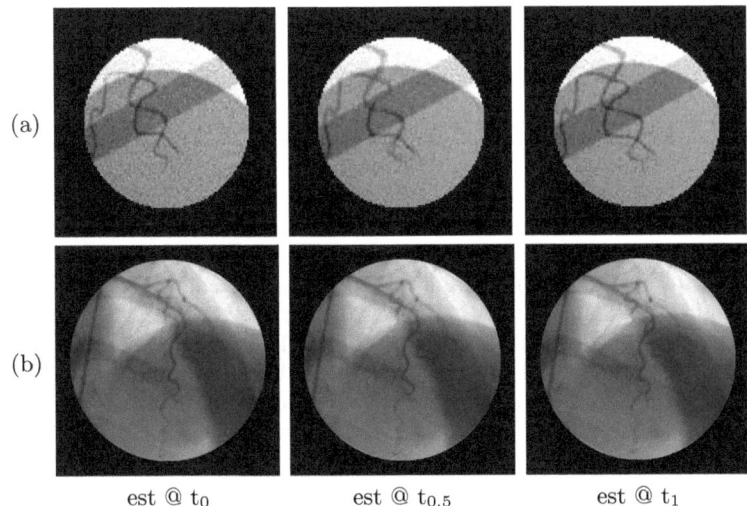

est @ t_0 est @ $t_{0.5}$ est @ t_1

Fig. 4. Frame interpolation using estimated layers and deformations. Row (a) shows results on synthetic data from Figure 2, and row (b) on clinical data from Figure 3. The center frame is estimated between t_0 and t_1.

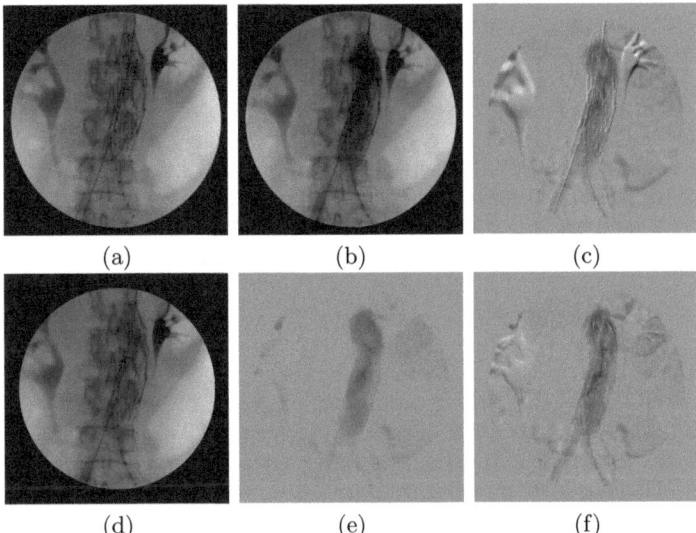

Fig. 5. DSA Results. (a) and (b) show initial (mask) frame and current frame, respectively. (c) show static subtraction. (d) is the estimated current frame (from layered registration) without residual layer. (e) shows DSA using frame (d). (f) shows subtraction using simple elastic registration between frames.

layer with a dynamic contrast model, and shown its effectiveness in correcting the motion artifacts in digital subtraction angiography.

The authors would like to acknowledge the support from GE Healthcare, which made this explorational research possible.

References

1. Auvray, V., Bouthemy, P., Liénard, J.: Joint motion estimation and layer segmentation in transparent image sequenc: application to noise reduction in x-ray image sequences. EURASIP J. Adv. Signal Process. 2009, 19:1–19:21 (2009)
2. Beck, A., Teboulle, M.: A fast iterative shrinkage-thresholding algorithm for linear inverse problems. SIAM Journal on Imaging Sciences 2(1), 183–202 (2009)
3. Beg, M.F., Miller, M.I., Trouv, A., Younes, L.: Computing large deformation metric mappings via geodesic flows of diffeomorphisms. IJCV 61(2), 139–157 (2005)
4. Chen, Y., Chang, T., Zhou, C., Fang, T.: Gradient domain layer separation under independent motion. In: ICCV, pp. 694–701. IEEE (2009)
5. Christensen, G.E., Rabbitt, R.D., Miller, M.I.: Deformable templates using large deformation kinematics. Transactions on Image Processing 5, 1435–1447 (1996)
6. Close, R., et al.: Accuracy assessment of layer decomposition using simulated angiographic image sequences. Transactions on Medical Imaging 20(10), 990–998 (2001)
7. Darrell, T., Simonecelli, E.: Nulling filters and the separation of transparent motions. In: Computer Vision and Pattern Recognition, pp. 738–739. IEEE (1993)
8. Jasper, J.: Role of digital subtraction fluoroscopic imaging in detecting intravascular injections. Pain Physician 6(3), 369–372 (2003)
9. Osher, S., et al.: An iterative regularization method for total variation-based image restoration. Multiscale Modeling & Simulation 4(2), 460–489 (2005)
10. Pingault, M., et al.: A robust multiscale b-spline function decomposition for estimating motion transparency. Tran. on Image Processing 12(11), 1416–1426 (2003)
11. Ramírez-Manzanares, A., Rivera, M., Kornprobst, P., Lauze, F.: A variational approach for multi-valued velocity field estimation in transparent sequences. In: Sgallari, F., Murli, A., Paragios, N. (eds.) SSVM 2007. LNCS, vol. 4485, pp. 227–238. Springer, Heidelberg (2007)
12. Rueckert, D., Aljabar, P., Heckemann, R.A., Hajnal, J.V., Hammers, A.: Diffeomorphic registration using B-splines. In: Larsen, R., Nielsen, M., Sporring, J. (eds.) MICCAI 2006, Part II. LNCS, vol. 4191, pp. 702–709. Springer, Heidelberg (2006)
13. Sarel, B., Irani, M.: Separating transparent layers through layer information exchange. In: Pajdla, T., Matas, J. (eds.) ECCV 2004. LNCS, vol. 3024, pp. 328–341. Springer, Heidelberg (2004)
14. Shizawa, M., Mase, K.: Simultaneous multiple optical flow estimation. In: International Conference on Pattern Recognition, vol. 1, pp. 274–278. IEEE (1990)
15. Stuke, I., et al.: Estimation of multiple motions using block matching and markov random fields. In: Proceedings of SPIE, vol. 5308, pp. 486–496 (2004)
16. Szeliski, R., Avidan, S., Anandan, P.: Layer extraction from multiple images containing reflections and transparency. In: CVPR, vol. 1, pp. 246–253. IEEE (2000)
17. Toro, J., Owens, F., Medina, R.: Using known motion fields for image separation in transparency. Pattern Recognition Letters 24(1), 597–605 (2003)
18. Wang, J., Adelson, E.: Representing moving images with layers. Transactions on Image Processing 3(5), 625–638 (1994)
19. Xiao, J., Shah, M.: Motion layer extraction in the presence of occlusion using graph cuts. Pattern Analysis and Machine Intelligence 27(10), 1644–1659 (2005)
20. Zhu, M., Chan, T.: An efficient primal-dual hybrid gradient algorithm for total variation image restoration. Tech. rep., CAM UCLA Tech. Rep. 08-34 (2008)

Fiber Connectivity Integrated Brain Activation Detection

Burak Yoldemir[1], Bernard Ng[2], Todd S. Woodward[3], and Rafeef Abugharbieh[1]

[1] Biomedical Signal and Image Computing Lab, The University of British Columbia, Canada
[2] Parietal Team, INRIA Saclay, France
[3] Department of Psychiatry, The University of British Columbia, Canada
buraky@ece.ubc.ca

Abstract. Inference of brain activation through the analysis of functional magnetic resonance imaging (fMRI) data is seriously confounded by the high level of noise in the observations. To mitigate the effects of noise, we propose incorporating anatomical connectivity into brain activation detection as motivated by how the functional integration of distinct brain areas is facilitated via neural fiber pathways. In this work, we formulate activation detection as a probabilistic graph-based segmentation problem with fiber networks estimated from diffusion MRI (dMRI) data serving as a prior. Our approach is reinforced with a data-driven scheme for refining the connectivity prior to reflect the fact that not all fibers are necessarily deployed during a given cognitive task as well as to account for false fiber tracts arising from limitations of dMRI tractography. Validating on real clinical data collected from 7 schizophrenia patients and 13 matched healthy controls, we show that incorporating anatomical connectivity significantly increases sensitivity in detecting task activation in controls compared to existing univariate techniques. Further, we illustrate how our model enables the detection of significant group activation differences between controls and patients that are missed with standard methods.

Keywords: activation detection, connectivity, dMRI, fMRI, random walker.

1 Introduction

Functional magnetic resonance imaging (fMRI) has become the primary modality for studying human brain activity. To map brain regions to function, standard analysis models the fMRI observations at each voxel as a linear combination of expected temporal responses using the general linear model (GLM) [1]. This univariate approach does not model the integrative property of the brain, which is known to facilitate brain function [2]. To ameliorate this serious limitation, the use of local neighbourhood information has been proposed to regularize activation detection [3, 4]. Although such methods help suppress false spatially-isolated activations by encouraging spatial continuity, they completely ignore long-range functional interactions. The incorporation of functional connectivity information into task activation detection has also been put forth [5], but the approach taken estimates both activation effects and functional connectivity from the same dataset, hence the information gain might be limited. Other works investigated the use of resting-state (RS) functional connectivity information to

J.C. Gee et al. (Eds.): IPMI 2013, LNCS 7917, pp. 135–146, 2013.
© Springer-Verlag Berlin Heidelberg 2013

inform task activation detection [6] as motivated by the similarity of RS networks and those engaged during task [7]. Given the typically strong noise in fMRI data, exploring other sources of information to regularize activation detection may be beneficial.

Incorporating anatomical information extracted from diffusion MRI (dMRI) data into the investigation of functional brain dynamics has attracted growing interest since functional synchronization between spatially distinct brain regions is enabled through neural fiber pathways [8, 9]. Most of the early work focused on direct comparisons of structural and functional connectivity information learned separately from dMRI and fMRI data [8, 9]. More recently, merits of multi-modal integration for joint anatomical and functional connectivity inference have been explored [10-12]. Promising results in these studies indicate benefits of multi-modal integration though the scope of this strategy has mostly been limited to connectivity estimation.

In this paper, we propose incorporating anatomical connectivity information into task activation detection. Given that fiber pathways serve as the physical substrate for functional interactions, we hypothesize that intrinsically connected brain areas would likely be in similar state, e.g. co-activate, during task [6]. Thus, informing activation detection with anatomical connectivity should presumably improve the detection sensitivity. For this, we employ the graph-theoretic random walker (RW) formulation [13], which easily permits such an integrated scheme for estimating activation probabilities. Posterior activation probabilities estimated by the RW formulation are guaranteed to be unique and globally-optimal [13], which makes RW an eminent choice. RW has been previously applied to task activation detection with functional connectivity taken as the prior [5]. Here, we investigate the implications of complementing task activation detection analysis with anatomical connectivity information. To infer group activation from posterior activation probabilities, we devise a permutation test with activation probabilities as attributes, which we empirically show to provide stronger control on false positive rate than simply comparing the posterior probability of being activated, not activated, and de-activated. On real data, we demonstrate that incorporating anatomical connectivity increases sensitivity in detecting group activation over using univariate techniques. We further show that our method is able to detect significant group activation differences between schizophrenia patients and healthy controls, which are missed by standard analysis approaches.

2   Method

We propose integrating anatomical connectivity into activation effect estimation to improve inference of activation states of brain regions from noisy observations. We use the RW formulation [13] (Section 2.1) to integrate anatomical connectivity learned through tractography (Section 2.2) with the activation likelihood of regions of interest (ROIs) computed using a mixture model applied to activation statistics maps (Section 2.3). Group activation inference is performed on the resulting posterior activation probabilities using a permutation test (Section 2.4). After estimating a group activation pattern, we iteratively refine the anatomical connectivity prior by removing the links between non-active brain regions and re-estimate the posterior activation probabilities until the detected activation pattern stabilizes (Section 2.5). An overview of our multi-modal task activation detection approach is shown in Fig.1.

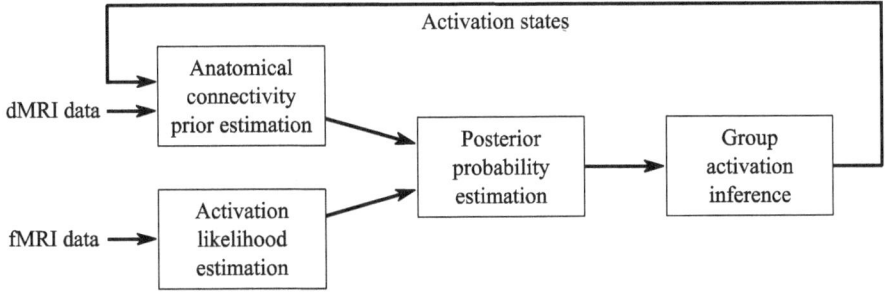

Fig. 1. Overview of proposed multi-modal task activation detection approach. Anatomical connectivity prior and activation likelihood estimates, i.e. label priors, are integrated under the RW formulation to find the posterior activation probabilities. A permutation test is applied on these probabilities to infer group activation. The anatomical connectivity prior is then iteratively refined based on the activation states of the brain regions until convergence.

2.1   Random Walker for Activation Estimation

RW is a graph-based image segmentation approach, in which graph nodes (vertices) correspond to image voxels and graph edges connecting neighbouring nodes are assigned weights reflecting node similarity. In its original formulation [14], RW labels nodes based on the probability that a random walker starting from each node will first reach a pre-labeled seed given edge weights that bias the paths. This requires user-specified seeds and does not utilize local observations at each vertex. Thus, in the context of activation detection with brain regions being the graph nodes and their interactions modeled through graph edges, this would require user-defined seeds for every functionally-disparate region and only functional interactions would be considered without accounting for activation effects. We thus adopt the formulation in [13], which overcomes the need for user interaction and integrates activation effects into the formulation as label priors. This is equivalent to adding a floating vertex for each label and connecting these floating vertices to every vertex in the original graph with label priors being the weights of the added edges [13]. In this formulation, posterior probabilities are calculated by the minimization of the following energy functional:

$$E(\mathbf{x}^s) = \mathbf{x}^{sT}\mathbf{L}\mathbf{x}^s + \sum_{k=1,k\neq s}^{K}\mathbf{x}^{kT}\mathbf{\Lambda}^k\mathbf{x}^k + (\mathbf{x}^s - 1)^T\mathbf{\Lambda}^s(\mathbf{x}^s - 1), \qquad (1)$$

where $\mathbf{x}^s$ is an $M\times1$ vector of unknown posterior probabilities of each ROI belonging to class s, $\mathbf{L}$ is an $M\times M$ weighted Laplacian matrix (Section 2.2), $\mathbf{\Lambda}^s$ is an $M\times M$ diagonal matrix having the prior probabilities of the ROIs belonging to class s on its diagonal (Section 2.3), K is the number of class labels, and M is the number of brain regions. The first term in (1) is a spatial term for modeling the interactions between graph vertices as characterized by $\mathbf{L}$. The second term denotes the aspatial component for modeling the local observations at the vertices. In our context of activation detection, the spatial term models the anatomical connectivity information and the aspatial term models the activation effects. The method can thus be thought of as grouping brain regions into classes via random walk on an augmented graph, where edges in the original graph are weighted by anatomical connectivity information and edges leading to the floating nodes are weighted by activation effects. Assuming equal weighting between the spatial and aspatial energy terms in (1), it has been shown [13] that the posterior probabilities can be found by solving:

$$\left(\mathbf{L} + \sum_{k=1}^{K} \mathbf{\Lambda}^k \right) \mathbf{x}^s = \mathbf{\lambda}^s, \tag{2}$$

where $\mathbf{\lambda}^s$ is an $M \times 1$ vector consisting of the diagonal elements of $\mathbf{\Lambda}^s$. Since $\mathbf{L}$ is positive semi-definite and $\mathbf{\Lambda}^k$ is strictly positive definite, their summation would be diagonally dominant. Hence, matrix inversion is possible for solving (2). Following [15], we set $K=3$ and define the class labels as deactive, nonactive, and active. For clarity, we explicitly denote the posterior probabilities for each class as $\mathbf{p}_D$, $\mathbf{p}_N$ and $\mathbf{p}_A$, corresponding to deactive, nonactive and active classes, respectively.

2.2   Anatomical Connectivity Prior Estimation

Let $\mathbf{D}$ be an $M \times M$ weighted adjacency matrix, where each element $\mathbf{D}_{ij}$ is an estimate of the anatomical connectivity between brain regions i and j, set to fiber count in this work. The corresponding $M \times M$ normalized Laplacian matrix, $\mathbf{L}$, of $\mathbf{D}$ is given by:

$$\mathbf{L}_{ij} = \begin{cases} 1 & \text{if } i = j \text{ and } d_j \neq 0 \\ -\dfrac{1}{\sqrt{d_i d_j}} & \text{if } i \text{ and } j \text{ are adjacent,} \\ 0 & \text{otherwise} \end{cases} \tag{3}$$

where $d_i = \Sigma_j \mathbf{D}_{ij}$ is the degree of node i. A major difficulty with tractography is resolving fiber crossing regions where accuracy of most algorithms is seriously affected. In [16], it was proposed that multiplying $\mathbf{D}$ by itself may help address this problem by generating multi-step fibers from parts of fibers that might be split at crossing regions:

$$\mathbf{D}^{MS} = \exp(\mathbf{D}) = \sum_{k=0}^{\infty} \frac{1}{k!} \mathbf{D}^k, \tag{4}$$

where $\exp(\,\cdot\,)$ denotes the matrix exponential. $\mathbf{D}^k = \mathbf{D}*\mathbf{D}*\mathbf{D}*\ldots$ and $\mathbf{D}^k_{ij}$ is the number of paths of length k connecting regions i and j. $\mathbf{D}^{MS}$ hence comprises all possible paths between each region pair, where indirect paths are more heavily penalized as these paths are potentially artifactual [16].

2.3   Activation Likelihood Estimation

To estimate the activation likelihoods, which are used as label priors $\mathbf{\lambda}^s$ in RW, we first apply the classical GLM [1] to compute the intra-subject activation statistics:

$$\mathbf{y}_j = \mathbf{X}\boldsymbol{\beta}_j + \mathbf{e}_j$$
$$\mathbf{t}_j = \hat{\boldsymbol{\beta}}_j / se(\hat{\boldsymbol{\beta}}_j), \tag{5}$$

where $\mathbf{y}_j$ is the $n{\times}1$ time course of ROI j, $\mathbf{X}$ is the $n{\times}r$ design matrix of expected responses, $\hat{\boldsymbol{\beta}}_j$ is an $r{\times}1$ vector containing estimates of the activation effects, $\boldsymbol{\beta}_j$, $\mathbf{e}_j$ is the $n{\times}1$ residual assumed to be white Gaussian noise after preprocessing, $se(\hat{\boldsymbol{\beta}}_j)$ is the standard error of $\hat{\boldsymbol{\beta}}_j$, $\mathbf{t}_j$ is the $r{\times}1$ vector of sought activation statistics, n is the number of time points, and r is the number of experimental conditions. Columns of the design matrix $\mathbf{X}$ are generated by convolving the canonical hemodynamic response function (HRF) with a boxcar time-locked to stimulus [1]. To compute the prior probabilities of ROIs belonging to each class, we fit a Gamma-Gaussian-Gamma (GGG) mixture model separately to the t-values of each condition, $\mathbf{t}^c$, i.e. c^{th} element of $\mathbf{t}_j$ assembled across all ROIs [15]. The Gaussian distribution models the nonactive state and the Gamma distributions model the deactive and active states:

$$\mathbf{t}_j^c \sim \pi_D \Gamma(k_D, \theta_D) + \pi_N N(\mu, \sigma) + \pi_A \Gamma(k_A, \theta_A), \tag{6}$$

where μ is the mean and σ is the standard deviation of the Gaussian component, k_D and k_A are the shape parameters, and θ_D and θ_A are the scale parameters of the deactivation (D) and activation (A) components, respectively. We employ the expectation-maximization (EM) algorithm [17] to estimate the model parameters separately for each experimental condition c with the probabilities of $\mathbf{t}^c$ given the parameter estimates used as the label priors λ^s. These label priors and the Laplacian matrix given in Section 2.2 are combined through (2) to estimate the posterior activation probabilities.

2.4   Group Activation Inference

The high dimensionality of fMRI data elicits a high risk of false detection. To infer group activation from activation statistics, such as t-values, several methods that control for false positive rate have been proposed, e.g. Bonferroni correction, Gaussian random field theory, max-t permutation test [18]. For group activation inference from posterior activation probability maps, most studies directly threshold the posterior activation probabilities at $1/K$, where K is the number of classes, arguing that activation inference from posterior activation probabilities does not suffer from false positives [19]. However, as we will empirically demonstrate in Section 4, directly thresholding the posterior probabilities is actually prone to false detection, necessitating a more rigorous activation inference method. To this end, we propose a permutation test for group inference from activation probabilities that controls for the false positive rate. Specifically, for each permutation, we first randomly select one third of the subjects and swap the posterior probabilities $\mathbf{p}_A$ and $\mathbf{p}_D$ of each selected subject. We note that this swap is done at the intra-subject level for all ROIs, hence the spatial pattern of the activation probabilities is preserved. Similarly, we swap $\mathbf{p}_A$ and $\mathbf{p}_N$ for another third of randomly selected subjects. We then compute the z-scores of $\mathbf{p}_A$ for each permutation across all subjects. This procedure is repeated 10,000 times to generate the null distribution of activation probabilities of each ROI. We assign the p-value for the activation likelihood of each ROI as the number of times the z-scores of permuted $\mathbf{p}_A$ are greater than the z-scores of the original $\mathbf{p}_A$ values divided by the total number of trials (in this case, 10,000). Under the null hypothesis that there is no activation, the z-score of the original $\mathbf{p}_A$ value of an ROI would lie around the mean of the generated null distribution, resulting in a non-significant p-value around 0.5. Finally, false discovery rate (FDR) [20] is applied to these p-values to account for multiple comparisons. As shown in Section 4 on a synthetic case, this permutation test offers a much lower false positive rate compared to posterior probability thresholding while keeping the true positive rate at the same (or even at a higher) rate.

2.5   Re-estimation of Group Activation Using Partial Connectome

Since some of the estimated fiber tracts might be false due to tractography errors and not all fibers are necessarily employed during a given cognitive task, we propose restricting the anatomical connectivity prior to the subset of fibers that are likely to be active by iteratively refining the original connectivity prior, $\mathbf{D}^{orig}$, as follows:

$$\mathbf{D}^{m+1} = \mathbf{D}^{task} + \frac{1}{\log(m+1)}\mathbf{D}^m, \tag{7}$$

$$\mathbf{D}_{ij}^{task} = \begin{cases} \mathbf{D}_{ij}^{orig} & \text{if } l_i^m \vee l_j^m = 1 \\ 0 & \text{if } l_i^m = l_j^m = 0 \end{cases}, \tag{8}$$

where $\mathbf{D}^m$ is the $M{\times}M$ partial adjacency matrix found in iteration m with $\mathbf{D}^1$ set to $\mathbf{D}^{orig}$. l_i^m is the estimated activation state of ROI i during iteration m with a value of 1 denoting activated and 0 denoting not activated or deactivated. We note that updating $\mathbf{D}^{orig}$ using the above scheme enables $\mathbf{D}^{orig}$ to gradually evolve as opposed to having its information from previous iterations completely discarded. The overall process proceeds by estimating the group activation map with $\mathbf{D}^1$ as the prior. We then refine $\mathbf{D}^1$ using (7) and (8), and repeat the process until the group activation map stabilizes.

3   Materials

After obtaining informed consent, fMRI data were collected from 13 healthy subjects (6 men, 7 women, mean age 27.46±6.38 years) and 7 schizophrenia patients (5 men, 2 women, mean age 30.57±10.08 years). Each subject was first presented with words in four different contexts: associating, hearing, solving and reading, during a non-scanned encoding session. The subjects were then presented the same set of words in a subsequent recall run during which fMRI data were acquired and subjects were asked to indicate the context in which the presented words were previously encountered. Image acquisition was performed on a Philips Achieva 3.0 T MRI scanner using a T2*-weighted gradient-echo spin pulse sequence with a repetition time of 2000 ms, an echo time of 30 ms, a flip angle of 90°, a field of view of 240×240 mm, and an in-plane resolution of 80×80 pixels. Each volume comprised 36 axial slices of 3 mm thickness with a 1 mm gap. Each scan lasted for 920 s, which tallies to 460 fMRI volumes. For each subject's data, motion correction and spatial normalization were performed using SPM8. The voxel time courses were then high-pass filtered to remove drifts and temporally whitened using an AR(1) model. For computing fiber count, we parcellated the brain into 500 ROIs [21] by applying Ward clustering [22] on voxel time courses concatenated across subjects. Voxel time courses within each ROI were averaged to generate ROI time courses.

dMRI data were collected from the same subjects using a Philips Achieva 3.0 T MRI scanner with a TR of 7500 ms, a TE of 54 ms, an EPI factor of 59, an FOV of 224×224 mm and an in-plane resolution of 256×256 pixels. Fifteen diffusion weighted volumes were acquired at a b-value of 800 s/mm^2 in addition to a volume with no diffusion sensitization. Each volume consisted of 72 slices of 2 mm thickness with no gap. Acquisition time was 480 s. We used FSL [23] for eddy current correction and MedINRIA [24] for diffusion tensor estimation and fiber tractography. To facilitate the computation of fiber count, we warped our functionally derived group parcel map to the B0 volume of each subject.

4   Results and Discussion

We first present the synthetic test performed to assess our proposed permutation test (Section 2.4) as compared to the posterior probability thresholding approach commonly employed in the literature [19]. For evaluation on real data, we compare the sensitivity of our proposed approach in detecting group activation in controls against that of univariate techniques. We then contrast our method against classical schemes in detecting group activation differences between schizophrenia patients and controls.

Synthetic Test of Group Inference Strategies. We performed a synthetic test carefully designed from activation probabilities calculated from the real data of healthy controls. Specifically, after estimating the group activation map with our approach, we used the highest one third of $\mathbf{p}_N$ among nonactive ROIs and the highest one third of $\mathbf{p}_A$ among active ROIs to generate a pseudo ground truth of nonactivation and activation probability distributions at the intra-subject level. These pseudo ground truth distributions are assumed to be Gaussian with means and standard deviations set to that of the respective thirds of $\mathbf{p}_N$ and $\mathbf{p}_A$. Out of a total of 100 synthetic datasets, each dataset comprised 13 subjects having 500 ROIs each, with 100 of them defined to be active. Random samples of $\mathbf{p}_N$ and $\mathbf{p}_A$ were drawn for each subject from the corresponding probability distributions. Deactivation probabilities were computed based on how posterior probabilities should sum to 1. Assessing group activation with the proposed permutation test resulted in a true positive rate (TP) of 0.819±0.038 and a false positive rate (FP) of 0.008±0.004, whereas thresholding $\mathbf{p}_A$ at 1/3 gave a TP of 0.374±0.049 and an FP of 0.097±0.015. One-sample t-tests among TPs and FPs of these two strategies declared the differences to be significant at $p<10^{-6}$, demonstrating superior sensitivity and specificity.

Detecting Group Activation in Controls. We compare the sensitivity of our method against classical GLM and against inferring group activation from the activation likelihoods given by the GGG mixture model. We further compare the effect of using $\mathbf{D}$ and $\mathbf{D}^{MS}$ as the anatomical connectivity estimates (Section 2.2). Fig. 2 shows the number of detected ROIs for different p-value thresholds. Our approach is denoted as RW for the first iteration where the full anatomical adjacency matrix is used, and RW_{it} for the following iterations with partial adjacency matrices. For the same specificity, our approach provided higher detection sensitivity than using the activation likelihoods given by the GGG mixture model, implicating the advantage of incorporating anatomical connectivity into activation detection. Iterating the procedure with refined anatomical connectivity estimates considerably improved detection. The procedure was iterated 100 times and for clarity, only the mean and standard deviations for the iterations with partial adjacency matrices were provided. It was observed that group activation map stabilized after 100 iterations, with only a couple of parcels changing labels in further iterations. This additional improvement provided by the refinement of the anatomical connectivity estimate suggests that only a subset of fibers is employed during a given task. Hence, isolating the utilized fibers can be beneficial. The improvement could also be partly due to removal of false fiber tracts arising from tractography errors. GLM (FDR corrected) provides more detection than our method at more liberal thresholds, but its performance varies considerably with p-value thresholds. In contrast, our method provides more consistent results across p-values. Comparing the results of using the original anatomical adjacency matrix versus the multi-step counterpart (denoted as RW-MS for the first, $RW\text{-}MS_{it}$ for the following iterations) suggests that some of the artifactual connections generated by the multi-step approach likely do not pertain to task activation.

Qualitatively, the ROIs detected across all experimental conditions in healthy controls largely match regions known to be involved in context memory tasks [25], which further validates our method. As shown in Fig. 3, the areas detected across all conditions include superior frontal gyrus, middle frontal gyrus, inferior frontal gyrus, supramarginal gyrus, precentral gyrus, postcentral gyrus, angular gyrus, lateral occipital cortex, occipital pole, cingulate gyrus, lingual gyrus, hippocampus and insula.

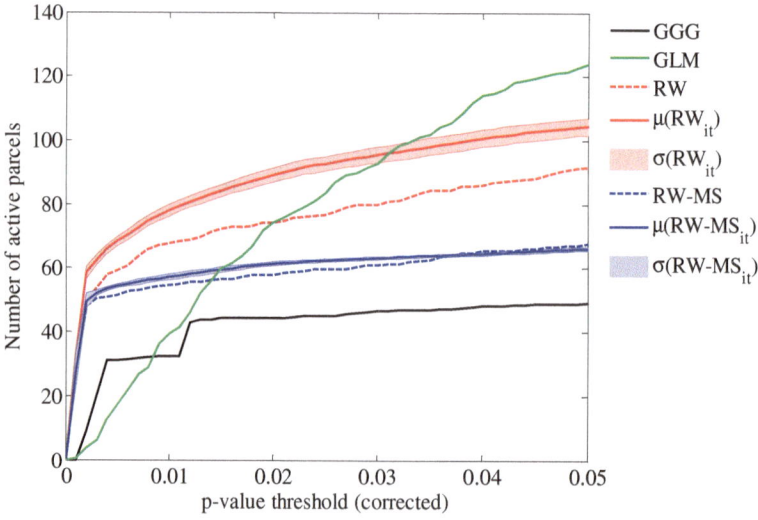

Fig. 2. Quantitative activation detection comparison

Detecting Differences between Patients and Controls. To assess the significant activation differences between schizophrenia patients and control subjects, we compared two different types of context memory recall: (1) self-other source information monitoring (did I say this word or did I hear it?) and (2) task information monitoring (did I produce a semantic associate of this word or did I read it?). Both types of context memory are thought to be impaired in schizophrenia. This comparison corresponds to the contrast between associating/reading and solving/hearing conditions. We employed a max-t permutation test [18] on the $\mathbf{p}_A$ values of the two groups

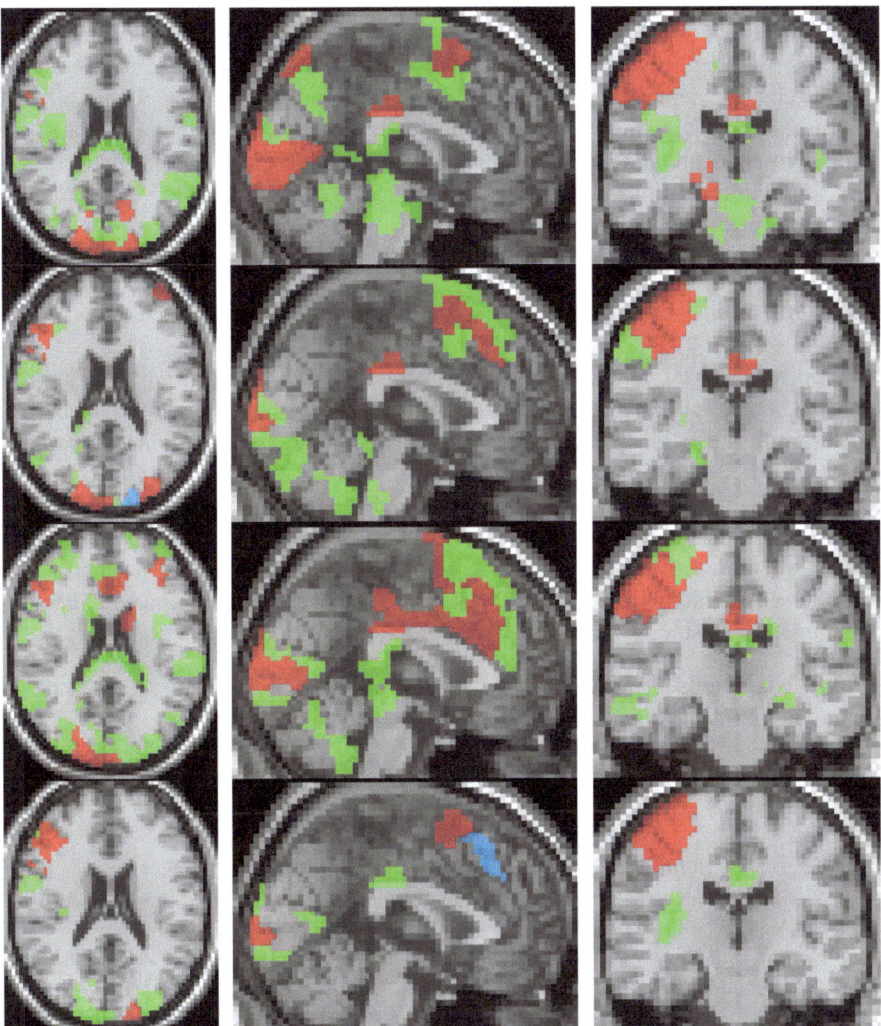

Fig. 3. Activation patterns detected at p-value < 0.05. Green=detected by RW only. Blue=detected by GGG only. Red=detected both by RW and GGG. Each row corresponds to an experimental condition, top-to-bottom: associating, hearing, solving, reading.

for this contrast and observed a significant difference (p<0.05, corrected) in the left hippocampus. Activity in this region was higher in the source monitoring condition for schizophrenia patients relative to controls but lower in the task monitoring condition relative to controls. Applying the same test on the results of GLM or GGG mixture modeling approach failed to detect any group differences up to p<0.2. The left hippocampus is involved in reactivation and association of stored semantic knowledge to consolidate new information into existing semantic frameworks [26-28]. The implication of the significant difference in the left hippocampus is that, aberrant activity in this region could lead to different manifestations of poor performance in context memory. Reduced activity during task monitoring could relate to the episodic memory impairments commonly observed in schizophrenia [29], which implies that underactivity in this region would lead to reduced reactivation of stored semantic knowledge for context memory. Increased activity during source monitoring could relate to the source memory impairments commonly observed in schizophrenia [30], such that overactivity in this region would lead to increased perceptual context for both self and other source information, leading to more difficulty in distinguishing between these two sources in context memory.

5 Conclusions

We proposed a novel fiber connectivity integrated approach for group activation inference. On real data of healthy subjects, we demonstrated that integrating dMRI and fMRI significantly increases sensitivity in detecting group activation compared to analyzing fMRI data alone. We further showed that incorporating a refined connectome comprising anatomical connections linked only to the estimated active brain regions results in improved performance over using the full estimated connectome. Finally, we presented novel findings in activation differences between healthy controls and schizophrenia patients that were missed with standard methods. Our multimodal integration strategy thus holds great promise for brain activity analysis.

Acknowledgements. This work is partly funded by NSERC and the Institute for Computing, Information and Cognitive Systems (ICICS) at UBC.

References

1. Friston, K.J., Holmes, A.P., Worsley, K.J., Poline, J.B., Frith, C.D., Frackowiak, R.S.J.: Statistical Parametric Maps in Functional Imaging: A General Linear Approach. Hum. Brain Mapp. 2, 189–210 (1995)
2. Rogers, B.P., Morgan, V.L., Newton, A.T., Gore, J.C.: Assessing Functional Connectivity in the Human Brain by fMRI. Magn. Reson. Imaging 25, 1347–1357 (2007)
3. Descombes, X., Kruggel, F., von Cramon, D.Y.: Spatio-Temporal fMRI Analysis Using Markov Random Fields. IEEE Trans. Med. Imaging 17, 1028–1039 (1998)
4. Penny, W.D., Trujillo-Barreto, N.J., Friston, K.J.: Bayesian fMRI Time Series Analysis with Spatial Priors. NeuroImage 24, 350–362 (2005)

5. Ng, B., Abugharbieh, R., Hamarneh, G., McKeown, M.J.: Random Walker Based Estimation and Spatial Analysis of Probabilistic fMRI Activation Maps. In: MICCAI fMRI Data Analysis Workshop, pp. 37–44 (2009)
6. Ng, B., Abugharbieh, R., Varoquaux, G., Poline, J.B., Thirion, B.: Connectivity-Informed fMRI Activation Detection. In: Fichtinger, G., Martel, A., Peters, T. (eds.) MICCAI 2011, Part II. LNCS, vol. 6892, pp. 285–292. Springer, Heidelberg (2011)
7. Smith, S.M., Fox, P.T., Miller, K.L., Glahn, D.C., Fox, P.M., Mackay, C.E., Filippini, N., Watkins, K.E., Toro, R., Laird, A.R., Beckmann, C.F.: Correspondence of the Brain's Functional Architecture During Activation and Rest. Proc. Natl. Acad. Sci. 106, 13040–13045 (2009)
8. Honey, C.J., Thivierge, J.P., Sporns, O.: Can Structure Predict Function in the Human Brain? NeuroImage 52, 766–776 (2010)
9. Damoiseaux, J.S., Greicius, M.D.: Greater than the Sum of its Parts: A Review of Studies Combining Structural Connectivity and Resting-State Functional Connectivity. Brain Struct. Funct. 213, 525–533 (2009)
10. Ng, B., Varoquaux, G., Poline, J.-B., Thirion, B.: A Novel Sparse Graphical Approach for Multimodal Brain Connectivity Inference. In: Ayache, N., Delingette, H., Golland, P., Mori, K. (eds.) MICCAI 2012, Part I. LNCS, vol. 7510, pp. 707–714. Springer, Heidelberg (2012)
11. Venkataraman, A., Rathi, Y., Kubicki, M., Westin, C.F., Golland, P.: Joint Modeling of Anatomical and Functional Connectivity for Population Studies. IEEE Trans. Med. Imaging 31, 164–182 (2012)
12. Chen, H., Li, K., Zhu, D., Zhang, T., Jin, C., Guo, L., Li, L., Liu, T.: Inferring Group-Wise Consistent Multimodal Brain Networks via Multi-view Spectral Clustering. In: Ayache, N., Delingette, H., Golland, P., Mori, K. (eds.) MICCAI 2012, Part III. LNCS, vol. 7512, pp. 297–304. Springer, Heidelberg (2012)
13. Grady, L.: Multilabel Random Walker Image Segmentation Using Prior Models. In: Proc. IEEE Comp. Soc. Conf. Comp. Vision Pattern Recog., vol. 1, pp. 763–770 (2005)
14. Grady, L.: Random Walks for Image Segmentation. IEEE Trans. Pattern Anal. Mach. Intell. 28, 1768–1783 (2006)
15. Hartvig, N.V., Jensen, J.L.: Spatial Mixture Modeling of fMRI Data. Hum. Brain Mapp. 11, 233–248 (2000)
16. Skudlarski, P., Jagannathan, K., Calhoun, V.D., Hampson, M., Skudlarska, B.A., Pearlson, G.: Measuring Brain Connectivity: Diffusion Tensor Imaging Validates Resting State Temporal Correlations. NeuroImage 43, 554–561 (2008)
17. Dempster, A.P., Laird, N.M., Rubin, D.B.: Maximum Likelihood from Incomplete Data via the EM Algorithm. J. R. Statist. Soc. B 39, 1–38 (1977)
18. Nichols, T., Hayasaka, S.: Controlling the Familywise Error Rate in Functional Neuroimaging: A Comparative Review. Stat. Methods Med. Research 12, 419–446 (2003)
19. Friston, K.J., Penny, W.: Posterior Probability Maps and SPMs. NeuroImage 19, 1240–1249 (2003)
20. Genovese, C.R., Lazar, N.A., Nichols, T.: Thresholding of Statistical Maps in Functional Neuroimaging Using the False Discovery Rate. NeuroImage 15, 870–878 (2002)
21. Thyreau, B., Thirion, B., Flandin, G., Poline, J.-B.: Anatomo-Functional Description of the Brain: A Probabilistic Approach. In: IEEE Int. Conf. Acoustics, Speech and Signal Proc., vol. 5, pp. 14–19 (2006)
22. Michel, V., Gramfort, A., Varoquaux, G., Eger, E., Keribin, C., Thirion, B.: A Supervised Clustering Approach for fMRI-based Inference of Brain States. Patt. Recog. 45, 2041–2049 (2012)

23. Smith, S.M., Jenkinson, M., Woolrich, M.W., Beckmann, C.F., Behrens, T.E.J., Johansen-Berg, H., Bannister, P.R., De Luca, M., Drobnjak, I., Flitney, D.E., Niazy, R., Saunders, J., Vickers, J., Zhang, Y., De Stefano, N., Brady, J.M., Matthews, P.M.: Advances in Functional and Structural MR Image Analysis and Implementation as FSL. NeuroImage 23, 208–219 (2004)
24. Toussaint, N., Souplet, J.C., Fillard, P.: MedINRIA: Medical Image Navigation and Research Tool by INRIA. In: MICCAI Workshop on Interaction in Medical Image Analysis and Visualization, pp. 1–8 (2007)
25. Wang, L., Metzak, P.D., Honer, W.G., Woodward, T.S.: Impaired Efficiency of Functional Networks Underlying Episodic Memory-for-Context in Schizophrenia. J. Neurosci. 30, 13171–13179 (2010)
26. Eichenbaum, H.: Conscious Awareness, Memory and the Hippocampus. Nat. Neurosci. 2, 775–776 (1999)
27. Henke, K., Weber, B., Kneifel, S., Wieser, H.G., Buck, A.: Human Hippocampus Associates Information in Memory. Proc. Natl. Acad. Sci. 96, 5884–5889 (1999)
28. Giovanello, K.S., Schnyer, D.M., Verfaellie, M.: A Critical Role for the Anterior Hippocampus in Relational Memory: Evidence from an fMRI Study Comparing Associative and Item Recognition. Hippocampus 14, 5–8 (2004)
29. Heinrichs, W., Zakzanis, K.K.: Neurocognitive Deficit in Schizophrenia: A Quantitative Review of the Evidence. Neuropsychology 12, 426–445 (1998)
30. Waters, F., Woodward, T.S., Allen, P., Aleman, A., Sommer, I.: Self-recognition Deficits in Schizophrenia Patients with Auditory Hallucinations: A Meta-analysis of the Literature. Schizophrenia Bulletin 38, 741–750 (2012)

Diffeomorphic Metric Mapping of Hybrid Diffusion Imaging Based on BFOR Signal Basis

Jia Du[1], A. Pasha Hosseinbor[3,4], Moo K. Chung[4,5], Barbara B. Bendlin[6],
Gaurav Suryawanshi[4], Andrew L. Alexander[3,4], and Anqi Qiu[1,2]

[1] Department of Bioengineering, National University of Singapore
[2] Clinical Imaging Research Center, National University of Singapore
[3] Department of Medical Physics, University of Wisconsin-Madison
[4] Waisman Laboratory for Brain Imaging and Behavior, University of Wisconsin-Madison
[5] Biostatistics and Medical Informatics, University of Wisconsin-Madison
[6] Department of Medicine, University of Wisconsin-Madison

Abstract. In this paper, we propose a large deformation diffeomorphic metric mapping algorithm to align multiple b-value diffusion weighted imaging (mDWI) data, specifically acquired via hybrid diffusion imaging (HYDI), denoted as LDDMM-HYDI. We adopt the work given in Hosseinbor et al. (2012) and represent the q-space diffusion signal with the Bessel Fourier orientation reconstruction (BFOR) signal basis. The BFOR framework provides the representation of mDWI in the q-space and thus reduces memory requirement. In addition, since the BFOR signal basis is orthonormal, the $\mathbf{L}^2$ norm that quantifies the differences in q-space signals of any two mDWI datasets can be easily computed as the sum of the squared differences in the BFOR expansion coefficients. In this work, we show that the reorientation of the q-space signal due to spatial transformation can be easily defined on the BFOR signal basis. We incorporate the BFOR signal basis into the LDDMM framework and derive the gradient descent algorithm for LDDMM-HYDI with explicit orientation optimization. Using real HYDI datasets, we show that it is important to consider the variation of mDWI reorientation due to a small change in diffeomorphic transformation in the LDDMM-HYDI optimization.

1   Introduction

In order to accurately reconstruct the diffusion signal and ensemble average propagator (EAP), a thorough exploration of q-space is needed, which requires multiple b-value diffusion weighted imaging (mDWI). MDWI can characterize more complex neural fiber geometries when compared to single b-value techniques like diffusion tensor imaging (DTI) or high angular resolution diffusion imaging (HARDI). Hybrid diffusion imaging (HYDI) [12] is a mDWI technique that samples the diffusion signal along concentric spherical shells in q-space, with the number of encoding directions increased with each shell to increase the angular resolution with the level of diffusion weighting. Originally, HYDI employed the fast Fourier transform (FFT) to reconstruct the EAP. However, the recent advent of analytical EAP reconstruction schemes, which obtain closed-form expressions of the EAP, obviate the use of the FFT in HYDI. One such technique successfully validated on HYDI datasets is Bessel Fourier orientation reconstruction (BFOR)

J.C. Gee et al. (Eds.): IPMI 2013, LNCS 7917, pp. 147–158, 2013.

[9]. MDWI techniques like HYDI, however, have not been widely used by clinicians and neuroscientists partially due to their relatively long acquisition times. In addition, there is a lack of fundamental image analysis tools, such as registration, that can fully utilize their information.

In the last decades, researchers have spent great efforts on developing registration algorithms to align diffusion tensors derived from DTI and orientation distribution functions (ODFs) derived from HARDI [e.g., [11,6]]. However, registration algorithms directly based on DWIs are few. The direct alignment of DWIs in q-space utilizes the full diffusion information, is independent of the choice of diffusion models and their reconstruction algorithms (e.g., tensor, ODF), and unifies the transformation to align the local diffusion profiles defined at each voxel of two brains [3,13,15]. Dhollander et al.[3] developed an algorithm that transforms the diffusion signals on a single shell of q-space and preserves anisotropic as well as isotropic volume fractions. Yap et.al [13] proposed to decompose the diffusion signals on a single shell of q-space into a series of weighted diffusion basis functions, reorient these functions independently based on a local affine transformation, and then recompose the reoriented functions to obtain the final transformed diffusion signals. This approach provides the representation of the diffusion signal and also explicitly models the isotropic component of the diffusion signals to avoid undesirable artifacts during the local affine transformation. Zhang et al. [15] developed a diffeomorphic registration algorithm for aligning DW signals on a single shell of q-space.

Only recently, Dhollander et al. [4] aligned DWIs on multiple shells of q-space by first estimating transformation using a multi-channel diffeomorphic mapping algorithm, in which generalized fractional anisotrophy (GFA) images computed from each shell were used as mapping objects, and then applying the transformation to DWIs in each shell using the DWI reorientation method in [3]. This approach neglected possible influences of the DWI reorientation on the optimization of the spatial transformation. Hsu et al. [10] generalized the large deformation diffeomorphic metric image mapping algorithm [7] to DWIs in multiple shells of q-space and considered the image domain and q-space as the spatial domain where the diffeomorphic transformation is applied to. The authors claimed that the reorientation of DWIs is no longer needed as the transformation also incorporates the deformation due to the shape differences in diffusion profiles in q-space. It is a robust registration approach with the explicit consideration of the large deformation in both the image domain and the q-space. However, its computational complexity and memory requirement are high.

In this paper, we propose a new large deformation diffeomorphic metric mapping (LDDMM) algorithm to align HYDI datasets, denoted as LDDMM-HYDI. In particular, we adopt the BFOR framework in representing the q-space signal. Unlike Hsu et al. [10], the BFOR signal basis provides the representation of the q-space signal and thus reduces memory requirement. In addition, since the BFOR signal basis is orthonormal, the $\mathbf{L}^2$ norm that quantifies the differences in q-space signals can be easily computed as the sum of the squared differences in the BFOR expansion coefficients. In this work, we will show that the reorientation of q-space signal due to spatial transformation can be easily defined on the BFOR signal basis. Unlike the work in [4], we will incorporate the BFOR signal basis into the LDDMM framework and derive the gradient descent algorithm for solving the LDDMM-HYDI variational problem with explicit orientation optimization. As shown below, the main contributions of this paper are:

1. to seek large deformation for aligning HYDI datasets based on the BFOR representation of mDWI.
2. to derive the rotation-based reorientation of the q-space signal via the BFOR signal basis. This is equivalent to applying Wigner matrix to the BFOR expansion coefficients, where Wigner matrix can be easily constructed by the rotation matrix (see Section 2.1).
3. to derive the gradient descent algorithm for the LDDMM-HYDI variational problem with the explicit orientation optimization. In particular, we provide a computationally efficient method for calculating the variation of Wigner matrix due to the small variation of the diffeomorphic transformation (see Section 2.4).
4. to show that the LDDMM-HYDI gradient descent algorithm does not involve the calculation of the BFOR signal bases and hence avoids the discretization in q-space.

2 Methods

According to the work in [9], the q-space diffusion signal, $S(\mathbf{x}, \mathbf{q})$, can be represented as

$$S(\mathbf{x}, \mathbf{q}) = \sum_{n=1}^{N_b} \sum_{j=1}^{N_Y} c_{nj}(\mathbf{x}) \Psi_{nj}(\mathbf{q}) , \tag{1}$$

where $\mathbf{x}$ and $\mathbf{q}$ respectively denote the image domain and q-space. $\Psi_{nj}(\mathbf{q})$ is the nj-th BFOR signal basis with its corresponding coefficient, $c_{nj}(\mathbf{x})$, at $\mathbf{x}$. $\Psi_{nj}(\mathbf{q})$ is given as

$$\Psi_{nj}(\mathbf{q}) = j_{l(j)} \left(\frac{\alpha_{nl(j)} |\mathbf{q}|}{\tau} \right) Y_j \left(\frac{\mathbf{q}}{|\mathbf{q}|} \right) . \tag{2}$$

Here, α_{nl} is the nth root of the lth order spherical Bessel (SB) function of the first kind j_l. τ is the radial distance in q-space at which the Bessel function goes to zero. Y_j are the modified real and symmetric spherical harmonics (SH) bases as given in [9]. $N_Y = \frac{(L+1)(L+2)}{2}$ is the number of terms in the modified SH bases of truncation order L, while N_b is the truncation order of radial basis. We refer readers to [9] for more details.

Using the fact that the BFOR signal basis is orthonormal, the $\mathbf{L}^2$-norm of $S(\mathbf{x}, \mathbf{q})$ can be easily written as

$$\|S(\mathbf{x}, \mathbf{q})\|_2 = \sqrt{\int_{\mathbf{x} \in \mathbb{R}^3} \int_{\mathbf{q} \in \mathbb{R}^3} S^2(\mathbf{x}, \mathbf{q}) d\mathbf{q} d\mathbf{x}} = \sqrt{\int_{\mathbf{x} \in \mathbb{R}^3} \sum_{n=1}^{N_b} \sum_{j=1}^{N_Y} c_{nj}(\mathbf{x})^2 d\mathbf{x}} . \tag{3}$$

2.1   Rotation-Based Reorientation of $S(\mathbf{x}, \mathbf{q})$

We now discuss the reorientation of $S(\mathbf{x}, \mathbf{q})$ when rotation transformation R is applied. We assume that the diffusion profile in each shell of q-space remains in the same shell after the reorientation. However, its angular profile in each shell of q-space is transformed according to the rotation transformation. Hence, we define

$$RS(\mathbf{x}, \mathbf{q}) = S\left(\mathbf{x}, |\mathbf{q}|R^{-1}\frac{\mathbf{q}}{|\mathbf{q}|}\right) .$$

According to the BFOR representation of $S(\mathbf{x}, \mathbf{q})$ in Eq. (1), we thus have

$$RS(\mathbf{x}, \mathbf{q}) = \sum_{n=1}^{N_b} \sum_{j=1}^{N_Y} c_{nj}(\mathbf{x}) j_{l(j)}\left(\frac{\alpha_{nl(j)}|\mathbf{q}|}{\tau}\right) Y_j\left(R^{-1}\frac{\mathbf{q}}{|\mathbf{q}|}\right) .$$

This indicates that the rotation reorientation of mDWI is equivalent to applying the rotation transformation to the real spherical harmonics, Y_j. According to the work in [8], the rotation of Y_j can be achieved by the rotation of their corresponding coefficients, yielding

$$RS(\mathbf{x}, \mathbf{q}) = \sum_{n=1}^{N_b} \left(\sum_{j=1}^{N_Y} \left(\sum_{j'=1}^{N_Y} M_{jj'} c_{nj'}(\mathbf{x}) \right) \right) j_{l(j)}\left(\frac{\alpha_{nl(j)}|\mathbf{q}|}{\tau}\right) Y_j\left(\frac{\mathbf{q}}{|\mathbf{q}|}\right), \quad (4)$$

where $M_{jj'}$ is the jj'th element of Wigner matrix $M(R)$ constructed based on R (see details in [8]). We can see that the same Wigner matrix is applied to c_{nj} at a fixed n. For the sake of simplicity, we rewrite Eq. (4) in the matrix form, i.e.,

$$RS(\mathbf{x}, \mathbf{q}) = \left(\mathbf{M}(R)\, \mathbf{c}(\mathbf{x})\right)^{\top} \boldsymbol{\Psi}(\mathbf{q}) ,$$

where $\mathbf{M}$ is a sparse matrix with N_b diagonal blocks of $M(R)$. $\mathbf{c}$ is a vector that concatenates coefficients $c_{nj'}$ in the order such that at a fixed n, $c_{nj'}$ corresponds to $M(R)$. $\boldsymbol{\Psi}(\mathbf{q})$ concatenates the BFOR signal basis.

2.2   Diffeomorphic Group Action on $S(\mathbf{x}, \mathbf{q})$

We define an action of diffeomorphisms $\phi : \Omega \to \Omega$ on $S(\mathbf{x}, \mathbf{q})$, which takes into consideration of the reorientation in q-space as well as the transformation of the spatial volume in Ω. Based on the rotation reorientation of $S(\mathbf{x}, \mathbf{q})$ in Eq. (4), for a given spatial location $\mathbf{x}$, the action of ϕ on $S(\mathbf{x}, \mathbf{q})$ can be defined as

$$\phi \cdot S(\mathbf{x}, \mathbf{q}) = S\left(\phi^{-1}(\mathbf{x}), R_{\phi^{-1}(\mathbf{x})}^{-1}\mathbf{q}\right)$$

$$= \left(\mathbf{M}\left(R_{\phi^{-1}(\mathbf{x})}\right) \mathbf{c}\left(\phi^{-1}(\mathbf{x})\right)\right)^{\top} \boldsymbol{\Psi}(\mathbf{q}) ,$$

where $R_{\mathbf{x}}$ can be defined in a way similar to the finite strain scheme used in DTI registration [1]. That is, $R_{\mathbf{x}} = (D_{\mathbf{x}}\phi D_{\mathbf{x}}^{\top}\phi)^{-\frac{1}{2}} D_{\mathbf{x}}\phi$, where $D_{\mathbf{x}}\phi$ is the Jacobian matrix of ϕ at $\mathbf{x}$. For the remainder of this paper, we denote this as

$$\phi \cdot S(\mathbf{x}, \mathbf{q}) = \left(\left(\mathbf{M}(R_{\mathbf{x}})\, \mathbf{c}(\mathbf{x})\right)^{\top}\right) \circ \phi^{-1}(\mathbf{x})\ \boldsymbol{\Psi}(\mathbf{q}) , \quad (5)$$

where $\circ$ indicates as the composition of diffeomorphisms.

2.3 Large Deformation Diffeomorphic Metric Mapping for HYDIs

The previous sections equip us with an appropriate representation of HYDI mDWI and its diffeomorphic action. Now, we state a variational problem for mapping HYDIs from one subject to another. We define this problem in the "large deformation" setting of Grenander's group action approach for modeling shapes, that is, HYDI volumes are modeled by assuming that they can be generated from one to another via flows of diffeomorphisms ϕ_t, which are solutions of ordinary differential equations $\dot{\phi}_t = v_t(\phi_t), t \in [0,1]$, starting from the identity map $\phi_0 = \texttt{Id}$. They are therefore characterized by time-dependent velocity vector fields $v_t, t \in [0,1]$. We define a metric distance between a target HYDI volume S_{targ} and a template HYDI volume S_{temp} as the minimal length of curves $\phi_t \cdot S_{\text{temp}}, t \in [0,1]$, in a shape space such that, at time $t = 1$, $\phi_1 \cdot S_{\text{temp}} = S_{\text{targ}}$. Lengths of such curves are computed as the integrated norm $\|v_t\|_V$ of the vector field generating the transformation, where $v_t \in V$, where V is a reproducing kernel Hilbert space with kernel k_V and norm $\| \cdot \|_V$. To ensure solutions are diffeomorphic, V must be a space of smooth vector fields. Using the duality isometry in Hilbert spaces, one can equivalently express the lengths in terms of m_t, interpreted as momentum such that for each $u \in V$, $\langle m_t, u \circ \phi_t \rangle_2 = \langle k_V^{-1} v_t, u \rangle_2$, where we let $\langle m, u \rangle_2$ denote the $\mathbf{L}^2$ inner product between m and u, but also, with a slight abuse, the result of the natural pairing between m and v in cases where m is singular (e.g., a measure). This identity is classically written as $\phi_t^* m_t = k_V^{-1} v_t$, where ϕ_t^* is referred to as the pullback operation on a vector measure, m_t. Using the identity $\|v_t\|_V^2 = \langle k_V^{-1} v_t, v_t \rangle_2 = \langle m_t, k_V m_t \rangle_2$ and the standard fact that energy-minimizing curves coincide with constant-speed length-minimizing curves, one can obtain the metric distance between the template and target volumes by minimizing $\int_0^1 \langle m_t, k_V m_t \rangle_2 dt$ such that $\phi_1 \cdot S_{\text{temp}} = S_{\text{targ}}$ at time $t = 1$. We associate this with the variational problem in the form of

$$J(m_t) = \inf\nolimits_{m_t : \dot{\phi}_t = k_V m_t(\phi_t), \phi_0 = \texttt{Id}} \int_0^1 \langle m_t, k_V m_t \rangle_2 dt + \lambda\, E(\phi_1 \cdot S_{\text{temp}}, S_{\text{targ}}), \quad (6)$$

where λ is a positive scalar. E quantifies the difference between deformed template $\phi_1 \cdot S_{\text{temp}}$ and target S_{targ}. Based on Eq. (3) and (5), E is expressed in the form of

$$E = \int_{\mathbf{x} \in \Omega} \left\| \left(\mathbf{M}(R_{\mathbf{x}})\, \mathbf{c}_{\text{temp}}(\mathbf{x}) \right) \circ \phi^{-1}(\mathbf{x}) - \mathbf{c}_{\text{targ}}(\mathbf{x}) \right\|_2^2 d\mathbf{x} . \quad (7)$$

2.4 Gradient of J with Respect to m_t

We now solve the optimization problem in Eq. (6) via a gradient descent method. The gradient of J with respect to m_t can be computed via studying a variation $m_t^\epsilon = m_t + \epsilon \tilde{m}_t$ on J such that the derivative of J with respect to ϵ is expressed in function of $\tilde{m}_t$. According to the general LDDMM framework derived in [7], we directly give the expression of the gradient of J with respect to m_t as

$$\nabla J(m_t) = 2 m_t + \lambda \eta_t , \quad (8)$$

where

$$\eta_t = \nabla_{\phi_1} E + \int_t^1 \left[\partial_{\phi_s}(k_V m_s) \right]^\top (\eta_s + m_s) ds , \quad (9)$$

Eq. (9) can be solved backward given $\eta_1 = \nabla_{\phi_1} E$. $\partial_{\phi_s}(k_V m_s)$ is the partial derivative of $k_V m_s$ with respect to ϕ_s.

In the following, we discuss the computation of $\nabla_{\phi_1} E$. We consider a variation of ϕ_1 as $\phi_1^\epsilon = \phi_1 + \epsilon h$ and denote the corresponding variation in $\mathbf{M}(R_\mathbf{x})$ as $\mathbf{M}(R_\mathbf{x}^\epsilon)$. Denote $\hat{\mathbf{c}}(\mathbf{x}) = \mathbf{M}(R_\mathbf{x})\mathbf{c}_{\text{temp}}(\mathbf{x})$ for the simplicity of notation. We have

$$
\left.\frac{\partial E}{\partial \epsilon}\right|_{\epsilon=0} = \int_{\mathbf{x}\in\Omega} \left.\frac{\partial \left\|(\mathbf{M}(R_\mathbf{x}^\epsilon)\mathbf{c}_{\text{temp}}(\mathbf{x}))\circ(\phi_1^\epsilon)^{-1}(\mathbf{x}) - \mathbf{c}_{\text{targ}}(\mathbf{x})\right\|_2^2}{\partial \epsilon}\right|_{\epsilon=0} d\mathbf{x} \qquad (10)
$$

$$
= \underbrace{2\int_{\mathbf{x}\in\Omega} \left\langle \hat{\mathbf{c}}(\mathbf{x})\circ\phi_1^{-1} - \mathbf{c}_{\text{targ}}(\mathbf{x}), \nabla_\mathbf{x}^\top \hat{\mathbf{c}}(\mathbf{x})\circ\phi_1^{-1}\left.\frac{\partial(\phi_1^\epsilon)^{-1}}{\partial \epsilon}\right|_{\epsilon=0}\right\rangle d\mathbf{x}}_{\text{term (A)}}
$$

$$
+ \underbrace{2\int_{\mathbf{x}\in\Omega}\left\langle \hat{\mathbf{c}}(\mathbf{x})\circ\phi_1^{-1} - \mathbf{c}_{\text{targ}}(\mathbf{x}), \left(\left.\frac{\partial\mathbf{M}(R_\mathbf{x}^\epsilon)\mathbf{c}_{\text{temp}}(\mathbf{x})}{\partial\epsilon}\right|_{\epsilon=0}\right)\circ\phi_1^{-1}\right\rangle d\mathbf{x}}_{\text{term (B)}} .
$$

As the calculation of Term (A) is straightforward, we directly give its expression, i.e.,

$$
\text{Term (A)} = -2\int_{\mathbf{x}\in\Omega}\left\langle (D_\mathbf{x}\phi_1)^{-\top}\nabla_\mathbf{x}\hat{\mathbf{c}}(\mathbf{x})\left(\hat{\mathbf{c}}(\mathbf{x}) - \mathbf{c}_{\text{targ}}(\phi_1(\mathbf{x}))\right) \det(D_\mathbf{x}\phi_1), h\right\rangle d\mathbf{x} .
$$
$$(11)$$

This term is similar to that in the scalar image mapping case. It seeks the optimal spatial transformation ϕ_t in the gradient direction of image $\hat{\mathbf{c}}(\mathbf{x})$ weighted by the difference between the template and target images.

The computation of Term (B) involves the differential of $\mathbf{M}(R_\mathbf{x})$ with respect to rotation matrix $R_\mathbf{x}$ and the variation of $R_\mathbf{x}^\epsilon$ with respect to the small variation of ϕ_1^ϵ. Let's first compute the derivative of $\mathbf{M}(R_\mathbf{x})$ with respect to rotation matrix $R_\mathbf{x}$. According to the work in [2], the analytical form of this derivative can be solved using the Euler angle representation of $R_\mathbf{x}$ but is relatively complex. Here, we consider Wigner matrix $\mathbf{M}(R_\mathbf{x})$ and the coefficients of the BFOR signal basis $\mathbf{c}_{\text{temp}}(\mathbf{x})$ together, which leads to a simple numeric approach for computing the derivative of $\hat{\mathbf{c}}(\mathbf{x}) = \mathbf{M}(R_\mathbf{x})\mathbf{c}_{\text{temp}}(\mathbf{x})$ with respect to rotation matrix $R_\mathbf{x}$, i.e., $\nabla_{R_\mathbf{x}}\hat{\mathbf{c}}(\mathbf{x})$. Assume $\tilde{R}_\mathbf{x} = e^{\delta U}R$, where $\delta U = \begin{bmatrix} 0 & -\delta\mu_3 & \delta\mu_2 \\ \delta\mu_3 & 0 & -\delta\mu_1 \\ -\delta\mu_2 & \delta\mu_1 & 0 \end{bmatrix}$ is a skew-symmetric matrix parameterized by $\delta\boldsymbol{\mu} = \begin{bmatrix} \delta\mu_1 & \delta\mu_2 & \delta\mu_3 \end{bmatrix}^\top$. From this construction, δU is the tangent vector at $R_\mathbf{x}$ on the manifold of rotation matrices and $\tilde{R}_\mathbf{x}$ is also a rotation matrix. Based on Taylor expansion, we have the first order approximation of $\mathbf{M}(\tilde{R}_\mathbf{x})\mathbf{c}_{\text{temp}}(\mathbf{x})$ as

$$
\mathbf{M}(\tilde{R}_\mathbf{x})\mathbf{c}_{\text{temp}}(\mathbf{x}) \approx \hat{\mathbf{c}}(\mathbf{x}) + \nabla_{R_\mathbf{x}}^\top \hat{\mathbf{c}}(\mathbf{x})\delta\boldsymbol{\mu} .
$$

Hence, we can compute $\nabla_{R_\mathbf{x}}\hat{\mathbf{c}}(\mathbf{x})$ as follows. Assume $\delta U_1, \delta U_2, \delta U_3$ to be skew-symmetric matrices respectively constructed from $[\delta\mu_1, 0, 0]^\top, [0, \delta\mu_2, 0]^\top, [0, 0, \delta\mu_3]^\top$. We have

$$
\nabla_{R_\mathbf{x}}\hat{\mathbf{c}}(\mathbf{x}) \approx \begin{bmatrix} \left(\mathbf{M}(e^{\delta U_1})\hat{\mathbf{c}}(\mathbf{x}) - \hat{\mathbf{c}}(\mathbf{x})\right)^\top/\delta\mu_1 \\ \left(\mathbf{M}(e^{\delta U_2})\hat{\mathbf{c}}(\mathbf{x}) - \hat{\mathbf{c}}(\mathbf{x})\right)^\top/\delta\mu_2 \\ \left(\mathbf{M}(e^{\delta U_3})\hat{\mathbf{c}}(\mathbf{x}) - \hat{\mathbf{c}}(\mathbf{x})\right)^\top/\delta\mu_3 \end{bmatrix} . \qquad (12)
$$

It is worth noting that this formulation significantly reduces the computational cost for $\nabla_{R_{\mathbf{x}}} \hat{\mathbf{c}}(\mathbf{x})$. Since $\delta \mu$ is independent of spatial location $\mathbf{x}$, $\mathbf{M}(e^{\delta U_1})$, $\mathbf{M}(e^{\delta U_2})$, and $\mathbf{M}(e^{\delta U_3})$ are only calculated once and applied to all $\mathbf{x}$.

We now compute the variation of $R_{\mathbf{x}}^{\epsilon}$ with respect to the small variation of ϕ_1^{ϵ}. This has been referred as exact finite-strain differential that was solved in [5] and applied to the DTI tensor-based registration in [14]. Here, we directly adopt the result from [14] and obtain

$$\frac{\partial R_{\mathbf{x}}^{\epsilon}}{\partial \epsilon}\bigg|_{\epsilon=0} = -F_{\mathbf{x}} \sum_{i=1}^{3} \left[\mathbf{r}_i \times (D_{\mathbf{x}} h^{\top})_i\right] , \qquad (13)$$

where $F_{\mathbf{x}} = -R_{\mathbf{x}}^{\top} \left(\text{trace}\left((D_{\mathbf{x}}\phi_1 D_{\mathbf{x}}^{\top}\phi_1)^{1/2}\right) \text{Id} - (D_{\mathbf{x}}\phi_1 D_{\mathbf{x}}^{\top}\phi_1)^{1/2} \right)^{-1} R_{\mathbf{x}}$. $\times$ denotes as the cross product of two vectors. $(A)_i$ denotes the ith column of matrix A. $\mathbf{r}_i = (R_{\mathbf{x}}^{\top})_i$.

Given Eq. (12) and (13), we thus have

$$\text{Term (B)} = -2 \int_{\mathbf{x} \in \Omega} \left\langle \hat{\mathbf{c}}(\mathbf{x}) \circ \phi_1^{-1} - \mathbf{c}_{\text{targ}}(\mathbf{x}), \left(\nabla_{R_{\mathbf{x}}} \hat{\mathbf{c}}^{\top}(\mathbf{x}) F_{\mathbf{x}} \sum_{i=1}^{3} \left[\mathbf{r}_i \times (D_{\mathbf{x}} h^{\top})_i\right]\right) \circ \phi_1^{-1} \right\rangle d\mathbf{x}$$

$$\qquad (14)$$

$$= -2 \int_{\mathbf{x} \in \Omega} \boldsymbol{\omega}_{\mathbf{x}}^{\top} \sum_{i=1}^{3} \left[\mathbf{r}_i \times (D_{\mathbf{x}} h^{\top})_i\right] d\mathbf{x}$$

$$= -2 \int_{\mathbf{x} \in \Omega} \sum_{i=1}^{3} \langle \boldsymbol{\omega}_{\mathbf{x}} \times \mathbf{r}_i, \nabla_{\mathbf{x}} h_i \rangle \, d\mathbf{x} ,$$

where

$$\boldsymbol{\omega}_{\mathbf{x}}^{\top} = \left(\nabla_{R_{\mathbf{x}}} \hat{\mathbf{c}}\left(\hat{\mathbf{c}}(\mathbf{x}) - \mathbf{c}_{\text{targ}}(\phi_1(\mathbf{x}))\right)\right)^{\top} F_{\mathbf{x}} \det\left(D_{\mathbf{x}}\phi_1\right) , \qquad (15)$$

and $h = \begin{bmatrix} h_1 & h_2 & h_3 \end{bmatrix}^{\top}$. $D_{\mathbf{x}} h$ is approximated as

$$D_{\mathbf{x}} h = \begin{bmatrix} \nabla_{\mathbf{x}} h_1^{\top} \\ \nabla_{\mathbf{x}} h_2^{\top} \\ \nabla_{\mathbf{x}} h_3^{\top} \end{bmatrix} \approx \frac{1}{2 \Delta d} \begin{bmatrix} h_{1,\mathbf{x}^{X+}} - h_{1,\mathbf{x}^{X-}} & h_{1,\mathbf{x}^{Y+}} - h_{1,\mathbf{x}^{Y-}} & h_{1,\mathbf{x}^{Z+}} - h_{1,\mathbf{x}^{Z-}} \\ h_{2,\mathbf{x}^{X+}} - h_{1,\mathbf{x}^{X-}} & h_{2,\mathbf{x}^{Y+}} - h_{2,\mathbf{x}^{Y-}} & h_{2,\mathbf{x}^{Z+}} - h_{2,\mathbf{x}^{Z-}} \\ h_{3,\mathbf{x}^{X+}} - h_{3,\mathbf{x}^{X-}} & h_{3,\mathbf{x}^{Y+}} - h_{3,\mathbf{x}^{Y-}} & h_{3,\mathbf{x}^{Z+}} - h_{3,\mathbf{x}^{Z-}} \end{bmatrix} ,$$

where $\{\mathbf{x}^{X+}, \mathbf{x}^{X-}, \mathbf{x}^{Y+}, \mathbf{x}^{Y+}, \mathbf{x}^{Z+}, \mathbf{x}^{Z-}\}$ are the neighbors of $\mathbf{x}$ in x, y, z directions, respectively. Δd is the distance of these neighbors to $\mathbf{x}$. Here, term (B) seeks the spatial transformation ϕ_t such that the local diffusion profiles of the template and target HYDIs have to be aligned.

In summary, we have

$$\frac{\partial E}{\partial \epsilon}\Big|_{\epsilon=0} \approx -2 \int_{\mathbf{x}\in\Omega} \Big\langle \left(D_{\mathbf{x}}\phi_1\right)^{-\top} \nabla_{\mathbf{x}}\hat{\mathbf{c}}(\mathbf{x})\Big(\hat{\mathbf{c}}(\mathbf{x}) - \mathbf{c}_{\mathrm{targ}}(\phi_1(\mathbf{x}))\Big) \det\left(D_{\mathbf{x}}\phi_1\right), h \Big\rangle d\mathbf{x}$$

(16)

$$-\frac{1}{\Delta d}\int_{\mathbf{x}\in\Omega}\sum_{k=1}^{3}\left\{\left\langle \boldsymbol{\omega}_{\mathbf{x}}\times\mathbf{r}_k, \begin{bmatrix} h_{k,\mathbf{x}^{X+}} \\ h_{k,\mathbf{x}^{Y+}} \\ h_{k,\mathbf{x}^{Z+}} \end{bmatrix}\right\rangle - \left\langle \boldsymbol{\omega}_{\mathbf{x}}\times\mathbf{r}_k, \begin{bmatrix} h_{k,\mathbf{x}^{X-}} \\ h_{k,\mathbf{x}^{Y-}} \\ h_{k,\mathbf{x}^{Z-}} \end{bmatrix}\right\rangle\right\}d\mathbf{x}.$$

Therefore, $\nabla_{\phi_1}E$ can be obtained from Eq. (16).

2.5 Numerical Implementation

We so far derive J and its gradient $\nabla J(m_t)$ in the continuous setting. In this section, we elaborate the numerical implementation of our algorithm under the discrete setting. Since HYDI DW signals were represented using the orthonormal BFOR signal bases, both the computation of J in Eq. (6) and the gradient computation in Eq. (16) do not explicitly involve the calculation $\boldsymbol{\Psi}(\mathbf{q})$. Hence, we do not need to discretize the q-space. In the discretization of the image domain, we first represent the ambient space, Ω, using a finite number of points on the image grid, $\Omega \cong \{(\mathbf{x}_i)_{i=1}^N\}$. In this setting, we can assume m_t to be the sum of Dirac measures, where $\alpha_i(t)$ is the momentum vector at $\mathbf{x}_i$ and time t. We use a conjugate gradient routine to perform the minimization of J with respect to $\alpha_i(t)$. We summarize steps required in each iteration during the minimization process below:

1. Use the forward Euler method to compute the trajectory based on the flow equation:

$$\frac{d\phi_t(\mathbf{x}_i)}{dt} = \sum_{j=1}^{N} k_V(\phi_t(\mathbf{x}_i), \phi_t(\mathbf{x}_j))\alpha_j(t) .$$

(17)

2. Compute $\nabla_{\phi_1(\mathbf{x}_i)}E$ based on Eq. (16).
3. Solve $\eta_t = [\eta_i(t)]_{i=1}^N$ in Eq. (9) using the backward Euler integration, where i indices $\mathbf{x}_i$, with the initial condition $\eta_i(1) = \nabla_{\phi_1(\mathbf{x}_i)}E$.
4. Compute the gradient $\nabla J(\alpha_i(t)) = 2\alpha_i(t) + \eta_i(t)$.
5. Evaluate J when $\alpha_i(t) = \alpha_i^{\mathrm{old}}(t) - \epsilon\nabla J(\alpha_i(t))$, where ϵ is the adaptive step size determined by a golden section search.

3 Experiments

In this section, we first illustrate the mapping results of HYDI datasets using LDDMM-HYDI and then evaluate the influence of the reorientation on the optimization of the diffeomorphic transformation, which is often neglected in existing DWI-based registration algorithms (e.g., [3,4]). Seven HYDI datasets used in this study consisted of 6 shells corresponding to b-values of 0, 300, 1200, 2700, 4800, and 7500 s/mm^2. We refer readers to [12] for more details on the HYDI acquisition. In our experiments, we

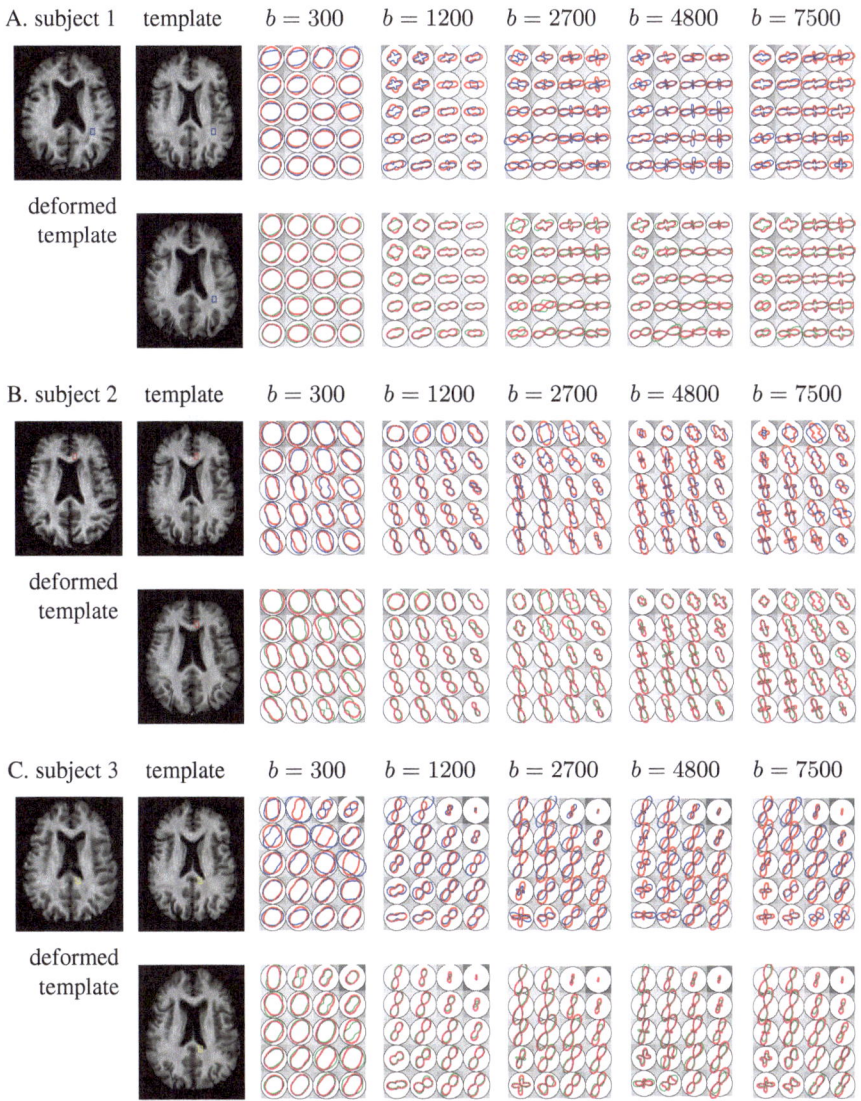

Fig. 1. Illustration of the LDDMM-HYDI mapping results. The first row of panels (A-C) illustrates the subject image, template image, the diffusion profiles at individual shells with b=300, 1200, 2700, 4800, and 7500 s/mm^2 in q-space, respectively. The second row of panels (A-C) illustrates the deformed template image after the LDDMM-HYDI mapping, the diffusion profiles at individual shells with b=300, 1200, 2700, 4800, and 7500 s/mm^2 in q-space, respectively. Red, blue, and green contours in the last five columns respectively illustrate the diffusion profiles of the subject, template, and deformed template. The closer the green contour to the red contour, the better the alignment. Note that the profile of diffusion weighted signals is shown in this figure. It is orthogonal to the fiber orientation.

represented HYDI DW signals using the BFOR signal basis with upto the fourth order modified SH bases and upto the sixth order spherical Bessel function. The corresponding BFOR expansion coefficients were used in the LDDMM-HYDI optimization.

Figure 1 shows the LDDMM-HYDI mapping results of three subjects. The last five columns respectively illustrate the geometric shapes of the diffusion signals at five shells of q-space in the brain regions with crossing fibers. Red, blue, and green contours respectively represent the shape of the diffusion signals from the subject, template, and deformed template. Visually, the diffusion profile at each shell can be matched well after the mapping. Table 1 lists the squared difference in the diffusion signals of the subjects and the template before and after the LDDMM-HYDI mapping at individual shells in q-space, suggesting the significant improvement in the alignment of DWIs after the mapping ($p < 0.05$).

We next evaluated the mapping accuracy of the LDDMM-HYDI algorithms with and without the computation of Term (B) in Eq. (10) during the optimization, where Term (B) seeks the diffeomorphic transformation such that the local diffusion profiles of the template and target HYDIs can be aligned. For this, we first computed the diffusion probability density functions (PDFs) of water molecules, i.e., the ensemble average propagator (EAP), using Fourier transform [9]. Then, we calculated the symmetrized Kullback-Leibler (sKL) divergence between the deformed template and target PDFs [6] in major white matter tracts. The smaller sKL metric indicates the better alignment between the deformed template and target images. The major white matter tracts evaluated in this study include corpus callosum (CC), corticospinal tract (CST), internal capsule (IC), corona radiata (CR), external capsule (EC), cingulum (CG), superior longitudinal fasciculus (SLF), and inferior fronto-occipital fasciculus (IFO). Table 2 lists the values of the mean and standard deviation of the sKL metric for each major white matter tract among six subjects when the LDDMM-HYDI algorithms with and without the Term (B) computation were respectively employed. These results suggest that the LDDMM-HYDI algorithm with the explicit orientation optimization (Term (B) computation) significantly improves the alignment in the major white matter tracts when compared to that without the explicit orientation optimization ($p < 0.05$).

Last, we generated the mDWI atlas by averaging the corresponding BFOR coefficients across seven subjects. For visualizing the neural fiber organization of this atlas, we constructed the EAP image based on the method in [9]. Figure 2 shows the diffusion profiles of this atlas at three layers of the EAP space.

Table 1. Evaluation of the LDDMM-HYDI mapping accuracy. The first row lists the squared difference in the diffusion signals of subjects and the template at each shell, while the second row lists that between subjects and the deformed template after the LDDMM-HYDI mapping. The numbers listed are the average and standard deviation values across six subjects.

	b=300	b=1200	b=2700	b=4800	b=7500
before LDDMM-HYDI	7.676(0.800)	5.475(0.318)	2.988(0.135)	2.533(0.071)	2.629(0.109)
after LDDMM-HYDI	2.675(0.143)	2.681(0.150)	1.775(0.071)	1.626(0.044)	1.516(0.047)

A. Atlas   B. $p = 5\mu m$ C. $p = 10\mu m$ D. $p = 15\mu m$

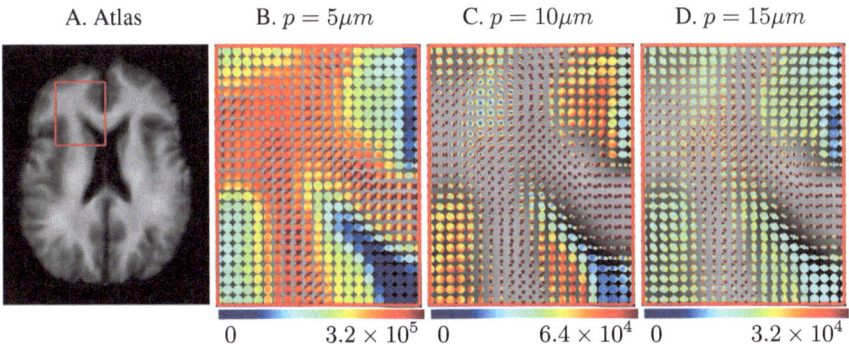

0   3.2×10^5 0 6.4×10^4 0 3.2×10^4

Fig. 2. HYDI atlas in the ensemble average propagator (EAP) space. Panel (A) shows the atlas in terms of zero displacement probability (Po), a scalar image defined in [9] based on EAP. Panels (B-D) respectively illustrate the diffusion profiles of the atlas at three given radii ($p = 5, 10, 15\mu m$) in the EAP space. The color indicates the values of EAP.

Table 2. Table lists the mean and standard deviation values of the symmetrized Kullback-Leibler (sKL) divergence of the diffusion probability density functions (PDFs) between the deformed template and target HYDIs in each major white matter tract. The second and third columns show the results obtained from the LDDMM-HYDI with and without the Term (B) computation. * denotes statistical significance indicating that the alignment obtained from the LDDMM-HYDI with the Term (B) computation is better than that obtained from the LDDMM-HYDI without the Term (B) computation at a significance level of 0.05. Abbreviation: CC-corpus callosum; CST-corticospinal tract; IC- internal capsule; CR-corona radiata; EC-external capsule, CG-cingulum, SLF-superior longitudinal fasciculus, and IFO-inferior fronto-occipital fasciculus.

	LDDMM-HYDI with Term (B)	LDDMM-HYDI without Term (B)
CST	0.598(0.265)	0.676(0.305)*
CC	0.407(0.180)	0.452(0.202)*
IC	0.425(0.189)	0.446(0.200)*
CR	0.368(0.163)	0.429(0.191)*
EC	0.476(0.212)	0.488(0.218)*
CG	0.504(0.223)	0.566(0.252)*
SLF	0.409(0.187)	0.527(0.241)*
IFO	0.518(0.229)	0.543(0.240)*

4 Conclusion

In this paper, we proposed the LDDMM-HYDI variational problem based on the BFOR signal basis representation of DWIs. We derived the gradient of this variational problem with the explicit computation of the mDWI reorientation and provided a numeric algorithm without a need of the discretization in q-space. Our results showed that the explicit orientation optimization is necessary as it improves the alignment of the diffusion profiles of HYDI datasets.

Acknowledgments. The work was supported by the Young Investigator Award at the National University of Singapore (NUSYIA FY10 P07), the National University of Singapore MOE AcRF Tier 1, Singapore Ministry of Education Academic Research Fund Tier 2 (MOE2012-T2-2-130), and NIH grants (MH84051, HD003352, AG037639, and AG033514).

References

1. Alexander, D., Pierpaoli, C., Basser, P., Gee, J.: Spatial transformation of diffusion tensor magnetic resonance images. IEEE Trans. on Medical Imaging 20, 1131–1139 (2001)
2. Cetingul, H., Afsari, B., Vidal, R.: An algebraic solution to rotation recovery in hardi from correspondences of orientation distribution functions. In: 2012 9th IEEE International Symposium on Biomedical Imaging (ISBI), pp. 38–41 (May 2012)
3. Dhollander, T., Van Hecke, W., Maes, F., Sunaert, S., Suetens, P.: Spatial transformations of high angular resolution diffusion imaging data in Q-space. In: MICCAI CDMRI Workshop, pp. 73–83 (2010)
4. Dhollander, T., Veraart, J., Van Hecke, W., Maes, F., Sunaert, S., Sijbers, J., Suetens, P.: Feasibility and advantages of diffusion weighted imaging atlas construction in Q-space. In: Fichtinger, G., Martel, A., Peters, T. (eds.) MICCAI 2011, Part II. LNCS, vol. 6892, pp. 166–173. Springer, Heidelberg (2011)
5. Dorst, L.: First order error propagation of the procrustes method for 3d attitude estimation. IEEE Transactions on Pattern Analysis and Machine Intelligence 27(2), 221–229 (2005)
6. Du, J., Goh, A., Qiu, A.: Diffeomorphic metric mapping of high angular resolution diffusion imaging based on riemannian structure of orientation distribution functions. IEEE Transactions on Medical Imaging 31(5), 1021–1033 (2012)
7. Du, J., Younes, L., Qiu, A.: Whole brain diffeomorphic metric mapping via integration of sulcal and gyral curves, cortical surfaces, and images. NeuroImage 56(1), 162–173 (2011)
8. Geng, X., Ross, T.J., Gu, H., Shin, W., Zhan, W., Chao, Y.P., Lin, C.P., Schuff, N., Yang, Y.: Diffeomorphic image registration of diffusion mri using spherical harmonics. IEEE Transactions on Medical Imaging 30(3), 747–758 (2011)
9. Hosseinbor, A.P., Chung, M.K., Wu, Y.C., Alexander, A.L.: Bessel fourier orientation reconstruction (bfor): An analytical diffusion propagator reconstruction for hybrid diffusion imaging and computation of q-space indices. NeuroImage 64, 650–670 (2013)
10. Hsu, Y.C., Hsu, C.H., Tseng, W.Y.I.: A large deformation diffeomorphic metric mapping solution for diffusion spectrum imaging datasets. NeuroImage 63(2), 818–834 (2012)
11. Raffelt, D., Tournier, J.D., Fripp, J., Crozier, S., Connelly, A., Salvado, O.: Symmetric diffeomorphic registration of fibre orientation distributions. NeuroImage 56(3), 1171–1180 (2011)
12. Wu, Y.C., Alexander, A.L.: Hybrid diffusion imaging. NeuroImage 36(3), 617–629 (2007)
13. Yap, P.T., Shen, D.: Spatial transformation of dwi data using non-negative sparse representation. IEEE Transactions on Medical Imaging 31(11), 2035–2049 (2012)
14. Yeo, B., Vercauteren, T., Fillard, P., Peyrat, J.M., Pennec, X., Golland, P., Ayache, N., Clatz, O.: Dt-refind: Diffusion tensor registration with exact finite-strain differential. IEEE Transactions on Medical Imaging 28(12), 1914–1928 (2009)
15. Zhang, P., Niethammer, M., Shen, D., Yap, P.-T.: Large deformation diffeomorphic registration of diffusion-weighted images. In: Ayache, N., Delingette, H., Golland, P., Mori, K. (eds.) MICCAI 2012, Part II. LNCS, vol. 7511, pp. 171–178. Springer, Heidelberg (2012)

Hyperbolic Harmonic Brain Surface Registration with Curvature-Based Landmark Matching

Rui Shi[1], Wei Zeng[2], Zhengyu Su[1], Yalin Wang[3], Hanna Damasio[4], Zhonglin Lu[5],
Shing-Tung Yau[6], and Xianfeng Gu[1]

[1] Department of Computer Science@Stony Brook University
[2] School of Computing & Information Sciences@Florida International University
[3] School of Computing, Informatics, and Decision Systems Engineering@Arizona State University
[4] Neuroscience@University of Southern California
[5] Department of Psychology@Ohio State University
[6] Mathematics Department@Harvard University
rshi@cs.stonybrook.edu, wzeng@cis.fiu.edu,
suzy.bryant@gmail.com, Yalin.Wang@asu.edu,
hdamasio@college.usc.edu, lu.535@osu.edu, yau@math.harvard.edu,
gu@cs.stonybrook.edu

Abstract. Brain Cortical surface registration is required for inter-subject studies of functional and anatomical data. Harmonic mapping has been applied for brain mapping, due to its existence, uniqueness, regularity and numerical stability. In order to improve the registration accuracy, sculcal landmarks are usually used as constraints for brain registration. Unfortunately, constrained harmonic mappings may not be diffeomorphic and produces invalid registration. This work conquer this problem by changing the Riemannian metric on the target cortical surface to a hyperbolic metric, so that the harmonic mapping is guaranteed to be a diffeomorphism while the landmark constraints are enforced as boundary matching condition. The computational algorithms are based on the Ricci flow method and hyperbolic heat diffusion. Experimental results demonstrate that, by changing the Riemannian metric, the registrations are always diffeomorphic, with higher qualities in terms of landmark alignment, curvature matching, area distortion and overlapping of region of interests.

1 Introduction

Morphometric and functional studies of human brain require that neuro-anatomical data from a population to be normalized to a standard template. The purpose of any registration methods is to find a map that assigns a correspondence from every point in a subject brain to a corresponding point in the template brain. Due to the anatomical fact, the mapping is required to be smooth and bijective, namely, diffeomorphic. Since cytoarchitectural and functional parcellation of the cortex is intimately related the folding of the cortex, it is important to ensure the alignment of the major anatomic features, such as sucal landmarks.

Harmonic mapping has been commonly applied for brain cortical surface registration. Physically, a harmonic mapping minimizes the "stretching energy", and produces

J.C. Gee et al. (Eds.): IPMI 2013, LNCS 7917, pp. 159–170, 2013.

smooth registration. The harmonic mappings between two hemsiphere cortical surfaces, which were modeled as genus zero closed surfaces, are guaranteed to be diffeomorphic, and angle-preserving [6]. Furthermore, all such kind of harmonic mappings differ by the Möbius transformation group. Numerically, finding a harmonic mapping is equivalent to solve an elliptic partial differential equation, which is stable in the computation and robust to the input noises.

Unfortunately, harmonic mappings with constraints may not be diffeomorphic any more, and produces invalid registrations with flips. In order to overcome this shortcoming, in this work we propose a novel brain registration method, which is based on hyperbolic harmonic mapping. Conventional registration methods map the template brain surface to the sphere or planar domain [6,7], then compute harmonic mappings from the source brain to the sphere or planar domain. When the target domains are with complicated topologies, or the landmarks, the harmonic mappings may not be diffeomrophic. In contrast, in our work, we slice the brain surfaces along the landmarks, and assign a unique hyperbolic metric on the template brain, such that all the boundaries become geodesics, harmonic mappings are established and guaranteed to be diffeomorphic.

In addition to the guaranteed diffeomorphism, we also addressed a curvature based landmark align method to obtain a geometric meaningful registration. i.e. it maps similarly shaped segments of sulcal curves to each other. We sample the landmark curves and record their curvature information, then use a Dynamic Time Warping algorithm (DTW) to align them together. This step achieves a geometric meaningful registration for landmarks compare to naive arc length interpolation.

In summary, the main contributions of the current work are as follows: First, introduce a novel brain registration method based on hyperbolic harmonic maps, the registration preserves all the merits of conventional harmonic brain registration methods, such as existence, uniqueness, regularity, numerical stability and so on. The new method overcomes the shortcomings of the conventional methods, such that the registration is guaranteed to be diffeomorphic. Second, develop a novel algorithm for computing harmonic mappings on hyperbolic metric using nonlinear heat diffusion method and Ricci flow. Third, develop a curvature based landmark matching method to achieve a geometric meaningful landmark registration. The paper is organized as follows: this section focuses on the motivation and introduction; next section briefly reviews the most related works; section 3 gives theoretic background for hyperbolic harmonic mapping; section 4 details the computational algorithms; section 5 reports our experimental results; section 6 summarizes the current work and points out future research directions.

2   Previous Works

In computer vision and medical imaging research, surface conformal parameterization with the Euclidean metric have been extensively studied [1,26,23]. Wang et al. [21] studied brain morphology with Teichmüller space coordinates where the hyperbolic conformal mapping was computed with the Yamabe flow method. Zeng [26] proposed a general surface registration method via the Klein model in the hyperbolic geometry where they used the inversive distance curvature flow method to compute the hyperbolic conformal mapping.

Various non-linear brain volume-based registration models [15,24] have been developed. However, early research [5,18] has demonstrated that surface-based approaches may offer advantages as a method to register brain images. To register brain surfaces, a common approach is to compute a range of intermediate mappings to some canonical parameter space [2,25]. A flow, computed in the parameter space of the two surfaces, then induces a correspondence field in 3D [7,17]. This flow can be constrained using anatomical landmark points or curves [8,10], by sub-regions of interest [13], by using currents to represent anatomical variation [3,20], or by metamorphoses [19]. There are also various ways to optimize surface registrations [12,16]. Overall, finding diffeomorphic mappings between brain surfaces is an important but difficult problem. In most cases, extra regulations, such as inverse consistency [9,16], have to be enforced to ensure a diffeomorphism. Since the proposed work offers a harmonic map based scheme for diffeomorphisms which guarantees a perfect landmark curve registration via enforced boundary matching, the novelty of the proposed work is that it facilitates diffeomorphic mapping between general surfaces with delineated landmark curves.

3   Theoretic Background

This section briefly introduces the theoretic foundations for the current work. We refer readers to [14] for more thorough exposition of harmonic maps, [26] for Ricci flow.

Hyperbolic Harmonic Map Suppose S is an oriented surface with a Riemannian metric g. One can choose a special local coordinates (x, y), the so-called *isothermal parameters*, such that $\mathbf{g} = \sigma(x, y)(dx^2 + dy^2) = \sigma(z)dzd\bar{z}$, where the complex parameter $z = x + iy, dz = dx + idy$. An atlas consisting of isothermal parameter charts is called an *conformal structure*. The *Gauss curvature* is given by $K(z) = -\frac{2}{\sigma(z)}\frac{\partial^2}{\partial z \partial \bar{z}} \log \sigma(z)$, where the complex differential operator $\frac{\partial}{\partial z} = \frac{1}{2}(\frac{\partial}{\partial x} + i\frac{\partial}{\partial y}), \frac{\partial}{\partial \bar{z}} = \frac{1}{2}(\frac{\partial}{\partial x} - i\frac{\partial}{\partial y})$. If $K(z)$ is -1 everywhere, then we say the Riemannian metric is *hyperbolic*. The Gauss-Bonnet theorem claims that the total Gauss curvature is a topological invariant $\int_S K(p)dp = 2\pi\chi(S)$, where $\chi(S)$ is the Euler-characteristic number. Given a mapping $f : (S_1, \mathbf{g}_1) \to (S_2, \mathbf{g}_2)$, z and w are local isothermal parameters on S_1 and S_2 respectively. $\mathbf{g}_1 = \sigma(z)dzd\bar{z}$ and $\mathbf{g}_2 = \rho(w)dwd\bar{w}$. Then the mapping has local representation $w = f(z)$ or denoted as $w(z)$.

Definition 1 (Harmonic Map). *The* harmonic energy *of the mapping is defined as* $E(f) = \int_S \rho(z)(|w_z|^2 + |w_{\bar{z}}|^2)dxdy$. *If f is a critical point of the harmonic energy, then f is called a* harmonic map.

The necessary condition for f to be a harmonic map is the Euler-Lagrange equation $w_{z\bar{z}} + \frac{\rho_w}{\rho} w_z w_{\bar{z}} \equiv 0$. The theory on the existence, uniqueness and regularity of harmonic maps have been thoroughly discussed in [14]. The following theorem lays down the theoretic foundation of our proposed method.

Theorem 1. [14] *Suppose $f : (S_1, \mathbf{g}_1) \to (S_2, \mathbf{g}_2)$ is a degree one harmonic map, furthermore the Riemann metric on S_2 induces negative Gauss curvature, then for each homotopy class, the harmonic map is unique and diffeomorphic.*

Ricci Flow Ricci flow deforms the Riemannian metric proportional to the curvature, such that the curvature evolves according to a heat diffusion process and eventually becomes constant everywhere.

Definition 2 (Ricci Flow). *Hamilton's surface Ricci flow is defined as* $\frac{dg_{ij}}{dt} = -2Kg_{ij}$.

Theorem 2 (Hamilton). *Let* $(S, \mathbf{g})$ *be compact. If* $\chi(S) < 0$, *then the solution to Ricci Flow equation exists for all* $t > 0$ *and converges to a metric of constant curvature.*

Given a surface with negative Euler-characteristic number, by running Ricci flow, a hyperbolic metric of the surface can be obtained. Then for each point $p \in S$, we can choose a neighborhood U_p and isometrically embed it onto the hyperbolic plane $\mathbb{H}^2$, $\phi_p : U_p \to \mathbb{H}^2$. (U_p, ϕ_p) is an isothermal coordinate chart, the collection of such charts $\{(U_p, \phi_p)|\forall p \in S\}$ forms a conformal structure of the surface.

Hyperbolic Space. In this work, we use the Poincaré's disk model for the hyperbolic plane $\mathbb{H}^2$, $\{z \in \mathbb{C}| |z| < 1\}$ with Riemannian metric $\rho(z)dzd\bar{z} = \frac{dzd\bar{z}}{(1-z\bar{z})^2}$. The geodesics are called *hyperbolic lines*. A hyperbolic line through two points p and q is a circular arc perpendicular to the unit circle. The hyperbolic rigid motions are Möbius transformations $\phi : z \to e^{i\theta}\frac{z-z_0}{1-\bar{z}_0 z}$. A *fixed point* p of a Möbius transformation ϕ satisfies $\phi(z) = z$. All the Möbius transformations in the current work have two fixed points z_1 and z_2, $z_1 = \lim_{n\to\infty} \phi^n(z), z_2 = \lim_{n\to\infty} \phi^{-n}(z)$, The *axis* of ϕ is the hyperbolic line through its fixed points. Given two non-intersecting hyperbolic lines γ_1 and γ_2, there exists a unique hyperbolic line τ orthogonal to both of them, and gives the shortest path connecting them. For each γ_k, there is a unique reflection ϕ_k whose axis is γ_k, then the axis of $\phi_2 \circ \phi_1^{-1}$ is τ. Another hyperbolic plane model is the Klein's disk model, where the hyperbolic lines coincide with Euclidean lines. The conversion from Poincare's disk model to Klein disk model is given by $z \to \frac{2z}{1+z\bar{z}}$.

Fundamental Group and Fuchs Group. Let S be a surface, all the homotopy classes of loops form the fundamental group (homotopy group), denoted as $\pi_1(S)$. A surface $\tilde{S}$ with a projection map $p : \tilde{S} \to S$ is called the *universal covering space* of S. The Deck transformation $\phi : \tilde{S} \to \tilde{S}$ satisfies $\phi \circ p = p$ and form a group $Deck(\tilde{S})$.

Let γ be a loop on the hyperbolic surface, then its homotopy class $[\gamma]$ corresponds to a unique Möbius transformation ϕ_γ. As the Gauss curvature of S is negative, in each homotopy class $[\gamma]$, there is a unique geodesic loop given by the axis of ϕ_γ.

Hyperbolic Pants Decomposition. As shown in Fig.2 (a) and (b), given a topological surface S, it can be decomposed to pairs of pants. Each pair of pants is a genus zero surface with three boundaries. If the surface is with a hyperbolic metric, then each homotopy class has a unique geodesic loop.

Suppose a pair of hyperbolic pants with three boundaries $\{\gamma_i, \gamma_j, \gamma_k\}$, which are geodesics. Let $\{\tau_i, \tau_j, \tau_k\}$ be the shortest geodesic paths connecting each pair of boundaries. The shortest paths divide the surface to two identical hyperbolic hexagons with right inner angles. When the hyperbolic hexagon with right inner angles is isometrically embedded on the Klein disk model, it is identical to a convex Euclidean hexagon.

4   Algorithms

We first explain our registration algorithm pipeline as illustrated in Alg. 1 and Fig. 1, then explain each step in details as following:

Algorithm 1. Brain Surface Registration Algorithm Pipeline

---

1. Slice the cortical surface along the landmark curves.
2. Compute the hyperbolic metric using Ricci flow.
3. Hyperbolic pants decomposition, isometrically embed them to Klein model.
4. Compute harmonic maps using Euclidean metrics between corresponding pairs of pants, with consistent curvature based boundary matching constraints computed by the DWT algorithm.
5. Use nonlinear heat diffusion to improve the mapping to a global harmonic map on Poincare disk model.

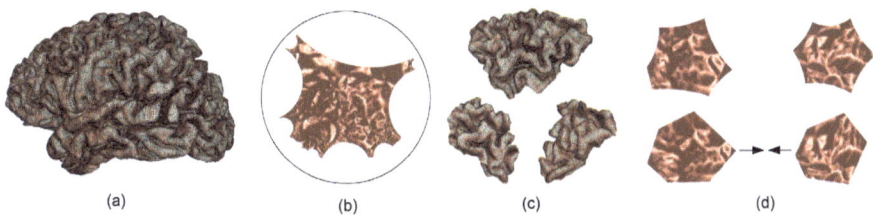

(a)   (b)   (c)   (d)

Fig. 1. Algorithm Pipeline (suppose we have 2 brain surface M and N as input): (a). One of the input brain models M, with landmarks being cut open as boundaries. (b). Hyperbolic embedding of the M on the Poincaré disk. (c). Decompose M into multiple pants by cuting the landmarks into boundaries, and each pant is further decomposed to 2 hyperbolic hexagons. (d). Hyperbolic hexagons on Poincaré disk become convex hexagons under the Klein model, then a one-to-one map between the correspondent parts of M and N can be obtained. Then we can apply our hyperbolic heat diffusion algorithm to get a global harmonic diffeomorphism.

1. Preprocessing The cortical surfaces are reconstructed from MRI images and represented as triangular meshes. The sucul landmarks are manually labeled on the edges of the meshes. Then we slice the meshes along the landmark curves, to form topological multiple connected annuli.

2. Discrete Hyperbolic Ricci Flow As the Euler characteristic numbers of the cortical surfaces are negative, they admit hyperbolic metrics. We treat each triangle as hyperbolic triangle and set the target Gauss curvature for each interior vertex to be zeros, and the target geodesic curvature for each boundary vertex to be zeros as well. We compute the hyperbolic metrics of the brain meshes using discrete hyperbolic Ricci flow method. For detailed discussion of the computational algorithm, one may refer to [26].

3. Hyperbolic Pants Decomposition In our work, the input surface is a genus zero surface with multiple boundary components $\partial S = \gamma_0 + \gamma_1 + \cdots \gamma_n$, moreover, the surface is with hyperbolic metric, and all boundaries are geodesics. The algorithm is as follows: choose arbitrary two boundary loops γ_i and γ_j, compute their product $[\gamma_i \cdot \gamma_j]$, if the product is homotopic to $[\gamma_k^{-1}]$, then choose other pair of boundary loops. Otherwise, suppose $[\gamma_i \cdot \gamma_k]$ is not homotopic to any boundary loop, compute its corresponding Möbius transformation, $\phi_{\gamma_i \gamma_j}$, and its fixed points $\phi_{\gamma_i \gamma_j}^{+\infty}(0)$ and $\phi_{\gamma_i \gamma_j}^{-\infty}(0)$. The hyperbolic line through the fixed points is the axis of the $\phi_{\gamma_i \gamma_j}$, which is the geodesic in $[\gamma_i \gamma_j]$. Slice the mesh along the geodesic, and repeat the process on each connected components, until all the connected components are pairs of pants. Figure 2 (c),(d) shows one example for the decomposition process. Alg. 2 gives the computational steps.

Algorithm 2. Hyperbolic Pants Decomposition

Input: Topological sphere M with B boundaries.
Output: Pants decomposition of M.
1. Put all boundaries γ_i of M into a queue Q.
2. If Q has < 3 boundaries, end; else goto Step 2.
3. Compute a geodesic loop γ' homotopic to $\gamma_i \cdot \gamma_j$
4. γ', γ_i and γ_j bound a pants patch, remove this pants patch from M. Remove γ_i and γ_j from Q. Put γ' into Q. Go to Step 1.

---

4. Initial Mapping Constructing with Dynamic Time Warping This step has several stages: first the pants are decomposed to hyperbolic hexagons and embed isometrically to the Poincaré disk; then convert the hexagons from Poincaré disk to Klein model; the final, also the most important step is to register the corresponding hexagons using Dynamic Time Warping (DTW) to achieve a geometric meaningful landmark matching and harmonic mapping for surface registration. The resultant piecewise harmonic mapping is the initial mapping. Fig 2 (e) shows the algorithm process.

For the first stage, we use the method described in the theory section to find the shortest path between two boundary loops. Assume a pair of hyperbolic pants M with three geodesic boundaries $\{\gamma_i, \gamma_j, \gamma_k\}$. On the universal covering space $\tilde{M}$, γ_i and γ_j are lifted to hyperbolic lines, $\tilde{\gamma}_i$ and $\tilde{\gamma}_j$ respectively. There are reflections $\tilde{\phi}_i$ and $\tilde{\phi}_j$, whose symmetry axis are $\tilde{\gamma}_i$ and $\tilde{\gamma}_j$. Then the axis of the Möbius transformation $\tilde{\gamma}_j \cdot \tilde{\gamma}_i^{-1}$ corresponds to the shortest geodesic path τ_k between γ_i and γ_j. In the second stage, each hyperbolic hexagon on the Poincaré disk is transformed to a convex hexagon in Klein's disk using $z \to \frac{2z}{1+z\bar{z}}$. The final step first register the correspondent landmarks, which are the boundaries of hyperbolic hexagon now, using DTW algorithm, then a planar harmonic map between two corresponding planar hexagons is established by $w_{z\bar{z}} \equiv 0$.

DTW algorithm [4] has being proved to be extremely efficient for detecting similar shapes with different phases. Given two curves $X = (x_1; x_2; ...x_N)$ and $Y = (y_1; y_2; ...y_M)$ represented by the sequences of vertices, DTW yields optimal matching solution in the $O(MN)$ time. Here the local cost function is defined as $c_{ij} = |MeanCurvature(x_i) - MeanCurvature(y_j)|$, and the global cost function is $C_{XY} = \sum_{l=1}^{L} c(x_{n_l}, y_{m_l})$. with L be the alignment path length. The result will align two curves according to their mean curvature distribution, which captures the geometry information. One thing worth mentioning is that to ensure the mapping between 2 curves is diffeomorphic, we locally turbulent the result if two vertices i and $i+1$ were mapped to one vertex j. For more detail about DTW algorithm we refer readers to [4].

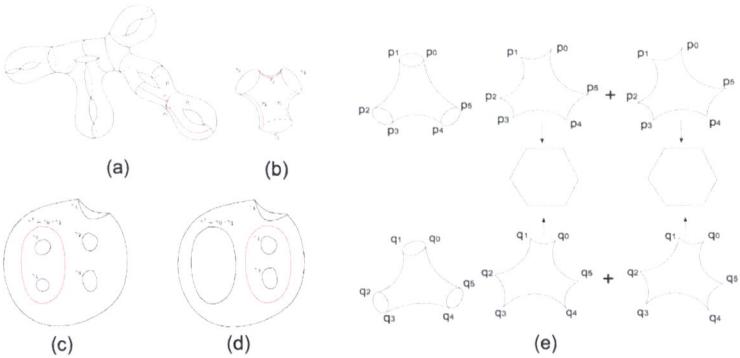

Fig. 2.

5. Non-linear Heat Diffusion Let $(S, \mathbf{g})$ be a triangle mesh with hyperbolic metric $\mathbf{g}$. Then for each vertex $v \in S$, the one ring neighboring faces form a neighborhood U_v, the union of U_v's cover the whole mesh, $S \subset \bigcup_{v \in S} U_v$. Isometrically embed U_v to the Poincaré's disk $\phi_v : U_v \rightarrow \mathbb{H}^2$, then $\{(U_v, \phi_v)\}$ form a conformal atlas. All the following computations are carried out on local charts of the conformal atlas. The computational result is independent of the choice of local parameters.

The initial mapping is diffused to form the hyperbolic harmonic map. Suppose $f : (S_1, \mathbf{g}_1) \rightarrow (S_2, \mathbf{g}_2)$ is the initial map, $\mathbf{g}_1$ and $\mathbf{g}_2$ are hyperbolic metrics. We compute the conformal atlases of S_1 and S_2, then choose local conformal parameters z and w for S_1 and S_2. The mapping f has local representation $f(z) = w$, or simply $w(z)$, then the non-linear diffusion is given by

$$\frac{dw(z,t)}{dt} = -\left[w_{z\bar{z}} + \frac{\rho_w(w)}{\rho(w)} w_z w_{\bar{z}}\right], \qquad (1)$$

where $\rho(w) = (1 - w\bar{w})^{-2}$. Suppose v_i is chosen to be a vertex on S_1, with local representation z_i, after diffusion, we get the local representation of its image $w(z_i)$.

Algorithm 3. Hyperbolic Heat Diffusion Algorithm

Input: Two surface models M, N with their hyperbolic metric C_M and C_N on Poincaré disk, the one-to-one correspondence (v_i, p_i) and a threshold ε. Here v_i is the vertex of mesh M, p_i is the 3D coordinate on mesh N.

Output: A new diffeomorphism (v_i, P_i).

1. For each vertex v_i of M that is not a landmark vertex, embed it's neighborhood onto Poincaré disk, in which v_i has coordinate z_i; do the same for p_i and note it's coordinate on Poincaré disk as w_i.

2. Compute $\frac{dw_i(z_i,t)}{dt}$ using equation (1).

3. Update $w_i = w_i + step\frac{dw_i(z_i,t)}{dt}$.

4. Compute new 3D coordinate P_i on N using the updated w_i, and repeat the above process until $\frac{w_i(z_i,t)}{dt}$ is less than ε.

Suppose $w(z_i)$ is inside a triangular face $t(v_i)$ of S_2, $t(v_i)$ has three vertices with local representation $[w_i, w_j, w_k]$, then we compute the *complex cross ratio*, which is given by $\eta(v_i) := [w(z_i), w_i, w_j, w_k] = \frac{(w(z_i)-w_i)(w_j-w_k)}{(w(z_i)-w_k)(w_j-w_i)}$. the image of v_i is then represented by the pair $[t(v_i), \eta(v_i)]$. Note that, all the local coordinates transitions in the conformal chart of S_1 and S_2 are Möbius transformations, and the cross ration η is invariant under Möbius transformation, therefore, the representation of the mapping $f : v_i \rightarrow [f(v_i), \eta(v_i)]$ is independent of the choice of local coordinates. Alg. 3 gives the process by steps. Notice that we may choose to apply the heat diffusion to the landmark vertices in order to get a soft landmark alignment.

5   Experimental Results

We implemented our algorithms using generic C++ on Windows, all the experiments are conducted on a laptop computer of Intel Core2 T6500 2.10GHz with 4GB memory.

Input Data. We perform the experiments on 24 brain cortical surfaces reconstructed from MRI images. Each cortical surface has about $150k$ vertices, $300k$ faces and used in some prior research [10]. On each cortical surfaces, a set of 26 landmark curves were manually drawn and validated by neuroanatomists. In our current work, we selected 10 landmark curves, including Central Sulcus, Superior Frontal Sulcus, Inferior Frontal Sulcus, Horizontal Branch of Sylvian Fissure, Cingulate Sulcus, Supraorbital Sulcus, Sup. Temporal with Upper Branch, Inferior Temporal Sulcus, Lateral Occipital Sulcus and the boundary of Unlabeled Subcortcial Region.

Registration Visualization. In Fig 3 we show the visualized registration result of 3 brain models, with one as target and 2 registered to it. We can see our algorithm shows a reasonable good result.

Landmark Curve Variation. For brain imaging research, it is important to achieve consistent local surface matching, e.g. landmark matching. We adapted a geometric quantitative measure of curve alignment error function to be the global cost function in section 4.4 $C_{XY} = \sum_{l=1}^{L} c(x_{n_l}, y_{m_l})$. For two curves $X = (x_1; x_2; ...x_N)$ and $Y = (y_1; y_2; ...y_M)$ represented by the sequences of vertices. Lower values indicate better geometric alignment for the curves. The DTW algorithm minimizes this error function while keeps the Hausdorff distance to be exactly zero. In Fig. 4 left we show the average histogram of curvature difference of aligned vertices on all 10 landmarks, from both the previous method [7] and our method.

Performance Evaluation and Comparison We compare our registration method with conventional cortical registration method based on harmonic mapping with Euclidean metric [22], where the template surface is conformally flattened to a planar disk, then the registration is obtained by a harmonic map from the source cortical surface to the disk with landmark constraints. Our experimental results show that by replacing Euclidean metric by hyperbolic metric on the source and target cortical surfaces, the quality of the registrations have been improved prominently.

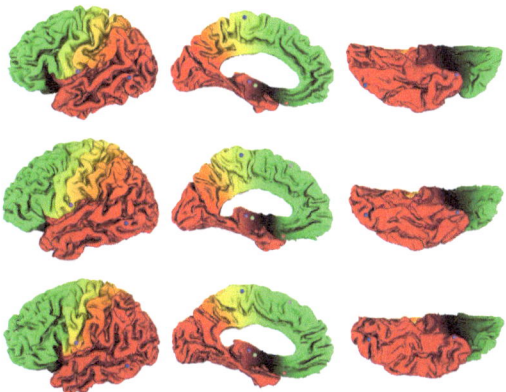

Fig. 3. First row: target brain surface from front, back and bottom view. Rest three rows: 2 brain models registered to the target model. The colored balls on the models show the detailed correspondence, as the balls with the same color are correspondent to each other.

5.1   Diffeomorphism

One of the most important advantages of our registration algorithm is that it guarantees the mapping between two surfaces to be diffeomorphic. We randomly choose one model as template and all others as source to compute the registration. For each registration, we compute the Jacobian determinant and measure the areas of flipped regions. The ratio between flipped area to the total area is collected to form the histogram shown in Fig.4 right. The horizontal axis shows the flipped area ratio, the vertical axis shows the number of registrations. The conventional method (blue bars) [22] produces a big flipped area ratio, even as much as 9%. In contrast, the flipped area ratios for all registrations obtained by the current method are exactly 0's.

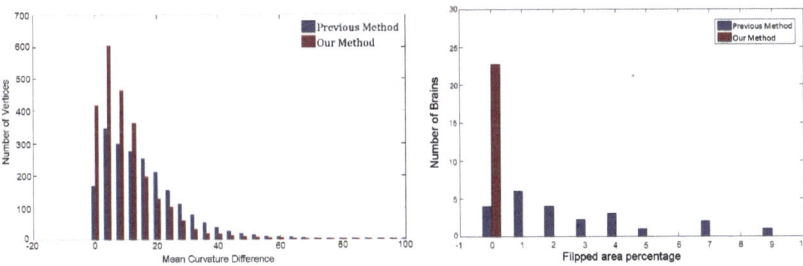

Fig. 4. Left: Landmark curvature difference of previous method and our method. Y axis is the vertex number on landmark that have the X amount of curvature difference. Right: Flipped area percentage of previous method and our method.

5.2   Curvature Maps

One method to evaluate registration accuracy is to compare the alignment of curvature maps between the registered models [11]. In this paper we calculated curvature maps using an approximation of mean curvature, which is the convexity measure. We quantified the effects of registration on curvature by computing the difference of curvature maps from the registered models. As Figure 5 left shows, we assign each vertex the curvature difference between its own curvature and the curvature of its correspondent point on the target surface, then build a color map according to the difference.

We use all 24 data sets for the experiment. First, one data set is randomly chosen as the template, then all others are registered to it. For each registration, we compute the curvature difference map. Then we compute the average of 23 curvature difference maps. The average curvature difference map is color encoded on the template, as shown in Fig.5 left. The histogram of the average curvature difference map is also computed, as shown in Fig.5 right. It is obvious that the current registration method produces less curvature errors than [22].

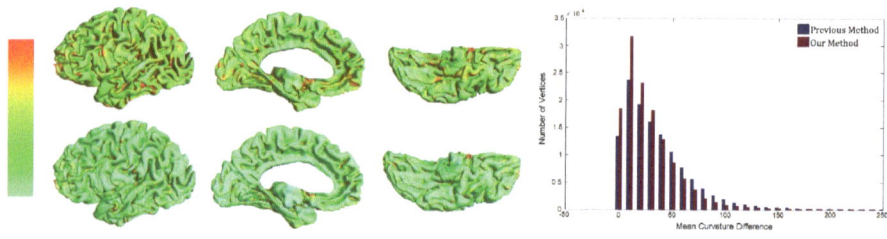

Fig. 5. Left: Curvature map difference of previous method (top row) and our method (bottom row). Color goes from green-yellow-red while the curvature difference increasing. Right: Average Curvature Map Difference of previous method and our method.

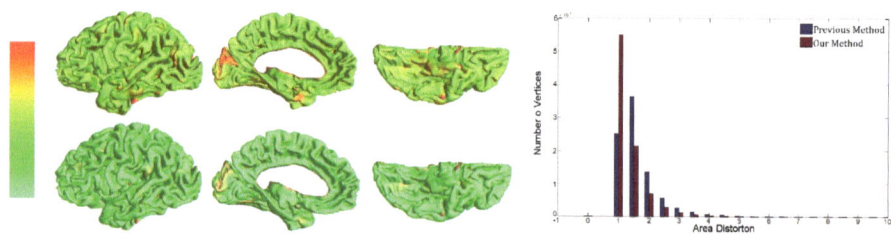

Fig. 6. Left: Average Area Distortion. Color goes from green-yellow-red while area distortion increasing. Right: Average Area Distortion of previous method and our method.

5.3   Local Area Distortion

Similarly, we measured the local area distortion induced by the registration. For each point p on the template surface, we compute its Jacobian determinant $J(p)$, and represent the local area distortion function at p as $\max\{J(p), J^{-1}(p)\}$. J can be approximated by the ratio between the areas of a face and its image. Note that, if the registration is not diffeomorphic, the local area distortion may go to ∞. Therefore, we add a threshold to truncate large distortions. Then we compute the average of all local area distortion functions induced by the 23 registrations on the template surface. The average local area distortion function on the template is color encoded as shown in Fig.6 left, the histogram is also computed in Fig.6 right. It can be easily seen that current registration method greatly reduces the local area distortions compare with [22].

6   Conclusion and Future Work

Conventional brain mapping method suffers from the fact that with the presence of landmark constraints, the registrations may not be bijective. This work introduces a novel registration algorithm, hyperbolic harmonic mapping with curvature based landmark matching, which completely solves this problem. The new method changes the metric on Cortical surfaces and greatly improves the registration quality. Experimental results demonstrate the current method always produces diffeomorphism, and outperforms some existing brain registration method in terms of curvature difference and local area distortion. In future, we will explore further the methodology of changing Riemannian metrics to improve efficiency and efficacy of different geometric algorithms.

References

1. Angenent, S., Haker, S., Tannenbaum, A., Kikinis, R.: Conformal geometry and brain flattening. In: Taylor, C., Colchester, A. (eds.) MICCAI 1999. LNCS, vol. 1679, pp. 271–278. Springer, Heidelberg (1999)
2. Bakircioglu, M., Joshi, S., Miller, M.I.: Landmark matching on brain surfaces via large deformation diffeomorphisms on the sphere. In: Proc. SPIE Medical Imaging, vol. 3661, pp. 710–715 (1999)
3. Durrleman, S., Pennec, X., Trouve, A., Thompson, P.M., Ayache, N.: Inferring brain variability from diffeomorphic deformations of currents: An integrative approach. Medical Image Analysis 12(5), 626–637 (2008)
4. Efrat, et al.: Curve matching, time warping, and light fields: New algorithms for computing similarity between curves. J. Math. Imaging Vis. (2007)
5. Fischl, B., Sereno, M.I., Dale, A.M.: Cortical surface-based analysis II: Inflation, flattening, and a surface-based coordinate system. NeuroImage 9(2), 195–207 (1999)
6. Gu, X., et al.: Genus zero surface conformal mapping and its application to brain surface mapping. IEEE Trans. Med. Imaging (2004)
7. Joshi, A.A., et al.: A parameterization-based numerical method for isotropic and anisotropic diffusion smoothing on non-flat surfaces. Trans. Img. Proc. (2009)
8. Joshi, S.C., Miller, M.I.: Landmark matching via large deformation diffeomorphisms. IEEE Trans. Image Process. 9(8), 1357–1370 (2000)

9. Leow, A., Yu, C.L., Lee, S.J., Huang, S.C., Nicolson, R., Hayashi, K.M., Protas, H., Toga, A.W., Thompson, P.M.: Brain structural mapping using a novel hybrid implicit/explicit framework based on the level-set method. NeuroImage 24(3), 910–927 (2005)
10. Pantazis, D., Joshi, A., Jiang, J., Shattuck, D.W., Bernstein, L.E., Damasio, H., Leahy, R.M.: Comparison of landmark-based and automatic methods for cortical surface registration. Neuroimage 49(3), 2479–2493 (2010)
11. Pantazis, D., Joshi, A.A., Jiang, J., Shattuck, D.W., Bernstein, L.E., Damasio, H., Leahy, R.M.: Comparison of landmark-based and automatic methods for cortical surface registration. NeuroImage 49(3), 2479–2493 (2009)
12. Pitiot, A., Delingette, H., Toga, A.W., Thompson, P.M.: Learning object correspondences with the observed transport shape measure. In: Taylor, C.J., Noble, J.A. (eds.) IPMI 2003. LNCS, vol. 2732, pp. 25–37. Springer, Heidelberg (2003)
13. Qiu, A., Miller, M.I.: Multi-structure network shape analysis via normal surface momentum maps. Neuroimage 42(4), 1430–1438 (2008)
14. Schoen, R.M., Yau, S.-T.: Lectures on harmonic maps. International Press, Mathematics (1997)
15. Shen, D., Davatzikos, C.: HAMMER: hierarchical attribute matching mechanism for elastic registration. IEEE Trans. Med. Imaging 21(11), 1421–1439 (2002)
16. Shi, Y., Morra, J.H., Thompson, P.M., Toga, A.W.: Inverse-consistent surface mapping with Laplace-Beltrami eigen-features. In: Prince, J.L., Pham, D.L., Myers, K.J. (eds.) IPMI 2009. LNCS, vol. 5636, pp. 467–478. Springer, Heidelberg (2009)
17. Thompson, P.M., Giedd, J.N., Woods, R.P., MacDonald, D., Evans, A.C., Toga, A.W.: Growth patterns in the developing human brain detected using continuum-mechanical tensor mapping. Nature 404(6774), 190–193 (2000)
18. Thompson, P.M., Toga, A.W.: A surface-based technique for warping 3-dimensional images of the brain. IEEE Trans. Med. Imag. 15(4), 1–16 (1996)
19. Trouvé, A., Younes, L.: Metamorphoses through Lie group action. Found. Comp. Math., 173–198 (2005)
20. Vaillant, M., Qiu, A., Glaunes, J., Miller, M.I.: Diffeomorphic metric surface mapping in subregion of the superior temporal gyrus. Neuroimage 34(3), 1149–1159 (2007)
21. Wang, Y., Dai, W., Gu, X., Chan, T.F., Toga, A.W., Thompson, P.M.: Studying brain morphology using Teichmüller space theory. In: IEEE 12th International Conference on Computer Vision, ICCV 2009, pp. 2365–2372 (September 2009)
22. Wang, Y., Gupta, M., Zhang, S., Wang, S., Gu, X., Samaras, D., Huang, P.: High resolution tracking of non-rigid motion of densely sampled 3d data using harmonic maps. Int. J. Comput. Vision 76(3), 283–300 (2008)
23. Wang, Y., Shi, J., Yin, X., Gu, X., Chan, T.F., Yau, S.T., Toga, A.W., Thompson, P.M.: Brain surface conformal parameterization with the Ricci flow. IEEE Trans. Med. Imaging 31(2), 251–264 (2012)
24. Yanovsky, I., Leow, A.D., Lee, S., Osher, S.J., Thompson, P.M.: Comparing registration methods for mapping brain change using tensor-based morphometry. Med. Image Anal. 13(5), 679–700 (2009)
25. Yeo, B.T., Sabuncu, M.R., Vercauteren, T., Ayache, N., Fischl, B., Golland, P.: Spherical demons: fast diffeomorphic landmark-free surface registration. IEEE Trans. Med. Imaging 29(3), 650–668 (2010)
26. Zeng, W., Samaras, D., Gu, X.: Ricci flow for 3d shape analysis. IEEE TPAMI 32, 662–677 (2010)

Geometric Tree Kernels: Classification of COPD from Airway Tree Geometry

Aasa Feragen[1,2], Jens Petersen[1], Dominik Grimm[2], Asger Dirksen[4],
Jesper Holst Pedersen[5], Karsten Borgwardt[2,3], and Marleen de Bruijne[1,6]

[1] Department of Computer Science, University of Copenhagen, Denmark
[2] Max Planck Institute for Intelligent Systems and Max Planck Institute for
Developmental Biology, Tübingen, Germany
[3] Zentrum für Bioinformatik, Eberhard Karls Universität Tübingen, Germany
[4] Lungemedicinsk Afdeling, Gentofte Hospital, Denmark
[5] Department of Cardiothoracic Surgery, Rigshospitalet, Denmark
[6] Erasmus MC - University Medical Center Rotterdam, The Netherlands
{aasa,phup,marleen}@diku.dk,
{aasa.feragen,dominik.grimm,karsten.borgwardt}@tuebingen.mpg.de
http://www.image.diku.dk/aasa

Abstract. *Methodological contributions:* This paper introduces a family
of kernels for analyzing (anatomical) trees endowed with vector valued
measurements made along the tree. While state-of-the-art graph and
tree kernels use combinatorial tree/graph structure with discrete node
and edge labels, the kernels presented in this paper can include geometric information such as branch shape, branch radius or other vector
valued properties. In addition to being flexible in their ability to model
different types of attributes, the presented kernels are computationally
efficient and some of them can easily be computed for large datasets
($N \sim 10.000$) of trees with $30 - 600$ branches. Combining the kernels
with standard machine learning tools enables us to analyze the relation
between disease and anatomical tree structure and geometry. *Experimental results:* The kernels are used to compare airway trees segmented from
low-dose CT, endowed with branch shape descriptors and airway wall
area percentage measurements made along the tree. Using kernelized hypothesis testing we show that the geometric airway trees are significantly
differently distributed in patients with Chronic Obstructive Pulmonary
Disease (COPD) than in healthy individuals. The geometric tree kernels
also give a significant increase in the classification accuracy of COPD
from geometric tree structure endowed with airway wall thickness measurements in comparison with state-of-the-art methods, giving further
insight into the relationship between airway wall thickness and COPD.
Software: Software for computing kernels and statistical tests is available
at http://image.diku.dk/aasa/software.php.

1 Introduction

Anatomical trees like blood vessels, dendrites or airways, carry information about
the organs they are part of, and if we can meaningfully compare anatomical

J.C. Gee et al. (Eds.): IPMI 2013, LNCS 7917, pp. 171–183, 2013.
© Springer-Verlag Berlin Heidelberg 2013

trees and measurements made along them, then we can learn more about aspects of disease related to the anatomical trees [11, 23]. For example, airway wall thickness is known to be a biomarker for Chronic Obstructive Pulmonary Disease (COPD), and in order to compare airway wall thickness measurements in different patients, a typical approach is to compare average airway wall area percentage measurements for given airway tree generations of particular subtrees [10, 11]. These approaches assume that measurements made in different locations of the lung are comparable on a common scale, which is not always the case [10, 11]. If we can compare tree structures attributed with measurements made along them in a way which respects the structure and geometry of the tree, then we can be more robustly compare measurements whose values are location sensitive. In this paper we present a family of kernels for comparing anatomical trees endowed with vector attributes, and use these to get a more detailed understanding of how COPD correlates with airway structure and geometry.

Related Work. Several approaches to statistics on attributed (geometric) trees have recently appeared, and some of them were applied to airway trees [7, 8, 16, 17]. These methods only consider branch length or shape and do not allow for using additional measurements along the airway tree, such as branch radius or airway wall area percentage. Moreover, these methods are computationally expensive [6], or need a set of leaf labels [8, 17], making them less applicable for general trees. Sørensen [20] treats the airway tree as a set of attributed branches which are matched and then compared using a dissimilarity embedding combined with a k-NN classifier. The matching introduces an additional computational cost and makes the approach vulnerable to incorrect matches.

Kernels are a family of similarity measures equivalent to inner products between data points implicitly embedded in a Hilbert space. Kernels are typically designed to be computationally fast while discriminative for a given problem, and often give nonlinear similarity measures in the original data space. Using the Hilbert space, many Euclidean data analysis methods are extended to kernels, such as classification [4] or hypothesis testing [9]. Kernels are popular because they give computational speed, modeling flexibility and access to linear data analysis tools for data with nonlinear behavior.

There are kernels available for structured data such as strings [5,13], trees [22], graphs [3, 19, 21] and point clouds [1]. The current state-of-the-art graph kernel in terms of scalability is the Weisfeiler-Lehman (WL) [19] kernel, which compares graphs by counting isomorphic labeled subtrees of a particular type and "radius" h. The WL scales linearly in h and the number of edges, but the scalability depends on algorithmic constructions for finite node label sets. Thus, the WL kernel, like most fast kernels developed in natural language processing and bioinformatics [5,13,22], does not generalize to vector-valued branch attributes.

Walk- and path based kernels [1,3,21], which reduce to comparing sub-walks or -paths of the graphs, are state-of-the-art among kernels which include continuous-valued graph attributes. Random walk-type kernels [1,21] suffer from several problems including tottering [15] and high computational cost. The shortest path kernel [3] by default only considers path length, and some of the kernels developed in this paper can be viewed as extensions of the shortest path kernel.

Contributions. We develop a family of kernels which are computationally fast enough to run on large datasets, and can incorporate any vectorial attributes on nodes[1], e.g., shape or airway wall measurements. Using the kernels in classification and hypothesis testing experiments, we show that classification of COPD can be substantially improved by taking geometry into account. This illustrates, in particular, that airway wall area percentage measurements made at different locations in the airway tree are not comparable on a common scale.

We compare the developed kernels to state-of-the-art methods. We see, in particular, that COPD can also be detected from combinatorial airway tree structure using state-of-the-art kernels on tree structure alone, but we show that these contain no more information than a branch count kernel, as opposed to the geometric tree kernels.

2   Geometric Trees and Geometric Tree Kernels

Anatomical trees like airways are *geometric trees*: they consist of both combinatorial tree structure and branch geometry (e.g., branch length or shape), where continuous changes in the branch geometry can lead to continuous transitions in the combinatorial tree structure. In addition to its geometric embedding, a geometric tree can be adorned with additional features measured along the tree, e.g., airway branch radius, airway wall thickness, airway wall thickness/branch radius, airway wall area percentage in an airway cross section, etc.

Definition 1. A *geometric tree* is a pair (T, x) where $T = (V, E, r)$ is a combinatorial tree with nodes V, root r and edges $E \subset V \times V$, and $x \colon V \to \mathbb{R}^n$ is an assignment of (geometric) attributes from a vector space $\mathbb{R}^n$ to the nodes of T, e.g. $3D$ position or landmark points. An *attributed geometric tree* is a triple (T, x, a) where (T, x) is a geometric tree and $a \colon x(T) \to \mathbb{R}^d$ is a map assigning a vector valued attribute $a(p) \in \mathbb{R}^d$ to each point $p \in x(T)$.

A common strategy for defining kernels on structured data such as trees, graphs or strings is based on combining kernels on sub-structures such as strings, walks, paths, subtrees or subgraphs [1, 3, 5, 13, 19, 21, 22]. These are all instances of the so-called *R-convolution kernels* by Haussler [12]. We shall use *paths* in trees as building blocks for defining kernels on trees.

Let (T, x) be a geometric tree. Given vertices $v_i, v_j \in V$ there is a unique path π_{ij} from v_i to v_j in the tree, defined by the sequence of visited nodes:

$$\pi_{ij} = \left[v_i, p^{(1)}(v_i), p^{(2)}(v_i), \ldots, w, \ldots, p^{(2)}(v_j), p^{(1)}(v_j), v_j \right],$$

where $p^{(0)}(v) = v$, $p^{(1)}(v) = p(v)$ is the parent node of v, more generally $p^{(k)}(v) = p(p^{(k-1)}(v))$, and w is the highest level common ancestor of v_i and v_j in T.

---

[1] Our formulation allows both node and edge attributes, as edge attributes are equivalent to node attributes on rooted trees: assign each edge attribute to its child node.

We call π_{ij} the *node-path* from v_i to v_j in T and for each j let the *node-rootpath* π_{jr} be the node-path from v_j to the root.

If the geometric node attributes $x(v): I \to \mathbb{R}^n$ denote embeddings of the edge $(v, p(v))$ into the ambient space $\mathbb{R}^n$, a continuous path $x_{ij}: [0, 1] \to \mathbb{R}^n$ can be defined, connecting the embedded nodes $x(v_i), x(v_j) \in \mathbb{R}^n$ along the embedded tree $x(V) \subset \mathbb{R}^n$. We call x_{ij} the *embedded path* from x_i to x_j in T.

Throughout the rest of this section, we shall define different kernels for pairs of trees T_1 and T_2, where $T_i = (V_i, E_i, r_i, x_i, a_i)$ are attributed geometric trees (including non-attributed geometric trees as a special case with $a_i \equiv 1$), $i = 1, 2$. All kernels defined in this section are positive semidefinite, as they are sums of linear and Gaussian kernels composed with known feature maps. This is a necessary condition for a kernel to be equivalent to an inner product in a Hilbert space [2], needed for the analysis methods used in Sec. 3.

2.1   Path-Based Tree Kernels

All-Pairs Path Kernels. The all-pairs path kernel is a basic path-based tree kernel. Given two geometric trees, it is defined as

$$K_a(T_1, T_2) = \sum_{\substack{(v_i, v_j) \,\in\, V_1 \times V_1, \\ (v_k, v_l) \,\in\, V_2 \times V_2}} k_p(p_{ij}, p_{kl}), \tag{2}$$

where k_p is a kernel defined on paths, and p_{ij}, p_{kl} are paths connecting v_i to v_j and v_k to v_l in T_1 and T_2, respectively – for instance, π_{ij} and π_{kl}, or x_{ij} and x_{kl}, as defined above. Note that if the path kernel k_p is a path length kernel, then the all-pairs path kernel is a special case of the shortest path kernel on graphs [3].

The kernel k_p should take large values on paths that are geometrically similar, and small values on paths which are not, giving a measure of the alignment of the two tree-paths p_{ij} and p_{kl}, making K_a an overall assessment of the similarity between the two geometric trees T_1 and T_2. The all-pairs path kernel is nice in the sense that it takes every possible choice of paths in the trees into account. It is, however, expensive: The computational cost is $\mathcal{O}(|V|^4) \cdot \mathcal{O}(k_p)$, where $|V| = \max\{|V_1|, |V_2|\}$ and $\mathcal{O}(k_p)$ is the cost of the path kernel k_p.

Rootpath Kernels. The computational complexity can be reduced by only considering rootpaths, giving a rootpath kernel K_r defined as:

$$K_r(T_1, T_2) = \sum_{v_i \in V_1, v_j \in V_2} k_p(p_{ir}, p_{jr}) \tag{3}$$

where k_p is a path kernel as before, and p_{ir} is the path from v_i to the root r. This reduces the computational complexity to $\mathcal{O}(|V|^2)\mathcal{O}(k_p)$.

2.2   Path Kernels

The modeling capabilities and computational complexity of the kernels K_a and K_r depend on the choices of path kernel k_p and path representation p.

Landmark Point Representation of Embedded Paths. From a shape modeling point of view, equidistantly sampled landmark points give a reasonable representation of a path through the tree. Representing paths by N equidistantly sampled landmark points $x_{ij} \in (\mathbb{R}^n)^N$, the path kernel $k_p = k_x$ is either a linear or Gaussian kernel:

$$k_x(x_{ij}, x'_{kl}) = \begin{cases} \langle x_{ij}, x'_{kl} \rangle & \text{(linear, i.e., dot product)} \\ e^{-\lambda \|x_{ij}-x'_{kl}\|_2^2} & \text{(Gaussian)} \end{cases} \tag{4}$$

for a scaling parameter λ which regulates the width of the Gaussian.

Node-Path Kernels. The landmark point kernels are expensive to compute (see Table 1). In particular, two embedded tree-paths may have large overlapping segments without having a single overlapping equidistantly sampled landmark point, as the distance between landmark points depends on the length of the entire path. Thus, most landmark points will only appear in one path, giving little opportunity for recursive algorithms or dynamic programming that take advantage of repetitive structure. To enable such approaches, we use node-paths.

Assume that $\pi^1 = [\pi^1(1), \pi^1(2), \dots, \pi^1(m)]$ and $\pi^2 = [\pi^2(1), \pi^2(2), \dots, \pi^2(l)]$ are node-paths in T_1, T_2, respectively, as defined above, that is, sequences of consecutive nodes $\pi^i(j) \in V_i$ in T_i. We define

$$k_\pi(\pi^1, \pi^2) = \begin{cases} \sum_{i=1}^{L} k_n \left(x_1(\pi^1(i)), x_2(\pi^2(i)) \right) & \text{if } |\pi^1| = |\pi^2| = L \\ 0 & \text{otherwise} \end{cases} \tag{5}$$

where k_n is a node kernel. In this paper $k_n(v_1, v_2)$ is either a linear kernel without/with additional attributes a_i:

$$\langle x_1(v_1), x_2(v_2) \rangle, \quad \langle x_1(v_1), x_2(v_2) \rangle \langle a_1(v_1), a_2(v_2) \rangle$$

or a Gaussian kernel with/without attributes a_i

$$e^{-\lambda_1 \|x_1(v_1)-x_2(v_2)\|^2}, \quad e^{-\lambda_1 \|x_1(v_1)-x_2(v_2)\|^2} \cdot e^{-\lambda_2 \|a_1(v_1)-a_2(v_2)\|^2},$$

where the Gaussian weight parameters are heuristically set to the inverse dimension of the relevant feature space, i.e., $\lambda_1 = \frac{1}{n}$ and $\lambda_2 = \frac{1}{d}$.

Now the node-rootpath tree kernel K_r can be rewritten as:

$$K_r(T_1, T_2) = \sum_{l=1}^{h} \sum_{v_1 \in V_1^l} \sum_{v_2 \in V_2^l} \sum_{i=1}^{l} k_n \left(x_1(\pi_1(i)), x_2(\pi_2(i)) \right), \tag{6}$$

where $h = \min\{\text{height}(T_i), i = 1, 2\}$. This can be reformulated as a weighted sum of node kernels, giving substantially improved computational complexity:

Proposition 7. *For each $l \le h$, let V_i^l be the set of vertices at level l in T_i. Then*

$$K_r(T_1, T_2) = \sum_{i=1}^{h} \sum_{v_1 \in V_1^l} \sum_{v_2 \in V_2^l} \langle \delta_{v_1}, \delta_{v_2} \rangle k_n(v_1, v_2), \tag{8}$$

where δ_{v_i} is an h-dimensional vector whose j^{th} coefficient counts the number of descendants of v_i at level j in T_i, respectively. The complexity of computing K_r is $\mathcal{O}(h \max_l |V^l|^2 (n+h))$.

When k_n is a linear kernel $\langle x_1(v_1), x_2(v_2) \rangle$ or $\langle x_1(v_1), x_2(v_2) \rangle \langle a_1(v_1), a_2(v_2) \rangle$, the kernel K_r can be further decomposed as

$$K_r(T_1, T_2) = \sum_{l=1}^{h} \langle \gamma(T_1, l), \gamma(T_2, l) \rangle,$$
$$\gamma(T_i, l) = \begin{cases} \sum_{v \in V_i^l} x_i(v) \otimes \delta(v), & \text{no } a_i \\ \sum_{v \in V_i^l} a_i(v) \otimes x_i(v) \otimes \delta(v), & \text{with } a_i \end{cases} \qquad (9)$$

at total complexity $\mathcal{O}(|V|hn) / \mathcal{O}(|V|hnd)$ (without/with attributes a_i). Here, $\otimes$ denotes the Kronecker product.

Proof. Eq. (8) follows from the fact that the terms $k_n(v_1, v_2)$ in kernel (6) will be counted once for every pair (w_1, w_2) of descendants of v_1 and v_2, respectively, which are at the same level. The descendant vectors $\delta(v_i)$ for all $v_i \in V_i$ can be precomputed using dynamical programming at computational cost $\mathcal{O}(|V|h)$, since $\delta(v) = [1, \oplus_{p(w)=v} \delta(w)]$, where $\oplus$ is defined as left aligned addition of vectors[2]. The cost of computing K_r is thus

$$\mathcal{O}(|V|h + h \max_l |V^l|^2 (h+n)) = \mathcal{O}(h \max_l |V^l|^2 (n+h)),$$

where $\mathcal{O}(n)$ is the cost of computing each node kernel $k_n(v_1, v_2)$.

To prove (8) without attributes a_i, let $x_1(v_1), x_2(v_2), \delta(v_1)$ and $\delta(v_2)$ be column vectors and use the Kronecker trick $(\langle a_i, a_j \rangle \langle b_i, b_j \rangle = \langle b_i \otimes a_i, b_j \otimes a_j \rangle)$:

$$K(T_1, T_2) = \sum_{l=1}^{h} \sum_{v_1 \in V_1^l} \sum_{v_2 \in V_2^l} \langle \delta(v_2), \delta(v_1) \rangle \langle x_1(v_1), x_2(v_2) \rangle$$
$$= \sum_{l=1}^{h} \langle \sum_{v_2 \in V_2^l} (x_2(v_2) \otimes \delta(v_2)), \sum_{v_1 \in V_1^l} x_1(v_1) \otimes \delta(v_1) \rangle$$
$$= \sum_{l=1}^{h} \langle \gamma(T_1, l), \gamma(T_2, l) \rangle.$$

The total complexity is thus $\mathcal{O}(\max_{l,i} |V_i^l| hn) + \mathcal{O}(|V|h) = \mathcal{O}(|V|hn)$. Similar analysis proves the attributed case. □

2.3   Pointcloud Kernels

Anatomical measurements can also be weighed by location using $3D$ position alone in a pointcloud kernel. The pointcloud kernel does not use the tree structure but treats each edges in the tree as a point and compares all points:

$$K_{PC}(T_1, T_2) = \sum_{e_1 \in E_1} \sum_{e_2 \in E_2} k_e(e_1, e_2) \qquad (10)$$

where k_e is a kernel on attributed edges. We use a Gaussian edge kernel (GPC):

$$k_e(e_1, e_2) = \underbrace{e^{-\lambda_1 \|x(e_1) - x(e_2)\|^2}}_{c_1} \underbrace{e^{-\lambda_2 \|a(e_1) - a(e_2)\|^2}}_{c_2}. \qquad (11)$$

---

[2] e.g., $[a, b, c] \oplus [d, e] = [a+d, b+e, c]$.

The kernel is designed to weight the contribution to the total kernel K_{PC} of the airway wall area percentage kernel value c_1 between edges e_1 and e_2 by the geometric alignment of the same edges, defined by the geometric kernel value c_2.

2.4 Baseline Kernels

The kernels presented in this paper are compared to a set of baseline kernels. Standard airway wall area percentage measurements are often compared by using an average measure over parts of the tree or a vector of average measures in chosen generations. We use two baseline airway wall area percentage kernels:

$$K_{AAW\%}(T_1, T_2) = e^{-\|\hat{a}_1 - \hat{a}_2\|^2}, \tag{12}$$

$$K_{AgAW\%}(T_1, T_2) = e^{-\|(\hat{a}_1)_{(3-6)} - (\hat{a}_2)_{(3-6)}\|^2} \tag{13}$$

where $\hat{a}_i$ is the average airway wall area percentage averaged over all centerline points in the tree, and $(\hat{a}_i)_{(3-6)}$ is a 4-dimensional vector of average airway wall area percentages averaged over all centerline points in generations $3 - 6$ in tree T_i. For these kernels (AAW%, AgAW%), linear versions were also computed (i.e. $e^{-\|w_1 - w_2\|^2}$ replaced with $\langle w_1, w_2 \rangle$), but the corresponding classification results are not reported as they were consistently weaker than the Gaussian kernels.

Airway segmentation is likely more difficult in diseased as opposed to healthy subjects, as also observed by [20]. In order to check whether the number of detected branches may be a bias in the studied kernels, we compare our kernels to a linear and a Gaussian branchcount kernel (LBC/GBC) defined by

$$K_{LBC}(T_1, T_2) = \sharp(V_1) \cdot \sharp(V_2), \quad K_{GBC}(T_1, T_2) = e^{-\|\sharp(V_1) - \sharp(V_2)\|^2}. \tag{14}$$

The linear kernel LBC is the most natural, since the Hilbert space associated to a linear kernel on $w \in \mathbb{R}^n$ is just $\mathbb{R}^n$. However, a linear kernel on 1-dimensional input cannot be normalized, as (15) produces a kernel matrix with entries $\equiv 1$, and the GBC kernel is used for comparison in Table 4 to show that the geometric tree kernels are, indeed, measuring something other than branch count.

Table 1. Computational complexities for the considered kernels. Trees are assumed to be embedded in $\mathbb{R}^n$ and admit additional vector valued measurements in $\mathbb{R}^d$.

	Embedded paths (m landmark points)	Node-path
All-paths	$\mathcal{O}(\|V\|^4 mn)$	$\mathcal{O}(\|V\|^2 h \max_l \|V^l\|^2 (n+h)$
Root-paths	$\mathcal{O}(\|V\|^2 mn)$	$\mathcal{O}(h \max_l \|V^l\|^2)(n+h)$
Attributed all-paths	N/A	$\mathcal{O}(h\|V\|^2 \max_l \|V^l\|^2)(n+d+h)$
Attributed root-paths	N/A	$\mathcal{O}(h \max_l \|V^l\|^2)(n+d+h)$
Attributed linear root-paths	N/A	$\mathcal{O}(\|V\|hnd)$
Pointcloud kernel	N/A	$\mathcal{O}(\|V\|^2 nd)$

Table 2. Runtime for selected kernels on a larger set of 9710 airway trees

Kernel	Linear root-node-path	Gaussian branchcount	average AW %	average generation AW %	Shortest path	Weisfeiler Lehman ($h = 10$)
Comp. time	46 m 43 s	23 m 3 s	0.87 s	1.61 s	42 m 26 s	59 m 23 s

Several state-of-the-art graph kernels were also used. The random walk kernel [21] did not finish computing within reasonable time. The shortest path kernel [3] was computed with edge number as path length, and the Weisfeiler-Lehman kernel [19] was computed with node degree as node label. Results are reported in Tables 2, 3 and 4.

3   Experiments

Analysis was performed on airway trees segmented from CT-scans of 1966 subjects from a national lung cancer screening trial. Triangulated mesh representations of the interior and exterior wall surface were found using an optimal surface based approach [18], and centerlines were extracted from the interior surface using front propagation [14]. As the resulting centerlines are disconnected at bifurcation points, the end points were connected using a shortest path search within an inverted distance map of the interior surface. The airway centerline trees were normalized using person height as an isotropic scaling parameter. Airway wall thickness and airway radius were estimated from the shortest distance from each surface mesh vertex to the centerline. The measurements were grouped and averaged along the centerline by each nearest landmark point.

Out of the 1966 participants, 980 were diagnosed with COPD level 1-3 based on spirometry, and 986 were symptom free. The minimal/maximal/average number of branches in an airway tree was 29/651/221.5, respectively.

3.1   Kernel Computation and Computational Time

The kernels listed in table 4 were implemented in Matlab [3] and computed on a 2.40GHz Intel Core i7-2760QM CPU with 32 GB RAM. Each kernel matrix was normalized to account for difference in tree size:

$$K_{\text{norm}}(T_1, T_2) = \frac{K(T_1, T_2)}{\sqrt{K(T_1, T_1) K(T_2, T_2)}}. \tag{15}$$

An exception was made for linear kernels between scalars (LBC and AAW%), since normalization such kernels results gives matrix coefficients $\equiv 1$.

Computation times for the different kernels used in the classification experiments in Section 3.3 on 1966 airway trees are shown in Table 4. To demonstrate

---

[3] Software: http://image.diku.dk/aasa/software.php; published software was used for SP, WL [19].

scalability, some of the kernels were ran on 9710 airways from a longitudinal study of the 1966 participants, see Table 2. The slower kernels were not included.

For classification and hypothesis testing, a set of 1966 airway trees from 1966 distinct subjects was used (980 diagnosed with COPD at scan time).

3.2   Hypothesis Testing: Two-Sample Test for Means

Let $\mathcal{X}$ denote a set of data objects. Given any positive semidefinite kernel $k\colon \mathcal{X} \times \mathcal{X}$ there exists an implicitly defined feature map $\phi\colon \mathcal{X} \to \mathcal{H}$ into a reproducing kernel Hilbert space $(\mathcal{H}, \langle\cdot\rangle)$ such that $k(x_1, x_2) = \langle\phi(x_1), \phi(x_2)\rangle$ for all $x_1, x_2 \in \mathcal{X}$ [2]. Hypothesis tests can be defined in $\mathcal{H}$ to check whether two samples $A, B \subset \mathcal{X}$ are implicitly embedded by ϕ into distributions on $\mathcal{H}$ that have, e.g., the same means $\mu_A = \mu_B$ [9]. Denote by $\hat{\mu}_A$ and $\hat{\mu}_B$ the sample means of $\phi(A)$ and $\phi(B)$ in $\mathcal{H}$, respectively; we use as a test statistic the distance

$$T(A, B) = \|\hat{\mu}_A - \hat{\mu}_B\|_{\mathcal{H}}$$

between the sample means and check the null hypothesis using a permutation test. Writing $|A| = a$ and $|B| = b$, we divide $\mathcal{X} = A \cup B$ into N random partitions A_i, B_i of size $|A_i| = a$ and $|B_i| = b$, $i = 1 \ldots N$, compute the test statistic T_i for each partition, and compare it with the statistic T_0 obtained for the original partition $\mathcal{X} = A \cup B$. An approximate p-value giving the probability of $\phi(A)$ and $\phi(B)$ coming from distributions with identical means $\mu_A = \mu_B$ is now given by $p = \frac{|\{T_i | T_i \geq T_0, i=1\ldots N\}|+1}{N+1}$. The T statistic can be computed from a kernel matrix since distances in $\mathcal{H}$ can be derived directly from the values of $k(\mathcal{X}, \mathcal{X})$ using the binomial formula:

$$\begin{aligned}
\|\hat{\mu}_A - \hat{\mu}_B\|^2 &= \langle \tfrac{1}{a}\sum_{i=1}^{a}\phi(a_i) - \tfrac{1}{b}\sum_{j=1}^{b}\phi(b_j), \tfrac{1}{a}\sum_{i=1}^{a}\phi(a_i) - \tfrac{1}{b}\sum_{j=1}^{b}\phi(b_j)\rangle \\
&= \tfrac{1}{a^2}\sum_{i=1}^{a}\sum_{m=1}^{a}\langle\phi(a_i), \phi(a_m)\rangle - \tfrac{2}{ab}\sum_{i=1}^{a}\sum_{j=1}^{b}\langle\phi(a_i), \phi(b_j)\rangle \\
&\quad + \tfrac{1}{b^2}\sum_{j=1}^{b}\sum_{n=1}^{b}\langle\phi(b_j), \phi(b_j n)\rangle \\
&= \tfrac{1}{a^2}\sum_{i=1}^{a}\sum_{m=1}^{a}k(a_i, a_m) - \tfrac{2}{ab}\sum_{i=1}^{a}\sum_{j=1}^{b}k(a_i, b_j) \\
&\quad + \tfrac{1}{b^2}\sum_{j=1}^{b}\sum_{n=1}^{b}k(b_j, b_n).
\end{aligned}$$

Using the test with selected kernels we show that healthy airways and COPD airways do not come from the same distributions (Table 3).

Table 3. Permutation tests for the means of the COPD patient and healthy subject samples. All permutation tests are made with 10.000 permutations.

Kernel	Gaussian pointcloud	Gaussian branchcount	Average AW-wall %	Generation-average AW-wall %
p-value	$9.99 \cdot 10^{-5}$	$9.99 \cdot 10^{-5}$	$9.99 \cdot 10^{-5}$	$9.99 \cdot 10^{-5}$
Kernel	Linear all-node-path	Linear Root-node-path	Shortest path	Weisfeiler Lehman
p-value	$9.99 \cdot 10^{-5}$	$9.99 \cdot 10^{-5}$	$9.99 \cdot 10^{-5}$	$9.99 \cdot 10^{-5}$

Table 4. Classification results for COPD on 1966 individuals, of which 893 have COPD

Kernel type	Mean class. accuracy	Kernel matrix computation time	Mean class. accuracy $K + K_{GBC}$
Rootpath, linear (3), (4)	$62.4 \pm 0.7\%$	9 h 9 m 20 s	$\mathbf{66.8 \pm 0.4\%}$
Rootpath, Gaussian (3), (4)	$\mathbf{64.9 \pm 0.4\%}$	6 h 53 m 21 s	$\mathbf{68.2 \pm 0.5\%}$
All-node-paths, linear (2), (5)	$62.0 \pm 0.6\%$	3 h 7 s	$63.2 \pm 0.5\%$
Root-node-path, linear (3), (5)	$61.8 \pm 0.7\%$	4 m 24 s	$62.9 \pm 0.8\%$
Root-node-path, Gaussian (3), (5)	$\mathbf{64.4 \pm 0.8\%}$	97 h 21 m 45 s	$\mathbf{64.9 \pm 0.6\%}$
Root-node-path, linear, a_i (3), (5) airway wall area % attribute	$58.6 \pm 0.6\%$	19 m 44 s	$62.3 \pm 0.8\%$
Pointcloud, Gaussian (10)	$\mathbf{64.4 \pm 0.6\%}$	18 h 40 m 26 s	$\mathbf{66.5 \pm 0.6\%}$
Branchcount, linear (14)	$62.3 \pm 1.0\%$	0.08 s	N/A
Branchcount, Gaussian	$63.3 \pm 0.4\%$	0.2	N/A
Linear kernel on % average airway wall area (12)	$56.2 \pm 0.6\%$	0.62 s	$63.3 \pm 0.5\%$
Gaussian kernel on average airway wall area %, generations $3-6$ (13)	$60.3 \pm 0.2\%$	0.35 s	$63.3 \pm 0.5\%$
Shortest path [3]	$62.6 \pm 0.4\%$	20 m 24 s	$63.4 \pm 0.4\%$
Weisfeiler Lehman ($h = 10$) [19]	$62.1 \pm 0.5\%$	14 m 40 s	$62.9 \pm 0.5\%$

3.3   COPD Classification Experiments

Based on the kernel matrices corresponding to the kernels described in Sec. 3.1 for a set of 1966 airway trees, classification into COPD/healthy was done using a support vector machine (SVM) [4]. The SVM slack parameter was trained using cross validation on 90% of the entire dataset, and tested on the remaining 10%. This experiment was repeated 10 times and the mean accuracies along with their standard deviations are reported in Table 4. All kernel matrices were combined with the GBC kernel matrix in order to check whether the kernels were, in fact, detecting something other than branch number.

4   Discussion

We have constructed a family of kernels that operate on geometric trees, and seen that they give a fast way to compare large sets of trees. We have applied the kernels to hypothesis testing and classification of COPD based on airway tree structure and geometry, along with state-of-the-art methods. We show that there is a connection between COPD and airway wall area percentage, and the COPD detected based on our weighted airway wall area percentage kernels is stronger than what can be found using average airway wall area percentage measurements over different airway tree generations, which is commonly done [10, 11].

Efficient kernels for trees with vector-valued node attributes are difficult to design because algorithmically, similarity of vector-valued attributes is more challenging to efficiently quantify than equality of discrete-valued attributes. Nevertheless, some of the defined kernels for vector-attributed trees are fast enough to be applied to large datasets from clinical trials.

Vector-valued attributes are important from a modeling point of view, as they allow inclusion of geometric information such as branch shape or clinical measurements in the trees. However, there is a tradeoff between computational speed and optimal use of the attributes. The efficient node paths are less robust than the embedded paths in airway segmentations with missing or spurious branches, and we observe a small drop in classification performance in Table 4. Rootpath kernels are introduced to improve computational speed. However, they do introduce a bias towards increased weighting of parts of the tree close to the root, which are contained in more root-paths. Gaussian local kernels perform significantly better than linear ones (Table 4), which is particularly pronounced in the pointcloud kernel. In convolution kernels based on quantification of substructure similarity rather than isomorphic substructure, all the dissimilar substructures are still contributing to the total value of the kernel, and the Gaussian local kernel downscales the effect of dissimilar substructures much more efficiently than the linear kernel. This is particularly pronounced in kernels that use geometric weighting of airway wall measurement comparison. Unfortunately, however, algorithmic constructions like the Kronecker trick (Prop. 7) do not work for the Gaussian kernels, which do not scale well to larger datasets.

Using hypothesis tests for kernels we show that the healthy and COPD diagnosed airway trees come from different distributions. Using SVM classification we show that COPD can be detected by kernels that depend on tree geometry, tree geometry attributed with airway wall area percentage measurements, or combinatorial airway tree structure. Another efficient detector of COPD is the number of branches detected in the airway segmentation. It is thus important to clarify that our defined kernels are not just sophisticated ways of counting the detected branches. Combining the GBC kernel with the other kernels improves classification performance of the geometrically informed tree and pointcloud kernels, showing that these kernels must necessarily contain independent information, and the connection between COPD and airway shape is more than differences in detected airway branch numbers. In contrast, graph kernels that only use the tree structure are not significantly improved by combination with the branch count kernel. Future work includes efficient ways of computing all-paths kernels with linear node attributes, efficient kernels for trees with errors in them, as well replacing the Gaussian local kernels with more efficient RBF type kernels.

Acknowledgements. This research was supported by the Danish Council for Independent Research | Technology and Production Sciences; the Lundbeck Foundation; AstraZeneca; The Danish Council for Strategic Research; Netherlands Organisation for Scientific Research; and the DFG project "Kernels for Large, Labeled Graphs (LaLa)".

References

1. Bach, F.R.: Graph kernels between point clouds. In: ICML, pp. 25–32 (2008)
2. Bishop, C.M.: Pattern Recognition and Machine Learning. Springer (2006)
3. Borgwardt, K.M., Kriegel, H.-P.: Shortest-path kernels on graphs. In: ICDM (2005)
4. Chang, C.-C., Lin, C.-J.: LIBSVM: A library for support vector machines. ACM Trans. Int. Syst. and Tech. 2, 27:1–27:27 (2011), Software available at http://www.csie.ntu.edu.tw/~cjlin/libsvm
5. Cortes, C., Haffner, P., Mohri, M.: Rational kernels: Theory and algorithms. JMLR 5, 1035–1062 (2004)
6. Feragen, A.: Complexity of computing distances between geometric trees. In: Gimel'farb, G., Hancock, E., Imiya, A., Kuijper, A., Kudo, M., Omachi, S., Windeatt, T., Yamada, K. (eds.) SSPR & SPR 2012. LNCS, vol. 7626, pp. 89–97. Springer, Heidelberg (2012)
7. Feragen, A., Hauberg, S., Nielsen, M., Lauze, F.: Means in spaces of tree-like shapes. In: ICCV (2011)
8. Feragen, A., Petersen, J., Owen, M., Lo, P., Thomsen, L.H., Wille, M.M.W., Dirksen, A., de Bruijne, M.: A hierarchical scheme for geodesic anatomical labeling of airway trees. In: Ayache, N., Delingette, H., Golland, P., Mori, K. (eds.) MICCAI 2012, Part III. LNCS, vol. 7512, pp. 147–155. Springer, Heidelberg (2012)
9. Gretton, A., Borgwardt, K.M., Rasch, M.J., Schölkopf, B., Smola, A.J.: A kernel two-sample test. JMLR 13, 723–773 (2012)
10. Hackx, M., Bankier, A.A., Genevois, P.A.: Chronic Obstructive Pulmonary Disease: CT quantification of airways disease. Radiology 265(1), 34–48 (2012)
11. Hasegawa, M., Nasuhara, Y., Onodera, Y., Makita, H., Nagai, K., Fuke, S.I., Ito, Y., Betsuyaku, T., Nishimura, M.: Airflow Limitation and Airway Dimensions in Chronic Obstructive Pulmonary Disease. Am. J. Respir. Crit. Care Med. 173(12), 1309–1315 (2006)
12. Haussler, D.: Convolution kernels on discrete structures. Technical report, Department of Computer Science, University of California at Santa Cruz (1999)
13. Leslie, C., Kuang, R.: Fast kernels for inexact string matching. In: Schölkopf, B., Warmuth, M.K. (eds.) COLT/Kernel 2003. LNCS (LNAI), vol. 2777, pp. 114–128. Springer, Heidelberg (2003)
14. Lo, P., van Ginneken, B., Reinhardt, J.M., de Bruijne, M.: Extraction of Airways from CT (EXACT'09). In: 2. Int. WS. Pulm. Im. Anal., pp. 175–189 (2009)
15. Mahé, P., Ueda, N., Akutsu, T., Perret, J.-L., Vert, J.-P.: Extensions of marginalized graph kernels. In: ICML (2004)
16. Miller, E., Owen, M., Provan, J.S.: Averaging metric phylogenetic trees (2012) (Preprint), http://arxiv.org/abs/1211.7046
17. Nye, T.M.W.: Principal components analysis in the space of phylogenetic trees. Ann. Statist. 39(5), 2716–2739 (2011)
18. Petersen, J., Nielsen, M., Lo, P., Saghir, Z., Dirksen, A., de Bruijne, M.: Optimal graph based segmentation using flow lines with application to airway wall segmentation. In: Székely, G., Hahn, H.K. (eds.) IPMI 2011. LNCS, vol. 6801, pp. 49–60. Springer, Heidelberg (2011)
19. Shervashidze, N., Schweitzer, P., van Leeuwen, E.J., Mehlhorn, K., Borgwardt, K.M.: Weisfeiler-Lehman graph kernels. JMLR 12, 2539–2561 (2011)
20. Sørensen, L., Lo, P., Dirksen, A., Petersen, J., de Bruijne, M.: Dissimilarity-based classification of anatomical tree structures. In: Székely, G., Hahn, H.K. (eds.) IPMI 2011. LNCS, vol. 6801, pp. 475–485. Springer, Heidelberg (2011)

21. Vishwanathan, S.V.N., Schraudolph, N.N., Kondor, R.I., Borgwardt, K.M.: Graph kernels. JMLR 11, 1201–1242 (2010)
22. Vishwanathan, S.V.N., Smola, A.J.: Fast kernels for string and tree matching. In: NIPS, pp. 569–576 (2002)
23. Washko, G.R., Dransfield, T., Estepar, R.S.J., Diaz, A., Matsuoka, S., Yamashiro, T., Hatabu, H., Silverman, E.K., Bailey, W.C., Reilly, J.J.: Airway wall attenuation: a biomarker of airway disease in subjects with COPD. J. Appl. Phys. 107(1), 185–191 (2009)

Segmenting the Papillary Muscles and the Trabeculae from High Resolution Cardiac CT through Restoration of Topological Handles

Mingchen Gao[1,*], Chao Chen[1,*], Shaoting Zhang[1], Zhen Qian[2], Dimitris Metaxas[1], and Leon Axel[3]

[1] CBIM Center, Rutgers University, Piscataway, NJ 08854
[2] 2 Piedmont Heart Institute, Atlanta, GA 30309
[3] New York University, 660 First Avenue, New York, NY 10016

Abstract. We introduce a novel algorithm for segmenting the high resolution CT images of the left ventricle (LV), particularly the papillary muscles and the trabeculae. High quality segmentations of these structures are necessary in order to better understand the anatomical function and geometrical properties of LV. These fine structures, however, are extremely challenging to capture due to their delicate and complex nature in both geometry and topology. Our algorithm computes the potential missing topological structures of a given initial segmentation. Using techniques from computational topology, e.g. persistent homology, our algorithm find topological handles which are likely to be the true signal. To further increase accuracy, these proposals are measured by the saliency and confidence from a trained classifier. Handles with high scores are restored in the final segmentation, leading to high quality segmentation results of the complex structures.

1 Introduction

Computed tomography (CT) is a very important imaging modality for diagnosing cardiovascular diseases. Compared with other imaging modalities (such as ultrasound and magnetic resonance imaging), CT is able to show detailed anatomic structures within the cardiac chambers [15]. Recent advances in CT technology allow a 320 multi-detector CT scanner to successfully capture the papillary muscles and trabeculae at a resolution which has not been reached before.

Most of the existing methods to perform cardiac segmentations [3,20,13] model the inner heart wall as a smooth surface, which does not include the papillary muscles and the trabeculae at all. Zheng *et al.* [20] proposed an algorithm to automatically segment the four chambers of the heart in four seconds. Ecabert *et al.* [5] presented a learning-based approach based on active shape model (ASM) for the segmentation of four chambers and major vessel trunks. Other models include, but are not limited to graph cut [7], atlas based segmentation [10] and local deformation [11].

---

* Both authors contributed equally to this work.

J.C. Gee et al. (Eds.): IPMI 2013, LNCS 7917, pp. 184–195, 2013.
© Springer-Verlag Berlin Heidelberg 2013

These methods, although proven to be successful in various situations, are not designed to accurately segment smaller, complex structures such as the papillary muscles and the trabeculae. Previous attempts [3,18] were able to capture the papillary muscle, but could not segment trabeculae with satisfying quality. Gao *et al.* [8] manually segmented one frame (at the end-diastole state) of an image sequence of a cardiac cycle, and then deformed the segmentation to match the other frames. Although their method focused on preserving the fine structures during the deformation, it only enforced consistency of geometry [17], not of topology. Accurately segmenting the complex structures of the papillary muscles and the trabeculae is still a challenging task. The reason is threefold. 1) The detailed structures are complex and small, making them hard to be distinguished from noise. 2) Some trabeculae go through the ventricle cavity and are very thin. Existing methods often fail to segment them due to the smoothness prior. 3) Such complex structures have a very different nature from other parts such as free wall and septum. Furthermore, trabeculae have a large variety of geometry and intensity even within the same cardiac image. This requires the segmentation method to be extremely adaptive in terms of parameters, making full automation very difficult.

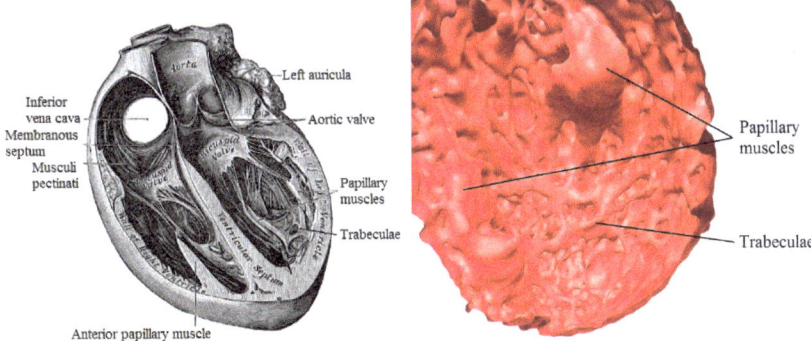

Fig. 1. Left: Left ventricle anatomy, picture from [9]. Right: Segmentation results represented as a 3D triangle mesh successfully captured the papillary muscle and the trabeculae.

Accurately segmenting the papillary muscles and the trabeculae is very important and of high interest to doctors. The functions of the papillary muscles and the trabeculae have still not been fully understood. Left ventricle anatomy is show in Fig. 1. The *papillary muscles* are attached to the valves via chordae tendineae. The *trabeculae* project from the inner surface of both ventricles of the heart. Some are completely attached to the wall of the heart. Others are fixed at both ends to the ventricular wall, but the intermediate section is freely mobile within the cavity, forming topological *handles*. There are a number of functional hypotheses for the trabeculation of the heart wall. High quality segmentations of such structures are useful for further investigating their functions, the mechanics of the heart [12] and geometrical properties of cardiac structures [13].

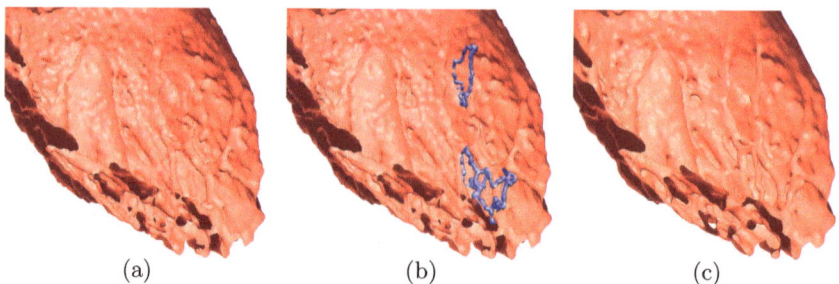

(a)   (b)   (c)

Fig. 2. Improvement of our method. (a) Baseline segmentation. (b) Proposed restoration handles. (c) Final segmentation.

In this paper, we propose a topological method to restore missing structures of a given segmentation, generated by any existing segmentation tool. It proposes hypotheses of where and how topological handles should be reestablished. On the basis of those topological proposals, a two-step screening is performed to select handles with higher confidence for structure restoration. Our algorithm evaluates each handle independently based on its saliency, rather than absolute intensities. Explicitly restoring selected handles makes the restoration adaptive to each trabecula, thus avoiding a universal threshold in the whole domain. Fig. 2 shows the improvements of our algorithm, with restored trabeculae highlighted. Quality of restored handles can be verified by comparing with the intensity function in Fig. 3.

Using topological information in image segmentation has been studied in both computer vision [2] and medical imaging [16]. As far as we know, in all previous methods, that use either random field energy models (MRF and CRF) [14] or deformable models [19], topological priors such as connectivity or handle-free are enforced as a segmentation constraint. In this paper, instead of enforcing the final segmentation to have an upper bound of the number of components or handles, we restore topological features, as long as we have high confidence in them.

2   Methodology

The algorithm flow is illustrated in Fig. 3. An initial segmentation is applied on the image and then we compute handles that need to be restored. Each handle is delineated by a thickened cycle, as illustrated in Fig. 3 (c). The segmentation is fixed accordingly, by enforcing these cycles to appear in the final segmentation.

In this section, we first state the desired properties for the cycles that we should use for handle restoration. Next, we build a connection to a theory of persistent homology [6] in the computational topology community. The output of persistent homology is a set of dots corresponding to handles that appear when we threshold the domain using a function value. Based on such theory, we design an algorithm to compute proposal cycles, each of which delineates

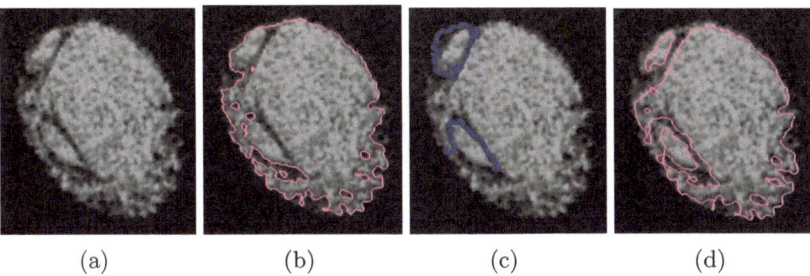

Fig. 3. A two-dimensional slice of the data on which we illustrate the workflow. (a) CT image. (b) Initial segmentation. (c) Proposed fixing cycles (partially occluded). (d) Final segmentation with handles restored.

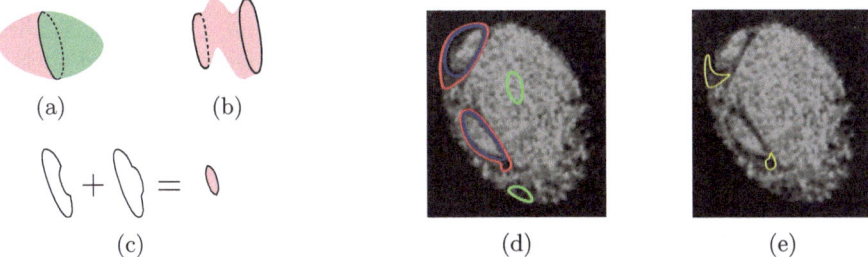

Fig. 4. (a) A given cycle is sealed by two different patches (pink and green). (b) The sum of two cycles is sealed by a tube shaped patch (pink), which delineates a way to deform between the two. (c) The mod-2 sum of two cycles, and a sealing patch. (d) Various cycles for a given function. (e) Sum of the corresponding blue and red cycles.

one handle. We conclude this section by explaining how to choose the promising candidates from all these proposals so that they satisfy the desired properties.

2.1 Intuition and the Desired Properties of Cycles for Handle Restoration

We start by introducing some terminology. A closed curve is called a *cycle*. The mod-2 sum (exclusive or) of a set of cycles is also called a *cycle*. A 2-manifold with boundary is called a surface *patch*. A patch c *seals* a cycle z if its boundary is z, formally, $\partial(c) = z$. When the sealed cycle is the sum of two cycles, the patch could be considered as the area swept through when we smoothly deform the first cycle into the second. In a 3D image, there could be infinitely many patches that seal a given cycle, and thus infinitely many ways to deform between cycles. See Fig. 4(a)-(c) for illustration.

Given a function defined on the image domain $f : \Omega \to \mathbb{R}$, $\Omega \subseteq \mathbb{R}^3$. To restore missing handles based on the image f, the two blue cycles in Fig. 4(d) are natural choices. Intuitively, a cycle is chosen if the intensity along it is low; yet the intensity between the corresponding handle and the wall is high. On the other hand, we need to propose a set of cycles such that any two of them would not delineate the same trabecula. Furthermore, each trabecula should be covered by a proposal. These intuitions lead to three properties need to be satisfied.

The set of cycles we select should satisfy the following properties. First, we require a high saliency for each selected cycle. A selected cycle z needs to go through points with relatively low function values, and any surface patch sealing this cycle has to have some points with relatively large function values. We measure the *saliency* of the cycle using the difference of maximal function values of the cycle and a sealing patch. There are infinitely many possible patches sealing a given cycle (Fig. 4(a)). Among them, we choose the patch whose maximal value is the smallest, formally,

$$\text{Saliency}(z) = \left(\min_{c:\partial(c)=z} \max_{p \in c} f(p) \right) - \max_{p \in z} f(p) \tag{1}$$

In Fig. 4(d), the blue and red cycles have high saliency, but green ones do not.

Second, we should not select several cycles that in fact correspond to the same trabeculae/handle. Any two selected cycles are required to have a large dissimilarity, i.e., the saliency of their mod-2 sum,

$$\text{Dissimilarity}(z_1, z_2) = \text{Saliency}(z_1 + z_2)$$

The dissimilarity between a cycle and zero is its saliency. In Fig. 4(d), there is a small dissimilarity between each blue cycle and the red cycle surrounding it. We should select only one of them. The sum of of the corresponding cycles, which are represented as yellow cycles in Fig. 4(e), have low saliency.

Third, we should exhaustively select all possible salient cycles. Any given cycle z should have a small dissimilarity from the set of selected cycles, Z, which is defined as the minimal dissimilarity between z and the mod-2 sum of a subset of Z,

$$\text{Dissimilarity}(z, Z) = \min_{Z' \subseteq Z} \text{Dissimilarity} \left(z, \sum_{z' \in Z'} z' \right)$$

This quantity lowerbounds the saliency of z itself since we allow Z' to be empty. Thus the dissimilarity is small if z has small saliency. In other words, any cycle z either has a low saliency, or has a good approximation from the given set Z, expressed as the sum of a subset $Z' \subseteq Z$.

2.2 Persistent Homology

In order to compute cycles that serve our purpose, we use persistent homology. The input of the tool is a topological space and a scalar function, e.g., the image domain Ω and the image function f. The output is a set of dots on $\mathbb{R}^2$ corresponding to a set of features.

For a given scalar value ℓ, we call the set of points with function value no greater than ℓ a *sublevel set*, formally, $\Omega_\ell = \{x \in \Omega \mid f(x) \leq \ell\}$. We study the topological changes of sublevel sets Ω_ℓ as the parameter ℓ increases from $-\infty$

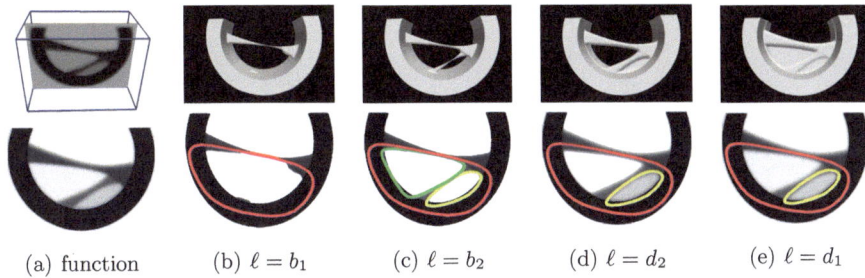

(a) function   (b) $\ell = b_1$ (c) $\ell = b_2$ (d) $\ell = d_2$ (e) $\ell = d_1$

Fig. 5. (a) Synthetic function. (b)-(e), Sublevel sets Ω_ℓ at time $b_1 < b_2 < d_2 < d_1$. Bottom row: 2D slices of the sublevel sets. We also show the intensity inside the sublevel sets. The red, yellow and green cycles are z_1, z_2 and z_3 respectively.

to $+\infty$, during which the sublevel set grows from empty to the whole domain Ω. For convenience, we say a topological event happens *at time ℓ_0* if it happens when we grow the sublevel set from $\Omega_{\ell_0-\epsilon}$ to Ω_{ℓ_0}.

In this paper, we focus on a specific kind of topological feature, handle. In Fig. 5, at time b_1, a new handle (delineated by the cycle z_1) is created. This handle is destroyed (becomes trivial) at time d_1. The two corresponding function values are called the *birth time* and *death time* of this topological feature. At time b_2 and d_2, another handle (delineated by the cycle z_2) is created and destroyed. For each handle, the difference between its death time and birth time is called the *persistence*.

All topological features are recorded in a *persistence diagram*. Each handle corresponds to a dot in $\mathbb{R}^2$, whose x and y coordinates are the birth and death times. The vertical or horizontal distance of a dot from the diagonal $x = y$ is its persistence. Fig. 6 is the persistence diagram of the synthetic function, with the two handles corresponding to two blue dots.

A justification of using the persistence diagram is its stability with regard to perturbations of the function [4]. Formally, the bottleneck distance between the diagrams of a function and the same function with added noise is upperbounded by the L_∞ norm of the noise, $\mathrm{dist}(\mathcal{D}_f, \mathcal{D}_{\hat{f}}) \leq \|f - \hat{f}\|_\infty = \|e\|_\infty$, where $\hat{f} = f + e$. In Fig. 6, after introducing noise e into the synthetic function, the persistence diagram could have many new dots with small persistence ($\leq \|e\|_\infty$). However, no large persistence dots are introduced or removed. The large persistence dots only move in the diagram by at most $2\|e\|_\infty$. In other words, noise in the image only introduces spurious handles that are destroyed right after creation.

In order to compute the persistence diagram, we first discretize the image domain into a *cubical complex* whose basic elements are *cells* of dimension zero to four, i.e., *vertices*, *edges*, *squares* and *cubes*, respectively. The set of vertices corresponds to the set of all voxels in the image. In Fig. 7(a), we show an example complex in 2D, with values of vertices specified. This discretization corresponds to the 4-/6-neighborhood for 2D/3D images, as defined in digital topology.

We build the *boundary matrix* of dimension d, whose columns and rows correspond to d-dimensional cells (d-cells) and d-dimensional cells ($(d-1)$-cells) respectively. Columns and rows are indexed from left to right and from

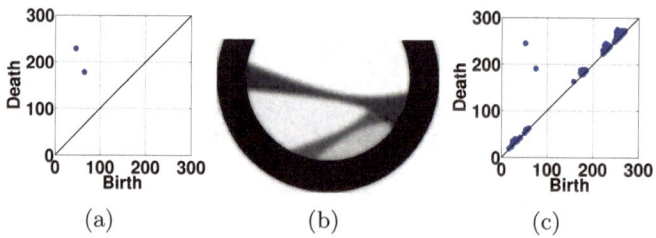

Fig. 6. (a) Persistence diagram of the synthetic function $\mathcal{D}_f$. (b) Perturbed function $\hat{f} = f + e$. (c) Persistence diagram of the perturbed function $\mathcal{D}_{\hat{f}}$.

top to bottom respectively, corresponding to cells sorted according to function values. An entry of the matrix is set to 1 if the corresponding $(d - 1)$-cell belongs to the boundary of the corresponding d-cell, and 0 otherwise. The one-dimensional boundary matrix is, in fact, the adjacency matrix of the underlying graph. For the example complex in Fig. 7(a), the sorted cells, and one-and-two-dimension boundary matrices are given in Fig. 7(b). Each column vector of the two-dimensional boundary matrix is a cycle, and the boundary of a 2-cell is a square. Since we use mod-2 addition, the sum of any set of columns is a cycle and the boundary of a patch which is the sum of the set of corresponding 2-cells. Columns of the boundary matrix span the space of all possible cycles of the discretized image domain Ω.

To compute the one-dimensional persistence diagram, which records features corresponding to handles, we apply a matrix reduction on the two-dimensional boundary matrix. Note that all additions are mod-2. We reduce columns of the matrix from left to right. For each column, we only use the columns on its left to reduce it. We start from the row index of the lowest nonzero entry of column i, called low(i). If this row index is equal to low(j) for some column j that has been reduced, we add column j to i, and thus reduce low(i). We repeat until low(i) is not the lowest nonzero entry of any column $j < i$, or column i becomes zero. In the former case, this reduced column corresponds to a handle in the persistence diagram, whose birth (resp. death) time is the function value of the cell low(i) (resp. the cell i). One property of the reduced matrix is that the lowest nonzero row index low($\cdot$) for all nonzero columns are unique. Fig. 7(c) shows an example of the reduced matrix, denoted by R. The edge low(i) and the square i are where the handle is created and destroyed, called the *creator* and *destroyer*.

2.3   Computing Proposal Cycles

We first compute one proposal cycle for each handle from the persistence diagram. For a handle that is born at time b and dies at d, we take a cycle that goes through the handle and lies within the sublevel set Ω_b. Furthermore, we choose a cycle which is sealed by a patch with the maximum function value d. For example, in Fig. 5, we choose z_1 for the handle born at b_1. For the handle born at b_2, we choose z_2 instead of z_3, because it is sealed up by a patch with

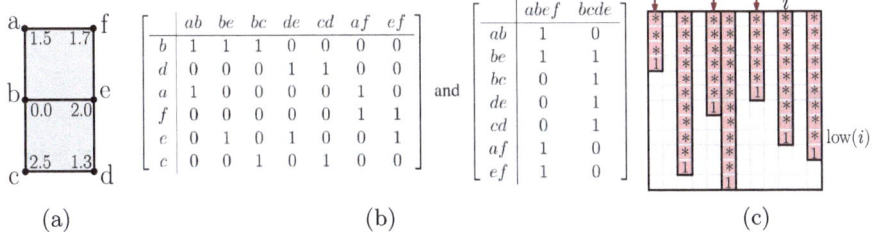

Fig. 7. (a) Example cubical complex, with function values given. (b) Boundary matrices of dimension one and two. (c) An indicative example of the reduced matrix R. This example does not correspond to boundary matrices in (b).

a maximum value d_2. We say the computed cycle *delineates* the corresponding handle. We denote by $\bar{Z}$ the set of all proposal cycles, delineating all handles that appeared in some sublevel sets. How to choose from them the salient ones will be discussed later.

To compute elements of $\bar{Z}$, we reuse the output of the algorithm for the persistence diagrams, in particular, the reduced matrix R (Fig. 7(c)). To compute a cycle for the handle corresponding to column i, collect the set of columns $R(*,j)$ on $R(*,i)$'s left such that $\text{low}(j) < \text{low}(i)$, e.g., the three marked columns in Fig. 7(c). These columns form a new matrix, $\widehat{R^i}$. The following theorem shows that any cycle that is the sum of the i-th column and a set of columns in $\widehat{R^i}$ is a valid cycle representing the handle corresponding to column i.

Theorem 1. $\forall x$, $y = R(*,i) + \widehat{R^i}x$ *is a cycle delineating the corresponding handle.*[1]

A delineating cycle may have freedom to wiggle within a handle, as long as it contains the creator edge $\text{low}(i)$. Thus we prefer computing a cycle with simple geometry.

Problem 1. *Compute* $y = R(*,i) + \widehat{R^i}x$ *with the minimal number of nonzero entries.*

Unfortunately, this problem is not only NP-hard, but also NP-hard to approximate within any constant. Alternatively, we propose a heuristic method to compute y as follows. Starting with the i-th column $y = R(*,i)$. Iterate through the row indices from $\text{low}(i) - 1$ to 1. For each row index k, if $y(k) \neq 0$, and $k = \text{low}(j)$ for some $j < i$, and adding $R(*,j)$ to y would reduce the number of nonzero entries, then add $R(*,j)$ to y.

Over the course of the algorithm, all used columns $R(*,j)$ will belong to $\widehat{R^i}$. So we always get a valid y. Furthermore, the number of nonzero entries of y monotonically decreases. The cycle gets shorter after each addition. In practice, the heuristic algorithm generates cycles that are reasonably simple. Trabeculae

---

[1] Theoretical proof is omitted due to limited space.

usually correspond to thin handles, which leave limited space for cycles to wiggle within.

2.4   Selecting Proposal Cycles Satisfying Desired Properties

From the set of all proposed cycles, $\bar{Z}$, we select the set of promising ones using a two level screening method. In the first level, we select cycles delineating handles with persistence not less than a threshold θ.

In fact, the saliency of each delineating cycle as defined in Equation (1) is equal to the persistence of the handle. We abuse notations and say a proposed cycle has the same birth time, death time and persistence as its corresponding handle. The following theorem guarantees that the selected set of cycles, namely, $Z_\theta = \{z \in \bar{Z} \mid \text{persistence}(z) \geq \theta\}$, satisfies the three desired properties we discussed in Section 2.1.

Theorem 2. *(A) Any cycle in Z_θ has a saliency at least θ;*
(B) The dissimilarity between any two cycles of Z_θ is at least θ;
(C) For any cycle z, its dissimilarity from Z_θ is at most θ.

Although high persistence cycles lead to salient handles that are more likely from trabeculae, in practice, the first screening would inevitable select certain wrong cycles. Therefore, we use a classifier with geometrical features as the second level screening.

3   Experiments

The proposed algorithm was employed on 6 cardiac CT image at the end diastolic state, where trabeculae structures are separated the most. The CT data were acquired on a 320-MDCT scanner, using a conventional ECG-gated contrast-enhanced CT angiography protocol. The imaging protocol parameters include: prospectively triggered, single-beat, volumetric acquisition; detector width 0.5 mm, voltage 120 KV, current $200 - 550$ mA.

We used the region competition algorithm [21] to initialize the segmentation. In order to focus on restoring the missed trabeculae, we decreased the function value of a voxel to zero if it was already segmented out. Handles which correspond to the structures that had been successfully captured would have birth time 0 and appear as dots on the y axis of the diagram (Fig. 8(a)). Their cycles were not be used for restoration. It took about 6 to 8 minutes on a commodity machine using 6 to 10 GB memory to compute the persistence diagram and cycles.

We used 5 out of 6 images for selecting persistence threshold, and training, and the remaining image for testing. We had human experts carefully examine proposal cycles and mark them as positive and negative, by studying the image function. (For example, the blue cycles in Fig. 3(c) are considered positive.) We performed the two level screening to select promising proposals. We empirically chose the persistence threshold. In Fig. 8(b) we plotted the number of positive and negative dots with persistence above a threshold, for one training image. We chose $\theta = 80$ so that we included all positive proposal cycles and a reasonable

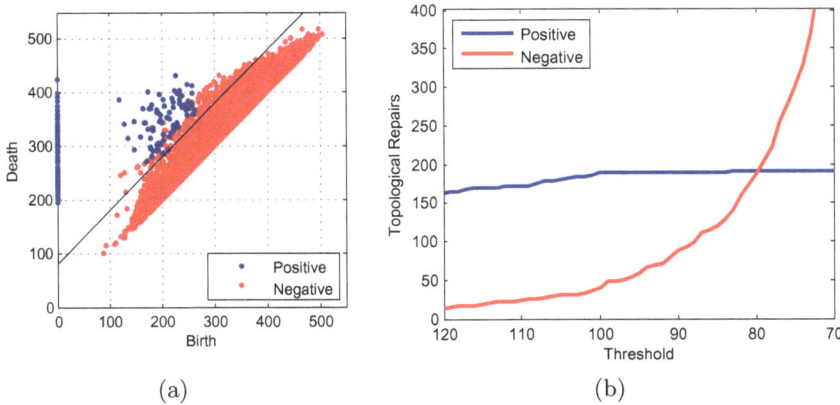

(a)   (b)

Fig. 8. (a) Persistence diagram of one cardiac image. The persistence threshold is marked as 80. (b) The relationship of persistence threshold and number of cycles.

number of negative ones from the training images. In the persistence diagram shown in Fig. 8(a), we drew the line $y = x + \theta$. All dots above this line were selected after the first level screening except the ones on the y axis. Notice the big variation of the birth and death times of positive dots. This implies that it is impossible to detect them using an universal intensity prior.

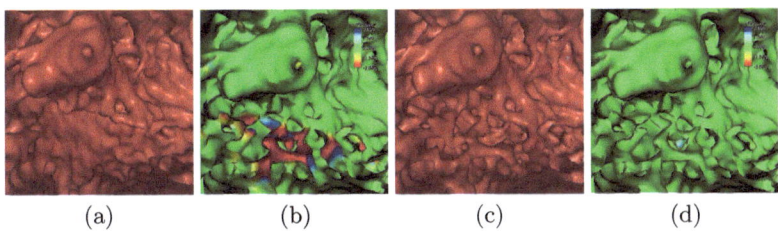

(a)   (b)   (c)   (d)

Fig. 9. (a) Baseline segmentation. (c) Proposed segmentation. (b)(d) Distance map from the pseudo-groundtruth to (a)(c) respectively.

Next we explain how to train the classifier for the second level. For all six images, we selected 458 positive out of 1095 proposals after persistence screening. Among those selected proposals, we used the ones from the five training images for training and 10-fold cross validation, and the ones belonging to the test image for testing. We used the LIBSVM toolbox [1] to train our classifier. Features used were birth time, death time, persistence, length of the cycle, and the relative position in the ventricle. We achieved 81.69% accuracy in the testing.

After promising proposals were selected, we generated the final segmentation by enforcing these cycles to be included. We reused the region competition algorithm with the same parameters so that the remaining parts of the final segmentation are the same as the initial one. Groundtruth is extremely difficult to get for this kind of data using manual segmentation. We generated the *pseudo-groundtruth* for the testing image by enforcing the human marked positive cycles. We compared the results of our method to that of a baseline segmentation generated using the region competition method (Fig. 9) by showing the distance from the pseudo-groundtruth to each result. Distance was represented by different colors. Green, red and blue represented accurate segmentation, over segmentation and under segmentation, respectively. The trabeculae missing from the baseline segmentation had greater error. Our segmentation, as shown in Fig. 9(b), successfully captured more trabeculae. The distance error of the initial segmentation is 0.2108 ± 0.4973 voxel, whereas our segmentation method has distance error 0.1101 ± 0.3679 voxel.

4 Conclusion

In this paper, we proposed a novel left ventricle segmentation method. Our segmentation approach is generic and could be applied to other topologically complicated segmentation problems with complex topological structures. It would be of theoretical interest if we build a quantitative relationship between the signal-noise ratio of the image and the stability of the persistent diagram.

Acknowledgement. This work is supported by NIH-R21HL88354-01A1, Multiscale Quantification of 3D LV Geometry from CT. The second author thanks Prof. Herbert Edelsbrunner for helpful discussions.

References

1. Chang, C.-C., Lin, C.-J.: LIBSVM: A library for support vector machines. ACM Transactions on Intelligent Systems and Technology 2, 27:1–27:27 (2011)
2. Chen, C., Freedman, D., Lampert, C.H.: Enforcing topological constraints in random field image segmentation. In: CVPR, pp. 2089–2096 (2011)
3. Chen, T., Metaxas, D., Axel, L.: 3D cardiac anatomy reconstruction using high resolution CT data. In: Barillot, C., Haynor, D.R., Hellier, P. (eds.) MICCAI 2004. LNCS, vol. 3216, pp. 411–418. Springer, Heidelberg (2004)
4. Cohen-Steiner, D., Edelsbrunner, H., Harer, J.: Stability of persistence diagrams. Discrete & Computational Geometry 37(1), 103–120 (2007)
5. Ecabert, O., Peters, J., Schramm, H., Lorenz, C., von Berg, J., Walker, M., Vembar, M., Olszewski, M., Subramanyan, K., Lavi, G., Weese, J.: Automatic model-based segmentation of the heart in CT images. TMI 27(9), 1189–1201 (2008)
6. Edelsbrunner, H., Harer, J.: Computational topology: an introduction. Amer. Mathematical Society (2010)
7. Funka-Lea, G., Boykov, Y., Florin, C., Jolly, M.-P., Moreau-Gobard, R., Ramaraj, R., Rinck, D.: Automatic heart isolation for CT coronary visualization using graph-cuts. In: ISBI, pp. 614–617 (April 2006)
8. Gao, M., Huang, J., Zhang, S., Qian, Z., Voros, S., Metaxas, D., Axel, L.: 4D cardiac reconstruction using high resolution CT images. In: Metaxas, D.N., Axel, L. (eds.) FIMH 2011. LNCS, vol. 6666, pp. 153–160. Springer, Heidelberg (2011)
9. Gray, H.: Anatomy of the human body. Lea & Febiger (1918)

10. Isgum, I., Staring, M., Rutten, A., Prokop, M., Viergever, M., van Ginneken, B.: Multi-atlas-based segmentation with local decision fusion-application to cardiac and aortic segmentation in CT scans. TMI 28(7), 1000–1010 (2009)
11. Jolly, M.-P.: Automatic segmentation of the left ventricle in cardiac MR and CT images. IJCV 70, 151–163 (2006)
12. Kulp, S., Gao, M., Zhang, S., Qian, Z., Voros, S., Metaxas, D., Axel, L.: Using high resolution cardiac CT data to model and visualize patient-specific interactions between trabeculae and blood flow. In: Fichtinger, G., Martel, A., Peters, T. (eds.) MICCAI 2011, Part I. LNCS, vol. 6891, pp. 468–475. Springer, Heidelberg (2011)
13. Lorenz, C., Berg, J.: A comprehensive shape model of the heart. Medical Image Analysis 10(4), 657–670 (2006)
14. Nowozin, S., Lampert, C.: Global connectivity potentials for random field models. In: CVPR, pp. 818–825 (2009)
15. Schoenhagen, P., Stillman, A., Halliburton, S., White, R.: CT of the heart: principles, advances, clinical uses. Cleveland Clinic Journal of Medicine 72(2), 127–138 (2005)
16. Ségonne, F., Pacheco, J., Fischl, B.: Geometrically accurate topology-correction of cortical surfaces using nonseparating loops. TMI 26(4), 518–529 (2007)
17. Shen, D., Herskovits, E., Davatzikos, C.: An adaptive-focus statistical shape model for segmentation and shape modeling of 3D brain structures. TMI 20(4), 257–270 (2001)
18. Spreeuwers, L., Bangma, S., Meerwaldt, R., Vonken, E., Breeuwer, M.: Detection of trabeculae and papillary muscles in cardiac MR images. Computers in Cardiology, 415–418 (September 2005)
19. Sundaramoorthi, G., Yezzi, A.: Global regularizing flows with topology preservation for active contours and polygons. TIP 16(3), 803–812 (2007)
20. Zheng, Y., Barbu, A., Georgescu, B., Scheuering, M., Comaniciu, D.: Four-chamber heart modeling and automatic segmentation for 3D cardiac CT volumes using marginal space learning and steerable features. TMI 27(11), 1668–1681 (2008)
21. Zhu, S., Yuille, A.: Region competition: Unifying snakes, region growing, and Bayes/MDL for multiband image segmentation. PAMI 18(9), 884–900 (1996)

Data-Driven Interactive 3D Medical Image Segmentation Based on Structured Patch Model

Sang Hyun Park[1], Il Dong Yun[2,*], and Sang Uk Lee[1]

[1] Electrical Engineering, ASRI, INMC, Seoul National University, Korea
shpark@cvl.snu.ac.kr, sanguk@snu.ac.kr
[2] Digital Information Engineering, Hankuk University of Foreign Studies, Korea
yun@hufs.ac.kr

Abstract. In this paper, we present a novel three dimensional interactive medical image segmentation method based on high level knowledge of training set. Since the interactive system should provide intermediate results to an user quickly, insufficient low level models are used for most of previous methods. To exploit the high level knowledge within a short time, we construct a structured patch model that consists of multiple corresponding patch sets. The structured patch model includes the spatial relationships between neighboring patch sets and the prior knowledge of the corresponding patch set on each local region. The spatial relationships accelerate the search of corresponding patch in test time, while the prior knowledge improves the segmentation accuracy. The proposed framework provides not only fast editing tool, but the incremental learning system through adding the segmentation result to the training set. Experiments demonstrate that the proposed method is useful for fast and accurate segmentation of target objects from the multiple medical images.

Keywords: interactive segmentation, 3D medical image, structured patch model, localized classifier.

1 Introduction

As creating an amount of medical images with the same modalities and properties, segmentation of desired objects from the multiple images becomes an important task for clinical studies and diagnosis of disease progression. Since the shapes and structures of an object in the medical images are generally maintained, many automatic methods [1–3] using prior knowledge of small number of training data have been proposed. However, most of them have struggled to obtain accurate segmentation for various clinical applications, because the medical images usually contain many vague boundaries and local variations of the same object. Therefore, an intelligent interactive segmentation method is inevitably preferable in the medical community [4].

---

* Corresponding author. This research was supported by the NRF of Korea funded by the Ministry of Education, Science and Technology (2010-0012006).

J.C. Gee et al. (Eds.): IPMI 2013, LNCS 7917, pp. 196–207, 2013.

The intelligent interactive method should satisfy two conditions: first, the method has to be fast enough to provide intermediate result to user. Second, the method has to provide flexible and accurate result even though small numbers of user interaction are given. The most interactive methods [5–8] have not satisfied the second condition due to the insufficient low level models depending on user inputs. On the other hand, the methods based on high-level knowledge require heavy computation, making harder to satisfy the first condition, to make and infer the model. Recently, Barnes *et al.* proposed the high level image editing method named PatchMatch [9] for image completion and reshuffling. Although the method satisfies the both conditions by finding dense patch correspondences, it is not applicable to the interactive segmentation because structural spatial relations, important for fast search and accurate segmentation, are not considered.

In this paper, we propose a novel 3D interactive segmentation method satisfying the both conditions by transferring the prior knowledge of similar patches from training sets to a target image with an assumption that the objects in medical images have common structure. Unlike the PatchMatch [9, 10], we construct a structured patch model which includes structural spatial relationships of adjacent patches within an image as well as multiple corresponding patch sets representing properties of local regions across images. The spatial relationships accelerate the patch search speed by constraining the positions of adjacent patches, while the prior knowledge of corresponding patch sets improves the segmentation accuracy by reflecting the properties of each local region. The proposed framework based on the structured patch model provides not only fast editing tool, but the incremental learning system through adding the segmentation result to the training set.

1.1   Related Work

Interactive Segmentation: There have been many interactive segmentation methods such as graph cut [5, 6, 11], random walk [7] and region growing [8]. The efficiency of methods has been further improved by constructing the fine models [12, 13], or incorporating the active learning scheme [4, 14]. However, high-quality user interactions are still required because the segmentation only depends on the low level cues which are insufficient to reflect various properties of the medical image. That is, most existing methods have focused on the single image segmentation based on the user input without prior knowledge. In this paper, we discuss how to incorporate the high level prior knowledge into interactive segmentation framework within a short time when training sets are given. Unlike the previous methods, the efficiency of proposed method is increased for multiple images segmentation.

Patch Matching: The strategy, finding out and using matches of similar patches, is relatively fast and flexible compared with the voxel level matching methods, e.g. non-rigid registration [15, 16]. Therefore, the strategy have been applied to various vision applications [9, 10, 17–19]. Especially, since the corresponding patches are likely to have the same labels, the method is applied to

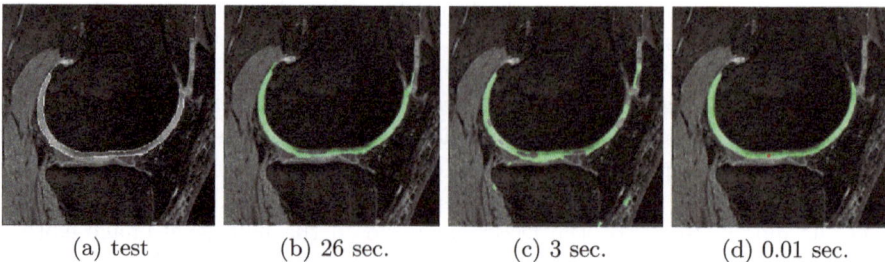

(a) test   (b) 26 sec.   (c) 3 sec.   (d) 0.01 sec.

Fig. 1. Transfer a label of training image to a test image (2D). (a) The test image and its ground truth boundary (white), (b) the transferred label (green) by the non-rigid registration method [15], (c) that by the PatchMatch [9], (d) that by the proposed method with few user input (red dot). The computational times are presented below the results.

semantic segmentation by constructing a graph of corresponding patches across a large image set [19]. In this paper, we expand the strategy to the interactive segmentation. In the proposed model, the corresponding patches are not only found across the training set, but the connection of the patch sets is also considered. Furthermore, multiple cues of each patch are learned for accurate segmentation unlike the previous methods which only transfer the label. Fig. 1 shows the difference of performance between the non-rigid registration method [15], the PatchMatch method [9] and the proposed method for the label transfer.

Patch Based Segmentation: There have been many patch based methods such as label fusion [1, 2] and localized classifier [20, 3]. Since the localized classifier can consider local variations by adaptively integrating the multiple cues, we adopt the method with some modifications to enforce the knowledge of user interactions and training patches. Unlike the previous methods which are only focused on automatic manner, effective 3D editing tool is provided in our framework by updating the patch correspondences of local regions. Furthermore, the computational time is accelerated because the search space is limited by an implicit patch structure without complicated alignment steps and all priors of patches are learned in training step.

2   Structured Patch Model

Unlike the PatchMatch-based methods which find the similar patches over an whole image without the structure information [18, 19], we find the exact nearest patch correspondence with the assumption that the medical images contain the same structural object. For example, if patches $P(v_j^i)$ and $P(v_{j'}^i)$, centered at voxels v_j^i and $v_{j'}^i$, are neighbor in a volume V^i, the corresponding patches $P(v_j^{i'})$ and $P(v_{j'}^{i'})$ of $P(v_j^i)$ and $P(v_{j'}^i)$ should be neighbor in another volume $V^{i'}$. Even though a patch more similar to $P(v_{j'}^i)$ than $P(v_{j'}^{i'})$ exists elsewhere in $V^{i'}$, $P(v_{j'}^{i'})$ next to $P(v_j^{i'})$ is determined as the most informative patch in our model.

2.1 Building Structured Patch Model

The structured patch model includes the connection of adjacent patches within an image and patch correspondences across images. To model this, the connection of neighboring patches are firstly constructed from a training set, then the corresponding patches are found from the other training sets. From m training sets $\mathbb{T} = \{T^i = (V^i, L^i) | i = 1, ..., m\}$ including the volume V^i and their manual label L^i, an initial set $T^{i'} = (V^{i'}, L^{i'})$ is randomly selected. From the surface $\xi(L^{i'})$ of $L^{i'}$, n voxels $\mathbf{v}^{i'} = \{v_j^{i'} | j = 1, ..., n\}$ are sampled with even distribution and the patches $\mathbf{P}^{i'} = \{P(v_j^{i'}) | j = 1, ..., n\}$ are constructed. Here, $\mathbf{v}^{i'}$ are sampled enough to overlap the adjacent patches (Details are listed in Sec. 5). Each patch has indices of the adjacent patches $\mathbf{N}_j = \{N_j(k) | k = 1, ..., l\}$ and their relative positions $\mathbf{r}_j^{i'} = \{r_j^{i'}(k) = p(v_{N_j(k)}^{i'}) - p(v_j^{i'}) | k = 1, ..., l\}$, where $p(v)$ denotes the position of voxel v and l is the number of adjacent patches.

The corresponding patches from another training set T^i are found by propagating $\mathbf{P}^{i'}$ to the relative positions of V^i. The propagation is started on the patch centered at the left-top point of L^i. First, we find the most similar patch with the starting patch among $\mathbf{P}^{i'}$. If the index of the most similar patch is j, the voxel v_j^i, the center of corresponding patch of $P(v_j^{i'})$, is searched near the left-top point within local search space Υ_j^i in V^i as:

$$v_j^i = \arg\max_{v \subset \Upsilon_j^i}(S(P(v), P(v_j^{i'}))), \tag{1}$$

where $S(\cdot, \cdot)$ denotes the similarity cost. After $P(v_j^i)$ is determined as the corresponding patch of $P(v_j^{i'})$, the adjacent patches of $P(v_j^{i'})$ are propagated to V^i. k^{th} adjacent patch $P(v_{N_j(k)}^{i'})$ is searched near the relative position $p(v_j^i) + r_j^{i'}(k)$ by (1). The propagation and the search are repetitively conducted until the all corresponding patches $\mathbf{P}^i$ of $\mathbf{P}^{i'}$ are determined. Since the search space is constrained by $\mathbf{r}_j^{i'}$, the propagation speed is accelerated even if the position of corresponding patch is exhaustively searched. The procedure is shown the upper row in Fig. 2.

The structured patch model $\mathbb{P} = \{\mathbf{P}^i | i = 1, ..., m\}$ is constructed by repeating the patch matching procedure to $m - 1$ training sets. Note that $\mathbf{P}^i$ represents the intra patch set from T^i, while $\mathbf{P}_j$ represents the corresponding inter patch set of jth local region across the training sets. The corresponding patch set reflects characteristics of the same local region of the training sets.

2.2 Adaptive Patch Propagation

Unlike the propagation of $\mathbf{P}^{i'}$ to V^i in the training step, that of the multiple patch sets $\mathbb{P}$ to a target volume V has to be conducted in the test step. Since the appropriate prior according to the local regions is different, we adaptively select the good corresponding patch on j^{th} local region from $\mathbf{P}_j$. The algorithm is started on few user input, e.g. a point near the object boundary. Although

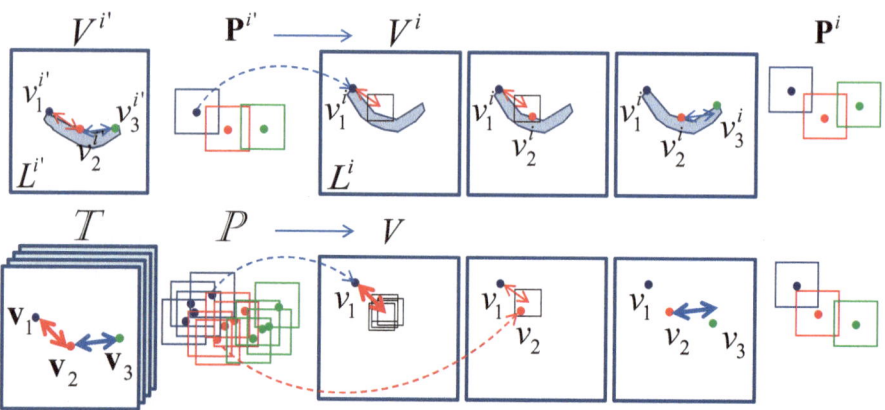

Fig. 2. Propagation and local search of the structured patch model. Upper row shows the propagation of $P^{i'}$ to V^i in the training step, while bottom row shows the propagation of $\mathbb{P}$ to V in the test step. The blue regions in upper row show labels and the points represent the center of patches. The neighboring point is searched from the local search space (black windows) near the relative positions (arrows).

the initial input can be automatically estimated by detection methods, we focus on the interactive system in this paper. We construct initial patch including the user input and find the most similar patch from $\mathbb{P}$ and its corresponding position by (1). Then, the adjacent patches are propagated. If the index of adjacent patch is j, the index i_{opt} of the best matching patch among $\mathbf{P}_j$ as well as the voxel v_j which is the center of corresponding patch of $P(v_j^{i_{opt}})$ in V is searched as:

$$(i_{opt}, v_j) = \arg\max_{v \subset \Upsilon_{j,i}}(S(P(v), P(v_j^i))). \tag{2}$$

That is, the patch $P(v_j)$ centered at v_j is localized in V and $P(v_j^{i_{opt}})$ is determined as the corresponding patch of $P(v_j)$. The adjacent patches are repetitively propagated to V by searching the best correspondences and the positions of adjacent patches near $p(v_j) + r_j^{i_{opt}}(k)$ within Υ_j as (2). The procedure is shown in the bottom row in Fig. 2. Finally, the positions of all patches are localized in V and its corresponding reference patch set $\tilde{\mathbf{P}}$ is obtained from $\mathbb{P}$. Note that the each element of $\tilde{\mathbf{P}}$ is referred by the difference training set.

2.3   Similarity Cost Function

The similarity cost $S(\cdot, \cdot)$ between patches can be computed by various functions. Among them, the normalized cross correlation (NCC) $S^{ncc}(\cdot, \cdot)$ and the overlapping cost, computed as $S^{ovl}(P(v_j^i), P(v_{j'}^{i'})) = \frac{|L_j^i \cap L_{j'}^{i'}|}{|L_j^i \cup L_{j'}^{i'}|}$, are used in the proposed method. Since the labels of two patches are required for computing $S^{ovl}(\cdot, \cdot)$, the overlapping cost is used for the training and editing steps. On the other hand, $S^{ncc}(\cdot, \cdot)$ is used for the test step.

2.4   Learning Multiple Cues

The patch provides informative cues of the local region. For each patch $P(v_j^i)$ including sub-volume V_j^i and sub-label L_j^i, we extract mean and variance of intensities of voxels inside V_j^i for computing NCC and the spatial information of neighboring patches for constraining the search space. Furthermore, we learn additional cues to construct a segmentation framework which is based on the conditional random field (CRF) model consisting of likelihood and smoothness terms. Details are as follow:

Multiple Cues Based on Localized Classifier. Inspired by the methods based on the localized classifier [20, 3], the likelihood of a voxel is determined by weighted sum of the probabilities regarding shape and appearance models. We use L_j^i and histograms H_j^f, H_j^b of voxel intensities of foreground (FG) and background (BG) labeled region as the shape model and the appearance model, respectively. The weight $w_j(v)$ between the shape and appearance probabilities is computed by the appearance confidence σ_j and the distance $d_j(v)$ from $\xi(L_j^i)$ as:

$$w_j(v) = 1 - \exp(-d_j^2(v)/\sigma_j). \tag{3}$$

When the voxel position is close to the surface and the appearances of FG and BG are distinguishable, $w_j(v)$ is decreased (the appearance cue is emphasized) and vice versa. σ_j is computed by sum of the difference between L_j^i and the FG probability regarding H_j^f and H_j^b. The detailed descriptions of σ_j and $w_j(v)$ are referred to [20].

Ratio between Likelihood and Smoothness. Since the CRF energy of small patch is sensitive to the ratio λ_j^i between the likelihood and smoothness terms, we estimate λ_j^i by using the shape of L_j^i. With observation that the result is likely to be over-smoothed when the surface is too large compared to the volume, e.g. thin parts, λ_j^i is computed by the ratio of FG volume $|L_j^i|$ and surface area $|\xi(L_j^i)|$ of L_j^i as: $\lambda_j^i = \lambda' \cdot \left(\frac{|L_j^i|}{|\xi(L_j^i)|} \right)$, where λ' is a parameter.

3   Segmentation Based on the Learned Priors

The voxel-labeling problem based on probabilistic models have been formulated as a pairwise CRF. We introduce two kinds of segmentation strategy based on the CRF model according to the learned priors $\tilde{\Theta} = \{\tilde{\theta}_j \supset \{\tilde{L}_j, \tilde{H}_j^f, \tilde{H}_j^b, \tilde{w}_j(v), \tilde{\lambda}_j\}|j = 1, ..., n\}$ of $\tilde{\mathbf{P}}$: one is based on patch-wise manner, while the other one is global manner.

For the patch-wise manner, the voxel-wise segmentation is conducted on each patch by using the learned prior $\tilde{\theta}_j$ and the user scribble U. The CRF energy on j^{th} patch is formulated as:

$$E(\mathbf{x}_j|\tilde{\theta}_j, U) = \sum_{v \in V_j} \phi(x_v|\tilde{\theta}_j, U) + \tilde{\lambda}_j \sum_{u,v \in \Gamma_j} |x_u - x_v| \cdot \exp \frac{|I(u) - I(v)|}{2\beta}, \tag{4}$$

where x_v is a random variable representing the label of voxel v in voxel set V_j and $\mathbf{x}_j$ is the label variable set of jth patch. $\phi(x_v|\tilde{\theta}_j, U)$ represents the likelihood term of single variables x_v when $\tilde{\theta}_j$ and U is given, while the exponential function represents the smoothness term between neighboring nodes (u, v) in neighbor set Γ_j. β is the average square-distance of intensities between adjacent voxels in V_j [5]. $\phi(x_v|\tilde{\theta}_j, U)$ is defined by the negative log of likelihood probability $Pr(v|\tilde{\theta}_j, U)$ as: $\phi\left(x_v|\tilde{\theta}_j, U\right) = -\log(Pr(v|\tilde{\theta}_j, U))$. If $U(v) = FG$ or BG, $Pr(v|\tilde{\theta}_j, U)$ is set as 1 or 0, respectively. If $U(v)$ is unknown,

$$Pr(v|\tilde{\theta}_j, U) = \tilde{w}_j(v)Pr(v|\tilde{L}_j) + (1 - \tilde{w}_j(v))Pr(v|\tilde{H}_j^f, \tilde{H}_j^b). \tag{5}$$

The probability $Pr(v|\tilde{L}_j)$ based on the reference label is computed as:

$$Pr(v|\tilde{L}_j) = \begin{cases} 1, & \text{if } \tilde{L}_j(v) = FG \\ 0, & \text{if } \tilde{L}_j(v) = BG \end{cases} \tag{6}$$

while $Pr(v|\tilde{H}_j^f, \tilde{H}_j^b)$ based on the appearance model is computed as:

$$Pr(v|\tilde{H}_j^f, \tilde{H}_j^b) = \frac{P(I(v)|\tilde{H}_j^f)}{P(I(v)|\tilde{H}_j^f) + P(I(v)|\tilde{H}_j^b)}, \tag{7}$$

where $I(v)$ denotes the intensity of v. Since the sub-modularity condition of (4) is satisfied, the optimal solution is obtained by the graph cut [5]. The patch-wise segmentations are aggregated on overlapping regions by averaging. Then, the voxels which have the higher averaging values than 0.5 are set as the foreground.

The procedure of global manner is similar with that of patch-wise segmentation. However, the likelihood probabilities of all patches are aggregated to a global likelihood by averaging the probabilities on overlapping regions before the patch-wise segmentation. The CRF energy model on the whole volume V is constructed by the global likelihood term and the smoothness term as:

$$E(\mathbf{x}|\tilde{\Theta}) = \sum_{v\in V} \phi(x_v|\tilde{\Theta}) + \lambda \sum_{u,v\in\Gamma} |x_u - x_v| \cdot \exp\frac{|I(u) - I(v)|}{2\beta}, \tag{8}$$

where $\mathbf{x}$ is label variable set in whole volume. Similarly, (8) is optimized by the graph cut [5]. The global method is faster than the patch-wise method because the max-flow algorithm of graph cut is conducted once. On the other hand, the result can be over-smoothed on vague regions or thin parts because λ_j^i according to the local shape is not considered.

4   Interactive Framework

Although most automatic methods have reduced the user effort, laborious slice-by-slice manual editing or post processing in a whole volume is required; the

---

Algorithm 1. Proposed framework based on the structured patch model

---

Input: the structured patch model $\mathbb{P}$ and a target volume V.
1: Adaptive patch propagation with few user input. (Sec. 2.2)
2: Segmentation by optimizing Eq. (8). (Sec. 3)
3: **Iterate** $4 \sim 6$ steps,
4:     Input the user scribbles U on false regions.
5:     Update the reference patches by Eq. (2) on local regions where the user
       scribbles are included.
6:     Segmentation on the local regions by optimizing Eq. (4). (Sec. 3)
7: **Until** the segmentation is satisfied.
8: (Optional) Add V and the result to $\mathbb{P}$ by the patch propagation (Sec. 2.1, 2.4)

---

intelligent editing process is not provided. On the other hand, the structured patch model provides the effective local editing framework by using the constructed corresponding patch sets.

The proposed framework is shown in Algorithm 1. Specifically, the framework is divided into the initial segmentation step and the editing step. The initial step is started from few user input near the boundary of a target object. $\mathbb{P}$ is set to the corresponding positions of the target volume by the adaptive propagation. Then, the initial result is obtained by the global segmentation. The editing step is started from the initial result. FG or BG scribbles are input on false parts by the user and the local regions (patches) including the scribbles are found. On those local regions, the corresponding reference patches and the positions are updated by (2) with the overlapping similarity cost between the labels and the user scribbles. The modified result is obtained by optimizing (4) which is computed by the updated reference patch and the user scribbles. The editing step is repeated until the segmentation is satisfied. After the segmentation is done, the test volume and its segmentation can be incrementally added to the training set by the propagation mentioned in Sec. 2.1 and 2.4.

In the proposed framework, the editing time takes less than few seconds because the editing is conducted on the small number of local regions. In addition, the updated reference patch guides the segmentation to true boundaries even though the user scribbles are roughly input.

5   Experiments

The structured patch model (SPM) was evaluated on various organs. First, we present quantitative validation for segmentation of femur and femoral cartilage from five knee MR images[1] with $384 \times 384 \times 160$ voxel dimensions and $0.36 \times 0.36 \times 0.70$ mm^3 resolutions. Two organs have very different properties: the femur is thick and cylindrical, while the femoral cartilage is thin and deformable. In

---

[1] The data were acquired from the Osteoarthritis Initiative
(http://www.oai.ucsf.edu).

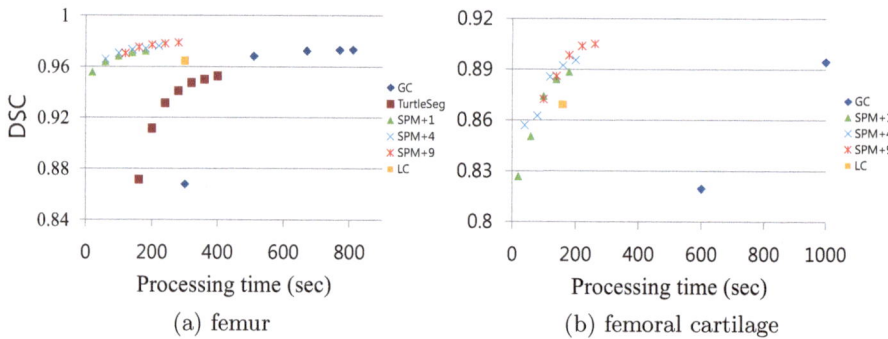

(a) femur   (b) femoral cartilage

Fig. 3. Comparisons of femur and femoral cartilage segmentation between the graph cut [5] (GC), the method based on active learning [4] (TurtleSeg), the automatic method based on localized classifier [3] (LC), and the proposed method (SPM+the number of training set). The graph shows the average DSC values versus the cumulative processing time (interaction time+computational time) of five test images. The interval of the points represents the processing time between iterations. In the case of cartilage, the result of TurtleSeg is not presented because the method does not work well within the several numbers of user delineations.

the proposed framework, the patch size was varied according to the object size to include the meaningful local region. We empirically set the patch size as $51 \times 51 \times 25$ for the femur and $31 \times 31 \times 15$ for the cartilage. The interval between the sampled points (center of the patches) was set to make the adjacent patches with $60 \sim 70$ percents overlap. Υ_j^i and Υ_j were set to one-third of the patch size. All experiments were conducted by the single core program on a PC with 2.93 GHz Intel Core i7 CPU, and 16GB of RAM.

The performance of SPM was compared with two interactive methods and an automatic method: the method based on 3D graph cut [11, 6] (GC), the method based on active learning [4] (TurtleSeg), and the automatic method based on localized classifier [3] (LC). The GC was conducted on cropping region near the target object because there were many BG regions having the similar appearance of the target object. The SPM was experimented regarding the different size of training set and the LC used nine images as the training sets. The segmentation accuracy was measured by Dice similarity coefficient (DSC) between the segmentation result S and ground truth R as: $\mathbf{dsc}(S, R) = \frac{2 \cdot |S \cap R|}{|S| + |R|}$.

Fig. 3 presents the comparisons of the accuracy versus the cumulative processing time including interaction time and computational time. Fig. 4 shows the difference of user inputs between the methods. The result of GC was converged to accurate result within few iterations. However, the interaction time between the iterations took long time because lots of scribbles should be input to prevent the result passing over true boundaries on vague regions or over-smoothing on thin parts. The TurtleSeg reduced the interaction time by providing the user with uncertain 2D planes. However, the improvement according to the user delineations was converged on rough segmentation. Furthermore, the method

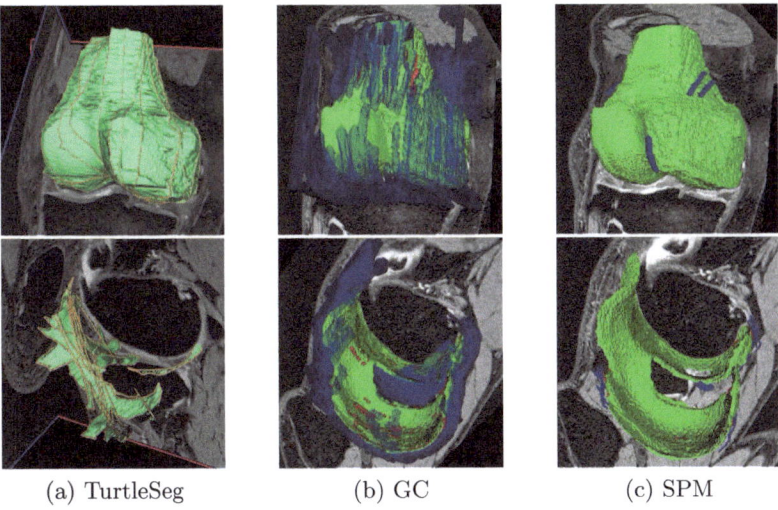

(a) TurtleSeg   (b) GC   (c) SPM

Fig. 4. Comparison of the user inputs between TurtleSeg [4], graph cut [5], and the proposed method. Green shows the segmentation result obtained by the user inputs, yellow lines represent the user delineations, and red and blue represent FG and BG scribbles, repectively.

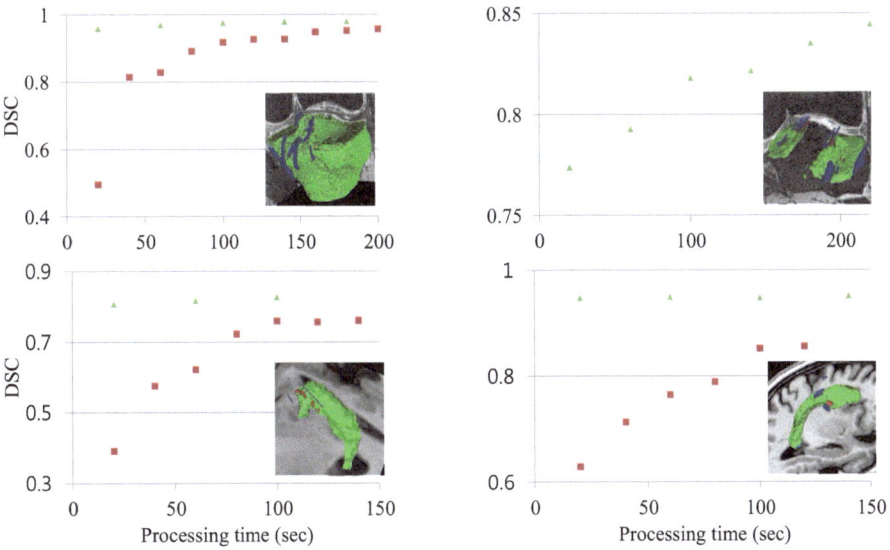

Fig. 5. Comparisons between SPM with one training set (green triangles) and Turtle-Seg (brown rectangles) for tibia, tibial cartilage, hippocampus, and ventricle. Figures inside the graphs show segmentation results and user scribbles of the proposed method.

required lots of delineations for the cartilage segmentation because its shape is very thin and deformable (Fig 4 (a)). On the other hand, the SPM obtained the accurate result, outperforming that of the LC method, within few processing time on both cases. For most cases, the SPM obtained better DSC than the LC method during the same processing time. As increasing the size of training set, the computational time of the initial step was increased while the performance of initial segmentation was enhanced.

For general purpose, the SPM with one training set was applied to the segmentation of other organs: tibia and tibial cartilage in the knee MRI, hippocampus and ventricle in the brain MRI[2]. The DSC versus the cumulative processing time was compared with TurtleSeg (Fig 5). The results imply that the SPM is applicable to various problems without many training sets and useful to the segmentation of multiple volumes more than two.

6 Discussion

Most previous methods usually focus on the automatic or interactive manners. The main contribution of the proposed framework is to provide the connection between the automatic and interactive strategies by using the SPM. The method largely reduces the laborious user efforts by automatically segmenting the most parts, which relatively easy to be inferred by the prior knowledge, in the initial step. The propagated patch structure provides the intelligent editing system by updating the patch models according to the user interaction.

Since the corresponding patch set represents the properties of the same local region, we expect that the SPM will be expanded more effective ways. First, the proposed framework can be combined with the active learning scheme to provide an user with the slices including uncertain local regions. It is useful for our framework because most errors on the editing step occur on small numbers of vague local regions. The uncertainty can be measured through the comparison between the priors such as L_j, σ_j of the reference patch and the segmentation. Second, local statistics and variations according to the pathological change can be modeled as increasing the size of training data. We have plan to cluster the similar patches and separately model the status of the cluster in each local region for managing the training patches. Third, the method can be expanded to the multi-object segmentation by using the optimization methods dealing with the multi-label problem. Finally, the algorithm can be parallelized because the same processes are repeated for multiple patches. The presented expansions are left to the future work.

References

1. Coupe, P., Manjon, J.V., Fonov, V., Pruessner, J., Robles, M., Collins, D.L.: Patch-based segmentation using expert priors: application to hippocampus and ventricle segmentation. Neuroimage 54(2), 940–954 (2011)

---

[2] The data were acquired from the Alzheimer's Disease Neuroimaging Initiative (http://www.loni.ucla.edu/ADNI).

2. Rousseau, F., Habas, P.A., Studholme, C.: Human brain labeling using image similarities. In: Proc. IEEE Conference on Computer Vision and Pattern Recognition (2011)
3. Lee, S., Park, S.H., Shim, H., Yun, I.D., Lee, S.U.: Optimization of local shape and appearance probabilities for segmentation of knee cartilage in 3-D MR images. Computer Vision and Image Understanding 115(12), 1710–1720 (2011)
4. Top, A., Hamarneh, G., Abugharbieh, R.: Active Learning for Interactive 3D Image Segmentation. In: Fichtinger, G., Martel, A., Peters, T. (eds.) MICCAI 2011, Part III. LNCS, vol. 6893, pp. 603–610. Springer, Heidelberg (2011)
5. Boykov, Y., Funka-Lea, G.: Graph cuts and efficient N-D image segmentation. International Journal of Computer Vision 70(2), 109–131 (2006)
6. Shim, H., Chang, S., Tao, C., Wang, J., Kwoh, C., Bae, K.: Knee cartilage: efficient and reproducible segmentation on high-spatial-resolution MR images with the semiautomated graph-cut algorithm method. Radiology 251(2), 548–556 (2009)
7. Grady, L.: Random walks for image segmentation. IEEE Transactions on Pattern Analysis and Machine Intelligence 28(11), 1768–1783 (2006)
8. Pohle, R., Toennies, K.D.: Segmentation of medical images using adaptive region growing. In: Proc. SPIE M.I. (2001)
9. Barnes, C., Shechtman, E., Finkelstein, A., Goldman, D.B.: PatchMatch: A randomized correspondence algorithm for structural image editing. In: Proc. SIGGRAPH (2009)
10. Barnes, C., Shechtman, E., Goldman, D.B., Finkelstein, A.: The generalized PatchMatch correspondence algorithm. In: Daniilidis, K., Maragos, P., Paragios, N. (eds.) ECCV 2010, Part III. LNCS, vol. 6313, pp. 29–43. Springer, Heidelberg (2010)
11. Shim, H., Kwoh, C., Yun, I., Lee, S., Bae, K.: Simultaneous 3-d segmentation of three bone compartments on high resolution knee mr images from osteoarthritis initiative (oai) using graph-cuts. In: Proc. SPIE M.I. (2009)
12. Rother, C., Kolmogorov, V., Blake, A.: "GrabCut" - Interactive foreground extraction using iterated graph cuts. In: Proc. SIGGRAPH (2004)
13. Mory, B., Ardon, R.: Non-euclidean image-adaptive radial basis functions for 3D interactive segmentation. In: Proc. International Conference on Computer Vision (2009)
14. Wang, D., Yan, C., Shan, S., Chen, X.: Active Learning for Interactive Segmentation with Expected Confidence Change. In: Lee, K.M., Matsushita, Y., Rehg, J.M., Hu, Z. (eds.) ACCV 2012, Part I. LNCS, vol. 7724, pp. 790–802. Springer, Heidelberg (2013)
15. Liu, C., Yuen, J., Torralba, A., Sivic, J., Freeman, W.T.: SIFT flow: Dense correspondence across different scenes. In: Forsyth, D., Torr, P., Zisserman, A. (eds.) ECCV 2008, Part III. LNCS, vol. 5304, pp. 28–42. Springer, Heidelberg (2008)
16. Glocker, B., Komodakis, N., Tziritas, G., Navab, N., Paragios, N.: Dense image registration through MRFs and efficient linear programming. Medical Image Analysis 12(6), 731–741 (2008)
17. Bleyer, M., Rhemann, C., Rother, C.: PatchMatch stereo - stereo matching with slanted support windows. In: Proc. BMVC (2011)
18. Zhang, H., Fang, T., Chen, X., Zhao, Q., Quan, L.: Partial similarity based nonparametric scene parsing in certain environment. In: Proc. IEEE Conference on Computer Vision and Pattern Recognition (2011)
19. Gould, S., Zhang, Y.: PATCHMATCHGRAPH: Building a graph of dense patch correspondences for label transfer. In: Fitzgibbon, A., Lazebnik, S., Perona, P., Sato, Y., Schmid, C. (eds.) ECCV 2012, Part V. LNCS, vol. 7576, pp. 439–452. Springer, Heidelberg (2012)
20. Bai, X., Wang, J., Simons, D., Sapiro, G.: Video snapcut: robust video object cutout using localized classifiers. In: Proc. SIGGRAPH (2009)

Sparse Deformable Models
with Application to Cardiac Motion Analysis

Yang Yu[1], Shaoting Zhang[1,*], Junzhou Huang[2],
Dimitris Metaxas[1], and Leon Axel[3]

[1] Department of Computer Science, Rutgers University, Piscataway, NJ, USA
[2] Computer Science and Engineering, University of Texas at Arlington, TX, USA
[3] Radiology Department, New York University, New York, NY, USA
shaoting@cs.rutgers.edu

Abstract. Deformable models have been widely used with success in medical image analysis. They combine bottom-up information derived from image appearance cues, with top-down shape-based constraints within a physics-based formulation. However, in many real world problems the observations extracted from the image data often contain gross errors, which adversely affect the deformation accuracy. To alleviate this issue, we introduce a new family of deformable models that are inspired from compressed sensing, a technique for efficiently reconstructing a signal based on its sparseness in some domain. In this problem, we employ sparsity to represent the outliers or gross errors, and combine it seamlessly with deformable models. The proposed new formulation is applied to the analysis of cardiac motion, using tagged magnetic resonance imaging (tMRI), where the automated tagging line tracking results are very noisy due to the poor image quality. Our new deformable models track the heart motion robustly, and the resulting strains are consistent with those calculated from manual labels.

1 Introduction

Deformable models have been widely used in computer vision [8], computer graphics [10] and medical image analysis [7]. They are able to solve diverse types of problems, such as, but not limited to, image segmentation [6], shape reconstruction [16], and motion tracking [11]. The name "deformable models" is derived from nonrigid body mechanics, which describes how elastic objects respond to applied forces. Starting from an initial shape, the model is deformed by two types of forces, i.e., internal and external forces. The internal forces limit the geometric flexibility of the shape, while the external forces drive the model to fit the observations. For example, in the initial active contour models [6], the internal forces are based on the first-order and second-order shape terms of the boundary. They regularize the length and the curvature of the underlying shape, to ensure a smooth shape result. The external forces drag the boundary to the positions that are more likely to be

---

* Corresponding author.

J.C. Gee et al. (Eds.): IPMI 2013, LNCS 7917, pp. 208–219, 2013.

edges. Because of the success of the active contours, many methods have been proposed since then to improve the performance of deformable models by modifying either the internal or external forces.

The internal forces usually enforce the smoothness characteristics of deformable models, such as the local continuity and curvature. 2D or 3D splines are widely used to constrain the image deformation [1]. B-spline [12] and nonuniform rational B-splines (NURBS) [17] define the model motion inside the object and on the boundary. They effectively reduce the degree of freedom for deformation and regularize the curvature on the deformation field. The Laplacian coordinate [15] is another well-known measurement for the local relative positions. Comparing with spline-based method, methods based on Laplacian coordinate allow more flexible shape representation. Sorkine et al. employed it to constrain the smoothness and local similarity of the 2D mesh deformation in geometry editing [15]. Shen et al. [14] decomposed the Laplacian coordinates into components in the perpendicular and tangential directions of the model, to formulate a detail-preserved internal force. Since the component of the perpendicular direction tends to shrink the model and eliminates the shape details, they proposed an internal force based on the tangential direction, to better approach the sharp features. In this paper, we apply the Laplacian coordinates on 3D volume models to enforce the smoothness not only on the surface, but also inside the models.

The external forces usually drive the model based on the control points extracted from low-level image information [13]. However, their positions may not be accurate, due to the noisy and/or weak image appearance cues. A general strategy to apply the external force is to minimize the distances between the control points extracted from image and the corresponding points on the initial model [15,20]. They used a Euclidean distance or $L2$ norm to measure the differences between the observations and the corresponding model control points. This assumes intrinsically that the errors of the control points follow a Gaussian distribution. Nevertheless, this is not always true in practice. They may contain not only Gaussian noise, but also some gross errors or outliers due to the erroneous tracking. Therefore, the accuracy of the traditional deformable models depends heavily on the control point accuracy. To improve the robustness of deformable models, Vogler et al. [18] explicitly modeled the distribution of control points, and considered the points rejected by the distribution as outliers. The local tracking results were first projected to the parameter space. Then they estimated a normal distribution based on the observations and rejected that with large Mahalanobis distance to the mean. Different from [18], our proposed deformable models implicitly handle the outliers with no elimination step. The influence of each local tracking observations is adaptively decided during the optimization process. The models are general enough for arbitrary deformable models with gross errors in the observations.

Inspired by the robust recovery power of the compressed sensing approach [3], we propose a new class of deformable models using sparse constraints. Recent research in compressed sensing shows that using an $L1$ norm can dramatically increase the probability of accurate signal recovery, even when there are both sparse outliers and moderate Gaussian noise [3]. Thus, we first propose a deformable model with only a $L1$ norm constraint, which is able to handle outliers robustly. However, when the variances of the Gaussian noise are large, solely using the $L1$ norm will cause overfitting problems because of its nature of pursuing the sparse structure [3]. Therefore, we further propose a deformable model using a hybrid norm constraint able to handle both the Gaussian errors and gross errors. We also generalize these two models in a unified formulation, named as Sparse Deformable Models. We apply the models to left ventricle (LV) motion analysis on mouse cardiac tagged MRI. The experiment results show that we can robustly track the mouse heart motions even based on inaccurate control point tracking results.

2   Methodology

Consider a set of points $\mathcal{V}$, where each point has a neighborhood structure[1], and a subset as control points $\mathcal{V}_c$ that are computed from the observations (e.g., image information). Let the homogeneous coordinate of the point i be denoted by $\mathbf{v}_i = [x_i, y_i, z_i, 1]^T$ and the position after deformation $\mathbf{v}'_i = [x'_i, y'_i, z'_i]^T$, where $i = 1, 2, \cdots, n$. We denote the coordinates of all the points after deformation as:

$$\mathbf{V}' = [\mathbf{v}'^T_1 \mathbf{v}'^T_2 \cdots \mathbf{v}'^T_n]^T.$$

The goal of our deformable models is to track the motion of the whole shape, given a set of control points. The deformation of each point i is parameterized by an affine 3×4 transformation matrix T_i. The unknown transformation parameters are organized in a $4n \times 3$ matrix:

$$T = [T_1 T_2 \cdots T_n]^T.$$

In our model, the internal forces preserve the local shape structure with the Laplacian coordinate, and the external forces minimize the difference between the shape and the control points with our proposed sparse constraints.

2.1   Internal Force

Our internal force ensures that the deformation matrices are similar among the neighborhood points. The similarity is measured based on the deformation they generate. Specifically, if we apply transformation matrices of neighboring points to the current one, the resulting displacements should be similar. For a point i, its displacement after applying its own transformation matrix T_i should be similar to applying its neighbor's transformation matrix T_j. Thus, the energy function of the internal force is:

$$E_{int} = \sum_{i \in \mathcal{V}} \sum_{j \in \mathcal{N}(i)} w_{ij} \|T_i \mathbf{v}_i - T_j \mathbf{v}_i\|^2_2, \tag{1}$$

---

[1] Mesh and meshless-based models are the most widely used shape representations. Our model works for both representations, and the neighborhood is defined by the connectivity for the mesh model, or the distance for the meshless model.

where $\|\cdot\|_2$ denotes the entry-wise matrix $L2$ norm[2], and weight w_{ij} is related to the distance between points i and j. Since this is a summation of the quadratic forms of the transformation matrices T_i, we can represent the energy function as a quadratic form of all the unknown transformations T. To do so, the point position $\mathbf{v}_i$ is encoded into matrix K_i as

$$K_i = M_i \otimes \mathbf{v}_i,$$

where $\otimes$ is the Kronecker product, and M_i is a $m_i \times n$ node-arc matrix of $\mathbf{v}_i$, where m_i is the number of its neighbors. For each neighbor $\mathbf{v}_j$, there is one row in M_i where the ith element is w_{ij} and the jth element is $-w_{ij}$, while the other elements are all zeros:

$$M_i = \begin{pmatrix} & \overset{i\text{th column}}{w_{ij}} & \cdots & \overset{j\text{th column}}{-w_{ij}} & \cdots \\ & \vdots & & \vdots & \end{pmatrix}, j \in \mathcal{N}(\mathbf{v}_i).$$

K_iT is the difference of the displacements based on different transformations of the neighborhood of point i. We concatenate the matrix K_i for all the points to form the matrix $K = [K_1^T K_2^T \cdots K_n^T]^T$. Thus, the energy function of the internal force (Eq.1) is formulated as:

$$E_{int} = \|KT\|_2^2. \tag{2}$$

2.2 External Force

Besides the shape constraint from the internal force, the deformable model also aims to match the observations. For example, a point i on the model is expected to fit to the given control point position $\mathbf{v}_i'$ after deformation T_i. We concatenate the point coordinates into an $n \times 4n$ sparse matrix:

$$D = \begin{bmatrix} \mathbf{v}_1^T & & & \\ & \mathbf{v}_2^T & & \\ & & \ddots & \\ & & & \mathbf{v}_n^T \end{bmatrix},$$

where $\mathbf{V}' = DT$ is the model deformation based on the transformation parameters T. We use a control point indicator c to select the rows of D and $\mathbf{V}'$ corresponding to the control points. Thus, the Laplacian deformable model (LDM) is defined as:

$$\arg\min_T \{\|KT\|_2^2 + \lambda\|D_cT - \mathbf{V}_c'\|_2^2\}, \tag{3}$$

where λ is the stiffness weight, which controls how much the model is able to deform to match the control points. Larger λ results in a better fitting, but the

---

[2] The matrix norms in the paper are all entry-wise norms.

deformed shape may not be smooth. The $L2$ norm is used as a penalty function in this formulation. As the standard norm on the Euclidean space, the $L2$ norm is the most widely used distance metric. However, it may not be the most proper metric in some applications, especially when there are gross errors or outliers.

The Sparse Prior Using $L1$ Norm. Gross errors are very common in some applications, such as the erroneous detections in a noisy image. The $L2$ norm follows a Gaussian distribution for residuals. It may overfit these sparse outliers, and hence reduce the deformation accuracy. It is desirable to produce a sparse solution that models the outliers. The $L0$ norm counts the number of non-zero elements and can model such sparse errors exactly. However, the $L0$ norm is non-convex, and solving an $L0$ norm problem is NP-hard. Recent developments in compressed sensing [3] show that minimizing an $L1$ norm problem can produce a nearly identical solution as using the $L0$ norm. Thus, we use convex relaxation to define a sparse deformable model based on the $L1$ norm as:

$$\arg \min_{T}\{\|KT\|_2^2 + \lambda\|D_c T - \mathbf{V}'_c\|_1\}. \tag{4}$$

The Sparse Prior Using Both $L1$ and $L2$ Norms. The sparsity constraint is useful in many applications, such as signal reconstruction and background subtraction. However, in most cases, the observations may still contain Gaussian errors with large variations. Using the $L1$ norm alone may not be able to handle them well [23]. Therefore, we combine both $L1$ and $L2$ norms and propose our sparse deformable models for general problems:

$$\arg \min_{T,\mathbf{e}}\{\|KT\|_2^2 + \lambda\left(\|D_c T - \mathbf{V}'_c - \mathbf{e}\|_2^2 + \gamma\|\mathbf{e}\|_1\right)\}, \tag{5}$$

where $\mathbf{e}$ represents the gross errors and is constrained by the $L1$ norm, and $\gamma \in [0,1]$ controls how sparse $\mathbf{e}$ is. The new model combines the advantages of both $L1$ and $L2$ norms. If γ is extremely large, $\mathbf{e}$ will be all zeros. Thus the model degenerates to a method with only an $L2$ norm, as in (3). It will be sensitive to any gross errors. If λ is extremely large and γ is small, the deformation errors will be approximately equal to $\mathbf{e}$. Thus the model is similar to models with only sparse constraints, as in (4). It will be robust to the outliers, but can not handle large Gaussian noise.

Optimization Framework. The above problem can be solved by the standard convex optimization algorithm, while we propose an effective iterative optimization algorithm that fully utilizes the special structure of the problem. The two variables T and $\mathbf{e}$ are optimized alternatively, with an analytical solution. The gross error $\mathbf{e}$ is initialized as zero. When $\mathbf{e}$ is fixed, the problem is reduced to the conventional $L2$ norm constraints.

$$\arg \min_{T}\{\|KT\|_2^2 + \lambda\|D_c T - \mathbf{V}'_c - \mathbf{e}\|_2^2\}, \tag{6}$$

It can be solved by least square minimization. Then T is fixed, and the optimization problems for each term e_i of the outlier $\mathbf{e}$ are independent:

$$\arg \min_{e_i}\{((D_cT)_i - \mathbf{V}'_{ci} - e_i)^2 + \gamma|e_i|\}, \tag{7}$$

where $(D_cT)_i$ is the ith element of the vector D_cT. The minimums for the two parts can be achieved at $(D_cT)_i - \mathbf{V}'_{ci}$ and 0 separately. Since both of them are convex, the minimum of the energy function must lie between them. Therefore, e_i has the same sign as $(D_cT)_i - \mathbf{V}'_{ci}$. After determining the sign of e_i, the problem reduces to a constrained quadratic function of e_i. The solution is:

$$e_i = \begin{cases} \max\{0, (D_cT)_i - \mathbf{V}'_{ci} - \gamma/2\} & \text{if } (D_cT)_i - \mathbf{V}'_{ci} \geq 0, \\ \min\{0, (D_cT)_i - \mathbf{V}'_{ci} + \gamma/2\} & \text{otherwise.} \end{cases} \tag{8}$$

The analytical solutions of the two sub-steps guarantee the energy monotonically decreases until the minimum is achieved. The convexity of the whole problem makes sure that this is the global solution of the problem.

2.3 Left Ventricle Motion Analysis

Tagged MRI (tMRI) offers a powerful non-invasive tool for making measurements of the beating heart that directly reflect its complex in vivo physiology. It has been widely used for the assessment of human heart diseases as well as in experimental heart disease models, as in mice. Compared to the human heart, the data acquisition from the mouse heart is more challenging for achieving adequate spatial and temporal resolutions. The mouse heart is about

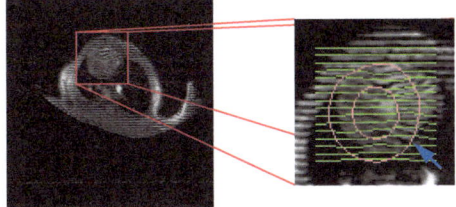

Fig. 1. Sample tagged SA image with tagging line tracking result

1000th the size of a human heart and beats much faster, at 400-600 beats per minute (bpm), than the human heart, with 60-80 bpm. Currently available MRI instruments for mouse imaging operate at a higher magnetic field strength (4.7T or above) than clinical MRI scanners, but they are still unable to provide temporal and spatial resolution in proportion with the mouse heart rate and size. Consequently, the tagging lines extracted from the mouse tMRI images contain more outliers than that from human data, as shown in Fig. 1.

MRI images are widely used for cardiac motion analysis [19]. In particular, the 3D characterization of the mouse cardiac mechanical function has been reported in [5,21,24]. However, all the prior methods assume that the tagging lines are manually labeled or correctly tracked. They cannot handle the tracking errors due to low image quality. To solve this problem, we employ our sparse deformable models to build an automatic strain analysis system based on tagged MRI images.

The system consists of four major components: 1) tagging line tracking, 2) control point tracking, 3) meshless model construction, and 4) meshless deformation. A Gabor filter bank [4] has been implemented to generate corresponding phase maps from low quality tagged MRI images. Then the 3D control points are tracked, based on the tagging lines and the contours of separate slices. The initial 3D meshless model of the end-diastole LV is built based on the sparse 2D contours [22]. First, a standard LV surface model, manually segmented from 3D CT data, is registered to the sample specified boundary using coherent point drift (CPD) [9]. Then a dense 3D point cloud is generated based on the fitted surface. When many LV surface samples are available, methods based on active shape models, like SPASM [2], are able to capture more model details. However, it is hard to collect enough training data in reality. Our method generate reasonable LV model with only one sample. Finally, the initial model is driven by the control points to track the LV movement along a cardiac cycle with our proposed sparse deformable model, and the motion strains are calculated locally based on the tracking result.

3   Experiments

3.1   Validations on Synthetic Data

We tested our sparse deformable models (SDM) on synthetic 3D volumes with known deformation. We first manually generated an LV volume model with the internal points evenly distributed on SA and LA directions. Twenty percent of SA slices with equal intervals were chosen as the control points. We then applied random global transformations, such as scaling, rotation and twisting, to the initial model. Two kinds of errors were applied to the deformed model to simulate the noisy tracking results. Gaussian noise was added to all control points, and a few points were selected randomly and large displacements were applied to them to simulate gross errors. Based on the displacements of the control points, we used the proposed sparse deformable models to reconstruct the displacements of the other points. The deformable models were tested under different parameters and different noise intensities. In each parameter setting, we randomly generated 1000 samples and calculated the mean and variance of deformation errors.

We first analyzed the relation between the deformation errors and the coefficient γ, reflecting the balance between the $L1$ and $L2$ norms (Fig. 2(a)). The sparse deformable models with both $L1$ and $L2$ norms were tested with different γ. The deformation error is large when γ is close to zero, and reduces dramatically when γ is a little larger. The combined norm is more like an $L1$ norm when γ is small. This may imply that SDM with the $L1$ norm alone cannot handle Gaussian error properly. As γ becomes even larger, the mean error increases again. It becomes stable when γ is large enough, and it is similar to the result using only the $L2$ norm. The results show that the sparse deformable models with combined norm outperform the other models that use only one type of norm. Theoretically, the model achieves the best result when the threshold γ is

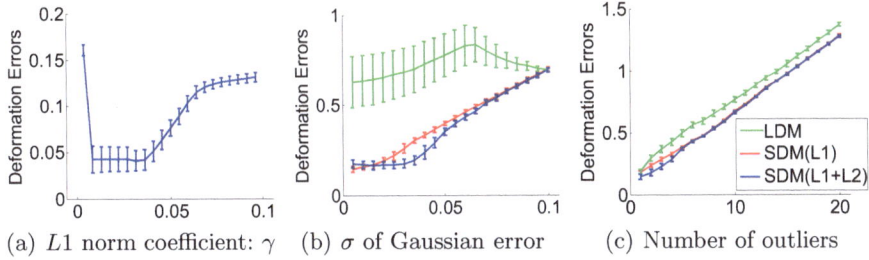

(a) $L1$ norm coefficient: γ (b) σ of Gaussian error   (c) Number of outliers

Fig. 2. (a) shows the deformation errors related to the coefficient γ of the $L1$ norm. (b) and (c) show the deformation errors of different deformable models. They are compared under different Gaussian noise variances and numbers of outliers, respectively. SDM with combined norm out-performs the other two most of the time, while SDM with the $L1$ norm is better when the Gaussian noise intensity is small.

similar to the variance of Gaussian noise. However, it is hard to measure the noise variance exactly in real data. We set it to one tenth of the median of the neighborhood distances empirically and the model shows good results.

We also tested our sparse deformable model under different noise intensities. First, we increased the variance of Gaussian noise with fixed outliers. In Fig. 2(b), SDM with $L1$ norm performs the best when the noise intensity is low. As the variance increases, SDM with combined norm out-performs the others. LDM is always the worst, due to the outliers. This experiment shows that our model is more stable with moderate Gaussian noise. Then we tested the models with different numbers of outliers. In Fig. 2(c), the errors of all models increase almost linearly with the number of outliers. SDM with combined norm, which is still the best among them, performs better than the SDM with $L1$ norm when there are a few outliers. They achieve similar errors when the outliers are dominant. Both of the experiments show that SDM with combined norm is more stable under different noisy conditions.

3.2 Left Ventricle Motion Analysis

We also tested our method on mouse myocardial strain analysis. The strain computation is especially sensitive to tracking outliers. Even when there are only a small amount of outliers on deformation, the strains on points near these outliers will be affected. To obtain ground truth, we manually labeled the tagging lines in each 2D image, and then used the tag motion to drive a 3D LV volume model based on finite element method (FEM). This method is accurate. However, manual labeling is a long and tedious task and FEM is not efficient. In this experiment, we used this method as reference, and compared our models using automatic tagging line tracking results that contain outliers. The results are compared between the LDM, SDM with only $L1$ norm and SDM with both $L1$

and $L2$ norms. Table 1 shows the deformation errors of different models on our 9 datasets. SDM with the combined norm has smaller average error than the others, owing to its robustness to outlier. Meanwhile, the results of SDM with $L1$ norm alone are much more unstable than other two methods. This may be because there is strong Gaussian noise in real data.

We also computed the myocardial strains over a cardiac cycle, which are commonly used to describe the strength of the heart motion. The strains are decomposed into radial, circumferential, and longitude directions, and the shear strains among them. Fig. 3 compares the strains generated with different deformable models on three mouse datasets. The

Table 1. Quantitative evaluation of deformation errors (Unit: mm)

Method	Average	Min	Max	Median
LDM	1.036	0.724	1.635	0.927
SDM, $L1$	2.107	0.437	3.580	2.069
SDM, $L1+L2$	0.482	0.341	0.719	0.469

rows correspond to different types of strains, and the columns correspond to different mice. Each figure contains the strains generated from different models in a cardiac cycle. The numbers of frames in the cardiac cycles may be different on each mouse because of the acquisition procedures. The first column is from a normal mouse, and the other two are from mice with myocardial infarction. We observe that the strains generated from the healthy mouse are larger than from the unhealthy ones. For each individual dataset, the strains generated from the automatically tracked tagging lines are more unstable than those from manually labeled ones, due to the tracking errors. The strains based on LDM are relatively smooth, but this method tends to underestimate the strains. The results from SDM with the $L1$ norm have the largest instability. This may be because of its nature to pursue the sparse solution. Since the control points contain not only outliers, but also strong Gaussian noise, the $L1$ norm cannot handle Gaussian noise stably. The results from SDM with the combined norm best match the reference strains. This shows that our model performs well in the LV motion tracking based on inaccurate control points.

In order to analyze the local heart motion properties, we also visualize the strains on the external and internal surfaces of the left ventricle. Since the points of the surface mesh are all in the initial volume model, where the strains are calculated, we use them as samples and linearly interpolate the strains on the LV surface. The circumferential strains are shown locally on the LV external and internal surfaces in Fig. 4. They indicate larger contraction near the endocardium than near the epicardium. The high strain area begins near the apical endocardium and extends quickly toward the base, which is similar to human hearts.

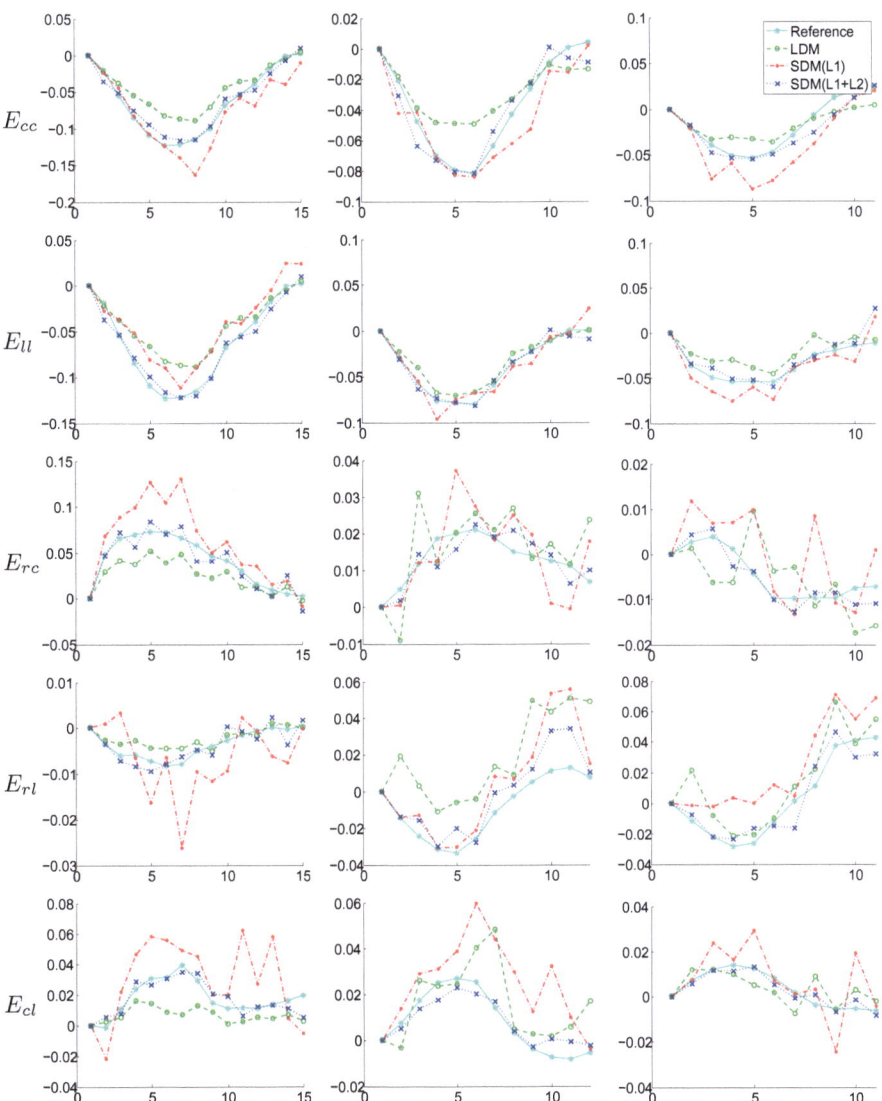

Fig. 3. Comparing the strains generated from different deformable models with the reference model in three mouse cardiac data. Each column represents one dataset, and each row represents one type of strain. In each figure, y-axis is the strain, and x-axis means the frame in a cardiac cycle.

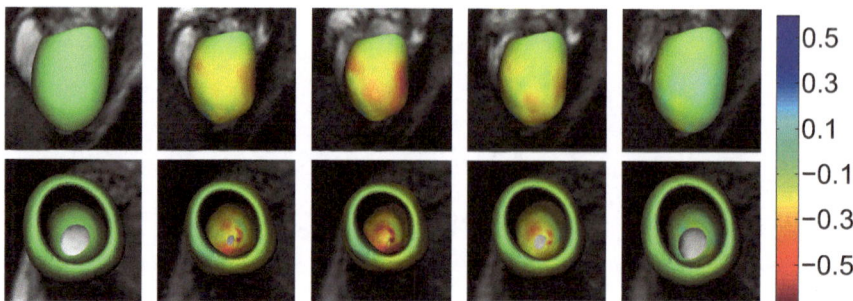

Fig. 4. The deformations of the left ventricle on a cardiac cycle are colored by the circumferential strain

4   Conclusions

In this paper, we introduce a group of sparse deformable models. Benefitted from the sparsity techniques, these deformable models are able to handle outliers or gross errors. Thus these models are robust when dealing with noisy images or tracking errors. We have validated these methods on both synthetic data and a cardiac motion tracking problem. Both qualitative and quantitative results demonstrate that our methods outperform and are more robust than previous ones. It is also noteworthy that the applications of our proposed methods are not limited to cardiac motion analysis. It is flexible enough for many other medical image problems.

In the future, we plan to extend the deformable models by using more constraints or priors. The left ventricle is conventionally separated into 17 segments. This inspires us to add group constraints to the current sparse model. The group sparsity and other structure sparsity constraints will further improve the robustness of the model. The current regularization term is only related to the external force based on noisy observations. It is easy to extend the other parts of the model. The problem for modeling arbitrary internal force is that the resulting model may not be a convex problem. The traditional finite difference method can be employed to find a local minimum, while the performance should then be further analyzed.

References

1. Amini, A., Chen, Y., Curwen, R., Mani, V., Sun, J.: Coupled B-snake grids and constrained thin-plate splines for analysis of 2-D tissue deformations from tagged MRI. IEEE Transactions on Medical Imaging 17(3), 344–356 (1998)
2. van Assen, H.C., Danilouchkine, M.G., Frangi, A.F., Ords, S., Westenberg, J.J., Reiber, J.H., Lelieveldt, B.P.: SPASM: A 3D-ASM for segmentation of sparse and arbitrarily oriented cardiac MRI data. Medical Image Analysis 10(2), 286–303 (2006)
3. Candes, E., Romberg, J., Tao, T.: Robust uncertainty principles: Exact signal reconstruction from highly incomplete frequency information. IEEE Transactions on Information Theory 52(2), 489–509 (2006)

4. Chen, T., Wang, X., Chung, S., Metaxas, D., Axel, L.: Automated 3D motion tracking using Gabor filter bank, robust point matching, and deformable models. IEEE Transactions on Medical Imaging 29(1), 1–11 (2010)
5. Chuang, J.S., Zemljic-Harpf, A., Ross, R.S., Frank, L.R., McCulloch, A.D., Omens, J.H.: Determination of three-dimensional ventricular strain distributions in gene-targeted mice using tagged MRI. MRM 64(5), 1281–1288 (2010)
6. Kass, M., Witkin, A., Terzopoulos, D.: Snakes: Active contour models. International Journal of Computer Vision 1(4), 321–331 (1988)
7. McInerney, T., Terzopoulos, D.: Deformable models in medical image analysis. In: MMBIA, pp. 171–180 (1996)
8. Metaxas, D.N.: Physics-based deformable models: Applications to computer vision, graphics, and medical imaging, 1st edn. Kluwer Academic Publishers (1996)
9. Myronenko, A., Song, X.: Point set registration: Coherent point drift. IEEE Transactions on Pattern Analysis and Machine Intelligence 32(12), 2262–2275 (2010)
10. Nealen, A., Müller, M., Keiser, R., Boxerman, E., Carlson, M.: Physically based deformable models in computer graphics. Computer Graphics Forum 25(4), 809–836 (2006)
11. Paragios, N., Deriche, R.: Geodesic active contours and level sets for the detection and tracking of moving objects. TPAMI 22(3), 266–280 (2000)
12. Radeva, P., Amini, A.A., Huang, J.: Deformable B-solids and implicit snakes for 3D localization and tracking of SPAMM MRI data. Computer Vision and Image Understanding 66(2), 163–178 (1997)
13. Shen, D., Davatzikos, C.: An adaptive-focus deformable model using statistical and geometric information. TPAMI 22(8), 906–913 (2000)
14. Shen, T., Huang, X., Li, H., Kim, E., Zhang, S., Huang, J.: A 3D Laplacian-driven parametric deformable model. In: ICCV, pp. 279–286 (2011)
15. Sorkine, O., Cohen-Or, D., Lipman, Y., Alexa, M., Rössl, C., Seidel, H.P.: Laplacian surface editing. In: SPG, pp. 175–184. ACM (2004)
16. Terzopoulos, D., Witkin, A., Kass, M.: Constraints on deformable models: Recovering 3D shape and nonrigid motion. Artificial Intelligence 36(1), 91–123 (1988)
17. Tustison, N., Amini, A.: Biventricular myocardial strains via nonrigid registration of AnFigatomical NURBS models. IEEE Transactions on Medical Imaging 25(1), 94–112 (2006)
18. Vogler, C., Goldenstein, S., Stolfi, J., Pavlovic, V., Metaxas, D.: Outlier rejection in high-dimensional deformable models. IVC 25(3), 274–284 (2007)
19. Wang, H., Amini, A.A.: Cardiac motion and deformation recovery from MRI: A review. IEEE Transactions on Medical Imaging 31(2), 487–503 (2012)
20. Wang, X., Chen, T., Zhang, S., Metaxas, D., Axel, L.: LV motion and strain computation from tMRI based on meshless deformable models. In: Metaxas, D., Axel, L., Fichtinger, G., Székely, G. (eds.) MICCAI 2008, Part I. LNCS, vol. 5241, pp. 636–644. Springer, Heidelberg (2008)
21. Young, A.A., French, B.A., Yang, Z., Cowan, B.R., Gilson, W.D., Berr, S.S., Kramer, C.M., Epstein, F.H.: Reperfused myocardial infarction in mice: 3D mapping of late gadolinium enhancement and strain. JCMR 8(5), 685–692 (2006)
22. Zhang, S., Wang, X., Metaxas, D., Chen, T., Axel, L.: Lv surface reconstruction from sparse tmri using laplacian surface deformation and optimization. In: ISBI 2009, pp. 698–701 (2009)
23. Zhang, S., Zhan, Y., Dewan, M., Huang, J., Metaxas, D.N., Zhou, X.S.: Towards robust and effective shape modeling: Sparse shape composition. Medical Image Analysis 16(1), 265–277 (2012)
24. Zhong, J., Liu, W., Yu, X.: Characterization of three-dimensional myocardial deformation in the mouse heart: An MR tagging study. JMRI 27(6), 1263–1270 (2008)

A Longitudinal Functional Analysis Framework for Analysis of White Matter Tract Statistics

Ying Yuan[1], John H. Gilmore[2], Xiujuan Geng[2], Martin A. Styner[2,3],
Kehui Chen[4], Jane-Ling Wang[5], and Hongtu Zhu[6,7]

[1] Department of Biostatistics, St. Jude Children's Research Hospital,
Memphis, TN 38105, USA
[2] Department of Psychiatry, and Biomedical Research Imaging Center, University of
North Carolina at Chapel Hill, Chapel Hill, NC 27599, USA
[3] Department of Computer Science, University of North Carolina at Chapel Hill,
Chapel Hill, NC 27599, USA
[4] Department of Statistics, University of Pittsburgh, PA 15260, USA
[5] Department of Statistics, University of California at Davis,CA 95616, USA
[6] Department of Biostatistics, University of North Carolina at Chapel Hill, Chapel
Hill, NC 27599, USA
[7] Biomedical Research Imaging Center, University of North Carolina at Chapel Hill,
Chapel Hill, NC 27599, USA

Abstract. Many longitudinal imaging studies have been/are being
widely conducted to use diffusion tensor imaging (DTI) to better understand white matter maturation in normal controls and diseased subjects.
There is an urgent demand for the development of statistical methods for
analyzing diffusion properties along major fiber tracts obtained from longitudinal DTI studies. Jointly analyzing fiber-tract diffusion properties
and covariates from longitudinal studies raises several major challenges
including (i) infinite-dimensional functional response data, (ii) complex
spatial-temporal correlation structure, and (iii) complex spatial smoothness. To address these challenges, this article is to develop a longitudinal
functional analysis framework (LFAF) to delineate the dynamic changes
of diffusion properties along major fiber tracts and their association with
a set of covariates of interest (e.g., age and group status) and the structure of the variability of these white matter tract properties in various
longitudinal studies. Our LFAF consists of a functional mixed effects
model for addressing all three challenges, an efficient method for spatially smoothing varying coefficient functions, an estimation method for
estimating the spatial-temporal correlation structure, a test procedure
with a global test statistic for testing hypotheses of interest associated
with functional response, and a simultaneous confidence band for quantifying the uncertainty in the estimated coefficient functions. Simulated
data are used to evaluate the finite sample performance of LFAF and
to demonstrate that LFAF significantly outperforms a voxel-wise mixed
model method. We apply LFAF to study the spatial-temporal dynamics
of white-matter fiber tracts in a clinical study of neurodevelopment.

J.C. Gee et al. (Eds.): IPMI 2013, LNCS 7917, pp. 220–231, 2013.
© Springer-Verlag Berlin Heidelberg 2013

1   Introduction

Many DTI studies have specifically focused on the region-of-interest (ROI) and voxel analyses of diffusion properties, such as fractional anisotropy (FA), to delineate white matter maturation and integrity along major fiber tracts in cross-sectional studies [1], [2], [3], [4], [5]. As discussed in [6], [7], [5], standard ROI and voxel-based analyses suffer from serious drawbacks, such as poor alignment quality and the identification of meaningful ROIs. To address these drawbacks, developing fiber-tract based analysis of diffusion properties have received much more attention recently [7], [8], [9], [6], [4], since major fiber tracts are much more objective, specific, and reliable ROIs compared with anatomically defined ROIs. Statistically, several functional regression models have been developed to analyze fiber-tract diffusion properties and covariates from cross-sectional studies [4], [5]. However, cross-sectional studies have limited power in characterizing individual white matter maturation compared with longitudinal studies.

Longitudinal DTI studies have been used to characterize individual change in diffusion properties over time and the effect of some covariates, such as gender, on the individual change in different age groups [10], [1], [11], [12]. A distinctive feature of longitudinal data is that measurements of the same individual usually exhibit positive correlation and the strength of the correlation decreases with the time separation. Ignoring temporal correlation structure in measures would likely influence subsequent statistical inference, such as increase in false positive and negative errors, which may lead to misleading scientific inference [13], [14]. Recently, linear and nonlinear mixed effects models have been used to explicitly account for the temporal correlation in the ROI analysis of longitudinal diffusion properties [14], [11], [12]. Moreover, in [1], a functional mixed effects model proposed by [15] is used to analyze fiber-tract diffusion properties from longitudinal studies. However, since the original mixed effects model in [15] was developed to model the data with functional responses(of time or distance) measured once for each subject, it is inappropriate to directly apply the method in [15] to longitudinally measured fiber-tract diffusion properties, which are essentially infinite-dimensional functional data measured across multiple time points instead of only one time point. These mixed effect models cannot be used to jointly analyze fiber-tract based diffusion properties and covariates from longitudinal studies due to at least three major challenges including (i) infinite-dimensional functional response data measured across time, (ii)complex spatial-temporal correlation structure, and (iii) complex spatial smoothness. According to the best of our knowledge, little has been done on the development of advanced statistical methods to address these challenges.

To fill up such gaps, we develop LFAF for the joint analysis of fiber-tract diffusion properties and covariates from longitudinal studies. Specifically, we propose a functional mixed effect model with two components: a multivariate varying-coefficient model for characterizing the dynamic association between fiber-tract diffusion properties and some covariates and a set of functional random effects for capturing complex spatial-temporal correlation structure. Our LFAF is closely related with a longitudinal functional principal component analysis in [16], but we make three major advances in formal statistical inference as follows. The first one is to develop an efficient estimation method to spatially smooth varying co-efficient functions, while accounting for spatial-temporal correlation structure. The second one is to propose a test procedure with a global test statistic for test-ing hypotheses of interest associated with functional response. The third one is to approximate a simultaneous confidence band for quantifying the uncertainty in the estimated coefficient functions. LFAF provides a rigorous analytical tool for characterizing the dynamic changes of functional response data and their association with a set of covariates.

2   Methodologies

To compare fiber-tract diffusion properties across subjects and populations, we use DTI atlas building with a group-wise longitudinal large deformation dif-feomorphic registration method followed by atlas fiber tractography and fiber parametrization as described in [1], [6] to extract DTI fibers and establish DTI fiber correspondence across all DTI datasets from different subjects at all time points. Since this method has been described in detail in [1], we do not include them here for the sake of space.

The aim of this paper is to present a longitudinal functional analysis pipeline for delineating the dynamic changes of fiber tract diffusion properties and their association with a set of covariates of interest, such as age. We discuss each step of LFAF below and will present the asymptotic properties of all estimators and the test statistic with detailed assumptions and proofs elsewhere.

Functional Mixed Effects Model. Consider a longitudinal study with n independent subjects. Let $s \in [0, L]$ be the arc length of any point on a specific fiber tract relative to a fixed end point of the fiber tract and $\{s_m : m = 1, \ldots, M\}$ a set of M grid points in $[0, L]$, where L is the longest arc length on the fiber tract. Let $y_{ij}(s)$ be a specific diffusion property measured at s and $\mathbf{x}_{ij}$ be a $p_x \times 1$ vector of covariates measured at time t_{ij} for the i-th subject for $j = 1, \cdots, r_i$ where r_i is the total number of time points for the subject i. A functional mixed model is given by

$$y_{ij}(s) = \mathbf{x}_{ij}^T B(s) + \mathbf{z}_{ij}^T \boldsymbol{\xi}_i(s) + \eta_{ij}(s) + \epsilon_{ij}(s), \tag{1}$$

where $\boldsymbol{\xi}_i(s)$ is $p_z \times 1$ vector of functional random effects, $\mathbf{z}_{ij}$ is a $p_z \times 1$ vector of covariates associated with $\boldsymbol{\xi}_i(s)$ and commonly a subvector of $\mathbf{x}_{ij}$, $\eta_{ij}(s)$ is a random function for subject i at time t_{ij}, $\epsilon_{ij}(s)$ is a measurement error, and $B(s) = (\beta_1(s), \ldots, \beta_{p_x}(s))^T$ is a $p_x \times 1$ vector of functions of s. Moreover, $\boldsymbol{\xi}_i(s)$ primarily characterizes the temporal variations and within-subject dependence, while $\eta_{ij}(s)$ characterizes individual curve variations from $\mathbf{x}_{ij}^T B(s) + \mathbf{z}_{ij}^T \boldsymbol{\xi}_i(s)$ and spatial dependence. It is also assumed that $\boldsymbol{\xi}_i(s)$, $\boldsymbol{\epsilon}_i(s) = (\epsilon_{i1}(s), \cdots, \epsilon_{ir_i}(s))^T$, and $\boldsymbol{\eta}_i(s) = (\eta_{i1}(s), \cdots, \eta_{ir_i}(s))^T$ are mutually independent and identical copies of $\mathrm{SP}(\mathbf{0}, \Sigma_\xi)$, $\mathrm{SP}(\mathbf{0}, \Sigma_\eta)$ and $\mathrm{SP}(\mu, \Sigma_\epsilon)$, respectively, where $\mathrm{SP}(\mu, \Sigma)$ denotes a stochastic process vector with mean function $\mu(s)$ and covariance function

$\Sigma(s,t)$. Moreover, $\epsilon_i(s)$ and $\epsilon_i(t)$ are assumed to be independent for $s \neq t$ and $\Sigma_\epsilon(s,t)$ takes the form of $\sigma_\epsilon(s)^2 \mathbf{1}(s=t)$, where $\mathbf{1}(\cdot)$ is an indicator function.

Initial Estimator of Varying Coefficient Functions. We use the local linear regression method and the weighted least squares estimation to estimate $B(s)$ [17]. Since the local linear regression method adapts automatically at the boundary points [17], it is ideal for dealing with scalar diffusion properties along fiber tracts with two ends. Specifically, for a specific bandwidth h, we estimate $B(s)$ by minimizing the following weighted least squares function

$$\sum_{i=1}^{n}\sum_{j=1}^{r_i}\sum_{m=1}^{M}\{y_{ij}(s_m) - \mathbf{x}_{ij}^T[B(s) + \dot{B}(s)(s_m - s)]\}^2 K_h(s_m - s),$$

where $K(s)$ is a kernel function and $K_h(s) = h^{-1}K(s/h)$. The optimal estimator of $B_j(s)$, denoted by $\hat{B}_j(s)$ is obtained at the optimal bandwidth selected by using a leave-one-curve-out cross-validation method.

Estimating Covariance Functions. The covariance structure of $y_i(s)$ plays a crucial role in our proposed inference procedure. We proposed the following estimation procedure to estimate the covariance functions in model (1).

- (I) Use the local constant regression method to estimate $\Sigma_\xi(s,t)$ and $\Sigma_\xi(s,t)$ for each pair $s \leq t$ [17], which yields the estimates $\tilde{\Sigma}_\xi(s,t)$ and $\tilde{\Sigma}_\eta(s,t)$.
- (II) Use the local constant regression method to smooth $\tilde{\Sigma}_\xi(s,t)$ to calculate $\hat{\Sigma}_\xi(s,t)$ across (s,t) and to smooth $\tilde{\Sigma}_\eta(s,t)$ for $s \neq t$ to calculate $\hat{\Sigma}_\eta(s,t)$ across (s,t).

The above procedure cannot guarantee that $\hat{\Sigma}_\xi(s,t)$ and $\hat{\Sigma}_\eta(s,t)$ are semipositive definite. We apply an adjustment procedure in [18] to transform $\hat{\Sigma}_\xi(s,t)$ and $\hat{\Sigma}_\eta(s,t)$ into semipositive definite covariance functions. Its key idea is to approximate the covariance functions by truncating the components corresponding to negative eigenvalues in the spectral representations of $\hat{\Sigma}_\xi(s,t)$ and $\hat{\Sigma}_\eta(s,t)$.

Refined Estimator of Varying Coefficient Functions. In the initial estimation of varying coefficient functions, it is assumed that there are no spatial-temporal correlations. At this stage, we refine the estimate of $B(\cdot)$ by incorporating the estimated spatial-temporal covariance functions for each subject. Let $\mathbf{X}_i = [\mathbf{x}_{i1} \cdots \mathbf{x}_{ir_i}]$ be a $p_x \times r_i$ matrix. We reestimate $B(s)$ by minimizing the following weighted least squares function

$$\sum_{i=1}^{n}\sum_{m=1}^{M}\{[\mathbf{y}_i(s_m) - \mathbf{X}_i^T(B(s) + \dot{B}(s)(s_m - s))]^T \hat{\Sigma}_{y,i}^{(1)}(s_m, s_m)^{-1/2}\}^{\otimes 2} K_h(s_m - s),$$

where $\hat{\Sigma}_{y,i}^{(1)}(s,t) = \mathbf{z}_{ij}^T \hat{\Sigma}_\xi(s,t)\mathbf{z}_{ij} + \hat{\Sigma}_\eta(s,t)$. We also select the bandwidth h by using the leave-one-curve-out cross-validation method.

Smoothing Individual Functions. Let $g_{ij}(s) = \mathbf{z}_{ij}^T \boldsymbol{\xi}_i(s) + \eta_{ij}(s)$ for all i, j. We also employ the local linear regression technique to estimate all individual functions $g_{ij}(s)$ [17]. Specifically, we estimate $g_{ij}(s)$ by minimizing the weighted least squares function given by

$$\sum_{m=1}^{M} [y_{ij}(s_m) - \mathbf{x}_{ij}^T \hat{B}(s_m) - (g_{ij}(s) + \dot{g}_{ij}(s)(s_m - s))]^2 K_h(s_m - s).$$

The optimal estimator, $\hat{g}_{ij}(s)$ is obtained at the optimal bandwidth selected by using the leave-one-out generalized cross-validation method.

Hypothesis Test. We test the null hypothesis $H_0 : CB(s) = \mathbf{b}_0(s)$ for all s against $H_1 : CB(s) \neq \mathbf{b}_0(s)$ by proposing a global test statistics $\mathbf{S}_n$, defined by

$$\mathbf{S}_n = \int_0^1 \mathbf{d}(s)^T \{C[\sum_{i=1}^{n} \mathbf{X}_i \hat{\mathcal{L}}_{y,i}^{(1)}(s,s)^{-1} \mathbf{X}_i^T]^{-1} C^T\}^{-1} \mathbf{d}(s) ds, \tag{2}$$

where $\mathbf{d}(s) = C\text{vec}(\hat{B}(s) - \text{bias}(\hat{B}(s))) - \mathbf{b}_0(s)$. Following [19], a smaller bandwidth leads to a smaller value of $\text{bias}(\hat{B}(s))$. Moreover, according to our simulation studies below, we have found that the effect of dropping $\text{bias}(\hat{B}(s))$ is negligible, and therefore we drop it from now on. The asymptotic distribution of $\mathbf{S}_n$ is very complicated and it is difficult to directly approximate the percentiles of $\mathbf{S}_n$ under the null hypothesis. Instead, we propose to use a resampling method to approximate the p-value of $\mathbf{S}_n$ as in [20], [5].

Simultaneous Confidence Bands. For a given significance level α, we construct a simultaneous confidence band for each $\beta_l(s)$ such that

$$P(\hat{\beta}_l^{L,\alpha}(s) < \beta_l(s) < \hat{\beta}_l^{U,\alpha}(s) \text{ for all } s \in [0,1]) = 1 - \alpha, \tag{3}$$

where $\beta_l^{L,\alpha}(s)$ and $\beta_l^{U,\alpha}(s)$ are the lower and upper limits of the confidence band. We develop a resampling method to approximate $C_l(\alpha)$ as in [20], [5].

3   A Real Example and Simulation Studies

A Real Example. We applied LFAF to investigate neonatal brain development in a longitudinal study consisting of 137 healthy infants (83 males and 54 females) with mean age at the baseline 297.89 days with SD: 13.9 days scanned at 2 week, 1 year, and 2 year. A 3T Allegra head-only MR system (Siemens Medical Solutions, Erlangen, Germany) was used to acquire all the images. The system was equipped with a maximal gradient strength of 40 mT/m and a maximal slew rate of 400 mT/(m · ms). The DTI images were obtained by using a single shot EPI DTI sequence with the following variables: TR/TE= 5200/73 ms, slice thickness= 2 mm, in-plane resolution= 2 × 2 mm^2 with eddy current compensation. In this study, two sequences with 6 or 42 non-collinear directions, respectively, were applied at the b-value of 1000 s/mm^2 with a reference scan ($b = 0$). When the sequence with 6 gradient directions was applied, to improve the signal-to-noise ratio of the images, a total of five scans were acquired and averaged. A weighted least squares estimation method were used to estimate diffusion tensors [21]. Then a DTI atlas building with a group-wise longitudinal large deformation diffeomorphic registration method followed by atlas fiber tractography and fiber parametrization as described in [1], [6] were used to extract DTI fibers and establish DTI fiber correspondence across all DTI datasets from different subjects at all time points. We chose the genu of the corpus callosum to illustrate our LFAF. Three diffusion properties were extracted along the selected fiber tracts including FA, RD, and AD, at each grid point and each time point for all 137 infants.

In this study, we have three specific aims. The first is to investigate the gender effect on the development of the fiber tract diffusion properties. The second is to investigate the number of gradient directions effect on the the fiber tract diffusion properties. The third is to delineate the development of fiber tract diffusion properties over time. As a graphical illustration, fractional anisotropy (FA), axial diffusivity (AD) and radial diffusivity (RD) values were plotted along the genu of the corpus callosum for all subjects within each age group (Fig. 1 (a)-(c)). They were also plotted for 35 selected subjects at a selected grid point (Fig. 1 (d)-(f)). An obvious increasing trend for the values of FA, and obvious decreasing trends for the values of RD and AD were observed at nearly all grid points, especially from neonate to the first year. It is also observed from Fig. 1 (a)-(c) that there is a random subject-to-subject variation in FA, RD and AD measures at each grid point along the two tracts. In addition, Fig. 1 (d)-(f) shows that there is a random subject-to-subject variation in the age effect on FA, RD and AD measures at the selected location. Thus, we use our functional mixed model to fit this dataset and to statistically test the gender, number of gradient directions and age effects on FA, RD and AD values along this tract.

We fit model (1) to the fiber-tract FA, RD and AD values from all 137 subjects, in which $\mathbf{x} = (1, \text{Dir}, \text{G}, \text{Age}_1, \text{Age}_2)^T$, $\mathbf{z} = (1, \text{Age}_1, \text{Age}_2)^T$ and Age_1 (or Age_2) is an indicator variable indicating whether a subject belongs to the first (or second) year age group. The coefficient functions related to Age_1 and Age_2 can be used to investigate whether there is some change from neonate to the first year of life, from the first year to the second year and from neonate to the second year. For the hypothesis testing, we constructed the global test statistic $\mathbf{S}_n$ to test the gender, number of gradient directions and age effects on FA, RD and AD values. We approximated the p-value of $\mathbf{S}_n$ using the resampling method with $G = 5,000$ replications. We also constructed the 95% simultaneous confidence bands for the functional coefficients $B(s)$.

Fig. 2 presents the estimated coefficient functions $B(s)$. The intercept functions describe the overall trend of the three diffusion properties. The coefficient functions of Age_1 and Age_2 for FA (the fourth and fifth rows in Fig. 2 (a)) are positive at all grid points, which indicates that FA increases from neonate to the first year and from neonate to the second year along the genu of the corpus

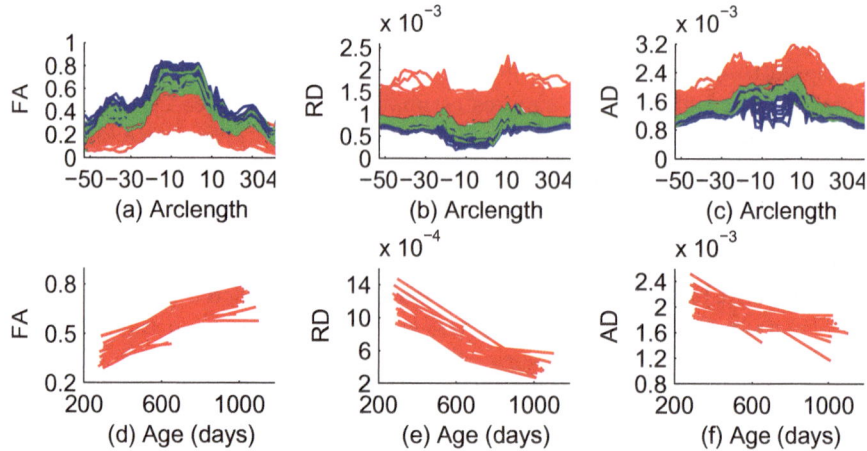

Fig. 1. FA (a), RD (b) and AD (c) values along the genu of the corpus callosum for all 137 subjects in each age group, with red, green and blue colors for neonate, one-year-old and two-year-old infants, separately. FA (d), RD (e) and AD (f) values varying across age at a selected location (arclength=-8.75) for the 35 selected subjects.

callosum, while the coefficients of Age_1 and Age_2 for RD and AD (the fourth and fifth rows in Fig. 2 (b) and (c)) are negative at all grid points, which indicates that RD and AD decrease from neonate to the first year and from neonate to the second year .

It is observed that the coefficients related to the number of gradient directions for FA (the second panel in Fig. 2 (a)) are positive in the central region of the tract, which indicates that compared with FA values obtained by DTI with 6 gradient directions, FA values with 42 gradient directions are larger in the central region of the tract while The coefficients of Dir for RD (the second panel in Fig. 2 (b)) are negative in the central regions, which indicates that compared with RD values obtained by DTI with 42 gradient directions, RD values with 6 gradient directions are larger in the central region of the tract.

Fig. 3 presents mean diffusion profiles along the tract at each age group. FA and AD values in the central region of the genu of the corpus callosum are larger compared to peripheral regions. RD values in the region close to mid-sagittal brain is smaller. They are consistent with general topological rules of white matter maturation as pointed in [1].

The hypothesis testing results show that there are significant age and number of gradient direction effects on FA, RD and AD values, which agrees with the findings in Fig. 2 (a)-(c). FA's, RD's and AD's are significantly different between neonate versus the first year, and between the first year versus the second year with p value $< .0001$, far smaller than 0.05 significance level. It is observed from Fig. 3 that mean FA values increase from neonate to the first year and then from the first year to the second year while mean RD and AD decreases from neonate to the first year and then from the first year to the second year at any

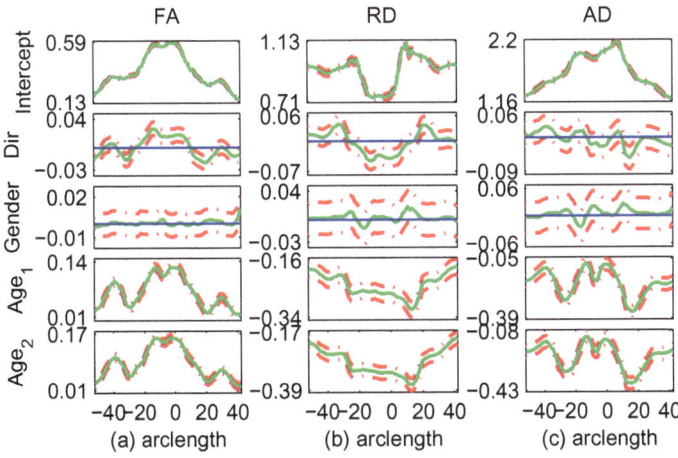

Fig. 2. 95% simultaneous confidence bands for varying coefficient functions for FA (a), RD (b) and AD (c) along the genu of the corpus callosum. The solid curves are the estimated coefficient functions, and the dashed curves are the 95% confidence bands. The thin horizontal line is the line crossing the origin.

grid point along the tract. Moreover, the change from the neonate to the first year is larger than that from the first year to the second year. In addition, the number of gradient directions was found to have the significant effect on FA, RD and AD values. It is shown in Fig. 3 that in general, FA values are smaller while RD and AD values are larger when 6 gradient directions instead of 42 gradient directions is used, especially in the central regions. No gender differences in FA, RD and AD were found for this tract.

Simulation Studies. We conducted a Monte Carlo simulation study to examine the finite sample performance of LFAF . At each point s_m along the genu, the noisy FA's are simulated according to the following model:

$$y_{ij}(s_m) = \mathbf{x}_{ij}^T B(s_m) + \tau_i g_{ij}(s_m) + \tau_{ij}(s_m)\epsilon_{ij}(s_m) \tag{4}$$

where τ_i and $\tau_{ij}(s_m)$ were independently generated from $N(0,1)$ random generators for $i = 1, \cdots, n$, $j = 1, \cdots, r_i$, and $m = 1, \cdots, M$. Specifically, we set $n = 137$, $M = 64$, $x_{ij} = (1, Dir_{ij}, G_i, Age_{ij})^T$ and $z_{ij} = (1, Age_{ij})^T$, where Dir_{ij}, G_i and Age_{ij}, respectively, denote the indicator of different numbers of gradient directions used, gender and age at MRI scanning. To mimic real imaging data, we applied our proposed LFAF method to FA's along the genu from all 137 infants in our clinical data to estimate $B(s)$ by $\hat{B}(s)$, $g_{ij}(s)$ by $\hat{g}_{ij}(s)$, and $\epsilon_{ij}(s)$ by $\hat{\epsilon}_{ij}(s)$. According to our real data analysis, the age effect is significant for our clinical data. So we fixed all functions in $B(s)$ at their corresponding functions in $\hat{B}(s)$ except that the fourth function of $B(s)$, denoted by $\beta_4(s)$, was set as c times the fourth column of $\beta_4(s)$ where c is set at different values in

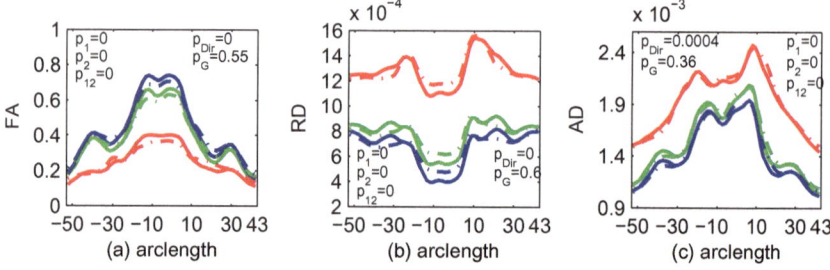

Fig. 3. Mean FA (a), RD (b) and AD (c) values along the genu of the corpus callosum and the gender, number of gradient directions and age effects on FA, RD and AD values. Solid lines are mean FA, RD and AD curves for the 42 gradient direction while the dashed lines are for the six gradient directions. Red, green and blue colors for neonate, one-year-old and two-year-old infants, separately. p_1 is the p value for the difference in the diffusion measure between neonate and the first year, p_2 is the p value for the difference in the diffusion measure between neonate and the second year, p_{12} is the p value for the difference between the first year and the second year, p_G is the p value for the gender effect, p_{Dir} is the p value for the effect of the number of gradient directions.

order to study the Type I and II error rates of our global test statistic in testing the age effect.

We have three aims in this simulation study. The first aim is to examine the coverage probabilities of the simultaneous confidence bands for all varying coefficient functions $\beta_l(s)$ for $l = 1, 2, 3, 4$ in $B(s)$. We only considered the simulated FA measures at $c = 0.1$ and constructed the 95% and 99% simultaneous confidence bands for all $\beta_l(s)$. Table 1 summarizes the empirical coverage probabilities based on 500 replications for $\alpha = 0.01$ and 0.05. The coverage probabilities are quite close to the prespecified confidence levels.

Table 1. Simulated coverage probabilities for varying coefficient functions in $B(s) = (\beta_l(s))$ based on 500 replications at the significance levels $\alpha = 0.01$ and 0.05

c	$\alpha = 0.01$				$\alpha = 0.05$			
	intercept $l=1$	Dir $l=2$	Gender $l=3$	Age $l=4$	intercept $l=1$	Dir $l=2$	Gender $l=3$	Age $l=4$
0.1	0.942	0.930	0.946	0.946	0.992	0.986	0.986	0.980

The second aim is to evaluate the Types I and II error rates of the global test statistic $\mathbf{S}_n$. In neuroimaging studies, some scientific questions require the assessment of the development of white matter across age. We formulated the questions as testing the null hypothesis $H_0 : \beta_4(s) = 0$ for all s along the genu against $H_1 : \beta_4(s) \neq 0$ for at least one s on the tract. We first fixed $c = 0$ to assess the Type I error rates for $\mathbf{S}_n$, and then set $c = 0.02, 0.04, 0.06, 0.08$, and

0.1 to examine the Type II error rates for $\mathbf{S}_n$ at different effect sizes. In order to evaluate the Types I and II error rates at different sample sizes, we let $n = 137$ and 70. For $n = 137$, the values of indicator of number of gradient directions, gender and age were set the same as the 137 subjects in our clinical study. For $n = 70$, we randomly chose 35 males and 35 females from the 137 subjects and used their values for indicator of number of gradient directions, gender and age to simulate the values of FA along the genu tract. We applied LFAF to the simulated FA measures along the genu and approximated the p-value of $\mathbf{S}_n$ by using the resampling method with $G = 500$. For each c, we set the significance level α at both 0.05 and 0.01 and used 500 replications to estimate the rejection rate of $\mathbf{S}_n$. At a fixed α, if the Type I rejection rate is smaller than α, then the test is conservative, whereas if the Type I rejection rate is greater than α, then the test is anticonservative, or liberal. Fig. 4 presents the rejection rates of $\mathbf{S}_n$ across all effect sizes at the two significance levels ($\alpha = 0.05$ or 0.01). It is observed that Type I error rates are well maintained with the values 0.048 and 0.01, respectively, at the two significance levels. In addition, the statistical power for rejecting the null hypothesis increases with the sample size, the effect size and the significance level, which is consistent with our expectation.

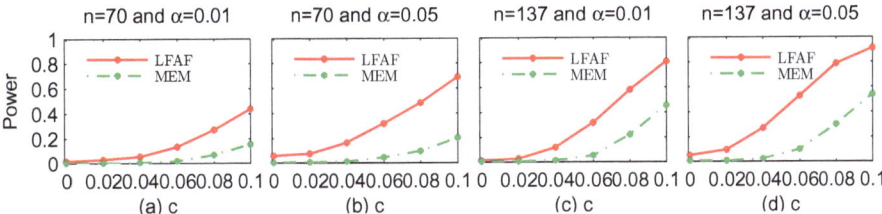

Fig. 4. Simulation study: Type I and Type II error rates as functions of c. Rejection rates of $\mathbf{S}_n$ based on the resampling method are calculated at six different values of the effect size c for sample size 70 and 137 at the 0.01 and 0.05 significance levels using LFAF and MEM.

The third aim is to show that LFAF outperforms mixed model. To this end, we first fitted linear mixed model at each s_m without separating $\eta_{ij}(s_m)$ from $\epsilon_{ij}(s_m)$. Then, we calculated the global testing statistic and approximated the p-values with the resampling method as in LFAF. Fig. 4 shows that the linear mixed model is much less powerful than LFAF.

4   Discussion

We presented a rigorous and efficient statistical method for analyzing longitudinally measured diffusion tensor properties along major white matter fiber tracts and showed that this method has the greater statistical power in detecting the effects of covariates of interest as is shown in Fig. 4 and the greater accuracy in characterizing the uncertainty in estimating coefficient functions as in Table 1. The proposed method was successfully applied to study the normal growth of white matter fiber tracts in the clinical study of neurodevelopment by revealing the complex spatiotemporal maturation patterns as the apparent changes in fiber tract diffusion properties. It can also be used to evaluate the time course of white matter disease induced by the treatment, such as high-dose chemotherapy, in clinical trials. Besides, because of its greater statistical power than voxelwise mixed effects methods, more significant findings could be obtained in the genome wide studies of the associations between the genetic markers with the white matter fiber tract phenotypes by using LFAF.

Acknowledgements. This work was partially supported by NIH grants RO1ES17240, MH091645, U54 EB005149, P30 HD03110, RR025747-01, P01CA142538-01, MH086633, MH064065, HD053000, and MH070890 to Dr. Zhu, NSF DMS 12-28369 and NSF DMS 09-06813 to Prof. Wang.

References

1. Geng, X., Gouttard, S., Sharma, A., Gu, H., Styner, M., Lin, W.: Quantitative tract-based white matter development from birth to age 2 years. NeuroImage 61, 542–557 (2012)
2. Ding, X.Q., Sun, Y., Braass, H., Illies, T., Zeumer, H., Lanfermann, H., Fiehler, J.: Evidence of rapid ongoing brain development beyond 2 years of age detected by fiber tracking. American Journal of Neuroradiology 29, 1261–1265 (2008)
3. Agosta, F., Henry, R.G., Migliaccio, R., Neuhaus, J., Miller, B.L., Dronkers, N.F., Brambati, S.M., Filippi, M., Ogar, J.M., Wilson, S.M., Gorno-Tempini, M.L.: Language networks in semantic dementia. Brain 133, 286–299 (2010)
4. Zhu, H., Styner, M., Tang, N., Liu, Z., Lin, W., Gilmore, J.H.: Frats: Functional regression analysis of dti tract statistics. IEEE Trans. Med. Imaging 29, 1039–1049 (2010)
5. Zhu, H., Kong, L., Li, R., Styner, M., Gerig, G., Lin, W., Gilmore, J.H.: Fadtts: Functional analysis of diffusion tensor tract statistics. NeuroImage 56, 1412–1425 (2011)
6. Goodlett, C.B., Fletcher, P.T., Gilmore, J.H., Gerig, G.: Group analysis of dti fiber tract statistics with application to neurodevelopment. NeuroImage 142, S133–S142 (2009)
7. Smith, S.M., Jenkinson, M., Johansen-Berg, H., Rueckert, D., Nichols, T.E., Mackay, C.E., Watkins, K.E., Ciccarelli, O., Cader, M.Z., Matthews, P.M., Behrens, T.E.: Tractbased spatial statistics: voxelwise analysis of multi-subject diffusion data. NeuroImage 31, 1487–1505 (2006)
8. O'Donnell, L.J., Westin, C.-F., Golby, A.J.: Tract-based morphometry for white matter group analysis. Neuroimage 45, 832–844 (2009)
9. Yushkevich, P.A., Zhang, H., Simon, T.J., Gee, J.C.: Structure-specific statistical mapping of white matter tracts. Neuroimage 41, 448–461 (2008)
10. Evans, A.C., Brain Development Cooperative Group: The nih mri study of normal brain development. NeuroImage 30, 184–202 (2006)

11. Lebel, C., Beaulieu, C.: Longitudinal development of human brain wiring continues from childhood into adulthood. The Journal of Neuroscience 31, 10937–10947 (2011)
12. Sadeghi, N., Prastawa, M., Fletcher, P.T., Wolff, J., Gilmore, J.H., Gerig, G.: Regional characterization of longitudinal dt-mri to study white matter maturation of the early developing brain. NeuroImage (in press, 2013)
13. Diggle, P., Heagerty, P., Liang, K.Y., Zeger, S.: Analysis of Longitudinal Data, 2nd edn. Oxford University Press, New York (2002)
14. Fitzmaurice, G.M., Laird, N.M., Ware, J.H.: Applied Longitudinal Analysis. Wiley, New York (2004)
15. Guo, W.: Functional mixed effects models. Biometrics 58, 121–128 (2002)
16. Greven, S., Crainiceanu, C., Caffo, B., Reich, D.: Longitudinal functional principal component analysis. Electron. J. Statist. 4, 1022–1054 (2010)
17. Wand, M.P., Jones, M.C.: Kernel Smoothing. Chapman and Hall, London (1995)
18. Hall, P., Muller, H.G., Yao, F.: Modelling sparse generalized longitudinal observations with latent gaussian processes. J. R. Statist. Soc. B 70, 703–723 (2008)
19. Fan, J., Zhang, W.: Simultaneous confidence bands and hypothesis testing in varying-coefficient models. Scand. J. Statist. 27(4), 715–731 (2000)
20. van der Vaar, A.W., Wellner, J.A.: Weak Convergence and Empirical Processes. Springer-Verlag Inc. (1996)
21. Basser, P.J., Mattiello, J., LeBihan, D.: MR diffusion tensor spectroscopy and imaging. Biophysical Journal 66, 259–267 (1994)

Groupwise Simultaneous Manifold Alignment for High-Resolution Dynamic MR Imaging of Respiratory Motion

Christian F. Baumgartner[1], Christoph Kolbitsch[1], Jamie R. McClelland[2], Daniel Rueckert[3], and Andrew P. King[1]

[1] Division of Imaging Sciences & Biomedical Engineering, King's College London, UK
[2] Centre for Medical Image Computing, University College London, UK
[3] Biomedical Image Analysis Group, Department of Computing, Imperial College London, UK
christian.baumgartner@kcl.ac.uk

Abstract. Respiratory motion is a complicating factor for many applications in medical imaging and there is significant interest in dynamic imaging that can be used to estimate such motion. Magnetic resonance imaging (MRI) is an attractive modality for motion estimation but current techniques cannot achieve good image contrast inside the lungs. Manifold learning is a powerful tool to discover the underlying structure of high-dimensional data. Aligning the manifolds of multiple datasets can be useful to establish relationships between different types of data. However, the current state-of-the-art in manifold alignment is not robust to the wide variations in manifold structure that may occur in clinical datasets. In this work we propose a novel, fully automatic technique for the simultaneous alignment of large numbers of manifolds with varying manifold structure. We apply the technique to reconstruct high-resolution and high-contrast dynamic 3D MRI images from multiple 2D datasets for the purpose of respiratory motion estimation. The proposed method is validated on synthetic data with known ground truth and real data. We demonstrate that our approach can be applied to reconstruct significantly more accurate and consistent dynamic images of the lungs compared to the current state-of-the-art in manifold alignment.

Keywords: Manifold learning, manifold alignment, MRI of the lungs, respiratory motion.

1 Introduction

Respiration is a complicating factor for many imaging techniques and image-guided interventions [10]. Motion caused by breathing is very complex with significant variations between respiratory cycles (inter-cycle variation), and also between inspiration and expiration (intra-cycle variation) [15,11].

Magnetic resonance imaging (MRI) offers an attractive means to image this complex motion because of its non-ionizing nature and high soft tissue contrast.

J.C. Gee et al. (Eds.): IPMI 2013, LNCS 7917, pp. 232–243, 2013.

Many attempts have been made to estimate and model respiratory motion from MRI [9,6], but the state-of-the-art is limited by current MRI technology. Dynamic 3D scans suffer from poor contrast in the lungs, low image resolution, and relatively long acquisition times, which can lead to motion blurring. Dynamic 2D scans, on the other hand, can be acquired in a shorter time frame, have excellent in-plane resolution and high contrast in the lungs due to the in-flow of unpolarised blood, but lack the coverage of 3D scans. This is illustrated in Fig. 1. In this paper we propose a novel technique, based on manifold alignment, for combining the excellent contrast of dynamic 2D scans with the full thorax coverage of dynamic 3D scans.

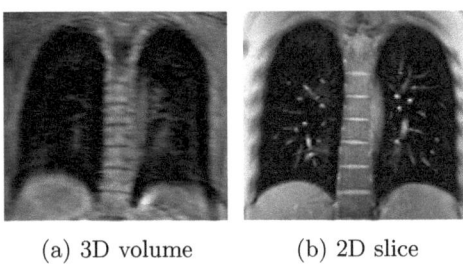

(a) 3D volume   (b) 2D slice

Fig. 1. Comparison of (a) a coronal slice through a dynamic 3D MRI volume; (b) a coronal dynamic 2D MRI slice. The 2D slice has much improved contrast inside the lungs due to the in-flow of unpolarised blood.

Manifold learning is a powerful tool for non-linear dimensionality reduction of complex high-dimensional data and various manifold learning algorithms such as locally linear embedding (LLE) [12] or Laplacian eigenmaps (LEM) [1] have been proposed. In recent years manifold learning was shown to be useful in the analysis of motion in medical images. Recent applications include the region-wise separation of cardiac and respiratory motion [2], retrospective reconstruction of respiratory-gated lung computed tomography volumes [4] and extraction of respiratory gating navigators from MRI and ultrasound images [16].

Manifold alignment can be used to establish correspondences between multiple related datasets, which are not directly comparable in high-dimensional space, but have a similar low-dimensional manifold structure. There are two general approaches to manifold alignment: 1) The datasets are embedded in a common low-dimensional space in a single *simultaneous* embedding, either with prior knowledge of corresponding points [5,18], or without such knowledge, e.g. Joint Manifold Representation (JMR) [13]; 2) The datasets are embedded *separately*, and are then transformed to the same coordinate system in a subsequent alignment step either with known correspondences using a shape matching technique like Procrustes analysis [17], or without known correspondences using simple normalisation [4].

Although manifold alignment has proved effective at solving synthetic problems in computer vision, such as aligning the manifolds of video images of rotating 3D objects [5,13], there have been very few applications of these techniques to real-world problems in medical imaging. To the best of our knowledge, the only such example is that by Bhatia et al. [2] who simultaneously aligned manifolds arising from different image patches in a hierarchical framework.

In this paper we show that the current state-of-the-art in manifold alignment is not robust to the wide variations in manifold structure which occur in real clinical images. We propose a novel method based on simultaneous group-wise embedding of datasets for the robust alignment of underlying manifolds without prior knowledge of correspondences. The method is demonstrated by retrospectively reconstructing dynamic high-resolution 3D MRI volumes from slice-by-slice 2D acquisitions. Such volumes can be used to estimate motion in the lungs, and have potential application in any scheme for which retrospective MRI-based respiratory motion estimates are required. One such application is the use of MRI data to motion-correct simultaneously acquired positron emission tomography (PET) data [14].

2   Theory

In the following we develop notation and theory for aligning the manifolds of large numbers of datasets by simultaneously embedding them in a groupwise framework.

2.1   Simultaneous Embedding of Two Datasets

In this section notation is established based on the example of simultaneously embedding two datasets. The derivations are conceptually similar to [5].

Given two high-dimensional datasets $\mathbf{X_1}, \mathbf{X_2}$, for each element $\mathbf{X}_i^{(1)}, \mathbf{X}_j^{(2)} \in \mathbb{R}^D$, we want to obtain the aligned embeddings $\mathbf{Y_1}, \mathbf{Y_2}$ with elements $\mathbf{Y}_i^{(1)}, \mathbf{Y}_j^{(2)} \in \mathbb{R}^d : d \ll D$. The total embedding error can be expressed as:

$$\phi_{tot}(\mathbf{Y_1}, \mathbf{Y_2}) = \phi_1(\mathbf{Y_1}) + \phi_2(\mathbf{Y_2}) + \mu \cdot \phi_{12}(\mathbf{Y_1}, \mathbf{Y_2}), \tag{1}$$

where ϕ_1, ϕ_2, are the *intra-dataset* embedding errors and ϕ_{12} is the *inter-dataset* embedding error. The weighting parameter μ regulates the influence of the inter-dataset error term. Increasing μ forces the embeddings to be closer together, but setting it too high may alter the natural manifold structure of the data.

In contrast to most related manifold alignment works, which extend LEM [2,13], here we chose a LLE-based intra-dataset error term. As will be discussed in Section 4, a LEM type cost function was also investigated, but extending LLE proved advantageous.

LLE tries to preserve locally linear relations of the high-dimensional data in the low-dimensional embeddings. It is assumed that each high-dimensional point can be reasonably well reconstructed as a linear combination of its k nearest neighbours. The optimal reconstruction weights W_{ij} for each point i from its respective neighbours j can be calculated in closed form as described in [12].

The intra-dataset embedding errors, ϕ_1, and ϕ_2, which preserve the local relations of the high-dimensional data can then be expressed as

$$\phi_m(\mathbf{Y_m}) = \sum_i \left(Y_i^{(m)} - \sum_{j\in\eta(i)} W_{ij}^{(m)} Y_j^{(m)} \right)^2, \quad m \in \{1,2\}, \tag{2}$$

where, for each dataset respectively, $\eta(i)$ is the neighbourhood of data point i.

For the inter-dataset error a different cost function is used. The embedding error of $\mathbf{Y_1}$, and $\mathbf{Y_2}$ is defined as

$$\phi_{12}(\mathbf{Y_1},\mathbf{Y_2}) = \sum_{i,j} \left(Y_i^{(1)} - Y_j^{(2)} \right)^2 U_{ij}, \tag{3}$$

where $U_{ij} = K(X_i^{(1)}, X_j^{(2)})$ is a (non-symmetric) similarity kernel. For high similarity values U_{ij} the error can only be minimised if $Y_i^{(1)}$, and $Y_j^{(2)}$ are close in the simultaneous embedding. The similarity kernel is application specific and may consist of a priori known labels [5,18], or image similarities [13].

With these choices of embedding error functions the minimisation of the whole cost function ϕ_{tot} can be rewritten in a single matrix expression,

$$\operatorname*{argmin}_{\mathbf{Y_1},\mathbf{Y_2}} Tr \left(\begin{bmatrix} \mathbf{Y_1} \\ \mathbf{Y_2} \end{bmatrix}^T \begin{bmatrix} \mathbf{M_1} + \mu\mathbf{D_1} & -\mu\mathbf{U} \\ -\mu\mathbf{U}^T & \mathbf{M_2} + \mu\mathbf{D_2} \end{bmatrix} \begin{bmatrix} \mathbf{Y_1} \\ \mathbf{Y_2} \end{bmatrix} \right), \tag{4}$$

where $\mathbf{D_1}$ and $\mathbf{D_2}$ are the row and column sums of $\mathbf{U}$ as diagonal matrices, i.e. $D_{ii}^{(1)} = \sum_j U_{ij}$ and $D_{jj}^{(2)} = \sum_i U_{ij}$, and $\mathbf{M_1}$ and $\mathbf{M_2}$, are the recentred reconstruction weight matrices $\mathbf{M_m} = (\mathbf{I} - \mathbf{W_m})^T (\mathbf{I} - \mathbf{W_m})$. This problem now has the same form as the standard LLE embedding [12], that is,

$$\operatorname*{argmin}_{\mathbf{V}} Tr(\mathbf{V}^T \mathbf{L} \mathbf{V}), \tag{5}$$

where $\mathbf{L}$ is the augmented matrix from Eq. (4) and $\mathbf{V}$ are the augmented embeddings. Under the constraint that $\mathbf{V}^T\mathbf{V} = \mathbf{I}$, the simultaneous aligned embedding is given by the second smallest to the $(d+1)$-th smallest eigenvectors of $\mathbf{L}$.

2.2 Groupwise Simultaneous Embedding of Multiple Datasets

Eq. (4) can be easily extended to three or more manifolds by further augmenting $\mathbf{V}$ and $\mathbf{L}$, as was described e.g. in [13]. However, this approach is not optimal for multiple reasons, in particular: 1) The problem becomes increasingly unstable when increasing the number of datasets $\mathbf{X_i}$; 2) The manifold structure may not be similar enough across all datasets to justify a simultaneous embedding of all of them.

To overcome these limitations, we propose a novel scheme to embed the datasets simultaneously in overlapping groups of two, producing a much more stable problem. For N high-dimensional inputs $\mathbf{X_1}, \ldots, \mathbf{X_N}$, the datasets are embedded in $N - 1$ groups $\mathcal{G}^{(p)}$. Each group contains the simultaneous embeddings of two datasets $\mathbf{X_p}$, and $\mathbf{X_{p+1}}$, i.e. $\mathcal{G}_1^{(p)} = \mathbf{Y_p}$, and $\mathcal{G}_2^{(p)} = \mathbf{Y_{p+1}}$. The groups are interleaved such that $\mathcal{G}_2^{(p)} = \mathcal{G}_1^{(p+1)}$. Fig. 2 shows an example of a groupwise embedding in $d = 2$ dimensions and the relations between the groups.

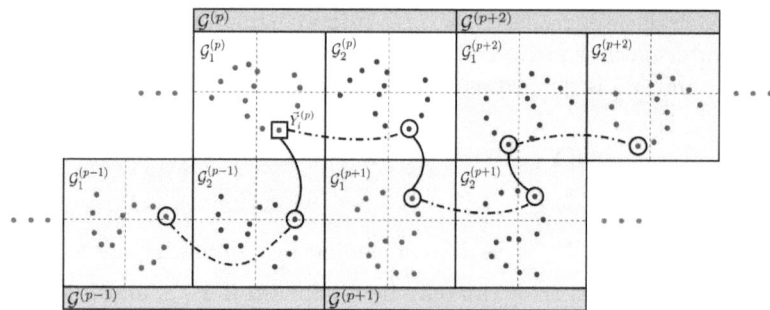

Fig. 2. Schematic illustration of groupwise manifold alignment. The curved lines illustrate the manifold connections through the group overlap (solid), or through aligned embedding (dotted).

By embedding the datasets in overlapping groups the manifolds are all aligned. The two members of each group are aligned due to the simultaneous embedding, and the connections to the next group are deterministically known through the group overlap. For example, consider an arbitrary embedded point i in manifold p, i.e. $\mathbf{Y}_i^{(p)}$ (labelled with a square in Fig. 2), which is embedded in the first member manifold of group $\mathcal{G}^{(p)}$, i.e. $\mathcal{G}_1^{(p)} = \mathbf{Y_p}$. Since within the group the manifolds are aligned, the closest neighbour on $\mathbf{Y_{p+1}} = \mathcal{G}_2^{(p)}$ can be found directly (see dotted lines in Fig. 2). The two points ($\mathbf{Y_p}$, and $\mathbf{Y_{p+1}}$) can be looked up in the neighbouring groups since $\mathcal{G}_1^{(p)} = \mathcal{G}_2^{(p-1)}$ and $\mathcal{G}_2^{(p)} = \mathcal{G}_1^{(p+1)}$ (see solid lines in Fig. 2). In this manner the corresponding embeddings on all manifolds can be found iteratively.

2.3   Inter-dataset Similarity Kernel Sparsification

Typically techniques that do not assume any a priori known correspondences evaluate the inter-dataset similarity kernel $U_{ij} = K(\mathbf{X}_i^{(r)}, \mathbf{X}_j^{(q)})$ (see Eq. 3) on all possible bipartite connections between two datasets. However, not all connections are desirable, and typically the graph is sparsified. The standard approach for sparsification is to keep only the k nearest neighbours for each data point. This may lead to unevenly distributed connectivities, which will distort the embedding. The JMR technique [13] instead performs an orthogonalisation step of the matrix representation of the full graph.

In this paper, we propose a sparsification technique based on a global bipartite maximum edge similarity (MES) matching. We calculate the matching in which every data point in $\mathbf{X_r}$ is connected to exactly one data point in $\mathbf{X_q}$, and the sum of similarities over the corresponding edges U_{ij} is maximised. Fig. 3 illustrates this process. The bipartite matching that maximises the similarity is highlighted in red. This is equivalent to a combinatorial optimisation problem and can be solved using the Hungarian method [8].

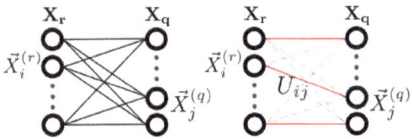

Fig. 3. Graph sparsification of similarity kernel. The left figure shows the fully connected graph, and the right figure shows the optimal one-to-one mapping.

The resulting graph can be written as a sparse matrix $\mathbf{U}$, which in every row and every column has exactly one non-zero entry, $0 < U_{ij} \leq 1$. The values represent the likelihood that the connection between $\boldsymbol{X}_i^{(r)}$ and $\boldsymbol{X}_j^{(q)}$ is correct.

3   Materials and Methods

In this section we show how our method can be used to reconstruct high-resolution 3D MRI volumes from sequentially acquired 2D MRI slices.

3.1   Application of Groupwise Manifold Alignment

We image the volume of interest by sequentially acquiring coronal slices at shifting slice positions. In order to sufficiently sample all respiratory states the volume is covered several times. The specific acquisition details will be given in Sec. 4.2.

The 2D MRI slices from different body positions are not directly comparable in high-dimensional image space. However, our hypothesis is that, because the underlying mechanics of respiratory motion are the same, the respiratory states at different slice positions lie on similar low-dimensional manifolds.

The low-dimensional representations are not intrinsically aligned. To overcome this we apply our novel groupwise manifold alignment algorithm. We define the 2D image data acquired at a slice position p as the high-dimensional input $\mathbf{X_p}$, and the i-th slice acquired at this position as $\boldsymbol{X}_i^{(p)}$. The groups are chosen such that neighbouring slices belong to the same group. Applying the algorithm we arrive at the aligned d-dimensional embeddings $\mathbf{Y_p}$ for each slice position, where the coordinates of the i-th acquired slice are given by $\boldsymbol{Y}_i^{(p)}$. Note that by virtue of the alignment the respiratory correspondences of $\boldsymbol{Y}_i^{(p)}$ to data from any other slice position are known. Since every $\boldsymbol{Y}_i^{(p)}$ is related to its original data slice $\boldsymbol{X}_i^{(p)}$ a volume can be reconstructed by looking up and combining the corresponding slices from other slice positions.

By reconstructing volumes from the corresponding embedded coordinates in the original acquisition order of the slices, a sequence of high-resolution 3D volumes, one for each time point of the acquisition, can be obtained.

3.2   Choice of Kernel

2D slices which represent different anatomical structures are not directly comparable in image space. However, neighbouring slices are similar to some degree. Since by design the similarity kernel K is only evaluated on neighbouring slices the $\mathcal{L}_2$-distance between images will serve as a reasonable measure. To obtain a similarity measure we define a Gaussian Kernel [1]

$$K(\boldsymbol{X}_i^{(r)}, \boldsymbol{X}_j^{(q)}) = \exp\left(-\frac{\tilde{\mathcal{L}}_2(\boldsymbol{X}_i^{(r)}, \boldsymbol{X}_j^{(q)})^2}{2\sigma^2} \right), \tag{6}$$

where $\tilde{\mathcal{L}}_2$ denotes the normalised $\mathcal{L}_2$-distance, such that the maximum distance is 1 and the minimum distance is 0. The parameter σ governs the kernel shape.

The $\mathcal{L}_2$-distance might be misleading even for neighbouring slices because a shift in space also causes a shift in the diaphragm, which might suggest a misleading change in respiratory position. By using the proposed MES sparsification (Section 2.3) this problem can be avoided. The sum over all the edges of the graph can only be maximised if those misleading connections are avoided.

4   Results

We evaluated our technique on two types of data: 2D MRI slices synthetically generated by extracting slices from warped high resolution 3D MRI volumes (7 volunteers), and real dynamic 2D MRI data (5 volunteers). The first made it possible to test our technique on realistic data with a known ground truth, whereas the second enabled us to test our technique on real data.

For both experiments we aligned the datasets originating from different slice positions using the simultaneous groupwise alignment method (SGA) proposed in this work, and also the JMR technique proposed in [13]. In addition, we performed the experiments on three variations of our technique, in order to evaluate each of the novelties of our proposed approach individually: SGA without groupwise embedding, i.e. with fully augmented matrices $\mathbf{V}$ and $\mathbf{L}$ (see Eq. 4) (SGA.FULL); SGA with a simple nearest neighbour sparsification instead of the proposed MES sparsification (SGA.NN); and SGA with a LEM-type cost function instead of the LLE cost function in Eq. 2 (SGA.LEM). For all examined techniques we empirically determined a good set of parameters before running the experiments. In particular, for all examined techniques we embedded the high-dimensional inputs into $d = 4$ dimensions, which proved to be sufficient to capture most intra- and inter-cycle breathing variations.

4.1   Experiments on Synthetic 2D Data

Fig. 4 illustrates the process of the synthetic data generation, from which we obtained realistic high-resolution coronal slices at different respiratory positions similar to those obtained by real slice-by-slice acquisitions from volunteers.

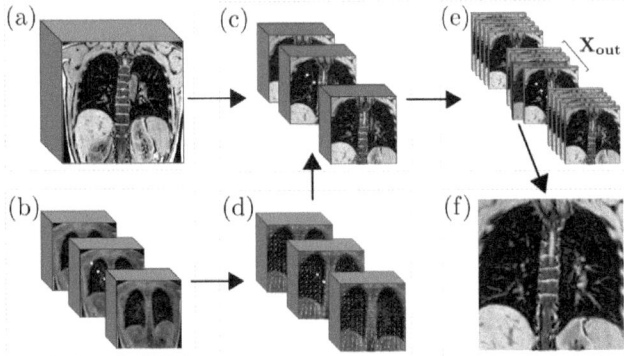

Fig. 4. Generation of synthetic data. A high-resolution breath-hold image such as that shown in (a) was warped to different respiratory states by generating motion fields (d) from 35 dynamic low-resolution volumes (b) [3]. A larger cross-section of a low-resolution volume is shown in Fig. 1a. Groups of slices from the synthetic high-resolution dynamics (c) obtained in this manner were combined to generate synthetic coronal slices with a realistic 2D dynamic slice thickness of 8 mm (e). A close-up of such a slice is shown in (f).

The high-resolution breath-hold volumes such as the one shown in Fig. 4a were acquired with a non-cardiac-triggered T1-weighted gradient echo sequence with an acquired image resolution of $1.5 \times 1.6 \times 1.5$ mm^3. The low-resolution dynamic volumes such as the ones shown in Fig. 4b were acquired with a cardiac-triggered T1-weighted gradient echo sequence with an acquired image resolution of $1.5 \times 4.1 \times 5$ mm^3, and typical acquisition time of 600 ms. Both scans were performed on a Philips Achieva 1.5T MRI scanner.

In order to estimate the performance of each of the manifold alignment approaches mentioned above we used a leave-out-one (LOO) cross validation framework. For each synthetic slice such as the one highlighted in red in Fig. 4e we left out the whole volume it belonged to (labelled by $\mathbf{X}_{out}$ in the same Figure), but not the highlighted slice itself. For the remaining volumes plus the highlighted slice we calculated the aligned embedding using each of the approaches, and reconstructed a volume around the highlighted slice as described in Section 3.1. This resulted in an approximation $\hat{\mathbf{X}}_{out}$ of the left-out volume $\mathbf{X}_{out}$. The reconstruction error was estimated by calculating the $\mathcal{L}_2$-distance, $\mathcal{L}_2(\hat{\mathbf{X}}_{out}, \mathbf{X}_{out})$, between the two volumes. This procedure was repeated for each of the slices originating from each of the warped volumes, and the mean and standard deviation of the $\mathcal{L}_2$-distance were computed as overall measures of accuracy. As the magnitudes of these errors varied widely between volunteers, before combining them we normalised the maximum error to 1 for each subject.

Fig. 5a shows the reconstruction errors for each of the tested techniques over all 7 volunteers. We grouped the reconstruction errors by region of origin of the input slice, i.e. anterior, medial, or posterior. The distribution of the error was symmetric but not normal. Therefore, we used a 1-tailed Wilcoxon signed

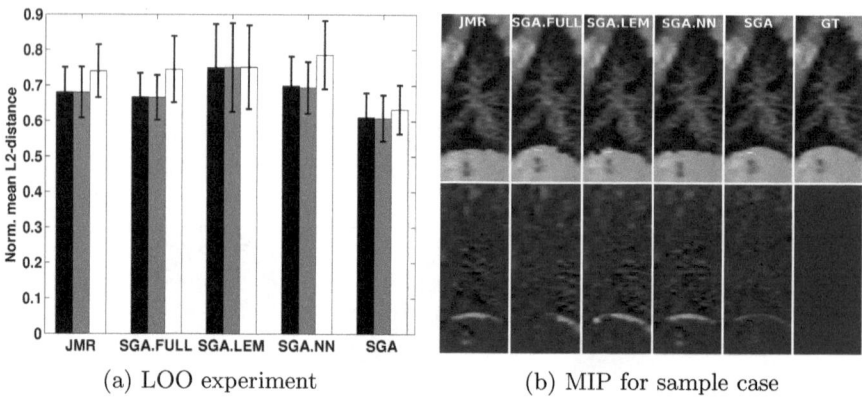

(a) LOO experiment   (b) MIP for sample case

Fig. 5. (a) Mean $\mathcal{L}_2$ distances of synthetic data reconstruction for the tested approaches for anterior (black), medial (grey), posterior (white) input slice regions, and (b) MIP of reconstructed volumes in sagittal direction (top), and their difference to the same MIP of the left out volume (bottom).

rank test and found a statistically significant improvement for SGA versus all compared techniques ($p < 0.001$). In the top row of Fig. 5b maximum intensity projections (MIP) over the right lung of reconstructed volumes for a sample volunteer at an arbitrary respiratory position are shown. The rightmost column contains the MIP of the ground truth (GT). The bottom row contains the differences between the top row and the GT MIP.

4.2   Experiments on Real Data

We validated our method on real dynamic MRI data acquired using the slice-by-slice acquisition protocol described in Sec. 3.1. To maximise vessel contrast, and to minimise cardiac motion, only one slice was acquired per heartbeat at systole. The acquisition time for each slice was 160 ms. The slice position was shifted for each acquisition and to cover the whole thorax typically 15-19 slice positions were needed. Each position was acquired 50 times resulting in an overall acquisition time of 13-16 minutes. The scans were carried out on a Phillips Achieva 3T MRI scanner using a T1-weighted gradient echo sequence with an acquired in-plane image resolution of 1.4×1.4 mm^2 and a slice thickness of 8 mm.

We used the manifold alignment techniques to embed the data from all slice positions and based on the respective embeddings reconstructed a volume for each slice. Thus, we obtained dynamic high-resolution volumes for each time point of the acquisition. We examined the same set of techniques as in the previous section, i.e. JMR, SGA.FULL, SGA.LEM, SGA.NN, and SGA.

Fig. 6a shows MIPs of reconstructed volumes through the right lung of a sample volunteer at a typical end-exhale position (top-row), and a typical end-inhale position (bottom-row).

In addition to reconstructing high-resolution dynamic volumes we evaluated the reconstruction consistency. For each acquired slice we reconstructed a

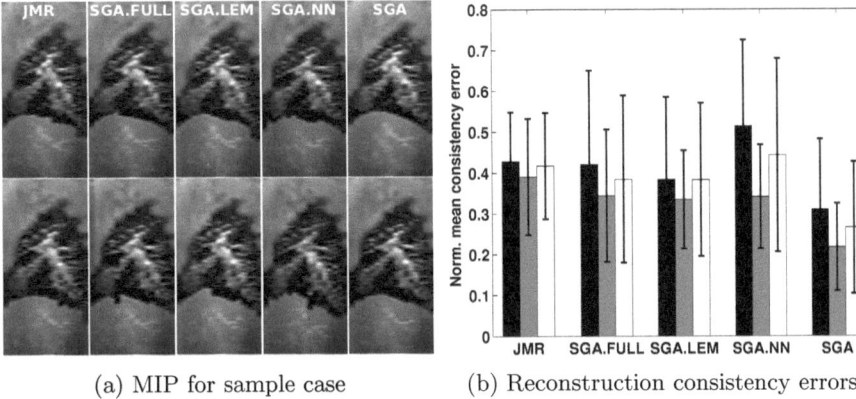

(a) MIP for sample case   (b) Reconstruction consistency errors

Fig. 6. (a) Sagittal MIP through reconstructed volumes from an input slice close to end-expiration (top row), end-inspiration (bottom row), and (b) consistency of reconstruction over different input slice positions for anterior (black), medial (grey), posterior (white) input slice regions for the five tested approaches.

volume $\mathbf{X}$, and for each slice in $\mathbf{X}$ we reconstructed a new volume $\hat{\mathbf{X}}_{\mathbf{s}}$. Ideally, $\hat{\mathbf{X}}_{\mathbf{s}}$ should be equal to $\mathbf{X}$. In practice, however, a different input slice position will give a different reconstruction. To estimate this reconstruction consistency we calculated the $\mathcal{L}_2$-distance, $\mathcal{L}_2(\hat{\mathbf{X}}_{\mathbf{s}}, \mathbf{X})$, for each slice of each reconstructed volume. The mean consistency errors for all the tested approaches are shown in Fig. 6b. In order to combine the mean errors of different subjects we normalised the errors for each subject as before. Again, we grouped the errors by body region of the input slice. Using a 1-tailed Wilcoxon signed rank test SGA's improvements over all other techniques were found to be statistically significant ($p < 0.001$).

5   Discussion and Conclusions

We have presented a novel, fully automatic approach for the simultaneous alignment of large numbers of related datasets based on an extension of LLE to groupwise simultaneous embeddings and a global, MES based optimisation of the inter-dataset kernel.

Applying the technique to the reconstruction of high-resolution dynamic MRI volumes from a slice-by-slice acquisition protocol gave better and more consistent results than the current state-of-the-art for manifold alignment with no known correspondences [13]. On synthetic data with a known GT our method yielded the most accurate reconstructions from all of the tested approaches. On real data our technique gave the most plausible and most consistent reconstructions. For all experiments the proposed method gave good reconstructions from input slices from anterior, medial and posterior body regions, which is important in forming a coherent dynamic sequence, as input slice positions will vary over time.

The experiments showed that each of the elements of the proposed technique, i.e. the MES sparsification, groupwise embedding, and extension of LLE instead of LEM were necessary for robust reconstructions. Generally, we noticed that LLE was better able to capture the subtle intra-, and inter-cycle breathing motion variations that occur in some subjects, than the commonly used LEM technique.

In this paper we investigated simultaneous manifold alignment approaches. Separate alignment without prior knowledge can be performed by simple normalisation [4]. However, this is only reliable for 1-dimensional embeddings, which may not be sufficient to capture all variations in the data.

A different approach to retrospective reconstruction of high-resolution volumes from a slice-by-slice acquisition protocol was proposed by von Siebenthal et al. [15]. The authors used an interleaved slice acquisition protocol where a navigator slice at a constant slice position was acquired before and after each data slice. Manually selected image features derived from the navigator slices were then matched retrospectively to reconstruct a volume. However, in this method only half of the data is actually used for reconstruction, which doubles the already long acquisition times. In contrast our method is fully automatic, doesn't require additional navigator slices and makes use of all the acquired data.

Slice-by-slice 2D acquisitions allow excellent image contrast and make it possible to image vessel structures inside the lungs which cannot be visualised using a dynamic 3D MRI acquisition protocol. These additional structures could be used to extract very detailed and reliable motion fields of the whole thorax, which would have potential application for motion correction of simultaneously acquired PET-MRI data. This could be achieved with minimal scanning overheads, since one slice per cardiac cycle is sufficient to retrospectively obtain high contrast volumes for the entire duration of a PET imaging session. Currently, the volumes only have a high in-plane resolution. Reducing the slice thickness is a natural extension of our work, but will increase acquisition times. PET imaging of the thorax typically takes 15-30 minutes which is sufficient time to acquire enough data for reconstructions which also have a high through-plane resolution.

The proposed technique also has potential application in MRI-guided treatments such as MRI-guided high-intensity focused ultrasound (HIFU) [7]. The aligned embeddings contain information about different respiratory motion states and can thus be seen as a motion model [10]. A volume can be generated from previously unseen data by acquiring a new slice at a convenient slice position and embedding it into its appropriate manifold. In MR-guided HIFU this could be applied for online updating of guidance information.

Acknowledgements. This work was funded by EPSRC programme grant EP/H046410/1. This research was supported by the National Institute for Health Research (NIHR) Biomedical Research Centre at Guy's and St Thomas' NHS Foundation Trust and King's College London. The views expressed are those of the authors and not necessarily those of the NHS, the NIHR or the Department of Health. This work was partly funded by the EU FP7 SUBLIMA project.

References

1. Belkin, M., Niyogi, P.: Laplacian eigenmaps and spectral techniques for embedding and clustering. Adv. Neur. In. 14, 585–591 (2001)
2. Bhatia, K.K., Rao, A., Price, A.N., Wolz, R., Hajnal, J., Rueckert, D.: Hierarchical manifold learning. In: Ayache, N., Delingette, H., Golland, P., Mori, K. (eds.) MICCAI 2012, Part I. LNCS, vol. 7510, pp. 512–519. Springer, Heidelberg (2012)
3. Buerger, C., Schaeffter, T., King, A.P.: Hierarchical adaptive local affine registration for fast and robust respiratory motion estimation. Med. Image Anal. 15(4), 551–564 (2011)
4. Georg, M., Souvenir, R., Hope, A., Pless, R.: Manifold learning for 4D CT reconstruction of the lung. In: Proc. IEEE CVPRW, pp. 1–8 (2008)
5. Ham, J., Lee, D., Saul, L.: Semisupervised alignment of manifolds. In: AI and Statistics, vol. 10, pp. 120–127 (2005)
6. King, A.P., Buerger, C., Tsoumpas, C., Marsden, P.K., Schaeffter, T.: Thoracic respiratory motion estimation from MRI using a statistical model and a 2-D image navigator. Med. Im. Anal. 16(1), 252–264 (2012)
7. Köhler, M.O., Denis de Senneville, B., Quesson, B., Moonen, C.T.W., Ries, M.: Spectrally selective pencil-beam navigator for motion compensation of MR-guided high-intensity focused ultrasound therapy of abdominal organs. Magn. Reson. Med. 66(1), 102–111 (2011)
8. Kuhn, H.W.: The Hungarian method for the assignment problem. Nav. Res. Logist. Q 2(1-2), 83–97 (1955)
9. Manke, D., Nehrke, K., Börnert, P.: Novel prospective respiratory motion correction approach for free-breathing coronary MR angiography using a patient-adapted affine motion model. Magn. Reson. Med. 50(1), 122–131 (2003)
10. McClelland, J.R., Hawkes, D.J., Schaeffter, T., King, A.P.: Respiratory motion models: A review. Med. Image Anal. 17(1), 19–42 (2013)
11. McClelland, J.R., Hughes, S., Modat, M., Qureshi, A., Ahmad, S., Landau, D.B., Ourselin, S., Hawkes, D.J.: Inter-fraction variations in respiratory motion models. Phys. Med. Biol. 56(1), 251–272 (2011)
12. Roweis, S.T., Saul, L.K.: Nonlinear dimensionality reduction by locally linear embedding. Science 290(5500), 2323–2326 (2000)
13. Torki, M., Elgammal, A., Lee, C.S.: Learning a joint manifold representation from multiple data sets. In: Proc. IEEE ICPR, pp. 1068–1071 (2010)
14. Tsoumpas, C., Mackewn, J.E., Halsted, P., King, A.P., Buerger, C., Totman, J.J., Schaeffter, T., Marsden, P.K.: Simultaneous PET–MR acquisition and MR-derived motion fields for correction of non-rigid motion in PET. Ann. Nucl. Med. 24(10), 745–750 (2010)
15. von Siebenthal, M., Székely, G., Gamper, U., Boesiger, P., Lomax, A., Cattin, P.: 4D MR imaging of respiratory organ motion and its variability. Phys. Med. Biol. 52(6), 1547–1564 (2007)
16. Wachinger, C., Yigitsoy, M., Rijkhorst, E.J., Navab, N.: Manifold learning for image-based breathing gating in ultrasound and MRI. Med. Im. Anal. 16(4), 806–818 (2011)
17. Wang, C., Mahadevan, S.: Manifold alignment using Procrustes analysis. In: Proc. ICML (2008)
18. Zhai, D., Li, B., Chang, H., Shan, S., Chen, X., Gao, W.: Manifold alignment via corresponding projections. In: Proc. BMVC, pp. 3–11 (2010)

Conformal Mapping via Metric Optimization with Application for Cortical Label Fusion

Yonggang Shi[1], Rongjie Lai[2], and Arthur W. Toga[1,*]

[1] Lab of Neuro Imaging, UCLA School of Medicine, Los Angeles, CA, USA
[2] Dept. of Mathematics, University of Southern California, Los Angeles, CA, USA
yshi@loni.ucla.edu

Abstract. In this paper we develop a novel approach for computing conformal maps between anatomical surfaces with the ability of aligning anatomical features and achieving greatly reduced metric distortion. In contrast to conventional approaches that focused on conformal maps to the sphere or plane, our method computes the conformal map between surfaces in the embedding space formed the intrinsically defined Laplace-Beltrami (LB) eigenfunctions. Utilizing the power of LB eigenfunctions as informative descriptors of global geometry, the conformal maps computed by our method can effectively align anatomical features on cortical surfaces. By computing such feature-aware conformal maps to a group-wisely optimal atlas surface, which is also computed with metric optimization in the LB embedding space, we develop a fully automated system for cortical labeling with the fusion of labels on a large number of atlas surfaces. In our experiments, we build our system with 40 labeled surfaces and demonstrate its excellent performance with leave-one-out cross validation. We also applied the automated labeling system to cortical surfaces reconstructed from MR scans of 50 patients with Alzheimer's disease (AD) and 50 normal controls (NC) to illustrate its robustness and effectiveness in clinical data analysis.

1 Introduction

Automated analysis of neuro-anatomical surfaces such as the cortex plays an important role in brain mapping research where the ultimate goal is to accurately align corresponding anatomical regions and detect changes across population and time. In this work, we develop a novel approach for computing conformal maps between anatomical surfaces via metric optimization in the Laplace-Beltrami (LB) embedding space of surfaces [1, 2]. Guided by the LB eigenfunctions, the conformal maps from our method have the nice property of being able to align anatomical features and having significantly reduced metric distortion. As a demonstration of these properties, we apply the conformal maps to develop an automated labeling system of gyral regions on cortical surfaces by fusing labels

---

* This work was in part supported by NIH grants K01EB013633, R01MH094343, and P41EB015922.

J.C. Gee et al. (Eds.): IPMI 2013, LNCS 7917, pp. 244–255, 2013.

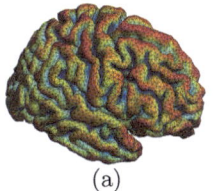
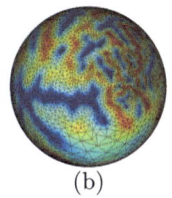
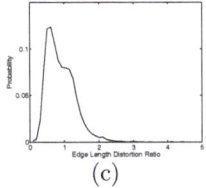

(a)   (b)   (c)

Fig. 1. Spherical conformal parameterization. (a) Cortical surface. (b) Projection of the cortical surface mesh onto the sphere with the conformal map to the sphere. (c) After surface area normalization, the distribution of the ratio of the length of corresponding edges in the mesh of (b) and (a).

from a large number of atlas surfaces. Cross-validation and application to clinical data analysis show that our method can achieve excellent performance.

Conformal maps were used successfully for medical shape analysis problems [3, 4], but the focus has typically been the mapping of surfaces to a canonical domain such as the sphere or plane. Because the canonical domains lack geometric similarity to anatomical surfaces, the conformal maps do not align anatomical features, but rather serve as a parameterization for downstream tasks such as registration [5]. While angles are preserved in conformal maps to canonical domains, large metric distortions are quite common. For example, we show in Fig. 1 the conformal map of a cortical surface to the unit sphere computed with the method in [4], where large variations of metric distortion can be seen clearly because of the geometric differences between the cortical surface and the sphere.

The eigen-system of the LB operator emerges recently as a novel way of studying anatomical shapes. It has been used for many surface classification and analysis works [6–8]. One important development is the embedding of a surface to a high dimensional space with eigenfunctions and the definition of rigorous distance measures[1, 2]. In particular, a surface mapping technique was proposed in the embedding domain with the optimization of conformal metrics[9]. In this work, we extend the method in [9] by establishing the connection between LB embedding and conformal maps, and thus developing a new way of computing conformal maps with metric optimization. As demonstrated in previous works [6–9], LB eigenfunctions are effective global descriptors of surface geometry. Minimizing distances in the embedding space is in effect the matching of these global descriptors, thus the conformal maps derived from metric optimization are *feature-aware* and can align geometric features on anatomical surfaces. Because of this property, there is no need of large metric distortion to match surfaces and the conformal maps generated by our method have greatly reduced metric distortions compared with maps to canonical domains.

Using the proposed metric optimization approach for computing conformal maps, we develop a new system to solve the challenging problem of automated cortical labeling [10–12]. Our cortical labeling system is based on the popular multi-atlas fusion approach in image segmentation [13–15]. Given a group of manually labeled surfaces, we first compute a group-wise atlas in the embedding space and align all individual atlas surfaces to it with metric optimization. To obtain the cortical labels of a new surface, we also perform metric optimization and align it with the group-wise atlas such that multi-atlas fusion can be performed using conformal maps between the subject surface and all individual atlas surfaces with labels. Note that we only need to compute one metric optimization to the group-wise atlas to obtain its conformal maps to all labeled surfaces. This allows the use of a large number of labeled surfaces in our system without significantly increasing the computational cost of the fusion process. In our experiment, we use cortical labels derived from the LPBA40 data set [16] to build the cortical labeling system. Leave-one-out cross-validation shows that our method can achieve accurate labeling of gyral regions. Application to 100 subjects from the Alzheimer's Neuro Imaging Initiative (ADNI) [17] demonstrates its effectiveness in population studies.

The rest of the paper is organized as follows. We first develop the metric optimization approach for conformal mapping in section 2. After that, the multi-atlas fusion system for cortical labeling is developed in section 3. Experimental results will be presented in section 4 to demonstrate the effectiveness of our method. Finally, conclusions are made in section 5.

2   Conformal Mapping via Metric Optimization

Let $(\mathcal{M}, g)$ be a genus-zero Riemannian surface where the metric g is the standard metric induced from $\mathbb{R}^3$. For a function $f : \mathcal{M} \to \mathbb{R}$, the LB operator on $\mathcal{M}$ with the metric g is defined as:

$$\Delta_{\mathcal{M}}^g f = \frac{1}{\sqrt{G}} \sum_{i=1}^{2} \frac{\partial}{\partial x_i} \left(\sqrt{G} \sum_{j=1}^{2} g^{ij} \frac{\partial f}{\partial x_j} \right) \tag{1}$$

where (g^{ij}) is the inverse matrix of $g = (g_{ij})$ and $G = \det(g_{ij})$. Because the spectrum of $\Delta_{\mathcal{M}}^g$ is discrete, its eigen-system is defined as

$$\Delta_{\mathcal{M}}^g f_n = -\lambda_n f_n \quad (n = 0, 1, 2, \cdots) \tag{2}$$

where λ_n and f_n are the n-th eigenvalue and eigenfunction, respectively. The set of eigenfunctions $\Phi = \{f_0, f_1, f_2, \cdots, \}$ form an orthonormal basis on the surface. Using the LB eigen-system, an embedding $I_{\mathcal{M}}^{\Phi} : \mathcal{M} \to l^2$ was proposed in [1]:

$$I_{\mathcal{M}}^{\Phi}(x) = \left(\frac{f_1(x)}{\sqrt{\lambda_1}}, \frac{f_2(x)}{\sqrt{\lambda_2}} \cdots, \frac{f_n(x)}{\sqrt{\lambda_n}}, \cdots \right) \quad \forall x \in \mathcal{M}. \tag{3}$$

This embedding has the nice property of being isometry invariant. Given two surfaces and their LB embeddings, a rigorous distance measure called *spectral l^2 distance* was proposed in [2].

Definition 1 (spectral l^2-distance). *Let $(\mathcal{M}_1, g_1)$ and $(\mathcal{M}_2, g_2)$ be two surfaces. For any given LB orthonormal basis Φ_1 of $\mathcal{M}_1$ and Φ_2 of $\mathcal{M}_2$, let*

$$d_{\Phi_1}^{\Phi_2}(x, \mathcal{M}_2) = \inf_{y \in \mathcal{M}_2} \|I_{\mathcal{M}_1}^{\Phi_1}(x) - I_{\mathcal{M}_2}^{\Phi_2}(y)\|_2 , \ \forall \ x \in \mathcal{M}_1$$

$$d_{\Phi_1}^{\Phi_2}(\mathcal{M}_1, y) = \inf_{x \in \mathcal{M}_1} \|I_{\mathcal{M}_1}^{\Phi_1}(x) - I_{\mathcal{M}_2}^{\Phi_2}(y)\|_2 , \ \forall \ y \in \mathcal{M}_2. \tag{4}$$

The spectral l^2-distance $d(\mathcal{M}_1, \mathcal{M}_2)$ between $\mathcal{M}_1$ and $\mathcal{M}_2$ independent of the choice of eigen-systems is defined as:

$d(\mathcal{M}_1, \mathcal{M}_2)$

$$= \inf_{\Phi_1 \in \mathcal{B}(\mathcal{M}_1), \Phi_2 \in \mathcal{B}(\mathcal{M}_2)} \max \left\{ \int_{\mathcal{M}_1} d^{\Phi_2}_{\Phi_1}(x, \mathcal{M}_2) \mathrm{d}_{\mathcal{M}_1}(x) , \int_{\mathcal{M}_2} d^{\Phi_2}_{\Phi_1}(\mathcal{M}_1, y) \mathrm{d}_{\mathcal{M}_2}(y) \right\}$$

where $\mathcal{B}(\mathcal{M}_1)$ and $\mathcal{B}(\mathcal{M}_2)$ denote the set of all possible LB basis on $\mathcal{M}_1$ and $\mathcal{M}_2$, and $\mathrm{d}_{\mathcal{M}_1}(x), \mathrm{d}_{\mathcal{M}_2}(y)$ are normalized area elements, i.e., $\int_{\mathcal{M}_1} \mathrm{d}_{\mathcal{M}_1}(x) = 1$ and $\int_{\mathcal{M}_2} \mathrm{d}_{\mathcal{M}_2}(y) = 1$.

Because all genus zero surfaces are conformally equivalent, we propose here to minimize the spectral l^2 distance as a new way to find conformal maps between surfaces. Given two surfaces $(\mathcal{M}_1, g_1)$ and $(\mathcal{M}_2, g_2)$, there exists a conformal metric wg_1, where $w : \mathcal{M}_1 \to \mathbb{R}^+$ is a positive function defined on $\mathcal{M}_1$, such that the LB embedding $I^{\Phi_1^*}_{\mathcal{M}_1}$ of $(\mathcal{M}_1, wg_1)$ under this new metric will be the same as the LB embedding $I^{\Phi_2^*}_{\mathcal{M}_2}$ of $\mathcal{M}_2$ because the LB embedding is completely determined by the metric, where Φ_1^* and Φ_2^* are the optimal basis that minimize the spectral l^2 distance. Because $(\mathcal{M}_1, g_1)$ and $(\mathcal{M}_1, wg_1)$ are conformal, and the two manifolds $(\mathcal{M}_1, wg_1)$ and $(\mathcal{M}_2, g_2)$ are isometric when the metric w is chosen so that the spectral l^2 distance is zero [2], we have a conformal map from $(\mathcal{M}_1, g_1)$ to $(\mathcal{M}_2, g_2)$ when we combine these maps. Let Id denote the identity map from $I^{\Phi_1^*}_{\mathcal{M}_1}$ to $I^{\Phi_2^*}_{\mathcal{M}_2}$, the conformal map $\mu : \mathcal{M}_1 \to \mathcal{M}_2$ from $\mathcal{M}_1$ to $\mathcal{M}_2$ is thus

$$\mu(x) = [I^{\Phi_2^*}_{\mathcal{M}_2}]^{-1} \circ Id \circ I^{\Phi_1^*}_{\mathcal{M}_1}(x) \quad \forall x \in \mathcal{M}_1 \tag{5}$$

where $[I^{\Phi_2^*}_{\mathcal{M}_2}]^{-1}$ is the inverse map of the embedding $I^{\Phi_2^*}_{\mathcal{M}_2}$.

To find the conformal map, the critical question is the selection of the metric w such that we can minimize $d(\mathcal{M}_1, \mathcal{M}_2)$. As a first step, we develop the numerical scheme to compute the LB eigen-system given the weighted metric. After that, an energy minimization scheme will be developed to find the optimal weight. Let $(\mathcal{M}, wg)$ denote a manifold $\mathcal{M}$ with the weight metric $\hat{g} = wg$. The LB operator with the new metric is then $\Delta_{\hat{g}} = \frac{1}{w}\Delta_g$ and its eigen-system is :

$$\Delta_{\hat{g}} f = -\lambda f. \tag{6}$$

For numerical computation, we represent $\mathcal{M} = (\mathcal{V}, \mathcal{T})$ as a triangular mesh with K vertices, where $\mathcal{V}$ and $\mathcal{T}$ are the set of vertices and triangles. At each vertex v_i, we denote its barycentric coordinate function as ϕ_i, and represent the weight function as $w = \sum_{j=1}^{N} \alpha_j \phi_j$, and $f = \sum_{k=1}^{N} \beta_k \phi_k$. By choosing $\eta = \phi_i$ as the test function, the weak form of (6) is:

$$\sum_{k=1}^{K} \beta_k \int_{\mathcal{M}} < \nabla \phi_i, \nabla \phi_k > d\mathcal{M} = \lambda \sum_{j=1}^{K} \sum_{k=1}^{K} \alpha_j \beta_k \int_{\mathcal{M}} \phi_i \phi_j \phi_k d\mathcal{M} \tag{7}$$

To find the eigen-system under the weighted metric, we only need to solve a generalized matrix eigen problem:

$$Q\beta = \lambda U(\alpha)\beta \qquad (8)$$

where the matrix Q and U are defined as:

$$Q_{ik} = \int_{\mathcal{M}} < \nabla\phi_i, \nabla\phi_k > d\mathcal{M} = \begin{cases} \frac{1}{2} \sum\limits_{v_j \in \mathcal{N}(v_i)} \sum\limits_{T_l \in \mathcal{N}(v_i, v_j)} \cot \theta_l^{i,j}, & \text{if } i = k; \\ -\frac{1}{2} \sum\limits_{T_l \in \mathcal{N}(v_i, v_k)} \cot \theta_l^{i,k}, & \text{if } v_k \in \mathcal{N}(v_i); \\ 0, & \text{otherwise.} \end{cases}$$

$$U_{ik}(\alpha) = \begin{cases} \alpha_i \sum\limits_{T_l \in \mathcal{N}(v_i)} \frac{|T_l|}{10} + \sum\limits_{j \in \mathcal{N}(v_i)} \alpha_j \sum\limits_{T_l \in \mathcal{N}(v_i, v_j)} \frac{|T_l|}{30} & \text{if } i = k \\ (\alpha_i + \alpha_k) \sum\limits_{T_l \in \mathcal{N}(v_i, v_k)} \frac{|T_l|}{30} + \sum\limits_{v_j \in \mathcal{N}(v_i) \cap \mathcal{N}(v_k)} \frac{\alpha_j |T_{i,j,k}|}{60} & \text{if } v_k \in \mathcal{N}(v_i) \quad (9) \\ 0 & \text{otherwise.} \end{cases}$$

where $|\cdot|$ denotes the area of a triangle, $\mathcal{N}(\cdot)$ and $\mathcal{N}(\cdot, \cdot)$ denote the neighborhood of vertices, and $T_{i,j,k}$ denotes the triangle formed by three vertices: v_i, v_j, v_k.

Because the definition of the spectral l^2 distance includes the max and inf operations, it is non-differentiable with respect to the weight w. To find the optimal weight w that minimizes the spectral l^2 distance of two surfaces $(\mathcal{M}_1, wg_1)$ and $(\mathcal{M}_2, g_2)$, we instead minimize a more tractable energy function. By solving the matrix eigenvalue problem in (8), we compute the eigenvalues and eigenfunctions of $\mathcal{M}_m(m = 1, 2)$ and denote them as $\lambda_{m,n}$ and $f_{m,n}$. Assuming no multiplicity in the eigenvalues, the eigenfunctions are determined up to sign. For numerical approximation, we choose up to the N-th eigenfunctions to define the embedding space, thus the set $\mathcal{B}(\mathcal{M}_m)$ can have 2^N different basis. To match these two surfaces in the embedding space, we minimize the following energy function with respect to the conformal metric w:

$$E(\omega, \Phi_1, \Phi_2) = \int_{\mathcal{M}_1} [d_{\Phi_1}^{\Phi_2}(\mathbf{x}, \mathcal{M}_2)]^2 d\mathcal{M}_1(\mathbf{x}) + \int_{\mathcal{M}_2} [d_{\Phi_1}^{\Phi_2}(\mathcal{M}_1, \mathbf{y})]^2 d\mathcal{M}_2(\mathbf{y}) \qquad (10)$$

When the energy equals zero, we can see that both distances have to be zero, thus the minimizer of the energy also minimizes the spectral l^2 distance. For numerical solution, we represent the surfaces as triangular meshes $\mathcal{M}_m = (\mathcal{V}_m, \mathcal{T}_m)(m = 1, 2)$. For the target surface, we fix its embedding by picking Φ_2 randomly from $\mathcal{B}(\mathcal{M}_2)$. For the surface $\mathcal{M}_1$, we start with uniform weight $w = 1$ and iteratively update Φ_1 and w to minimize E. At each iteration, we first compute the eigensystem and search Φ_1 from $\mathcal{B}(\mathcal{M}_1)$ to minimize E. With the current basis Φ_1 and Φ_2 for embedding, we denote $Id_1(\mathcal{V}_1) = A\mathcal{V}_2$ and $Id_2(\mathcal{V}_2) = B\mathcal{V}_1$ as the nearest point maps from $I_{\mathcal{M}_1}^{\Phi_1}$ to $I_{\mathcal{M}_2}^{\Phi_2}$, and vice versa. Given these two maps, we write the energy in discrete form as:

$$E(\omega) = \sum_{n=1}^{N} \left(\frac{1}{S(\mathcal{M}_1)} \left(\frac{f_{1,n}}{\sqrt{\lambda_{1,n}}} - \frac{Af_{2,n}}{\sqrt{\lambda_{2,n}}} \right)^T U_1 \left(\frac{f_{1,n}}{\sqrt{\lambda_{1,n}}} - \frac{Af_{2,n}}{\sqrt{\lambda_{2,n}}} \right) \right.$$

$$\left. + \frac{1}{S(\mathcal{M}_2)} \left(\frac{f_{2,n}}{\sqrt{\lambda_{2,n}}} - \frac{Bf_{1,n}}{\sqrt{\lambda_{1,n}}} \right)^T U_2 \left(\frac{f_{2,n}}{\sqrt{\lambda_{2,n}}} - \frac{Bf_{1,n}}{\sqrt{\lambda_{1,n}}} \right) \right) \qquad (11)$$

where $S(\mathcal{M}_1)$ and $S(\mathcal{M}_2)$ are the surface area of $\mathcal{M}_1$ and $\mathcal{M}_2$, the matrices U_1 and U_2 are defined in (9) with uniform weight, i.e., the standard metric induced from $\mathbb{R}^3$. Using the eigen-derivatives with respect to the weight functions, we can update the weight function w in the gradient descent direction as:

$$
\begin{aligned}
\frac{dw}{dt} = -2 \sum_{n=1}^{N} & \left[\frac{1}{S_1} \left(\frac{1}{\sqrt{\lambda_{1,n}}} \frac{\partial f_{1,n}}{\partial w} - \frac{\partial \lambda_{1,n}}{\partial w} \frac{(f_{1,n})^T}{2 \sqrt[3/2]{\lambda_{1,n}}} \right) U_1 \left(\frac{f_{1,n}}{\sqrt{\lambda_{1,n}}} - \frac{A f_{2,n}}{\sqrt{\lambda_{2,n}}} \right) \right. \\
& \left. - \frac{1}{S_2} \left(\frac{\partial f_{1,n}}{\partial w} \frac{B^T}{\sqrt{\lambda_{1,n}}} - \frac{\partial \lambda_{1,n}}{\partial w} \frac{(B f_{1,n})^T}{2 \sqrt[3/2]{\lambda_{1,n}}} \right) U_2 \left(\frac{f_{2,n}}{\sqrt{\lambda_{2,n}}} - \frac{B f_{1,n}}{\sqrt{\lambda_{1,n}}} \right) \right]
\end{aligned}
\tag{12}
$$

where $\frac{\partial \lambda_{1,n}}{\partial w}$ and $\frac{\partial f_{1,n}}{\partial w}$ are the derivatives of the eigen-system with respect to the conformal metric. By repeating the above steps for searching Φ_1 and updating w, we minimize the energy function until convergence. The final conformal map is then obtained by the composition of the embedding $I_{\mathcal{M}_1}^{\Phi_1}$, the nearest point map Id_1 and the inverse map $[I_{\mathcal{M}_2}^{\Phi_2}]^{-1}$ as defined in (5).

3   Application for Multi-atlas Cortical Labeling

In this section, we develop an automated cortical labeling system using conformal maps computed from metric optimization. Given a set of P individual atlas surfaces $\mathcal{M}_1, \mathcal{M}_2, \cdots, \mathcal{M}_P$ with manually delineated labels, we first compute a group-wise atlas surface that minimizes its distance to all surfaces. After that, a multi-atlas fusion scheme is developed to automatically assign labels to unknown cortical surfaces.

3.1   Group-Wise Atlas Construction

The group-wise atlas $(\mathcal{M}^*, w^*g)$ we want to compute has the smallest average distance to all individual atlas surfaces. Theoretically we can choose $\mathcal{M}^*$ as any genus zero surface because they are conformally equivalent. In practice, we pick $\mathcal{M}^*$ as the individual atlas surface that has the smallest distance to all other surfaces to speed up convergence. Our goal is to find the optimized metric w^*g that minimizes the following energy function:

$$
E(w^*) = \sum_{p=1}^{P} \int_{\mathcal{M}^*} \left[d_{\Phi^*}^{\Phi_p}(x, \mathcal{M}_p) \right]^2 d\mathcal{M}^*(x) + \sum_{p=1}^{P} \int_{\mathcal{M}_p} \left[d_{\Phi^*}^{\Phi_p}(\mathcal{M}^*, x) \right]^2 d\mathcal{M}_i(x)
\tag{13}
$$

where Φ^* and Φ_p are the LB basis for $\mathcal{M}^*$ and $\mathcal{M}_p(p = 1, \cdots, P)$.

To numerically compute the group-wise atlas, we follow a similar approach as in section 2 for metric optimization. For each surface $\mathcal{M}_p$, we compute its eigen-system and obtain the set $\mathcal{B}(\mathcal{M}_p)$ for LB basis. At each iteration, we compute the eigen-system of $(\mathcal{M}^*, w^*g)$ and denote them as (λ_n, f_n). The basis for each surface is then updated to minimize the energy and we denote them as $(\lambda_{p,n}, f_{p,n})$ for $\mathcal{M}_p$. The gradient descent flow for the metric is then

$$\frac{dw^*}{dt} = -2 \sum_{p=1}^{P} \sum_{n=1}^{N} \left[\frac{1}{S(\mathcal{M})} \left(\frac{1}{\sqrt{\lambda_n}} \frac{\partial f_n}{\partial w^*} - \frac{\partial \lambda_n}{\partial w^*} \frac{(f_n)^T}{2 \sqrt[3/2]{\lambda_n}} \right) U \left(\frac{f_n}{\sqrt{\lambda_n}} - \frac{A_p f_{p,n}}{\sqrt{\lambda_{p,n}}} \right) \right. \quad (14)$$

$$\left. - \frac{1}{S(\mathcal{M}_p)} \left(\frac{\partial f_n}{\partial w^*} \frac{B_p^T}{\sqrt{\lambda_n}} - \frac{\partial \lambda_n}{\partial w^*} \frac{(B_p f_n)^T}{2 \sqrt[3/2]{\lambda_n}} \right) U_p \left(\frac{f_{p,n}}{\sqrt{\lambda_{p,n}}} - \frac{B_p f_n}{\sqrt{\lambda_n}} \right) \right]$$

where $S(\cdot)$ denote the area of surface, U and U_p are defined as in (9) for $\mathcal{M}^*$ and $\mathcal{M}_p$, respectively. The interpolation matrix A_p, and B_p are used to represent the nearest point map between $\mathcal{M}^*$ and $\mathcal{M}_p$ in the embedding space. By repeating the above steps until convergence, we obtain the group-wise atlas $(\mathcal{M}^*, w^*g)$.

3.2 Fusion of Cortical Labels

Let $L_p : \mathcal{M}_p \to \mathcal{Z}$ denote the labels defined on the individual atlas surface, where $\mathcal{Z}$ is a set of discrete labels. Let $I_{\mathcal{M}^*}^{\Phi^*}$ denote the LB embedding of the group-wise atlas $(\mathcal{M}^*, w^*g)$. Using the metric optimization approach, we compute the optimized embedding $I_{\mathcal{M}_p}^{\Phi_p}$ for each surface $\mathcal{M}_p$ that minimizes the distance to $I_{\mathcal{M}^*}^{\Phi^*}$. For a new surface $\mathcal{M}_S$, we also compute its optimal metric w_S such that the distance between its LB embedding $I_{\mathcal{M}_S}^{\Phi_S}$ and $I_{\mathcal{M}^*}^{\Phi^*}$ is minimized. As a result, the LB embeddings of the subject surface and individual atlas surfaces are all aligned and the conformal maps $\mu_p : \mathcal{M}_S \to \mathcal{M}_p$ can be defined easily:

$$\mu_p = [I_{\mathcal{M}_p}^{\Phi_p}]^{-1} \circ Id_p \circ I_{\mathcal{M}_S}^{\Phi_S} \quad (15)$$

where Id_p denote the nearest point map from $I_{\mathcal{M}_S}^{\Phi_S}$ to $I_{\mathcal{M}_p}^{\Phi_p}$.

Using these maps, we fuse the labels from $\mathcal{M}_p(p = 1, \cdots, P)$ with weighted voting to generate gyral labels on $\mathcal{M}_S$. Let $v_i \in \mathcal{M}_S$ be the i-th vertices, and $\mathcal{N}_\Gamma(v_i)$ be the Γ-ring neighborhood of v_i. The correlation coefficient between the mean curvature $\kappa(\mathcal{N}_\Gamma(v_i))$ of $\mathcal{N}_\Gamma(v_i)$ and the mean curvature $\kappa(\mu_p(\mathcal{N}_\Gamma(v_i)))$ of its map on $\mathcal{M}_p$ is computed as:

$$C_p = corr(\kappa(\mathcal{N}_\Gamma(v_i)), \kappa(\mu_p(\mathcal{N}_\Gamma(v_i)))) \quad (16)$$

For each label $\mathcal{Z}_q \in \mathcal{Z}$, its weight is calculated as $W_q = \sum_{L_p(\mu_p(\mathcal{V}_i))==\mathcal{Z}_q} C_p$ and the label of v_i is

$$L(v_i) = Z_{q^*} \quad \text{where} \quad q^* = \arg\max_q W_q. \quad (17)$$

By applying the label fusion approach to all vertices on $\mathcal{M}_S$, we obtain the label map for the whole cortical surface.

4   Experimental Results

In this section, we present experimental results in cortical surface analysis to demonstrate our conformal mapping method with metric optimization. For all experiments, we choose the first $N = 6$ eigenfunctions, and use $\Gamma = 4$ as the size of vertex neighborhood for weight computation in label fusion.

4.1   Conformal Maps between Cortical Surfaces

In the first experiment, we apply our metric optimization approach to compute the conformal map between two cortical surfaces. The source surface $\mathcal{M}_1$ and the target surface $\mathcal{M}_2$ are plotted in Fig. 2(a) and (b). With the iterative algorithm developed in section 2, the energy is minimized as plotted in Fig. 2(c). The final metric w for $\mathcal{M}_1$ is plotted in Fig. 2(d). We can see that it intuitively captures the geometric differences between the two surfaces. For example, the metric w is less than one in the inferior temporal gyral region and shows that $\mathcal{M}_1$ needs to shrink here to match corresponding region on $\mathcal{M}_2$. To illustrate the effect of the metric optimization process on matching geometric features, we plotted the 3rd and 6th eigenfunction of $\mathcal{M}_1$ and $\mathcal{M}_2$ in Fig. 3. As highlighted in regions enclosed by the dashed ellipses, the metric optimization process lead to much better match of eigen-

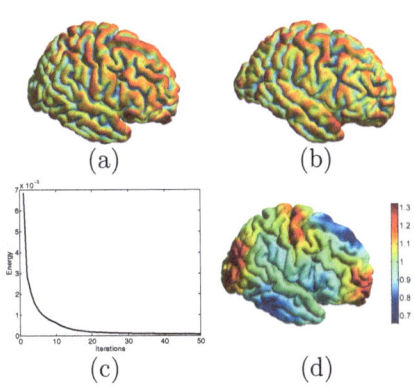

Fig. 2. The computation of the feature-aware conformal map from the source surface $\mathcal{M}_1$ (a) to the target surface $\mathcal{M}_2$ (b). Both surfaces are color coded with their mean curvature. (c) The energy function decreases with the iterative metric optimization process. (d) The optimized metric w on the source surface $\mathcal{M}_1$.

functions in corresponding areas of the cortical surfaces.

In Fig. 4(a), we plotted the projection of the mesh structure of $\mathcal{M}_1$ onto $\mathcal{M}_2$ using the conformal map, i.e., $\mu(\mathcal{M}_1)$, where the mean curvature of $\mathcal{M}_1$ is also carried over to color code the surface $\mu(\mathcal{M}_1)$. By examining the mean curvature map with the sulcal and gyral pattern of $\mathcal{M}_2$, we can see the conformal map very well matches the folding patterns of the surface. Comparing the regular mesh structure in Fig. 4(a) with that of Fig. 1(b), we can see metric distortion is greatly reduced as compared with the spherical map. More quantitatively, we plotted the distribution of angle difference and edge length ratio between $\mu(\mathcal{M}_1)$ and $\mathcal{M}_1$. Compared with the plot in Fig. 1(c), we can see the distribution of the edge length ratio here is centered around one. This clearly shows that the conformal map computed from our method only very well preserves the angle, but also greatly reduces metric distortion.

4.2   Multi-atlas Fusion with LPBA40 Data

In the second experiment, we build the multi-atlas cortical labeling system using the publicly available LPBA40 data [16], which is a set of 40 MR images with manually labeled regions. We first applied a reconstruction method [18] to extract the triangular mesh representation of the cortical surfaces. In this work, we only use

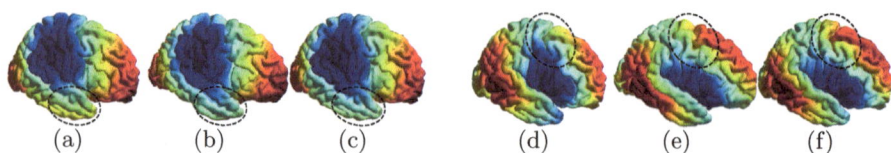

Fig. 3. Metric optimization results in better match of eigen-functions between $\mathcal{M}_1$ and $\mathcal{M}_2$. (a)$f_{1,3}$ on $\mathcal{M}_1$. (b) $f_{2,3}$ on $\mathcal{M}_2$. (c) $f_{1,3}$ after metric optimization. (d)$f_{1,6}$ on $\mathcal{M}_1$. (e) $f_{2,6}$ on $\mathcal{M}_2$. (c) $f_{1,6}$ after metric optimization. Here $f_{m,n}$ denote the n-th eigenfunction on $\mathcal{M}_m$.

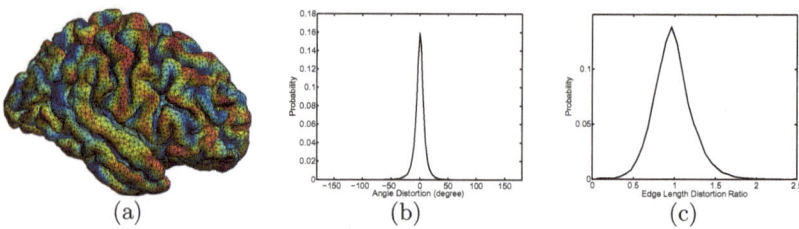

Fig. 4. Angle and metric distortion in the conformal map. (a) Projection of the triangular mesh of $\mathcal{M}_1$ onto $\mathcal{M}_2$ with the conformal map. (b) Angle distortion distribution. (c) Edge length distortion ratio distribution.

the left hemisphere of each image because the two hemispheres are intrinsically similar. A set of 24 gyral labels are projected onto the cortical surfaces to generate the 40 labeled individual atlas surfaces as plotted in Fig. 5 (a). A group-wise atlas is computed with the algorithm in section 3.1 using the 40 cortical surfaces and the result is plotted in the center of Fig. 5 (a), where the surface is color coded with the optimized metric. We also applied multi-dimensional scaling (MDS) analysis to the individual atlas surfaces and the group-wise atlas and projected them onto a 2D plane shown in Fig. 5(b), where the spectral l^2 distance between surfaces are used in MDS analysis. From this plot we can see that the group-wise atlas moves the initial surface, which provides the geometric representation for the atlas, toward a more centralized location in this population.

Using the 40 labeled surfaces, we validated our multi-atlas fusion algorithm in section 3.2 with leave-one-out cross-validation. Note that the group-wise atlas serves only as a *geometric* target for aligning LB embeddings and does not contain label information, thus it is fixed during the cross-validation. For each surface, we obtain its label by fusing the labels from the other 39 surfaces, and the Dice coefficient is computed for each gyral region by comparing with the manual labels. By repeating this process 40 times, we obtain the mean and standard deviation of Dice coefficients for each of the 24 gyral regions and show them collectively as bar plots in Fig. 5(c). The average Dice coefficient is 0.82 across all regions and surfaces. In an extensive validation study [19], for both state-of-the-art surface-based and volume-based registration methods, the mean Dice is below 0.8 on the same data. This shows that our method is able to achieve excellent performance in automated cortical labeling.

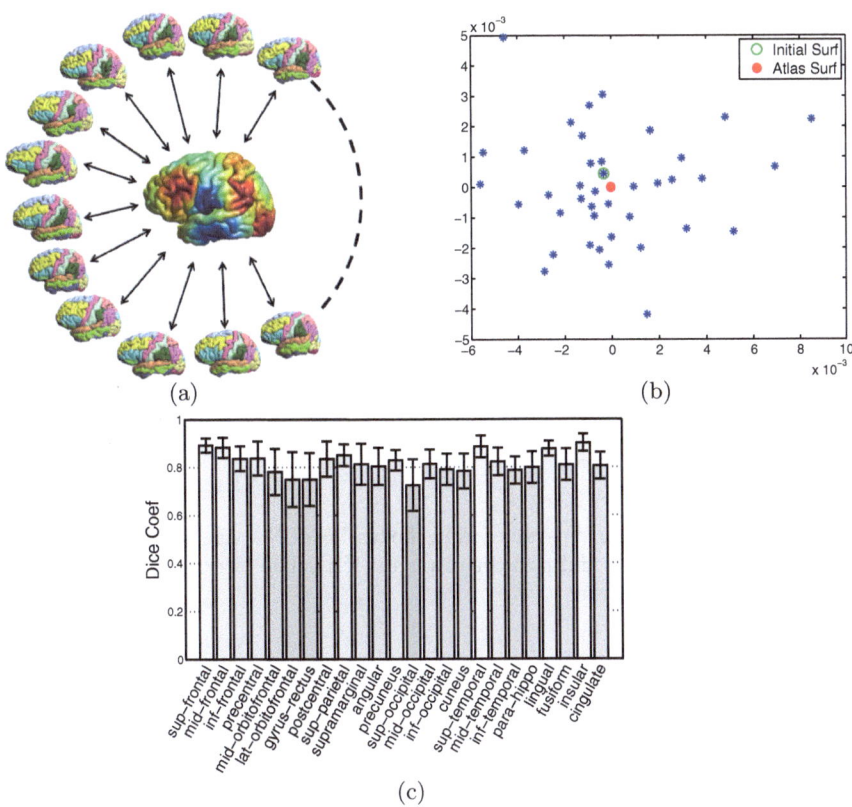

Fig. 5. Multi-atlas fusion for cortical labeling. (a) All labeled surfaces are mapped to the embedding space with metric optimization to match the group-wise atlas shown in the center. (b) A multi-dimensional scaling (MDS) illustration of the surfaces and their group-wise atlas surface. (c) Bar plots of Dice coefficients of the 24 gyral regions in leave-one-out cross-validation.

4.3 Results from ADNI Data

In the third experiment, we applied the cortical labeling system in the second experiment to MR scans from 50 AD patients and 50 NCs of the ADNI study[17]. Both the left and right hemispherical cortical surfaces are reconstructed with the method in [18]. The labeling system is fully automated and there is no need of any special handling for the left and right hemisphere because the metric optimization process is based on intrinsic geometry. For all 100 scans, our system successfully generated the gyral labels. As a demonstration, we plotted the results on three subjects in Fig. 6. We can see that excellent labeling performances were achieved on both hemispheres.

Using the average gray matter thickness in each gyral region as the statistical variable, we applied t-tests to all gyral regions to locate group differences between AD and NC. For both hemispheres, the map of p-values from the t-test on

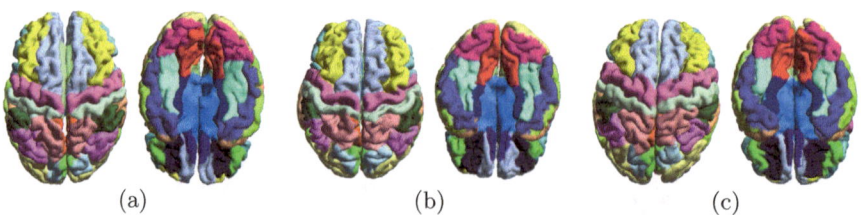

Fig. 6. Three examples of labeling from the ADNI data are shown in (a), (b) and (c). The superior and inferior view of each case are plotted.

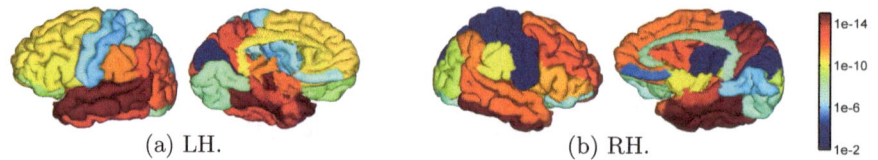

Fig. 7. Gyrus-based map of p-values from the testing of NC versus AD group differences on left hemisphere (LH) and right hemisphere (RH). The lateral and medial views are plotted in each hemisphere.

each gyrus are plotted in Fig. 7. We can see highly significant group differences were detected in regions that are consistent with previous findings in the literature such as gyri in the temporal lobe and precuneus. This demonstrates the effectiveness of our method in detecting population differences, and its potential in large scale studies.

5   Conclusions

In this paper, we developed a novel approach for computing conformal maps between anatomical surfaces and successfully demonstrated its application in automated cortical labeling. Our method is based on the optimization of conformal metrics in the LB embedding space and is able to align global geometric features as guided by the LB eigen-functions. The proposed method is general and we will investigate its application in mapping high-genus surfaces in future work. We will also apply it to study other anatomical structures such as hippocampus and perform more extensive validations on the cortical labeling algorithm.

References

1. Rustamov, R.M.: Laplace-Beltrami eigenfunctions for deformation invariant shape representation. In: Proc. Eurograph. Symp. on Geo. Process., pp. 225–233 (2007)
2. Lai, R., Shi, Y., Scheibel, K., Fears, S., Woods, R., Toga, A., Chan, T.: Metric-induced optimal embedding for intrinsic 3D shape analysis. In: Proc. CVPR, pp. 2871–2878 (2010)

3. Hurdal, M.K., Stephenson, K.: Cortical cartography using the discrete conformal approach of circle packings. NeuroImage 23, S119–S128 (2004)
4. Gu, X., Wang, Y., Chan, T.F., Thompson, P.M., Yau, S.T.: Genus zero surface conformal mapping and its application to brain surface mapping. IEEE Trans. Med. Imag. 23(8), 949–958 (2004)
5. Wang, Y., Lui, L.M., Chan, T.F., Thompson, P.M.: Optimization of brain conformal mapping with landmarks. In: Duncan, J.S., Gerig, G. (eds.) MICCAI 2005, Part II. LNCS, vol. 3750, pp. 675–683. Springer, Heidelberg (2005)
6. Reuter, M., Wolter, F., Peinecke, N.: Laplace-Beltrami spectra as Shape-DNA of surfaces and solids. Computer-Aided Design 38, 342–366 (2006)
7. Qiu, A., Bitouk, D., Miller, M.I.: Smooth functional and structural maps on the neocortex via orthonormal bases of the Laplace-Beltrami operator. IEEE Trans. Med. Imag. 25(10), 1296–1306 (2006)
8. Shi, Y., Lai, R., Morra, J., Dinov, I., Thompson, P., Toga, A.: Robust surface reconstruction via Laplace-Beltrami eigen-projection and boundary deformation. IEEE Trans. Med. Imag. 29(12), 2009–2022 (2010)
9. Shi, Y., Lai, R., Gill, R., Pelletier, D., Mohr, D., Sicotte, N., Toga, A.W.: Conformal metric optimization on surface (CMOS) for deformation and mapping in Laplace-Beltrami embedding space. In: Fichtinger, G., Martel, A., Peters, T. (eds.) MICCAI 2011, Part II. LNCS, vol. 6892, pp. 327–334. Springer, Heidelberg (2011)
10. Fischl, B., van der Kouwe, A., Destrieux, C., Halgren, E., Sagonne, F., Salat, D.H., Busa, E., Seidman, L.J., Goldstein, J., Kennedy, D., Caviness, V., Makris, N., Rosen, B., Dale, A.M.: Automatically parcellating the human cerebral cortex. Cerebral Cortex 14(1), 11–22 (2004)
11. Wan, J., Carass, A., Resnick, S., Prince, J.: Automated reliable labeling of the cortical surface. In: Proc. ISBI, pp. 440–443 (2008)
12. Yeo, B., Sabuncu, M., Vercauteren, T., Ayache, N., Fischl, B., Golland, P.: Spherical demons: Fast diffeomorphic landmark-free surface registration. IEEE Trans. Med. Imag. 29(3), 650–668 (2010)
13. Rohlfing, T., Brandt, R., Menzel, R., Maurer Jr., C.R.: Evaluation of atlas selection strategies for atlas-based image segmentation with application to confocal microscopy images of bee brains
14. Sabuncu, M., Yeo, B., Van Leemput, K., Fischl, B., Golland, P.: IEEE Trans. Med. Imag. 29(10), 1714–1729 (2010)
15. Wang, H., Suh, J., Das, S., Pluta, J., Craige, C., Yushkevich, P.: Multi-atlas segmentation with joint label fusion. IEEE Trans. Pattern Anal. Machine Intell. (2012), doi:10.1109/TPAMI.2012.143
16. Shattuck, D., Mirza, M., Adisetiyo, V., et al.: Construction of a 3D probabilistic atlas of human brain structures. NeuroImage 39(3), 1064–1080 (2008)
17. Mueller, S., Weiner, M., Thal, L., Petersen, R.C., Jack, C., Jagust, W., Trojanowski, J.Q., Toga, A.W., Beckett, L.: The Alzheimers disease neuroimaging initiative. Clin. North Am. 15, 869–877, xi–xii (2005)
18. Shi, Y., Lai, R., Toga, A.: Cortical surface reconstruction via unified Reeb analysis of geometric and topological outliers in magnetic resonance images. IEEE Trans. Med. Imag. (2012), doi:10.1109/TMI.2012.2224879
19. Klein, A., Ghosh, S.S., Avants, B., Yeo, B., Fischl, B., Ardekani, B., Gee, J.C., Mann, J., Parsey, R.V.: Evaluation of volume-based and surface-based brain image registration methods. NeuroImage 51, 214–220 (2010)

A Novel Sparse Group Gaussian Graphical Model for Functional Connectivity Estimation

Bernard Ng[1,2], Gaël Varoquaux[1], Jean Baptiste Poline[1], and Bertrand Thirion[1]

[1] Parietal Team, Neurospin, INRIA Saclay, France
[2] FIND Lab, Stanford University, United States
bernardyng@gmail.com

Abstract. The estimation of intra-subject functional connectivity is greatly complicated by the small sample size and complex noise structure in functional magnetic resonance imaging (fMRI) data. Pooling samples across subjects improves the conditioning of the estimation, but loses subject-specific connectivity information. In this paper, we propose a new sparse group Gaussian graphical model (SGGGM) that facilitates joint estimation of intra-subject and group-level connectivity. This is achieved by casting functional connectivity estimation as a regularized consensus optimization problem, in which information across subjects is aggregated in learning group-level connectivity and group information is propagated back in estimating intra-subject connectivity. On synthetic data, we show that incorporating group information using SGGGM significantly enhances intra-subject connectivity estimation over existing techniques. More accurate group-level connectivity is also obtained. On real data from a cohort of 60 subjects, we show that integrating intra-subject connectivity estimated with SGGGM significantly improves brain activation detection over connectivity priors derived from other graphical modeling approaches.

Keywords: brain connectivity, fMRI, Gaussian graphical model, regularized consensus optimization, sparse inverse covariance estimation.

1 Introduction

Accumulating evidence suggests that a prominent effect of neurological diseases is abnormal alterations in functional connectivity [1, 2], which is fundamental to brain function. In recent years, functional magnetic resonance imaging (fMRI) has become the primary means for investigating this integrative property of the brain. Particularly relevant to clinical applications is the discovery of synchronized, ongoing brain activity even when a person is at rest [3]. The sets of brain areas that show such synchronized activity during resting state (RS) are broadly conceptualized as networks. These RS networks have been shown to display high resemblance to those evoked by task [4], thus demonstrating the presence of important structures in RS connectivity patterns that reflect brain organization [3]. This finding has significant implications for studying diseased populations, since patients often have trouble performing certain tasks, but have much less difficulties lying at rest in the scanner.

J.C. Gee et al. (Eds.): IPMI 2013, LNCS 7917, pp. 256–267, 2013.
© Springer-Verlag Berlin Heidelberg 2013

Inference of functional connectivity from RS-fMRI data is commonly performed by computing the Pearson's correlation between the observations of different brain areas. Due to the small sample size and the complex noise structure in RS-fMRI data, reliable estimation of intra-subject functional connectivity is extremely challenging [1, 5]. Also, Pearson's correlation cannot distinguish whether two brain areas are directly connected or indirectly connected through a third area [1]. This distinction is crucial if one is interested in the underlying connection structure of the brain [6]. To improve correlation estimation given limited noisy samples, a number of techniques based on l_2 and l_1 regularization has been proposed. l_2 regularization amounts to adding a scaled identity matrix to the sample covariance matrix for reducing estimation errors and improving the conditioning, which in turn enables stable matrix inversion [7]. The implication of being able to stably invert a covariance matrix is that elements of the inverse covariance matrix are proportional to partial correlations, which accounts for indirect influences [6]. The drawback of l_2 regularization is that it is limited to uniform shrinkage of the off diagonal elements [5]. This limitation can be mitigated using a l_1 regularization approach [5], commonly referred to as sparse Gaussian graphical model (SGGM), in which sparsity is imposed on the inverse covariance estimates to learn the partial correlation structure in a data-driven fashion. Imposing sparsity also helps reduce estimation errors. In the context of functional connectivity estimation, enforcing sparsity conforms to past findings that the connection structure of the brain is, in fact, sparse [1].

In settings where the number of parameters is greater than the number of samples, which is typical for single-subject RS-fMRI data, accurate correlation estimation is far from trivial even with l_2 and l_1 regularization. To this end, we have previously proposed extending SGGM by exploiting anatomical connectivity [8] as well as commonalities across subjects [5]. Alternatively, a more widely-used approach is to pool data across subjects [9] by either averaging their correlation matrices or concatenating their RS-fMRI time courses to increase the number of samples. Although this approach sacrifices subject-specific information, it generates group-level correlation estimates, which are useful for population comparisons.

The optimal way for deriving a representative group correlation matrix, while accounting for inter-subject variability, is still an open question. Approaches based on Bayesian networks that enable learning of conditional independence structure, i.e. brain connection structure, common across subjects have been proposed, but these approaches do not scale well with increasing number of brain areas [6]. Recently, a probabilistic model that enables integration of fMRI and diffusion MRI (dMRI) has been put forth [9], but this model assumes each brain connection is independent, which complicates the separation of direct connections from indirect connections [1].

In this paper, we propose a sparse group Gaussian graphical model (SGGGM) that permits joint estimation of intra-subject and group-level functional connectivity. We cast the estimation as a regularized consensus optimization problem [10], in which each subject's data is modeled as a GGM with intra-subject inverse covariance matrices tied across subjects by a sparse latent group inverse covariance matrix. Commonalities across subjects are thus exploited in handling noise and the problem of limited samples in each subject's data. The general idea of aggregating information across subjects is akin to SGGM with group Lasso [5]. The difference is that SGGGM encourages intra-subject inverse covariance estimates to be *similar* to a sparse latent group inverse covariance estimate but does not impose all intra-subject inverse covariance estimates to have exactly the same sparsity pattern, i.e. the same connection structure. We show on simulated data with similar sample-to-parameter ratio as in real fMRI experiments that SGGGM significantly outperforms state-of-the-art covariance estimation techniques at both intra-subject and group level. Moreover, we illustrate on real data from a cohort of 60 subjects that incorporating intra-subject connectivity estimated using SGGGM significantly increases sensitivity in brain activation detection over connectivity computed with other widely-used methods.

2   Methods

The goal of this work is to address the challenge of reliable inverse covariance estimation under the setting where the number of samples is much less than the number of parameters and the samples are contaminated by strong noise. The state-of-the-art method for estimating a well-conditioned sparse inverse covariance matrix under this setting is SGGM, which we summarize in Section 2.1. We then describe our proposed model, SGGGM, for coalescing information across subjects in jointly estimating intra-subject and group-level inverse covariance matrices in Section 2.2. A quantitative scheme for validation is discussed in Section 2.3.

2.1   Sparse Gaussian Graphical Model

Given a $d{\times}d$ sample covariance matrix, $\mathbf{S}$, in which the samples are drawn from a multivariate Gaussian distribution, estimating a well-conditioned sparse invariance covariance matrix, $\hat{\mathbf{\Lambda}}$, can be formulated as the following optimization problem [11]:

$$\min_{\mathbf{\Lambda}>0} tr(\mathbf{S\Lambda}) - logdet(\mathbf{\Lambda}) + \lambda \parallel \mathbf{\Lambda} \parallel_1, \tag{1}$$

in which we search over the space of $d{\times}d$ positive definite matrices, $\mathbf{\Lambda} > 0$, to minimize the negative log-likelihood of a multivariate Gaussian distribution, $l(\mathbf{\Lambda}) = tr(\mathbf{S\Lambda}) - logdet(\mathbf{\Lambda})$, while promoting a sparse estimate, $\hat{\mathbf{\Lambda}}$, by minimizing the l_1-norm of the off diagonal elements, which we denote as $\parallel\mathbf{\Lambda}\parallel_1$. The level of sparsity is governed by λ, which can be selected in a data-driven manner through cross-validation (Section 2.2). In the context of functional connectivity estimation, $\mathbf{S}$ corresponds to the correlation matrix estimated from the RS-fMRI time courses of d brain areas of a given subject. (1) can be efficiently solved using algorithms, such as QUadratic Inverse Covariance (QUIC) [11] and Alternating Direction Method of Multipliers (ADMM) [10]. The latter algorithm is described in the next section.

2.2   Sparse Group Gaussian Graphical Model

Given N $d{\times}d$ sample covariance matrices, $\mathbf{S}^s$, where s is the subject index, we post the joint estimation of intra-subject inverse covariance, $\hat{\mathbf{\Lambda}}^s$, and group-level inverse covariance, $\hat{\mathbf{\Lambda}}^G$, as a regularized consensus optimization problem [10].

Regularized Consensus Optimization. For the case in which the solution is restricted to reside in the space of positive definite matrices, the regularized consensus optimization problem written in the unconstrained form is given by [10]:

$$\min_{\mathbf{\Lambda}^s>0,\,\mathbf{\Lambda}^G>0} J(\mathbf{\Lambda}^G)+\sum_{s=1}^{N}l_s(\mathbf{\Lambda}^s)+\frac{\rho}{2}\|\mathbf{\Lambda}^s-\mathbf{\Lambda}^G\|_F^2. \tag{2}$$

The intuition behind (2) is that each $\mathbf{\Lambda}^s$ should explain its own observations as encouraged through the individual loss, $l_s(\mathbf{\Lambda}^s)$, but to handle noise and the issue of limited samples in each subject's data, commonalities across subjects are exploited by penalizing deviations of $\mathbf{\Lambda}^s$ from $\mathbf{\Lambda}^G$, as imposed by minimizing $\|\mathbf{\Lambda}^s - \mathbf{\Lambda}^G\|^2_F$ where $\|\cdot\|_F$ denotes the Frobenius norm. The degree of this penalty is governed by ρ. For learning inverse covariance, we set $l_s(\mathbf{\Lambda}^s)$ to $tr(\mathbf{S}^s\mathbf{\Lambda}^s) - logdet(\mathbf{\Lambda}^s)$ as in the SGGM formulation and $J(\mathbf{\Lambda}^G)$ to $\lambda\|\mathbf{\Lambda}^G\|_1$ for enforcing sparsity. We use ADMM to solve (2).

ADMM. Given initial $\mathbf{\Lambda}^s(0)$, $\mathbf{\Lambda}^G(0)$, and $\mathbf{U}^s(0)$, the overall idea of ADMM is to alternatingly update these matrices by minimizing the augmented Lagrangian [10]:

$$L_\rho(\mathbf{\Lambda}^s,\mathbf{\Lambda}^G,\mathbf{U}^s)=J(\mathbf{\Lambda}^G)+\sum_{s=1}^{N}\left(l_s(\mathbf{\Lambda}^s)+\mathbf{U}^s(\mathbf{\Lambda}^s-\mathbf{\Lambda}^G)+\frac{\rho}{2}\|\mathbf{\Lambda}^s-\mathbf{\Lambda}^G\|_F^2\right), \tag{3}$$

where $\mathbf{U}^s$ is a $d{\times}d$ Lagrangian multiplier matrix. With $\mathbf{\Lambda}^G$ and $\mathbf{U}^s$ fixed, we find the update for $\mathbf{\Lambda}^s$ by minimizing $L_\rho(\mathbf{\Lambda}^s, \mathbf{\Lambda}^G(k), \mathbf{U}^s(k))$ over $\mathbf{\Lambda}^s$:

$$\mathbf{\Lambda}^s(k+1)=\arg\min_{\mathbf{\Lambda}^s>0} l_s(\mathbf{\Lambda}^s)+\frac{\rho}{2}\|\mathbf{\Lambda}^s-\mathbf{\Lambda}^G(k)+\mathbf{U}^s(k)\|_F^2, \tag{4}$$

where $l_s(\mathbf{\Lambda}^s) = tr(\mathbf{S}^s\mathbf{\Lambda}^s) - logdet(\mathbf{\Lambda}^s)$ for inverse covariance estimation and k denotes the iteration number. For this choice of $l_s(\mathbf{\Lambda}^s)$, there is an analytic solution for $\mathbf{\Lambda}^s(k+1)$ [10], computed by taking the derivative of (4) and setting that to zero, which gives:

$$\rho\mathbf{\Lambda}^s-(\mathbf{\Lambda}^s)^{-1}=\rho(\mathbf{\Lambda}^G(k)-\mathbf{U}^s(k))-\mathbf{S}^s. \tag{5}$$

Since all matrices in (5) are symmetric, the right hand side can be decomposed into $\mathbf{Q}\mathbf{\Gamma}\mathbf{Q}^{\mathrm{T}}$, where $\mathbf{Q}$ is the eigenmatrix of $\rho(\mathbf{\Lambda}^G(k) - \mathbf{U}^s(k)) - \mathbf{S}^s$, and $\mathbf{\Gamma}$ is a diagonal matrix containing the eigenvalues, γ_i. Multiplying both side by $\mathbf{Q}^{\mathrm{T}}$ and $\mathbf{Q}$, results in:

$$\rho\tilde{\mathbf{\Lambda}}^s - (\tilde{\mathbf{\Lambda}}^s)^{-1} = \mathbf{\Gamma}, \tag{6}$$

where $\tilde{\mathbf{\Lambda}}^s = \mathbf{Q}^{\mathrm{T}}\mathbf{\Lambda}^s\mathbf{Q}$. An elegant way for solving (6) is to assume $\tilde{\mathbf{\Lambda}}^s$ is a diagonal matrix, which amounts to finding $\tilde{\mathbf{\Lambda}}_{ii}^s$ such that $\rho\,\tilde{\mathbf{\Lambda}}_{ii}^s - 1/\tilde{\mathbf{\Lambda}}_{ii}^s = \gamma_i$, solution of which is given by the quadratic formula. $\mathbf{\Lambda}^s = \mathbf{Q}\,\tilde{\mathbf{\Lambda}}^s\,\mathbf{Q}^{\mathrm{T}}$ is thus a solution of (4).

After computing $\mathbf{\Lambda}^s(k+1)$ for all subjects, we fix $\mathbf{\Lambda}^s$ and $\mathbf{U}^s$, and find the update for $\mathbf{\Lambda}^G$ by minimizing $L_\rho(\mathbf{\Lambda}^s(k+1), \mathbf{\Lambda}^G, \mathbf{U}^s(k))$ over $\mathbf{\Lambda}^G$:

$$\mathbf{\Lambda}^G(k+1) = \underset{\mathbf{\Lambda}^G > 0}{\arg\min}\; J(\mathbf{\Lambda}^G) + \sum_{i=1}^N \frac{\rho}{2} \| \mathbf{\Lambda}^s(k+1) - \mathbf{\Lambda}^G + \mathbf{U}^s(k) \|_F^2 . \tag{7}$$

where $J(\mathbf{\Lambda}^G) = \lambda\|\mathbf{\Lambda}^G\|_1$ to impose sparsity. Since (7) is exactly the proximal operator of $J(\mathbf{\Lambda}^G)$, $\mathbf{\Lambda}^G(k+1)$ can be found by element-wise soft thresholding [10]:

$$\mathbf{\Lambda}_{ij}^G(k+1) = \left(\overline{\mathbf{\Lambda}}_{ij}(k+1) + \frac{\overline{\mathbf{U}}_{ij}(k)}{\rho} - \frac{\lambda}{N\rho} \right)_+ - \left(-\overline{\mathbf{\Lambda}}_{ij}(k+1) - \frac{\overline{\mathbf{U}}_{ij}(k)}{\rho} - \frac{\lambda}{N\rho} \right)_+ , \tag{8}$$

where $(a)_+ = a$ if $a > 0$ and $(a)_+ = 0$ if $a \leq 0$. $\overline{\mathbf{\Lambda}}_{ij}$ and $\overline{\mathbf{U}}_{ij}$ denote the subject average of $\mathbf{\Lambda}_{ij}^s$ and $\mathbf{U}_{ij}^s$, respectively.

Finally, we fix $\mathbf{\Lambda}^s$ and $\mathbf{\Lambda}^G$, and minimize $L_\rho(\mathbf{\Lambda}^s(k+1), \mathbf{\Lambda}^G(k+1), \mathbf{U}^s)$ over $\mathbf{U}^s$ to find an update for $\mathbf{U}^s$. The solution is given by:

$$\mathbf{U}^s(k+1) = \mathbf{U}^s(k) + \rho(\mathbf{\Lambda}^s(k+1) - \mathbf{\Lambda}^G(k+1)) . \tag{9}$$

(4), (7), and (9) are repeated until convergence. We highlight that (4) is separable across subjects. Thus, the estimation of $\mathbf{\Lambda}^s$ can be distributed over multiple processors, in which the computational cost of each $\mathbf{\Lambda}^s$ estimation is approximately that of an eigenvalue decomposition, i.e. $O(d^3)$. For initialization, we set $\mathbf{U}^s(0)$ to $0_{d\times d}$ and $\mathbf{\Lambda}^G(0)$ to the subject average inverse covariance, with each subject's inverse covariance estimated using oracle approximating shrinkage (OAS), which is an l_2 regularization technique with a closed-form solution for the optimal shrinkage parameter [7]. We note that for $N = 1$, (1) and (2) are equivalent, thus the above procedures can be directly applied for pure single-subject sparse inverse covariance estimation.

Convergence Criteria. We adopt the convergence criteria in [10], which are based on the differences between the intra-subject inverse covariance estimates and their means, $\|\mathbf{R}(k)\|_F < \varepsilon_{\mathrm{pri}}$, and the differences between the mean inverse covariance of two consecutive iterations, $\|\mathbf{Q}(k)\|_F < \varepsilon_{\mathrm{dual}}$, as summarized below:

$$\| \mathbf{R}(k) \|_F^2 = \sum_{s=1}^{N} \| \mathbf{\Lambda}^s(k) - \overline{\mathbf{\Lambda}}(k) \|_F^2, \ \| \mathbf{Q}(k) \|_F^2 = N\rho^2 \| \overline{\mathbf{\Lambda}}(k) - \overline{\mathbf{\Lambda}}(k-1) \|_F^2, \tag{10}$$

$$\varepsilon_{\mathrm{pri}} = d\varepsilon_{\mathrm{abs}} + \varepsilon_{\mathrm{rel}} \max\{\| \overline{\mathbf{\Lambda}}(k) \|_F, \| \mathbf{\Lambda}^G(k) \|_F\}, \tag{11}$$

$$\varepsilon_{\mathrm{dual}} = d\varepsilon_{\mathrm{abs}} + \varepsilon_{\mathrm{rel}} \| \rho\overline{\mathbf{U}}(k) \|_F. \tag{12}$$

Both $\varepsilon_{\mathrm{abs}}$ and $\varepsilon_{\mathrm{rel}}$ are set to 10^{-4} in this work. We note that one would normally prefer finding solutions with $\varepsilon_{\mathrm{abs}}$ and $\varepsilon_{\mathrm{rel}}$ being as small as computationally practical. However, in the present context of functional connectivity estimation, we anticipate inter-subject differences, thus setting $\varepsilon_{\mathrm{abs}}$ and $\varepsilon_{\mathrm{rel}}$ too low could falsely force all subjects to have overly-similar intra-subject connectivity estimates.

Parameter Selection. SGGGM requires setting two parameters: λ and ρ. Since the estimated connection structure highly depends on λ, we employ cross validation in combination with a refined grid search strategy similar to the approach we have taken in [8] to find the optimal λ. We proceed by first selecting a range of λ and temporally splitting the data into K folds. We then estimate $\mathbf{\Lambda}^G$ on $K - 1$ training folds and compute the log data likelihood of the left-out test fold given $\mathbf{\Lambda}^G_{\mathrm{train}}$ for each λ, i.e. $\Sigma_s(logdet(\mathbf{\Lambda}^G_{\mathrm{train}}) - tr(\mathbf{S}^s_{\mathrm{test}}\mathbf{\Lambda}^G_{\mathrm{train}}))$. We define the optimal λ as the one that gives the largest average log data likelihood across folds. We then search within a refined range around the optimal λ and repeat the procedure. The initial λ range is set as $[\lambda_{\max}/100, \lambda_{\max}]$, where $\lambda_{\max} = \max|\overline{\mathbf{S}}_{ij}|, i \neq j$ is the value beyond which off-diagonal elements of $\mathbf{\Lambda}^G$ are shrunk to 0. $\overline{\mathbf{S}}_{ij}$ denotes the mean sample covariance across subjects. For each refinement level, we evenly distribute 5 grid points on a logarithm scale to cover the λ range. K is set to 3, and we refine the search 3 times within the interval defined by the two grid points adjacent to the optimal λ found at the previous refinement level. For ρ, we fix it to 1 to ensure convergence [10] as well as to reduce the computation load arising from nesting the λ search into an internal cross-validation loop. We defer investigation of efficient means for joint selection of λ and ρ to future work.

2.3   Validation

We base our validation on increased sensitivity in group activation detection by using our recently proposed model that permits incorporation of connectivity into the estimation of activation effects [12]. The rationale is that connectivity estimates that better reflect the intrinsic wiring of the brain would presumably result in higher detection. By using this validation scheme, *quantitative* comparison of different connectivity estimation techniques is facilitated. We summarized below our model in [12]:

$$\mathbf{Y}^s \sim N(\mathbf{A}^s \mathbf{X}^s, \mathbf{V}_1^s) = \frac{1}{|2\pi\mathbf{V}_1^s|^{\frac{n}{2}}} \exp\left(\frac{-tr((\mathbf{Y}^s - \mathbf{A}^s \mathbf{X}^s)^T \mathbf{V}_1^{s^{-1}} (\mathbf{Y}^s - \mathbf{A}^s \mathbf{X}^s))}{2}\right) \quad (13)$$

$$\mathbf{A}^s \sim MN(0, \mathbf{V}_2^s, \alpha\mathbf{X}^s\mathbf{X}^{s^T}) = \frac{|\alpha\mathbf{X}^s\mathbf{X}^{s^T}|^{\frac{d}{2}}}{|2\pi\mathbf{V}_2^s|^{\frac{m}{2}}} \exp\left(-\frac{\alpha}{2} tr(\mathbf{X}^{s^T} \mathbf{A}^{s^T} \mathbf{V}_2^{s^{-1}} \mathbf{A}^s \mathbf{X}^s)\right), \quad (14)$$

where $\mathbf{Y}^s$ is a $d{\times}n$ matrix containing task fMRI time courses of d brain areas of subject s. $\mathbf{X}^s$ is a $m{\times}n$ matrix with m regressors along the rows for modeling the expected task-evoked responses [13]. $\mathbf{A}^s$ is a $d{\times}m$ activation effect matrix to be estimated. $\mathbf{V}_1^s$ and $\mathbf{V}_2^s$ are $d{\times}d$ covariance matrices of $\mathbf{Y}^s$ and $\mathbf{A}^s$, respectively. $\mathbf{X}^s\mathbf{X}^{sT}$ models the correlations between the m experimental conditions. $MN(0,\mathbf{V}_2^s,\alpha\mathbf{X}^s\mathbf{X}^{sT})$ denotes the matrix normal distribution, which serves as a conjugate prior of (13). The influence of this prior on $\mathbf{A}$ is governed by α, which can be optimized by maximizing model evidence [12]. We assume $\mathbf{V}_1^s = I_{d{\times}d}$ as conventionally done, and $\mathbf{V}_2^s$ is where we inject our RS connectivity estimates. We note that all parameters in the model can be estimated in a data-driven manner without any manual interventions [12], thus providing an objective framework for evaluating different connectivity estimation methods.

3   Materials

3.1   Synthetic Data

For validation, we created 100 synthetic datasets with a sample-to-parameter ratio similar to that in a typical fMRI connectivity study. Specifically, each dataset comprised 10 subjects with 500 regional time courses of 186 time samples, and was generated as follows. First, we created a random 500×500 sparse positive definite matrix, $\mathbf{\Lambda}^G$, with 20% of the elements being non-zero to approximately match the sparsity level observed when we applied SGGM to the real data. $\mathbf{\Lambda}^G$ corresponds to the group inverse covariance matrix, representative of the 10 subjects. We then randomly drew 10 positive definite matrices, $\mathbf{\Lambda}^s$, $s = 1$ to 10, from $Wishart(\mathbf{\Lambda}^G, v)$, where v is the degrees of freedom set to ten times the number of parameters, i.e. 10×500×499/2, to ensure that $\mathbf{\Lambda}^s$ is well-conditioned for matrix inversion. $\mathbf{\Lambda}^s$ corresponds to the inverse covariance matrix of each subject s, which was used to generate regional time courses by drawing samples from $N(0, \mathbf{\Sigma}^s)$, where $\mathbf{\Sigma}^s$ is the matrix inverse of $\mathbf{\Lambda}^s$.

3.2   Real Data

60 healthy subjects were recruited and scanned at multiple centers. Each subject was asked to perform 10 language, computation, and sensorimotor tasks similar to those in [14], as fMRI data were acquired over a duration of ~5 min. ~7 min of RS-fMRI data were also collected. Scanning was performed using 3T scanners from multiple manufacturers with TR = 2200 ms, TE = 30 ms, and flip angle = $75°$. The task fMRI data were corrected for slice timing and head motions, temporally detrended, and spatially normalized using the SPM8 software. The RS-fMRI data were similarly preprocessed except we applied a band-pass filter with cutoff frequencies at 0.01 and 0.1 Hz. White matter and cerebrospinal fluid confounds were regressed out from the gray matter voxel time courses. To create a finer brain parcellation than provided by standard brain atlases (< 150 regions), we divided the brain into 500 parcels by concatenating RS-fMRI time courses across subjects and applying Ward clustering [15]. We then averaged the voxel time courses within each parcel to generate parcel time courses. These time courses were normalized by subtracting the mean and dividing by the standard deviation to account for scanner variability across imaging centers.

4   Results and Discussion

To investigate the gain of jointly estimating intra-subject and group-level connectivity under a unified model, we compared SGGGM against a number of state-of-the-art techniques on both synthetic and real data. Contrasted methods at the intra-subject level include SGGM [1] and OAS [7]. We excluded Pearson's correlation, since it does not provide an invertible correlation matrix when the number of parameters is greater than the number of samples, which is the case for our real data and quite generally in fMRI-based functional connectivity analysis. At the group level, we examined different ways of computing the mean from the SGGM and OAS intra-subject connectivity estimates as well as SGGM and OAS applied to concatenated observations across subjects. Specifically, we considered the conventionally-used Euclidean mean, $\Sigma_s \Lambda^s / N$, and the Log-Euclidean mean [16], $expm(\Sigma_s logm(\Lambda^s)/N)$, where $expm(\cdot)$ and $logm(\cdot)$ denote matrix exponential and matrix logarithm, respectively. The reason for using Log-Euclidean mean is that Λ^s lives on the space of positive definite matrices, which is not a vector space. Applying $logm(\cdot)$ preserves the spectral characteristics of the input matrices, which avoids the undesirable "swelling effect" observed with Euclidean mean [16]. We note that when estimating group connectivity by concatenating observations across subjects, it is important to normalize the subjects' observations by subtracting the mean and dividing by the standard deviation to reduce inter-subject variability.

4.1   Synthetic Data Results

To assess the accuracy of the contrasted inverse covariance estimation methods, we computed the affine invariant distance [16] between the estimates and ground truth:

$$d(\hat{\Lambda}, \Lambda_{\text{gnd}}) = \| \, logm(\Lambda_{\text{gnd}}^{-1/2} \hat{\Lambda} \Lambda_{\text{gnd}}^{-1/2}) \|_F^2 \,, \tag{15}$$

where $\hat{\Lambda}$ denotes the estimated inverse covariance of a given method and Λ_{gnd} is the ground truth inverse covariance. The results are summarized in Fig. 1. At intra-subject level, SGGGM significantly outperformed SGGM and OAS, which demonstrates the benefits of incorporating group information into intra-subject inverse covariance estimation when the subjects belong to the same population. At the group level, using SGGGM also resulted in significantly more accurate inverse covariance estimates. Interestingly, using concatenated observations performed better than Euclidean and Log-Euclidean means. We speculate the reason is that the increased number of samples by concatenating observations improves the conditioning of the estimation, whereas using subject means amounts to averaging poorly estimated intra-subject inverse covariance matrices. The higher accuracy achieved with SGGM over OAS for the case where observations are concatenated is also likely due to a similar reason, in which the increased sample size enables SGGM to more accurately learn the support, i.e. the sparsity pattern, of the ground truth inverse covariance matrix.

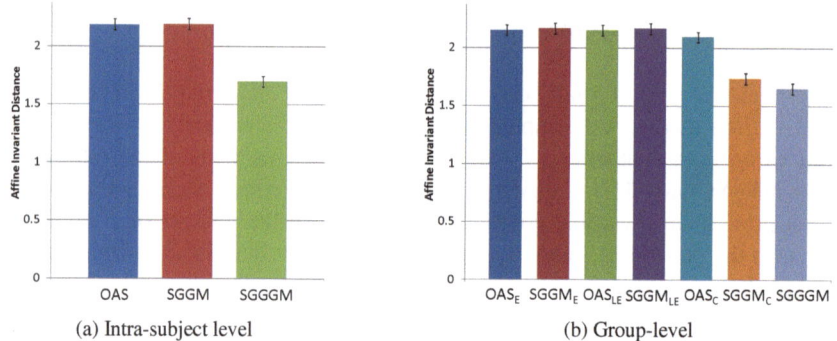

(a) Intra-subject level   (b) Group-level

Fig. 1. Synthetic data results. Subscripts "$_E$", "$_{LE}$", and "$_C$" denote estimation with Euclidean mean, Log-Euclidean mean, and concatenated observations. Using SGGGM resulted in significantly more accurate inverse covariance estimates than the contrasted methods.

4.2 Real Data Results

Validation on real data is greatly complicated by the lack of ground truth. To safely base our validation on increased sensitivity in brain activation detection, we employed the max-t permutation test [17] to enforce strict control on false positive rate. With detection sensitivity in group activation being the validation criterion, using a common group connectivity prior or even injecting group information into intra-subject connectivity estimation could bias the results. To remove this bias, we first randomly permuted the rows and columns of a given estimated connectivity matrix, $\hat{\Lambda}$, and computed the percentage of parcels found to be activated. This percentage indicates the amount of detections that could be obtained given the same set of estimated connectivity values but with the connection structure randomized. This process was repeated 50 times with the maximum difference in the percentages of detected parcels between the permuted cases and that obtained with ordinary least square (OLS), i.e. standard univariate analysis without any prior [13], subtracted from the original percentage of detected parcels found with $\hat{\Lambda}$. This procedure was applied for all methods that used group information in the connectivity estimation. To test the generality of SGGGM, we examined the mean detection rate averaged over the 10 experimental conditions and 21 contrasts of interest between these conditions.

Quantitative results obtained by incorporating intra-subject connectivity priors into task activation detection are shown in Fig. 2(a). OLS is also plotted to serve as a baseline. Using SGGGM significantly increased detection sensitivity over SGGM and OAS for a typical p-value range of 0 to 0.05. Significance is declared based on a permutation described in [8]. Our results thus indicate that there are commonalities across subjects that can be exploited to improve intra-subject connectivity estimation. Denoting group-level connectivity estimation using SGGM and OAS with Euclidean mean, Log-Euclidean mean, and concatenated observations as $SGGM_E$, OAS_E, $SGGM_{LE}$, OAS_{LE}, $SGGM_C$, and OAS_C in Fig. 2(b), SGGGM was found to significantly outperform $SGGM_E$, OAS_E, and $SGGM_{LE}$. SGGGM also resulted in slightly more detections than OAS_{LE} and similar performance compared to $SGGM_C$ and OAS_C. Overall, our results show that SGGGM provides relevant priors for activation detection at both intra-subject and group level.

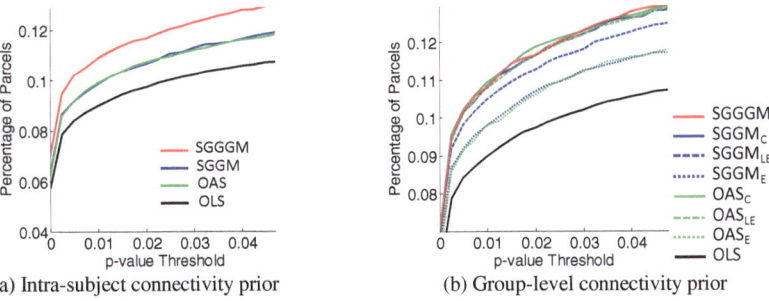

(a) Intra-subject connectivity prior   (b) Group-level connectivity prior

Fig. 2. Real data results. Percentage of parcels with significant activation averaged across contrasts v.s. p-value thresholds displayed. Subscripts "$_E$", "$_{LE}$", and "$_C$" denote group connectivity estimation with Euclidean mean, Log-Euclidean mean, and concatenated observations.

Qualitative results obtained by incorporating intra-subject connectivity priors are shown in Fig. 3. We did not include the group connectivity prior results due to space limitation. Areas in red are parcels detected with SGGGM only. The other coloured areas are parcels detected by SGGGM as well as one or more of the contrasted methods (OLS, OAS, and SGGM). For the task in which subjects performed calculations following auditory instructions, only SGGGM detected the right auditory thalamus (Fig. 3(a)), which is responsible for relaying information to the auditory cortex. For the case where the calculations to be performed was visually presented, SGGGM detected a much wider extent of the dorsal anterior cingulate cortex (Fig. 3(b)), which is involved with executive processing and attention. Moreover, for the task in which subjects listened to sentences, only SGGGM detected the right Broca's area (Fig. 3(c)), which is associated with processing of subtle features in speech, e.g. prosody.

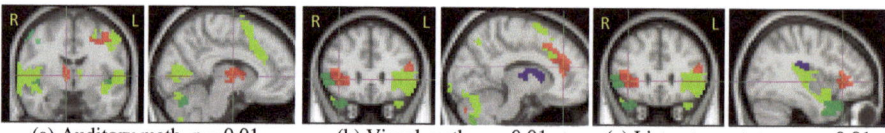

(a) Auditory math, $p = 0.01$ (b) Visual math, $p = 0.01$ (c) Listen to sentences, $p = 0.01$

Fig. 3. Activation maps with intra-subject connectivity priors. Red = detected by SGGGM only. Other colours indicate areas detected by SGGGM and one or more of the contrasted methods.

5   Conclusions

We proposed a new sparse graphical model for joint estimation of intra-subject and group-level functional connectivity. We showed on synthetic data that SGGGM provides significantly more accurate inverse covariance estimates than state-of-the-art techniques at both the intra-subject and group level. We also demonstrated on real data that incorporating intra-subject connectivity priors learned from SGGGM results in higher sensitivity in activation detection compared to SGGM and OAS. Based on our results, a couple of insights can be drawn. First, sample size appears to be the limiting factor to functional connectivity estimation, as suggested by the improvements obtained by concatenating observations in contrast to using subject means. Thus, concatenating data across subjects, while appropriately accounting for inter-subject variability, could be a compelling strategy if only group connectivity is of interest. Moreover, since more sensitive activation detection can be achieved by incorporating a group connectivity prior, one can envision building a functional connectivity atlas by applying SGGGM to datasets from a large cohort of subjects and using the resulting connectivity estimate as a generic prior for future activation studies.

Acknowledgements. This work was supported by the Genim ANR-10-BLAN-0128 grant, NSERC, and the Berkeley-INRIA-Stanford grant. The data were acquired within the IMAGEN project. Jean Baptiste Poline was partly funded by the IMAGEN project, which receives funding from the E.U. Community's FP6, LSHM-CT-2007-037286. This manuscript reflects only the authors' views and the Community is not liable for any use that may be made of the information contained therein.

References

1. Huang, S., Li, J., Sun, L., Ye, J., Fleisher, A., Wu, T., Chen, K., Reiman, E.: Learning Brain Connectivity of Alzheimer's Disease by Sparse Inverse Covariance Estimation. Neuroimage 50, 935–949 (2010)

2. Delbeuck, X., Van der Linden, M., Collette, F.: Alzheimer's Disease as a Disconnection Syndrome? Neuropsychol. Rev. 13, 79–92 (2003)
3. Fox, M.D., Raichle, M.E.: Spontaneous Fluctuations in Brain Activity Observed with Functional Magnetic Resonance Imaging. Nat. Rev. Neurosci. 8, 700–711 (2007)
4. Smith, S.M., Fox, P.T., Miller, K.L., Glahn, D.C., Fox, P.M., Mackay, C.E., Filippini, N., Watkins, K.E., Toro, R., Laird, A.R., Beckmann, C.F.: Correspondence of the Brain's Functional Architecture During Activation and Rest. Proc. Natl. Acad. Sci. 106, 13040–13045 (2009)
5. Varoquaux, G., Gramfort, A., Poline, J.B., Thirion, B.: Brain Covariance Selection: Better Individual Functional Connectivity Models Using Population Prior. In: Advances in Neural Information Processing Systems, vol. 23, pp. 2334–2342 (2010)
6. Smith, S.: The Future of fMRI Connectivity. NeuroImage 62, 1257–1266 (2012)
7. Chen, Y., Wiesel, A., Eldar, Y.C., Hero, A.O.: Shrinkage Algorithms for MMSE Covariance Estimation. IEEE Trans. Sig. Proc. 58, 5016–5029 (2010)
8. Ng, B., Varoquaux, G., Poline, J.-B., Thirion, B.: A Novel Sparse Graphical Approach for Multimodal Brain Connectivity Inference. In: Ayache, N., Delingette, H., Golland, P., Mori, K. (eds.) MICCAI 2012, Part I. LNCS, vol. 7510, pp. 707–714. Springer, Heidelberg (2012)
9. Venkataraman, A., Rathi, Y., Kubicki, M., Westin, C.F., Golland, P.: Joint Modeling of Anatomical and Functional Connectivity for Population Studies. IEEE Trans. Med. Imaging 31, 164–182 (2012)
10. Boyd, S., Parikh, N., Chu, E., Peleato, B., Eckstein, J.: Distributed Optimization and Statistical Learning via the Alternating Direction Method of Multipliers. Found. Trend Mach. Learn. 3, 1–122 (2010)
11. Hsieh, C.J., Sustik, M.A., Dhillon, I.S., Ravikumar, P.: Sparse Invers Covariance Matrix Estimation Using Quadratic Approximation. In: Advances in Neural Information Processing Systems, vol. 24, pp. 2330–2338 (2011)
12. Ng, B., Abugharbieh, R., Varoquaux, G., Poline, J.B., Thirion, B.: Connectivity-Informed fMRI Activation Detection. In: Fichtinger, G., Martel, A., Peters, T. (eds.) MICCAI 2011, Part II. LNCS, vol. 6892, pp. 285–292. Springer, Heidelberg (2011)
13. Friston, K.J., Holmes, A.P., Worsley, K.J., Poline, J.B., Frith, C.D., Frackowiak, R.S.J.: Statistical Parametric Maps in Functional Imaging: A General Linear Approach. Hum. Brain Mapp. 2, 189–210 (1995)
14. Pinel, P., Thirion, B., Meriaux, S., Jober, A., Serres, J., Le Bihan, D., Poline, J.B., Dehaene, S.: Fast Reproducible Identification and Large-scale Databasing of Individual Functional Cognitive Networks. BioMed. Central Neurosci. 8, 91 (2007)
15. Michel, V., Gramfort, A., Varoquaux, G., Eger, E., Keribin, C., Thirion, B.: A Supervised Clustering Approach for fMRI-based Inference of Brain States. Patt. Recog. 45, 2041–2049 (2012)
16. Arsigny, V., Fillard, P., Pennec, X., Ayache, N.: Fast and Simple Calculus on Tensors in the Log-Euclidean Framework. In: Duncan, J., Gerig, G. (eds.) MICCAI 2005, Part I. LNCS, vol. 3749, pp. 115–122. Springer, Heidelberg (2005)
17. Nichols, T., Hayasaka, S.: Controlling the Familywise Error Rate in Functional Neuroimaging: a Comparative Review. Stat. Methods Med. Research 12, 419–446 (2003)

Joint Co-segmentation and Registration of 3D Ultrasound Images

Raphael Prevost[1,2], Remi Cuingnet[1], Benoit Mory[1], Jean-Michel Correas[3],
Laurent D. Cohen[2], and Roberto Ardon[1]

[1] Philips Research Medisys, Suresnes, France
[2] CEREMADE UMR 7534, Universite Paris Dauphine, Paris, France
[3] Adult Radiology Department, Necker Hospital, Paris, France

Abstract. Contrast-enhanced ultrasound (CEUS) allows a visualization of the vascularization and complements the anatomical information provided by conventional ultrasound (US). However, these images are inherently subject to noise and shadows, which hinders standard segmentation algorithms. In this paper, we propose to use simultaneously the different information coming from 3D US and CEUS images to address the problem of kidney segmentation. To that end, we introduce a generic framework for joint co-segmentation and registration that seeks objects having the same shape in several images. From this framework, we derive both an ellipsoid co-detection and a model-based co-segmentation algorithm. These methods rely on voxel-classification maps that we estimate using random forests in a structured way. This yields a fast and fully automated pipeline, in which an ellipsoid is first estimated to locate the kidney in both US and CEUS volumes and then deformed to segment it accurately. The proposed method outperforms state-of-the-art results (by dividing the kidney volume error by two) on a clinically representative database of 64 images.

Keywords: co-segmentation, registration, kidney, random forests, ultrasound, contrast-enhanced ultrasound.

1 Introduction

1.1 Clinical Setting

Contrast-enhanced ultrasound (CEUS) consists in acquiring a ultrasound image after injecting in the patient's blood a contrast agent made of gas-filled microbubbles. Since those bubbles have a different acoustic response from the tissues, they can be isolated and images showing only the blood flow can be generated [1]. This modality is particularly valuable for visual assessment of the functioning of highly vascularized organs like kidneys. Yet, analysis of such images can be very challenging and literature on their segmentation is limited.

In [13], we proposed a method to detect and segment kidneys in 3D CEUS images. While we provided an automated pipeline, failures were reported in several cases and user interactions were needed to obtain a satisfying result. Yet,

J.C. Gee et al. (Eds.): IPMI 2013, LNCS 7917, pp. 268–279, 2013.

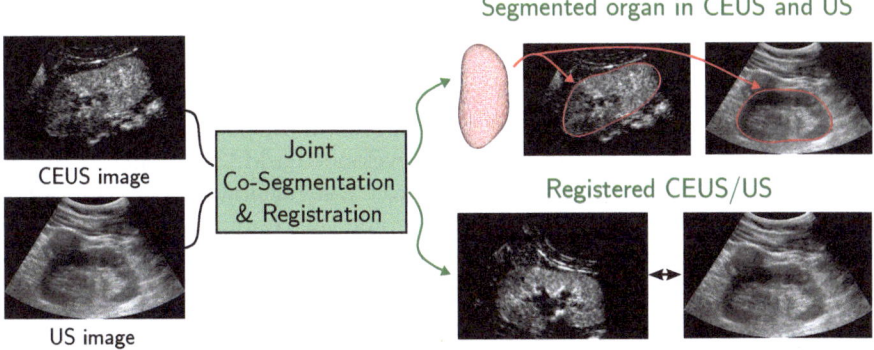

Fig. 1. Joint co-segmentation and registration. Given two different non-aligned images of the same object, the proposed method aims at segmenting this object in both images as well as estimating a rigid transformation between them.

because of shadowing effects, pathologies and restricted field of view, parts of the kidney may be hardly visible in the image. In such cases even expert users may have difficulty delineating the true boundary of the organ by solely relying on the CEUS images. In clinical routine every CEUS acquisition is preceded by a conventional US acquisition to locate the kidney. Hence, the latter could be used to complement the CEUS image and thus cope with missing and corrupted information. However, automated kidney segmentation in 3D US images is also an open issue. Martin-Fernandez and Alberola-Lopez [8] tackled this problem but their method requires a manual initialization. For both US and CEUS segmentation are equally challenging, we propose to address them simultaneously by performing kidney co-segmentation in the two images.

1.2   Related Work on Co-segmentation and Registration

Co-segmentation often denotes the task of finding an object in each image that shares the same appearance but not necessarily the same shape [16]. Here we look for the exactly same organ in two images but with a different appearance. As simultaneous acquisition of US and CEUS is not possible on current 3D imaging systems, the two images are in arbitrary referentials and need to be aligned. However, standard iconic registration methods are not adapted since visible structures, apart from the kidney itself, are completely different in US and CEUS. Co-segmentation shall therefore help registration, just as registration helps co-segmentation. This calls for a method that jointly performs these two tasks (see Figure 1).

Although segmentation and registration are often seen as two separate problems, several approaches have already been proposed to perform them simultaneously. Most of them rely on an iconic registration guiding the segmentation (e.g. [17,12,7]). Yet they assume that the segmentation is known in one of the images, which is not the case in our application of co-segmentation. Moreover, as stated before, CEUS/US intensity-based registration is bound to fail since visible structures does not correspond to each other. Instead of registering the images themselves, Wyatt et al. [18] developped a MAP formulation to perform registration on label maps resulting from a segmentation step. However no shape model is enforced and noise can degrade the results. In [19], Yezzi et al. introduced a variational framework that consists in a feature-based registration in which the features are actually the segmenting active contours.

In this paper, we aim at extending both the kidney detection and segmentation in a 3D CEUS image presented in [13] to a pair of 3D CEUS and US images. To that end, we develop a generic joint co-segmentation and registration framework inspired by [19]. This results in a fully automated pipeline to obtain both an improved kidney segmentation in CEUS and US images and a registration of them.

The article is structured as follows. Section 2 describes the generic framework and its application to two consecutive algorithms. Both rely on an appearance characterization of the kidney in ultrasound images that is learnt using random forest in an original structured way (Section 3). Results of the proposed co-segmentation method on a challenging clinical database are presented in Section 4. Finally, Section 5 provides some discussion and concludes the paper.

2   Joint Co-segmentation and Registration

2.1   Generic Implicit Variational Framework

Segmentation consists in finding an optimal two-phase (inside and outside) partitioning of a given image $I : \Omega \to \mathbb{R}^+$. In implicit methods, this partitioning is defined using the sign of an implicit function $\phi : \Omega \to \mathbb{R}$. In [13], two variational methods are developed to respectively detect and segment the kidney. They both consist in seeking ϕ as the minimum of functional of the following generic form

$$E_I(\phi) = \int_\Omega f(\phi(\mathbf{x})) \, r_I(\mathbf{x}) \, d\mathbf{x} + \mathcal{R}(\phi) \tag{1}$$

where f is a real-valued function and $r_I(\mathbf{x})$ denotes a pointwise score on whether $\mathbf{x}$ looks like an interior or exterior voxel in the image I. This is a standard setting in which the optimal implicit function ϕ must achieve a trade-off between an image-based term and a regularization term $\mathcal{R}$. For example, the seminal method of Chan and Vese [3] falls in this framework with $f = H$ the Heaviside function and $r_I(\mathbf{x}) = (I(\mathbf{x}) - c_{int})^2 - (I(\mathbf{x}) - c_{ext})^2$ with c_{int} and c_{ext} denoting mean intensities inside and outside the target object.

We are interested in the case where a pair of images $I_1 : \Omega_1 \to \mathbb{R}$ and $I_2 : \Omega_2 \to \mathbb{R}$ of the same object are available. If those images were perfectly aligned, the energy in Eq (1) can be straightforwardly generalized to perform co-segmentation:

$$E_{I_1,I_2}(\phi) = \int_{\Omega_1} f(\phi(\mathbf{x})) \, (r_{I_1}(\mathbf{x}) + r_{I_2}(\mathbf{x})) \, d\mathbf{x} + \mathcal{R}(\phi) \,. \tag{2}$$

Unfortunately, such an assumption rarely holds in medical applications unless the two images are acquired simultaneously. A more realistic hypothesis is to assume that the target object, segmented by ϕ, is not deformed between the two acquisitions, but only undergoes an unknown rigid transformation $\mathcal{G}_r$. The co-segmentation energy thus reads

$$E_{I_1,I_2}(\phi, \mathcal{G}_r) = \int_{\Omega_1} f(\phi(\mathbf{x})) \, r_{I_1}(\mathbf{x}) \, d\mathbf{x} + \int_{\Omega_2} f(\phi \circ \mathcal{G}_r(\mathbf{x})) \, r_{I_2}(\mathbf{x}) \, d\mathbf{x} + \mathcal{R}(\phi) \,. \tag{3}$$

Note that, after a variable substitution, it can be equivalently written

$$E_{I_1,I_2}(\phi, \mathcal{G}_r) = \int_{\Omega_1} f(\phi(\mathbf{x})) \, (r_{I_1}(\mathbf{x}) + r_{I_2} \circ \mathcal{G}_r^{-1}(\mathbf{x})) \, d\mathbf{x} + \mathcal{R}(\phi) \,. \tag{4}$$

Minimizing E_{I_1,I_2} with respect to ϕ and $\mathcal{G}_r$ simultaneously can be therefore interpreted as performing jointly segmentation (via ϕ) and rigid registration (via $\mathcal{G}_r$). This generalizes a more common co-segmentation approach (e.g. [5]) where the images are first aligned in a preprocessing step. Note that for clarity, we only consider two images but all equations can be generalized straightforwardly to an arbitrary number of images.

In the following, we apply this framework to (i) a robust ellipsoid detection [13] and (ii) implicit template deformation [10] to build a completely automated workflow for kidney segmentation in CEUS and US images. Note that the kidney, which is surrounded by a tough fibrous renal capsule, is a rigid organ. The hypothesis of non-deformation is therefore justified.

2.2   Robust Ellipsoid Co-detection

In [13], we proposed to detect the kidney in CEUS images as an ellipsoid. For that purpose, we developed a variational framework to achieve fast and robust ellipsoid detection. Any ellipsoid can be implictly represented by a function $\phi_{\mathbf{c},\mathbf{M}} : \Omega \to \mathbb{R}$ such that $\phi_{\mathbf{c},\mathbf{M}}(\mathbf{x}) = 1 - (\mathbf{x} - \mathbf{c})^T \mathbf{M} (\mathbf{x} - \mathbf{c})$, where $\mathbf{c} \in \mathbb{R}^3$ denotes the ellipsoid center and $\mathbf{M}$ is a symmetric positive-definite matrix. The ellipsoid interior is then the zero superlevel set of $\phi_{\mathbf{c},\mathbf{M}}$. Given a probability map $p : \Omega \to [0,1]$ of the target object, defined at each pixel, the detection is sought as the smallest ellipsoid that includes most of the pixels $\mathbf{x}$ with high probability $p(\mathbf{x})$. To limit the influence of possible false positives pixels, a weighting function $w : \Omega \to [0,1]$ acting on p is also estimated. We thus proposed to solve the following problem

$$\min_{\mathbf{c},\mathbf{M},w} E_{det}(\mathbf{c},\mathbf{M},w) = - \int_{\Omega} \phi_{\mathbf{c},\mathbf{M}}(\mathbf{x})\, p(\mathbf{x})\, w(\mathbf{x})\, d\mathbf{x} \tag{5}$$

$$+ \mu \cdot \left(\int_{\Omega} p(\mathbf{x})\, w(\mathbf{x})\, d\mathbf{x} \right) \cdot \log \left(\frac{\mathcal{V}ol(\mathbf{M})}{|\Omega|} \right)$$

with $\quad \mathcal{V}ol(\mathbf{M}) = \dfrac{4\pi}{3} \sqrt{\det \mathbf{M}^{-1}} \quad$ the ellipsoid volume.

Such a setting falls into the framework described in Eq (1) :

- with $f = Id$ and $r_I = -pw$ in the image-based term. r_I is then highly negative at voxels that have a high probability and are not outliers. To minimize the energy, such pixels must be inside the ellipsoid i.e. where ϕ is positive.
- with $\mathcal{R}(\phi_{\mathbf{c},\mathbf{M}}) = \mathcal{R}(\mathbf{M}) = \mu \cdot \int_{\Omega} pw \cdot \log \left(\frac{\mathcal{V}ol(\mathbf{M})}{|\Omega|} \right)$ as a regularization term that penalizes the volume of the ellipsoid. The rationale behind the logarithm is statistical: the energy in Eq (5) is closely related to maximum likelihood estimation of a Gaussian distribution. Factor $\int_{\Omega} pw$ normalizes the contribution of such a term, while μ denotes a trade-off parameter set to $\frac{1}{2}$ in 2D and $\frac{2}{5}$ in 3D (see [13]).

Expanding this algorithm to another image with a given probability p_2 requires the introduction of another weighting function w_2. Following Eq (3), we can now define the co-detection energy as

$$E_{co-det}(\mathbf{c},\mathbf{M},w_i,\mathcal{G}_r) = - \int_{\Omega} \phi_{\mathbf{c},\mathbf{M}}\, p_1\, w_1 \;-\; \int_{\Omega} \phi_{\mathbf{c},\mathbf{M}} \circ \mathcal{G}_r\, p_2\, w_2$$

$$+ \mu \left(\int_{\Omega} p_1 w_1 + p_2 w_2 \right) \log \left(\frac{\mathcal{V}ol(\mathbf{M})}{|\Omega|} \right)$$

with $\quad \mathcal{V}ol(\mathbf{M}) = \dfrac{4\pi}{3} \sqrt{\det \mathbf{M}^{-1}} \quad$ the ellipsoid volume. $\tag{6}$

To facilitate the resolution of such a problem, $\mathcal{G}_r$ - as a rigid transformation - can be decomposed into a rotation and a translation. We can therefore equivalently write the energy as a function of the ellipsoid center $\mathbf{c}_2$ in the second image and the rotation matrix $\mathbf{R}$:

$$E_{co-det}(\mathbf{c}_i, w_i, \mathbf{R}, \mathbf{M}) = - \int_{\Omega} \phi_{\mathbf{c}_1,\mathbf{M}}(\mathbf{x})\, p_1(\mathbf{x})\, w_1(\mathbf{x})\, d\mathbf{x} \tag{7}$$

$$- \int_{\Omega} \phi_{\mathbf{c}_2,\mathbf{R}^T\mathbf{M}\mathbf{R}}(\mathbf{x})\, p_2(\mathbf{x})\, w_2(\mathbf{x})\, d\mathbf{x}$$

$$+ \mu \left(\int_{\Omega} p_1 w_1 + p_2 w_2 \right) \log \left(\frac{\mathcal{V}ol(\mathbf{M})}{|\Omega|} \right)$$

Minimization of such functional is done in an alternate three-step process:

1. The statistical interpretation still holds for the ellipsoids centers and matrix: minimizers c_1^* and c_2^* are weighted centroids while minimizer $\mathbf{M}^*$ is related to the weighted covariance matrix of pixels coming from both images.

2. The unknown matrix $\mathbf{R}$ accounts for the possible rotation between the two images and can be parametrized by a vector of angles $\Theta \in \mathbb{R}^3$. A gradient descent is peformed at each iteration to minimize the energy with respect to Θ.
3. The weights w_1 and w_2 are finally updated as indicator functions (up to a slight dilation) of the current ellipsoid estimates.

The complete minimization strategy is summarized in Algorithm 1. This algorithm is computationally efficient : closed-form solutions are available (except for $\mathbf{R}$) and the process, though iterative, usually converges in very few iterations.

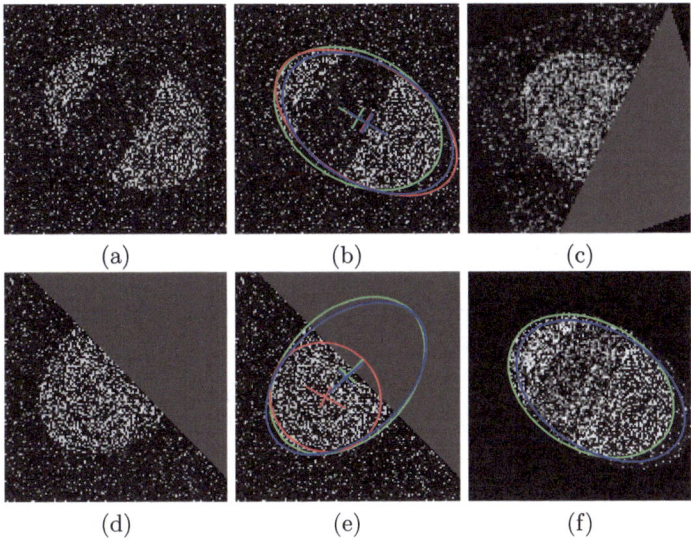

Fig. 2. Ellipse detection on two synthetic images with p_1 (a) and p_2 (d). Detected ellipses with their center and main axes are shown in (b) and (e) for independent ellipse detection (red) and proposed method for co-detection (blue) compared to the ground truth (green). (c) Second image registered with the estimated transform $\mathcal{G}_r^{-1}$. (f) Combination of image terms $w_1 p_1 + (w_2 p_2) \circ \mathcal{G}_r^{-1}$ used for ellipse estimation at convergence.

Figure 2 shows an example of ellipse co-detection in synthetic images, where the probability of belonging to the target object is the image intensity. Despite the noise, the simulated shadow and the reduced field-of-view effect, the co-detection algorithm provides a good estimate on the ellipse position, size and orientation in both images.

2.3 Co-segmentation via Implicit Template Deformation

The previously detected ellipsoid is not a precise segmentation of the kidney, but can be used as an initialization for a more elaborate segmentation method, namely template deformation [14,10].

Algorithm 1. Robust ellipsoid co-detection algorithm

---

initialization $\forall\, \mathbf{x} \in \Omega,\ w_1(\mathbf{x}) \leftarrow 1,\ w_2(\mathbf{x}) \leftarrow 1$

repeat

    // Estimation of centers $\mathbf{c}_1$ and $\mathbf{c}_2$ and matrix $\mathbf{M}$

    $\mathbf{c}_1 \leftarrow \frac{1}{\int_\Omega p_1 w_1} \int_\Omega p_1(\mathbf{x})\, w_1(\mathbf{x})\, \mathbf{x}\, dx$

    $\mathbf{c}_2 \leftarrow \frac{1}{\int_\Omega p_2 w_2} \int_\Omega p_2(\mathbf{x})\, w_2(\mathbf{x})\, \mathbf{x}\, dx$

    $\mathbf{M}^{-1} \leftarrow \frac{2}{\mu \int_\Omega p_1 w_1 + p_2 w_2} \Big(\int_\Omega p_1(\mathbf{x})\, w_1(\mathbf{x})\, (\mathbf{x} - \mathbf{c}_1)\, (\mathbf{x} - \mathbf{c}_1)^T dx$

                        $+ \int_\Omega p_2(\mathbf{x})\, w_2(\mathbf{x})\, \mathbf{R}\, (\mathbf{x} - \mathbf{c}_2)\, (\mathbf{x} - \mathbf{c}_2)^T\, \mathbf{R}^T dx \Big)$

    // Update of the rotation matrix $\mathbf{R}$ by gradient descent with time step Δt

    repeat

    | $\mathbf{R}(\Theta) \leftarrow \mathbf{R}\left(\Theta - \Delta t\, \nabla_\Theta E_{co-det}(\Theta)\right)$

    until *convergence*;

    // Update of the weighting functions w_1 and w_2 for each $\mathbf{x} \in \Omega$

    if $(\mathbf{x} - \mathbf{c})^T \mathcal{M}\, (\mathbf{x} - \mathbf{c}) \leq 1 - \mu \log\left(\frac{\mathcal{V}ol(\mathbf{M})}{|\Omega|}\right)$ **then**

      $\lfloor\ w_1(\mathbf{x}) \leftarrow 1$ **else** $w_1(\mathbf{x}) \leftarrow 0$

    if $(\mathbf{x} - \mathbf{c}_2)^T \mathbf{R}^T \mathbf{M} \mathbf{R}\, (\mathbf{x} - \mathbf{c}_2) \leq 1 - \mu \log\left(\frac{\mathcal{V}ol(\mathbf{M})}{|\Omega|}\right)$ **then**

      $\lfloor\ w_2(\mathbf{x}) \leftarrow 1$ **else** $w_2(\mathbf{x}) \leftarrow 0$

until *convergence*;

Template deformation is a model-based segmentation framework that represents the segmented object as a deformed initial function (called template). In an implicit setting [10], this segmentation is represented by the zero-level set of a function $\phi : \Omega \to \mathbb{R}$ defined as $\phi = \phi_0 \circ \psi$, where ϕ_0 is the implicit template and the transformation $\psi : \Omega \to \Omega$ becomes the unknown of the problem. ψ is sought as a minimum of the following energy

$$E_{seg}(\psi) = \int_\Omega H(\phi_0 \circ \psi)\, r_I(\mathbf{x})\, d\mathbf{x} + \mathcal{R}(\psi)\ . \tag{8}$$

where H is the Heaviside function (i.e. $H(x) = 1$ if $x > 0$, otherwise 0) and r_I an image-based term negative (resp. positive) at pixels likely to be inside (resp. outside) the target object. The template ϕ_0 acts as a shape prior and the transformation ψ that ϕ_0 undergoes is penalized via $\mathcal{R}$. In order to define this regularization term, this transformation is decomposed as $\psi = \mathcal{L} \circ \mathcal{G}$ where

- $\mathcal{G}$ is a global transformation that accounts for the pose and scale of the segmentation. It is defined through a vector of parameters (typically in $\mathbb{R}^7$ for a 3D similarity);
- $\mathcal{L}$ is a non-rigid local deformation, expressed using a displacement field $\mathbf{u}$ such that $\mathcal{L}(\mathbf{x}) = \mathbf{x} + (\mathbf{u} * K_\sigma)(\mathbf{x})$. K_σ is a Gaussian kernel that provides built-in smoothness.

This decomposition allows $\mathcal{R}$ to be pose-invariant and constrains only the non-rigid deformation : $\mathcal{R}(\psi) = \mathcal{R}(\mathcal{L}) = \int_\Omega \|\mathcal{L} - Id\|^2 = \int_\Omega \|\mathbf{u} * K_\sigma\|^2$. Penalizing the magnitude of the displacement field allows to control the deviation of the segmentation from the initial shape prior.

Implicit template deformation, as previously described, is part of the framework defined in Eq. (1) with $f = H$. We can therefore extend it to co-segmentation using Eq. (3) by considering the following functional:

$$
E_{co-seg}(\mathcal{L}, \mathcal{G}, \mathcal{G}_r) = \int_{\Omega} H(\phi_0 \circ \mathcal{L} \circ \mathcal{G}) \, r_{I_1}(\mathbf{x}) \, d\mathbf{x}
$$
$$
+ \int_{\Omega} H(\phi_0 \circ \mathcal{L} \circ \mathcal{G} \circ \mathcal{G}_r) \, r_{I_2}(\mathbf{x}) \, d\mathbf{x} + \frac{\lambda}{2} \|\mathcal{L} - Id\|_2^2 \ . \qquad (9)
$$

In our application, the template ϕ_0 is defined as the implicit representation of the detected ellipsoid $\phi_{\mathbf{c}_1, \mathcal{M}}$. $\mathcal{G}$ and $\mathcal{L}$ are initially set to the identity while $\mathcal{G}_r$ is initialized with the previously estimated registering transformation: $\mathcal{G}_r(\mathbf{x}) = \mathbf{R}\,(\mathbf{x} + \mathbf{c}_1 - \mathbf{c}_2)$. As in [13], the image-terms are defined as $r_{I_i} = \Delta p_i$ where Δ denotes the Laplacian operator and p_i the kidney probability in image i. The energy E_{co-seg} is then minimized with respect to the parameters of $\mathcal{G}$, $\mathcal{G}_r$ and each component of the vector field $\mathbf{u}$, through a gradient descent.

3   Learning Kidney Appearance Using Random Forests

The previously described algorithms rely on functions p_I that associate to each voxel $\mathbf{x}$ of the image I a probability to belong to the kidney. In CEUS images, bright areas indicate the presence of contrast agent which is mainly localized in the kidney. Therefore we can directly use the normalized intensity of the image as a probability term, i.e. $p_{CEUS} = \frac{I_{CEUS}}{\max I_{CEUS}}$.

However, the kidney appearance has a much higher variability in US images, although their structure is consistent: kidneys are always composed of a bright sinus surrounded by a darker parenchyma (see Figure 3). As intensity itself is not reliable enough, we chose to combine multiple image features using decision forests [2] to obtain a class posterior map p_{US}. Recent work [11,9,6,4,20] demonstrated that adding contextual information allows to improve spatial consistency and thus classification performance. Here we propose to exploit the kidney structure in a simple yet efficient way. Similarly to the auto-context framework introduced by Tu et al. [15], contextual information is included by using two classifiers in cascade. A first classification (kidney vs background) is performed in each voxel using a decision forest. Then we use these class posterior probabilities as additional input of a second random forest that will give the final kidney probability p_{US}.

The features used for the first decision forest were the intensity of the image and its Laplacian at the considered voxel as well as at its neighbors' within a $7 \times 7 \times 7$ local patch, at three different scales ($\sigma = 2, 4, 6$ mm). Intensities were normalized in each patch. For the second forest, we added the estimated class posterior as additional channels. Each forest was composed of 10 trees with maximum depth 15.

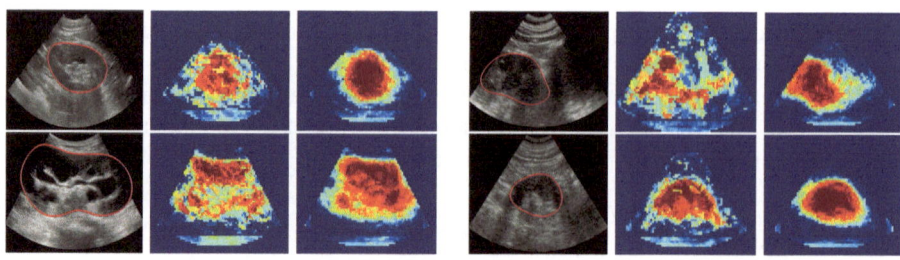

Fig. 3. Kidney appearance in US images (denoted in red). Left: original images showing the high variability of the database. Middle: kidney probability given by the first classifier. Right: final kidney probablity p_{US}.

4   Experiments and Validation

4.1   Material

Our database is composed of 64 couples of CEUS and US volumes acquired from 35 different patients. This set is clinically representative as different ultrasound probes were used, with different fields of view, on both diseased and healthy kidneys. The volumes size was $512 \times 510 \times 256$ voxels with varying spatial resolutions ($0.25 \times 0.25 \times 0.55$ mm in average). The CEUS acquisitions have been performed a few seconds after injection of 2.4 mL of Sonovue (Bracco, Italy) contrast agent. Kidney segmentation made by an expert was available for each image as a ground truth. The proposed method was implemented in C++ and the average overall computational time was around 20 seconds on a standard computer (Intel Core i5 2.67 Ghz, 4GB RAM).

4.2   Validation on the Learnt Kidney Appearance in US Images

The patient database was split into two groups. Results on the whole dataset were then obtained using a two-fold cross-validation. Figure 4 shows the ROC and Precision-Recall curves, as well as a boxplot of the Dice coefficients obtained by thresholding the kidney probabilities computed (i) by the first decision forest and (ii) using the auto-context approach with another forest in cascade. The latter provides better kidney probabilities with respect to all reported statistics. In particular, Dice coefficients are significantly improved, with a p-value $< 10^{-4}$ (in this paper, all p-values were obtained for the Wilcoxon signed-rank test after Bonferroni correction). Indeed, taking into account structural information helps for example in distinguishing the kidney sinus from the background or the parenchyma from shadows, and allows a more spatially coherent classification (see Figure 3).

4.3   Validation on the Kidney Co-segmentation

In all CEUS/US couples, kidneys were co-detected using Section 2.2 as an initialization for the co-segmentation algorithm of Section 2.3. For comparison, we

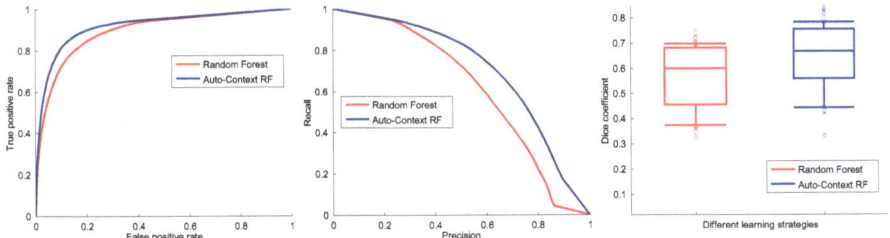

Fig. 4. Comparison of classification results for the single decision forest and the auto-context approach. (Left) ROC Curve. (Middle) Precision-Recall curve. (Right) Boxplot of the Dice coefficients (p-value $< 10^{-4}$).

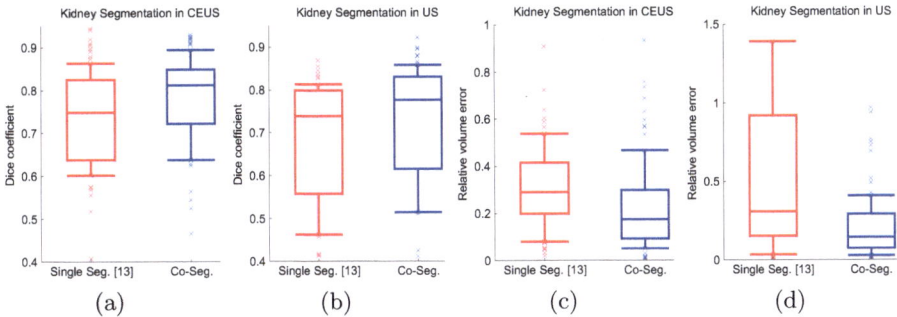

Fig. 5. Boxplots of segmentation results for kidney segmentation in US and CEUS images, in terms of Dice coefficients (a-b) and relative volume error (c-d). The proposed co-segmentation compares favorably to independent segmentation following [13], with a p-value $< 10^{-4}$.

also segmented the kidney following [13] independently in each modality, which is state-of-the-art for CEUS segmentation. Validation was performed by comparing the segmentation result and the ground truth in both US and CEUS images. Dice coefficients and relative error on the measured kidney volume are reported in Figure 5. Using simultaneously the complementary information from US and CEUS images significantly improves the segmentation accuracy in both modalities. More specifically, the median Dice coefficient is increased from 0.74 to 0.81 in CEUS (p-value $< 10^{-4}$) and 0.73 to 0.78 in US (p-value $< 10^{-4}$). Furthermore, the proposed approach provides more reliable clinical information as the median error on the kidney volume is almost divided by two in CEUS (29% versus 15%) and in US (25% versus 13%). Figure 6 shows the joint co-segmentation and registration results for one case. Independent segmentation fails in both US and CEUS images because of the kidney lesion (indicated by the yellow arrow), that looks like the background in CEUS but like the kidney in US. Conversely, the proposed co-segmentation manages to overcome this difficulty by combining information from the two modalities. Furthermore, for this example, one can assess the estimated registration by comparing the location of the lesion in the two modalities. Results on another case were also displayed in Figure 1.

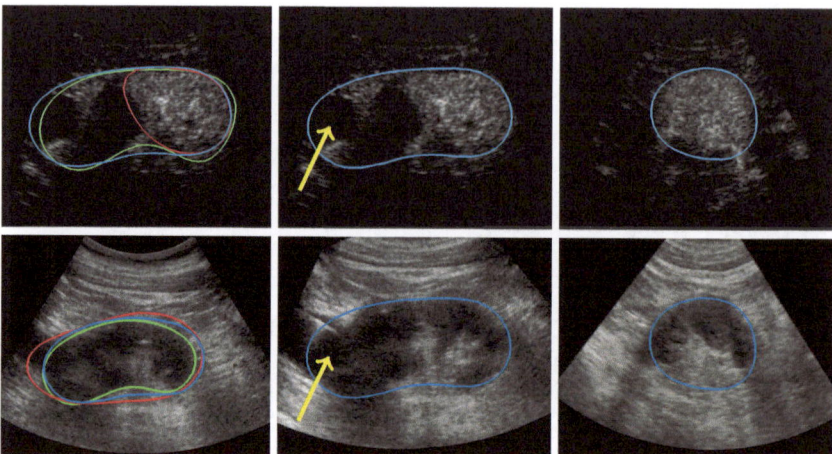

Fig. 6. Example of joint co-segmentation and registration for a CEUS (top) and a US (bottom) images. (Left) Comparison of independent segmentations (red) and the proposed co-segmentation (blue) with respect to the ground truths (green). (Middle, Right) Two views of the registered volumes that can be assessed by considering the position of the lesion (yellow arrow).

5   Conclusion

In this paper, we introduced a novel framework to jointly perform co-segmentation and registration by seeking the same object in different images. This allowed to significantly improve state-of-the-art results of kidney segmentation in CEUS images by simultaneously taking into account complementary information coming from the available US image. A global CEUS/US registration is also available as a side outcome. The full pipeline is automated and computationally efficient for 3D images.

The genericity of our joint co-segmentation and registration framework is three-fold. First, it can be applied to a large class of variational problems, as shown here with ellipsoid detection and model-based segmentation methods. Second, it can be used for any kind of image: in this paper, we used dedicated classifiers for kidney in US/CEUS images but our approach can be plugged on top of any pixelwise classifier. Finally, we presented co-segmentation in two images but generalization to an arbitrary number of images is straightforward. This paves the way for organ tracking application in 3D+T sequences, which we are currently investigating. We also plan to extend the current framework by considering a non global transformation between images in order to cope with deformable organs.

References

1. Albrecht, T., et al.: Guidelines for the use of contrast agents in ultrasound. Ultraschall Med. 25(4), 249–256 (2004)
2. Breiman, L.: Random forests. Machine Learning 45(1), 5–32 (2001)
3. Chan, T.F., Vese, L.A.: Active contours without edges. IEEE TIP 10(2), 266–277 (2001)

4. Glocker, B., Pauly, O., Konukoglu, E., Criminisi, A.: Joint classification-regression forests for spatially structured multi-object segmentation. In: Fitzgibbon, A., Lazebnik, S., Perona, P., Sato, Y., Schmid, C. (eds.) ECCV 2012, Part IV. LNCS, vol. 7575, pp. 870–881. Springer, Heidelberg (2012)
5. Han, D., Bayouth, J., Song, Q., Taurani, A., Sonka, M., Buatti, J., Wu, X.: Globally optimal tumor segmentation in PET-CT images: A graph-based co-segmentation method. In: Székely, G., Hahn, H.K. (eds.) IPMI 2011. LNCS, vol. 6801, pp. 245–256. Springer, Heidelberg (2011)
6. Kontschieder, P., Bulò, S.R., Criminisi, A., Kohli, P., Pelillo, M., Bischof, H.: Context-sensitive decision forests for object detection. In: Proceedings of NIPS, pp. 440–448 (2012)
7. Lu, C., Duncan, J.S.: A coupled segmentation and registration framework for medical image analysis using robust point matching and active shape model. In: IEEE Workshop on MMBIA, pp. 129–136 (2012)
8. Martin-Fernandez, M., Alberola-Lopez, C.: An approach for contour detection of human kidneys from ultrasound images using Markov random fields and active contours. MedIA 9(1), 1–23 (2005)
9. Montillo, A., Shotton, J., Winn, J., Iglesias, J.E., Metaxas, D., Criminisi, A.: Entangled decision forests and their application for semantic segmentation of CT images. In: Székely, G., Hahn, H.K. (eds.) IPMI 2011. LNCS, vol. 6801, pp. 184–196. Springer, Heidelberg (2011)
10. Mory, B., Somphone, O., Prevost, R., Ardon, R.: Real-time 3D image segmentation by user-constrained template deformation. In: Ayache, N., Delingette, H., Golland, P., Mori, K. (eds.) MICCAI 2012, Part I. LNCS, vol. 7510, pp. 561–568. Springer, Heidelberg (2012)
11. Payet, N., Todorovic, S.: 2-Random Forest Random Field. In: Proceedings of NIPS 2010 (2010)
12. Pohl, K.M., Fisher, J., Grimson, W.E.L., Kikinis, R., Wells, W.M.: A Bayesian model for joint segmentation and registration. NeuroImage 31(1), 228–239 (2006)
13. Prevost, R., Mory, B., Correas, J.-M., Cohen, L.D., Ardon, R.: Kidney detection and real-time segmentation in 3D contrast-enhanced ultrasound images. In: Proceedings of IEEE ISBI, pp. 1559–1562 (2012)
14. Saddi, K., Chefd'hotel, C., Rousson, M., Cheriet, F.: Region-based segmentation via non-rigid template matching. In: Proceedings of ICCV, pp. 1–7 (2007)
15. Tu, Z., Bai, X.: Auto-context and its application to high-level vision tasks and 3D brain image segmentation. IEEE TPAMI 32(10), 1744–1757 (2010)
16. Vicente, S., Kolmogorov, V., Rother, C.: Cosegmentation revisited: Models and optimization. In: Daniilidis, K., Maragos, P., Paragios, N. (eds.) ECCV 2010, Part II. LNCS, vol. 6312, pp. 465–479. Springer, Heidelberg (2010)
17. Wang, F., Vemuri, B.C.: Simultaneous registration and segmentation of anatomical structures from brain MRI. In: Duncan, J.S., Gerig, G. (eds.) MICCAI 2005. LNCS, vol. 3749, pp. 17–25. Springer, Heidelberg (2005)
18. Wyatt, P.P., Noble, J.A.: MAP MRF joint segmentation and registration. In: Dohi, T., Kikinis, R. (eds.) MICCAI 2002, Part I. LNCS, vol. 2488, pp. 580–587. Springer, Heidelberg (2002)
19. Yezzi, A., Zöllei, L., Kapur, T.: A variational framework for integrating segmentation and registration through active contours. MedIA 7(2), 171–185 (2003)
20. Zikic, D., Glocker, B., Konukoglu, E., Criminisi, A., Demiralp, C., Shotton, J., Thomas, O.M., Das, T., Jena, R., Price, S.J.: Decision Forests for Tissue-Specific Segmentation of High-Grade Gliomas in Multi-channel MR. In: Ayache, N., Delingette, H., Golland, P., Mori, K. (eds.) MICCAI 2012, Part III. LNCS, vol. 7512, pp. 369–376. Springer, Heidelberg (2012)

Deformable Modeling Using a 3D Boundary Representation with Quadratic Constraints on the Branching Structure of the Blum Skeleton

Paul A. Yushkevich[1] and Hui Gary Zhang[2],[*]

[1] Penn Image Computing and Science Laboratory (PICSL), Department of Radiology, University of Pennsylvania, Philadelphia, USA
[2] Centre for Medical Image Computing, Department of Computer Science, University College London, London, United Kingdom

Abstract. We propose a new approach for statistical shape analysis of 3D anatomical objects based on features extracted from skeletons. Like prior work on medial representations [7,15,9], the approach involves deforming a template to target shapes in a way that preserves the branching structure of the skeleton and provides intersubject correspondence. However, unlike medial representations, which parameterize the skeleton surfaces explicitly, our representation is boundary-centric, and the skeleton is implicit. Similar to prior constrained modeling methods developed 2D objects [8] or tube-like 3D objects [13], we impose symmetry constraints on tuples of boundary points in a way that guarantees the preservation of the skeleton's topology under deformation. Once discretized, the problem of deforming a template to a target shape is formulated as a quadratically constrained quadratic programming problem. The new technique is evaluated in terms of its ability to capture the shape of the corpus callosum tract extracted from diffusion-weighted MRI.

1 Introduction

The *Blum skeleton* [2] is a geometrical construct that provides a powerful set of features for quantifying the symmetric properties of geometric objects, particularly those derived from biomedical imaging. Although the skeleton, or *medial axis*, was originally described by Blum [2] in the plane (defined as the set of connected curves formed by the centers of maximal inscribed disks a 2D object), the concept and the definition of the skeleton naturally extend to 3D. The skeleton of a 3D object, also called the *medial scaffold*, consists of surfaces, which are formed by the centers of all maximal inscribed balls (MIBs) in the object. We give a more formal definition in Sec. 2.1, and Fig. 1 provides an illustration.

The Blum skeleton is used frequently in image and shape analysis because it captures important salient properties of natural objects [9]. For instance, the curvature of the skeleton can be used to characterize how an object bends locally,

---

[*] This research was supported by NIH grants R01-AG037376, R01-NS065347 and R01-EB014346.

J.C. Gee et al. (Eds.): IPMI 2013, LNCS 7917, pp. 280–291, 2013.
© Springer-Verlag Berlin Heidelberg 2013

particularly for tube-like or sheet-like objects. Each point on the skeleton is associated with the radius of the corresponding MIB, and the radius function provides a way to measure the local thickness of tube and sheet-like objects. Since many of the commonly studied organs in the human body are sheet-like or tube-like (cerebral cortex, many white matter tracts, myocardium, heart valves, etc.), such measures of thickness and bending are commonly sought in biomedical applications, e.g., to characterize the effects of disease on organs and tissues. Even objects that are not sheet-like (e.g., the hippocampus) have been analyzed using features derived from skeletons [10,3].

The use of skeleton-derived geometric features in statistical shape analysis is complicated by the fact that the composition of the medial axis/scaffold into curves and surfaces, known as *branching structure*, is almost always different for multiple instances of a given class of geometric objects (e.g., the hippocampi of different individuals). A very small deformation to the boundary of an object, such as adding a bump on the surface, can change the medial branching structure. This variability in branching makes it challenging to find correspondences between medial axes/scaffolds of different instances and to apply the standard tools of statistical shape analysis. In some cases, this challenge can be overcome by pruning smaller branches heuristically until, for each instance, the medial axis/scaffold is reduced to a common branching structure [3]. An alternative approach that allows features derived from skeletons to be used for statistical shape analysis is based on the deformable modeling framework. A template is deformed to optimally match each instance in a class of objects, with deformations constrained to preserve the medial branching structure of the template. The match between each deformed template and the instance it is approximating is not perfect, but in many problems, the mismatch is on the order of the other errors involved in imaging-based morphometry, and thus an acceptable price to pay for preserving homology between skeleton-derived features. Such medially-constrained deformable modeling methods can be divided into two rough groups: (1) methods that model the medial axis/scaffold of the deformable template explicitly, and (2) methods that impose geometric constraints on the boundary of the deformable template. In the first class are the the Pizer et al. m-rep method [7], and derivative techniques such as continuous m-rep [15,12]. These methods explicitly describe the medial scaffold of the deformable template, and derive the boundary of the model algorithmically. Examples from the second class of methods include symmetry-seeking tubular models by Terzopoulos et al. [13], skeleton-constrained 2D level set methods [8], and linked-surface deformable modeling techniques (e.g., [16]).

Among these medially-constrained deformable modeling methods, few have sought to adhere strictly to "true" 3D Blum medial geometry, which, we would argue, takes away from the interpretability of the skeleton-derived features in shape analysis applications. For instance, the original m-rep approach does not model medial scaffolds with multiple branches as such; instead, it models complex objects using subfigures attached to the boundaries of parent figures [7]. Coupled surface methods frequently model surfaces as parallel or constrained to be a certain minimal distance apart [16], constraints that are not directly related to how skeletons are defined. Continuous m-rep methods [15,12], which describe the medial scaffold parametrically and derive the boundary by inverting the skeletonization process, have been successful at creating 3D deformable models that adhere to Blum geometry. However, they suffer from the inherent challenges that arise from trying to explicitly parameterize medial scaffolds, which are, essentially, singularities. For instance, near the free edges of the medial scaffold (see Fig. 1), inverse skeletonization is asymptotic: an infinitesimal step along the medial scaffold maps to a big step on the boundary. Behavior along creases (curves along which medial surfaces join) is also asymptotic and challenging to model. Most difficult of all is to model endpoints of creases parametrically. In fact, just one paper by Terriberry et al. [12] has claimed this capability, and has only demonstrated it with a static example. To our knowledge, the ability to deform templates adhering to 3D Blum geometry to target data has not been demonstrated for templates with multiple branches.[1]

The main contribution of this paper is to propose a new paradigm for Blum-adherent 3D deformable medial modeling, which bridges these two classes of deformable modeling techniques. Our goals are closest to those of m-rep methods (to allow statistical analysis of skeleton-derived features across populations of objects), but our approach is closer to symmetry-seeking models by Terzopoulos et al. [13] and skeletally coupled level sets by Sebastian et al. [8]. It is the boundary of the deformable template that is modeled parametrically, while the medial scaffold is defined implicitly. Similar to [13,8], constraints are imposed on the boundary parameterization to ensure that deformation does not change the medial branching structure of the template. Unlike [8], which is 2D, and [13], which imposes tubular symmetries, our approach is used to model arbitrary 3D shapes, including those with branching medial scaffolds. An additional contribution of this paper is to formulate the problem deformable modeling with medial constraints as a quadratically constrained quadratic programing (QCQP) problem, leading to efficient, albeit non-convex, optimization.

2   Methods

2.1   3D Medial Geometry Background

We use the term *object* to refer to a set $S \subset \mathbb{R}^n$ that is homologous to a closed ball and has a smooth boundary, denoted ∂S. A ball B is a *maximal inscribed ball (MIB)* in S if $B \subset S$ and there exists no other ball $B' \subset S$ such that $B \subset B'$. Every point on ∂S belongs to exactly one MIB. The Blum [2] *medial axis transform (MAT)* of S is the transformation that maps each point $\mathbf{x} \in \partial S$ to the center of the MIB containing $\mathbf{x}$. The terms *medial scaffold, medial axis* or *skeleton* are used to describe the range of this mapping, i.e., the set of centers

---

[1] Sun et al. [11] developed a myocardium model with three surfaces joining along a crease, but they did not model the myocardium as a closed surface, which simplified Blum geometry at crease endpoints.

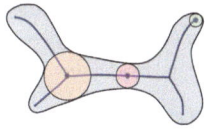 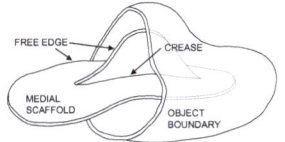

Fig. 1. Left: the medial axis of a 2D object, with examples of MIBs tangent to the boundary at one, two and three points. Right: an illustration of a 3D object, half of which has been cut away to reveal the medial scaffold. The medial scaffold consists of surface patches that join along crease curves and terminate at free edge curves.

of all MIBs in S. Generically, the medial scaffold consists of one or more surface patches. Curves that are shared by multiple surface patches in the medial scaffold are called *creases*. The remaining boundaries of these surface patches are called *free edges* (see Figure 1).

Each MIB in S is tangent to ∂S at one or more points. Thus, the MAT is a many-to-one mapping. In fact, most MIBs in S are tangent to ∂S at two points. Centers of these bitangent MIBs lie on the interiors of the surface patches that form the medial scaffold of S. Centers of MIBs tangent to ∂S at three points form the creases of the medial scaffold. Centers of MIBs that are tangent to ∂S at only one point form the free edges of the medial scaffold. These MIBs have a higher order of tangency with ∂S, i.e., the radius of such MIB is the reciprocal the larger of the principal curvatures to ∂S at the point of tangency. As shown by Giblin [4], two more types of MIB tangency occur generically, corresponding to junctions of creases and free edges, and to crease-crease intersections.

2.2 Derivation of Medial Constraints on the Boundary

We begin by deriving a constraint on the boundary of a deformable template that ensures that the branching structure of the template's medial axis is preserved under deformation. We say that two points $x_1, x_2 \in \partial S$ are *medially linked* if they belong to the same MIB in S, or, equivalently, $\text{MAT}(x_1) = \text{MAT}(x_2)$. Our method is based on the fact that transformations of S that preserve medial links also preserve the branching structure of the medial scaffold. More formally,

Theorem 1. *Let S be an object in $\mathbb{R}^3$. Let $\Phi : \mathbb{R}^3 \to \mathbb{R}^3$ be a bijective and differentiable transformation. Let $S' = \{x \in \mathbb{R}^3 : \Phi^{-1}(x) \in S\}$. Suppose that Φ "preserves medial links", i.e., for any two points $x_1, x_2 \in \partial S$, the points $\Phi(x_1)$ and $\Phi(x_2)$ are medially linked in S' if and only if x_1 and x_2 are medially linked in S. Then the MAT of S' is homeomorphic to the MAT of S.*

Proof. We outline the proof due to limited space. The proof involves constructing a mapping Ψ between the MAT of S' and the MAT of S, as follows. Let m be a point on the MAT of S, then let $X \in \partial S$ be the non-empty set of points where the MIB centered at m is tangent to ∂S. Let $X' = \{x \in \mathbb{R}^3 : \Phi^{-1}(x) \in X\}$. If X has only one element, let $\Psi(m)$ be the center of the MIB containing the sole point in X'. If X has multiple elements, any two of them are medially linked, and thus any two elements in X' are medially linked. Thus, there exists an MIB that is tangent to $\partial S'$ at all points in X'. Let $\Psi(\mathbf{m})$ be the center of that MIB. Proof by contradiction can be used to show that Ψ is bijective and continuous.

Next, we write down the sufficient conditions for transformation Φ to preserve medial links. It is a trivial fact that a ball with center $\mathbf{m} \in S$ and radius R is tangent to ∂S at the point $\mathbf{x}$ if and only if $\mathbf{m} = \mathbf{x} - R\mathbf{N}$, where $\mathbf{N}$ is the unit outward normal to ∂S at $\mathbf{x}$. It is also simple to show that such a ball is a MIB in S if $\forall \mathbf{y} \in \partial S$, $\|\mathbf{y} - \mathbf{m}\| \geq R$. From these observations, we conclude that two points $\mathbf{x}_1, \mathbf{x}_2 \in \partial S$ are medially linked if and only if there exists $R > 0$ such that $\mathbf{x}_1 - R\mathbf{N}_1 = \mathbf{x}_2 - R\mathbf{N}_2$ and $\|\mathbf{y} - (\mathbf{x}_1 - R\mathbf{N}_1)\| \geq R$ for all $\mathbf{y} \in \partial S$.

2.3   Medially-Constrained Model Fitting – Continuous Formulation

We first formulate the problem of fitting a medially-constrained template to a target object in the continuous case. In the following section, the continuous problem is discretized and solved numerically. Let the object S be a template, whose MAT has the desired branching structure, and let $\mathcal{T}$ be a target object. The goal is to deform S, making it as similar as possible to $\mathcal{T}$, while maintaining the branching structure of the MAT of S after deformation.

   Let U be some parametric domain (e.g., the unit sphere), and $\mathbf{x} : U \to \partial S$ be a smooth bijective map that provides a global parameterization of ∂S. Let $\mathcal{L} \subset U \times U$ be the set of all parameter value pairs $(\mathbf{u}, \mathbf{v})$, such that $\mathbf{u} \neq \mathbf{v}$ and $\mathbf{x}(\mathbf{u})$ and $\mathbf{x}(\mathbf{v})$ are medially linked in S. Let $\mathcal{D}$ be the set of diffeomorphic transformations of $\mathbb{R}^3$ and let $\mathcal{F}_{\mathcal{L}}^+$ be the set of all bounded continuous positive real-valued functions on $\mathcal{L}$. For any $\Phi \in \mathcal{D}$, let $S_\Phi = \{\mathbf{x} \in \mathbb{R}^3 : \Phi^{-1}(\mathbf{x}) \in S\}$, let $\mathbf{x}_\Phi(\mathbf{u}) = \Phi(\mathbf{x}(\mathbf{u}))$, and let $\mathbf{N}_\Phi(\mathbf{u})$ be the unit outward normal vector to ∂S_Φ at $\mathbf{x}_\Phi(\mathbf{u})$. Let μ be some measure of dissimilarity between two objects in $\mathbb{R}^3$ (e.g., mean closest-point distance) and let ρ be some measure of irregularity of a transformation (e.g., bending energy). *The continuous medially-constrained deformable modeling problem seeks to find a transformation $\Phi^* \in \mathcal{D}$ that satisfies*

$$\Phi^* = \underset{\Phi \in \mathcal{D}, R \in \mathcal{F}_{\mathcal{L}}}{\arg\min} \ \mu(\mathcal{T}, S_\Phi) + \rho(\Phi), \tag{1}$$

subject to the following two conditions:

$$\mathbf{x}_\Phi(\mathbf{u}) - R(\mathbf{u}, \mathbf{v})\,\mathbf{N}_\Phi(\mathbf{u}) = \mathbf{x}_\Phi(\mathbf{v}) - R(\mathbf{u}, \mathbf{v})\,\mathbf{N}_\Phi(\mathbf{v}) \qquad \forall (\mathbf{u}, \mathbf{v}) \in \mathcal{L}, \tag{2}$$

$$\|\mathbf{x}_\Phi(\mathbf{w}) - [\mathbf{x}_\Phi(\mathbf{u}) - R(\mathbf{u}, \mathbf{v})\,\mathbf{N}_\Phi(\mathbf{u})]\,\| \geq R(\mathbf{u}, \mathbf{v}) \qquad \forall (\mathbf{u}, \mathbf{v}) \in \mathcal{L}, \mathbf{w} \in U. \tag{3}$$

The constraints (2,3) guarantee that $\mathbf{x}_\Phi(\mathbf{u})$ and $\mathbf{x}_\Phi(\mathbf{v})$ are medially linked, and hence the that Φ preserves the branching structure of the MAT of S under deformation. Conversely, any $\Phi \in \mathcal{D}$ that preserves the branching structure of the MAT of S under deformation must satisfy (2,3). Since transformations that preserve MAT branching do exist, we conclude that the minimization problem above is not over-constrained and solutions can be found, in theory. In practice, however, we must discretize and simplify the problem to find solutions.

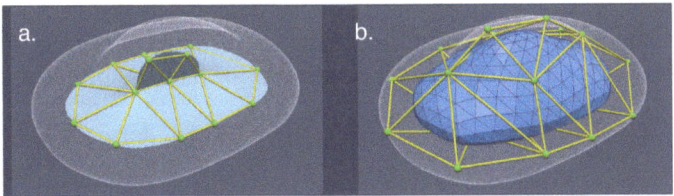

Fig. 2. Illustration of the template building process. **a.** The boundary of a reference object (transparent white surface), its medial scaffold (opaque cyan surfaces), and the coarse mesh formed by points sampled from the creases and free edges of the medial scaffold (green points and yellow tubes). **b.** The coarse mesh inflated onto the boundary of the reference object (green points and yellow tubes) and a fine mesh obtained by applying Loop subdivision [6] to the coarse mesh.

2.4 Medially-Constrained Model Fitting – Discrete Formulation

In the discrete implementation, we model the boundary of the deforming template as a triangular mesh, i.e., a piecewise linear surface with triangular elements. We consider this mesh to be an approximation of a continuous boundary surface, and impose medial linkage constraints (2,3) on tuples of mesh vertices, along with additional constraints on mesh quality. We then deform the mesh to maximize similarity with a target object as well as mesh regularity.

Encoding Medial Links. Let N_b be the number of vertices in the mesh describing the boundary of the deforming template, and let $\mathbf{x}_i$ denote the position of each vertex $i \in [1, N_b]$. Medial links between vertices are encoded by assigning a *medial link index* $M_i \in \mathbb{N}$ to each vertex. Any two vertices i, j such that $M_i = M_j$ are considered medially linked. Some of the vertices are not medially linked to any other vertex (corresponding to free edges of medial scaffolds) and some vertices are medially linked to more than one vertex (corresponding to creases on the medial scaffold). Furthermore, the mesh is constructed in such a way that each triangle on the mesh is linked to exactly one other triangle as follows: if vertices (i, j, k) form a triangle, then there exists exactly one other triangle (i', j', k') in the mesh for which $M_i = M_{i'}$, $M_j = M_{j'}$ and $M_k = M_{k'}$.

How can such meshes be constructed? The approach we use is to take a reference object whose medial scaffold has the desired branching structure. We then define a coarse triangle mesh on the medial scaffold, with vertices sampled along creases and free edges (Fig. 2a). Each triple of connected points is included as a triangular face twice, facing in different directions. The result is a mesh of spherical topology that is infinitely thin, as if shrink-wrapped around the medial scaffold. We then "inflate" the resulting mesh onto the boundary of the reference object (Fig. 2b). The medial link index of each vertex on the coarse inflated mesh is just the index of the vertex on the coarse medial mesh from which it originated. Lastly, we apply Loop subdivision [6] to the inflated coarse mesh, resulting in a finer mesh (blue object in Fig. 2b). It is simple to adjust the Loop subdivision scheme to generate medial link indices consistent with the encoding above.

General Problem Formulation. Once a mesh conforming to the above requirements is created, the problem of deforming it to target objects is defined as a constrained optimization problem. The general form of the problem is

$$\xi^* = \underset{\xi \in \mathbb{R}^{N_v}}{\arg \min} f(\xi) \quad \text{subj. to} \quad \alpha_c \le g_c(\xi) \le \beta_c \quad \text{for } c \in [1, N_c], \qquad (4)$$

where f is the objective being minimized, and g_c are constraint functions, N_v is the number of variables and N_c is the number of constraints. The objective function captures the dissimilarity between the deforming mesh and the target object, as well as the irregularity of the deforming template. The constraints incorporate conditions derived from (2) and (3) that ensure that vertices with the same medial link index are medially linked, and well as additional conditions that ensure mesh quality. The vector of variables ξ includes the vertex coordinates $\mathbf{x}_i$, as well as a large number of additional "helper" variables introduced in order to make all constraints quadratic. The terms forming the objective and the constraints are described in the next few paragraphs.

Medial Linkage Constraints. We impose constraints to ensure that any two vertices (i, j) for which $M_i = M_j$ satisfy discrete versions of the conditions of medial linkage (2) and (3). Let $k = M_i = M_j$. The first condition has the form $\mathbf{x}_i - R_k \mathbf{N}_i = \mathbf{x}_j - R_k \mathbf{N}_j$, where R_k is included as an additional variable in the optimization (analogous to R in the continuous case), and $\mathbf{N}_i$ is the approximation of the unit normal vector to the boundary at $\mathbf{x}_i$. The computation of $\mathbf{N}_i$ requires taking a square root, which would make the constraint non-quadratic. Instead of computing $\mathbf{N}_i$ directly, we add it as an additional variable in the optimization, and impose additional constraints on $\mathbf{N}_i$ that are quadratic:

$$\mathbf{N}_i^t \mathbf{N}_i = 1; \qquad \mathbf{N}_i^t (\mathbf{x}_{,1})_i = 0; \qquad \mathbf{N}_i^t (\mathbf{x}_{,2})_i = 0 \qquad \forall i \in [1, N_b],$$

where $(\mathbf{x}_{,1})_i$ and $(\mathbf{x}_{,2})_i$ are a pair of non-parallel vectors in the tangent plane to the boundary at $\mathbf{x}_i$. Such a pair of vectors can be approximated as weighted sums of vertices in the one-ring neighborhood of i using a scheme described by Loop [6], with the weights dependent only on the valence of the vertex i.

Note that we have not yet defined any constraint on R_k for vertices that are not medially linked to any other vertex. In the continuous case, we did not have to deal with such points, since MIBs that have a single point of tangency with the boundary are limit cases of MIBs with double tangency [2,4]. In the discrete case, we need to deal with these vertices explicitly. Recall from Sec. 2.1 that the radius of a singly tangent MIB is the reciprocal of the larger principal curvature of the boundary at the point of tangency. This leads to the constraint $R_k \cdot \kappa_{i,2} = 1$, where $\kappa_{i,2}$ is the approximation of the larger principal curvature at $\mathbf{x}_i$, and $k = M_i$. The approximation of $\kappa_{i,2}$ is not quadratic but, as we did above for the normal vector, we introduce additional variables and constraints to the optimization problem to keep all constraints quadratic. The added variables are the elements of the first fundamental form, the elements of the shape operator, and the principal curvatures. We omit the details due to space limitations.

The condition that mirrors (3) has the form $\|\mathbf{x}_j - (\mathbf{x}_i - R_k \mathbf{N}_i)\|^2 \geq R_k^2$, where $k = M_i$, for all pairs of vertices i and j. These constraints are quadratic in the variables $\mathbf{x}, \mathbf{N}$ and R. However, there are $O(N_b^2)$ constraints, which does not scale well for larger meshes. Fortunately, in practice, if often suffices to relax this constraint just to the vertices j that are in the one-ring neighborhood of i. Analogous relaxation of a global non self-intersection condition is used in continuous m-reps (i.e., positive medial-boundary Jacobian condition) [15].

Mesh quality constraints. For the approximations of the unit normal and principal curvature on a triangular mesh to be accurate, the triangular elements must not be degenerate. We introduce additional constraints on the minimal angle of each boundary triangle, and on the minimum dihedral angle between adjacent triangles. As before, we introduce additional variables into the optimization problem, such as the area of each triangle, the unit normal to each triangle, and the length of each edge, and relate these variables to each other and the vertex coordinates using quadratic constraints.

Similarity to Target Shape. The objective function f consists of a similarity and regularization terms. The similarity term is based on the iterative closest point (ICP) algorithm. At the beginning of optimization, we match each vertex in the template mesh to the closest point on $\partial \mathcal{T}$, the boundary of the target object $\mathcal{T}$. We also match points on $\partial \mathcal{T}$ to the closest locations on the template. We then minimize the sum of squared distances between the matched points. Specifically, for each vertex i, let $\mathbf{y}_i$ be the point on $\mathcal{T}$ that is closest to $\mathbf{x}_i$ at the start of the optimization. Likewise, for a set of N_s regularly sampled points $\mathbf{z}_j$ on $\partial \mathcal{T}$, let $\mathbf{z}'_j$ be the closest point on the template mesh, not necessarily a vertex. Let $\{\mathbf{x}_{i_{j,1}}, \mathbf{x}_{i_{j,2}}, \mathbf{x}_{i_{j,3}}\}$ be the triangle containing $\mathbf{z}'_j$, and let $w_{j,1}, w_{j,2}, w_{j,3}$ be the barycentric coordinates of $\mathbf{z}'_j$ in it. We formulate the objective function as

$$f(\xi) = \frac{1}{N_b} \sum_{i=1}^{N_b} \|\mathbf{x}_i - \mathbf{y}_i\|^2 + \frac{1}{N_s} \sum_{i=1}^{N_s} \|\mathbf{z}_j - \sum_{d=1}^{3} w_{j,d} \mathbf{x}_{i_{j,d}}\|^2 + \rho(\xi), \qquad (5)$$

where ρ is the regularization term, discussed below. As in ICP, the matching and optimization are alternated for several iterations until convergence.

Regularization. Regularization is implemented using Loop subdivision surfaces. Recall that the template mesh is initially generated by Loop subdivision from a coarse mesh. We define the regularization penalty to be the residual between the deforming template mesh and the best approximation of the deforming mesh by a Loop subdivision surface. Specifically, let $\hat{\mathbf{x}}_q$ be the vertices in the coarse mesh, for $j \in [1, N_q]$. Applying Loop subdivision creates a new set of vertices, with the coordinate of the i-th vertex in the subdivided surface given by $\sum_{q \in Q(i)} W_{iq} \hat{\mathbf{x}}_q$, where $Q(i)$ is the set of vertices in the coarse mesh that contribute to the coordinates of the i-th vertex, and W_{iq} are the coefficients from the subdivision scheme, which depend only on the structure of the coarse mesh. We add the vertices $\hat{\mathbf{x}}_q$ as additional variables to the optimization problem. We then define the regularization penalty as the total squared residual $\rho(\xi) = \lambda_\rho \sum_i^{N_b} \|\mathbf{x}_i - \sum_{j \in Q(i)} W_{ij} \hat{\mathbf{x}}_j\|^2$, where λ_ρ is the weight given to the regularization term (set to 1 in our experiments). Since Loop subdivision surfaces are smooth, penalizing the residual to the closest fitting Loop subdivision surface imposes smoothness on the template.

Numerical Solution. The optimization problem for deformable modeling with preservation of medial links involves a large number of variables ($\mathbf{x}_i, \mathbf{N}_i, \mathbf{R}_k, \kappa_{i,2}, \hat{\mathbf{x}}_j$ and several others) and a large number of constraints. However, the constraints and the objective function are quadratic in the variables, i.e., have the form $f(\xi) = \xi^t A_0 \xi + b_0^t \xi$ and $g_k(\xi) = \xi^t A_k \xi + b_k^t$, where the matrices A_0 and A_k are sparse. Although the matrices A_q are not positive definite, and thus a global solution can not be guaranteed, the optimization problem can be solved efficiently using interior point methods. Our implementation uses the Ipopt method [14].

3   Experiments and Results

Corpus Callosum Tract Shape Analysis. The goal of this experiment is to demonstrate that the proposed deformable model can accurately capture the shape of the corpus callosum (CC) across a cohort of subjects. To demonstrate this, we first automatically label the CC using atlas-based segmentation, and then fit a deformable medial model to each segmentation, allowing subsequent shape analysis using skeleton-derived features. We focus on the CC because its shape in 3D is non-trivial, and because skeleton-derived features have proved useful for joint analysis of microscopic and macroscopic properties of sheet-like white matter tracts extracted from diffusion MRI [17]. We use diffusion tensor imaging (DTI) data from 51 subjects (ages 29-82, mean 70.0±7.1, 30 females and 21 males) in the IXI brain MRI database (http://biomedic.doc.ic.ac.uk/brain-development). We label the CC in each subject using atlas-based segmentation, with the IXI aging DTI template [17] serving as the atlas. Specifically, we register each subject to the template using the DTI-TK deformable registration algorithm [18], then use the resulting deformation field to map the binary segmentation of the CC from the atlas into the subject space.

Deformable medial modeling proceeds as follows. We manually construct an initial CC mesh that encodes medial links between boundary vertices. We then fit this mesh to the boundary of the CC segmentation in the IXI atlas using our ICP algorithm, creating a template that satisfies medial linkage conditions. Fitting this template to each subject is performed in three steps. First, the template is initialized close to the subject's CC by applying the deformation computed by DTI-TK to its vertices. This deformation does not preserve medial linkage conditions. Second, we apply the ICP algorithm to fit the deformed template to the subject's CC segmentation, obtaining a mesh that closely fits the CC shape and satisfies medial linkage conditions. Finally, we refine the fitted mesh using one level of Loop subdivision, and perform one more stage of ICP-style fitting, obtaining a dense mesh satisfying the medial linkage conditions and

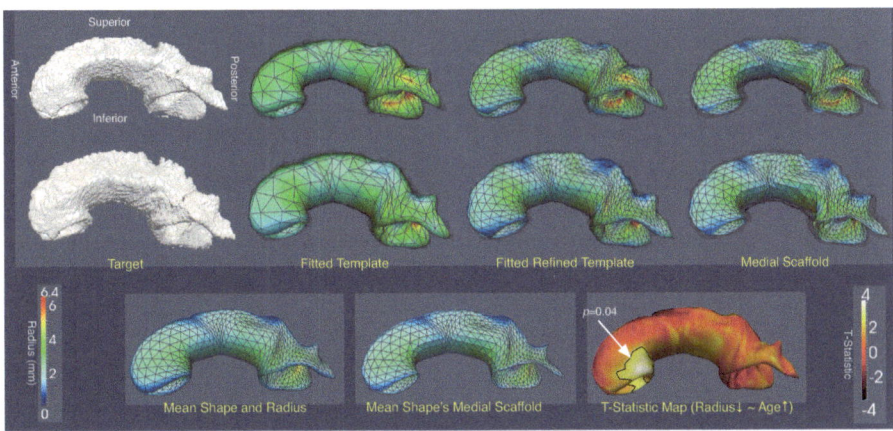

Fig. 3. Results from CC fitting experiment. The top two rows show two examples (third-worst and third-best fitting quality) of templates fitted to atlas-based CC segmentations. The columns show the target surface, the template fitted using ICP, the last-stage fitted subdivided template, and the medial scaffold of the latter. The bottom row shows the Procrustes mean of the fitted models, its medial scaffold (computed by applying ICP-style fitting to the Procrustes mean), and the t-statistic map for the age-related thinning hypothesis. The significant cluster ($p = 0.04$) is outlined.

closely matching the subjects' CC segmentations. The meshes have the same number of vertices and triangles, which enables point-wise statistical analysis of MAT-derived features. We use the radius values R_k at the vertices of the fitted meshes as a thickness feature, and use a general linear model to test the cross-sectional hypothesis that the thickness of the CC decreases as age increases. To control for multiple comparisons, we use cluster-level permutation testing [5].

Results. The results of the fitting are illustrated in Fig. 3. The template meshes initially fitted to subject CC segmentations have 410 vertices and 816 triangles. The corresponding constrained optimization problem has 11320 variables, 10116 equality constraints and 3744 inequality constraints. The Jacobian of the constraints is 99.91% sparse, and the Hessian of the Lagrangian is 99.95% sparse. Optimization was successful in 50 of the 51 subjects, converging to a local minimum of f and satisfying all the constraints within the tolerance of 10^{-8}. In one subject, it failed to satisfy the constraints in the 200 steps allowed. For the rest of the subjects, each ICP iteration required an average of 16.5 optimization steps to converge, taking an average of 42 s on a single 2.2GHz Intel CPU core. The number of ICP iterations was fixed at 5 for each subject. After fitting, the root mean squared (RMS) distance from the fitted template boundary to the boundary of the subject's CC segmentation was 0.89 ± 0.04 mm on average, and the average distance from the segmentation to the template boundary was 1.16 ± 0.05 mm. The subdivided meshes fitted at the last stage have 1634 vertices, 3264 triangles, 42712 variables, 38988/14832 equality/inequality constraints, 99.98%

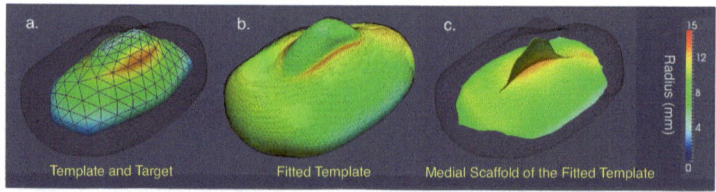

Fig. 4. Fitting a medially constrained template with a fin-like medial scaffold to a target object. The boundary of the target object is rendered as a dark gray wireframe in all three views. **a.** The template before the fitting, colored by the radius value R_k. **b.** The template after fitting. **c.** The medial scaffold of the fitted template.

Jacobian and 99.99% Hessian sparsity. ICP required an average of 21.5 optimization steps and 297 s to converge. [2] The RMS template-to-segmentation and segmentation-to-template distances were 0.70 ± 0.04 mm and 0.92 ± 0.05 mm, respectively. Statistical analysis using an *a priori* cluster T-score threshold of $t = 2.0$ and 10000 permutations revealed one significant cluster ($p = 0.04$) where age correlated negatively with thickness, located in the anterior of the CC (the genu). Such a finding is consistent with the literature, e.g., [1].

Proof of Concept for Branching Medial Scaffolds. While the medial scaffold in the CC template has only one surface, the strength of the method is that it is as easily applied to scaffolds with branches. In this pilot experiment, we fit a "fin-like" medial scaffold illustrated in Fig. 2 to a target shape. The target shape is produced by warping the reference shape in Fig. 2 based on a landmark transformation. The ICP algorithm is then used to fit the template to the target shape. Fig. 4 shows the template in relation to the target object before and after the fitting. The medial scaffold of the fitted model is also shown.

4   Discussion and Conclusions

We presented a new way to fit deformable models to surface and image data with preservation of medial branching structure. The method shows promise for modeling objects whose medial scaffolds have multiple branches, although additional experiments are needed to establish its utility for modeling complex branching shapes in medical imaging data, e.g., the myocardium. The scalability of the method is limited by the need to solve very large sparse linear systems, but for many anatomical structures, meshes having on the order of 1000 vertices should be sufficient to meet modeling needs. The number of empirical parameters in the method is small and performance on real-data is robust, making the method practical for shape analysis applications.

---

[2] Computation time is dominated by solving sparse systems, and in theory, time should scale with the number of non-zero elements in the sparse matrices, which is less than $4\times$ for the refined mesh. The $9\times$ increase in time may be due to memory limitations.

References

1. Bastin, M.E., Maniega, S.M., Ferguson, K.J., Brown, L.J., Wardlaw, J.M., MacLullich, A.M.J., Clayden, J.D.: Quantifying the effects of normal ageing on white matter structure using unsupervised tract shape modelling. Neuroimage 51(1), 1–10 (2010)
2. Blum, H.: A transformation for extracting new descriptors of shape. In: Models for the Perception of Speech and Visual Form. MIT Press (1967)
3. Bouix, S., Pruessner, J.C., Louis Collins, D., Siddiqi, K.: Hippocampal shape analysis using medial surfaces. Neuroimage 25(4), 1077–1089 (2005)
4. Giblin, P.J., Kimia, B.B.: On the intrinsic reconstruction of shape from its symmetries. IEEE T. Pattern Anal. 25(7), 895–911 (2003)
5. Hayasaka, S., Nichols, T.E.: Combining voxel intensity and cluster extent with permutation test framework. Neuroimage 23(1), 54–63 (2004)
6. Loop, C.T.: Smooth subdivision surfaces based on triangles. Master's thesis, Department of Mathematics, University of Utah, Salt Lake City (1987)
7. Pizer, S.M., Fletcher, P.T., Joshi, S., Thall, A., Chen, J.Z., Fridman, Y., Fritsch, D.S., Gash, A.G., Glotzer, J.M., Jiroutek, M.R., Lu, C., Muller, K.E., Tracton, G., Yushkevich, P., Chaney, E.L.: Deformable m-reps for 3D medical image segmentation. Int. J. Comput. Vision 55(2), 85–106 (2003)
8. Sebastian, T.B., Tek, H., Crisco, J.J., Kimia, B.B.: Segmentation of carpal bones from CT images using skeletally coupled deformable models. Med. Image Anal. 7(1), 21–45 (2003)
9. Siddiqi, K., Pizer, S.: Medial representations: mathematics, algorithms and applications, vol. 37. Springer (2008)
10. Styner, M., Gerig, G., Lieberman, J., Jones, D., Weinberger, D.: Statistical shape analysis of neuroanatomical structures based on medial models. Med. Image Anal. 7(3), 207–220 (2003)
11. Sun, H., Frangi, A.F., Wang, H., Sukno, F.M., Tobon-Gomez, C., Yushkevich, P.A.: Automatic Cardiac MRI Segmentation Using a Biventricular Deformable Medial Model. In: Jiang, T., Navab, N., Pluim, J.P.W., Viergever, M.A. (eds.) MICCAI 2010, Part I. LNCS, vol. 6361, pp. 468–475. Springer, Heidelberg (2010)
12. Terriberry, T.B., Gerig, G.: A Continuous 3-D Medial Shape Model With Branching. In: International Workshop on Mathematical Foundations of Computational Anatomy MFCA 2006, in Conjunction with MICCAI 2006 (2006)
13. Terzopoulos, D., Witkin, A., Kass, M.: Symmetry-seeking models and 3D object reconstruction. Int. J. Comput. Vision 1(3), 211–221 (1988)
14. Wächter, A., Biegler, L.T.: On the implementation of an interior-point filter line-search algorithm for large-scale nonlinear programming. Mathematical Programming 106, 25–57 (2006)
15. Yushkevich, P.A., Zhang, H., Gee, J.: Continuous medial representation for anatomical structures. IEEE Trans. Med. Imaging 25(2), 1547–1564 (2006)
16. Zeng, X., Staib, L.H., Schultz, R.T., Duncan, J.S.: Segmentation and measurement of the cortex from 3-D MR images using coupled-surfaces propagation. IEEE Trans. Med. Imaging 18(10), 927–937 (1999)
17. Zhang, H., Awate, S.P., Das, S.R., Woo, J.H., Melhem, E.R., Gee, J.C., Yushkevich, P.A.: A tract-specific framework for white matter morphometry combining macroscopic and microscopic tract features. Med. Image Anal. (May 2010)
18. Zhang, H., Yushkevich, P.A., Alexander, D.C., Gee, J.C.: Deformable registration of diffusion tensor MR images with explicit orientation optimization. Med. Image Anal. 10(5), 764–785 (2006)

Sparse Projections
of Medical Images onto Manifolds

George H. Chen, Christian Wachinger, and Polina Golland

Massachusetts Institute of Technology, Cambridge MA 02139, USA
{georgehc,wachinger,polina}@csail.mit.edu

Abstract. Manifold learning has been successfully applied to a variety of medical imaging problems. Its use in real-time applications requires fast projection onto the low-dimensional space. To this end, out-of-sample extensions are applied by constructing an interpolation function that maps from the input space to the low-dimensional manifold. Commonly used approaches such as the Nyström extension and kernel ridge regression require using all training points. We propose an interpolation function that only depends on a small subset of the input training data. Consequently, in the testing phase each new point only needs to be compared against a small number of input training data in order to project the point onto the low-dimensional space. We interpret our method as an out-of-sample extension that approximates kernel ridge regression. Our method involves solving a simple convex optimization problem and has the attractive property of guaranteeing an upper bound on the approximation error, which is crucial for medical applications. Tuning this error bound controls the sparsity of the resulting interpolation function. We illustrate our method in two clinical applications that require fast mapping of input images onto a low-dimensional space.

1   Introduction

Manifold learning maps high-dimensional data to a low-dimensional manifold and has recently been successfully applied to a variety of applications. Specifically in medical imaging, manifold learning has been used in segmentation [24], registration [12,15], computational anatomy [11], classification [6,22], detection [20], and respiratory gating [10,23]. But to the best of our knowledge, little work has been done using manifold learning for medical imaging applications that require fast projections onto a low-dimensional space.

In this paper, we demonstrate a method that achieves fast projection of input data onto a low-dimensional manifold by constructing a projection function that only depends on a small subset of the training data. Our method is a sparse variant of kernel ridge regression [18] and can be interpreted as an interpolation function optimized to only use a few of the training data. Furthermore, the construction of the interpolation function guarantees an upper bound on an interpolation error for training data. The error is measured in terms of the average squared Euclidean distance between the predicted points of the interpolator

J.C. Gee et al. (Eds.): IPMI 2013, LNCS 7917, pp. 292–303, 2013.

versus those of kernel ridge regression using all the points. As our interpolator has no parametric model for the data points, its complexity is driven by the complexity of the training data and the bound on the approximation error.

Related Work on Out-of-Sample Extensions. Manifold learning is a specific case of nonlinear dimensionality reduction and refers to a host of different algorithms [13]. In medical image analysis, manifold learning is used to construct a low-dimensional space for images in which subsequent statistical analysis (regression, classification, etc.) is performed. Many manifold learning techniques do not construct a mapping of the entire input space but only of the training points. For these methods, estimating a new point's location in the low-dimensional space is performed via an out-of-sample extension [5], with Nyström extensions commonly used. For certain manifold learning methods, a Nyström extension is a special case of kernel ridge regression [19], and for both the Nyström extension and kernel ridge regression, the resulting interpolation function for mapping a new input point to the low-dimensional space depends on all training data. Thus, we need to compare a new point to all training data points, which is computationally expensive for volumetric images, especially if the number of input data used to learn the manifold is large.

Our work is most similar to reduced rank kernel ridge regression [7], which also approximates kernel ridge regression by only using a small number of input training points. Reduced rank kernel ridge regression greedily selects training points to minimize a particular cost function. Specifically, the algorithm incrementally adds a training point that causes the largest decrease in overall cost. Different criteria could be used for when the greedy procedure is terminated such as if a pre-specified desired number of training points to use is reached or if the overall cost drops below a pre-specified desired error tolerance. Importantly, for medical applications, the latter criterion is more directly connected to the error analysis of the whole processing pipeline. Our approach also requires the user to specify a desired error tolerance but uses a different cost function. Rather than using a greedy approach to select which training points to add, we solve a convex optimization problem implied by our cost function. We remark that the proposed cost function also differs from that of support vector regression [9], which essentially achieves sparsity via excluding training points that map sufficiently close to the estimated function. Our cost is more lenient, asking that an average error be small rather than asking that an error be small for each individual training point.

Contributions. For high-dimensional input points $x_1, x_2, \ldots, x_n \in \mathbb{R}^d$ and their low-dimensional representations $y_1, y_2, \ldots, y_n \in \mathbb{R}^p$ as computed by any manifold learning algorithm, we propose a convex program for constructing an out-of-sample extension that guarantees a bound on the approximation error. Formally, if $\widehat{f} : \mathbb{R}^d \to \mathbb{R}^p$ is the out-of-sample extension function estimated via kernel ridge regression, then the sparse projection function $\widetilde{f} : \mathbb{R}^d \to \mathbb{R}^p$ constructed by our algorithm satisfies

$$\frac{1}{n} \sum_{i=1}^{n} \|\widehat{f}(x_i) - \widetilde{f}(x_i)\|_2^2 \leq \varepsilon^2, \tag{1}$$

where $\|\cdot\|_2$ denotes the Euclidean norm, $\varepsilon > 0$ is a pre-specified error tolerance, and $\widetilde{f}$ depends only on a small subset of $x_1, \ldots, x_n$. The size of the subset, i.e., the sparsity of the resulting function $\widetilde{f}$, depends on tolerance ε and training pairs $(x_1, y_1), \ldots, (x_n, y_n)$. Finding the smallest such subset is NP-hard. We instead consider a convex relaxation with sparsity induced by a mixed ℓ_1/ℓ_2 norm. While the proposed sparse approximation to kernel ridge regression can be used more generally for other multivariate regression tasks, we restrict our focus in this paper to out-of-sample extensions for manifold learning.

We apply our method to two medical imaging applications that require a fast projection onto a low-dimensional space. The first application is respiratory gating in ultrasound, where we assign the breathing state to each ultrasound frame during the acquisition in real-time. The second application is the estimation of a patient's position in a magnetic resonance imaging (MRI) scanner while the patient is being moved to a target location.

2   Background

Our method builds heavily on kernel ridge regression [18], reviewed below. We also briefly discuss the result that a Nyström extension is a special case of kernel ridge regression under certain conditions [19]. As a consequence, our sparse approximation to kernel ridge regression also contains a sparse approximation to the widely used Nyström extension.

Kernel Ridge Regression. Let $\mathbb{H}$ be a family of functions mapping $\mathbb{R}^d$ to $\mathbb{R}$ such that $\mathbb{H}$ is a reproducing kernel Hilbert space (RKHS) [1] with kernel function $\mathbb{K}: \mathbb{R}^d \times \mathbb{R}^d \to \mathbb{R}$. Given points $x_1, \ldots, x_n \in \mathbb{R}^d$ and $y_1, \ldots, y_n \in \mathbb{R}^p$, we assume that there exists a function $f^* = (f_1^*, \ldots, f_p^*) \in \mathbb{H}^p$ such that for each i, we have $y_i = f^*(x_i) + w_i$ for some noise term $w_i \in \mathbb{R}^p$. Kernel ridge regression seeks an estimate $\widehat{f}$ of function f^* by solving

$$\widehat{f} = \operatorname*{argmin}_{(f_1, \ldots, f_p) \in \mathbb{H}^p} \sum_{j=1}^{p} \left\{ \sum_{i=1}^{n} (Y_{ij} - f_j(x_i))^2 + \lambda \|f_j\|_{\mathbb{H}}^2 \right\}, \tag{2}$$

where matrix $Y \in \mathbb{R}^{n \times p}$ contains data point y_i as its i-th row, constant $\lambda > 0$ controls the amount of regularization, and $\|\cdot\|_{\mathbb{H}}$ is the norm induced by the inner product of $\mathbb{H}$. The solution of optimization problem (2) is

$$\widehat{f}(\cdot) = \sum_{i=1}^{n} \mathbb{K}(\cdot, x_i)\widehat{\alpha}_i, \tag{3}$$

where $\widehat{\alpha}_i$ refers to the i-th row of n-by-p matrix

$$\widehat{\alpha} = (K + \lambda I_{n \times n})^{-1} Y, \tag{4}$$

matrix $K \in \mathbb{R}^{n \times n}$ is given by $K_{ij} = \mathbb{K}(x_i, x_j)$, and $I_{n \times n}$ is the n-by-n identity matrix [18].

Nyström Extension. The Nyström method approximates a certain type of eigenfunction problem and is used for out-of-sample extensions in manifold learning [5]. For manifold learning algorithms that assign the low-dimensional coordinates directly from the eigenvectors of K, e.g., Isomap [21], locally linear embeddings [17], and Laplacian eigenmaps [4], we can derive the Nyström extension as a special case of kernel ridge regression with $\lambda = 0$. Specifically, with eigendecomposition $K = \Phi \Lambda \Phi^{-1}$, where $\Lambda = \mathrm{diag}(\lambda_1, \lambda_2, \ldots, \lambda_n)$ and $\lambda_1 \geq \lambda_2 \geq \cdots \geq \lambda_n$, we consider when the low-dimensional embedding is given by $Y = \Phi_\ell$, the matrix consisting of the first ℓ columns of Φ. If we use $\phi^{(j)}$ to denote the j-th column of Φ, then with $\lambda = 0$ and $Y = \Phi_\ell$, eq. (4) reduces to

$$\widehat{\alpha} = K^{-1} Y = \Phi \Lambda^{-1} \Phi^{-1} \Phi_\ell = \Phi \Lambda^{-1} \begin{bmatrix} I_{\ell \times \ell} \\ \mathbf{0} \end{bmatrix} = \left[\tfrac{1}{\lambda_1} \phi^{(1)} \mid \tfrac{1}{\lambda_2} \phi^{(2)} \mid \cdots \mid \tfrac{1}{\lambda_\ell} \phi^{(\ell)} \right].$$
(5)

Letting $\phi_i^{(j)}$ refer to the i-th element of $\phi^{(j)}$, and substituting eq. (5) into eq. (3), we see that, for a new point $x \in \mathbb{R}^d$, the j-th element of $\widehat{f}(x)$ is given by

$$\widehat{f}_j(x) = \sum_{i=1}^n \mathbb{K}(x, x_i) \widehat{\alpha}_{ij} = \sum_{i=1}^n \mathbb{K}(x, x_i) \left(\frac{1}{\lambda_j} \phi_i^{(j)} \right) = \frac{1}{\lambda_j} \sum_{i=1}^n \phi_i^{(j)} \mathbb{K}(x, x_i), \quad (6)$$

which is the formula for the low-dimensional embedding of x using the Nyström extension [5]. Importantly, kernel function $\mathbb{K}$ depends on the choice of a manifold learning algorithm [5]. The above relationship shows that for certain manifold learning algorithms, kernel ridge regression is a richer model for out-of-sample extensions than the Nyström extension.

3   Sparse Approximation to Kernel Ridge Regression

We now present our method. We seek an interpolation function $\widetilde{f} : \mathbb{R}^d \to \mathbb{R}^p$ within a family of functions $\mathbb{G} = \{f(\cdot) = \sum_{i=1}^n \mathbb{K}(\cdot, x_i)\alpha_i : \alpha \in \mathbb{R}^{n \times p}\}$, with many vectors $\alpha_i \in \mathbb{R}^p$ equal to zero while ensuring that upper bound (1) holds. In particular, we formulate a convex optimization problem where $\alpha \in \mathbb{R}^{n \times p}$ is the only decision variable; solving this problem yields $\widetilde{\alpha}$ that implies a sparse approximation $\widetilde{f}$ to the kernel ridge regression solution $\widehat{f}$.

Because we optimize over functions in $\mathbb{G}$, upper bound (1) can be simplified by noting that $\sum_{i=1}^n \|\widehat{f}(x_i) - f(x_i)\|_2^2 = \|K\widehat{\alpha} - K\alpha\|_F^2$, where $\|\cdot\|_F$ denotes the Frobenius norm, and $\widehat{\alpha}$ is given by eq. (4). In fact, $\widehat{f}(x_i)$ and $f(x_i)$ are given by the i-th rows of $K\widehat{\alpha}$ and $K\alpha$, respectively. Thus, bound (1) can be rewritten as $\|K\widehat{\alpha} - K\alpha\|_F^2 \leq n\varepsilon^2$. Satisfying this constraint while encouraging the number of nonzero vectors α_i to be small can be achieved by solving the following convex optimization problem:

$$\widetilde{\alpha} = \operatorname*{argmin}_{\alpha \in \mathbb{R}^{n \times p}} \sum_{i=1}^n \|\alpha_i\|_2 \quad \text{s.t.} \quad \|K\widehat{\alpha} - K\alpha\|_F^2 \leq n\varepsilon^2. \tag{7}$$

By minimizing the mixed ℓ_1/ℓ_2 norm of α, we encourage each vector α_i to either consist of all zeros or all non-zero entries [2]. Note that if $p = 1$ and we instead ask for the sparsest solution possible, then the objective function becomes the ℓ_0 norm (i.e., the number of nonzero elements) of α, and the optimization problem itself becomes NP-hard [14].

To solve optimization problem (7), we reduce it to solving many instances of its unconstrained Lagrangian form for which there is already a fast solver. Specifically, by Lagrangian duality and convexity, solving optimization problem (7) is equivalent to solving the dual problem

$$\max_{\xi \geq 0} \min_{\alpha \in \mathbb{R}^{n \times p}} \left\{ \sum_{i=1}^{n} \|\alpha_i\|_2 + \xi \big(\|K\widehat{\alpha} - K\alpha\|_F^2 - n\varepsilon^2 \big) \right\} = \sup_{\xi > 0} \xi \left[g(1/\xi) - n\varepsilon^2 \right], \quad (8)$$

where ξ is a Lagrange multiplier, and

$$g(\gamma) = \min_{\alpha \in \mathbb{R}^{n \times p}} \left\{ \|K\widehat{\alpha} - K\alpha\|_F^2 + \gamma \sum_{i=1}^{n} \|\alpha_i\|_2 \right\}. \quad (9)$$

For a fixed ξ, we can compute $g(1/\xi)$ efficiently using the fast iterative shrinkage-thresholding algorithm (FISTA) [3]. Moreover, from a standard result of Lagrangian duality, dual problem (8) maximizes a concave function, which in this case is only over scalar variable ξ. Thus, we can efficiently solve the right hand side of (8) by making as many calls to FISTA as needed to achieve the desired accuracy in estimating ξ. Given the final estimated value $\widetilde{\xi}$ of ξ, we recover solution $\widetilde{\alpha}$ by seeking $\alpha \in \mathbb{R}^{n \times p}$ that yields $g(1/\widetilde{\xi})$ in eq. (9).

Once the coefficient matrix $\widetilde{\alpha}$ is obtained, the interpolation function $\widetilde{f}$ is uniquely defined:

$$\widetilde{f}(\cdot) = \sum_{i=1}^{n} \mathbb{K}(\cdot, x_i)\widetilde{\alpha}_i. \quad (10)$$

The number of nonzero $\widetilde{\alpha}_i \in \mathbb{R}^p$ vectors depends on error tolerance ε, regularization parameter λ, the kernel function $\mathbb{K}$, and the data itself. We refer to the data points x_i corresponding to nonzero $\widetilde{\alpha}_i$ as *support vectors*. As we observe empirically in the next section, decreasing parameters ε and λ each generally produce more support vectors used in projection. This is not surprising: increasing ε increases the size of the feasible set in optimization problem (7), allowing for potentially more candidate solutions $\widetilde{\alpha}$. Meanwhile, as $\lambda \to \infty$, the coefficient matrix $\widehat{\alpha}$ for kernel ridge regression, defined in eq. (4), approaches $\widehat{\alpha} = \frac{1}{\lambda}Y$, which goes to 0 for large λ. As a result, $\widetilde{\alpha}$ also gets pushed to 0.

We can choose the similarity kernel $\mathbb{K}$ to match the specific choice of manifold learning algorithm used to embed the training data. This allows us to provide a sparse approximation to the Nyström extension as discussed in Section 2. Alternatively, our method is applicable to any kernel $\mathbb{K}$, regardless of the manifold learning algorithm used for training.

Lastly, we note that solving the convex program (8) to obtain $\widetilde{\alpha}$ incurs an offline, one-time cost. During testing, we use the resulting sparse interpolator (10) whose computational cost is directly proportional to the number of support vectors. Our interpolator will always be at least as fast to compute as that of kernel ridge regression that uses all the training points as support vectors and corresponds to the special case of our interpolator where $\varepsilon = 0$.

4   Results

We apply our sparse interpolator to synthetic data (a Swiss roll), respiratory gating in ultrasound, and MRI classification. We report the number of support vectors as a proxy for computational speed since wall-clock time is directly proportional to the number of support vectors. Furthermore, the datasets we use are still relatively small for the scenarios our method intends to address, making wall-clock time for the experiments we run not reflective of real use. However, our empirical results suggest that our method can work with larger datasets since the number of support vectors scales not with the size of the training dataset but instead with the complexity of the training data's low-dimensional embedding.

For synthetic data, we use Hessian eigenmaps [8] for manifold learning, which, to the best of our knowledge, does not have a known Nyström extension. For the two experiments on real data, we use Laplacian eigenmaps [4] for manifold learning and construct our sparse interpolator using the same kernel function as the one used for Laplacian eigenmap's Nyström extension [5]:

$$\mathbb{K}(x, x') = \frac{W(x, x')}{\sqrt{\sum_{i=1}^{n} W(x, x_i) \sum_{j=1}^{n} W(x', x_j)}}, \tag{11}$$

where $W : \mathbb{R}^d \times \mathbb{R}^d \to \mathbb{R}_+$ is a heat kernel given by $W(x, x') = e^{-\|x-x'\|_2^2/t}$ if $\|x - x'\|_2 \leq \tau$ and 0 otherwise, for some pre-specified temperature t and nearest-neighbor threshold τ — both parameters chosen based on the application of interest. We can also find the k nearest neighbors rather than defining nearest neighbors to be within a ball of radius τ. With kernel function (11), constructing our sparse interpolator with $\lambda = 0$ and $\varepsilon = 0$ yields Laplacian eigenmap's Nyström extension that uses all the training points. We do not use the same manifold learning algorithm for all datasets; the choice of manifold learning algorithm depends on the dataset and the application of interest.

4.1   Synthetic Data

We apply our method to a Swiss roll with $n = 1000$ points, shown in Fig. 1(a). First, we compute low-dimensional representations $y_1, \ldots, y_n \in \mathbb{R}^2$ using Hessian eigenmaps [8] with a 7-nearest-neighbor graph. We construct our sparse interpolator using kernel function $\mathbb{K}(x, x') = \exp(-\|x - x'\|_2^2/\sigma^2)$. To probe the behavior of our interpolator, we vary kernel ridge regression parameter λ, kernel width σ, and error tolerance ε. Fig. 1 reports the resulting number of support vectors and illustrates results for one setting of the parameters.

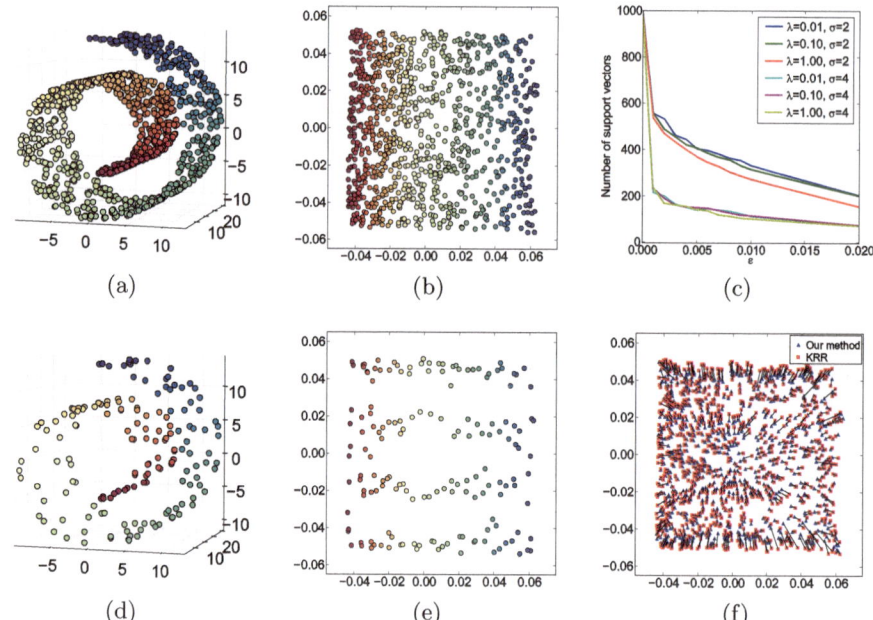

Fig. 1. Results for a Swiss roll with $n = 1000$ points: (a) the original 3D data points; (b) their 2D embedding; (c) the number of support vectors as a function of error tolerance ε for various λ and σ. For the remaining panels (d)-(f), we fix $\lambda = 0.1$, $\sigma = 4$, and $\varepsilon = 0.003$: (d) the 161 support vectors found; (e) our approximated 2D embedding of support vectors; (f) a comparison of 2D embeddings from our method and kernel ridge regression (lines show correspondences).

We observe that the support vectors are not uniformly sampled in the input space nor on the learned 2D manifold. Instead, they appear along the boundaries or form a skeleton within the learned manifold. We also observe in Fig. 1(f) that the largest discrepancies in the predicted point locations between our sparse interpolator and kernel ridge regression occur along the boundaries. Unsurprisingly, increasing kernel width σ reduces the number of support vectors needed to achieve the same error tolerance ε as each support vector has broader spatial influence in the input space. Furthermore, increasing kernel ridge regression regularization parameter λ also reduces the number of support vectors, as discussed in Section 3.

By repeating this experiment using a Swiss roll with $n = 2000$, $n = 3000$, and $n = 4000$ points, we empirically find that for a variety of parameter settings λ, σ, and ε, the number of support vectors remains roughly constant as n grows large. For example, with $\lambda = 0.1$, $\sigma = 4$, and $\varepsilon = 0.003$, we obtain 161, 174, 163, and 170 support vectors for $n = 1000, 2000, 3000, 4000$ points respectively. This suggests that the number of support vectors to depend on the low-dimensional embedding's complexity and not on the dataset size n.

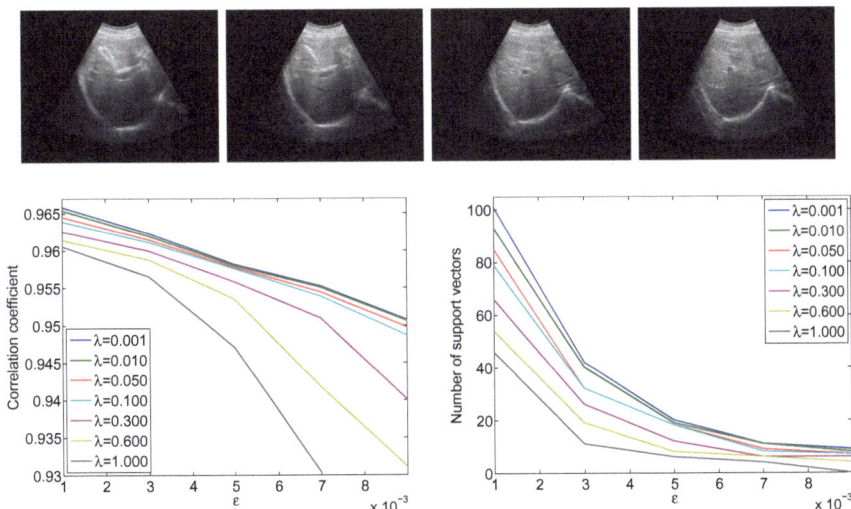

Fig. 2. Ultrasound gating. Top: Ultrasound images of the liver over time (abdomen, right upper quadrant). Bottom left: Correlation coefficient vs. error tolerance ε. Bottom right: The number of support vectors vs. error tolerance ε. Both figures in the bottom report results for different values of kernel ridge regression regularization parameter λ.

4.2 Respiratory Gating of Ultrasound Images

Respiratory gating tracks a patient's breathing cycle, which has numerous applications such as 4D imaging, radiation therapy, and image mosaicing [16]. Manifold learning has been used for highly accurate respiratory gating of ultrasound images [23], where 4D data reconstruction was achieved with retrospective gating, i.e., the gating was calculated after the data acquisition was finished. We extend this work to attain real-time gating. A small number of breathing cycles are acquired and used as input for manifold learning to construct the respiratory signal, as is done for retrospective gating. The new incoming stream of ultrasound images is then gated by performing an out-of-sample extension.

We conduct experiments on five 2D ultrasound image sequences of the human liver acquired during free breathing; example images are shown in Fig. 2. Each sequence contains 640×480-pixel images and vary in length between 298 and 371 frames captured at 33 Hz. For a given image sequence, we use each image in the sequence as an input data point for learning a 1D manifold with Laplacian eigenmaps [4]; we use a 9-nearest-neighbor graph with an associated heat kernel of temperature $t = 10$. The 1D embedding learned using an entire sequence of images serves as a reference signal for evaluating our sparse out-of-sample extension versus kernel ridge regression as the baseline. In what follows, we compare the 1D embedding of our sparse out-of-sample extension to the reference signal by computing a correlation coefficient between them. We use kernel ridge regression as a baseline method. Here we train on the first 200 frames and test

Table 1. Results for respiratory gating on ultrasound images. For each image sequence, we show the number of frames it contains, the correlation coefficient (CC) for kernel ridge regression (KRR) and our sparse interpolator, and the number of support vectors (SV's). Parameter values: $\lambda = 0.1$, $\varepsilon = 0.001$.

Data	# Frames	Learning on first 200 frames			Learning on entire data		
		CC (KRR)	CC (sparse)	# SV's	CC (KRR)	CC (sparse)	# SV's
Seq. 1	354	96.5%	96.4%	79	99.9%	96.9%	73
Seq. 2	335	97.7%	97.5%	99	99.9%	98.6%	100
Seq. 3	298	98.3%	97.8%	51	99.3%	98.9%	61
Seq. 4	371	99.7%	99.4%	53	99.6%	99.7%	45
Seq. 5	298	99.0%	98.7%	41	99.9%	99.5%	50

on the remaining frames. We then compare the results with those obtained by training on all frames, as would be done for retrospective gating.

We first examine the influence of parameters ε and λ on the resulting interpolator. Training on the first 200 images of one of the ultrasound image sequences, we compute the correlation coefficient with the reference signal and the number of support vectors versus the error tolerance ε (Fig. 2). As expected, smaller error tolerance ε requires more support vectors but also leads to a higher correlation coefficient with respect to the reference signal. Also, a higher kernel ridge regression regularization parameter λ leads to fewer support vectors. However, stronger regularization also leads to lower correlation coefficients. These results suggest a natural tradeoff between the accuracy and the computational cost of the projection operation.

In the next experiment, we use $\lambda = 0.1$ and $\varepsilon = 0.001$. Training on the first 200 frames and testing on the rest of the frames, we report the correlation coefficients and the number of support vectors in Table 1. The number of support vectors for kernel ridge regression is 200 in this case. We then repeat the experiment, training on all the frames. In this case, the number of support vectors for kernel ridge regression is the length of the sequence. We achieve a high correlation for all sequences, with a comparable performance between our sparse interpolator and kernel ridge regression. Comparing the number of support vectors when training on the first 200 frames vs. training on all the frames, we note that the number of support vectors stays roughly the same for a given image sequence. This again suggests that the number of support vectors depends on the low-dimensional embedding's complexity and not the training set size.

4.3 Patient Position Estimation Using MRI

The radio frequency power in magnetic resonance imaging leads to tissue heating and has to be monitored by measuring the specific absorption rate, which depends on the position of the patient in the scanner. For current high-resolution scanners, this imposes restrictions because either fewer slices can be acquired

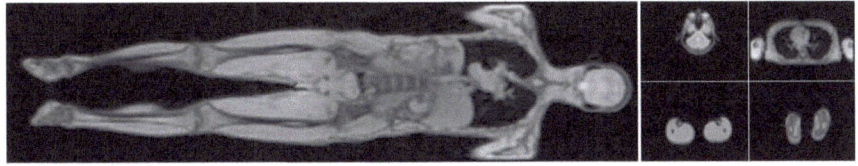

Fig. 3. Left: Coronal plane of MRI scan showing the entire patient. Right: Axial slices on which manifold learning is performed.

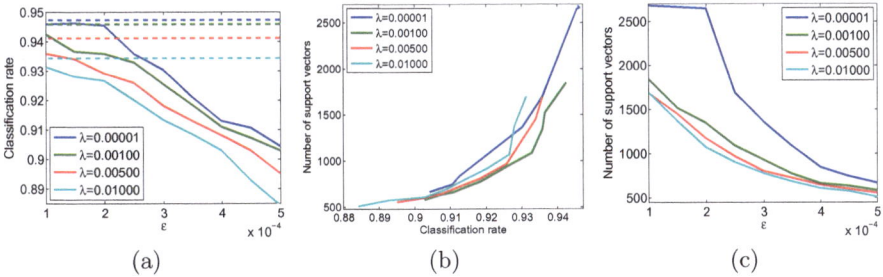

(a)   (b)   (c)

Fig. 4. Leave-one-out classification results for MRI data: (a) classification rate vs. ε for our sparse out-of-sample extension (solid line) and kernel ridge regression (dotted line) (b) the number of support vectors vs. classification rate; (c) the number of support vectors vs. error tolerance ε. All figures report results for different values of kernel ridge regression regularization parameter λ.

or the in-plane resolution has to be reduced. Manifold learning can be used to estimate the position of the patient in the scanner [22].

First, low-resolution images are acquired while the bed that the patient lies on moves inside the scanner. The images are embedded in a low-dimensional space, where each axial image is associated with a body part (head, neck, lung, etc.) using a nearest-neighbor classifier. By knowing which slices correspond to which body parts, we can estimate the position of the patient in the scanner. It is important that the estimation be done in real-time to provide the position information before the high-resolution scan starts. In this application, we can apply manifold learning offline on a large database of scans. Then during the actual scan, we use an out-of-sample extension to project the acquired slices into the low-dimensional space. For large training datasets, it may be difficult to meet the time requirements with kernel ridge regression. Consequently, the reduction to a small set of support vectors offers a substantial advantage.

We run experiments on 13 whole body scans, such as the example shown in Fig. 3. A medical expert assigned an anatomical label (head, neck, lung, abdomen, upper leg, and lower leg) to each of the axial slices (64×64 pixels). We apply Laplacian eigenmaps to embed the high dimensional slices in a two-dimensional space; we use a 40-nearest-neighbor graph with a heat kernel of temperature $t = 49$. To predict the anatomical label of an axial image, we perform nearest-neighbor classification in the learned low-dimensional space. We repeat this classification procedure for different values of error tolerance ε ranging from 1×10^{-4} to 5×10^{-4}.

We compare the classification performance of embeddings obtained from our sparse interpolator and kernel ridge regression. Fig. 4(a) reports leave-one-out classification performance for different values of error tolerance ε. The classification rates for kernel ridge regression are provided for comparison; they do not change for different values of ε. Figs. 4(b) and 4(c) characterize the sparsity of the interpolation function constructed by reporting the number of support vectors as a function of the classification rate and error tolerance ε. The total number of frames used in this experiment is 2697, which corresponds to the number of support vectors for kernel ridge regression. We observe a clear correlation between error tolerance ε and the classification performance. Smaller values of ε lead to better classification performance but require more support vectors. Thus, we can trade off computational speed with classification performance by tuning parameters λ and ε to be as large as possible while maintaining a classification rate above a minimum tolerated threshold.

5   Conclusion

We derived a novel method for multivariate regression that approximates kernel ridge regression, where the final estimated interpolation function depends only on a subset of the original input points acting as support vectors. Our approach provides a guarantee on the approximation error for training data. We applied our method as an out-of-sample extension for manifold learning, illustrating applications to respiratory gating and MRI classification.

Turning toward nonlinear dimensionality reduction more generally, many widely used algorithms are computationally expensive for massive datasets. Thus, ideally we would like to find support vectors first, before applying dimensionality reduction. Our results suggest that the support vectors for interpolation may not be uniformly sampled in the input space. This invites the question of how to non-uniformly sample training data in the input space and adjust a dimensionality reduction algorithm accordingly to account for the geometry of these samples.

Acknowledgements. We thank Siemens Healthcare for image data. This work was funded in part by the National Alliance for Medical Image Computing (grant NIH NIBIB NAMIC U54-EB005149) and the National Institutes of Health (grants NIH NCRR NAC P41-RR13218 and NIH NIBIB NAC P41-EB-015902).

References

1. Aronszajn, N.: Theory of reproducing kernels. Trans. AMS (1950)
2. Bach, F.R., Jenatton, R., Mairal, J., Obozinski, G.: Optimization with sparsity-inducing penalties. Foundations and Trends in Machine Learning (2012)
3. Beck, A., Teboulle, M.: A fast iterative shrinkage-thresholding algorithm for linear inverse problems. SIAM Journal on Imaging Sciences (2009)
4. Belkin, M., Niyogi, P.: Laplacian eigenmaps and spectral techniques for embedding and clustering. In: NIPS (2002)

5. Bengio, Y., Paiement, J.F., Vincent, P., Delalleau, O., Roux, N.L., Ouimet, M.: Out-of-sample extensions for LLE, Isomap, MDS, eigenmaps, and spectral clustering. In: NIPS (2004)
6. Bhatia, K.K., Rao, A., Price, A.N., Wolz, R., Hajnal, J., Rueckert, D.: Hierarchical manifold learning. In: Ayache, N., Delingette, H., Golland, P., Mori, K. (eds.) MICCAI 2012, Part I. LNCS, vol. 7510, pp. 512–519. Springer, Heidelberg (2012)
7. Cawley, G.C., Talbot, N.L.C.: Reduced rank kernel ridge regression. Neural Processing Letters (2002)
8. Donoho, D.L., Grimes, C.: Hessian eigenmaps: New locally linear embedding techniques for high-dimensional data. PNAS (2003)
9. Drucker, H., Burges, C.J.C., Kaufman, L., Smola, A.J., Vapnik, V.: Support vector regression machines. In: NIPS (1997)
10. Georg, M., Souvenir, R., Hope, A., Pless, R.: Manifold learning for 4d ct reconstruction of the lung. In: CVPR Workshops (2008)
11. Gerber, S., Tasdizen, T., Joshi, S., Whitaker, R.: On the manifold structure of the space of brain images. In: Yang, G.-Z., Hawkes, D., Rueckert, D., Noble, A., Taylor, C. (eds.) MICCAI 2009, Part I. LNCS, vol. 5761, pp. 305–312. Springer, Heidelberg (2009)
12. Hamm, J., Davatzikos, C., Verma, R.: Efficient large deformation registration via geodesics on a learned manifold of images. In: Yang, G.-Z., Hawkes, D., Rueckert, D., Noble, A., Taylor, C. (eds.) MICCAI 2009, Part I. LNCS, vol. 5761, pp. 680–687. Springer, Heidelberg (2009)
13. van der Maaten, L.J.P., Postma, E.O., van den Herik, H.J.: Dimensionality reduction: A comparative review. Tilburg University Technical Report (2008)
14. Natarajan, B.K.: Sparse Approximate Solutions to Linear Systems. SIAM J. Comput. (1995)
15. Rohde, G.K., Wang, W., Peng, T., Murphy, R.F.: Deformation-based nonlinear dimension reduction: Applications to nuclear morphometry. In: ISBI (2008)
16. Rohlfing, T., Maurer Jr., C.R., O'Dell, W.G., Zhong, J.: Modeling liver motion and deformation during the respiratory cycle using intensity-based free-form registration of gated MR images. In: Medical Imaging: Visualization, Display, and Image-Guided Procedures (2001)
17. Roweis, S.T., Saul, L.K.: Nonlinear dimensionality reduction by locally linear embedding. Science (2000)
18. Saunders, C., Gammerman, A., Vovk, V.: Ridge regression learning algorithm in dual variables. In: ICML (1998)
19. Schölkopf, B., Smola, A.J.: Learning with Kernels: Support Vector Machines, Regularization, Optimization, and Beyond. MIT Press (2001)
20. Suzuki, K., Zhang, J., Xu, J.: Massive-training artificial neural network coupled with laplacian-eigenfunction-based dimensionality reduction for computer-aided detection of polyps in ct colonography. IEEE TMI (2010)
21. Tenenbaum, J.B., de Silva, V., Langford, J.C.: A global geometric framework for nonlinear dimensionality reduction. Science (2000)
22. Wachinger, C., Mateus, D., Keil, A., Navab, N.: Manifold learning for patient position detection in MRI. In: ISBI (2010)
23. Wachinger, C., Yigitsoy, M., Navab, N.: Manifold learning for image-based breathing gating with application to 4D ultrasound. In: Jiang, T., Navab, N., Pluim, J.P.W., Viergever, M.A. (eds.) MICCAI 2010, Part II. LNCS, vol. 6362, pp. 26–33. Springer, Heidelberg (2010)
24. Zhang, Q., Souvenir, R., Pless, R.: On Manifold Structure of Cardiac MRI Data: Application to Segmentation. In: CVPR (2006)

Efficient 3D Multi-region Prostate MRI Segmentation Using Dual Optimization

Wu Qiu[1], Jing Yuan[1], Eranga Ukwatta[1,2], Yue Sun[1,2],
Martin Rajchl[1,2], and Aaron Fenster[1,2]

[1] Robarts Research Institue
[2] Department of Biomedical Engineering,
Western University, London, Ontario, Canada
wqiu@imaging.robarts.ca

Abstract. Efficient and accurate extraction of the prostate, in particular its clinically meaningful sub-regions from 3D MR images, is of great interest in image-guided prostate interventions and diagnosis of prostate cancer. In this work, we propose a novel multi-region segmentation approach to simultaneously locating the boundaries of the prostate and its two major sub-regions: the central gland and the peripheral zone. The proposed method utilizes the prior knowledge of the spatial region consistency and employs a customized prostate appearance model to simultaneously segment multiple clinically meaningful regions. We solve the resulted challenging combinatorial optimization problem by means of convex relaxation, for which we introduce a novel spatially continuous flow-maximization model and demonstrate its duality to the investigated convex relaxed optimization problem with the region consistency constraint. Moreover, the proposed continuous max-flow model naturally leads to a new and efficient *continuous max-flow based* algorithm, which enjoys great advantages in numerics and can be readily implemented on GPUs. Experiments using 15 T2-weighted 3D prostate MR images, by inter- and intra-operator variability, demonstrate the promising performance of the proposed approach.

Keywords: 3D Prostate MRI, Zonal Segmentation, Convex Optimization.

1 Introduction

Prostate cancer is a major health problem in the western world, with one in six men affected during their lifetime [1]. In diagnosing prostate cancer, transrectal ultrasound (TRUS) guided biopsies have become the gold standard. However, the accuracy of the TRUS guided biopsy relies on and is limited by the fidelity. Magnetic resonance (MR) imaging is an attractive option for guiding and monitoring such interventions due to its superior visualization of not only the prostate, but also its substructure and the surrounding tissues [2,3]. The fusion of 3D TRUS and MRI provides an effective way to target biopsy needles in 3D TRUS images toward regions of the prostate containing MR identified suspicious lesions,

J.C. Gee et al. (Eds.): IPMI 2013, LNCS 7917, pp. 304–315, 2013.

which is regarded as an alternative to the more expensive and inefficient MRI-based prostate biopsy [4] and the less accurate conventional 2D TRUS-guieded prostate biopsy. The prostate consists of four zones: peripheral zone (PZ), central zone (CZ), transition zone (TZ), and fibromuscular stroma [5]. During guidance of the biopsy, the prostate is usually considered to have two visible zones on MRI: the *central gland* (CG) and the *peripheral zone* (PZ). The CG is assumed to be the outer contour of the prostate minus the PZ [6]. The reason for segmenting these regions is that up to 80% of prostate cancer are located within the PZ [7]. Thus, the ability to superimpose the 3D TRUS image used to guide the biopsy onto the pre-segmented regions of interest in MRI is highly desired in a fused 3D TRUS/MRI guided biopsy system. Computer aided diagnosis (CAD) techniques for prostate cancer can also benefit from the correct interpretation of the zonal anatomy of the prostate since the occurrence and appearance of cancer is dependent on its zonal location [8,9]. Furthermore, the ratio of CG volume to whole prostate gland (WG) can be used to monitor prostate hyperplasia [10].

Many studies have focused their efforts on whole prostate segmentation from in 3D MR images, especially in T2-weighted (T2w) 3D MR images, see [11] for a review of the existing literature. However, only a few studies focused on prostate zonal segmentation in 3D MRI. Allen *et al.* [12] proposed a method for automatic delineation of prostate boundaries and the CG. Unfortunately, the authors limited their segmentation to the middle region of the prostate (where T2w contrast permits accurate segmentation), and ignored the apex and base of the gland. Yin *et al.* [13] proposed an automated CG segmentation algorithm based on Layered Optimal Graph Image Segmentation of Multiple Objects and Surfaces (LOGISMOS). The test set indicated that their approach obtained a mean Dice Similarity Coefficient (DSC) of 80% for CG. The first paper about segmenting the prostate into the PZ and CG was proposed by Makni *et al.* [14]. The authors proposed a modified version of the evidential C-means algorithm to cluster voxels into their respective zones incorporating the spatial relation between voxels in 3D multispectral MR images including a T2w image, a diffusion weighted image (DWI), and a contrast enhanced MRI (CEMRI). The obtained mean DSCs were 87% for the central gland and 76% for the peripheral zone. More recently, Litjens *et al.* [15] proposed a pattern recognition method to classify the voxels using anatomical, intensity and texture features in multispectral MR images. Their method obtained a DSC of 89% for the central gland and 75% for the peripheral zone. However, in [14] and [15], the segmentation of prostate peripheral zone relies on the manual segmentation of the whole prostate gland. In [15], the authors additionally stated that they also developed an atlas-based method to segment the prostate zones at the same time without a manual whole prostate mask. Unfortunately, the method failed to give any favourable results. Moreover, there are no further details about that method reported in that study.

In this work, we propose a new global optimization-based multi-region segmentation approach to delineating the whole prostate gland (WG) and its subregions: the central gland (CG) and peripheral zone (PZ) simultaneously from the input 3D T2w prostate MR image. The proposed method adapts the prior

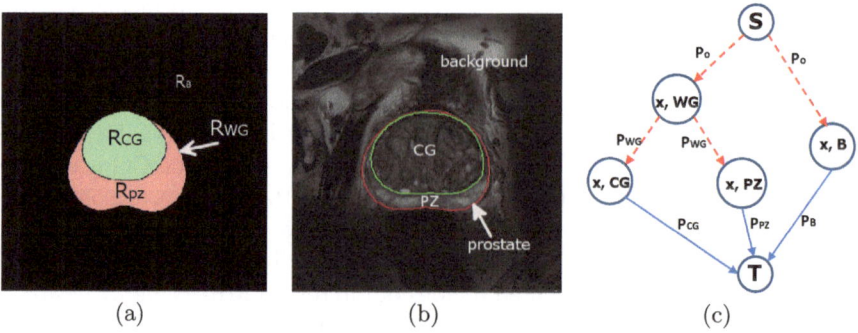

Fig. 1. Proposed layout of anatomically consistent regions (a) and contours overlaid on a T2w prostate MRI slice (b). The prostate region $\mathcal{R}_B$ is divided into two subregions: central gland $\mathcal{R}_{CG}$ and peripheral zone $\mathcal{R}_{PZ}$ and is mutually distinct from the background R_B. (c) shows the proposed spatially continuous flow-maximization scheme.

knowledge of the spatial region consistency to the segmentation of the three prostate-associate regions. We solve the introduced challenging combinatorial optimization problem by means of convex relaxation, for which we propose a novel spatially continuous flow-maximization model and demonstrate its duality to the studied convex relaxed optimization problem with the region consistency constraint. The proposed *continuous max-flow model* directly leads to a new and efficient *continuous max-flow based* algorithm, which enjoys great advantages in numerics and can be readily implemented on GPUs. Experiments over 15 T2-weighted 3D prostate MRIs, by inter- and intra-operator variability, demonstrate the promising performance of the proposed approach.

To our best knowledge, this paper reports the first study on simultaneously extracting the three clinically meaningful regions of prostate: WG, CG and PZ, from 3D T2w MRIs. A similar continuous max-flow based method [16] was proposed in parallel to address the segmentation of cardiac scar tissues from a single Late-Enhancement Cardiac MR Image.

2   Method

We aim to segment a given 3D T2w prostate MR image $I(x)$ into the prostate region $\mathcal{R}_{WG}$ and its two mutually distinct sub-regions: the central gland $\mathcal{R}_{CG}$ and the peripheral zone $\mathcal{R}_{PZ}$, where $\mathcal{R}_B$ denotes the background (see Figure 1(a)), i.e.

$$\Omega = \mathcal{R}_{WG} \cup \mathcal{R}_B, \quad \mathcal{R}_{WG} \cap \mathcal{R}_B = \emptyset, \qquad (1)$$

where the two spatially coherent sub-regions: the R_{CG} and R_{PZ} constitute the whole prostate region $\mathcal{R}_{WG}$ such that

$$\mathcal{R}_{WG} = \mathcal{R}_{CG} \cup \mathcal{R}_{PZ}; \quad \mathcal{R}_{CG} \cap \mathcal{R}_{PZ} = \emptyset. \qquad (2)$$

The typical T2w prostate MR image shows that each of the zones $\mathcal{R}_{CG}$ and $\mathcal{R}_{PZ}$ of $\mathcal{R}_{WG}$ has a distinct intensity appearance, hence constituting the complex/inhomogeneous appearance model of the prostate region $\mathcal{R}_{WG}$. This fact makes it challenging to directly extract the correct boundaries of $\mathcal{R}_{WG}$ from the given MRI without taking such region-associated inhomogeneity into account.

We introduce a new multi-region segmentation approach to accurately and efficiently extract $\mathcal{R}_{WG}$ and its sub-regions $\mathcal{R}_{CG}$ and $\mathcal{R}_{PZ}$ simultaneously from the input T2w MR volume, which encodes the complex intensity appearance of prostate by its two visually independent sub-regions and integrate such region consistency prior into the associate optimization problem. In particular, we solve the introduced combinatorial optimization problem by means of convex relaxation, for which we propose a new continuous max-flow model and demonstrate its duality to the investigated convex relaxation problem. The introduced continuous max-flow model directly derives a new multiplier-based algorithm, which enjoys great numerical advantages in simplicity and efficiency.

2.1   Multi-region Segmentation Model and Convex Relaxation

Given the volume image $I(x)$, let $\pi_i(I(x))$, $i \in L(:= \{CG, PZ, B\})$, be the intensity probability density function (PDF) of the respective region $\mathcal{R}_i$. In practice, such intensity PDF models provide a global descriptor of the objects of interest in statistics, which can be learned from either sampled pixels or given training datasets. The appearance models of the two prostate sub-regions $\mathcal{R}_{CG}$ and $\mathcal{R}_{PZ}$ are distinct from each other and, in combination, represent a proper appearance description of the entire prostate region $\mathcal{R}_{WG}$. [17] showed that such a composite intensity appearance model was more accurate than the often-used mixture appearance model [18] in practice.

We therefore define the cost function $D_i(x)$, where $i \in L$, of labeling each pixel x to be in the prostate sub-region $\mathcal{R}_{CG}$, $\mathcal{R}_{PZ}$ or the background region $\mathcal{R}_B$ by the log-likelihood of the respective PDF, i.e.

$$D_i(x) = -\log\left(\pi_i(I(x))\right), \quad i \in L.$$

Consequently, the total labeling cost of segmenting the input prostate MRI $I(x)$ into multiple regions: $\mathcal{R}_{WG} \cup \mathcal{R}_B := \{\mathcal{R}_{CG} \cup \mathcal{R}_{PZ}\} \cup \mathcal{R}_B$ can be formulated by

$$\sum_{i \in L} \int_{\mathcal{R}_i} D_i(x)\, dx.$$

In this work, we propose to partition the given volume image $I(x)$ by achieving the minimum of the total labeling cost and area such that

$$\min_{\mathcal{R}_{WG}, \mathcal{R}_B, \mathcal{R}_{CG}, \mathcal{R}_{PZ}} \quad \sum_{i \in L} \int_{\mathcal{R}_i} D_i(x)\, dx + \sum_{i \in WG \cup L} \int_{\partial \mathcal{R}_i} ds \qquad (3)$$

subject to the constraints of the region layout (1) and (2).

Let $u_i(x) \in \{0,1\}$, $i \in \{WG, CG, PZ, B\}$, be the indicator or labeling function of the corresponding region $\mathcal{R}_i$, such that

$$u_i(x) := \begin{cases} 1, & \text{where } x \text{ is inside } \mathcal{R}_i \\ 0, & \text{otherwise} \end{cases} , \quad i \in \{WG, CG, PZ, B\}.$$

Then, we can identically rewrite the region constraint (1) as

$$u_{WG}(x) + u_B(x) = 1, \quad \forall x \in \Omega \tag{4}$$

and the constraints (2) of the prostate sub-regions by

$$u_{CG}(x) + u_{PZ}(x) = u_{WG}(x), \quad \forall x \in \Omega. \tag{5}$$

Therefore, the optimization problem (3) can be reformulated in terms of the labeling functions $u_i(x) \in \{0,1\}$, $i \in \{WG, CG, PZ, B\}$, as follows

$$\min_{u(x) \in \{0,1\}} \sum_{i \in L} \langle u_i, D_i \rangle + \sum_{i \in WG \cup L} \int_{\Omega} g(x) |\nabla u_i(x)| \, dx \tag{6}$$

subject to the labeling constraints (4) and (5), where $g(x) \geq 0$ gives the edge weight function and each weighted total-variation function of (6) measures the weighted area of the corresponding surface $\partial \mathcal{R}_i$, $i \in WG \cup L$.

In this study, we solve the challenging combinatorial optimization problem (6) by its convex relaxation:

$$\min_{u(x) \in [0,1]} \sum_{i \in L} \langle u_i, D_i \rangle + \sum_{i \in WG \cup L} \int_{\Omega} g(x) |\nabla u_i(x)| \, dx \tag{7}$$

subject to the linear equality constraints (4) and (5). The binary-valued labeling funtion $u_i(x) \in \{0,1\}$, $i \in WG \cup L$, in (3) is relaxed into the convex-set constraint $u_i(x) \in [0,1]$ in (7). Given the convex energy function of (7) and the linear equality constraints (4) and (5), the complicated combinatorial optimization problem (6) is therefore reduced to its convex optimization version (7).

2.2 Dual Optimization Model

Now we introduce the new continuous max-flow approach to solving the proposed *convex relaxed optimization problem* (7) efficiently, which relies on the following flow configuration (similar as [19,20]), see Fig. 1(c):

– We add two terminals s and t as the source and sink of the flows, the two image copies Ω_{WG} and Ω_B (w.r.t. $\mathcal{R}_{WG}$ and $\mathcal{R}_B$) and the two image copies Ω_{CG} and Ω_{PZ} (w.r.t. the prostate sub-regions $\mathcal{R}_{CG}$ and $\mathcal{R}_{PZ}$).
– We link the source s to the same position x of Ω_{WG} and Ω_B, along which an unconstrained source flow $p_o(x)$ is defined. We link any $x \in \Omega_{WG}$ to the same position x at each of Ω_{CG} and Ω_{PZ}, along which an unconstrained prostate flow $p_{WG}(x)$ is defined. In addition, we link each pixel x of Ω_B and $\Omega_{CG,PZ}$ to the

sink t, along which the respective sink flow $p_i(x)$, $i \in L$, is given.
– Additionally, the spatial flow $q_i(x)$, $i \in WG \cup L$, is specified at any x within
the image domain Ω_i.

Based upon the above settings of flows, we propose a novel *continuous max-flow model*, which maximizes the total flow streaming from the source s, i.e.

$$\max_{p,q} \quad \int_\Omega p_o(x)\, dx \tag{8}$$

subject to
– *Flow capacity constraints*: the sink flows $p_i(x)$, $i \in L$ suffice:

$$p_i(x) \le D_i(x), \quad i \in L, \tag{9}$$

and the spatial flows $q_i(x)$, $i \in WG \cup L$ suffice:

$$|q_i(x)| \le g(x), \quad i \in WG \cup L. \tag{10}$$

– *Flow conservation constraints*: the total flow residue vanishes at each x of the image domain Ω_{WG} or Ω_B, i.e.

$$G_i(x) := \big(\operatorname{div} q_i - p_o + p_i \big)(x) = 0, \quad i \in \{WG, B\}; \tag{11}$$

and the total flow residue also vanishes at each x of Ω_{CG} or Ω_{PZ}, i.e.

$$G_i(x) := \big(\operatorname{div} q_i - p_{WG} + p_i \big)(x) = 0, \quad i \in \{CG, PZ\}. \tag{12}$$

Now we introduce the multiplier functions $u_i(x)$ to the flow conservation constraints of (11) and (12) in the *continuous max-flow model* (8) , which results in the *primal-dual model* equivalen to (8):

$$\max_{p,q} \min_u \quad L(u; p, q) := \int_\Omega p_o(x)\, dx + \sum_{i \in WG \cup L} \langle u_i, G_i \rangle \tag{13}$$

subject to (9) and (10).

Through analysis, we can prove the duality between the introduced three optimization models (8), (13) and (7):

Proposition 1. *The continuous max-flow model* (8), *the primal-dual model* (13) *and the* convex relaxed optimization model (7) *are dual (equivalent) to each other, i.e.,*

$$(8) \iff (13) \iff (7).$$

Its proof is omitted due to the limited space.

2.3 Duality-Based Algorithm

By Prop. 1, it is easy to see that the *convex relaxed optimization model* (7) can be solved equally by computing the *continuous max-flow model* (8). Moreover, by the *primal-dual model* (13) which is equivalent to the (8), the labeling functions $u_i(x)$, $i \in WG \cup L$, work as the multipliers to the corresponding linear equalities (11) and (12) of flow conservation, and the energy function of (13) is just the associated Lagrangian function of the *continuous max-flow model* (8). Hence, an efficient *continuous max-flow algorithm* can be derived upon the augmented multiplier algorithmic scheme [21], which iteratively optimizes the associated augmented Lagrangian function:

$$\max_{p,q} \min_{u} L_c(u; p, q) := L(u; p, q) - \frac{c}{2} \sum_{i \in WG \cup L} \|G_i\|^2$$

subject to the flow capacity constraints (9) and (10), where $L(u; p, q)$ is the Lagrangian function (13). Typically, each k-th iteration of the algorithm maximizes the $L_c(u; p, q)$ over the flow functions p and q subject to the flow constraints (9) and (10), and simply updates the labeling functions $u_i(x)$, $i \in WG \cup L$, afterwards (the detailed algorithimic scheme is similar as in [19,20] and omitted here due to the limited space).

3   Experiments and Results

Image Acquisition. We applied the proposed continuous max-flow algorithm on 15 T2w MR images acquired using a body coil. Subjects were scanned at 3 Tesla with a GE Excite HD MRI system (Milwaukee, WI, USA). All images were acquired at $512 \times 512 \times 36$ voxel with spacing of $0.27 \times 0.27 \times 2.2$ mm^3.

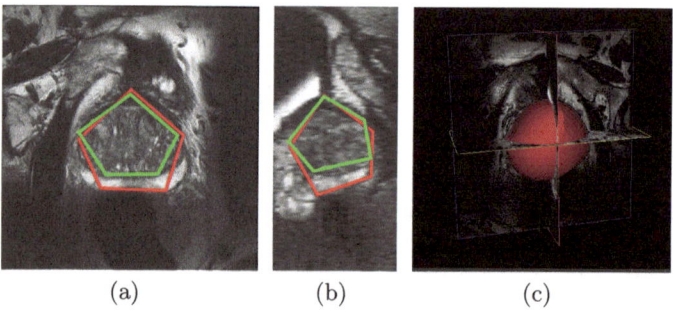

(a)   (b)   (c)

Fig. 2. Initialization scheme. (a) Axial view, (b) Sagital view, (c) orthogonal view overlapped with an initial WG surface. Initial polygon generated by user-selected points for WG (red), and CG (green).

Initialization. The segmentation is initialized by two closed surfaces, which are used to approximate the CG and WG boundaries, respectively. Each of these surfaces is constructed via a thin-plate spline fitting with the positioning of ten to twelve initial points on the prostate or CG surface: half on the axial view and half of the points on the sagittal view. Figure 2 shows example initializations for

WG and CG surfaces, respectively. The smooth closed surface approximates the prostate shape and provides a reasonably good initialization condition (see [22] for more details). The original input volume image is cropped by enlarging the bounding box of the initial WG surface by 30 voxels in each component direction in order to speed up computations. The initial PDFs for each region R_{WG}, R_B, R_{CZ} and R_{PZ}, are calculated based on the user-initialized surfaces, respectively.

Evaluation Metrics. We evaluated the proposed segmentation method by comparing the algorithm to manual segmentation results using Dice similarity coefficient (DSC), the mean absolute surface distance (MAD) and the maximum absolute surface distance (MAXD) [23,24]. Each prostate image was sub-divided into three regions, base, mid-gland and apex, according to the apex-base axis of the manual segmented prostate surface (respectively 0.3, 0.4, 0.3 of the length of the base-apex axis) [25]. All validation metrics were calculated for the entire prostate gland, central gland and peripheral zone in the three respective regions. In addition, the coefficient-of-variation (CV) [26] of DSC was used to evaluate the intra- and inter-observer variability of our method.

Accuracy. Table. 1 shows the segmentation result for 15 patient images using the proposed method. In average the DSC was $89.1 \pm 3.3\%$ for the whole prostate gland, $82.3 \pm 2.9\%$ for the central gland, and $69.3 \pm 6.8\%$ for the peripheral zone. More specifically, our method is capable of generating good segmentation accuracy for the base-, mid- and apex-section of CG and WG. DSCs for the base-

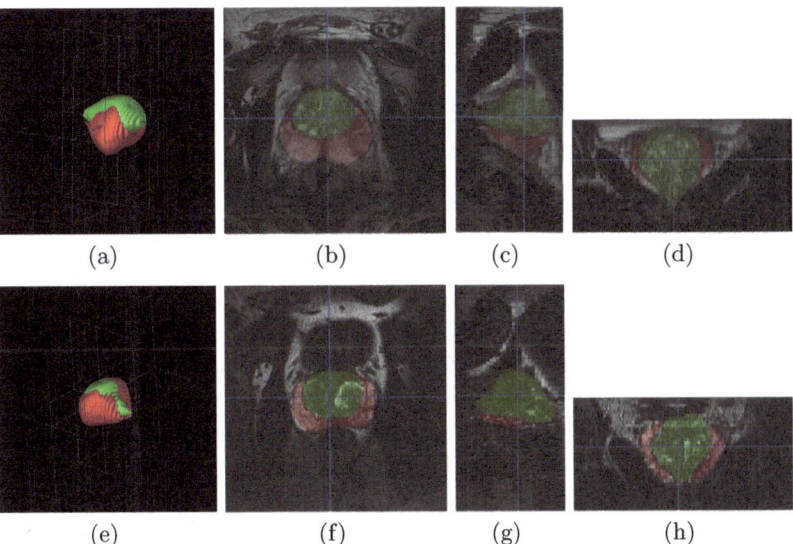

(a)   (b)   (c)   (d)

(e)   (f)   (g)   (h)

Fig. 3. Segmentation result of two prostates. Column 1 to column 4: resulting surface, axial view, sagittal view, and coronal view, respectively. Red: the segmented PZ, green: the segmented CG.

Table 1. Overall segmentation accuracy for 15 patient images

	DSC (%)			
	total	base	mid	apex
PZ	69.3 ± 6.8	54.7 ± 20.8	81.8 ± 5.0	60.1 ± 12.2
CG	82.3 ± 2.9	81.1 ± 2.9	92.0 ± 2.5	68.0 ± 8.1
WG	89.1 ± 3.3	84.5 ± 3.3	94.5 ± 1.6	87.2 ± 5.0

	MAD (voxels)			
	total	base	mid	apex
PZ	2.5 ± 0.8	4.4 ± 3.0	2.0 ± 0.7	2.2 ± 1.6
CG	2.9 ± 1.0	3.3 ± 1.5	3.5 ± 2.2	3.7 ± 1.4
WG	1.7 ± 0.5	2.6 ± 1.6	2.2 ± 0.9	1.8 ± 0.7

	MAXD (voxels)			
	total	base	mid	apex
PZ	20.8 ± 14.0	35.4 ± 24.6	15.0 ± 12.6	15.2 ± 9.6
CG	15.0 ± 15.5	17.0 ± 16.0	15.3 ± 15	19.6 ± 9.9
WG	7.9 ± 3.9	13.8 ± 10.4	10.8 ± 4.3	17.9 ± 6.9

and apex-PZ are comparably low and have large standard deviation (54.7±20.8% and 60.1 ± 12.2%, respectively) since the segmentation for these two regions is more challenging even for radiologists using manual segmentation due to the low degree of recognition of such a thin structure interfered by partial volume effects and unclear boundaries between the zones. However, a DSC of 81.8 ± 5.0% for mid-PZ is favourable, which could meet clinical requirements. In addition, the evaluation results of MAD and MAXD are provided in Table. 1, which provides similar consistent information to DSC.

Reproducibility. Ten images were randomly selected for evaluating the reproducibility of the proposed method. The entire PZ, CG, and WG for each prostate were taken into account instead of their separate sections (apex, mid and base). Each image was segmented five times by the same observer for assessing intra-observer variability in terms of DSC. Figure 4(a) depicts the results for the intra-observer variability. A mean coefficient-of-variation (CV) of 9.25%, 1.63%, and 3.36% was found for PZ, CG, and WG, respectively. To evaluate the variability introduced by manual initialization, ten images were also segmented by other three blinded users. The proposed method initialized by the three users yielded a mean CV of 9.43%, 1.71%, and 3.47% for PZ, CG, and WG, respectively (Fig. 4(b)). It can be seen that the proposed method has low variability of both intra- and inter-observer segmentation for CG and WG, but the observer variability is higher for PZ.

Computation Time. The proposed *continuous max-flow algorithm* was implemented on GPUs (CUDA, NVIDIA Corp., Santa Clara, CA) and the user

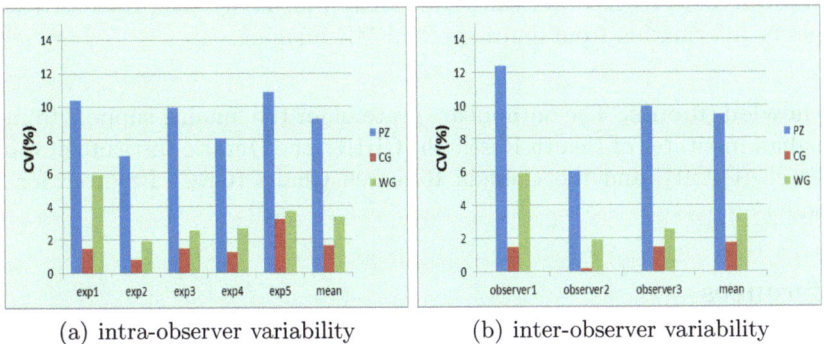

(a) intra-observer variability   (b) inter-observer variability

Fig. 4. Result of intra- and inter-observer variabilities in terms of the coefficient-of-variation (CV) of DSC

interface in Matlab (Natick, MA). The experiments were conducted on a Windows desktop with an Intel i7-2600 CPU (3.4 GHz) and a GPU of NVIDIA Geforce 580X. The segmentation time was calculated as the mean run time of five repeated segmentations for each 3D MR image: for each patient image, the proposed algorithm took 5 ± 0.5s in addition to 35 ± 5s for initialization, and resulted in less than 1 minute in total to segment one image volume.

4   Discussion and Conclusion

In this work, we propose and evaluate a new convex optimization-based multi-region segmentation approach to simultaneously extracting the boundaries of prostate and its component zones from the input 3D prostate T2w MRI, which addresses the challenge of segmenting multiple prostate regions in a numerically sound and efficient manner. The introduced algorithm shows reliable performance results with minimal user interactions using 15 patient images and suggests itself for use in 3D TRUS/MR image guided prostate interventions and computer aided diagnosis of prostate cancer.

The experiments showed that the proposed approach was capable of jointly segmenting different prostate zones with promising accuracy, intra- and inter-observer variability. In terms of accuracy, DSCs of $69.3\pm6.8\%$ and $82.3\pm2.9\%$ for PZ and CG yielded by our methods were lower than $75.0\pm7.0\%$ and $89.0\pm3.0\%$ reported in [15] or $76.0\pm6.0\%$ and $87.0\pm4.0\%$ reported in [14]. However, both methods of [15,14] made use of multi-spectral MR information and relied on the manual segmentation of WG as initialization. Moreover, comparing to those methods, the proposed method required fewer user interactions in practice.

On the other hand, the proposed method can provide good segmentation accuracy for PZ, CG, and WG in the mid-prostate section, which is highly desirable during image-guided prostate interventions and cancer diagnosis. To further improve the segmentation accuracy in the basal and apical regions, future studies will focus on incorporating additional prior knowledge, such as texture, shapes or information from multi-spectral MR imaging.

Acknowledgments. The authors are grateful for the funding support from the Canadian Institutes of Health Research (CIHR), the Ontario Institute of Cancer Research (OICR), and the Canada Research Chairs (CRC) Program for this work.

References

1. Siegel, R., Naishadham, D., Jemal, A.: Cancer statistics, 2012. CA: A Cancer Journal for Clinicians 62(1), 10–29 (2012)
2. Leslie, S., Goh, A., Lewandowski, P.M., Huang, E.Y.H., de Castro Abreu, A.L., Berger, A.K., Ahmadi, H., Jayaratna, I., Shoji, S., Gill, I.S., Ukimura, O.: 2050 contemporary image-guided targeted prostate biopsy better characterizes cancer volume, gleason grade and its 3d location compared to systematic biopsy. The Journal of Urology 187(4, suppl.), e827 (2012)
3. Doyle, S., Feldman, M.D., Tomaszewski, J., Madabhushi, A.: A boosted bayesian multiresolution classifier for prostate cancer detection from digitized needle biopsies. IEEE Trans. Biomed. Engineering 59(5), 1205–1218 (2012)
4. Beyersdorff, D., Winkel, A., Hamm, B., Lenk, S., Loening, S.A., Taupitz, M.: MR imaging-guided prostate biopsy with a closed MR unit at 1.5 T: initial results. Radiology 234(2), 576–581 (2005)
5. McNeal, J.E.: The zonal anatomy of the prostate. The Prostate 2(1), 35–49 (1981)
6. Villeirs, G., De Meerleer, G.: Magnetic resonance imaging (mri) anatomy of the prostate and application of mri in radiotherapy planning. European Journal of Radiology 63(3), 361–368 (2007)
7. Haffner, J., Potiron, E., Bouyé, S., Puech, P., Leroy, X., Lemaitre, L., Villers, A.: Peripheral zone prostate cancers: location and intraprostatic patterns of spread at histopathology. The Prostate 69(3), 276–282 (2009)
8. Reinsberg, S., Payne, G., Riches, S., Ashley, S., Brewster, J., Morgan, V., et al.: Combined use of diffusion-weighted mri and 1h mr spectroscopy to increase accuracy in prostate cancer detection. American Journal of Roentgenology 188(1), 91–98 (2007)
9. Kitajima, K., Kaji, Y., Fukabori, Y., Yoshida, K., Suganuma, N., Sugimura, K.: Prostate cancer detection with 3 t mri: Comparison of diffusion-weighted imaging and dynamic contrast-enhanced mri in combination with t2-weighted imaging. Journal of Magnetic Resonance Imaging 31(3), 625–631 (2010)
10. Kirby, R., Gilling, P.: Fast facts: benign prostatic hyperplasia. Health Press Limited (2011)
11. Ghose, S., Oliver, A., Martí, R., Lladó, X., Vilanova, J., Freixenet, J., Mitra, J., Sidibé, D., Meriaudeau, F.: A survey of prostate segmentation methodologies in ultrasound, magnetic resonance and computed tomography images. Computer Methods and Programs in Biomedicine 108(1), 262–287 (2012)
12. Allen, P., Graham, J., Williamson, D., Hutchinson, C.: Differential segmentation of the prostate in mr images using combined 3d shape modelling and voxel classification. In: 3rd IEEE International Symposium on Biomedical Imaging: Nano to Macro, pp. 410–413. IEEE (2006)

13. Yin, Y., Fotin, S., Periaswamy, S., Kunz, J., Haldankar, H., Muradyan, N., Turkbey, B., Choyke, P.: Fully automated 3d prostate central gland segmentation in mr images: a logismos based approach. In: SPIE, p. 83143B (2012)

14. Makni, N., Iancu, A., Colot, O., Puech, P., Mordon, S., Betrouni, N., et al.: Zonal segmentation of prostate using multispectral magnetic resonance images. Medical Physics 38(11), 6093 (2011)

15. Litjens, G., Debats, O., van de Ven, W., Karssemeijer, N., Huisman, H.: A pattern recognition approach to zonal segmentation of the prostate on MRI. In: Ayache, N., Delingette, H., Golland, P., Mori, K. (eds.) MICCAI 2012, Part II. LNCS, vol. 7511, pp. 413–420. Springer, Heidelberg (2012)

16. Rajchl, M., Yuan, J., White, J.A., Nambakhsh, C.M.S., Ukwatta, E., Li, F., Stirrat, J., Peters, T.M.: A fast convex optimization approach to segmenting 3D scar tissue from delayed-enhancement cardiac MR images. In: Ayache, N., Delingette, H., Golland, P., Mori, K. (eds.) MICCAI 2012, Part I. LNCS, vol. 7510, pp. 659–666. Springer, Heidelberg (2012)

17. Delong, A., Gorelick, L., Schmidt, F.R., Veksler, O., Boykov, Y.: Interactive segmentation with super-labels. In: Boykov, Y., Kahl, F., Lempitsky, V., Schmidt, F.R. (eds.) EMMCVPR 2011. LNCS, vol. 6819, pp. 147–162. Springer, Heidelberg (2011)

18. Yuan, J., Qiu, W., Ukwatta, E., Rajchl, M., Sun, Y., Fenster, A.: An efficient convex optimization approach to 3D prostate MRI segmentation with generic star shape prior. In: Prostate MR Image Segmentation Challenge, MICCAI (2012)

19. Yuan, J., Bae, E., Tai, X.-C., Boykov, Y.: A continuous max-flow approach to potts model. In: Daniilidis, K., Maragos, P., Paragios, N. (eds.) ECCV 2010, Part VI. LNCS, vol. 6316, pp. 379–392. Springer, Heidelberg (2010)

20. Yuan, J., Bae, E., Tai, X.: A study on continuous max-flow and min-cut approaches. In: CVPR 2010 (2010)

21. Bertsekas, D.P.: Nonlinear Programming. Athena Scientific (September 1999)

22. Hu, N., Downey, D.B., Fenster, A., Ladak, H.M.: Prostate boundary segmentation from 3D ultrasound images. Med. Phys. 30(7), 1648–1659 (2003)

23. Qiu, W., Yuan, J., Ukwatta, E., Tessier, D., Fenster, A.: Rotational-slice-based prostate segmentation using level set with shape constraint for 3D end-firing TRUS guided biopsy. In: Ayache, N., Delingette, H., Golland, P., Mori, K. (eds.) MICCAI 2012, Part I. LNCS, vol. 7510, pp. 537–544. Springer, Heidelberg (2012)

24. Qiu, W., Yuan, J., Ukwatta, E., Tessier, D., Fenster, A.: Prostate segmentation in 3d TURS using convex optimization with shape constraint. In: SPIE, Medical Imaging (2013)

25. Mahdavi, S.S., Moradi, M., Wen, X., Morris, W.J., Salcudean, S.E.: Evaluation of visualization of the prostate gland in vibro-elastography images. Medical Image Analysis 15(4), 589–600 (2011)

26. Zou, K.H., McDermott, M.P.: Higher-moment approaches to approximate interval estimation for a certain intraclass correlation coefficient. Statistics in Medicine 18(15), 2051–2061 (1999)

Locality Preserving Non-negative Basis Learning with Graph Embedding

Yasser Ghanbari[1], John Herrington[2], Ruben C. Gur[3],
Robert T. Schultz[2], and Ragini Verma[1,*]

[1] Section of Biomedical Image Analysis, University of Pennsylvania, Philadelphia, PA
{Yasser.Ghanbari,Ragini.Verma}@uphs.upenn.edu
[2] Center for Autism Research, Children's Hospital of Philadelphia, Philadelphia, PA
{herringtonj,schultzrt}@mail.chop.edu
[3] Brain Behavior Laboratory, Department of Psychiatry, University of Pennsylvania,
Philadelphia, PA
gur@mail.med.upenn.edu

Abstract. The high dimensionality of connectivity networks necessitates the development of methods identifying the connectivity building blocks that not only characterize the patterns of brain pathology but also reveal representative population patterns. In this paper, we present a non-negative component analysis framework for learning localized and sparse sub-network patterns of connectivity matrices by decomposing them into two sets of discriminative and reconstructive bases. In order to obtain components that are designed towards extracting population differences, we exploit the geometry of the population by using a graph-theoretical scheme that imposes locality-preserving properties as well as maintaining the underlying distance between distant nodes in the original and the projected space. The effectiveness of the proposed framework is demonstrated by applying it to two clinical studies using connectivity matrices derived from DTI to study a population of subjects with ASD, as well as a developmental study of structural brain connectivity that extracts gender differences.

Keywords: Connectivity analysis, non-negative matrix factorization, locality-preserving dimensionality reduction, graph embedding.

1 Introduction

Computational techniques applied to neuroimaging data have helped unveil the underlying structural or functional differences between groups of interest, e.g. patients and healthy controls. Altered brain connectivity has recently gained a lot of attention in investigating the origin of many brain disorders such as

* The authors acknowledge support for this work, from the following grants: NIH - MH092862 (PI: R. Verma), MH089983 & MH089924 (PI: R. Gur), Pennsylvania Department of Health (SAP # 4100042728, SAP # 4100047863, PI: R. Schultz) and IDDRC (P30 HD026979, PI: M. Yudkoff).

J.C. Gee et al. (Eds.): IPMI 2013, LNCS 7917, pp. 316–327, 2013.

autism spectrum disorder (ASD) [1] and in developmental studies [2]. Hence, advanced techniques of brain connectivity analysis are emerging as a powerful tool in pathological studies of brain disorders. Such tools quantify the connectivity between two regions of interest in DTI, fMRI, EEG, or MEG by calculating tractography [3], mutual information, or synchronization [1] measures.

A number of established analysis methods are available for studying the underlying brain structure via a succinct representation. A successful analysis methodology must possess a means of identifying relevant sub-networks providing an interpretable representation of the brain connectivity, while also facilitating the statistical analysis that describes how this representation is affected by disease. The traditional approaches, i.e. principal and independent components analysis (PCA and ICA) used for investigating brain networks [4] provide dimensionality reduction but may lack physiological interpretability.

Recently, non-negative matrix factorization (NMF) and its alternatives have received extensive attention and proven effective in providing an interpretable set of bases characterizing multivariate data. After being first introduced by Lee and Seung [5], NMF has been successfully employed in many applications such as signal processing, pattern recognition, and medical imaging [6–10]. This was later extended to enforce higher sparseness by adding certain regularization terms [11]. NMF's part-based representation of image data, as well as non-negativity constraints on both the bases and coefficients, facilitates interpretability, and its small size of the basis set categorizes NMF among the unsupervised dimensionality reduction techniques. Although the unsupervised methods are useful in interpretation due to their positivity and sparsity, they do not necessarily provide discriminative bases, only bases which best reconstruct the original data.

The approach taken here is a decomposition of connectivity matrices into interpretable basis components while enforcing positivity of both the components and coefficients. Such a decomposition maintains the interpretation of each component as a network connectivity matrix and the coefficients associated with these components as activations of those networks, while providing a succinct low dimensional representation of the population amenable to statistical analysis. We split the components into two sets of *discriminative* and *reconstructive* bases, which are learned during the optimization process by a graph embedding scheme.

The reconstructive basis set is modeled by minimizing the Frobenius norm of the reconstruction error matrix. To reach our discriminatory basis components, we create two graphs in the high dimensional space of connectivity elements (we call them high dimensional points here): A graph of nearest neighbors to maintain representatives of nearby high dimensional points as close as possible after dimensionality reduction, and a second graph connecting distant high dimensional points to maintain the long distance between their representatives in the projected space. Accounting for the geometrical information in the unsupervised projective NMF helps us categorize the non-negative basis set into discriminative (i.e. providing group differences) and reconstructive (i.e. providing low reconstruction error) components.

The two capabilities of low reconstruction error and good discrimination are unified into minimizing one objectives function by using a gradient descent approach with guaranteeing the positivity of bases and their coefficients.

While the method is generalizable to any type of non-negative connectivity matrix, in this work we apply it to structural connectivity networks computed from Diffusion Tensor Imaging (DTI) data from two different populations of subjects with autism spectrum disorder (ASD) and a developmental study. When NMF is combined with the geometrical information, we show that the discriminative bases are grouped in the discriminative set and dominant bases gather in the reconstructive set.

2   Methods

We hypothesize that each connectivity matrix obtained from the brain connectivity network of a subject, is a linear combination of several fundamental connectivity matrices called connectivity components. Due to the symmetry of connectivity matrices, a vector of all elements of the upper triangular part of any connectivity matrix is considered as the representative of that matrix, and is used as an observation vector $\boldsymbol{x}_i$ for the corresponding subject i. To compute the connectivity components whose mixture approximately constructs the observed connectivity matrices, a matrix factorization model is used as $\boldsymbol{X} = \boldsymbol{W}\boldsymbol{\Phi} + \boldsymbol{\epsilon}$, where $\boldsymbol{\epsilon}$ represents the residual error matrix, columns of $\boldsymbol{X} = [\boldsymbol{x}_1, \boldsymbol{x}_2, \ldots, \boldsymbol{x}_n] \in \mathbb{R}^{m \times n}$, i.e. $\boldsymbol{x}_i$ ($1 \leq i \leq n$), are the connectivity matrix representatives, and columns of $\boldsymbol{W} = [\boldsymbol{w}_1, \boldsymbol{w}_2, \ldots, \boldsymbol{w}_p] \in \mathbb{R}^{m \times p}$, i.e. $\boldsymbol{w}_j$ ($1 \leq j \leq p$), are representative of the normalized basis connectivity components, i.e. the upper triangular elements of the matrix of the corresponding connectivity component. These components ($\boldsymbol{w}_j$) are then mixed by the elements of each column of the loading matrix $\boldsymbol{\Phi} = [\boldsymbol{\varphi}_1, \boldsymbol{\varphi}_2, \ldots, \boldsymbol{\varphi}_n] \in \mathbb{R}^{p \times n}$ to approximate the corresponding column of $\boldsymbol{X}$ [7, 10], i.e. $\boldsymbol{x}_i \approx \sum_{j=1}^{p} \Phi_{ji}\boldsymbol{w}_j$; $1 \leq i \leq n$.

2.1   Unsupervised Learning of Projective Non-negative Bases

Inspired by [12], we assume that $\boldsymbol{\Phi}$ is the projection of $\boldsymbol{X}$ onto $\boldsymbol{W}$, i.e. $\boldsymbol{\Phi} = \boldsymbol{W}^T\boldsymbol{X}$, the non-negativity constraint on the elements of $\boldsymbol{W}$ and $\boldsymbol{\Phi}$ makes our non-negative component analysis an optimization problem of minimizing the cost function $F(\boldsymbol{W}) = \|\boldsymbol{X} - \boldsymbol{W}\boldsymbol{W}^T\boldsymbol{X}\|^2$ with respect to $\boldsymbol{W}$, where $\|.\|$ represents the matrix norm. Considering the Frobenius norm, the minimization problem can be denoted by

$$\min_{\boldsymbol{W} \geq 0} F_1(\boldsymbol{W}) = \min_{\boldsymbol{W} \geq 0} trace\left\{\left(\boldsymbol{X} - \boldsymbol{W}\boldsymbol{W}^T\boldsymbol{X}\right)\left(\boldsymbol{X} - \boldsymbol{W}\boldsymbol{W}^T\boldsymbol{X}\right)^T\right\}. \quad (1)$$

2.2   Locality Preserving Bases with Graph Embedding

In order to impose locality preserving properties, we split the set of projective bases into two sets of $\boldsymbol{W} = [\hat{\boldsymbol{W}}, \tilde{\boldsymbol{W}}]$ in which $\hat{\boldsymbol{W}} = [\boldsymbol{w}_1, \ldots, \boldsymbol{w}_q] \in \mathbb{R}^{m \times q}$ ($q < p$)

captures the *discriminative* basis components while $\tilde{W} = [w_{q+1}, \ldots, w_p] \in \mathbb{R}^{m \times (p-q)}$ is the complimentary space containing the *reconstructive* basis components which minimizes the reconstruction error together with $\hat{W}$. Thus, the coefficient matrix is also split into $\boldsymbol{\Phi} = \begin{bmatrix} \hat{\boldsymbol{\Phi}} \\ \tilde{\boldsymbol{\Phi}} \end{bmatrix} = \begin{bmatrix} \hat{W}^T \\ \tilde{W}^T \end{bmatrix} X$. A proper modeling of such intent would provide at most q of those bases which are likeliest to provide discrimination to belong to $\hat{W}$.

Assuming that the two-group multivariate m-dimensional points, e.g. connectivity elements of patients and controls, lie on a manifold, we would like the basis components captured in $\hat{W}$ to be discriminative, meaning that they should group the p-dimensional coefficients corresponding to the similar (i.e. nearby) m-dimensional points close to each other while keeping the p-dimensional coefficients corresponding to dissimilar (i.e. far) m-dimensional points as far as possible after dimensionality reduction. In this section, we propose a model to satisfy such goals.

To clarify the general idea behind our mathematical modeling given later in this section, suppose that the m-dimensional points of two groups lie on a manifold, as illustrated in Fig. 1(a), and are to be projected into a $p=2$ dimensional space with $q = 1$ discriminative and $p - q = 1$ reconstructive basis. Therefore, between the two orthogonal bases $\overrightarrow{x}$ and $\overrightarrow{y}$, it is desirable for $\hat{W}$ to include $\overrightarrow{y}$ (which is the most discriminative), while $\tilde{W}$ is to include $\overrightarrow{x}$ (which would have the best reconstruction together with $\hat{W}$). Since $\hat{W}$ defines our discriminatory space, it is supposed to provide clustering of coefficients. In order to get the 1-dimensional projections (i.e. coefficients) of m-dimensional points clustered in the 1-dimensional space, we need to keep projections of nearby m-dimensional points as close as possible. This can be obtained by taking advantage of an intrinsic k-nearest-neighbor graph [6]. However, due to the unsupervised nature of our approach, $\hat{W}$ may pick up $\overrightarrow{x}$ which keeps points closer to each other than $\overrightarrow{y}$, and therefore unfavorably merge the two present groups together. To inhibit this, we incorporate a second graph to keep the projections of the distant m-dimensional points as far as possible. Then, we impose the reconstructive basis $\tilde{W}$ to keep the projections of the distant m-dimensional points close to each other, i.e. imposing $\tilde{W}$ to pick up $\overrightarrow{x}$. This will prevent the discriminatory basis from picking up $\overrightarrow{x}$ because it is already picked by $\tilde{W}$ and also because there is some degrees of inherent orthogonality [12] in the bases for the best reconstruction. As a result, the discriminatory basis picks up hyperplanes which maintain coefficients of nearby m-dimensional points together but keeps coefficients of distant points as far as possible, i.e. in this example $\hat{W}$ will be $\overrightarrow{y}$.

There are a variety of approaches that can characterize separability of multivariate data-points. Most of such techniques can be unified in the framework of graph embedding [6]. Let $G = \{X, S\}$ be an undirected weighted graph of n vertices, i.e. data points x_i, with a symmetric similarity matrix $S \in \mathbb{R}^{n \times n}$ with

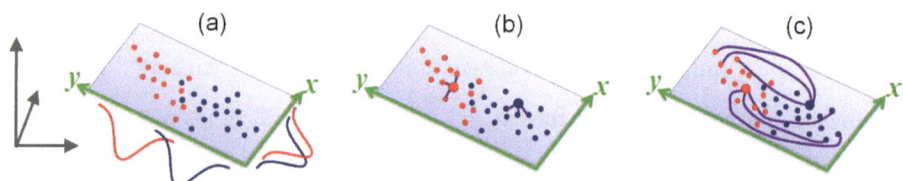

Fig. 1. Illustration of a two-group multivariate point distribution on a manifold in the m-dimensional space. (a) The point distribution when projected into the direction $\vec{x}$ or $\vec{y}$. (b) The 3-nearest-neighbor graph of two selected magnified points. (c) The 3-farthest-point graph of the same two selected points as in b.

non-negative elements corresponding to the edge weight of the graph ($\boldsymbol{S}$ has zero diagonal elements). The Laplacian matrix $\boldsymbol{L}$ of the graph is then defined by

$$\boldsymbol{L} = \boldsymbol{D} - \boldsymbol{S}, \quad D_{ii} = \sum_{j=1}^{n} S_{ij}, \; \forall i. \tag{2}$$

In order for the bases in $\hat{\boldsymbol{W}}$ to provide discriminatory information, we would like the resulting coefficients of nearby $\boldsymbol{x}_i$ points to stay close to each other when projected into $\hat{\boldsymbol{W}}$. To satisfy such intent, we first construct a k-nearest-neighbor graph $\hat{G} = \{\boldsymbol{X}, \hat{\boldsymbol{S}}\}$ of the m-dimensional points $\boldsymbol{x}_i$, as illustrated in Fig. 1(b), in which the edge weight of neighbor points $\boldsymbol{x}_i$ and $\boldsymbol{x}_j$ is defined by

$$\hat{S}_{ij} = e^{-\frac{\|\boldsymbol{x}_i - \boldsymbol{x}_j\|^2}{\hat{\sigma}^2}}, \tag{3}$$

where $\hat{\sigma}$ is a scaling parameter. In this scheme, $\hat{S}_{ij}$ is non-zero, if and only if $\boldsymbol{x}_i$ is among the k-nearest-neighbors of $\boldsymbol{x}_j$ or vice versa, i.e. $\hat{\boldsymbol{S}}$ is sparse and symmetric. Hence, minimizing the following cost function will preserve coefficients ($\hat{\varphi}_i$) of the nearby points as close as possible.

$$\min_{\boldsymbol{W} \geq 0} F_2(\boldsymbol{W}) = \min_{\hat{\boldsymbol{W}} \geq 0} \sum_{i=1}^{n} \sum_{j=1}^{n} \|\hat{\varphi}_i - \hat{\varphi}_j\|^2 \hat{S}_{ij} = \min_{\hat{\boldsymbol{W}} \geq 0} trace \left\{ \hat{\boldsymbol{\Phi}} \hat{\boldsymbol{L}} \hat{\boldsymbol{\Phi}}^T \right\}. \tag{4}$$

According to the equation (4), if data-points $\boldsymbol{x}_i$ and $\boldsymbol{x}_j$ are close, their graph edge weight S_{ij} will be large, and therefore, the cost function $F_2(\hat{\boldsymbol{W}})$ gets minimized only if the corresponding coefficients $\hat{\varphi}_i$ and $\hat{\varphi}_j$ remain close.

As explained earlier, to avoid the issue of merging the two groups by $\hat{\boldsymbol{W}}$, we introduce the graph of k-farthest points $\tilde{G} = \{\boldsymbol{X}, \tilde{\boldsymbol{S}}\}$ where, as illustrated in Fig. 1(c), each point $\boldsymbol{x}_i$ is connected by a non-zero weighted edge to its k most distant points in the m-dimensional space by

$$\tilde{S}_{ij} = e^{-\frac{\|\boldsymbol{x}_i - \boldsymbol{x}_j\|^2}{\tilde{\sigma}^2}}, \tag{5}$$

where $\tilde{\sigma}$ is a scaling parameter. $\tilde{S}_{ij}$ is non-zero, if and only if $\boldsymbol{x}_i$ is among the k-farthest points of $\boldsymbol{x}_j$ or vice versa, i.e. $\tilde{\boldsymbol{S}}$ is sparse and symmetric. With a similar rationale as in the nearest-neighbor graph $\hat{G}$, we exploit this graph $\tilde{G}$ to impose $\tilde{\boldsymbol{W}}$ to keep the representative coefficients $(\tilde{\varphi}_i)$ of the the farthest points as close as possible in the lower dimensional space. This is performed by minimizing

$$\min_{\boldsymbol{W} \geq 0} F_3(\boldsymbol{W}) = \min_{\tilde{\boldsymbol{W}} \geq 0} \sum_{i=1}^{n} \sum_{j=1}^{n} \|\tilde{\varphi}_i - \tilde{\varphi}_j\|^2 \tilde{S}_{ij} = \min_{\tilde{\boldsymbol{W}} \geq 0} trace\left\{\tilde{\boldsymbol{\Phi}} \tilde{\boldsymbol{L}} \tilde{\boldsymbol{\Phi}}^T\right\}. \quad (6)$$

This will lead to resolve the aforementioned issue, and thereby $\hat{\boldsymbol{W}}$ will gain discriminatory properties by picking up the projection direction than maintains the original nearby points as close as possible while keeping the distant points as far as possible.

2.3   Objective Function

To achieve the above three objectives of (1), (4), and (6), the final objective function is to minimize $F(\boldsymbol{W}) = F_1(\boldsymbol{W}) + \lambda\,(F_2(\boldsymbol{W}) + F_3(\boldsymbol{W}))$, and according to the projective properties of the model, i.e. $\boldsymbol{\Phi} = \boldsymbol{W}^T \boldsymbol{X}$, the final objective function can be rewritten as follows

$$F(\boldsymbol{W}) = trace\left\{\left(\boldsymbol{X} - \boldsymbol{W}\boldsymbol{W}^T\boldsymbol{X}\right)\left(\boldsymbol{X} - \boldsymbol{W}\boldsymbol{W}^T\boldsymbol{X}\right)^T\right\} +$$
$$\lambda\left(trace\left\{\hat{\boldsymbol{W}}^T\boldsymbol{X}\hat{\boldsymbol{L}}\boldsymbol{X}^T\hat{\boldsymbol{W}}\right\} + trace\left\{\tilde{\boldsymbol{W}}^T\boldsymbol{X}\tilde{\boldsymbol{L}}\boldsymbol{X}^T\tilde{\boldsymbol{W}}\right\}\right), \quad (7)$$

where λ is a tunable parameter to balance the two terms of reconstruction error norm and graph embedding.

2.4   Optimization Solution

Minimizing the objective function of the equation (7) with non-negativity constraints of $\boldsymbol{W}$ yields the optimal projective bases among which q likeliest discriminative ones are obtained in $\hat{\boldsymbol{W}}$. To minimize our objective function, we use a gradient descent approach, i.e. updating $W_{ij} = W_{ij} - \eta_{ij}\frac{\partial F}{\partial W_{ij}}$ with a positive step-size η_{ij}, where

$$\frac{\partial F}{\partial \boldsymbol{W}} = -4\left(\boldsymbol{X}\boldsymbol{X}^T\boldsymbol{W}\right) + 2\left(\boldsymbol{W}\boldsymbol{W}^T\boldsymbol{X}\boldsymbol{X}^T\boldsymbol{W}\right) + 2\left(\boldsymbol{X}\boldsymbol{X}^T\boldsymbol{W}\boldsymbol{W}^T\boldsymbol{W}\right)$$
$$+ \left[2\lambda\boldsymbol{X}\hat{\boldsymbol{L}}\boldsymbol{X}^T\hat{\boldsymbol{W}}\,,\,2\lambda\boldsymbol{X}\tilde{\boldsymbol{L}}\boldsymbol{X}^T\tilde{\boldsymbol{W}}\right]. \quad (8)$$

Regarding that $\hat{\boldsymbol{L}} = \hat{\boldsymbol{D}} - \hat{\boldsymbol{S}}$ and $\tilde{\boldsymbol{L}} = \tilde{\boldsymbol{D}} - \tilde{\boldsymbol{S}}$, and the fact that both $\boldsymbol{D}$ and $\boldsymbol{S}$ matrices have non-negative elements, our non-negativity constraint is guaranteed by positive initialization of $\boldsymbol{W}$ and applying the step-size as follows:

$$\eta_{i,j} = \frac{\frac{1}{2}W_{ij}}{(\boldsymbol{WW^T XX^T W})_{ij} + (\boldsymbol{XX^T WW^T W})_{ij} + \left[\lambda \boldsymbol{X\hat{D}X^T \hat{W}} \ , \ \lambda \boldsymbol{X\tilde{D}X^T \tilde{W}}\right]_{ij}}.$$
(9)

This results in the a multiplicative updating solution as

$$W_{ij} = W_{ij} \frac{\left(2\boldsymbol{XX^T W} + \lambda \left[\boldsymbol{X\hat{S}X^T \hat{W}} \ , \ \boldsymbol{X\tilde{S}X^T \tilde{W}}\right]\right)_{ij}}{\left(\boldsymbol{WW^T XX^T W} + \boldsymbol{XX^T WW^T W} + \lambda \left[\boldsymbol{X\hat{D}X^T \hat{W}} \ , \ \boldsymbol{X\tilde{D}X^T \tilde{W}}\right]\right)_{ij}}.$$
(10)

For stability of the convergence, at each iteration, each column of $\boldsymbol{W}$ is normalized by $\boldsymbol{w}_i = \frac{\boldsymbol{w}_i}{\|\boldsymbol{w}_i\|_2}$. Starting with initial random positive elements on $\boldsymbol{W}$, the iterative procedure will converge to the desired $\boldsymbol{W} \geq 0$, whose first q columns are likeliest discriminative bases and the rest are the reconstructive ones.

2.5   Scaling Parameter of Graph Edge Weights

The parameters $\hat{\sigma}$ and $\tilde{\sigma}$ in equations (3) and (5) are a scaling measure of similarity between two points. Such scaling parameters are commonly set by trial and error, but this approach requires manual intervention and is time-consuming [13]. We propose to set the scaling parameter of the graph $\hat{G}$ by

$$\hat{\sigma} = \frac{1}{n} \sum_{i=1}^{n} \hat{\delta}_i \ ; \quad \hat{\delta}_i = \|\boldsymbol{x}_i - \hat{\boldsymbol{x}}_{i,k}\|_2 \ ,$$
(11)

where $\hat{\boldsymbol{x}}_{i,k}$ is the most distant point among the k-nearest neighbors of $\boldsymbol{x}_i$.

This results in a suitable scaling measure because $\hat{\delta}_i$ becomes large for the outliers and small for the points near the center of each distribution in the high dimensional space. The average of the $\hat{\delta}_i$s is dominated by the edges of the points around the center of population distributions, because the number of points around the distribution center exceeds the number of outliers. With the same rationale, the scaling parameter of the graph $\tilde{G}$ is set by

$$\tilde{\sigma} = \frac{1}{n} \sum_{i=1}^{n} \tilde{\delta}_i \ ; \quad \tilde{\delta}_i = \|\boldsymbol{x}_i - \tilde{\boldsymbol{x}}_{i,k}\|_2 \ ,$$
(12)

where $\tilde{\boldsymbol{x}}_{i,k}$ is the least distant point among the k-farthest points to $\boldsymbol{x}_i$.

2.6   Group Analysis Model

As stated by equation $\boldsymbol{X} \approx \boldsymbol{W\Phi}$, the n connectivity observations, i.e. $\boldsymbol{x}_i : 1 \leq i \leq n$, in the matrix $\boldsymbol{X}$ are approximated by

$$[\boldsymbol{x}_1, \boldsymbol{x}_2, \ldots, \boldsymbol{x}_n] \approx [\boldsymbol{w}_1, \boldsymbol{w}_2, \ldots, \boldsymbol{w}_p] \begin{bmatrix} \Phi_{11} & \Phi_{12} & \ldots & \Phi_{1n} \\ \vdots & \vdots & & \vdots \\ \Phi_{p1} & \Phi_{p2} & \ldots & \Phi_{pn} \end{bmatrix}.$$
(13)

Each observation vector per subject i is thus, approximately reconstructed by

$$x_i \approx \sum_{j=1}^{p} \Phi_{ji} w_j = \sum_{j=1}^{p} \left(w_j^T x_i \right) w_j \; ; \; 1 \le i \le n. \tag{14}$$

Thereby, the presence of each component w_j in the corresponding connectivity vector of a subject x_i, is characterized by the corresponding coefficients Φ_{ji}. Let us suppose, with no loss of generality, that the first n_1 elements are from the first group (e.g. population of patients) and the remaining $n_2 = n - n_1$ from the second group (e.g. controls). Therefore, the statistical significance between the set of $\{\Phi_{ji} : 1 \le i \le n_1\}$ and $\{\Phi_{ji} : n_1 + 1 \le i \le n\}$ describes the importance of the corresponding connectivity basis w_j in differentiating the two groups, which can be verified by a two-sample t-test.

3   Results

The proposed method above provides a linear framework of dimensionality reduction yielding two sets of discriminative and reconstructive network components. The reconstructive basis set is expected to show the primary sub-networks of the overall connectivity which are dominant based on their magnitude of coefficients representing their average activation within the population.

The discriminatory set of basis components are expected to show localized sparse sub-networks which represent population clustering and differentiate the two groups but do not contribute considerably in reconstruction of the original connectivity matrices. These two basis sets help us understand the primary global dominant networks as well as pattern-based discriminatory sub-networks characterizing population differences.

In order to show the effectiveness of our method, we examine it over two separate datasets of DTI connectivity matrices. We will obtain the reconstructive bases as well as pattern-based discriminative bases, and examine the differences between the two groups pooled. Similar to the feature extraction problem, the number of bases (i.e. p and q) is population dependent; however, we show that with relatively small numbers for p and q, we obtain stable group differences.

Dataset Demographics. Our first dataset consisted of 83 children, 24 ASD and 59 typically developing (TD), all male, aged 6-18 years (mean=12.9, SD=3.0 in ASD, and mean=11.6, SD=3.2 in TD). A standard t-test showed that the age difference between the two groups was not statistically significant. Our second dataset is a developmental study consisting of 595 subjects with 262 males and 333 females. Subjects are aged 8-22 years (mean=14.9, SD=3.2 in males, and mean=15.4, SD=3.3 in females). A standard t-test showed that there was no significant age difference between the genders.

Establishing Structural Connectivity. DTI data was acquired for each subject and brain extraction was performed on each diffusion-weighted volume and used in computing a fractional anisotropy (FA) volume. Cortical parcellation and sub-cortical segmentation was carried out for each subject using Freesurfer. For the developmental study, a total of 95 ROIs from the Desikan atlas [14] were extracted to represent the nodes of the structural network, comprising 68 cortical regions and 27 sub-cortical structures. In the ASD study, 79 ROIs were extracted comprising 68 cortical regions and 11 sub-cortical structures.

The seed region was limited to the GM-WM boundary of each ROI for reliable tracking. The seed regions were then transferred to the diffusion space via intra-subject affine coregistration between T1 and FA volumes, to act as node labels. Probabilistic tractography [3] was performed on all the subjects with 5000 streamline fibers sampled per voxel. The result was a 79×79 (in ASD) or 95×95 (in developmental) matrix of weighted connectivity values, where each (i, j) element represents the conditional probability of a pathway between regions i and j, normalized by the active surface area of the ROI i. This matrix was treated as a weighted, undirected symmetric network of each subject.

3.1 Connectivity Analysis in ASD

The 79×79 connectivity matrix of each subject was vectorized to their $m = 3081$ upper triangular elements. In order to compute the bases and their linearly projected coefficients, we used a three-nearest-neighbor graph for $\hat{G}$ as well as a 3-farthest-point graph for $\tilde{G}$ (i.e. $k = 3$) and correspondingly calculated their graph edge weights and node strengths, i.e. S and D. Also, the tuning parameter was set to $\lambda = 1$. We used $p = 5$ for the number of bases with $q = 2$. The iterative procedure of equation (10) was performed and the two discriminative as well as three reconstructive bases learned are shown in Fig. 2.

A statistical group analysis, as described in Sect. 2.6, was performed over the resulting projective coefficients of each w_i basis, i.e. Φ_{ji}. The two-sample t-test is applied to the coefficients of each basis from the pooled population of AST–TD subjects and the p−values and t−values are given in Table 1, as well as the average of the coefficients in the entire population as a ranking criterion of their activation magnitude in the population. The average values here are scaled down similarly for all bases due to their large values.

It is observed that the discriminatory bases are quite sparse with localized patterns, as expected. The large average of the reconstructive coefficients shows that those bases are playing the main role in reconstructing the overall connectivity while the small coefficients in the discriminative bases confirm that they do not play a significant role in the reconstruction but are important in distinguishing the two groups. The statistical significance of the discriminative basis (a) in Fig. 2 shows distinct connectivity deficiencies in inter-hemisphere subcortical and parietal connections in children with ASD, as well as in short-range frontal connections with other nearby cortical and subcortical regions. The significance of the reconstructive basis (c) also shows that the brain is slightly deficient in children with autism in the overall short-range intra-hemisphere connectivity.

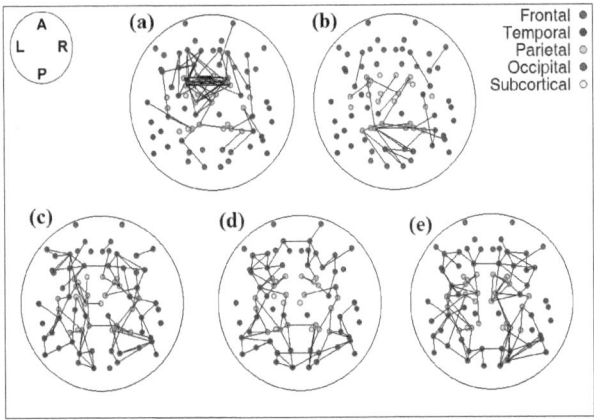

Fig. 2. The $p = 5$ connectivity bases (ASD study) learned by the proposed method. (a)–(b) are the $q = 2$ discriminatory, and (c)–(e) are the three reconstructive bases.

3.2   Connectivity Analysis in the Developmental Study

The $m = 4465$-length vectors of the upper triangular part of the 95×95 connectivity matrices were used for basis learning. Similar to the ASD dataset, we used a three-nearest-neighbor graph for $\hat{G}$, as well as a 3-farthest-point graph for $\tilde{G}$ (i.e. $k = 3$) and correspondingly calculated their graph matrices, S and D. Also, the tuning parameter was similarly set to $\lambda = 1$. We applied our method with $p = 10$ basis components with the first $q = 6$ bases forming the set of discriminatory ones. The resulting bases are shown in Fig. 3.

The statistical group analysis results of the resulting coefficients of each basis are given in Table 2, as well as the average of the coefficients in the entire population. The average values here are scaled down similarly for all bases.

According to the statistics of the coefficients, it is seen from the discriminative set of bases in the top row of Fig. 3 that the discriminative bases are sub-networks of connectivity which mostly show strong group differences in both males and females. Males show stronger intra-hemisphere inter-cortical connectivity structure (see Fig. 3(a), (b), (d)) whereas women are distinguished by their stronger

Table 1. Statistical group analysis of the coefficients of the ASD-TD bases

Component label	Pooled ASD-TD average coefficients	ASD-TD group p-value	ASD-TD group t-value
a	0.6	0.002	-3.3
b	0.4	0.96	-0.1
c	5.5	0.02	-2.5
d	5.8	0.44	-0.8
e	5.7	0.16	-1.4

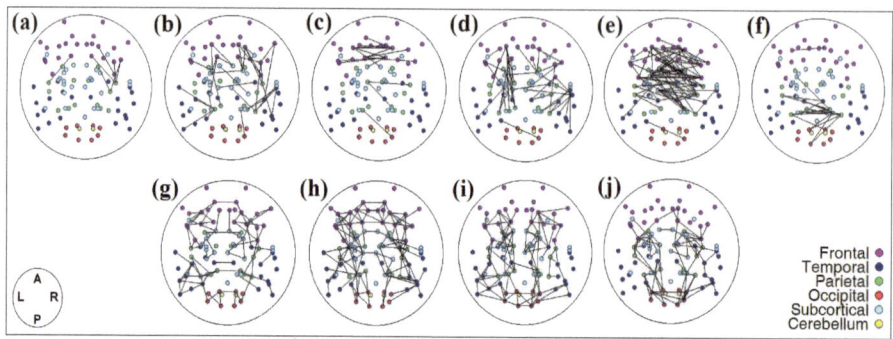

Fig. 3. The $p = 10$ connectivity bases (developmental study) learned by the proposed method. (a)–(f) are the $q = 6$ discriminatory, and (g)–(j) are the 4 reconstructive bases.

Table 2. Statistical group analysis of the developmental basis coefficients

Component label	Pooled Male-Female average coefficients	Male-Female group p–value	Male-Female group t–value
a	0.15	9.8e-12	+7.0
b	0.17	1.5e-6	+4.9
c	0.10	1.6e-3	-3.2
d	0.13	1.2e-2	+2.5
e	0.17	0.56	-0.59
f	0.21	0.69	+0.39
g	4.1	6.1e-14	+7.7
h	4.2	2.5e-9	+6.1
i	4.4	4.2e-15	+8.1
j	3.6	3.0e-12	+7.1

inter-hemisphere connectivity specially in the frontal regions (e.g. see Fig. 3(c)). Also, the four reconstructive bases at the bottom row of this figure show that the overall dominant brain connectivity is a collection of short-range connections which are stronger towards the male.

4   Conclusion

We have presented a novel technique for extracting the discriminative sub-networks of a population via graph embedding. This maps the connectivity patterns of the population onto a lower dimensional space to ease subsequent population statistics. Our method consists of basis learning which simultaneously minimizes the reconstruction error, as well as provides discriminative bases which identify group differences in the presence of non-negativity constraints over both bases and coefficients. The method was evaluated on two datasets of connectivity analysis, one in a study of ASD which revealed significant inter-hemisphere connectivity deficiencies in a set of interpretable connections as part of a discriminatory basis. The second developmental dataset also showed dominant intra-hemisphere connectivity in males while the inter-hemisphere frontal connectivity appeared stronger in females. The presented technique represents a framework, that is in principle capable of handling other types of non-negative functional or structural connectivity networks from any modality for statistical group analysis. Its linearity makes our technique attractive for the unsupervised feature selection applications as well.

References

1. Vissers, M., Cohen, M., Geurts, H.: Brain connectivity and high functioning autism: a promising path of research that needs refined models, methodological convergence, and stronger behavioral links. Neurosci. Biobehav. Rev. 36(1), 604–625 (2012)
2. Dennis, E.L., Jahanshad, N., et al.: Development of brain structural connectivity between ages 12 and 30: A 4-tesla diffusion imaging study in 439 adolescents and adults. Neuroimage 64, 671–684 (2013)
3. Behrens, T.E.J., Johansen-Berg, H., et al.: Non-invasive mapping of connections between human thalamus and cortex using diffusion imaging. Nat. Neurosci. 6(7), 750–757 (2003)
4. Calhoun, V., Kiehl, K., Pearlson, G.: Modulation of temporally coherent brain networks estimated using ICA at rest and during cognitive tasks. Hum. Brain Mapp. 29(7), 828–838 (2008)
5. Lee, D.D., Seung, H.S.: Learning the parts of objects by non-negative matrix factorization. Nature 401(6755), 788–791 (1999)
6. Yan, S., Xu, D., Zhang, B., Zhang, H.J., Yang, Q., Lin, S.: Graph embedding and extensions: a general framework for dimensionality reduction. IEEE Trans. Pattern Anal. Mach. Intell. 29(1), 40–51 (2007)
7. Batmanghelich, N., Taskar, B., Davatzikos, C.: Generative-discriminative basis learning for medical imaging. IEEE Trans. Med. Imaging 31(1), 51–69 (2011)
8. Wang, C., Yan, S., Zhang, L., Zhang, H.: Non-negative semi-supervised learning. Journal of Machine Learning Research 5, 575–582 (2009)
9. Berry, M.W., Browne, M., Langville, A.N., Pauca, V.P., Plemmons, R.J.: Algorithms and applications for approximate nonnegative matrix factorization. Computational Statistics and Data Analysis 52, 155–173 (2007)
10. Yang, Z., Oja, E.: Linear and nonlinear projective nonnegative matrix factorization. IEEE Trans. Neural Netw. 21(5), 1734–1749 (2010)
11. Hoyer, P.O.: Non-negative matrix factorization with sparseness constraints. The Journal of Machine Learning Research 5, 1457–1469 (2004)
12. Ghanbari, Y., Bloy, L., Batmanghelich, K., Roberts, T.P.L., Verma, R.: Dominant component analysis of electrophysiological connectivity networks. In: Ayache, N., Delingette, H., Golland, P., Mori, K. (eds.) MICCAI 2012, Part III. LNCS, vol. 7512, pp. 231–238. Springer, Heidelberg (2012)
13. Manor, L.Z., Perona, P.: Self-tuning spectral clustering. In: Advances in Neural Information Processing Systems, pp. 1601–1608 (2005)
14. Desikan, R., Sgonne, F., et al.: An automated labeling system for subdividing the human cerebral cortex on MRI scans into gyral based regions of interest. NeuroImage 31, 968–980 (2006)

Hierarchical Discriminative Framework
for Detecting Tubular Structures in 3D Images

Dirk Breitenreicher[1], Michal Sofka[1], Stefan Britzen[2], and Shaohua K. Zhou[1]

[1] Imaging and Computer Vision, Siemens Corporation,
Corporate Technology, Princeton, NJ, USA
[2] Imaging & Therapy Systems, Siemens Healthcare, Forchheim, Germany

Abstract. Detecting tubular structures such as airways or vessels in medical images is important for diagnosis and surgical planning. Many state-of-the-art approaches address this problem by starting from the root and progressing towards thinnest tubular structures usually guided by image filtering techniques. These approaches need to be tailored for each application and can fail in noisy or low-contrast regions. In this work, we address these challenges by a two-layer model which consists of a low-level likelihood measure and a high-level measure verifying tubular branches. The algorithm starts by computing a robust measure of tubular presence using a discriminative classifier at multiple image scales. The measure is then used in an efficient multi-scale shortest path algorithm to generate candidate centerline branches and corresponding radii measurements. Finally, the branches are verified by a learning-based indicator function that discards false candidate branches. The experiments on detecting airways in rotational X-ray volumes show that the technique is robust to noise and correctly finds airways even in the presence of imaging artifacts.

1 Introduction

Accurate and efficient detection of tree-like structures such as airways or vessels in 3D medical images is important for accurate diagnosis, treatment monitoring, and surgical planning [1,5,8]. The segmentation of such structures is challenging due to noise, imaging artifacts, pathologies, and low-resolution of images (see Fig. 1 for examples). Despite these challenges, the segmented trees are required to be complete and have low number of false branches to make the results accurate for diagnostic and interventional procedures [5,9,15]. In this paper, we propose an efficient algorithm that addresses the challenges above and produces accurate tree detection. This is achieved by discriminative techniques to design a reliable measure of tubularness and to verify candidate branches of the detected tree.

State-of-the-art techniques can be roughly categorized into top-down and bottom-up. Top-down approaches start at a root point and propagate the tree segmentation into distant branches, for example by region growing [2,9]. These algorithms obtain the segmentation by energy-based image filtering techniques [3,7,13] which evaluate manually tuned cost functions at certain image locations. Strong assumptions on the filter design (e.g. sampling pattern) make it difficult to adapt these algorithms for detecting tubular structures that have high variability of thickness or direction. Furthermore, sophisticated

J.C. Gee et al. (Eds.): IPMI 2013, LNCS 7917, pp. 328–339, 2013.

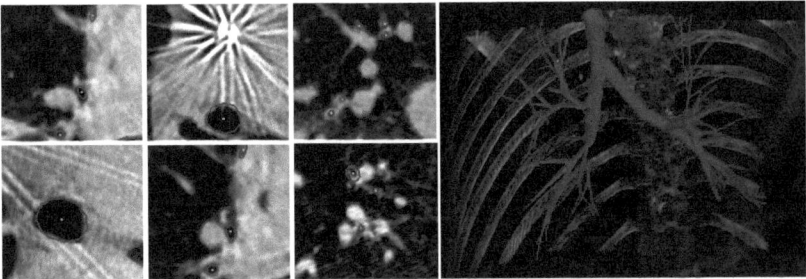

Fig. 1. Accurate detection of airways in rotational X-ray volumes is challenging due to the varying size and context of airways, low signal-to-noise ratio, and presence of imaging artifacts.

stopping criteria are necessary to prevent leaking of the segmentation in regions of high noise, especially when segmenting thin structures and structures of low-contrast.

Bottom-up approaches show much more promise [18] and this strategy is also taken in this paper. These algorithms use the likelihood of each voxel belonging to a tubular structure and introduce a tubular *neighborhood* through a global graph of voxel locations. The tree structure is found through the global optimization on the neighborhood graph that uses candidate source nodes and pre-determined sink node to search for candidate branches. Bifurcations, noisy and low-contrast regions are handled through optimization and graph constraints. Termination criteria are naturally defined by the global optimum of the graph. The challenge is the global optimization which becomes computationally prohibitive with large image sizes.

In this work, we present a novel bottom-up algorithm for detecting centerlines and approximate radii of tubular structures. The algorithm relies on a two-layer model which consists of a low-level likelihood measure and a high-level measure verifying tubular branches. The algorithm starts by computing a robust measure of tubular presence using a discriminative classifier at multiple image scales. The classifier responses are then used to identify a number of candidate source points likely belonging to a centerline. The root of the tubular tree (sink) is found in the coarsest scale as a candidate with the highest probability. In the next step, candidate centerline paths from the source points towards the sink are obtained using multi-scale variant of the Dijkstra's shortest path algorithm. Finally, the candidate paths are verified using a learned branch classifier and combined in a centerline tree.

The proposed two-layer model makes it possible to efficiently search for tubular structures in large 3D images. This is because the algorithm only uses the most reliable candidate points (determined at the first layer) to search for centerline paths towards the root. Although a large number of points (several thousand) is used initially, many of them do not yield valid centerlines. These are discarded by the classifier at the second layer which validates the candidate centerline paths.

We will show on a dataset of rotational X-ray volumes, that the algorithm effectively detects centerlines of airway trees. Out of all detected centerline points, 74.0% are detected within 4 mm of the ground truth tree centerlines and only 14.3% are detected more than 10 mm away. The final detection speed is 1.5 minutes per volume. The results satisfy clinical requirements and suggest that the approach is suitable for practical use. To the best of our knowledge, this is the first algorithm ever proposed for detecting airway centerlines in rotational X-ray volumes. Extension of the algorithm to other tree-like structures in other modalities should be possible by retraining the classifiers.

The paper is organized as follows. After a brief overview of the relevant literature in Sect. 2, the discriminative tubular model is presented in Sect. 3. The two layers of the model are explained in Sect. 3.1 and Sect. 3.2. The experiments on rotational X-ray volumes of the lung are shown in Sec. 4. We conclude the paper in Sect. 5.

2   Related Work

Many centerline extraction algorithms focus on the design of the measure of tubularness at each location. These techniques use intensity values directly, or compute their first or second order derivatives at various locations of a sampling pattern [3,4,7,13]. Such approaches are typically not robust to noise, imaging artifacts, or high variability of tubular sizes and orientations. Furthermore, applying standard multi-scale analysis might not always be possible due to memory and runtime requirements. Finally, some algorithms aggregate measures via a voting mechanism to increase robustness [12,21] but it is not clear how to extract tubular centerlines from the voting maps.

The robustness of centerline detectors have been recently improved by applying machine learning techniques. These algorithms model the tubular pattern directly and use discriminative classifiers on features describing low-level image characteristics [5,10,20]. The classifier responses are then used in a region growing algorithm to find the tree segmentations. However, classification solely based on low-level features can have errors due to the absence of contextual information [19].

One approach to model context is to define a graphical model [6,17] which captures the relationships between neighboring locations. These algorithms can be computationally expensive, especially for large volumetric datasets. Standard algorithms used for optimization such as graph cuts or belief propagation can no longer be applied. Another approach is to sample the classification map directly [19] or according to a rotational invariant sampling pattern [17]. The former approach is similar to steerable features which sample the appearance using a regular grid [20]. In our model, we also incorporate context similar to [19,20] but instead of using densely sampled grid, our sampling pattern is specific to centerline branches and thus directly incorporates prior knowledge.

Our model has two layers: The first layer models the uncertainty of classifying individual voxels and the second layer decides about tubular branches. A similar idea was used in [6] to segment natural images. The first layer of the hierarchy encodes pixel-wise labeling and the second layer captures relative configuration of objects or parts. However, the distributions are modeled as conditional random fields which are not suitable for tubular objects due to the induced graph topology.

3   Discriminative Tree Detection

Our tree detection algorithm comprises (1) a robust low-level measure of tubularness computed at multiple scales, (2) an efficient bottom-up search strategy, and (3) a reliable

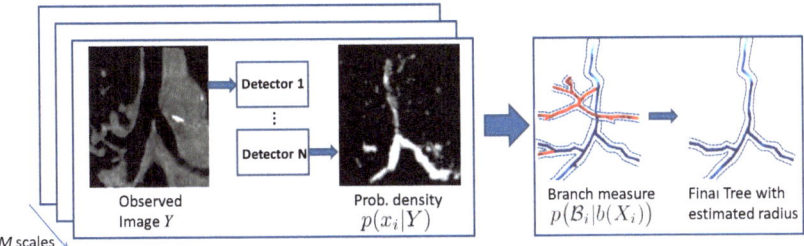

Fig. 2. Automatic detection of tubular structures. In Layer 1 (Sect. 3.1), the density $p(x_i|Y)$ is obtained using N detectors at each of the M scales. In Layer 2 (Sect. 3.2), the candidate centerlines are verified using the branch measure $p(\mathcal{B}_i|b(X_i))$ to compose the final centerline tree.

branch verification. The low-level measure indicates the presence of a tubular structure at each voxel location. The measure is determined by a discriminative classifier trained on a large annotated database of images (Sect. 3.1). The likelihood measure is used in a multi-scale centerline extraction procedure based on Dijkstra's shortest path search. This step produces promising candidate branches of a tree (Sect. 3.2). The candidate branches are verified using a discriminative classifier which prunes false branch candidates while preserving true branches. Finally, an approximate tube radius is estimated at each centerline point. The algorithm stages are shown in Fig. 2.

Let each tubular tree be composed of constituent tubular structures. The centerlines of tubular structures are detected using a hierarchical model as follows. Let $\mathcal{C} = \{\mathcal{B}_1, \ldots, \mathcal{B}_n\}$ denote a centerline composed of branches $\mathcal{B}_i$, $i = 1, \ldots, n$. Each branch $\mathcal{B}_i$ consists of centerline points $X_i = x_1, x_2, \ldots, x_n$. In our case, $x_i = \{x_l, x_s\}$ denotes a point location x_l and size (radius) x_s. The observations Y are obtained by extracting features for each centerline point x_i from an image neighborhood at scale x_s surrounding location x_l.

The goal of the centerline extraction is to obtain $\mathcal{C}^*$ maximizing the posterior probability $p(\mathcal{C}|Y)$ over all centerlines $\mathcal{C}$. Clearly, this optimization is computationally involved in most practical situations due to the large space of centerlines. Therefore, we consider a posterior approximation which is based on the assumption that the branches are pairwise independent:

$$p(\mathcal{B}_1, \ldots, \mathcal{B}_n|Y) = \prod_{i=1}^{n} p(\mathcal{B}_i|Y) . \qquad (1)$$

Although this assumption ignores the connectivity of branches $\mathcal{B}_i$, we will show that (1) empirically yields accurate centerline detections.

Next, since each branch $\mathcal{B}_i$ consists of centerline points $X_i \in \mathcal{X}$, we can write (1) as

$$p(\mathcal{B}_i|Y) = \sum_{X_i \in \mathcal{X}} p(\mathcal{B}_i|X_i)p(X_i|Y) , \qquad (2)$$

where $p(X_i|Y)$ refers to the posterior distribution of centerline points given image observations. Inferring the optimal set of branches from (2) is possible using e.g. Monte

Carlo sampling strategies [14]. However, in our setting, the large domain of $\mathcal{X}$ prohibits the application of exhaustive sampling.

In order to efficiently find the optimal set of branches, we propose a two layer model, inspired by the hierarchical field applied to segmentation of natural images [6]. The optimal configuration and the uncertainty obtained from $p(X_i|Y)$ at the first layer is propagated to the second layer. The second layer infers the centerline from branch candidates and their corresponding uncertainties. The overall algorithm is shown in Fig. 2.

Formally, let the probability density at each site x_i be represented as

$$b_i(x_i) = p(x_i|Y) \tag{3}$$

and the set of branch probabilities be expressed as

$$b(X_i) = \{b_i(x_i)\}_{x_i \in X_i} . \tag{4}$$

Then, the optimal configuration X_i^* of tubular centerline points can be obtained by site-wise maximization of $b(X_i)$. As a consequence, we can approximate (2) [6] by

$$p(\mathcal{B}_i|Y) \approx p(\mathcal{B}_i|b(X_i)) . \tag{5}$$

Both layers, i.e. the computation of the branch location probabilities in (4) and the inference of branches in (5), will be described in detail next.

3.1   Layer 1: Multi-scale Voxel-Wise Detection

In this section, we describe how to estimate the conditional density $p(x_i|Y)$. This term determines the likelihood of a voxel location being a tubular structure given observations. We train a Probabilistic Boosting Tree classifier (PBT) [16], that has nodes composed of AdaBoost classifiers trained to select features that best discriminate between positive and negative examples of the tubular structures. Let us now define a random variable $y \in \{-1, +1\}$, where $y = +1$ indicates presence and $y = -1$ absence of the tubular structure. The PBT classifier is trained to select features that best discriminate between positive and negative samples. We can then evaluate the probability of a tubular structure being detected as $\mathrm{p}(y_i = +1|x_i, Y)$ and therefore rewrite the density as

$$p(x_i|Y) = p(y_i = +1|x_i, Y) . \tag{6}$$

The classifiers are extracted for M different scale levels which correspond to the sizes of tubular structures. This multi-scale setup has several advantages compared to a classifier trained at a single scale. First, it provides more accurate results by training more focused classifier since the structures at each scale have different anatomical context (see Fig. 1). Second, robustness is improved since the feature parameters are adjusted for each scale level rather than using one set of parameters for all tubular structure sizes. Third, no special treatment is necessary to ensure uniform distribution of samples of different tubular sizes which would otherwise be needed since a typical tree contains more thin than thick branches.

The classifiers at each scale level use 3D Haar features. The advantage of Haar features (apart from being efficient to compute) is that they form a basis and can approximate first and second order differential operators with only few basis elements. As such they can naturally mimic more complicated features such as Hessian or Flux [7,13].

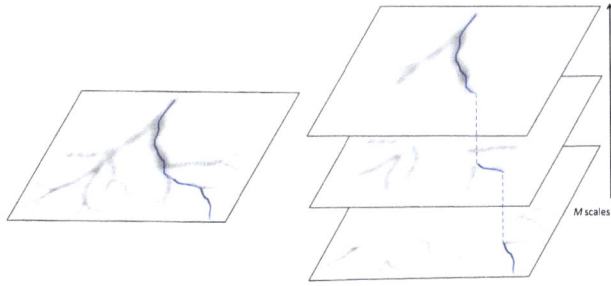

Fig. 3. In the standard Dijkstra's algorithm (left), the shortest path (blue) is obtained using a single level (which could be composed from multiple scales) by tracing the high probability regions (black and dark grey). In the multi-scale variant (right), the tracing is performed over multiple scales M. The cost penalties on scale changes make it possible to avoid exploring unnecessary regions which results in faster computation and higher robustness.

3.2   Layer 2: Branch Measure

The conditional density of the branch $p(\mathcal{B}_i|b(X_i))$ is estimated using a set of candidate branches and the associated branch probabilities (4). The candidate branches are extracted by the shortest path tracing algorithm as follows.

Let a candidate centerline branch originate from a source vertex s of G and terminate at the root vertex v (both automatically determined as described below). We associate each voxel with a vertex and we assume that each voxel is connected by an edge to its 18 neighbors. Let c be a nonnegative cost assigned to each edge and computed from the voxel-wise classifiers specific for each scale M using (4) as: $c = \left(1 - b_i(x_i)\right)^2$. The single-source shortest path is then computed by finding, for a vertex v reachable from s, the minimum-cost path from s to v. We perform the search by a multi-scale variant of Dijkstra's shortest path algorithm as illustrated in Fig. 3. Since the tubular size along the path generally increases, we set the costs to 0 and ∞ for switching from a fine to a coarse level and from coarse to fine, respectively. This way, the centerline branches $\mathcal{B}_i$ are extracted by following high values of b_i over M scales.

The source vertex points are generated as follows. The probability density maps obtained from (6) are combined by computing the maximum over scales. The combined map is used as input to a skeletonization algorithm [11]. The skeleton points serve as source point samples which might contain many false centerline points but cover all branches. The sink vertex point is computed as the point with the highest probability after applying skeletonization at the coarsest level. This is robust due to the distinctiveness of the trachea. The shortest path is found between each source point s and a vertex point v (which can be the root point or any previously detected centerline point). This way, bifurcations are handled simply by connecting branches.

Each branch is assigned a probability using the density $p(\mathcal{B}_i|b(X_i))$ from (5). Only high probability branches are kept and merged into the final centerline tree. The density $p(\mathcal{B}_i|b(X_i))$ is obtained from a discriminative classifier similar to (6). As features, we extract various statistics from $\mathcal{B}_i$, i.e. the average, minimum and maximum intensity and likelihood, histogram distributions of the local intensity and likelihood, distribution of the tubularness measures from [4], and the distribution of scale values, which all focus on the local context of $\mathcal{B}_i$. The most discriminative features were average intensity (used 17% of the time), average likelihood (14%), and minimum likelihood (8%). From the distributions, tubular features were used most often. To introduce characteristics which take the entire branch into account, we extract a piece-wise linear approximation $\mathcal{L}$ of $\mathcal{B}_i$ up to a given accuracy and use the number of piecewise elements in $\mathcal{L}$, the minimum, maximum, and average angular change between elements in $\mathcal{L}$, and the absolute length of $\mathcal{L}$.

4 Experiments

Before discussing the experiments, the training procedure is first described in Sect. 4.1. The experimental evaluation in Sect. 4.2 starts by a comparison of various features used as a measure of tubularness (Layer 1), which includes learning-based techniques. The next experiments compare qualitatively and quantitatively the detected centerlines to ground truth. Finally, a set of testing images is used to compute statistics of overall centerline detection errors and radius deviations.

4.1 Training the Tubular Model

Experts annotated a database of medical images by connecting airway centers and assigning approximate airway radii while navigating the visualization planes of each image. The annotated database is leveraged to train both layers of the tubular model. The Layer 1 is trained at $M = 3$ scale levels. At the three levels, the diameter of tubular structures are 1.5 to 3.5 mm, 3.0 to 7.0 mm, and 6.0 to 30.0 mm to handle thin, medium and large airways respectively. At each scale level, we train a sequence of $N = 3$ Probabilistic Boosting Tree (PBT) classifiers [16] using a tree depth of 3 and 10 weak learners at each level.

To train the branch measure at Layer 2, we generate the set of positive samples (true branches) and negative samples (false positives) as follows. First, we run Layer 1 detection on a separate training dataset and obtain source points as described in Sect. 3.2. The source points are used to run tracing by applying Dijkstra's shortest path. This way, we obtain set of branch samples. The samples are labeled as positives, if they have no more than 7 centerline points outside (with 1 voxel tolerance) of the ground truth tubular structure. Otherwise, they are labeled as negatives. The samples are used to train the branch measure $p(\mathcal{B}_i|b(X_i))$ using PBT classifiers with tree depth of 4 and 20 weak learners at each level.

4.2 Airway Trees in Rotational X-Ray

Our data set consists of 49 rotational X-ray volumes of the lung acquired by an Axiom Artis imaging system from Siemens. The system is useful during interventions since it provides full 3D acquisition at lower radiation and faster scanning time compared to standard CT but the images are noisy and contain various imaging artifacts.

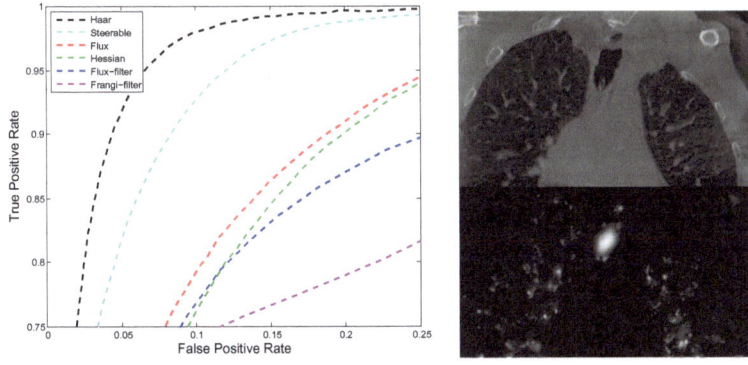

Fig. 4. ROC plots computed for the voxel classification using $p(x_i|Y)$ from Layer 1. The plots are computed for the learning-based classification (using Haar, steerable [20], flux [7], and intensity Hessian features) and for the filter-based techniques using flux filter [7] and Frangi filter [4]. Learning-based classification using Haar features performs the best. Example of a response combined over scales is shown for one coronal slice on the right.

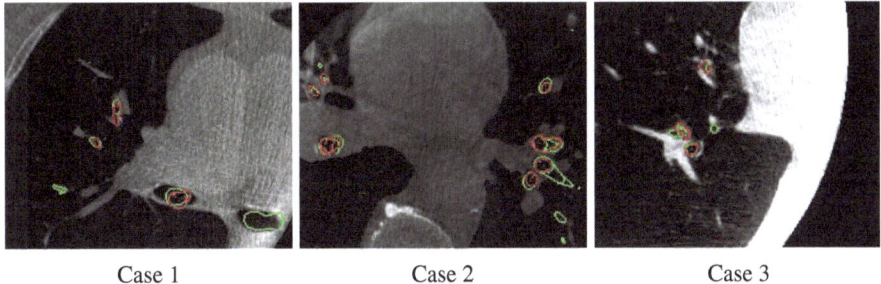

Case 1   Case 2   Case 3

Fig. 5. Detection result (red) on unseen cases. Ground truth annotation is marked as green. Note that since the intersection of the airways and the visualization plane can have various angles, the boundaries are not always circular. The image on the right only contains one lobe. All images show high level of noise.

The volumes have resolution $0.40 \times 0.49 \times 0.49$ mm^3 and average size of $512 \times 512 \times 275$. A total of 36 volumes are used for training and 13 for testing (selected randomly).

The first experiment evaluates the performance of Layer 1 (Fig. 4). The model was trained as described in Sect. 4.1 and applied to unseen cases. The resulting probability density (6) was thresholded at various levels between 0 and 1. This produced voxel-wise classification of airways. We compared learning-based classification (using Haar, steerable [20], flux [7], and intensity Hessian features) and filter-based techniques (using flux filter [7] and Frangi filter [4]). Learning-based classification using Haar features performs the best. Although Haar features are simpler than tube-specific filters, combination of different Haar types in the classification can learn complex patterns.

The next experiments compares the detected centerlines to the ground truth annotation. This is done by computing for each centerline point the Hausdorff distance to the

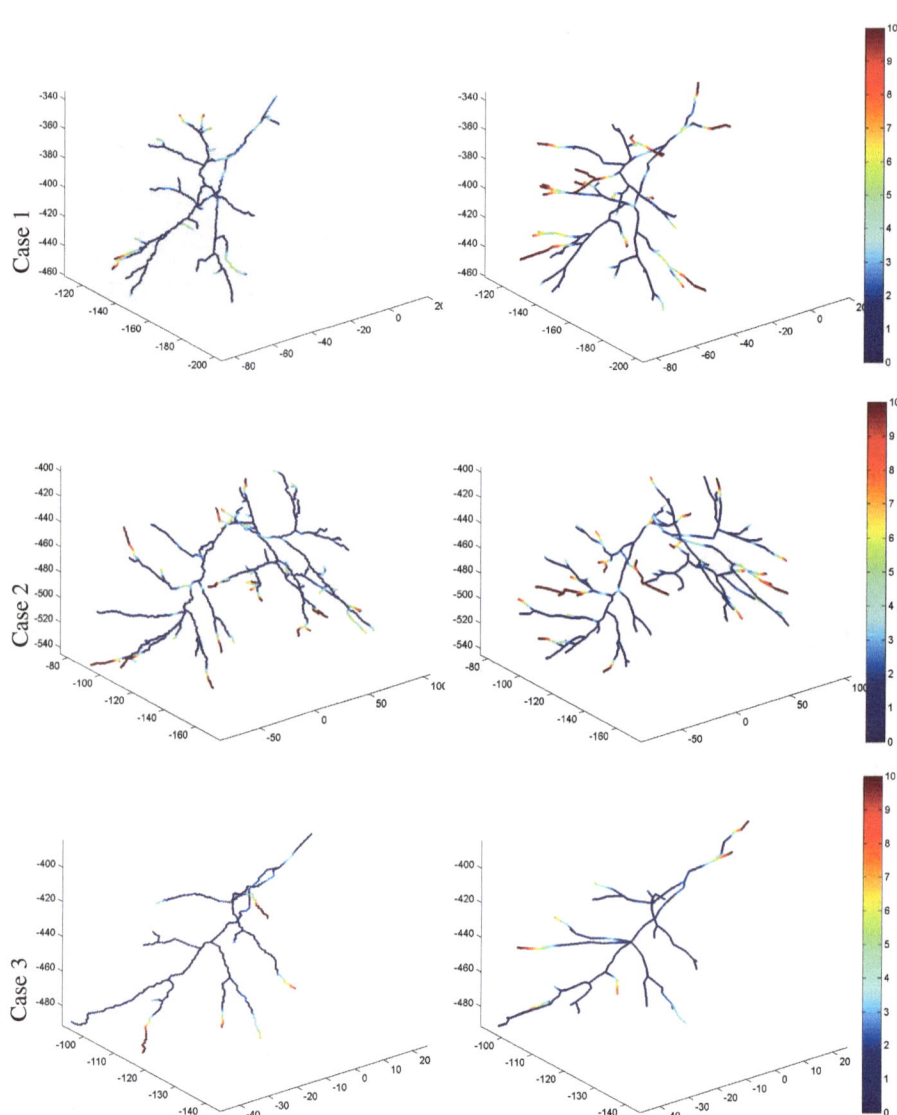

Fig. 6. Tree detection result (left) compared to ground truth annotation (right) on images from Fig. 5. Color reflects the point-wise Hausdorff distance of each centerline point to the reference tree. For the left column, the reference tree is ground truth and for the right column, the reference tree is the detection. Note the agreement of the detection and ground truth as evidenced by low number of red branches on the left (low false positives) and on the right (low false negatives). Case 3 had only image acquisition of one lobe.

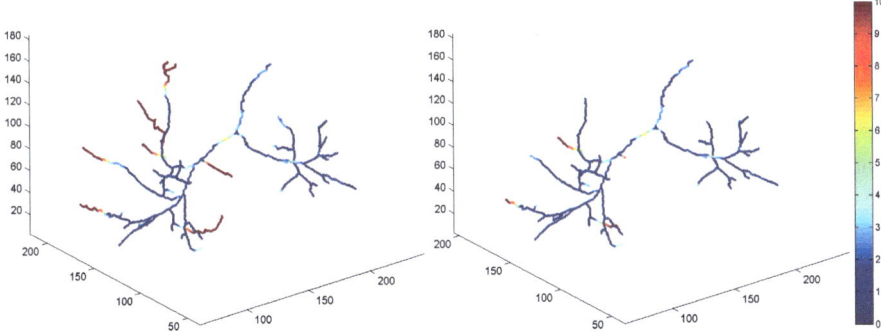

Fig. 7. Example of branch pruning using the proposed branch measure. For the automatically detected tree (left) false branch candidates (red) are rejected to obtain a verified estimate (right).

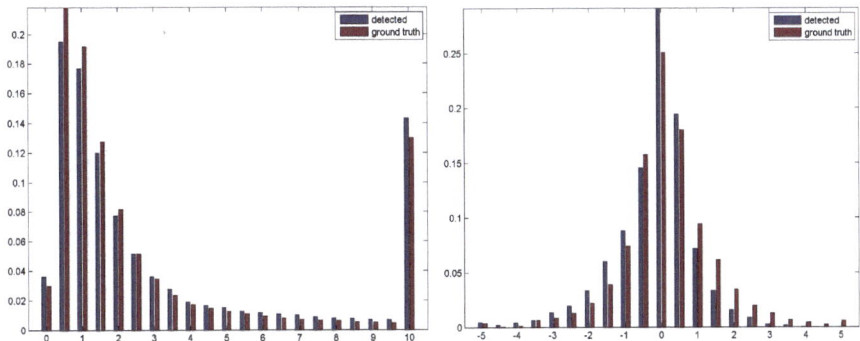

Fig. 8. Overall detection errors summarized as a histogram of Hausdorff distances for all testing cases. The left plot shows the relative distribution of distances from the detected result to ground truth (blue) and vice versa (red). The right plot shows the corresponding errors of tubular radius estimation.

ground truth centerline tree. The distance is shown on the detected tree by color coding the centerlines. This shows, for each point and branch on the detected tree, how far it is w.r.t. the ground truth tree (evaluating true positives and false positives). The same procedure is repeated for each ground truth centerline point by computing Hausdorff distances to the detected tree. This evaluates false negatives. Fig. 6 shows example results for the cases in Fig. 5. Overall, there is a good agreement of the detected tree and the ground truth tree. Both trees show only several points marked as red demonstrating low false positive and false negative detection, respectively. This is possible by the proposed branch measure which uses many candidate centerlines (and their uncertainties) to reject false positives (Fig. 7).

The final experiment shows quantitative evaluation of all detected centerlines. As before, we compute the Hausdorff distance for each centerline point on the detected and on the ground truth tree, respectively. The distances are then plotted in two histograms, one for the detected and one for the ground truth tree (Fig. 8). The plots show that 40.8% of detections are within 1 mm, 60.5% within 2 mm, and 74.0% of all centerline points are within 4 mm of the ground truth. There are only 14.3% centerline points detected more than 10 mm from the ground truth. Correspondingly, there are 44.0%, 65.0%, and 77.8% ground truth centerline points within 1, 2, and 4 mm of detected centerlines, respectively. Only 13.0% ground truth centerline points are more than 10 mm from the detected tree. The detected centerlines have radius error within 1 mm of ground truth for 79.1% points. Please note, that this strict evaluation is performed at the centerline level rather than the branch level as in [5], for example. Despite that, the results suggest that the algorithm is suitable for clinical setting, e.g. for bronchoscopic navigation [5,15], since most detected centerlines are within the airway boundaries.

The tree extraction algorithm is efficient. Computing the multi-scale likelihood maps takes on average 1.5 minutes per volume on Intel Xeon 2.67 GHz computer. Significant improvement is possible by computing the maps only in local regions determined from the neighborhood surrounding the source and sink points. The candidate branches are extracted in less than 1 second on average. Finally, the branches are verified in less than 1 second on average yielding fast overall computational speed.

5   Conclusion

In this work, we presented a discriminative approach for automatic detection of tubular structures from volumetric datasets. The algorithm is robust and efficient thanks to the two-layer model of tubular centerlines and associated tubular sizes. Layer 1 provides an indication of how likely a particular voxel location belongs to a tubular structure. The most likely locations and the automatically determined tree root are used to find candidate centerline branches using a multi-scale variant of Dijkstra's shortest path algorithm. The candidate branches are verified at Layer 2 by a discriminative branch measure.

The algorithm was evaluated on a challenging dataset of rotational X-ray volumes of the lung – the first reported technique for this type of dataset. The airway centerlines were accurately detected with as much as 77.8% centerline points being within 4 mm of correponding ground truth annotation and with radius error of less than 1 mm for 79.1% of the points.

Our future work will focus on improving accuracy, especially for thin structures. This will require feature computation at a subvoxel level which will pose a challenge in keeping the computational speed fast. In addition, we will explore the use of tree-prior information to further boost the robustness and accuracy. We also plan to design an additional data-driven boundary refinement step to improve the accuracy of tubular radius estimation. Finally, we would like to verify the algorithm on other applications, e.g. detecting vessels in liver scans.

References

1. Barbu, A., Bogoni, L., Comaniciu, D.: Hierarchical part-based detection of 3D flexible tubes: Application to CT colonoscopy. In: Larsen, R., Nielsen, M., Sporring, J. (eds.) MICCAI 2006. LNCS, vol. 4191, pp. 462–470. Springer, Heidelberg (2006) 328
2. Bauer, C., Pock, T., Sorantin, E., Bischof, H., Beichel, R.: Segmentation of interwoven 3D tubular tree structures utilizing shape priors and graph cuts. Med. Image Anal. 14(2), 172–184 (2010) 328

3. Benmansour, F., Cohen, L.D.: Tubular structure segmentation based on minimal path method and anisotropic enhancement. Int. J. Comput. Vision 92, 192–210 (2011) 328, 330

4. Frangi, A.F., Niessen, W.J., Vincken, K.L., Viergever, M.A.: Multiscale vessel enhancement filtering. In: Wells, W.M., Colchester, A., Delp, S. (eds.) MICCAI 1998. LNCS, vol. 1496, p. 130. Springer, Heidelberg (1998) 330, 334, 335

5. Graham, M., Gibbs, J., Cornish, D., Higgins, W.: Robust 3-D airway tree segmentation for image-guided peripheral bronchoscopy. IEEE T. Med. Imaging 29, 982–997 (2010) 328, 330, 338

6. Kumar, S., Hebert, M.: A hierarchical field framework for unified context-based classification. In: Proc. Int. Conf. Comput. Vision (2005) 330, 332

7. Lesage, D., Angelini, E., Bloch, I., Funka-Lea, G.: Design and study of flux-based features for 3D vascular tracking. In: Proc. Int. Symp. Biomed. Imaging (2009) 328, 330, 332, 335

8. Lesage, D., Angelini, E., Bloch, I., Funka-Lea, G.: A review of 3D vessel lumen segmentation techniques: Models, features and extraction schemes. Med. Image Anal. 13(6), 819–845 (2009) 328

9. Lo, P., Sporring, J., Ashraf, H., Pedersen, J.J., de Bruijne, M.: Vessel-guided airway tree segmentation: A voxel classification approach. Med. Image Anal. 14(4), 527–538 (2010) 328

10. Ochs, R., Goldin, J., Abtin, F., Kim, H., Brown, K., Batra, P., Roback, D., McNitt-Gray, M., Brown, M.: Automated classification of lung bronchovascular anatomy in CT using AdaBoost. Med. Image Anal. 11, 315–324 (2007) 330

11. Palágyi, K., Sorantin, E., Balogh, E., Kuba, A., Halmai, C., Erdohelyi, B., Hausegger, K.: A sequential 3D thinning algorithm and its medical applications. In: Insana, M.F., Leahy, R.M. (eds.) IPMI 2001. LNCS, vol. 2082, pp. 409–415. Springer, Heidelberg (2001) 333

12. Rouchdy, Y., Cohen, L.: A geodesic voting method for the segmentation of tubular tree and centerlines. In: Proc. Int. Symp. on Biomed. Imaging, pp. 979–983 (2011) 330

13. Schuh, A., Kaftan, J.N., Tietjen, C., O'Donnell, T.P.: Sparse axes-aligned MFlux. In: Workshop on Comp. and Vis. for (Intra-) Vascular Imaging (2011) 328, 330, 332

14. Sofka, M., Zhang, J., Zhou, S., Comaniciu, D.: Multiple object detection by sequential Monte Carlo and hierarchical detection network. In: Proc. Int. Conf. Comput. Vision and Pattern Recogn., San Francisco, CA, June 13-18 (2010) 332

15. Steger, T., Hosbach, M.: Navigated bronchoscopy using intraoperative fluoroscopy and preoperative CT. In: Proc. Int. Symp. on Biomed. Imaging, pp. 1220–1223 (2012) 328, 338

16. Tu, Z.: Probabilistic boosting-tree: learning discriminative models for classification, recognition, and clustering. In: Proc. Int. Conf. Comput. Vision (2005) 332, 334

17. Tu, Z., Bai, X.: Auto-context and its application to high-level vision tasks and 3D brain image segmentation. IEEE Trans. Pattern Anal. Machine Intelligence 32, 1744–1757 (2010) 330

18. Türetken, E., Benmansour, F., Fua, P.: Automated reconstruction of tree structures using path classifiers and mixed integer programming. In: Proc. Int. Conf. Comput. Vision and Pattern Recogn., pp. 566–573. IEEE (2012) 329

19. Wolf, L., Bileschi, S.: A critical view of context. Int. J. Comput. Vision (2006) 330

20. Zheng, Y., Loziczonek, M., Georgescu, B., Zhou, S.K., Vega-Higuera, F., Comaniciu, D.: Machine learning based vesselness measurement for coronary artery segmentation in cardiac CT volumes. In: Proc. SPIE (2011) 330, 335

21. Zhou, J., Chang, S., Metaxas, D., Axel, L.: Vascular structure segmentation and bifurcation detection. In: Proc. Int. Symp. on Biomed. Imaging, pp. 872–875 (2007) 330

Joint Fractional Segmentation and Multi-tensor Estimation in Diffusion MRI

Xiang Hao and P. Thomas Fletcher

Scientific Computing and Imaging Institute, University of Utah, Salt Lake City, UT

Abstract. In this paper we present a novel Bayesian approach for fractional segmentation of white matter tracts and simultaneous estimation of a multi-tensor diffusion model. Our model consists of several white matter tracts, each with a corresponding weight and tensor compartment in each voxel. By incorporating a prior that assumes the tensor fields inside each tract are spatially correlated, we are able to reliably estimate multiple tensor compartments in fiber crossing regions, even with low angular diffusion-weighted imaging (DWI). Our model distinguishes the diffusion compartment associated with each tract, which reduces the effects of partial voluming and achieves more reliable statistics of diffusion measurements. We test our method on synthetic data with known ground truth and show that we can recover the correct volume fractions and tensor compartments. We also demonstrate that the proposed method results in improved segmentation and diffusion measurement statistics on real data in the presence of crossing tracts and partial voluming.

1 Introduction

Diffusion-weighted imaging (DWI) is a magnetic resonance imaging (MRI) modality that can measure the directional diffusion of water in tissue. In diffusion tensor imaging (DTI) a second-order model of diffusion within a voxel is estimated from the DWI data. While the diffusion tensor is an elegant description of anisotropic diffusion in white matter, it is limited to representing only one tract in each imaging voxel. At several regions of the brain, two or more white matter tracts are passing through each other, such as the intersection of the corona radiata and the corpus callosum. In addition, some white matter tracts are mixed with gray matter or cerebrospinal fluid (CSF) at the boundary, such as the corpus callosum and lateral ventricles. In these cases, a single diffusion tensor is incapable of distinguishing between multiple diffusion compartments.

It has been shown that partial volume effects and underestimation of diffusion measurements occur in crossing areas [1,9,8]. For example, Alexander et al. [1] show that the trace of the diffusion tensor will tend to be underestimated in presence of partial voluming, and Metzler-Baddeley et al. [8] show that CSF-based partial volume artifacts have a larger impact for tensors with smaller fractional anisotropy (FA). What's more, underestimation of diffusion tensor measurements could bias statistics of diffusion measurements, providing misleading results in clinical studies. Although the partial volume effects might

J.C. Gee et al. (Eds.): IPMI 2013, LNCS 7917, pp. 340–351, 2013.

be detected during the DTI analysis [13], it cannot resolve the partial volume effects completely, and other methods that can correct the partial volume effects are needed. High-angular resolution diffusion imaging (HARDI) (see [2] for a review) has been introduced as a means of distinguishing multiple diffusion compartments. Several multi-compartment models of diffusion have been introduced, such as the multi-tensor [12] and ball-and-stick [3] models. However, one drawback to HARDI is the increased imaging time required, which has been a barrier to its introduction in clinical studies.

Several works have proposed correcting the partial volume effects using low-angular resolution images (approximately 30 gradient directions). Pasternak et al [10] used a smooth regularization to reduce partial volume effects using multi-tensor fitting and showed that the regularization can help solve ill-posedness, but they only test their methods on two fiber crossings. Landman et al [7] used a multi-tensor model and compressed sensing to solve the fiber crossing using low angular DWI, but they use a set of basis directions to map the multiple tensor model to lower dimensionality, which could bias the estimated tensors.

None of these methods combine multiple compartment estimation with white matter tract segmentation, which is often a primary goal of DWI analysis. In this paper, we propose a method that jointly solves the tract segmentation and multi-tensor model estimation problem. In each voxel our model assigns a fractional weight to each fiber tract indicating the proportion of that voxel that belongs to the given tract. These weights also serve as the volume fractions in the multi-tensor model for that voxel, linking the segmentation to the diffusion estimation problem. We impose a Markov random field (MRF) spatial prior to take advantage of spatial redundancy during the estimation and to regularize the multi-tensor field. To the best of our knowledge, ours is the first model that combines fractional segmentation of white matter with multi-tensor estimation. We compare our method with state-of-the-art binary segmentations of white matter tracts, which sometimes under- or over-segment tracts. We demonstrate that the fractional weights can improve statistical analysis of derived measurements, such as fractional anisotropy (FA), by appropriately weighting the data associated with a particular tract. Using synthetic data with known ground truth, as well as real DWI brain data, we show that our method improves tract segmentations, distinguishes multiple tissue compartments, and provides better diffusion estimates even when using only 12 gradient directions.

2   Fractional Segmentation and Multi-tensor Estimation

In this section we propose a Bayesian approach to simultaneously estimate both the fractional segmentation of white matter tracts and the multi-tensor diffusion model. Our goal is to estimate the volume fractions and diffusion tensors in such a way that the DWI signal from the estimated multi-tensor model matches the measured DWI signal and the estimated tensor compartments in each tract are spatially smooth. This leads to a maximum a posteriori (MAP) estimation approach, in which the log posterior is

$$\log p(\theta|S) \propto \log p(S|\theta) + \log p(\theta),$$

where θ represents the parameters of the model, namely, the multi-tensor field and volume fractions, and S is the original DWI signal. The likelihood, $p(S|\theta)$, models the fit of the multi-tensor model in each voxel to the DWI signal, and the prior, $p(\theta)$, is a Markov Random Field (MRF) smoothness prior on the multi-tensor field. We now describe both the likelihood and prior in detail.

2.1   Likelihood - The Data Attachment Term

To model multiple diffusion compartments within a voxel, whether from crossing white matter fiber tracts or mixtures of white matter with CSF or gray matter, we use a multi-tensor model of the given DWI signals. The multi-tensor model uses n tensor compartments, D_i, and each tensor compartment is associated with a nonnegative volume fraction f_i to model the DWI signals S_j as

$$S_j(x) = S_0(x) \sum_{i=1}^{n} f_i(x)e^{-bg_j^T D_i(x)g_j}, \text{ with } \sum_{i}^{n} f_i = 1, \tag{1}$$

where b is the b-value, S_0 is the baseline image, g_j is the j-th gradient encoding direction. In contrast to the usual multi-tensor model, we also associate each volume fraction f_i to a white matter tract segmentation. That is, we want to segment the DWI image into n white matter tracts, where $f_i(x)$ represents the fraction of the voxel at position x that is occupied by fibers in the ith tract.

   Now, assuming the DWI signal is corrupted by additive, i.i.d. Gaussian noise, our log-likelihood is the following DWI signal matching term:

$$\log p(S_j|f_i, D_i) \propto - \int_{\Omega} \sum_{j=1}^{m} \left(S_0(x) \sum_{i=1}^{n} f_i(x)e^{-bg_j^T D_i(x)g_j} - S_j(x) \right)^2 dx.$$

This noise model could be replaced with a Rician noise likelihood or a non-central chi-distribution for multichannel MRI. Conceptually this would not change the underlying methodology, but rather make the estimation procedure slightly more complicated. The Gaussian likelihood is a simplifying approximation.

2.2   The Markov Random Field Prior

Inside a white matter tract, it is reasonable to think that the tensors field should be spatially correlated, i.e., the tensor field flows smoothly inside a white matter tract. Thus we incorporate a MRF prior on the tensor fields inside each tract, given by

$$p(D_i) = \frac{1}{Z} e^{-U(D_i)}, \text{ and } U(D_i) = \lambda \int_{\Omega} \sum_{i}^{n} \phi(D_i(x))dx,$$

where Z is a normalization constant, λ is a weighting parameter, and $\phi(D_i(x))$ is a function that measures the correlation of tensors in the ith tract, around x.

With a uniform prior on the fractions, f_i, and by combining the log-likelihood term with the prior, we end up minimizing the energy

$$E(f_i, D_i) = \int_\Omega \left(\sum_{j=1}^{m} \left(S_0(x) \sum_{i=1}^{n} f_i(x) e^{-bg_j^T D_i(x) g_j} - S_j(x) \right)^2 + \lambda \sum_{i}^{n} \phi(D_i(x)) \right) dx.$$

We use the full six-component tensor model to represent D_i, but we want to emphasize that D_i could be any other diffusion model, such as the ball-and-stick model. In addition, we use $\phi(D_i(x)) = \|\nabla D_i(x)\|^2 = \sum_{p,q} \sum_{y \in N(x)} (D_i^{pq}(y) - D_i^{pq}(x))^2$, where N(x) is a neighborhood around x, and D_i^{pq} represents component in the pth row and the qth column of the matrix D_i, but it could be generalized to other functions for measuring the smoothness of D_i.

2.3   Optimizing f_i and D_i

We use a gradient descent algorithm to compute f_i and D_i. The partial derivative of E respect to f_i is

$$\frac{\partial E}{\partial f_i} = 2 S_0(x) \sum_{j=1}^{m} \left(e^{-bg_j^T D_i(x) g_j} \cdot \left(S_0(x) \sum_{i=1}^{n} f_i(x) e^{-bg_j^T D_i(x) g_j} - S_j(x) \right) \right),$$

and the partial derivative of E respect to D_i^{pq} is

$$\frac{\partial E}{\partial D_i^{pq}} = \left(\sum_{j=1}^{m} 2 \left((S_0(x) \sum_{i=1}^{n} f_i(x) e^{-bg_j^T D_i(x) g_j} - S_j(x)) f_i e^{-bg_j^T D_i(x) g_j} S_0(x) \right. \right.$$
$$\left. \left. \cdot (-bg_j^p g_j^q) \right) + 4 \cdot \lambda \sum_{y \in N(x)} (D_i^{pq}(x) - D_i^{pq}(y)) \right) \cdot \psi(p, q),$$

where g_j^p represents the pth element of the vector g_j, and $\psi(p, q) = 1$ if $p = q$ and $\psi(p, q) = 2$ if $p \neq q$. Special care is required in the update of f_i. In every iteration of our gradient descent algorithm, we project the computed gradient of E with respect to f_i onto the constraint hyperplane defined by $\sum_{i=1}^{n} f_i = 1$. To ensure that the f_i remain positive, we also need to project the gradient on the simplex boundary defined by the constraints $f_i \geq 0$ when necessary. Then we do a line search to compute the optimal step size for updating f_i.

To initialize our gradient descent, we first compute binary segmentations for each of $n - 1$ tracts of interest. The nth label is reserved as a "background" label that does not belong to any of the tracts. The binary segmentations just need to roughly capture the tracts, which could be done by several methods. We use a front-propagation geodesic segmentation [5,6], which uses a Riemannian metric derived from the diffusion tensor field and constructs white matter tracts as geodesics connecting two regions-of-interest (ROI) on the resulting manifold. These geodesics have the desirable property that they tend to follow the main eigenvectors of the tensors, yet still have the flexibility to deviate from these directions when it results in lower costs. This makes such methods more robust to noise and also allows them to pass through crossing regions. After segmenting the $n-1$ tracts of interest, for each voxel inside the predefined image mask, if no segmentations include the voxel, we initialize f_n as 1, and D_n as the weighted least squares estimate of a single-tensor model. Otherwise, we initialize the fractions f_i equally amongst all segmentations that intersect at the voxel, and we initialize all corresponding tensors D_i in that voxel with the same weighted least-squares estimate of a single-tensor model at that voxel.

2.4   Path Regression Along the Segmented Tracts

Our estimated fraction f_i can also be used to improve statistical summaries of the diffusion data along segmented tracts. Here we demonstrate an example of the use of these fractions in nonparametric regression along a tract. Let $\{x_i\}$ be the collection of voxel locations within a segmented tract. Each voxel has an associated parameter, $s_i = s(x_i) \in [0, 1]$, which denotes the arc-length parameter along the pathway at the spatial location x_i [5]. Denote by d_i a data value at the location x_i. This data may be a full diffusion tensor, or a derived measure, such as FA or MD. We compute a continuous description of the data as a function of s using a nonparametric kernel regression,

$$y(s) = \frac{\sum_i^N d_i f_i G(s - s_i, \sigma)}{\sum_i^N f_i G(s - s_i, \sigma)},$$

where $G(\mu, \sigma)$ denotes a Gaussian kernel with mean μ and standard deviation σ. In the kernel regression, in addition to the Gaussian kernel, each data value is weighted by the fraction f_i, which makes our regression more robust to partial voluming since our fractional segmentation will appropriately assign small f_i to data values influenced by partial voluming. The function y defined above gives a continuous average of the data along the pathway, which can be used to quantify the diffusion measurement along a pathway as shown in Figure 2.

3   Results

In this section we demonstrate the advantages of the fractional segmentations and improvements in multi-tensor estimations computed by our method on both synthetic and real data. On synthetic data with ground truth, we test our method on both low and high angular DWI and compare it with the multi-tensor model estimation implemented in Camino [4] using HARDI. Our measure of quality is the root mean square error (RMSE) between the estimated volume fractions/tensors and true volume fractions/tensors. In addition, we also show that our method improves the diffusion measurement statistics. On real data, we demonstrate that the proposed method results in improved segmentation and diffusion measurement statistics in crossing tracts and in the presence of partial voluming. To visualize the fractional segmentation, we convert our fractional segmentation to a color-coded RGB image, where each color component is set to a corresponding volume fraction. For visualization purposes, tensors with weight lower than 0.2 are not shown.

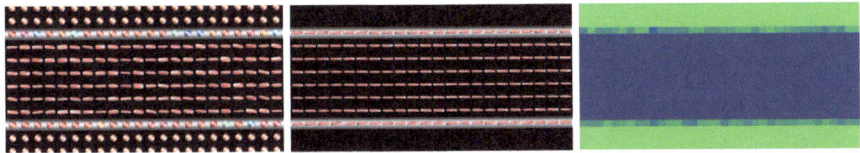

Fig. 1. Left: synthetic white matter tract with partial volume effects at the boundary (shown in white). Middle: our estimated tensors. Right: our fractional segmentation. We subsample the tensor field by a factor of two both horizontally and vertically in order to visualize it.

3.1   Correcting Partial Volume Effect

To test the ability of our method to correct partial volume effects, we generated one white matter tract whose boundary is mixed with isotropic tensors as shown in Figure 1. The ground truth is a straight white matter tract with width 8 voxels and length 38 voxels, mixed with isotropic diffusion tensors at the boundary (shown in white in Figure 1) with equal volume fractions in the multi-tensor model (1). The sphere tensors used to simulate CSF have eigenvalue $(3,3,3)\times10^{-3}$mm^2/s. The tensors in the white matter tract have eigenvalue $(1.6,0.4,0.4)\times10^{-3}$mm^2/s. Using the mixed tensor field, we generate DWIs with 12 gradient directions and slightly blur the DWIs to simulate the point spread function (PSF) arising from imaging. We corrupt the DWIs with Rician noise to get a SNR of 20 (left picture of Figure 1).

Our estimated white matter tensor field is in the middle picture of Figure 1. As we can see, the estimated tensor field can recover the true white matter tensor from the mixed tensors at the boundary. In addition, our estimation algorithm denoises tensors in the interior. Our color-coded fractional segmentation is shown in the right panel of Figure 1. In this example, the segmented white matter tract is the blue channel and the exterior is the green channel. The boundary is correctly assigned a 50% mixture of both compartments. The RMSE of our fractional segmentation of the white matter tract is 7.74×10^{-2}, and the RMSE of our estimated tensors is 5.22×10^{-5}.

In the left two pictures of Figure 2, we do a regression analysis of the FA in the segmented tracts with $\sigma = 0.1$ as mentioned in Section 2.4, where the x-axis is the arc-length position along the tract. We first plot the FA values as points. The color is coded by the volume fractions: solid blue denotes 0, and solid red denotes 1, so the binary segmentation values are always shown in red. The regression along the tract is shown in black and the ground truth is shown as a dashed green line. It is clear that the partial volume effects bias the regression in the binary segmentations. In our method, the FA values are more tightly distributed around the ground truth, due to the reduction of the partial volume effects and the denoising from our spatial prior.

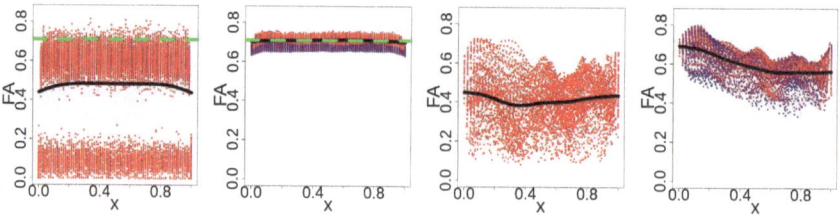

Fig. 2. Left two pictures: FA regression of simulated straight tract using binary and fractional segmentations, respectively. Ground truth is shown in green and the regression is shown in black. Right two pictures: FA regression of arcuate fasciculus from binary and fractional segmentations, respectively.

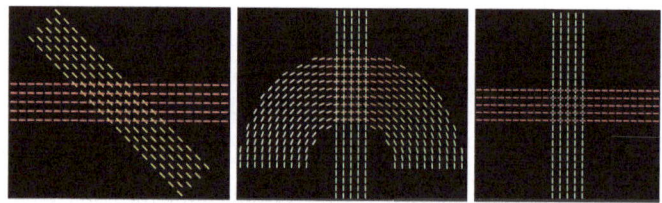

Fig. 3. Generated fiber crossing data. Left: 45° crossing. Middle: a curved tract crossing with a straight tract. Right: three orthogonal tracts crossing. We subsample the tensor field by a factor of three both horizontally and vertically in order to visualize it.

3.2   Fiber Crossing White Matter Tracts

To test the performance of the our method in the presence of multiple white matter tracts crossing, we generate three fiber crossing tensor fields that have similar properties to many white matter tracts in the brain. They are 1) two bars crossing at the center of the image at an angle of 45°, 2) a curved tract crossing with a bar, and 3) three orthogonal bars crossing at the center of the image. We show a center slice of each tensor field in Figure 3.

The tensors in each white matter tract have eigenvalues $(1.6, 0.4, 0.4) \times 10^{-3} \mathrm{mm}^2/\mathrm{s}$. We generate two sets of DWI datasets, one with 12 gradient directions and the other with 64 gradient directions. Each voxel of the generated crossing DWI at the crossing area was computed based on the multi-tensor model (1), and we use $b = 1000 \mathrm{s}/\mathrm{mm}^2$ for both datasets. The true fractions in the crossing regions for the three data sets are (0.4, 0.6), (0.4, 0.6), and (0.3, 0.3, 0.4), respectively. In addition, the DWI was corrupted by Rician noise to simulate SNR of 20.

In Figure 4, we show the estimated tensors from our method and Camino. We test Camino only on noisy 64-direction DWI (shown in the last column of Figure 4) because Camino cannot estimate a multi-tensor model from only 12 gradient directions (it estimates each voxel independently). However, we can test our method on both noisy 64-direction DWI and 12-direction DWI because our

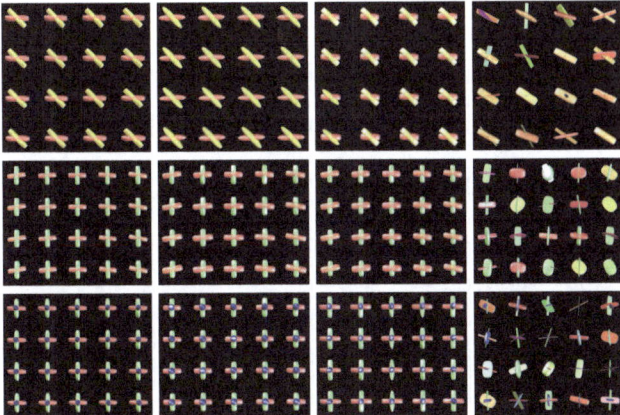

Fig. 4. Estimated tensors of the crossing region for the three crossing datasets: Top row is for the 45° crossing, Middle row is for the curved tract crossing, and the Bottom row is for the three orthogonal tracts crossing. 1st column: our estimated tensors from noiseless 12-direction DWI. 2nd column: our estimated tensors from noisy 64-direction DWI. 3rd column: our estimated tensors from noisy 12-direction DWI. Last column: estimated tensors from Camino using noisy 64-direction DWI.

spatial prior utilizes information from multiple neighboring voxels. On the first column of Figure 4, we test our method on noiseless 12-direction DWI to show that we can recover multiple tensors, even when the solution is underdetermined at single voxels because of our spatial prior. On the second and third column, we test our method on noisy 64-direction DWI and noisy 12-direction DWI. The results are much improved over those from Camino, and our method works slightly better on 64-direction DWI since it has more information. The results from Camino are shown in the last column of Figure 4. We gave Camino the advantage of a map of the correct number of tensor compartments in each voxel, but did not provide this extra information to our algorithm.

We also show our fractional segmentation in Figure 5. Since the weights computed from Camino do not correspond to segmentations, we solve a correspondence problem by minimizing the angles between estimated tensors from Camino and the true tensors. After the optimal order is found, we use the corresponding weights as the fractional segmentation. Outside the crossing region, as we mentioned earlier, we tell Camino the number of tensors, so Camino always has the true weights outside. The finding is consistent with the case for tensor estimation. On the noiseless data, the error between our solution and the true solution is close to zero as shown is Table 1. On the noisy data, the solution of our method is worse when we use the 12-direction DWI than the one using the 64-direction DWI, but generally our results are fairly good for all three cases, and they look better than Camino inside the crossing regions.

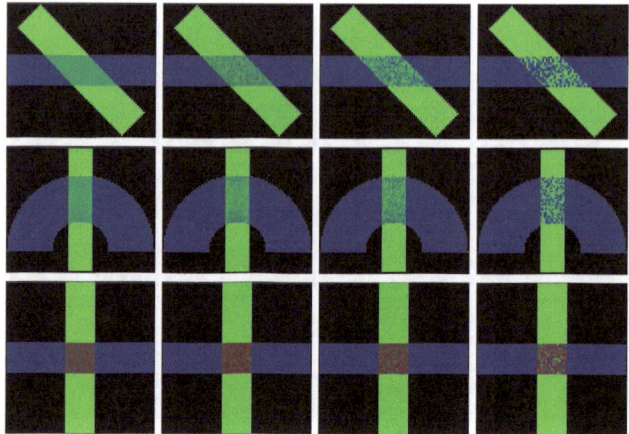

Fig. 5. Estimated fractional segmentations. The order is the same as Figure 4.

Table 1. RMSE of the estimated volume fractions and tensor compartments of our method (first three rows) and Camino using noisy DWI with 64 directions (last row)

	45° Crossing		Curved Crossing		Three Crossing	
	Weight	Tensor	Weight	Tensor	Weight	Tensor
Clean 12-dir	$1.16E{-}04$	$5.61E{-}07$	$1.44E{-}02$	$2.97E{-}05$	$1.33E{-}05$	$1.12E{-}07$
Noisy 64-dir	$7.38E{-}02$	$1.39E{-}04$	$4.89E{-}02$	$1.38E{-}04$	$5.16E{-}02$	$2.09E{-}04$
Noisy 12-dir	$8.37E{-}02$	$1.54E{-}04$	$6.18E{-}02$	$1.63E{-}04$	$5.71E{-}02$	$3.07E{-}04$
Camino	$2.6E{-}01$	$4.40E{-}03$	$2.34E{-}01$	$2.89E{-}03$	$1.45E{-}01$	$3.14E{-}03$

In Table 1, we do a quantitative comparison of our method and Camino. Since we give Camino the true weight outside the crossing regions, to do a better comparison, we compute the RMSE of the estimated volume fractions only inside the crossing region, but we compute the RMSE of tensors in the whole white matter tracts. As shown in the Table, the RMSE of our method is much smaller than the RMSE of Camino, and our method works best on the noiseless data, but when there is noise, our method has smaller RMSE when using DWI with more gradient directions.

3.3   Real Data

We now show the results of our method with $\lambda = 10^9$ applied on a DWI of a volunteer. DWI data were acquired on a Siemens Trio 3.0 Tesla Scanner with an 8-channel, receive-only head coil. DWI was performed using a single-shot, spin-echo, EPI pulse sequence and SENSE parallel imaging (undersampling factor of 2). Diffusion-weighted images were acquired in 12 non-collinear diffusion encoding directions with diffusion weighting factor b=1000 s/mm^2 in addition

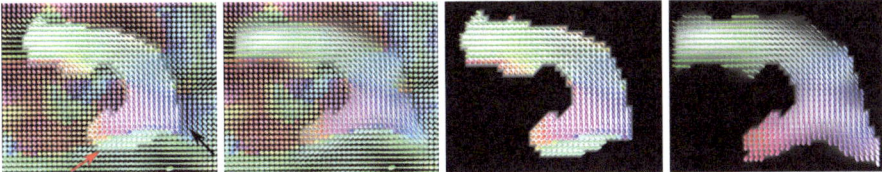

Fig. 6. The binary segmentation is shown on the 1st and 3rd columns and our fractional segmentation is shown on the 2nd and 4th columns. The overlay tensor fields are the DTI tensor field except for the last one, where our estimated tensors are displayed.

to a single reference image (b=0). Data acquisition parameters included the following: contiguous (no-gap) fifty 2.5mm thick axial slices with an acquisition matrix of 128 x 128 over a FOV of 256 mm (2 x 2 mm^2 in-plane resolution), 4 averages, repetition time (TR) = 7000 ms, and echo time (TE) = 84 ms. Eddy current distortion and head motion were corrected using an automatic image registration program [11]. Distortion-corrected DW images were interpolated to 1 x 1 x 1 mm^3 voxels, and six tensor elements were calculated using weighted least squares. The tensor upsampling is done only for the purposes of numerical computations on the voxel grid; a finer grid results in higher numerical accuracy.

In Figure 6, we test our method on the arcuate fasciculus of the brain. In the 1st and 3rd pictures, we show the initial binary segmentation and the DTI tensor field. As we can see, the binary segmentation over-segments the tract since it includes many voxels (red arrow) below the tract which should be inside the inferior longitudinal fasciculus. In addition, it also under-segments the tract, missing the blue area on the lower right of image (black arrow), which should be included in the segmentation. On the 2nd column, we overlay the DTI tensor field on our fractional segmentation to demonstrate that our segmentation corrects the errors from the binary segmentation. In the last picture, we overly our estimated tensors on top of our segmentation. We can see that our segmentation reduces partial voluming effect at the boundary of tract and has lower weights at the border of the arcuate fasciculus and inferior longitudinal fasciculus, where the tensors from the two different tracts are mixed together. In addition, our segmentation also includes the blue area, which the binary segmentation missed.

In the right two pictures of Figure 2, we do a similar regression analysis as mentioned in Section 3.1. We can see the FA values are more tightly distributed on the right picture than the left one, which is a sign of possible reduction of partial volume effects as shown in Section 3.1. What's more, it may improve statistical power in clinical studies by reducing the within-subject variance.

We also test our method on a brain region with complex white matter organization as shown in Figure 7. In this brain region, we segment three white matter tracts as our binary input of our method. These three tracts are one branch from the corpus callosum, the corticospinal tract, and the superior longitudinal fasciculus. In the top row of Figure 7, we compare the DTI model with the proposed method. In the 1st and 3rd pictures, we overlay DTI tensor field on the

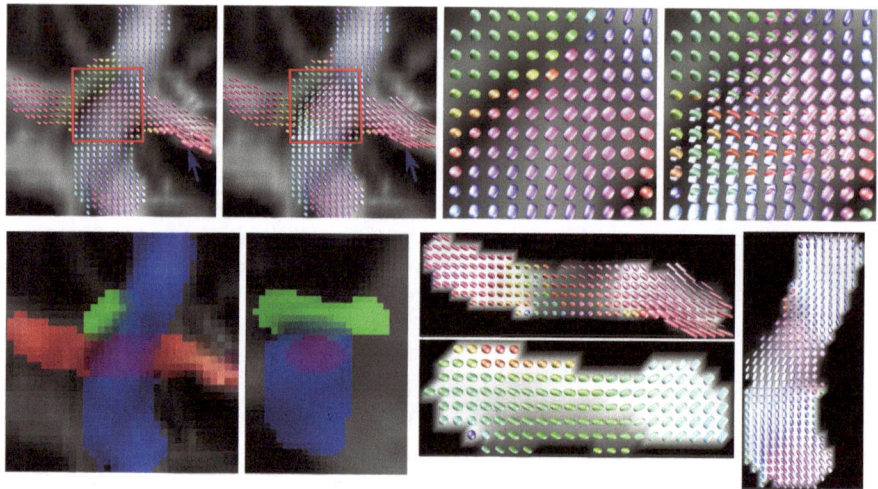

Fig. 7. 1st row: the DTI field, our estimated multi-tensor field and their closer views of the crossing region (inside the red box). 2nd row: our fractional segmentation.

FA background and its closer view of the crossing region. In the 2nd and 4th pictures, we show our estimated tensors and a closer view of the same crossing region. As we can see, the DTI model can not tell the different fibers inside a voxel. However, it is clear that our method can estimate multiple tensor compartments in the crossing region and also reduce the isotropic partial voluming of the estimated tensors in the corpus callosum (blue arrow). Our fractional segmentation is shown in the 2nd row of Figure 7, where we overlay our color-coded fractional segmentation on the top of FA background on the left two pictures and we overlay the estimated tensor compartments on the corresponding fractional segmentation on the right three pictures. We can see that the tensors in each white matter tract are spatially consistent due to our spatial prior, and the fractional segmentation is biologically reasonable.

4   Conclusion and Future Work

We present a Bayesian approach for joint fractional segmentation of white matter tracts and multi-tensor estimation in DWI. Our method can reliably estimate multiple tensor compartments in fiber crossing regions even with low angular DWI. There are three areas we have identified as potential future work. First, our noise model could be replaced with a Rician noise likelihood. Second, we can use an anisotropic spatial prior [14] instead of the isotropic spatial prior to prevent blurring across the whiter matter tracts. Finally, we plan to investigate the sensitivity of our current gradient-based optimization to the initial binary segmentation and explore stochastic optimization schemes.

Acknowledgements. We would like to thank Dr. Janet Lainhart for providing the image data, funded by NIH Grant R01 MH080826. This work was supported by NIH Grant R01 MH084795.

References

1. Alexander, A.L., Hasan, K.M., Lazar, M., Tsuruda, J.S., Parker, D.L.: Analysis of partial volume effects in diffusion-tensor MRI. MRM 45(5), 770–780 (2001)
2. Assemlal, H.-E., Tschumperl, D., Brun, L., Siddiqi, K.: Recent advances in diffusion MRI modeling: Angular and radial reconstruction. MedIA 15(4), 369–396 (2011)
3. Behrens, T.E.J., Woolrich, M.W., Jenkinson, M., Johansen-Berg, H., Nunes, R.G., Clare, S., Matthews, P.M., Brady, J.M., Smith, S.M.: Characterization and propagation of uncertainty in diffusion-weighted MR imaging. MRM 50, 1077–1088 (2003)
4. Cook, P.A., Bai, Y., Gilani, N.S., Seunarine, K.K., Hall, M.G., Parker, G.J., Alexander, D.C.: Camino: Open-source diffusion-MRI reconstruction and processing. In: ISMRM, p. 2759 (May 2006)
5. Fletcher, P.T., Tao, R., Jeong, W.-K., Whitaker, R.T.: A volumetric approach to quantifying region-to-region white matter connectivity in diffusion tensor MRI. In: Karssemeijer, N., Lelieveldt, B. (eds.) IPMI 2007. LNCS, vol. 4584, pp. 346–358. Springer, Heidelberg (2007)
6. Hao, X., Whitaker, R.T., Fletcher, P.T.: Adaptive riemannian metrics for improved geodesic tracking of white matter. In: Székely, G., Hahn, H.K. (eds.) IPMI 2011. LNCS, vol. 6801, pp. 13–24. Springer, Heidelberg (2011)
7. Landman, B.A., Wan, H., Bogovic, J.A., Bazin, P.-L., Prince, J.L.: Resolution of crossing fibers with constrained compressed sensing using traditional diffusion tensor MRI. NeuroImage 59, 2175–2186 (2012)
8. Metzler-Baddeley, C., O'Sullivan, M.J., Bells, S., Pasternak, O., Jones, D.K.: How and how not to correct for CSF-contamination in diffusion MRI. NeuroImage 59(2), 1394–1403 (2012)
9. Oouchi, H., Yamada, K., Sakai, K., Kizu, O., Kubota, T., Ito, H., Nishimura, T.: Diffusion anisotropy measurement of brain white matter is affected by voxel size: underestimation occurs in areas with crossing fibers. AJNR 28(6), 1102–1106 (2007)
10. Pasternak, O., Assaf, Y., Intrator, N., Sochen, N.: Variational multiple-tensor fitting of fiber-ambiguous diffusion-weighted magnetic resonance imaging voxels. Magnetic Resonance Imaging 26(8), 1133–1144 (2008)
11. Rohde, G., Barnett, A., Basser, P., Marenco, S., Pierpaoli, C.: Comprehensive approach for correction of motion and distortion in diffusion-weighted MRI. MRM 51, 103–114 (2004)
12. Tuch, D.S., Reese, T.G., Wiegell, M.R., Makris, N., Belliveau, J.W., Wedeen, V.J.: High angular resolution diffusion imaging reveals intravoxel white matter fiber heterogeneity. MRM 48(4), 577–582 (2002)
13. Vos, S.B., Jones, D.K., Viergever, M.A., Leemans, A.: Partial volume effect as a hidden covariate in DTI analyses. NeuroImage 55(4), 1566–1576 (2011)
14. Wang, Z., Vemuri, B.C., Chen, Y., Mareci, T.H.: A constrained variational principle for direct estimation and smoothing of the diffusion tensor field from complex dwi. IEEE Transactions on Medical Imaging 23(8), 930–939 (2004)

Retrospective Estimation of the Susceptibility Driven Field Map for Distortion Correction in Echo Planar Imaging

Hiroyuki Takeda and Boklye Kim

Department of Radiology, University of Michigan, Ann Arbor, MI, USA
{htakeda,boklyek}@umich.edu

Abstract. Echo planar imaging (EPI) sequence used for acquiring functional MRI (fMRI) time series data provides the advantage of high temporal resolution, but also is highly sensitive to the magnetic field inhomogeneity resulting in geometric distortions. A static field-inhomogeneity map measured before or after the fMRI scan to correct for such distortions does not account for magnetic field changes due to the head motion during the time series acquisition. In practice, the field map dynamically changes with head motion during the scan and leads to variations in the geometric distortion. We model in this work the field inhomogeneity with the object and the scanner dependent terms. The object-specific term varies with the object's magnetic susceptibility and orientation, i.e., head position with respect to B_0. Thus, the simple transformation of the acquired field may not yield an accurate field map. We assume that the scanner-specific field remains unchanged and independent of the head motion. Our approach in this study is to retrospectively estimate the object's magnetic susceptibility (χ) map from an observed high-resolution static field map using an estimator derived from a probability density function of non-uniform noise. This approach is capable of finding the susceptibility map regardless of the wrapping effect. A dynamic field map at each head position can be estimated by applying a rigid body transformation to the estimated χ-map and the 3-D susceptibility voxel convolution (SVC) which is a physics-based discrete convolution model for computing χ-induced field inhomogeneity.

Keywords: Echo planar imaging, geometric distortion correction, field inhomogeneity, susceptibility map.

1 Introduction

While echo planar imaging (EPI) is widely used in functional MRI for brain activation analysis, the measured k-space samples are sensitive to the magnetic field inhomogeneity resulting in geometric distortions of the acquired images [1]. The field map dynamically changes with head motion during the scan, and such changing field map leads considerable variations not only in geometric distortions but also in voxel intensities from one image to another, which negatively impacts the performance of the activation analysis in functional magnetic resonance imaging (fMRI).

J.C. Gee et al. (Eds.): IPMI 2013, LNCS 7917, pp. 352–363, 2013.

Magnetic susceptibility (χ)-induced local field variation due to the human anatomy, mainly the air in the sinus interfaced with tissue and bone, induces the local B0 field inhomogeneity, which is the cause of geometric distortion and signal loss. Such χ–induced local field variation is hard to compensate mechanically by the scanner especially with the presence of motion during fMRI time series acquisitions using the EPI sequence. In practice, the field map dynamically changes with the presence of head motion during the fMRI scan, and such changes lead to variations in geometric distortion. Conventionally, a static field map can be obtained from the phase difference of an image pair acquired at different echo times [2-4]. Approximating a dynamic field map by applying rigid body transformations to an observed static field map may not be sufficient in the presence of significant head rotations with respect to the B0 field since the field inhomogeneity may change nonlinearly [5]. We consider that the acquired field map is comprised of the object-specific, χ-induced, and the system-specific, non-χ-induced components. The χ-induced field inhomogeneity term varies with the object's orientation with respect to B0 while the system-specific field term depends mainly on the bulk changes in the applied static field. For the estimation of a χ-induced field map subject to head rotation at a specific image acquisition time, we first estimate the χ-map from a measured static field map and transform the object-specific χ-map using the estimated the head motion parameters [6-8] and reconstruct a new field map [5, 9] using the susceptibility voxel convolution (SVC) technique [10, 11]. We present in this work the estimation of the χ-induced and non-χ-induced field map, termed system-specific herein, components in human brain data to be used for the computation of dynamic field maps in EPI time series.

The χ-induced field (ΔB_χ) may be the dominant component of the field inhomogeneity changes and approximately expressed as a convolution of the object-specific χ-map with the SVC kernel (h) (i.e., $\Delta B_\chi = B_0 \cdot h * \chi$ where B_0 is the strength of the applied magnetic field) [10, 11]. The previous and commonly used approach for the χ-induced field map estimation is by deconvolution of the measured field map (ΔB) with the SVC kernel [5, 12-27]. Such deconvolution approach in χ-map estimation poses following difficulties:

- The measured field map (ΔB) often suffers from wrapping effects due to large susceptibility value changes in the phase difference $\theta \in (-\pi, \pi]$ between the two complex-valued images acquired at different echo times (T_{E1} and T_{E2}), i.e. $\theta = \frac{1}{\gamma} \Delta B (T_{E2} - T_{E1})$ where γ is the gyromagnetic ratio [28].
- Other than the χ-induced field inhomogeneity, there are other sources of error from the non-χ–induced, system specific magnetic field component [29].
- Noise variance on the acquired phase difference map θ or the local signal-to-noise ratio (SNR) depends on the local signal intensity (i.e., the magnitude of the complex-valued image voxels) causing spatially-varying variance of the noise [30-32].
- The deconvolution process may produce significant ringing/streak artifacts and amplify the phase noise due to the zero fills in the SVC kernel [5, 12-27].

Some of the previous studies on the χ-map estimation employ unwrapping techniques [30-40], and high-pass filtering [18-21, 24, 25, 27, 41] to remove the wrapping effects and the system-specific inhomogeneous field term, respectively. Then, the weighted least square estimator with an appropriate (smoothing) regularization is used to estimate the χ-map [5, 15-27], where the weights are computed from either the estimation of the local noise variance or local signal magnitudes. Though the potential of the SVC deconvolution approach could be demonstrated, the statistical theory behind the approach is not well utilized in those previous works. Consequently, the performance of the SVC deconvolution approach could not be fully exploited because the unwrapping process may cause additional errors [5, 15-27] or their weighting functions would not quite rely on the property of the noise that the phase data θ carry [5, 15-27]. Some of the methods require masking out the surrounding air region and the skull part of the human head manually in advance, where noise and wrapping effects are severe [16, 19-22, 24-27].

In our work, for the deconvolution approach we take advantage of multiple receiver coils, each of which has non-uniform, complex-valued, sensitivity and provides a separate phase difference map rather than using the combined data. Estimating one χ-map out of multiple datasets is always preferable in terms of SNR. Besides, combining the given phase data from multiple coil channels can introduce additional averaging or combination errors depending on the method used, i.e., sum of squares or Roemer [42].

In this study, in lieu of the previous approaches, we explicitly show appropriate terms in modeling the field homogeneity and an effective probability density function (PDF) of the noise. Using the PDF of the given phase data our estimator penalizes less reliable samples by giving smaller weights for computing the χ-map of the object. Note that, though it was convenient, Gaussian noise does not really represent the noise distribution in the phase domain [30-32], therefore a weighting function is necessary to suppress undesired effects caused by the less reliable phase samples [5, 15-27]. Furthermore, our estimator derived from the PDF is capable of finding a χ-map regardless of phase wrapping effects. Finally, we take into account the scanner-specific, non-χ-induced, field in order to estimate a χ-map accurately [5]. The scanner-specific field component may be identified by scanning a homogeneous head phantom and we introduce regularizations which effectively suppress noise and other artifacts.

This paper is structured as follows. In Section 2, we introduce and derive a χ-map estimator based on our data model and the PDF of the noise ridden on the phase difference map. In Section 3, we show our results from simulation and real MRI scan data, and conclude our paper in Section 4.

2   Susceptibility Map Estimation

A field inhomogeneity map ΔB is obtained from a pair of complex-valued images I_{TE1} and I_{TE2} acquired at different echo times, T_{E1} and T_{E2}, using a dual-echo or multi-echo sequence, by taking the phase difference θ as

$$\theta(\mathbf{r})[rad] = \angle\{\bar{I}_{TE1}(\mathbf{r}) \cdot I_{TE2}(\mathbf{r})\} = \gamma \Delta B(\mathbf{r}) \Delta T_E - 2\pi n(\mathbf{r}) + \eta(\mathbf{r}) \qquad (1)$$

where $\mathbf{r} = [x, y, z, q]$ is the coordinate of the phase difference map, i.e. the 3-D spatial coordinate and the coil channel index, q, γ is the gyromagnetic ratio, $-2\pi n$ represents the wrapping effect with some integer $n(\mathbf{r})$ due to the angle operation and $\theta(\mathbf{r})$ stays in the range of $(-\pi, \pi]$ and $\Delta T_E = T_{E2} - T_{E1}$. The field inhomogeneity map ΔB, model may be comprised of three components: (i) the object's χ-induced field ΔB_χ, which can be computed by the susceptibility voxel convolution (SVC) as $\Delta B_\chi = B_0 \cdot h * \chi$ where h is the three dimensional SVC kernel, (ii) the higher order field perturbation ΔB_e induced by the object's susceptibility and (iii) the system-specific, non-χ-induced, field ΔB_{sys}. We denote the field inhomogeneity map $\Delta B = B_0 \cdot h * \chi + \Delta B_e + \Delta B_{\text{sys}}$ and rewrite the data model (1) as

$$\theta(\mathbf{r}) = \gamma \Delta T_E B_0 \cdot h(\mathbf{r}) * \chi(\mathbf{r}) + \theta_e(\mathbf{r}) + \theta_{\text{sys}}(\mathbf{r}) - 2\pi\, n(\mathbf{r}) + \epsilon(\mathbf{r}), \qquad (2)$$

where $\theta_e(\mathbf{r}) = \gamma \Delta T_E \Delta B_e(\mathbf{r})$ and $\theta_{\text{sys}}(\mathbf{r}) = \gamma \Delta T_E \Delta B_{\text{sys}}(\mathbf{r})$. We assume that ΔB_e is smooth across the space and ΔB_{sys} is dependent mainly on the system and stays constant for a given magnet system. Modeling and estimating the ΔB_e and ΔB_{sys} terms are not like any other existing methods that handle those terms by applying a low-pass filter [19, 41].

Often noise is assumed to be Gaussian and consequently necessitates noise variance estimation for each phase sample prior to the χ-map estimation. However, the multiplication of voxel intensities in the angle operation in the phase map alters the property of the noise carried by the image voxels. In this work, we introduce an approximated probability density function of ϵ. Assuming that the noise ridden on the two images I_{TE1} and I_{TE2} is i.i.d. zero-mean complex Gaussian noise with variance of σ^2, where $\sigma^2 \ll var(I_{TE2})$, we can approximately express the PDF of η in (1) as (q.v. Appendix for the derivation),

$$p\big(\eta(\mathbf{r})\big) \propto \exp\{\kappa(\mathbf{r}) \cdot \cos\eta(\mathbf{r})\} \quad \text{where} \quad \kappa(\mathbf{r}) \approx \frac{|I_{TE1}(\mathbf{r})|^2 |I_{TE2}(\mathbf{r})|^2}{(|I_{TE1}(\mathbf{r})|^2 + |I_{TE2}(\mathbf{r})|^2)\sigma^2 + \sigma^4}. \qquad (3)$$

It is advantageous that the term $2\pi n$ appeared in (1) has no effect in $\cos(\cdot)$ and the term κ as a weight function, although it is rather related to the reciprocal of the variance of the PDF, eliminates noisy data (i.e. phase samples in the air region and the region where the coil sensitivity is low) by penalizing with small weights.

Having introduced the data model (2) and the noise PDF (3), we have the following maximum likelihood estimator for the χ-map and θ_e with regularizations as

$$\max_{\chi, \theta_e} \Big[\textstyle\sum_{\text{for all } \mathbf{r}} \kappa(\mathbf{r}) \cdot \cos\{\theta(\mathbf{r}) - \gamma \Delta T_E B_0 \cdot h(\mathbf{r}) * \chi(\mathbf{r}) - \theta_e(\mathbf{r}) - \tilde{\theta}_{\text{sys}}(\mathbf{r})\}$$
$$- \textstyle\sum_{i=\{x,y,z\}} \{\mu_1 |Y_i(\mathbf{r}) * \theta_e(\mathbf{r})|^2 + \mu_2 |\Gamma_i(\mathbf{r}) * \chi(\mathbf{r})|\}\Big], \qquad (4)$$

where μ_1 and μ_2 are the regularization parameters for θ_e and χ, respectively, and Γ_i and Y_i are the convolution kernel function of the first and second derivatives, respectively, along i-axis for $i = \{x, y, z\}$. We chose the kernel functions assuming that the secondary field perturbation component θ_e is piecewise smooth and the χ-map is piecewise constant across the space. We estimate χ and θ_e by the steepest descent method iteratively. We initialize χ by first making a binary image of the body tissue and air from I_{TE1}. We initialize θ_e with residuals, i.e. $\hat{\theta}_e^{(0)} = \theta - \gamma \Delta T_E B_0 \cdot h *$ $\hat{\chi}^{(0)} - \tilde{\theta}_{sys}$ where $\hat{\chi}^{(0)}$ is the initial χ-map estimate. As for the system-specific component θ_{sys}, we obtain the phase difference map empirically from a pair image of a homogeneous phantom in advance, and smoothen it by the polynomial fitting method for the system-specific component $\tilde{\theta}_{sys}$.

3   Experiments

Images were acquired from a Philips 3T MRI Ingenia system (Beth, Netherlands). We estimated the system-specific field component $\theta_{sys} (= \gamma \Delta T_E \Delta B_{sys})$ which includes scanner's shimming with a bulk homogeneous object. Using a sphere phantom filled with a homogeneous agar gel (diameter = 22 cm), we empirically estimated θ_{sys}. Using a multiecho sequence, I_{TE1} and I_{TE2} were acquired with $\Delta T_E = 2.0$ ms and image resolution $2 \times 2 \times 2$ mm^3. In Fig 1, the phase image of I_{TE1}, one of the image pair measured from one of the 13 coils (a) and the computed phase difference map (b) from the pair are shown. Each coil exhibits distinct coil sensitivity and we estimated all data from 13 channels. Also the system-specific field component was explicitly estimated using data from all receiver coils. Assuming that the field is smooth across the space, we estimated $\tilde{\theta}_{sys}$ with the global polynomial fitting [43] as shown in Fig 1(f). The plots in Fig 2 show the middle cross sections along x, y, z-axes of the acquired phase difference image (circles) and the smoothed phase difference image (solid lines). We assume that the system specific field stays stable for the given MRI scanner [5].

Human brain data were acquired from the same scanner using the same sequence and acquisition parameters as the phantom data. The phase and phase difference images from the first (out of 13) receiver coil are shown in Fig 3(a) and (b), respectively. Fig 3(c) shows the phase difference image after removing the estimated system-specific field, i.e. $\angle(\bar{I}_{TE1} \cdot I_{TE2}) - \tilde{\theta}_{sys}$ (rad). Using our proposed estimator (4), the χ-map of the human head and ΔB_e were estimated as shown in Fig 4 (b) and (c), respectively. We note that the estimated perturbation field ΔB_e includes the error caused by the structure of the human head outsides the field of view.

As a comparison, we generated a susceptibility map, χ_{ICBM} by registering a discrete brain atlas data from the International Consortium of Brain Mapping (ICBM) [44] on to the magnitude image of I_{TE1}. The discrete images are segmented into four different parts, air, born, fat, and brain tissues (i.e., white/gray matter, CSF, vessel). Then a theoretical χ-map, χ_{ICBM}, of a human brain was created by filling in the literature susceptibility values to specific segmented structures as shown in Fig 4(a). The susceptibility values $\chi_{air} = 0.4 \times 10^{-6}$, $\chi_{bone} = -8.86 \times 10^{-6}$, $\chi_{fat} = -7.5 \times 10^{-6}$, and $\chi_{tissue} = -9.05 \times 10^{-6}$ were used [11, 45]. . The χ-induced fields, B_x and B_{ICBM}, were computed by applying the SVC to both the estimated susceptibility map $\hat{\chi}$ and χ_{ICBM}, respectively,as shown in Fig 4(d) and (e): (left) the computed χ-induced field (kHz) using χ_{ICBM}; (center) the computed field using $\hat{\chi}$; (right) the difference image. Both χ-maps exhibit typical strong local inhomogeneous field structures caused by the frontal sinus, the sphenoid sinus, the nasal passage, and the ear canal. These are the critical part of the field map estimation because of the severe geometric distortions in EPI around the air/tissue and air/bone interfaces.

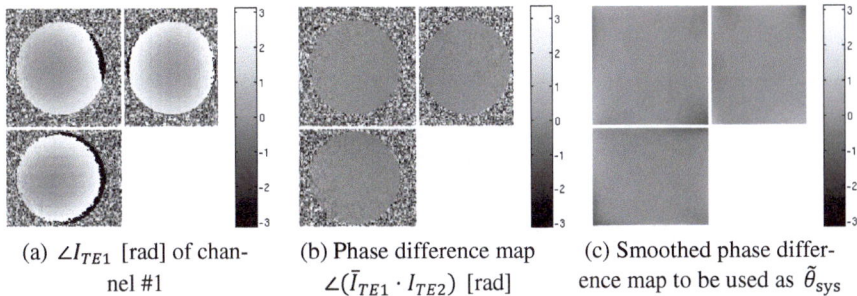

(a) $\angle I_{TE1}$ [rad] of channel #1

(b) Phase difference map $\angle(\bar{I}_{TE1} \cdot I_{TE2})$ [rad]

(c) Smoothed phase difference map to be used as $\tilde{\theta}_{sys}$

Fig. 1. The estimation of the system-specific field component (θ_{sys}) using a homogeneous phantom: (a) the phase of one of the image pair, I_{TE1}, (b) the phase difference map from the image pair which is assumed to be the system-specific component $\theta_{sys} = \angle(\bar{I}_{TE1} \cdot I_{TE2}) = \gamma \Delta T_E \Delta B_{sys}$ of the coil channel #1, and (c) the smoothed phase difference map ($\tilde{\theta}_{sys}$) by the global (3-D) polynomial fitting.

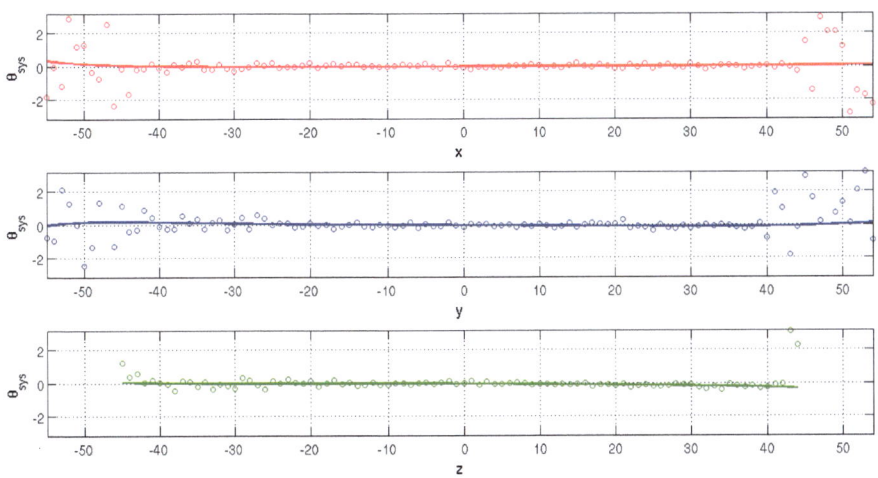

Fig. 2. Middle cross sections comparing the phase difference maps from the homogeneous phantom data (circles) and the smoothed phase difference map by the global polynomial fitting (solid lines)

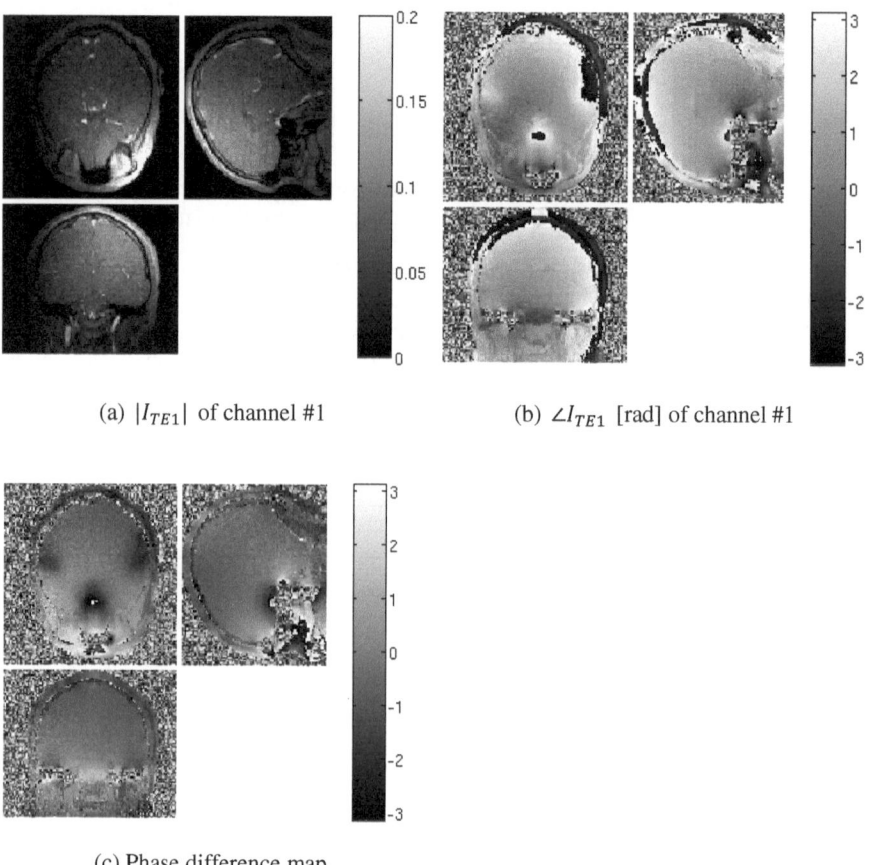

(a) $|I_{TE1}|$ of channel #1

(b) $\angle I_{TE1}$ [rad] of channel #1

(c) Phase difference map
$\angle(\bar{I}_{TE1} \cdot I_{TE2}) - \tilde{\theta}_{sys}$ [rad]

Fig. 3. Human brain data: (a) the magnitude and (b) phase images, I_{TE1}, (c) the phase difference map from the image pair I_{TE1} and I_{TE2}, after the system-specific component $\tilde{\theta}_{sys}$, estimated using the homogeneous phantom, was subtracted

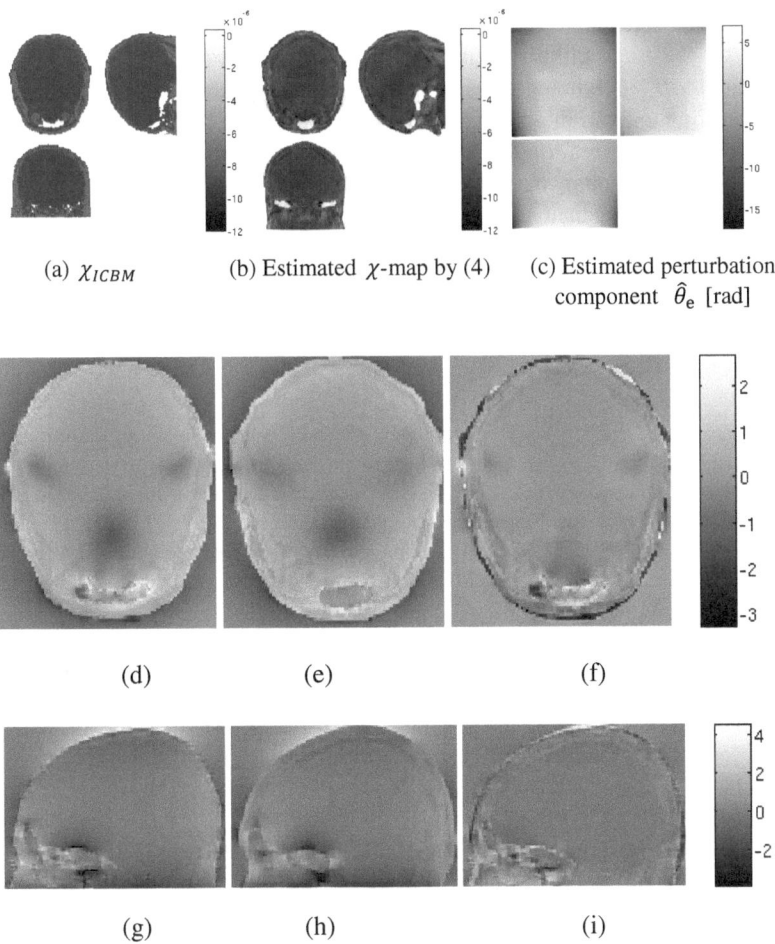

(a) χ_{ICBM} (b) Estimated χ-map by (4)   (c) Estimated perturbation
component $\hat{\theta}_e$ [rad]

(d)   (e)   (f)

(g)   (h)   (i)

Fig. 4. The estimated susceptibility map: (a) χ-map generated by filling the literature values in the registered ICBM image on to I_{TE1}, (b) the estimated χ-map by (4), (c) the estimated perturbation error component $\hat{\theta}_e$ by (4). Comparisons of the computed χ-induced field maps (kHz) at the middle transverse (top) and sagittal (bottom) planes. (d, g) The χ-map generated from ICBM and (e, h) estimated from the static field map, and (f, i) the difference image.

4   Conclusion and Future Works

The proposed method estimates a susceptibility-induced field map from a measured static field map. It does not require segmentation or pulse sequence modifications, and may yield dynamic field maps that address nonlinear changes due to head rotations. We introduced an effective probability density function of the non-uniform

noise in the phase difference images and investigated a method to empirically meas
ure non-χ-induced field inhomogeneities and characterized their magnitudes. The
experiments presented showed that the proposed estimator provided a reasonable
estimate of the susceptibility-map by successfully separating the susceptibility-
induced field ΔB_x and the perturbation error field component ΔB_e. The χ -induced
field map estimate from the human brain was close to the theoretical field map computed from using the brain atlas.   Possible sources of error may be the registration
error between the human data and the ICBM brain atlas.   The effects of non-χ-
induced field inhomogeneities, i.e., ΔB_{sys} and ΔB_e, in image distortion and reconstruction along with the motion induced χ-induced field changes need to be assessed
for the use of the estimated χ-map in time series data reconstruction.

References

1. Edelman, R.R., Wielopolski, P., Schmitt, F.: Echo-Planar MR Imaging. Radiology 192(3),
   600–612 (1994)
2. Jezzard, P., Balaban, R.S.: Correction for Geometric Distortion in Echo Planar Images
   from B0 Field Variations. Magnetic Resonance in Medicine 34, 65–73 (1995)
3. Zeng, H., Constable, R.T.: Image Distotion Correction in EPI: Comparison of Field Mapping With Point Spread Function Mapping. Magnetic Resonance in Medicine 48, 137–146
   (2002)
4. Hsu, Y., Han, C., Tseng, W.I.: Correction for Susceptibility-Induced Distrotion in Echo-
   Planar Imaging Using Field Maps and Model-Based Point Spread Function. IEEE Transactions on Medical Imaging 28(11), 1850–1857 (2009)
5. Yeo, D.T.B., Fessler, J.A., Kim, B.: Motion Robust Magnetic Susceptibility and Field Inhomogeneity Estimation Using Regularized Image Restoration Techniques for fMRI. In:
   Metaxas, D., Axel, L., Fichtinger, G., Székely, G. (eds.) MICCAI 2008, Part I. LNCS,
   vol. 5241, pp. 991–998. Springer, Heidelberg (2008)
6. Kim, B., Yeo, D.T.B., Bhagalia, R.: Comprehensive Mathematical Simulation of Functional Magnetic Resonance Imaging Time Series Including Motion-Related Image Distortion and Spin Saturation Effect. Magnetic 26, 147–159 (2008)
7. Viola, P., Wells III, W.M.: Alignment by Maximization of Mutual Information. International Journal of Computer Vision 24(2), 137–154 (1997)
8. Pluim, J.P.W., Maintz, J.B.A., Viergever, M.A.: Mutual-Information-Based Registration of
   Medical Images: A Survey. IEEE Transactions on Medical Imaging 22(8), 986–1004
   (2003)
9. Poynton, C., Jenkinson, M., Whalen, S., Golby, A.J., Wells III, W.: Fieldmap-Free Retrospective Registration and Distortion Correction for EPI-Based Functional Imaging. In: Metaxas, D., Axel, L., Fichtinger, G., Székely, G. (eds.) MICCAI 2008, Part II. LNCS,
   vol. 5242, pp. 271–279. Springer, Heidelberg (2008)
10. Salomir, R., de Senneville, B.D., Moonen, C.T.: A Fast Calculation Method for Magnetic
    Field Inhomogeneity due to an Arbitrary Distribution of Bulk Susceptibility. Concepts in
    Magnetic Resonance Part B: Magnetic Resonance Engineering 19B(1), 26–34 (2003)
11. Yoder, D.A., Zhao, Y., Paschal, C.B., Fitzpatrick, J.M.: MRI Simulator with Object-
    Specific Field Map Calculations. Magnetic Resonance Imaging 22, 315–328 (2004)

12. Weisskoff, R.M., Kiihne, S.: MRI Susceptometry: Image-Based Measurement of Absolute Susceptibility of MR Contrast Agents and Human Blood. Magnetic Resonance in Medicine 24, 375–383 (1992)
13. Beuf, O., Briguet, A., Lissac, M., Davis, R.: Magnetic Resonance Imaging for the Determination of Magnetic Susceptibility of Materials. Journal of Magnetic Resonance B-112(0120), 111–118 (1996)
14. Wang, Z.J., Li, S., Haselgrove, J.C.: Magnetic Resonance Imaging Measurement of Volume Magnetic Susceptibility Using a Boundary Condition. Journal of Magnetic Resonance 140, 477–481 (1999)
15. Liu, T., Spincemaille, P., de Rochefort, L., Kressler, B., Wang, Y.: Calculation of Susceptibility Through Multiple Orientation Sampling (COSMOS): A Method for Conditioning the Inverse Problem from Measured Magnetic Field Map to Susceptibility Source Image in MRI. Magnetic Resonance in Medicine 61, 196–204 (2009)
16. Schafer, A., Wharton, S., Bowtell, R.: Calculation of Susceptibility Maps from Phase Image Data. In: Proceedings of International Society for Magnetic Resonance in Medicine, vol. 16 (2008)
17. Morgan, J., Irarrazaval, P.: Efficient Solving for Arbitrary Susceptibility Distributions using Residual Difference Fields. In: Proceedings of International Society for Magnetic Resonance in Medicine, vol. 15 (2007)
18. Kressler, B., De Rochefort, L., Liu, T., Spincemaille, P., Jiang, Q., Wang, Y.: Nonlinear Regularization for Per Voxel Estimation of Magnetic Susceptibility Distributions from MRI Field Maps. IEEE Transactions on Medical Imaging 39(2), 273–281 (2010)
19. de Rochefort, L., Liu, T., Kressler, B., Liu, J., Spincemaille, P.: Quantitative Susceptibility Map Reconstruction from MR Phase Data Using Bayesian Regularization: Validation and Application to Brain Imaging. Magnetic Resonance in Medicine 63, 194–206 (2010)
20. Wharton, S., Bowtell, R.: Whole-Brain Susceptibility Mapping at High Field: A Comparision of Multiple- and Single-Orientation Methods. NeuroImage 53, 515–525 (2010)
21. Liu, T., Liu, J., De Rochefort, L., Spincemaille, P., Khalidov, L., Robert Ledoux, J., Wang, Y.: Morphology Enabled Dipole Inversion (MEDI) from a Single-Angle Acquisition: Comparison with COSMOS in Human Brain Imaging. Magnetic Resonance in Medicine 66, 777–783 (2011)
22. Liu, T., Spincemaille, P., De Rochefort, L., Wong, R., Prince, M., Wang, Y.: Unambiguous Identification of Superparamagnetic Iron Oxide Particles through Quantitative Susceptibility Mapping of the Nonlinear Response to Magnetic Fields. Magnetic REsonance Imaging 28, 1383–1389 (2010)
23. Grabner, G., Trattnig, S., Barth, M.: Filtered Deconvolution of a Simulated and an In Vivo Phase Model of the Human Brain. Journal of Magnetic Resonance Imaging 32, 289–297 (2010)
24. Liu, T., Wisnieff, C., Lou, M., Chen, W., Spincemaille, P., Wang, Y.: Nonlinear Formulation of the Magnetic Field to Source Relationship for Robust Quantitative Susceptibility Mapping. Magnetic Resonance in Medicine (2012)
25. Tang, J., Neelavalli, J., Cheng, Y.N., Buch, S., Haacke, E.M.: Improving Susceptibility Mapping using a Threshold-Based K-space/Image Domain Iterative Reconstruction Approach. Magnetic REsonance in Medicine (2012)
26. Liu, T., Xu, W., Spincemaille, P., Avestimehr, A.S., Wang, Y.: Accuracy of the Morphology Enabled Dipole Inversion (MEDI) Algorithm for Quantitative Susceptibility Mapping in MRI. IEEE Transactions on Medical Imaging 31(3), 816–824 (2012)
27. Wu, B., Li, W., Guidon, A., Liu, C.: Whole Brain Susceptibility Mapping Using Compressed Sensing. Magnetic Resonance in Medicine 67, 137–147 (2012)

28. Liang, Z.-P., Lauterbur, P.C.: Principles of Magnetic Resonance Imaging: A Signal Processing Perspective. Wiley-IEEE Press, Piscataway, NJ (1999)
29. Jenkinson, M., Wilson, J.L., Jezzard, P.: Perturbation Method for Magnetic Field Calculations of Nonconductive Objects. Magnetic Resonance in Medicine 52, 471–477 (2004)
30. Lee, J., Hoppel, K.W., Mango, S.A., Miller, A.R.: Intensity and Phase Statistics of Multilook Polarimetric and Interferometric SAR Imagery. IEEE Transactions on Geoscience and Remote Sensing 32(5), 1017–1028 (1994)
31. Ho, K., Kahn, J.: Exact Probability Density Function for Phase Mesaturement Interferometry. Journal of the Optical Society of America 12, 1984–1989 (1995)
32. Leitao, J.M.N., Figueiredo, M.A.T.: Absolute Phase Image Reconstruction: A Stochastic Nonlinear Filtering Approach. IEEE Transactions on Image Processing 7(6), 868–882 (1998)
33. Goldstein, R.M., Zebken, H.A., Werner, C.L.: Satellite Rader Interferometry: Two-Dimensional Phase Unwrapping. Radio Science 23(4), 713–720 (1988)
34. Chiglia, D.C., Pritt, M.D.: Two-Diumensional Phase Unwrapping: Theory, Algorithms and Software. Wiley-Interscience, New York (1998)
35. Bagher-Ebadian, H., Jiang, Q., Ewing, J.R.: A Modified Fourier Based Phase Unwrapping Algorithm with an Application to MRI venography. Journal of Magnetic Resonance Imaging 27(3), 649–652 (2008)
36. Dias, J.B., Leitao, J.N.: The ZpiM algorithm: A Method for Interferometric Image Reconstruction in SAR/SAS. IEEE Transactions on Image Processing 11(4), 408–422 (2002)
37. Abdul-Rahman, H.S., Gdeisat, M.A., Burton, D.R., Lalor, M.J., Lilley, F., Moore, C.J.: Fast and Robust Three-Dimensional Best Path Phase Unwrapping Algorithm. Applied Optics 46(26), 6623–6635 (2007)
38. Jenkinson, M.: Fast, Automated, N-Dimensional Phase-Unwrapping Algorithm. Magnetic Resonance in Medicine 49, 193–197 (2003)
39. Volkov, V.V., Zhu, Y.: Deterministic Phase Unwrapping in the Presence of Noise. Optics Letters 28(22), 2156–2158 (2003)
40. Truong, T., Clymer, B.D., Chakeres, D.W., Schmalbrock, P.: Three-Dimensional Numerical Simulations of Susceptibility-Induced Magnetic Field Inhomogeneities in the Human Head. Magnetic Resonance Imaging 20, 759–770 (2002)
41. Wharton, S., Schafer, A., Bowtell, R.: Susceptibility Mapping in the Human Brain Using Threshold-Based k-Space Division. Magnetic Resonance in Medicine 63, 1292–1304 (2010)
42. Roemer, P.B., Edelstein, W.A., Hayes, C.E., Souza, S.P., Mueller, O.M.: The NMR Phase Array. Magnetic Resonance in Medicine 16, 192–225 (1990)
43. Horowitz, J.L.: Semiparametric and Nonparametric Methods in Econometrics. Springer Series in Statistics. Springer, Evanston (2009)
44. Holmes, C.J., Hoge, R., Collins, L., Woods, R., Toga, A.W., Evans, A.C.: Enhancement of MR Images using Registration for Signal Averaging. Journal of Computer Assisted Tomography 22(2), 324–333 (1998)
45. Schenck, J.F.: The Role of Magnetic Susceptibility in Magnetic Resonance Imaging: MRI Magnetic Compatibility of the First and Second Kinds. Medical Physics 23(6), 815–850 (1996)

Appendix

Assuming that both images I_{TE1} and I_{TE2} carry *i.i.d.* complex white Gaussian noise ϵ with standard deviation σ, they can be expressed as

$$I_{TE1}(\mathbf{r}) = f(\mathbf{r}) + \varepsilon_1(\mathbf{r})$$
$$I_{TE2}(\mathbf{r}) = a(\mathbf{r})f(\mathbf{r})e^{j\theta(\mathbf{r})} + \varepsilon_2(\mathbf{r})$$

where $f(\mathbf{r})$ is the noise free complex-valued image of I_{TE1}, $a(\mathbf{r})$ is the intensity scaling (real-valued) function due to the free induction decay from T_{E1} to T_{E2}, $\theta(\mathbf{r})$ is the phase difference map between I_{TE1} and I_{TE2}, and $\varepsilon_1(\mathbf{r})$ and $\varepsilon_2(\mathbf{r})$ are noise, i.e. $\varepsilon_1, \varepsilon_2 \sim \mathcal{CN}(0, \sigma^2)$. Then, we can express the product of I_{TE2} and the complex conjugate of I_{TE1} as g:

$$g(\mathbf{r}) = \bar{I}_{TE1}(\mathbf{r}) \cdot I_{TE2}(\mathbf{r})$$
$$= a|f|^2 e^{j\theta} + |f|^2 \left(\frac{af}{\bar{f}} e^{j\theta} \bar{\varepsilon}_1 + \frac{\bar{f}}{f} \varepsilon_2 \right) + \bar{\varepsilon}_1 \varepsilon_2$$
$$= a(\mathbf{r})|f(\mathbf{r})|^2 e^{j\theta} + \epsilon(\mathbf{r}).$$

where the variance ς^2 of ϵ is voxel intensity dependent:

$$\varsigma^2(\mathbf{r}) = \text{var}\{\epsilon(\mathbf{r})\} = |f|^2(1 + a^2)\sigma^2 + \sigma^4.$$

When $|f|^2 \ll \sigma^2$, the noise ϵ can be assumed to be Gaussian (Note: strictly speaking, it is a mixture of Gaussian and normal product distribution), we approximately express the PDF of ϵ as

$$p(\epsilon) = p(\Re\{\epsilon\}, \Im\{\epsilon\})$$
$$\approx \frac{1}{2\pi\varsigma^2} \exp\left[-\frac{1}{2\varsigma^2}(\Re\{g\} - a|f|^2 \cos\theta)^2 - \frac{1}{2\varsigma^2}(\Im\{g\} - a|f|^2 \sin\theta)^2 \right]$$
$$= \frac{1}{2\pi\varsigma^2} \exp\left[-\frac{1}{2\varsigma^2}\{|g|^2 + a^2|f|^4 - 2a|f|^2|g|\cos(\theta - \angle g)\} \right]$$
$$= \frac{1}{2\pi\varsigma^2} \exp\left[-\frac{|g|^2 + a^2|f|^4}{2\varsigma^2} \right] \cdot \exp\left[\underbrace{\frac{a|f|^2|g|}{\varsigma^2}}_{\kappa} \underbrace{\cos(\theta - \angle g)}_{\eta} \right].$$

Therefore, for small σ^2, we have the approximated PDF of η as

$$p(\eta(\mathbf{r})) \propto \exp\{\kappa(\mathbf{r}) \cdot \cos\eta(\mathbf{r})\} \quad \text{with} \quad \kappa(\mathbf{r}) \approx \frac{|I_{TE1}(\mathbf{r})|^2|I_{TE2}(\mathbf{r})|^2}{(|I_{TE1}(\mathbf{r})|^2 + |I_{TE2}(\mathbf{r})|^2)\sigma^2 + \sigma^4}.$$

Group-Wise Cortical Correspondence via Sulcal Curve-Constrained Entropy Minimization

Ilwoo Lyu[1], Sun Hyung Kim[2], Joon-Kyung Seong[4], Sang Wook Yoo[5],
Alan C. Evans[6], Yundi Shi[2], Mar Sanchez[7],
Marc Niethammer[1,3], and Martin A. Styner[1,2]

[1] Dept. of Computer Science, University of North Carolina, Chapel Hill, NC, USA
{ilwoolyu,styner}@cs.unc.edu
[2] Dept. of Psychiatry, University of North Carolina, Chapel Hill, NC, USA
[3] BRIC, University of North Carolina, Chapel Hill, NC, USA
[4] Dept. of Biomedical Engineering, Korea University, Seoul, South Korea
[5] Dept. of Computer Science, KAIST, Daejeon, South Korea
[6] Montreal Neurological Institute, McGill University, Montreal, Quebec, Canada
[7] Yerkes National Primate Research Center, Emory University, Atlanta, GA, USA

Abstract. We present a novel cortical correspondence method employing group-wise registration in a spherical parametrization space for the use in local cortical thickness analysis in human and non-human primate neuroimaging studies. The proposed method is unbiased registration that estimates a continuous smooth deformation field into an unbiased average space via sulcal curve-constrained entropy minimization using spherical harmonic decomposition of the spherical deformation field. We initialize a correspondence by our pair-wise method that establishes a surface correspondence with a prior template. Since this pair-wise correspondence is biased to the choice of a template, we further improve the correspondence by employing unbiased ensemble entropy minimization across all surfaces, which yields a deformation field onto the iteratively updated unbiased average. The specific entropy metric incorporates two terms: the first focused on optimizing the correspondence of automatically extracted sulcal landmarks and the second on that of sulcal depth maps. We also propose an encoding scheme for spherical deformation via spherical harmonics as well as a novel method to choose an optimal spherical polar coordinate system for the most efficient deformation field estimation. The experimental results show evidence that the proposed method improves the correspondence quality in non-human primate and human subjects as compared to the pair-wise method.

Keywords: Group-wise correspondence, Sulcal curves, Spherical harmonics, Entropy minimization, Cortical thickness.

1 Introduction

Group analysis of cortical properties such as cortical thickness is an important task for monitoring brain growth, investigating anatomic connectivity, and discovering cortical disease patterns. A prerequisite to such tasks is to establish a

J.C. Gee et al. (Eds.): IPMI 2013, LNCS 7917, pp. 364–375, 2013.

consistent cortical correspondence across a population of subject cortices. However, the high variability of the cortical folding patterns provides a significant challenge to the computation of such an inter-subject cortical correspondence over the entire cortical surface.

There have been two main approaches to the cortical correspondence computation, based either on volume images or on cortical surface models. A cortical correspondence is more likely to be enhanced via surface registration on a cortical surface model due to its geometric property preservation of the cortex, while volume-based approaches using only image intensities are hard to sufficiently characterize the cortical regions for a localized vertex or voxel-wise analysis. Moreover, since the choice of invariant features across a population is essential for a consistent correspondence, folding patterns along central sulcal fundic regions can be used as features due to their relatively reduced variability. Studies on sulcal fundic region recognition and sulcal folding pattern analysis were presented in [6,11,5].

Several researchers proposed cortical registration via a spherical mapping to the template space in a pair-wise registration manner [14,13,8]. In [3], an iterative registration scheme was introduced, which updates the initial template for better correspondence establishment. The study presented by Van Essen [12] even applied to non-human primate subjects. Lyu et al. [4] also proposed a spherical mapping that uses spherical harmonic decomposition for correspondence interpolation by taking advantage of its convenient, global representation of the deformation field. In general, however, these pair-wise registration methods are inherently biased to the template surface, which is undesirable for the group analysis purpose.

To take account of variance of the cortical properties over pair-wise methods, Cates et al. [1] proposed particle-based registration on cortical surface models without using a template model or prior information. Later, Oguz et al. [7] further enhanced the particle-based registration by incorporating curvature features, showing the improved correspondence via the analysis of cortical thickness over the entire cortical surface. However, these methods did not incorporate gyral/sulcal patterns nor did they provide explicit estimation of a deformation field between subjects, rather with a particle-based correspondence that implicitly defines a deformation model without guarantee of topology preservation.

In this paper, we propose a fully automatic group-wise cortical correspondence method evaluated on both macaque and human cortical surfaces. We initially compute a pair-wise correspondence to the given template surface and further improve the correspondence across a population via ensemble entropy minimization without employing any template surface. In particular, we use spherical harmonic decomposition to continuously represent the correspondence over the entire cortical surface by using a metric that incorporates errors over sulcal landmarks and sulcal depth maps. We also propose a novel spherical polar coordinate system to avoid a distorted representation of the deformation field. In summary, the main novelties presented here are: 1) group-wise cortical correspondence using an explicit deformation field, 2) optimal pole selection for a smooth

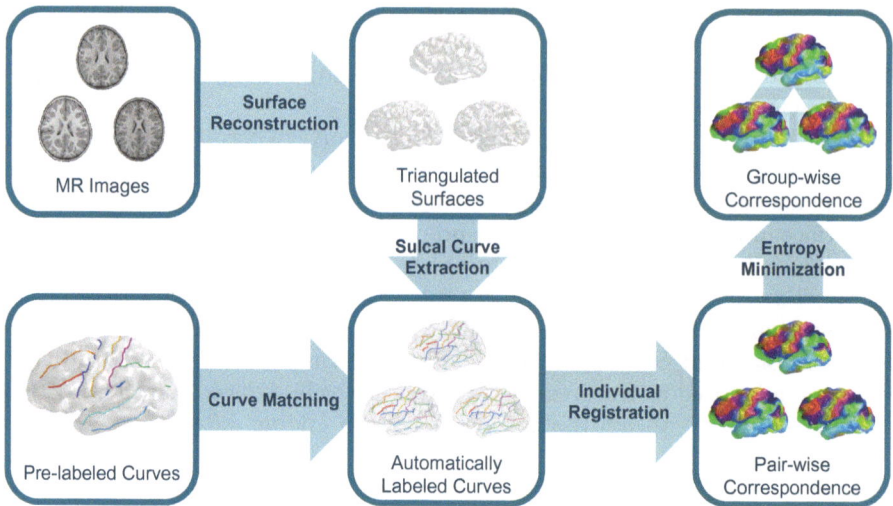

Fig. 1. Schematic overview of the proposed method

deformation field representation, and 3) application in both non-human primate and human data. Figure 1 illustrates an overview of our pipeline.

2   Method

2.1   Preprocessing

Surface Reconstruction. Raw MR images are registered into the standardized stereotaxic space using a rigid transformation. The registered images are corrected for intensity nonuniformity resulting from inhomogeneities in the magnetic field. The inner- and outer-surfaces are automatically extracted by the Constrained Laplacian-based Automated Segmentation with Proximities (CLASP) algorithm [2]. We use the middle cortical surface models with a triangulated mesh of 40,962 vertices in the native space. Each vertex of the surface models is then homeomorphically transformed onto the common unit sphere using a deformable surface model [2]. After surface reconstruction, we compute sulcal depth maps via geodesic distances from the gyral crowns as proposed in [10].

Landmark Correspondence. We use automatic sulcal curve extraction [11] and automatic sulcal curve labeling [5] to extract a set of labeled sulcal curves. In particular, the unlabeled sulcal curves (consisting of ordered sets of points) are extracted from the triangulated surface, and then pre-labeled sulcal curves in the template are employed to label matched (corresponding) sulcal curves in the subject, while discarding minor and extraneous curves. This labeling method further establishes a point-by-point correspondence across these sulcal curves called sulcal landmarks in the remainder of this paper.

2.2   Sulcal Curve-Constrained Pair-Wise Correspondence

Problem Definition. For two given triangulated cortical surfaces (template and subject), we denote Ω_{temp} and Ω_{subj} as the template and subject surfaces. Our goal is to estimate a continuous mapping function of the cortical correspondence $M : \mathbb{R}^3 \to \mathbb{R}^3$ such that

$$u = M(v) , \tag{1}$$

where $u \in \Omega_{\text{temp}}$ and $v \in \Omega_{\text{subj}}$ are the corresponding points.

Consistent Displacement Encoding Scheme. To take advantage of the well-known spherical parametrization, we map all vertices of the cortical surfaces onto the common unit sphere by using an invertible spherical mapping $\psi : \mathbb{R}^3 \to \mathbb{S}^2$ established in the preprocessing stage. Note that this spherical mapping generally does not establish an appropriate correspondence. We then locally encode the deformation as change in local spherical polar angles of elevation $\Delta\theta$ and azimuth $\Delta\phi$. It can be easily observed that the same length of geodesic distances provides different angular differences close to the equator as compared to closer to the pole. To avoid such inconsistency and thus to provide a consistent arclength encoding, we propose a locally normalized coordinate system. For this local normalization, let $\psi_{\text{temp}}(p)$ and $\psi_{\text{subj}}(q)$ be the mapped corresponding sulcal landmarks from the template and the subject, respectively. First, we find a rotation matrix $\mathbf{R}_q$ with an angle ($\leq 90°$) along the longitude circle passing through $\psi_{\text{subj}}(q)$ and the two poles, such that $\psi_{\text{subj}}(q)$ is exactly located on the equator. By applying $\mathbf{R}_q$ to $\psi_{\text{temp}}(p)$ and $\psi_{\text{subj}}(q)$, we then compute normalized angular displacements $\Delta\theta$ and $\Delta\phi$. As sulcal landmarks are described by spherical polar coordinates, we denote an operator $\odot$ that rotates these landmarks with a rotation matrix defined in a Cartesian coordinate system. Thus, the local landmark displacement at a point i (θ_i, ϕ_i) on the unit sphere is represented as a vector $\mathbf{d}_i = \mathbf{R}_{q_i} \odot \psi_{\text{temp}}(p_i) - \mathbf{R}_{q_i} \odot \psi_{\text{subj}}(q_i) = [\Delta\theta_i, \Delta\phi_i]^T$ (see Fig. 2a).

Initial Deformation Field. To find an initial deformation field of the entire surface, we compute least squares fitting of spherical harmonics to displacements of the sulcal landmarks established in the sulcal labeling step. This fitting is standard spherical harmonic decomposition of the spherical signals ($\Delta\theta$ and $\Delta\phi$). At a point (θ, ϕ) on the sphere, the spherical harmonic basis function of degree l and order m $(-l \leq m \leq l)$ is given by

$$Y_l^m(\theta, \phi) = \sqrt{\frac{2l+1}{4\pi} \frac{(l-m)!}{(l+m)!}} P_l^m(\cos\theta) e^{im\phi} , \tag{2}$$

$$Y_l^{-m}(\theta, \phi) = (-1)^m Y_l^{m*}(\theta, \phi) , \tag{3}$$

where Y_l^{m*} denotes the complex conjugate of Y_l^m and P_l^m is the associated Legendre polynomial

$$P_l^m(x) = \frac{(-1)^m}{2^l l!} (1 - x^2)^{\frac{m}{2}} \frac{d^{(l+m)}}{dx^{(l+m)}} (x^2 - 1)^l . \tag{4}$$

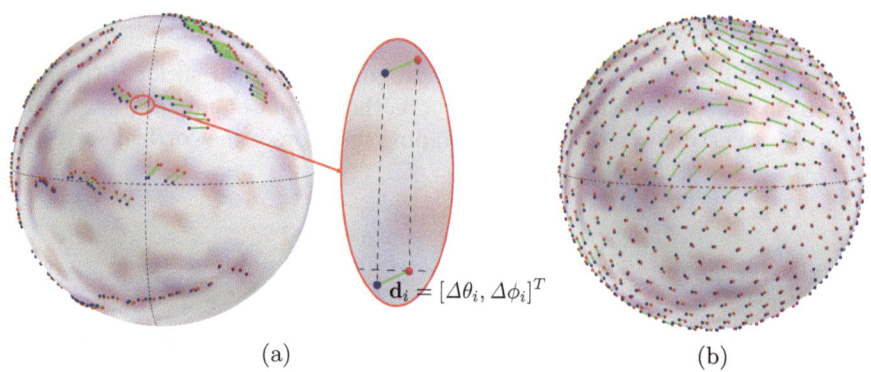

Fig. 2. Displacement encoding (a) and estimated deformation field (sampling of a continuous representation) with sulcal depth maps (b). A spherical displacement is encoded as change in spherical angles after rotation onto the equator for consistent arclength encoding, which avoids a distorted displacement representation. The deformation field is estimated by interpolation using spherical harmonic decomposition.

Since the spherical harmonic basis functions are defined in the complex domain, we use a real form of the functions defined by

$$
Y_{l,m} = \begin{cases} \frac{1}{\sqrt{2}}(Y_l^m + (-1)^m Y_l^{-m}) & m > 0, \\ Y_l^0 & m = 0, \\ \frac{1}{\sqrt{2}i}(Y_l^{-m} - (-1)^m Y_l^m) & m < 0. \end{cases} \tag{5}
$$

Given spherical harmonic decomposition of degree k, we have $(k+1)^2$ spherical harmonic basis functions at a given point on the sphere. To avoid a rank deficient problem, we assume that the number n of the landmarks is larger than $(k+1)^2$. The coefficients can then be estimated by standard least squares fitting:

$$
\mathbf{C} = \left(\mathbf{YY^T}\right)^{-1}\mathbf{YD^T}, \tag{6}
$$

where $\mathbf{D} = [\mathbf{d}_1, \mathbf{d}_2, \cdots, \mathbf{d}_n]$ and $\mathbf{Y}$ is a $(k+1)^2$-by-n matrix that incorporates the spherical harmonic basis functions. Once the coefficients of the spherical harmonic decomposition are determined, for $\forall v \in \Omega_{\text{subj}}$, its deformed position in the template space is easily reconstructed by the mapping function $\hat{M}$:

$$
\hat{u} = \hat{M}(v) = \psi_{\text{temp}}^{-1}(\mathbf{R}_v^T \odot (\mathbf{R}_v \odot \psi_{\text{subj}}(v) + \mathbf{C}^T \cdot \mathbf{Y}_v)), \tag{7}
$$

where $\mathbf{Y}_v$ is a column vector of the spherical harmonic basis functions at $\psi_{\text{subj}}(v)$ and $\mathbf{R}_v$ is a rotation matrix that puts $\psi_{\text{subj}}(v)$ on the equator. Figure 2b shows an example of the estimated deformation field.

This spherical harmonic decomposition of the deformation field is hierarchical and orthonormal. We employ the hierarchy in that the initial deformation field is computed via low degree ($k = 5$) fitting of sulcal landmarks and higher degree representations are used in the optimization stage.

Optimization. Since the initial coefficients are determined only by sulcal land-marks, the cortical correspondence is potentially biased to the specific sulcal fundic regions selected in the sulcal labeling step as well as affected by minor mislabeling errors. For improved correspondence establishment, we further formulate a metric that incorporates sulcal landmark errors and differences between sulcal depth maps via normalized cross correlation over the entire cortical surface. To regularize the impact of sulcal landmark errors, we define a weighting function f under the Gaussian assumption. Specifically, incorporating d_{min} as voxel size, sulcal landmark errors below d_{min} are ignored and have the maximum at distance d_{max}, chosen 10–20 times larger than d_{min}, as follows.

$$f(d) = 2 \int_{d_{min}}^{d} \frac{I(d)}{\sigma\sqrt{2\pi}} \exp\left\{-\frac{1}{2}\left(\frac{x - d_{min}}{\sigma}\right)^2\right\} dx , \tag{8}$$

$$I(d) = \begin{cases} 1 & d \geq d_{min} , \\ 0 & \text{otherwise} , \end{cases} \tag{9}$$

where $6 \cdot \sigma = d_{max} - d_{min}$. Now, we define $L(\cdot, \cdot) = f(\eta \cdot \text{arclen}(\cdot, \cdot))$ as a regularized arclength, where η is a ratio of the geodesic distance between two points on the unit sphere and on the template surface. In practice, it can be approximated by a ratio of the triangle size under the assumption that the template surface consists of uniform triangles. The resulting overall cost function like an M-estimator is thus formulated with a regularization factor w by letting an operator $\otimes$ denote the normalized cross correlation between two sulcal depth maps:

$$\hat{\mathbf{C}} = \underset{\mathbf{C}}{\text{argmin}} \left[w\left\{\frac{1}{n}\sum_{i=1}^{n} L(p_i, \hat{p}_i)\right\} + (1 - w)\left\{\frac{1}{2}\left(1 - SD(\{u\}) \otimes SD(\{\hat{u}\})\right)\right\} \right] , \tag{10}$$

where $SD(\cdot)$ is a sulcal depth map reconstructed from a set of vertices. The optimization procedure employs the NEWUOA optimizer [9] for minimizing $\mathbf{C}$. In our experiment, we empirically set $w = 0.5$.

Optimal Pole Selection. The proposed spherical polar coordinate system does not force the direction of displacements to be invariant to locations. Depending on rotation to the equator, two identical displacements are likely to have a different sign in polar angles if they are computed on opposite sites with respect to the pole. This can yield a deformation field with abrupt sign changes close to the pole. A proper choice of the pole $\mathbf{e}$ can significantly minimize this issue and yield smooth deformation fields. The presence of non-smooth deformation will generally lead to high magnitude coefficients in the high-frequency harmonic basis functions. Based on this observation, we employ a coefficient sum-based metric that weighs higher frequency coefficients stronger:

$$\hat{\mathbf{e}} = \underset{\mathbf{e}}{\text{argmin}} \sum_{l=0}^{k} \sum_{m=-l}^{l} (l + 1) \cdot \left(|c_{\theta_{l,m}}| + |c_{\phi_{l,m}}|\right) , \tag{11}$$

where c_θ and c_ϕ are coefficients for elevation and azimuth displacements. As this metric possibly has local minima, we initialize the optimization with multiple initial guesses spread across the sphere and select the minimum as the final pole.

2.3   Extension to Group-Wise Correspondence

While our pair-wise method provides adequate registration results (see Sect. 3), we propose here the use of group-wise registration to further improve these results as well as to remove the template selection bias inherent to pair-wise registration. A group-wise correspondence is computed independently from the template and thus is expected to perform more stably across a population of surfaces. We propose to use entropy minimization to establish a group-wise correspondence. Our group-wise correspondence method incorporates entropy terms computed over the landmark distribution and sulcal depth maps.

Problem Definition. For N given triangulated cortical surfaces mapped onto the unit sphere, each of which has the same number n of the common corresponding points, we let Ω_i denote the ith subject surface, $i = 1, \cdots, N$. The goal is to estimate continuous mapping functions of the cortical correspondence $M_i : \mathbb{S}^2 \to \mathbb{S}^2$ across subjects such that

$$M_1(v^1) = M_2(v^2) = \cdots = M_N(v^N) , \qquad (12)$$

where $v^i \in \Omega_i$ are the corresponding points across subjects. Let $\mathbf{x}(M_i(v^i))$ be a column vector of the corresponding points of the ith subject deformed by M_i, i.e., $\mathbf{x}(M_i(v^i)) = [M_i(v_1^i), \cdots, M_i(v_n^i)]^T$. As described in [7], we assume that $\mathbf{x}(M_i(v^i))$ is an instance of a random variable $\mathbf{X}$, drawn from a probability density function. The amount of the information of $\mathbf{X}$ is denoted by entropy $H[\mathbf{X}]$, and the minimization problem is then formulated as follows.

$$\{\hat{M}_1, \cdots, \hat{M}_N\} = \operatorname*{argmin}_{\{M_1, \cdots, M_N\}} H[\mathbf{X}] , \qquad (13)$$

which drives mapped/deformed corresponding points closer to each other.

Entropy of Landmark Errors. We employ the pair-wise correspondence (Sect. 2.2) as initialization for the proposed group-wise method. As the sulcal labeling procedure yields varying parts of sulcal curves being labeled, we constrain the set of sulcal landmarks only those that have a full correspondence across all cortical surfaces. A key step for entropy computation is the density estimation of corresponding sulcal landmarks. However, appropriate density estimation on the sphere can be computationally demanding since it involves geodesic distance computation. Similar to [7] for efficiency, we assume that the initial mapping well centralizes corresponding sulcal landmarks, which allows a mapping from the spherical space to the Euclidean space $\mathbb{S}^2 \to \mathbb{R}^3$ under the assumption of the proximity of the landmarks. We compute the average over corresponding sulcal landmarks, which is rescaled to the sphere, and the landmarks are projected onto the tangential plane at that approximated mean to enable Euclidean statistics.

Entropy of Sulcal Depth. Since sulcal landmarks are sparsely distributed over the sphere and also likely possess minor mislabeling, we employ additional entropy computation over sulcal depth maps densely sampled across the surface. For a given point u on the sphere, we find a point $v^i \in \Omega_i$ such that $u = M_i(v^i)$. Once M_i is given, v^i forms a correspondence with its deformed corresponding points that are located at u on the sphere. Let $sd(\cdot)$ denote the sulcal depth at a query point. Ideally, there will be little difference in sulcal depth across the corresponding points if the mapping is well established, that is, $sd(v^1) \cong \cdots \cong sd(v^N)$. By uniform icosahedron subdivision-based spherical sampling of u, the sulcal depth agreement is straightforwardly plugged into the entropy minimization problem.

Entropy Minimization. We model $\mathbf{x}(M_i(v^i))$ as an instance of $\mathbf{X}$ such that

$$\mathbf{x}(M_i(v^i)) = \left[T_{\bar{v}_1}(M_i(v_1^i)), \cdots, T_{\bar{v}_n}(M_i(v_n^i)), SD(\{M_i(v^i)\})\right]^T, \quad (14)$$

where $T_{\bar{v}}(\cdot)$ denotes the projection of a point onto the tangential plane at the approximated mean $\bar{v}$ over the corresponding sulcal landmarks. For the density estimation, we assume a multivariate Gaussian distribution with covariance Σ and therefore, the entropy is obtained by

$$H[\mathbf{X}] \approx \frac{1}{2} \ln |\Sigma| = \frac{1}{2} \sum \ln \lambda, \quad (15)$$

where λ are the eigenvalues of Σ. By letting $\bar{\mathbf{x}}$ be the sample mean and $\mathbf{Z} = [\mathbf{x}(M_1(v^1))-\bar{\mathbf{x}}, \cdots, \mathbf{x}(M_N(v^N))-\bar{\mathbf{x}}]$, the sample covariance is given by $\frac{1}{N-1}\mathbf{Z}\mathbf{Z}^T$. In practice, however, the eigendecomposition of the sample covariance is an intractable task for the large dimension of $\mathbf{X}$ ($\gg N$). As stated in [7], we instead compute the eigenvalues of $\frac{1}{N-1}\mathbf{Z}^T\mathbf{Z}$ in the dual space. The optimization uses the NEWUOA optimizer [9] for solving the entropy cost function.

3   Experimental Results

We applied the proposed method on both non-human primate and human subjects to evaluate the established correspondence quality. Since there exists no ground-truth of the cortical correspondence, we made comparisons with the initial spherical mapping and the pair-wise method via analysis on cortical thickness as well as the agreement with manually labeled sulcal curves.

3.1   Macaque Cortical Surfaces

We used the same data set as that in [4]. 18-month-old macaques were imaged under anesthesia at the Yerkes Imaging Center (Emory University, GA) on a 3T Siemens Trio scanner with an 8-channel phase array trans-receiving volume coil. T_1-weighted scans were acquired using a 3D MP-RAGE sequence with GRAPPA at a high resolution of $0.6\,mm \times 0.6\,mm \times 0.6\,mm$ (TR $= 3,000\,ms$,

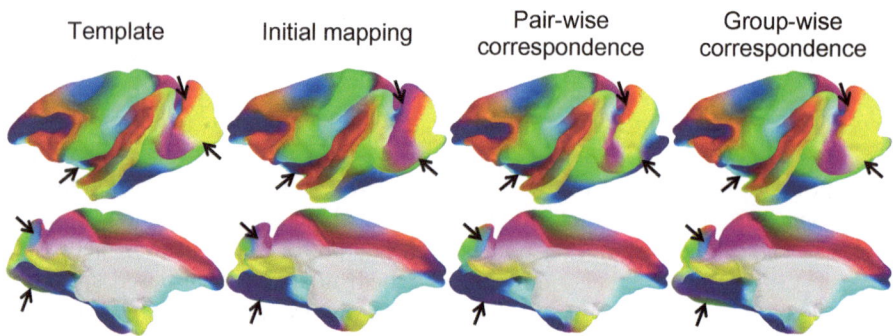

Fig. 3. Visual comparison of correspondence results. The colored template surface (*first column*) is propagated to a selected, representative example surface via initial spherical mapping (*second*), pair-wise correspondence (*third*), and group-wise correspondence (*fourth*). The arrows indicate areas of visual differences across the correspondence methods.

$TE = 3.33\,ms$, flip angle $= 8°$, matrix $= 192 \times 192$). In the experiment, we randomly selected a single subject as a template with its 11 manually labeled sulcal curves: central sulcus, arcuate sulcus, principal sulcus, superior temporal sulcus, intraparietal sulcus, lunate sulcus, inferior occipital sulcus, occipitotemporal sulcus, cingulate sulcus, parieto-occipital fissure, and sylvian fissure.

We further established a sulcal curve-based color mapping across the cortical surfaces to provide a visual quality assessment of the established correspondence by propagation of the colorized template surface to other subjects. To generate the reference colorized surface, a unique RGB color was assigned to each sulcal curve, and then each RGB channel was interpolated to the entire surface via spherical harmonic decomposition. In Fig. 3, the proposed group-wise method shows qualitative improvement over the pair-wise correspondence.

3.2   Human Cortical Surfaces

Pediatric 2-year-old subjects were acquired on a 3T Siemens Trio scanner at a resolution of $1.0\,mm \times 1.0\,mm \times 1.0\,mm$ with T_1-(160 slices, $TR = 2400\,ms$, $TE = 3.16\,ms$, flip angle $= 8°$, matrix $= 256 \times 256$) and T_2-weighted (160 slices, $TR = 3200\,ms$, $TE = 499\,ms$, flip angle $= 120°$, matrix $= 256 \times 256$) scans. We used 10 subjects chosen at random from the scans acquired as part of the Infant Brain Imaging Study (IBIS) network[1] at four different sites (University of North Carolina, University of Washington, Washington University in Saint Louis, and The Children's Hospital of Philadelphia). We randomly selected a single subject as a template, and an expert manually labeled 13 major curves on the template surface: superior temporal sulcus (STS), inferior temporal sulcus (ITS), collateral sulcus (ColS), central sulcus (CS), precentral sulcus (PrCS), postcentral sulcus

---

[1] http://www.ibis-network.org

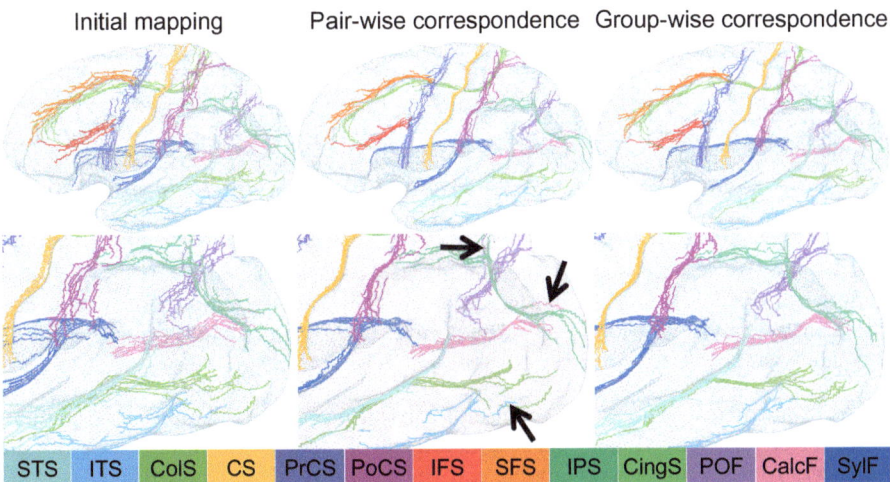

Fig. 4. Sulcal curve agreement by initial spherical mapping (*left*), pair-wise correspondence (*middle*), and group-wise correspondence (*right*). The arrows indicate improved agreement in the group-wise as compared to the pair-wise correspondence.

(PoCS), inferior frontal sulcus (IFS), superior frontal sulcus (SFS), intraparietal sulcus (IPS), cingulate sulcus (CingS), parieto-occipital fissure (POF), calcarine fissure (CalcF), and sylvian fissure (SylF) (see Fig. 4). Only left hemispheres were used in the experiment. For a visual assessment, all major curves were also manually labeled on the 9 remaining subjects.

We applied a leave-one-out cross-validation technique for evaluation of the optimal pole selection. We removed a single sulcus from each individual subject during registration and measured landmark (reconstruction) errors between the removed sulcus reconstructed by the deformation field and its corresponding one in the template. Figure 5 shows the smaller average reconstruction errors for the optimal pole and the reduced coefficient load of the azimuth displacement for the high-frequency harmonic basis functions by the proposed pole selection.

For quantitative evaluation of the correspondence quality, we first measured cross-subject variance estimates of sulcal depth over all vertices of the entire surface across subjects. However, such an evaluation is biased, as sulcal depth is employed in the cost function. We further used variance estimates of cortical thickness as well as a visual assessment of manually labeled sulcal curves for unbiased evaluation. Note that the manually labeled sulcal curves were not used during processing in our pipeline, which implies that the evaluation is independent of the automatically labeled curves. In Table 1 the statistical analysis indicates superior performance of our method for variance of sulcal depth and cortical thickness measures, with significant differences to both the initial mapping and the pair-wise method, revealed by Student's t-test ($p < 0.0001$). Visually, the mapped major sulcal curves shows improved agreement in several regions as compared to the pair-wise correspondence as shown in Fig. 4.

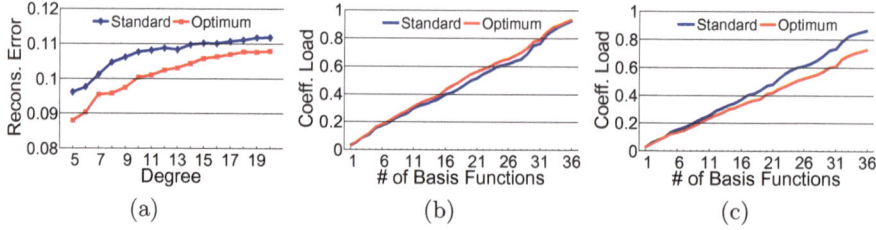

Fig. 5. Reconstruction errors (a) and cumulative coefficient load for elevation (b) and azimuth (c) displacements. No major differences are observed for the elevation displacements, whereas for the azimuth displacements, the total amount of the coefficient load significantly decreases for the optimal pole selection.

Table 1. Statistical analysis of variance of cortical properties. The proposed method shows better variance estimates of sulcal depth and of cortical thickness with significant differences to both the initial mapping and the pair-wise method ($p < 0.0001$).

Method	Sulcal Depth (mm^2)		Cortical Thickness (mm^2)	
	Mean	SD	Mean	SD
Initial	1.9234	1.1300	0.5003	0.3925
Pair-wise	1.5014	0.9759	0.4948	0.3799
Group-wise	**1.3181**	**0.9446**	**0.4741**	**0.3616**

4   Conclusion

We presented an automatic group-wise cortical correspondence method that estimates a smooth continuous deformation field using entropy minimization of sulcal landmarks and sulcal depth maps. In our experiment, the proposed method outperformed the pair-wise method in non-human subjects via a visual assessment and in human subjects via quantitative analysis and visual comparisons. To enable enhanced spherical harmonic decomposition of the deformation field, we also proposed a consistent displacement encoding scheme and an optimal pole selection strategy. In the experiment, the optimal pole selection showed smaller reconstruction errors and more efficient encoding of the deformation field.

The proposed method allows the inclusion of additional information such as DTI-based connectivity akin to [7]. Furthermore, any prior information such as lobar labeling, surface colorization, etc. can be straightforwardly propagated from the template. In this way, inter-subject variability of cortical properties defined in the template space could be incorporated into the entropy minimization.

It is noteworthy that our proposed method is sensitive to the quality of the automatic labeling of sulcal curves, as mislabeled sulcal curve will negatively influence the established correspondence. In our experiment, the proposed method has (qualitatively) shown to be quite resilient to errors in sulcal labeling if the large majority of sulcal curves within the same class are correctly identified. In our future work, we will extend this method to include robust estimators of entropy for the sulcal curves to reduce the influence of such errors.

Acknowledgments. This work was funded by the National Institutes of Health (NIH) under Grant Nos. R01 MH091645-02, U54 EB005149, P50 MH078105-01A2S1, P50 MH078105-01, P50 MH100029, and P30 HD003110.

References

1. Cates, J., Fletcher, P., Styner, M., Shenton, M., Whitaker, R.: Shape modeling and analysis with entropy-based particle systems. In: Karssemeijer, N., Lelieveldt, B. (eds.) IPMI 2007. LNCS, vol. 4584, pp. 333–345. Springer, Heidelberg (2007)
2. Kim, J., Singh, V., Lee, J., Lerch, J., Ad-Dab'bagh, Y., MacDonald, D., Lee, J., Kim, S., Evans, A.: Automated 3-d extraction and evaluation of the inner and outer cortical surfaces using a laplacian map and partial volume effect classification. NeuroImage 27(1), 210–221 (2005)
3. Lyttelton, O., Boucher, M., Robbins, S., Evans, A.: An unbiased iterative group registration template for cortical surface analysis. NeuroImage 34(4), 1535–1544 (2007)
4. Lyu, I., Kim, S., Seong, J., Yoo, S., Evans, A., Shi, Y., Sanchez, M., Niethammer, M., Styner, M.: Cortical correspondence via sulcal curve-constrained spherical registration with application to macaque studies. In: Ourselin, S., Haynor, D. (eds.) Medical Imaging 2013: Image Processing, vol. 8669, pp. 86692X-1–86692X-7. SPIE (2013)
5. Lyu, I., Seong, J., Shin, S., Im, K., Roh, J., Kim, M., Kim, G., Kim, J., Evans, A., Na, D., Lee, J.: Spectral-based automatic labeling and refining of human cortical sulcal curves using expert-provided examples. NeuroImage 52(1), 142–157 (2010)
6. Mangin, J., Riviere, D., Cachia, A., Duchesnay, E., Cointepas, Y., Papadopoulos-Orfanos, D., Scifo, P., Ochiai, T., Brunelle, F., Régis, J.: A framework to study the cortical folding patterns. NeuroImage 23, S129–S138 (2004)
7. Oguz, I., Niethammer, M., Cates, J., Whitaker, R., Fletcher, T., Vachet, C., Styner, M.: Cortical correspondence with probabilistic fiber connectivity. In: Prince, J.L., Pham, D.L., Myers, K.J. (eds.) IPMI 2009. LNCS, vol. 5636, pp. 651–663. Springer, Heidelberg (2009)
8. Park, H., Park, J., Seong, J., Na, D., Lee, J.: Cortical surface registration using spherical thin-plate spline with sulcal lines and mean curvature as features. Journal of Neuroscience Methods 206(1), 46–53 (2012)
9. Powell, M.: The newuoa software for unconstrained optimization without derivatives. In: Large-Scale Nonlinear Optimization, vol. 83, pp. 255–297 (2006)
10. Robbins, S.: Anatomical standardization of the human brain in euclidean 3-space and on the cortical 2-manifold. Ph.D. thesis, McGill University (2004)
11. Seong, J., Im, K., Yoo, S., Seo, S., Na, D., Lee, J.: Automatic extraction of sulcal lines on cortical surfaces based on anisotropic geodesic distance. NeuroImage 49(1), 293–302 (2010)
12. Van Essen, D.: Surface-based approaches to spatial localization and registration in primate cerebral cortex. NeuroImage 23, S97–S107 (2004)
13. Yeo, B., Sabuncu, M., Vercauteren, T., Ayache, N., Fischl, B., Golland, P.: Spherical demons: Fast diffeomorphic landmark-free surface registration. IEEE Trans. Med. Imaging 29(3), 650–668 (2010)
14. Zou, G., Hua, J., Muzik, O.: Non-rigid surface registration using spherical thin-plate splines. In: Ayache, N., Ourselin, S., Maeder, A. (eds.) MICCAI 2007, Part I. LNCS, vol. 4791, pp. 367–374. Springer, Heidelberg (2007)

Diffeomorphic Spectral Matching
of Cortical Surfaces

Herve Lombaert[1], Jon Sporring[1,2], and Kaleem Siddiqi[1]

[1] Centre for Intelligent Machines, McGill University, Montreal
[2] eScience Center, Computer Science, University of Copenhagen, Denmark

Abstract. Accurate matching of cortical surfaces is necessary in many neuroscience applications. In this context diffeomorphisms are often sought, because they facilitate further statistical analysis and atlas building. Present methods for computing diffeomorphisms are based on optimizing flows or on inflating surfaces to a common template, but they are often computationally expensive. It typically takes several hours on a conventional desktop computer to match a single pair of cortical surfaces having a few hundred thousand vertices. We propose a very fast alternative based on an application of spectral graph theory on a novel association graph. Our symmetric approach can generate a diffeomorphic correspondence map within a few minutes on high-resolution meshes while avoiding the sign and multiplicity ambiguities of conventional spectral matching methods. The eigenfunctions are shared between surfaces and provide a smooth parameterization of surfaces. These properties are exploited to compute differentials on highly folded cortical surfaces. Diffeomorphisms can thus be verified and invalid surface folding detected. Our method is demonstrated to attain a vertex accuracy that is at least as good as that of FreeSurfer and Spherical Demons but in only a fraction of their processing time. As a practical experiment, we construct an unbiased atlas of cortical surfaces with a speed several orders of magnitude faster than current methods.

1 Introduction

The cerebral cortex is the center of many important functional activities, including vision and perception, and these are often studied by establishing properties which hold across a large population. These studies thus require fast and accurate algorithms for cortical surface matching are often sought. Early approaches based on volumetric comparisons [1] ignore the complex geometry of cortical folds, and therefore, produce misaligned cortical areas [2]. Recent surface-based approaches either optimize flows on surfaces [3,4,5] or inflate cortical surfaces to a spherical template [6,7,8]. Methods that "flow" surfaces into one another, such as LDDMM [9] and Currents [10,11], provide an elegant mathematical framework that guarantees diffeomorphic deformations between surfaces, i.e., they provide smooth and invertible correspondence maps. However, these methods are computationally expensive and typically require several hours on a conventional desktop

J.C. Gee et al. (Eds.): IPMI 2013, LNCS 7917, pp. 376–389, 2013.

computer to process meshes containing a few thousand vertices. On the other hand, spherical methods, such as FreeSurfer [6] and Spherical Demons [8], establish correspondences on simplified spherical models of the cortex. They handle the complexity of the cortical folds by exploiting metrics that are derived from the original surfaces, such as sulcal depth and mean curvature. Unfortunately, in these approaches, the surfaces need to be inflated to spheres via an expensive process [12]. They too require a few hours to process high-resolution meshes. Current methods may therefore be computationally prohibitive for neuro-studies that involve several thousands of individuals.

Spectral graph theory [13] offers a fast alternative where surfaces containing several hundred thousand vertices can be matched within minutes on a conventional computer [14,15]. Spectral methods facilitate the correspondence problem by matching shapes in the spectral domain. Their spectral representations are in fact invariant to isometry, i.e., two shapes with identical geodesic distances between points have identical spectral representations. However, perturbations in shape isometry, such as expansion and compression of surfaces, change these spectral representations, and thus, alter the matching accuracy. This has limited the use of spectral methods in matching coarse hierarchical structures [16] or in defining global metrics for shape analysis [17]. Previous work attempted to correct these spectral representations with rigid [18] and nonrigid transformations [19,14,15]. In addition, a vertex accuracy of up to 88% of FreeSurfer's performance is achieved in [14] by embedding additional information, such as sulcal depth, in extra dimensions to the spectral representations. However, these extended representations may no longer be smooth and, consequently, the correspondence maps are not guaranteed to be diffeomorphic.

This paper proposes a new accurate surface matching approach that retains the speed advantage of spectral matching methods while guaranteeing diffeomorphic correspondence maps between cortical models of several hundred thousand vertices. Our method exploits a novel association graph that is formed with two meshes and a preliminary correspondence map generated from conventional spectral matching. The spectral decomposition of this unique association graph creates a shared set of eigenvectors that enables a direct comparison between meshes. This contrasts with the conventional spectral methods that produce two separate sets of eigenvectors, and thus, need to handle ambiguities inherent to the sign and multiplicity of eigenvectors, as well as perturbations in isometry. Additionally, the eigenvectors computed with our method provide a smooth parameterization of surfaces. We exploit this property to compute differentials on highly curved cortical surfaces. More precisely, we define a novel Jacobian operator on surfaces to verify diffeomorphisms of correspondence maps and to detect invalid folding of surfaces. Our new diffeomorphic method is demonstrated to produce, in only 350 seconds on a conventional laptop computer (2.53GHz Intel Core 2 Duo), a vertex accuracy that is at least as good as that of FreeSurfer and Spherical Demons. We finally show that our method can be used to construct accurate and unbiased atlases with a significant speed advantage over current competing methods.

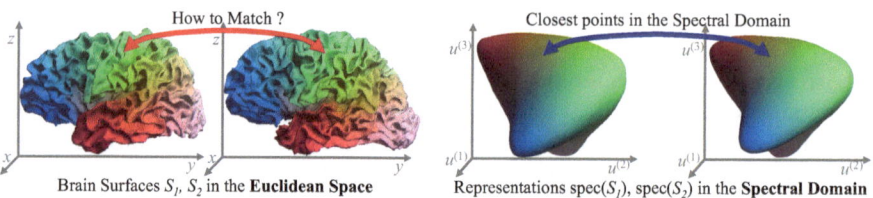

Fig. 1. Spectral matching – Correspondences are made using spectral representations of surfaces (built with Laplacian eigenmodes). To aid visualization, equivalent points have a unique color on the above surfaces (rgb = $u^{(1,2,3)}$).

2   Spectral Matching

We begin by reviewing the basic concepts for matching two shapes with spectral methods.

Graph Laplacian. Let us build the graph $\mathcal{G} = \{\mathcal{V}, \mathcal{E}\}$ from the set of vertices (with position x) and edges of a surface model S. We may define the $|V| \times |V|$ *weighted adjacency* matrix W in terms of node affinities, e.g., $w_{ij} = \|x_i - x_j\|^{-2}$ if $\exists\, e_{ij} \in \mathcal{E}$ (the inverse distance between neighboring points) or 0 otherwise. The diagonal *node degree* matrix D is the sum of all point affinities $d_i = \sum_j W_{ij}$. The *general Laplacian operator* on a graph was formulated in [20] as a $|V| \times |V|$ matrix with the form $\mathcal{L} = G^{-1}(D - W)$ where G is the diagonal *node weighting* matrix ($G = I$, $G = D$ or any meaningful node weighting). It was found [14,15] that setting higher weights on gyral points produces better cortical matchings, e.g., the node weighting, $g_i = \exp(-h_i)$, is the exponential of the sulcal depth h_i (computed with FreeSurfer) at point i.

Spectral Coordinates. The spectral decomposition of the graph Laplacian $\mathcal{L} = U \Lambda U^{-1}$ provides the eigenvalues $\Lambda = \mathrm{diag}(\lambda_0, \lambda_1, \ldots, \lambda_{|V|})$ and the associated eigenvectors $U = \left(u^{(0)}, u^{(1)}, \ldots, u^{(|V|)}\right)$, where $u^{(\cdot)}$ is a column of U. The values of $u^{(\cdot)}$ depict in fact a vibration mode of the shape S, which is a surface function, [13], and thus, the term *eigenmode* is used. These eigenmodes must be additionally corrected for their sign ambiguity, multiplicity, and perturbation in isometry (see [14,15] for more details). We denote as the *spectral representation*, spec(S), a k-dimensional embedding of the shape S where a point has the *spectral coordinates* defined as $u^{(1,\ldots,k)}$, which is a row of the truncated matrix U^k.

Spectral Matching with Vertex Accuracy. The correspondence problem is to match a point x_i on S_1, with $y_{c(i)}$ on S_2. The map $c : x_i \mapsto y_{c(i)}$ (also denoted here as $S_1 \mapsto S_2 \circ c$) is established with pairs of closest points (u, v) between spectral representations spec(S_1) and spec(S_2), as illustrated in Fig. 1. However, in order to achieve vertex accuracy in cortical surface matching, [14,15] proposed to incorporate extra information, such as sulcal depth h, in extended

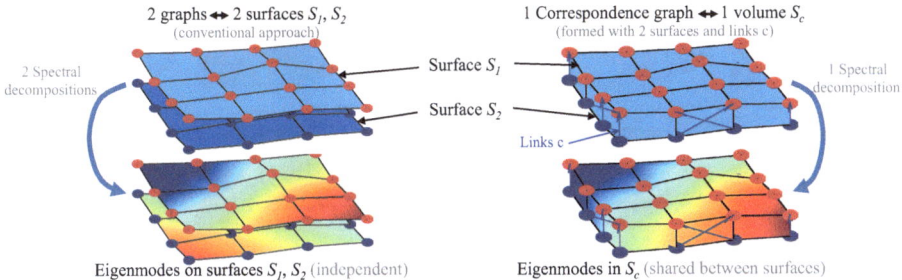

Fig. 2. Correspondence Graph – *Left*: Conventional spectral matching decomposes 2 independent graphs (built from 2 surfaces) – *Right*: Our approach decomposes 1 correspondence graph (built from one volumetric entity formed with the surfaces and a map c between them). Note that in our approach eigenmodes (u, v) do match without the explicit handling of their sign flips, reordering or changes in isometry. They are smooth even if c is irregular (shown here with many-to-one and crossing links c).

spectral representations where point coordinates are then (u, h). The map $c(i) = \arg\min_j \|(u_i, h_i)_{S_1} - (u_j, h_j)_{S_2}\|^2$ is solved with a simple nearest-neighbor search between these extended representations. Unfortunately, this incorporation of extra information creates discontinuities in the correspondence map in the sense that neighbors in space may no longer be neighbors in the extended spectral representations.

3 Diffeomorphic Spectral Matching

We now show that the spectral decomposition of a novel associative graph provides the ability to compute diffeomorphic maps between two surfaces.

3.1 Correspondence Graph

We define the *correspondence graph* $\mathcal{G}_c = \{\mathcal{V}_{1,2}, \mathcal{E}_{1,2,c}\}$ as the union of the set of vertices and edges of two surfaces $S_{1,2}$ with an initial set of correspondence links c between both surfaces. The initial map c, not necessarily dense, may be computed with a conventional spectral matching methods. We used [14] since it is optimized for cortical matching. This correspondence graph is a 2-split graph, where each surface is a separable set, and has its $|\mathcal{V}_1 \cup \mathcal{V}_2| \times |\mathcal{V}_1 \cup \mathcal{V}_2|$ weighted adjacency matrix in the form:

$$W_c = \begin{bmatrix} W_1 & W_{12} \\ W_{21} & W_2 \end{bmatrix}, \tag{1}$$

where W_1 and W_2 are the weighted adjacency matrices of both surfaces and W_{12}, W_{21} are the weighted adjacency matrices defined by the links c between surfaces, i.e., $w_{ij} = \|x_i - x_j\|^{-2}$ if nodes (i, j) or (j, i) are connected. The graph Laplacian operator $\mathcal{L}_c$ of $\mathcal{G}_c$ is defined as previously. Such a graph is illustrated in Fig. 2 where surfaces have been simplified to small patches to ease illustration.

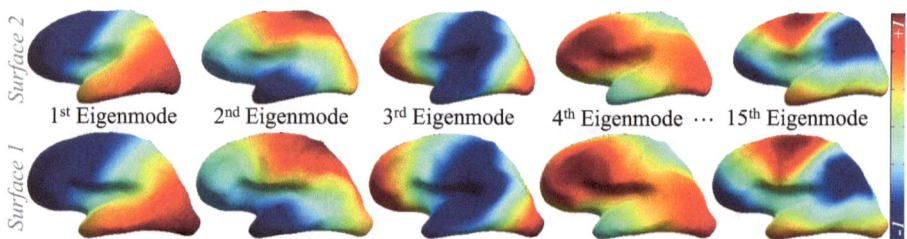

Fig. 3. Spectral Decomposition of the Correspondence Graph – One graph is decomposed (rather than two as in conventional methods). This produces a smooth and shared parameterization (u, v) (color-coded between $[-1, +1]$) between surfaces. This prevents handling sign flips, reordering and corrections in isometry of (u, v). The principal eigenmodes are shown on smoothed meshes to aid visualization.

Shared Parameterization. The graph $\mathcal{G}_c$ embeds both surfaces within one single entity S_c, which is a double layered graph that represents two cortical surfaces interconnected with c. The spectral decomposition, $\mathcal{L}_c = U_c \Lambda_c U_c^{-1}$, therefore provides one orthonormal basis of the whole entity S_c. This contrasts with conventional spectral matching methods that produce two independent sets of eigenmodes. Moreover, each eigenmode $u_c^{(\cdot)}$, a $|\mathcal{V}_1 \cup \mathcal{V}_2|$ column vector of U_c, is separable back into two functions: $u^{(\cdot)}$, the first $|\mathcal{V}_1|$ values of $u_c^{(\cdot)}$, is a surface function on S_1, and $v^{(\cdot)}$, which is the last $|\mathcal{V}_2|$ values of $u_c^{(\cdot)}$, is a surface function on S_2 (illustrated in Fig. 3). They share in fact the same eigenvalue and represent the same vibration mode. There is therefore no need to correct for a sign flip between $u^{(\cdot)}$ and $v^{(\cdot)}$, nor to reorder the set of eigenmodes or correct for perturbations in isometry since the surface functions $u^{(\cdot)}$ and $v^{(\cdot)}$ are derived from the same single entity and not from two independent surfaces.

Smooth Parameterization. Courant's nodal line theorem [21,22,23] demonstrates that any n^{th} eigenmode of the graph Laplacian has the remarkable property of being *smooth* and *monotonous* between at most n poles of vibrations. This phenomenon is observed on Fig. 3 where $u^{(1)}$ and $u^{(2)}$ have two poles (red and blue spots), $u^{(3)}$ has three poles, $u^{(4)}$ has four poles, and so on.

Since S_c always remains one single double-layered entity, the function $u^{(\cdot)}$ varies smoothly within the global shape formed by S_c (as illustrated in Fig. 2 *right*, both $u^{(1)}$ and $v^{(1)}$ always increase smoothly in the same direction even if c has crossing links). The coordinate system formed by $u^{(1,\dots,k)}$ and $v^{(1,\dots,k)}$ provides, therefore, a smooth parameterization within the entity S_c and is shared between surfaces $S_{1,2}$.

Differentiable Space. We further consider each eigenmode $u^{(\cdot)}$ as continuous and differentiable between the discrete values at the mesh nodes. This is motivated by the fact that the graph Laplacian approximates the Laplace-Beltrami operator on Riemannian manifolds [24]. Since the mesh nodes associate a smooth spectral coordinate with a position in space, $u \mapsto x$ on S_1 and $v \mapsto y$ on S_2, it is possible to model the positions of points on S_1 and S_2 that have equal spectral coordinates, using any type of differentiable interpolation. We chose the Gaussian kernel for its regularity (differentiable in C^∞) and asymptotic behavior [25]. For instance, the node i on S_1 has its equivalent point on S_2 with position:

$$y'_i = \frac{\sum_{j \in \mathcal{N}_{\psi(i)}} \omega_{ij} y_j}{\sum_{j \in \mathcal{N}_{\psi(i)}} \omega_{ij}}, \tag{2}$$

where $\mathcal{N}_{\psi(i)}$ is the set of neighboring nodes of $\psi(i)$ on S_2; $\psi(i)$ is the node on S_2 with the closest spectral coordinate to u_i (the mapping ψ is found as previously with a nearest-neighbor search $\psi(i) = \arg\min_j \|u_i - v_j\|^2$); and ω_{ij} is the spectral similarity, e.g, $\omega_{ij} = \exp\left(-\|v_i - v_j\|^2/2\sigma^2\right)$. This simple modeling scheme creates a k-D differentiable space $\mathcal{S}^k$ between S_1 and S_2.

Diffeomorphic Mapping. The differentiable space $\mathcal{S}^k$ allows us to establish symmetric correspondences between surfaces by locating points on S_1 and S_2 that have equal spectral coordinates, $\phi_{1\mapsto2} : x_i \mapsto y'_i$ using Eq. 2 and conversely $\phi_{2\mapsto1} : y_j \mapsto x'_j$. Such a mapping prevents an invalid folding of space (crossing of links is avoided since $\mathcal{S}^k$ is monotonous between poles of vibration) as well as the collapse of space (many-to-one correspondences are prevented since equivalent points (x_i, y'_i) have unique spectral coordinates). The mapping ϕ between $S_{1,2}$ is consequently diffeomorphic (ϕ is smooth, bijective, and invertible $\phi_{1\mapsto2}^{-1} = \phi_{2\mapsto1}$).

Jabocian Operator on Surfaces. The continuous spectral parameterization (u, v) may be used to compute differentials on the curved space defined by $S_{1,2}$. We express the correspondence map ϕ in terms of (u, v) with $\phi_u : u_i \mapsto v'_i$ and define its Jacobian matrix as $J(\phi_u) = \left(\frac{\partial \phi_{u^{(1)}}}{\partial u^{(1)}} \cdots \frac{\partial \phi_{u^{(1)}}}{\partial u^{(k)}}; \cdots; \frac{\partial \phi_{u^{(k)}}}{\partial u^{(1)}} \cdots \frac{\partial \phi_{u^{(k)}}}{\partial u^{(k)}} \right)$ where $\partial \phi_{u_i^{(\cdot)}}$ and $\partial u_i^{(\cdot)}$ are estimated in the neighborhood $\mathcal{N}_i$ using Taylor series approximation for central differences. Its determinant is simply denoted as the Jacobian $|J|$. To illustrate, two equivalent surface elements on $S_{1,2}$ may appear flipped in space, and thus, generate a negative Jacobian $|J(\phi)|$ when it is expressed in Cartesian coordinates, while in fact, these vectors may have been always pointing outwards from the surface. Expressing the variations in the spectral coordinates generates in this case a positive Jacobian $|J(\phi_u)|$. We, therefore, propose to study the variations of a surface map ϕ using the Jacobian matrix $J(\phi_u)$ expressed in terms of spectral coordinates (u, v).

Objective Function. The initial map c is generated using [14], which minimizes $E_c = (u_{S_1} - u_{S_2} \circ c)^2 + (h_{S_1} - h_{S_2} \circ c)^2$. To summarize our method, c is reused to build the correspondence graph $\mathcal{G}_c$, whose spectral decomposition creates a differentiable parameterization $(u, v)_{S_c}$ in $\mathrm{spec}(S_c)$. A symmetric and diffeomorphic map ϕ is then found by minimizing $E_\phi = (u_{S_c} - v_{S_c} \circ \phi)^2$ via simple nearest-neighbor searches.

3.2   Unbiased Atlas Construction

The computation of an average shape typically relies on an iterative evolution of an initial reference shape [26,27,27]. This process may, however, be biased by the choice of the initial reference [28]. We define the average cortical surface S_0 as the geometric mean of all surfaces in a dataset $\mathscr{S}$. The position of its vertices is defined with $\bar{x}_i = \frac{1}{|\mathscr{S}|} \sum_{t \in \mathscr{S}} x_i'^{(t)}$, where $x_i'^{(t)}$ is the interpolated position of point i on surface S_t, computed with Eq. 2. This requires the computation of mappings $\{\phi_{0 \mapsto t}\}_{t \in \mathscr{S}}$, as well as an initial reference surface S_0^{init}.

Transitivity. Since ϕ is diffeomorphic, it is also transitive [29]. The composition of mappings $\phi_{s \mapsto t} \circ \phi_{t \mapsto u}$, from S_s to S_t to S_u, is therefore identical to the mapping $\phi_{s \mapsto u}$, from S_s to S_u. This transitive relation implies that the mapping from the initial reference $\phi_{0 \mapsto t}$ is equivalent to the composition with any other intermediate mapping, $\phi_{0 \mapsto t} = \phi_{0 \mapsto s} \circ \phi_{s \mapsto t}$, and the average position $\bar{x}_i$ is consequently unbiased to the choice of S_0^{init} since the mapping $\phi_{0 \mapsto t}$ could be composed with any intermediate surface S_s in the dataset. Our diffeomorphic spectral method, therefore, has the advantage that it constructs an unbiased atlas with a direct, one-step, approach (without the need for an iterative evolution of S_0^{init} [28]).

4   Results

We begin our validation by verifying the key properties of our method and then assess its matching accuracy using synthetic and real cortical surfaces. Our dataset consists of 16 real cortical surfaces ranging from 109k to 174k vertices with an average resolution of 0.88mm, generated from MRI.

4.1   Verifying Properties of Our Method

We verify through a series of simple experiments that our method produces *a)* a shared parameterization between surfaces, *b)* diffeomorphic mappings from irregular (i.e., non-smooth) correspondences, and *c)* mappings that maintain transitivity.

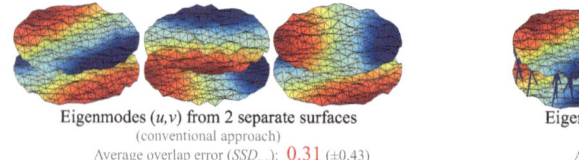

Eigenmodes (u,v) from 2 separate surfaces
(conventional approach)
Average overlap error ($SSD_{u,v}$): 0.31 (±0.43)

Eigenmodes (u,v) from 1 correspondence graph
(our approach gives stable (u,v))
Average overlap error ($SSD_{u,v}$): 0.01 (±0.01)

Fig. 4. Shared Parameterization – Surfaces show eigenmodes $(u^{(1)}, v^{(1)})$ color-coded between $[-1, +1]$. The eigenmodes computed on separate surfaces may not overlap on them (*left*), whereas the spectral decomposition of 1 correspondence graph produces a common set of eigenmodes (*right*). 3 samples out of 1000 are shown. Overlap errors are measured with $SSD_{u,v}$.

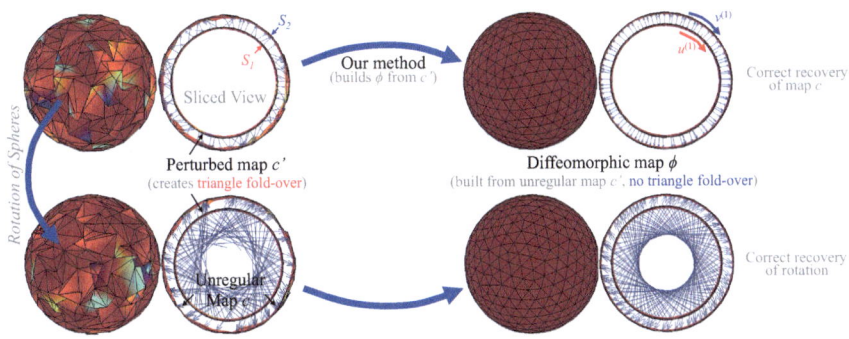

Fig. 5. Diffeomorphic Mapping — An arbitrary and randomly perturbed correspondence map c (seen in the sliced views) folds over triangles on a sphere (blue indicates a face normal pointing inward), whereas the diffeomorphic map generated from c (by decomposing $\mathcal{G}_c$) recovers the original correspondences c and guarantees no folding of space by ϕ. The mapping ϕ is therefore diffeomorphic since (u, v) is smooth and bijective between surfaces.

Shared Parameterization. We study the stability of eigenmodes on circular shapes. Since these shapes have ambiguous axes of symmetry, $\mathrm{spec}(S_1)$ and $\mathrm{spec}(S_2)$ should differ by an arbitrary rotation on disks. However, $\mathrm{spec}(S_c)$ should theoretically produce a shared set of eigenmodes (u, v) between surfaces. We use two uniform meshes of a disk, whose node positions have been perturbed with Gaussian noise (this perturbs isometry between disks). Their ground truth correspondence map is defined as their direct overlap, $c(i) = i$. This mapping c is then perturbed with Gaussian noise $c'(i) = \arg\min_j \|(y_i + \text{noise}) - y_j\|^2)$ (as shown in Fig. 4). Firstly, we generate $u = \mathrm{spec}(S_1)$ and $v = \mathrm{spec}(S_2)$ for both disks. This is the conventional spectral matching approach. Secondly, we generate $(u, v) = \mathrm{spec}(S_c)$ using the correspondence graph formed by c'. We repeat the experiment a thousand times and measure the overlap $SSD_{u,v} = \sum_{i \in S_1} \|u_i - v_i\|^2$. As expected, (u, v) rotates arbitrarily on the disks when they are computed separately. The worst overlap among the thousand samples gives $SSD_{u,v} = 0.95$. In contrast, (u, v) demonstrate a better overlap when decomposing the correspondence graph. The worst overlap, at $SSD_{u,v} = 0.05$, actually still produces aligned eigenmodes (Fig. 4). The decomposition of a correspondence graph is therefore demonstrated to generate a stable set (u, v) of eigenmodes that is in common between surfaces.

Diffeomorphic Mapping. We now verify the smoothness of correspondence maps by testing for folding of the triangulation between S_1 and $S_2 \circ \phi$. We use two uniform models $S_{1,2}$ of a sphere and rotate them arbitrarily. The face normals on both models are all initially pointing outward. We use the direct mapping $c(i) = i$ between $S_{1,2}$ as ground truth. We randomly perturb it as in the previous experiment (see slice view in Fig. 5). A discontinuity in c' is detected with a triangle fold-over (we check if a face normal points inward from the sphere). We generate a diffeomorphic map ϕ by decomposing the correspondence

Distance between transitive compositions $S_{1\to2\to3}$ and $S_{1\to3}$ (should be identical)

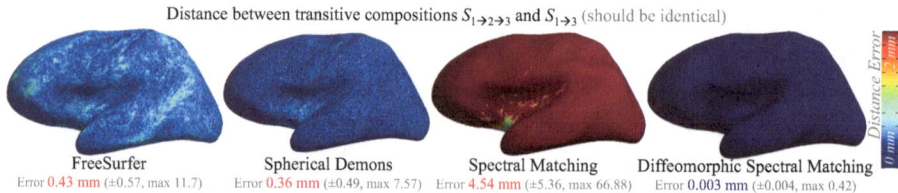

FreeSurfer	Spherical Demons	Spectral Matching	Diffeomorphic Spectral Matching
Error 0.43 mm (±0.57, max 11.7)	Error 0.36 mm (±0.49, max 7.57)	Error 4.54 mm (±5.36, max 66.88)	Error 0.003 mm (±0.004, max 0.42)

Fig. 6. Transitive Mapping – The average distance error between 4,096 (16^3) composed surfaces $S_1 \circ \phi_{1\mapsto2} \circ \phi_{2\mapsto3}$ and $S_1 \circ \phi_{1\mapsto3}$. FreeSurfer and the Spherical Demons have an error below the mesh resolution (0.88mm). The non-diffeomorphic spectral matching fails to achieve transitivity since it does not generate diffeomorphic maps. The new diffeomorphic spectral matching demonstrates transitivity with an error of 0.00292(±0.00432) mm.

graph formed with c' and check if any face normal points inward. We repeat the experiment a thousand times with random perturbation of c and random rotations of spheres. Each time, ϕ is found to be identical to c (a one-to-one map) and no triangle fold-over is observed across the experiment (smooth map). The map ϕ produced by our method is, therefore, demonstrated to be diffeomorphic (smooth and bijective).

Transitive Mapping. We check for transitivity of our correspondence maps using real cortical surfaces. We first compute all 256 correspondence maps ϕ between all pairs of cortical surfaces with four methods: FreeSurfer (FS) [6], Spherical Demons (SD) [8], Spectral Matching (SM) [14], and our diffeomorphic spectral matching. We then generate pairs of surfaces $S_1 \circ \phi_{1\mapsto2} \circ \phi_{2\mapsto3}$ and $S_1 \circ \phi_{1\mapsto3}$ using all 4,096 (16^3) possible compositions $\phi_{1\mapsto2} \circ \phi_{2\mapsto3}$ (using Eq. 2 and compositions of vertex indexing). We finally verify transitivity by measuring the distances between equivalent points (x, y) on composed surfaces, $\mathrm{sqrt}(\sum_{i \in S_1} \|x_{\phi_{1\mapsto2}\circ\phi_{2\mapsto3}}(i) - y_{\phi_{1\mapsto2\mapsto3}}(i)\|^2)$ (Fig. 6). The non-diffeomorphic SM did not satisfy transitivity with an error of 4.54 mm, i.e., $S_{1\mapsto2\mapsto3} \neq S_{1\mapsto3}$. FS and SD demonstrated transitivity with errors of 0.43mm, 0.36mm (below the mesh resolution of 0.88mm) while our method produced a lower error of 0.003mm, i.e., $S_{1\mapsto2\mapsto3} \approx S_{1\mapsto3}$.

4.2   Validating Correspondence Maps

We now assess the matching accuracy by testing for robustness to deformation and we compare our method with FreeSurfer and Spherical Demons.

Robustness to Deformation. The matching accuracy is evaluated in this synthetic experiment by monitoring the difference between the computed map ϕ and the ground truth $c(i) = i$, while increasing the level of deformation of the surface. A surface is deformed with the transformation $z' = (1-\alpha)z$. This simulated head compression creates a controlled environment that does not produce any triangle fold-over, nor any intersecting face. We deform all 16 cortical surfaces

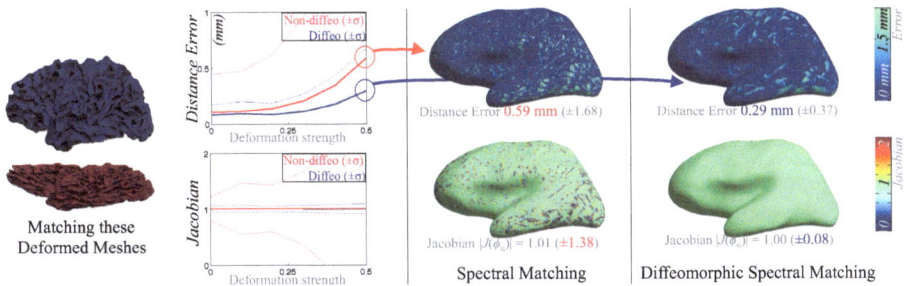

Fig. 7. Robustness to Deformation – We monitor the correspondence error between two meshes while increasing the deformation strength. The errors at maximal deformation (in mm) and the Jacobian of the correspondence map are shown. Our diffeomorphic spectral matching produces smaller errors and smoother correspondence maps.

by varying $\alpha \in [0; 0.5]$ and observe the differences between conventional spectral matching [14] and our diffeomorphic method. At maximal deformation $\alpha = 0.5$, SM gives an average error of 0.58mm (± 1.68) while our method gives an error of 0.29mm (± 0.08). The Jacobian $|J(\phi_u)|$ is strikingly different in both methods (Fig. 7): SM produces negative Jacobians (non-smooth map, breaking diffeomorphism) with an average $|J(\phi_u)| = 1.01(\pm 1.38)$, while our method gives strictly positive Jacobian (i.e., always diffeomorphic) with $|J(\phi_u)| = 1.00(\pm 0.08)$.

Benchmark with FreeSurfer and Spherical Demons. A ground truth mapping between real cortical surfaces is unfortunately unknown. However, the widely used FreeSurfer and Spherical Demons methods, can be used as a benchmark for evaluating the matching accuracy of our method. Our dataset has for all surfaces a labeling of cortical parcellations [30]. We verify how our method aligns these parcellations between individuals and compare these overlaps with the performance of FS, SD and SM. We measure the Dice overlap ($2|A \cap B|/(|A|+|B|)$) for 12 major parcellations between all 256 pairs of cortices (Fig. 8) and found an average Dice overlap of 0.84 (± 0.08) for FS (one matching took 3 hours), 0.85 (± 0.07) for SD (one matching took 2 hours), 0.82 (± 0.08) for SM (one matching took 250 seconds), and 0.83 (± 0.08) for our method (one matching took 350 seconds). Timing was measured on a 2.53GHz Core 2 Duo laptop with 8GB of RAM. The matching accuracy of spectral methods is arguably similar, achieving 99% accuracy of FS and SD, but they have a clear speed advantage. Clearly, conventional SM produces highly irregular, or non-smooth, maps with an average Jacobian of $|J(\phi_u)| = 1.61(\pm 1.00)$. This is observed as holes and island patches in the projected parcels in Fig. 8. Our method has the notable advantage of producing diffeomorphic maps with strictly positive and smooth $|J(\phi_u)| = 1.00(\pm 0.12)$.

4.3 Building Unbiased Atlases

We conclude by building atlases of cortical surfaces and verify that their constructions are unbiased to an initial reference. To do so, an arbitrary initial reference

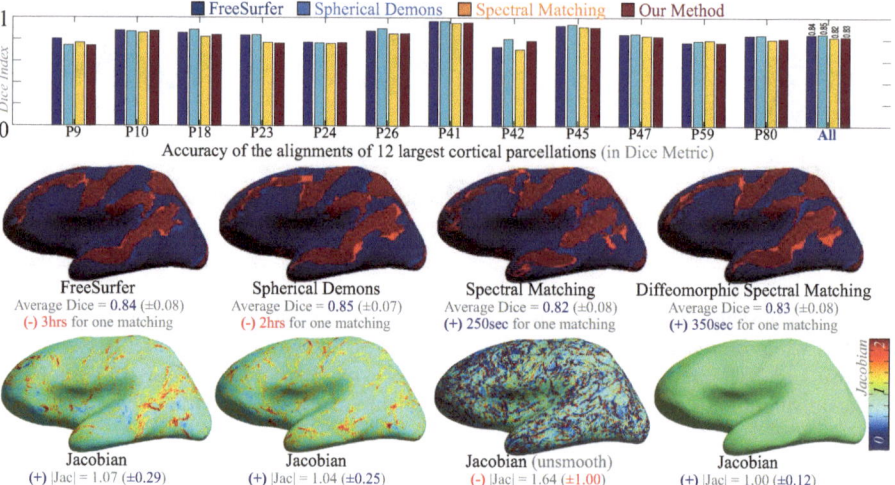

Fig. 8. Accuracy of Parcellation Alignments – Bar plot on *Top*: Average accuracy of 256 alignments of cortical parcellations (measured with Dice Index), using FreeSurfer (dark blue), Spherical Demons (light blue), Spectral Matching (yellow), and our Diffeomorphic Spectral Matching (red) – *Middle*: One example showing the alignment of 12 major parcellations (light blue for first cortex, light red for projected second cortex) – *Bottom*: Determinant of Jacobian (conventional spectral matching produces non-smooth maps). Our method yields similar accuracy than the state-of-the-art but in a fraction of its time.

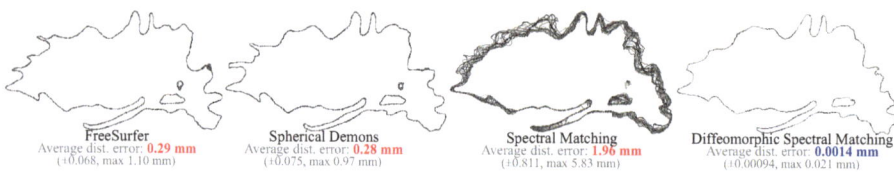

Fig. 9. Unbiased Atlas Construction – Overlap of 16 average shapes computed from 16 different initial references using FS, SD, SM, and our method. To aid visualization, surface contours are of the same slice. Our method produces average shapes that are unbiased to the initial reference (all contours overlap with a variability of 0.001mm).

is first defined as one of the cortical surfaces in the dataset, e.g., $S_0^{\text{init}} = S_1$. All surfaces are then matched to this reference and the atlas is built using the average position $\bar{x}$ of all mapped points as described in Sec. 3.2. We build 16 different atlases by iterating $S_0^{\text{init}} = S_i$. The bias to the initial reference is evaluated by measuring the average standard deviation of the distances between equivalent points across all 16 different atlases. This measures the variability of distances between atlas boundaries. We find a boundary variability of 0.29mm (± 0.07) for FS, 0.28mm (± 0.08) for SD, 1.96mm (± 0.81) for SM, and 0.0014mm (± 0.0009) for our method. Fig. 9 shows the contour overlays of all 16 atlases and shows that our method produces stable atlases that are unbiased to the choice of initial reference, i.e., they all overlap.

5   Conclusion

Our method contributes to the challenging problem of cortical matching. First, we enhanced current spectral approaches to achieve diffeomorphism, and second, we provided a very fast algorithm that has a vertex accuracy comparable to FreeSurfer and Spherical Demons, in fact, 20 times faster with equivalent accuracy. Besides the clear speed advantage, we tackled the diffeomorphic matching problem with a direct, one-step approach that fundamentally contrasts with current iterative solutions. Our smooth and bijective correspondences are found via simple nearest-neighbor searches in the spectral domain rather than with an optimization of flows or with an inflation of surfaces to spheres. In fact, these current iterative approaches, including the LDDMM, could even reuse our diffeomorphic maps as initialization, and perhaps, gain speed and accuracy. Our method currently relies on an initial correspondence map c. We used the map generated from [14], which allowed us to obtain our high-accuracy maps. Our spectral approach can also be regarded as an action that builds a diffeomorphic map ϕ from an irregular map c. In this context, it would be interesting to see how our method performs with other maps. For instance, c could be built from fast graph matching methods [31,32] or even from manual pairing of surface landmarks. Moreover, our approach may also be related to methods based on the heat kernel [33], however, we do not exploit their multiscale properties. To conclude, our new diffeomorphic spectral matching method provides a fast and accurate alternative to current methods specialized for cortical matching.

Acknowledgments. The authors would like to thank Stanley Durrleman and BT Thomas Yeo for helpful comments, and Jonathan Polimeni for suggestions and for providing data. Funding is from the Fonds de Recherche du Québec (FRQNT) and and the Natural Sciences and Engineering Research Council of Canada (NSERC).

References

1. Talairach, J., Szikla, G., Tournoux, P., Prosalentis, A., Bordas-Ferrier, M., Covello, L., Iacob, M., Mempel, E.: Atlas stereotaxique du telencephale. Masson (1967)
2. Amunts, K., Malikovic, A., Mohlberg, H., Schormann, T., Zilles, K.: Brodmann's areas 17 and 18 brought into stereotaxic space-where and how variable? NeuroImage (2000)
3. Drury, H., Van Essen, D., Joshi, S., Miller, M.: Analysis and comparison of areal partitioning schemes using 2-D fluid deformations. NeuroImage 3 (1996)
4. Van Essen, D., Drury, H.: Structural and functional analyses of human cerebral cortex using a surface-based atlas. Neuroscience 17(18) (1997)
5. Thompson, P., Toga, A.W.: A surface-based technique for warping three-dimensional images of the brain. TMI 15(4) (1996)

6. Fischl, B., Sereno, M.I., Tootell, R.B., Dale, A.M.: High-resolution intersubject averaging and a coordinate system for cortical surface. Human Brain Mapping 8 (1999)

7. Fischl, B., Rajendran, N., Busa, E., Augustinack, J., Hinds, O., Yeo, T., Mohlberg, H., Amunts, K., Zilles, K.: Cortical folding patterns and predicting cytoarchitecture. Cereb. Cortex 18(8) (2007)

8. Yeo, T., Sabuncu, M., Vercauteren, T., Ayache, N., Fischl, B., Golland, P.: Spherical demons: fast diffeomorphic landmark-free surface registration. TMI 29(3) (2010)

9. Beg, F., Miller, M., Trouvé, A., Younes, L.: Computing large deformation metric mappings via geodesic flows of diffeomorphisms. IJCV 61 (2005)

10. Vaillant, M., Glaunès, J.: Surface matching via currents. In: Christensen, G.E., Sonka, M. (eds.) IPMI 2005. LNCS, vol. 3565, pp. 381–392. Springer, Heidelberg (2005)

11. Durrleman, S., Pennec, X., Trouvé, A., Ayache, N.: Statistical models of sets of curves and surfaces based on currents. MedIA 13(5) (2009)

12. Segonne, F., Pacheco, J., Fischl, B.: Geometrically accurate Topology-Correction of cortical surfaces using nonseparating loops. TMI 26(4) (2007)

13. Chung, F.: Spectral Graph Theory. AMS (1997)

14. Lombaert, H., Grady, L., Polimeni, J.R., Cheriet, F.: Fast brain matching with spectral correspondence. In: Székely, G., Hahn, H.K. (eds.) IPMI 2011. LNCS, vol. 6801, pp. 660–673. Springer, Heidelberg (2011)

15. Lombaert, H., Grady, L., Polimeni, J.R., Cheriet, F.: FOCUSR: Feature Oriented Correspondence using Spectral Regularization - A Method for Accurate Surface Matching. TPAMI (2012)

16. Reuter, M.: Hierarchical shape segmentation and registration via topological features of Laplace-Beltrami eigenfunctions. IJCV (2009)

17. Niethammer, M., Reuter, M., Wolter, F.-E., Bouix, S., Peinecke, N., Koo, M.-S., Shenton, M.E.: Global Medical Shape Analysis Using the Laplace-Beltrami Spectrum. In: Ayache, N., Ourselin, S., Maeder, A. (eds.) MICCAI 2007, Part I. LNCS, vol. 4791, pp. 850–857. Springer, Heidelberg (2007)

18. Mateus, D., Horaud, R., Knossow, D., Cuzzolin, F., Boyer, E.: Articulated shape matching using Laplacian eigenfunctions and unsupervised registration. In: CVPR (2008)

19. Jain, V., Zhang, H.: Robust 3D shape correspondence in the spectral domain. In: CSMA (2006)

20. Grady, L., Polimeni, J.R.: Discrete Calculus: Applied Analysis on Graphs for Computational Science. Springer (2010)

21. Courant, R., Hilbert, D.: Methods of Mathematical Physics. Wiley (1989)

22. Tlusty, T.: A relation between the multiplicity of the second eigenvalue of a graph Laplacian, Courant's nodal line theorem and the substantial dimension of tight polyhedral surfaces. Linear Algebra 16 (2010)

23. Colin de Verdiere, Y.: Multiplicités des valeurs propres. Laplaciens discrets et laplaciens continus. Rendiconti di Matematica 13(7) (1993)

24. Belkin, M., Niyogi, P.: Convergence of Laplacian eigenmaps. In: NIPS (2006)

25. Nielsen, M., Andresen, P.R.: Feature displacement interpolation. In: ICIP (1998)

26. Studholme, C., Cardenas, V.: A template free approach to volumetric spatial normalization of brain anatomy. Pattern Recogn. Lett. 25(10) (2004)

27. Zöllei, L., Learned-Miller, E., Grimson, W., Wells, W.: Efficient population registration of 3D data. In: Liu, Y., Jiang, T.-Z., Zhang, C. (eds.) CVBIA 2005. LNCS, vol. 3765, pp. 291–301. Springer, Heidelberg (2005)

28. Guimond, A., Meunier, J., Thirion, J.P.: Average brain models: A convergence study. CVIU 77(2) (2000)
29. Christensen, G., Johnson, H.: Invertibility and transitivity analysis for nonrigid image registration. J. Elec. Im. 12(1) (2003)
30. Fischl, B., van der Kouwe, A., Destrieux, C., Halgren, E., Segonne, F., Salat, D.H., Busa, E., Seidman, L.J., Goldstein, J., Kennedy, D., Caviness, V., Makris, N., Rosen, B., Dale, A.M.: Automatically parcellating the human cerebral cortex. Cereb. Cortex 14(1) (2004)
31. Gold, S., Rangarajan, A.: A graduated assignment algorithm for graph matching. TPAMI 18(4) (1996)
32. Zheng, Y., Doermann, D.: Robust point matching for nonrigid shapes by preserving local neighborhood structures. TPAMI 28(4) (2006)
33. Ovsjanikov, M., Mérigot, Q., Mémoli, F., Guibas, L.: One point isometric matching with the heat kernel. Computer Graphics Forum 29(5) (2010)

The Non-Local Bootstrap – Estimation of Uncertainty in Diffusion MRI

Pew-Thian Yap*, Hongyu An, Yasheng Chen, and Dinggang Shen

Department of Radiology and Biomedical Research Imaging Center (BRIC)
The University of North Carolina at Chapel Hill, U.S.A.
{ptyap,hongyu_an,yasheng_chen,dgshen}@med.unc.edu

Abstract. Diffusion MRI is a noninvasive imaging modality that allows for the estimation and visualization of white matter connectivity patterns in the human brain. However, due to the low signal-to-noise ratio (SNR) nature of diffusion data, deriving useful statistics from the data is adversely affected by different sources of measurement noise. This is aggravated by the fact that the sampling distribution of the statistic of interest is often complex and unknown. In situations as such, the bootstrap, due to its distribution-independent nature, is an appealing tool for the estimation of the variability of almost any statistic, without relying on complicated theoretical calculations, but purely on computer simulation. In this work, we present new bootstrap strategies for variability estimation of diffusion statistics in association with noise. In contrast to the residual bootstrap, which relies on a predetermined data model, or the repetition bootstrap, which requires repeated signal measurements, our approach, called the *non-local bootstrap* (NLB), is non-parametric and obviates the need for time-consuming multiple acquisitions. The key assumption of NLB is that local image structures recur in the image. We exploit this self-similarity via a multivariate non-parametric kernel regression framework for bootstrap estimation of uncertainty. Evaluation of NLB using a set of high-resolution diffusion-weighted images, with lower than usual SNR due to the small voxel size, indicates that NLB is markedly more robust to noise and results in more accurate inferences.

1 Introduction

Diffusion magnetic resonance imaging (MRI) [16] reveals spectacular details of brain tissue micro-structures through observation of water diffusion patterns. It therefore captures vital information that is of paramount importance for *in vivo* investigation of white matter and connectivity alterations that are associated with brain diseases, development, and aging [24, 27–30]. However, the noisy nature of diffusion MRI data adversely affects the estimation precision of quantities such as local fiber orientations, which will eventually introduce uncertainty in important applications such as white matter fiber tractography. The impact of noise can be large, especially in high angular resolution diffusion imaging (HARDI), where relatively high diffusion weightings (i.e, b-values) are employed for increasing angular contrast.

---

* Corresponding author.

J.C. Gee et al. (Eds.): IPMI 2013, LNCS 7917, pp. 390–401, 2013.

Considerable efforts have been directed to modeling the variability caused by noise [8, 13]. However, the models used often assume normality and are yet to be verified in complex situations where various noise sources, such as physiologic variation, scanner instability, and imaging noise, might be simultaneously involved. The distributions of these types of noise are non-normal and cannot be adequately modeled using simple models that rely on the normality assumption. To avoid unrealistic assumptions, an appealing alternative is to use the bootstrap method.

The bootstrap method is a non-parametric procedure for estimating the statistical properties of a population from a limited number of measurement samples, without prior assumptions about the population distribution [6]. It was designed to replace complex and often inaccurate approximations to uncertainty measures with computer simulation based on real data [2]. For instance, the bootstrap has been shown to be capable of accurately estimating the true uncertainty in fiber orientations [14]. The repetition bootstrap and the residual bootstrap are two commonly used bootstrap techniques in medical image analysis. The repetition bootstrap [17, 18] depends on repeated measurements of signal for each diffusion-sensitizing gradient, a requirement which might be difficult to fulfill with limited acquisition time. On the other hand, the residual bootstrap [2, 15] is a model-based approach that resamples the residuals of a linear regression model that is fitted to the data. Since the residual bootstrap does not require repeated measurements, it can be applied to data that are acquired under clinically realistic scan times. However, since it relies on a model, the model needs to describe the signal measurements adequately so that the error terms across all diffusion gradients will have a common mean of zero. Extra care should also be taken so that the model does not overfit the signal, especially in noisy conditions, causing misleading reduction in variability.

In this work, we introduce novel non-parametric bootstrap strategies that will allow bootstrap samples to be generated from a single image without requiring repeated signal measurements as well as predetermined data models. Our approach hinges on the observation that local imaging information recurs in an image. This self-similarity implies that imaging information coming from spatially distant (non-local) regions can be exploited for more effective estimation of statistics of interest. In what follows, we will first show that estimation using non-local information can be seen as a non-parametric regression problem with a multivariate predictor variable that captures local neighborhood information and a univariate or multivariate response variable that is related to the statistic of interest. Based on this regression-based formulation, we then show that the uncertainty of the statistic can be estimated with bootstrap samples generated using case resampling or residual resampling. We will demonstrate with empirical evidence that the proposed bootstrap strategies are significantly more robust to noise and yields inferences that are markedly more accurate.

2   Approach

We will first discuss how the non-local estimation problem can be recast as a non-parametric kernel regression problem. We will then show how this regression-based formulation can be used to compute bootstrap estimates of the variability of statistics of concern.

2.1 Non-Local Estimation as Non-parametric Kernel Regression

Let $\mathbf{Z} = [(\mathbf{x}_1, \mathbf{y}_1), \dots, (\mathbf{x}_n, \mathbf{y}_n)]$ be a sample of n independent observations of bivariate random variable $(\mathbf{X}, \mathbf{Y})$. $\mathbf{X}$ is a $\mathbb{R}^{d_X}$-valued predictor random variable and $\mathbf{Y}$ is a $\mathbb{R}^{d_Y}$-valued response random variable. The regression function of $\mathbf{Y}$ on $\mathbf{X}$ is

$$m(\mathbf{x}) = \mathrm{E}(\mathbf{Y}|\mathbf{X} = \mathbf{x}). \tag{1}$$

The problem is to obtain an estimate of $m(\mathbf{x})$, $\hat{m}(\mathbf{x})$, using the n observations, such that $\hat{m}(\mathbf{x})$ tends to $m(\mathbf{x})$ as $n \to \infty$.

Nadaraya [21] and Watson [26] proposed to estimate $m(\mathbf{x})$ as a locally weighted average, using a kernel as a weighting function. The Nadaraya-Watson estimator is

$$\hat{m}_{\mathbf{H}}(\mathbf{x}) = \frac{\sum_{i=1}^n K_{\mathbf{H}}(\mathbf{x} - \mathbf{x}_i) \mathbf{y}_i}{\sum_{i=1}^n K_{\mathbf{H}}(\mathbf{x} - \mathbf{x}_i)}, \tag{2}$$

where $K_{\mathbf{H}}(\cdot) = |\mathbf{H}|^{-1} K(\mathbf{H}^{-1} \cdot)$ is a multivariate kernel function with symmetric positive-definite bandwidth matrix $\mathbf{H}$ [11]. $K(\mathbf{u})$ satisfies

$$\text{①}\ K(\mathbf{u}) \geq 0,\ \forall \mathbf{u}; \quad \text{②} \int K(\mathbf{u}) d\mathbf{u} = 1; \quad \text{③} \int \mathbf{u} K(\mathbf{u}) d\mathbf{u} = 0;$$
$$\text{④} \int \mathbf{u}\mathbf{u}^{\mathsf{T}} K(\mathbf{u}) d\mathbf{u} = \mu_2(K)\mathbf{I},\ \mu_2(K) < \infty. \tag{3}$$

The first and second requirements ensure that, when used for density estimation, the kernel results in a density estimate that is indeed a probability density function (i.e., non-negative with unit integral). The third requirement ensures that the expected value of the random variable computed from the estimated distribution is equal to the average of the observations. The last requirement ensures that the estimation bias is bounded. The estimation of $m(\mathbf{x})$ can be improved by employing locally weighted least squares regression, as shown in [23].

The estimator can be derived by noting that estimates of the unknown joint density function $f(\mathbf{x}, \mathbf{y})$ of $\mathbf{X}$ and $\mathbf{Y}$ and density function $f(\mathbf{x})$ of $\mathbf{X}$ can be obtained via kernel density estimation as

$$\hat{f}_{\mathbf{H},\mathbf{H}'}(\mathbf{x}, \mathbf{y}) = \frac{1}{n} \sum_{i=1}^n K_{\mathbf{H}}(\mathbf{x} - \mathbf{x}_i) K_{\mathbf{H}'}(\mathbf{y} - \mathbf{y}_i), \quad \hat{f}_{\mathbf{H}}(\mathbf{x}) = \frac{1}{n} \sum_{i=1}^n K_{\mathbf{H}}(\mathbf{x} - \mathbf{x}_i). \tag{4}$$

These, together with the fact that

$$\mathrm{E}(\mathbf{Y}|\mathbf{X}) = \int \mathbf{y} f(\mathbf{y}|\mathbf{x}) d\mathbf{y} = \int \mathbf{y} \frac{f(\mathbf{x}, \mathbf{y})}{f(\mathbf{x})} d\mathbf{y}, \tag{5}$$

lead to (2). From the theory of kernel density estimation, it is known that $\hat{f}(\mathbf{x}, \mathbf{y})$ and $\hat{f}(\mathbf{x})$ converge asymptotically ($n \to \infty$, $\mathbf{H} \to 0$, $n\mathbf{H} \to \infty$) to the true densities of the underlying distribution.

Determining the non-local means [1] can be recast as a regression problem with voxel neighborhoods as the predictor and the corresponding central voxels as the response. The mean estimates are non-local as in principle they are computed from voxels throughout the image, not limited by physical distance. For instance, if we let $\mathbf{x}_1 \ldots, \mathbf{x}_n$ be the intensity values of voxel blocks throughout the image ($d_X = \#$ voxels in each block, assuming each voxel is scalar-valued) and $\mathbf{y}_1, \ldots, \mathbf{y}_n$ be the intensity values of the corresponding central voxels ($d_Y = 1$), then, if $\mathbf{x}$ is the neighborhood intensity values of a voxel located at $\mathbf{p}$, $\hat{m}_{\mathbf{H}}(\mathbf{x})$ in (2) becomes the non-local mean at voxel location $\mathbf{p}$. This important observation, in addition to allowing us to improve non-local estimation using different kernel regression estimators that have been vastly studied [9], also provides the underpinning of the bootstrap strategies that will be discussed next. Before proceeding, we would like to highlight the fact that there is nothing in the regression framework that limits $\mathbf{X}$ and $\mathbf{Y}$ to random variables representing image intensity values; they can in fact be any features that are derived from the image. This regression framework also provides an explanation as to why non-local means denoising produces good white 'method noise' [1].

2.2 Non-Local Bootstrap Strategies

Bootstrap methods depend on the notion of *bootstrap samples*. Having observed a random sample of size n from a distribution with cumulative density function F (or probability density function f),

$$F \to (\mathbf{z}_1, \ldots, \mathbf{z}_n), \tag{6}$$

the *empirical distribution function* $\hat{F}$ is defined to be the discrete distribution that puts probability $1/n$ on each $\mathbf{z}_i$. The arrow notation ($\to$) indicates that the sample values are outcomes of independent and identically distributed random variables, each with distribution function F, i.e., $\mathbf{z}_i \overset{\text{i.i.d.}}{\sim} F$. A bootstrap sample is defined as a random sample of size n, $\mathbf{Z}^* = (\mathbf{z}_1^*, \mathbf{z}_2^*, \ldots, \mathbf{z}_n^*)$, that is drawn from $\hat{F}$, i.e.,

$$\hat{F} \to (\mathbf{z}_1^*, \mathbf{z}_2^*, \ldots, \mathbf{z}_n^*). \tag{7}$$

The star ($*$) notation indicates that $\mathbf{Z}^*$ is not the actual dataset $\mathbf{Z}$, but rather a randomized version of $\mathbf{Z}$ obtained via resampling with replacement. Generation of a significant amount of bootstrap samples allows us to estimate the sampling distribution of a statistic T, which can be used to make inferences about a population parameter θ. If we denote the estimate $\hat{\theta} = t(\mathbf{Z})$, for each bootstrap sample we can compute a *bootstrap replication* of $\hat{\theta}$,

$$\hat{\theta}^* = t(\mathbf{Z}^*), \tag{8}$$

a collection of which gives us an estimate of the sampling distribution of $\hat{\theta}$.

Recasting the non-local estimation problem in the form of kernel regression allows us to devise a number of bootstrap strategies for the estimation of the variability of statistics computed from the image. Out of the many possibilities, we will introduce here two non-local bootstrap strategies.

Case-Resampling Non-Local Bootstrap (CR-NLB): The first bootstrap scheme that we propose is called the *case-resampling non-local bootstrap* (CR-NLB). Recall from the discussion in the previous section that $\hat{m}_{\mathbf{H}}(\mathbf{x})$ is the regression function for $\mathbf{Y}$ with respect to $\mathbf{X}$. If $\mathbf{p}_1, \ldots, \mathbf{p}_n$ denote the spatial locations of all voxels in an image, with corresponding neighborhood $\mathbf{x}_1, \ldots, \mathbf{x}_n$, then $\hat{m}_h(\mathbf{x}_1), \ldots, \hat{m}_{\mathbf{H}}(\mathbf{x}_n)$ are the non-local means at these locations. Determining the variability of the non-local means can hence be interpreted as determining the variability of the regression function. One way to achieve this is by resampling with replacement from the sample $\mathbf{Z} = [(\mathbf{x}_1, \mathbf{y}_1), \ldots, (\mathbf{x}_n, \mathbf{y}_n)]$ to generate bootstrap sample $\mathbf{Z}^* = [(\mathbf{x}_{i_1}, \mathbf{y}_{i_1}), \ldots, (\mathbf{x}_{i_n}, \mathbf{y}_{i_n})]$, where $(i_1, \ldots, i_n)$ is a random sample of integers from 1 to n. For each bootstrap sample $\mathbf{Z}^*$, we generate a bootstrap replication of $\hat{m}_{\mathbf{H}}(\mathbf{x})$, denoted as $\hat{m}_{\mathbf{H}}^*(\mathbf{x})$. To estimate the standard error of $\hat{m}_{\mathbf{H}}(\mathbf{x})$, the bootstrap algorithm works by drawing a large number (B) of independent bootstrap samples $\mathbf{Z}_1^*, \ldots, \mathbf{Z}_B^*$, evaluating the corresponding bootstrap replications, and computing the empirical standard deviation of the replications. Note that bootstrap statistics of quantities other than the mean can be determined similarly.

CR-NLB is similar to the conventional repetition bootstrap as applied in [18]; but the 'repeated measurements' are now coming from non-local regions with voxel neighborhoods that are similar to the neighborhood of a voxel of interest. Since n is typically very large (possibly a few hundreds of thousands), the small sample size problem is now less of an issue. This approach does not rely on any assumptions regarding residuals of the sample with respect to the regression function and is hence less susceptible to difficulties caused by residual heteroscedasticity. But if the residuals are indeed homoscedastic, a residual resampling approach, discussed next, is a viable alternative.

Residual-Resampling Non-Local Bootstrap (RR-NLB): The second bootstrap scheme is called the *residual-resampling non-local bootstrap* (RR-NLB). RR-NLB resamples the residuals of the observations $\mathbf{Z} = [(\mathbf{x}_1, \mathbf{y}_1), \ldots, (\mathbf{x}_n, \mathbf{y}_n)]$ with respect to the regression curve $\hat{m}_{\mathbf{H}}(\mathbf{x})$, i.e.,

$$\mathbf{r}_i = \mathbf{y}_i - \hat{m}_{\mathbf{H}}(\mathbf{x}_i). \qquad (9)$$

The residuals will not necessarily have zero mean; so to let the resampled residuals reflect the behavior of the true observation errors, they should first be recentered as $\tilde{\mathbf{r}}_i = \mathbf{r}_i - \bar{\mathbf{r}}$, where $\bar{\mathbf{r}} = \frac{1}{n} \sum_i^n \mathbf{r}_i$. The residuals can be further corrected for leverage [5] by dividing each recentered residual by $\sqrt{1 - g_i}$, where $g_i = K_{\mathbf{H}}(\mathbf{0})/\sum_{j=1}^n K_{\mathbf{H}}(\mathbf{x}_i - \mathbf{x}_j)$. Each bootstrap sample is generated via

$$\mathbf{Z}^* = [(\mathbf{x}_1, \hat{m}_{\mathbf{H}}(\mathbf{x}_1) + \tilde{\mathbf{r}}_{i_1}), \ldots, (\mathbf{x}_n, \hat{m}_{\mathbf{H}}(\mathbf{x}_n) + \tilde{\mathbf{r}}_{i_n})], \qquad (10)$$

where $(i_1, \ldots, i_n)$, as before, is a random sample of integers from 1 to n. This bootstrap strategy allows residuals to be used from throughout the whole image, giving us a great deal more information at our disposal.

If $\mathbf{Y}$ is multivariate, as in the case of diffusion MRI where each voxel can be seen as containing a vector of signal measurements corresponding to different diffusion-sensitizing directions, a more confined sampling approach can be employed by limiting the sampling within each voxel to capture more localized and subtle variation. That is, assuming homoscedasticity across elements of the residual vector, we can generate a bootstrap sample via

$$\mathbf{Z}^* = [(\mathbf{x}_1, \hat{m}_{\mathbf{H}}(\mathbf{x}_1) + \tilde{\mathbf{r}}_1^*), \ldots, (\mathbf{x}_n, \hat{m}_{\mathbf{H}}(\mathbf{x}_n) + \tilde{\mathbf{r}}_n^*)], \qquad (11)$$

where in this case, if we use $[\cdot]^{(k)}$ to denote the k-th element of a vector and if $\tilde{\mathbf{r}}_i = [\tilde{\mathbf{r}}_i^{(1)}, \ldots, \tilde{\mathbf{r}}_i^{(d_Y)}]^{\mathrm{T}}$, then $\tilde{\mathbf{r}}_i^* = [\tilde{\mathbf{r}}_i^{(j_1)}, \ldots, \tilde{\mathbf{r}}_i^{(j_{d_Y})}]^{\mathrm{T}}$, with $(j_1, \ldots, j_{d_Y})$ being a random sample of integers from 1 to d_Y. The residual is recentered differently from above as $\tilde{\mathbf{r}}_i^{(j)} = \mathbf{r}_i^{(j)} - \bar{r}_i$, where $\bar{r}_i = \frac{1}{d_Y} \sum_{j=1}^{d_Y} \mathbf{r}_i^{(j)}$. This approach is similar to the conventional residual bootstrap [2] but does not require a predetermined model. We will use this formulation in the experiments so that comparison can be made with respect to the conventional residual bootstrap [2].

2.3 Kernel and Bandwidth

A variety of kernel functions are possible in general [9]. Consistent with non-local means [1], we use a Gaussian kernel, i.e.,

$$K(\mathbf{u}) = \frac{1}{\sqrt{2\pi}} \exp\left(-\frac{1}{2}\mathbf{u}^{\mathrm{T}}\mathbf{u}\right), \tag{12}$$

and hence

$$K_{\mathbf{H}}(\mathbf{u}) = |\mathbf{H}|^{-1} K(\mathbf{H}^{-1}\mathbf{u}) = \frac{1}{\sqrt{2\pi}|\mathbf{H}|} \exp\left(-\frac{1}{2}\mathbf{u}^{\mathrm{T}}\mathbf{H}^{-2}\mathbf{u}\right). \tag{13}$$

The choice of $\mathbf{H}$ is dependent on the application. For simplicity, we require equal bandwidth h in all dimensions, corresponding to $\mathbf{H} = h\mathbf{I}$. If different bandwidths are needed, we can set $\mathbf{H} = \mathrm{diag}(h_1, \ldots, h_d)$. We can also set $\mathbf{H} = \mathbf{\Sigma}^{-\frac{1}{2}}$, the covariance matrix of the data. Using such a bandwidth matrix corresponds to a transformation of the data to obtain an identity covariance matrix.

The choice of h depends upon a trade-off between the bias and variance of the estimate of the regression function: a small h gives small bias and large variance, whereas a large h results in the opposite. We determine h based on the fact that, in non-local estimation, we are mainly interested in voxels with neighborhoods that ideally differ only by noise. That is, if the standard deviation of the noise is σ_{noise}, following [3] we set $h = \sigma_{\mathrm{noise}} \sqrt{d_X}$. The noise level σ_{noise} can be estimated globally as shown in [19] or spatial-adaptively as shown in [20]; we implemented the former for simplicity.

2.4 Application to Uncertainty Estimation in Diffusion MRI

The non-local bootstrap strategies described above can be applied to uncertainty estimation in diffusion MRI data. To do this, we have to first define the predictor vector $\mathbf{x}$ and the response vector $\mathbf{y}$. Since, as noted in [4], noise will interfere with block matching in non-local estimation, we average the signal measurements across gradient directions for increased signal-to-noise ratio (SNR). More specifically, for each voxel $\mathbf{p}$, we define a predictor vector $\mathbf{x}$ based on the corresponding local neighborhood: $[\langle S(\mathbf{g}, \mathbf{p}(1)) \rangle_{\mathbf{g}}, \ldots, \langle S(\mathbf{g}, \mathbf{p}(k)) \rangle_{\mathbf{g}}, \ldots]^{\mathrm{T}}$, where $\langle S(\mathbf{g}, \mathbf{p}) \rangle_{\mathbf{g}}$ denotes the averaging of diffusion-weighted signal $S(\mathbf{g}, \mathbf{p})$ over gradient direction $\mathbf{g} \in \mathcal{G}$. Here, $\mathbf{p}(k) \in \mathcal{N}(\mathbf{p})$, with $\mathcal{N}(\mathbf{p})$ denoting the neighborhood of $\mathbf{p}$. If the noise level for the measured signal is σ_{noise}, the noise level for the average signal is $\sigma_{\mathrm{noise}}/\sqrt{|\mathcal{G}|}$, where $|\mathcal{G}|$ denotes the total number of gradient directions. The response vector $\mathbf{y}$ is simply defined as the signal vector at location $\mathbf{p}$.

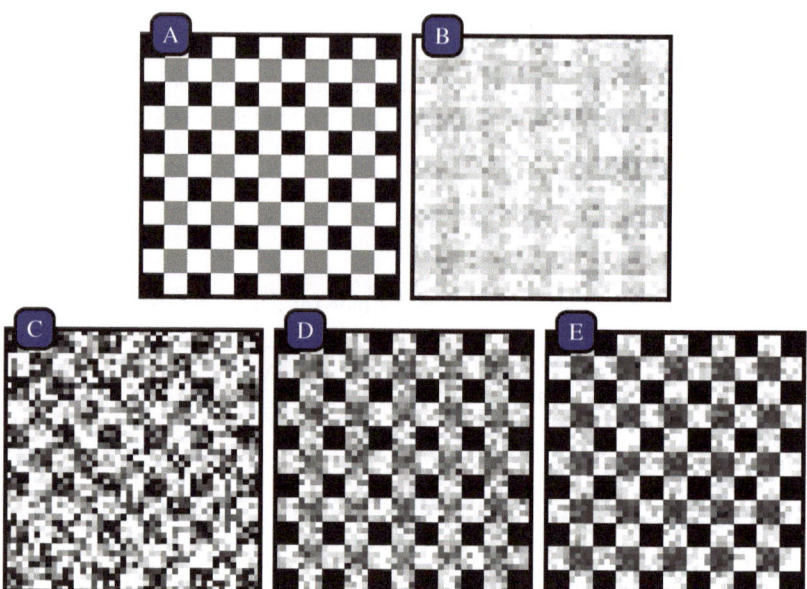

Fig. 1. Synthetic Data. Exemplar results for $\sigma_{noise} = 100$. (A) The anisotropy image of the noise-free DWI phantom. (B) The anisotropy image of a noisy realization of the phantom. Average ϕ-images over 10 noisy realizations of the phantom for (C) RR-B, (D) CR-NLB, and (E) RR-NLB.

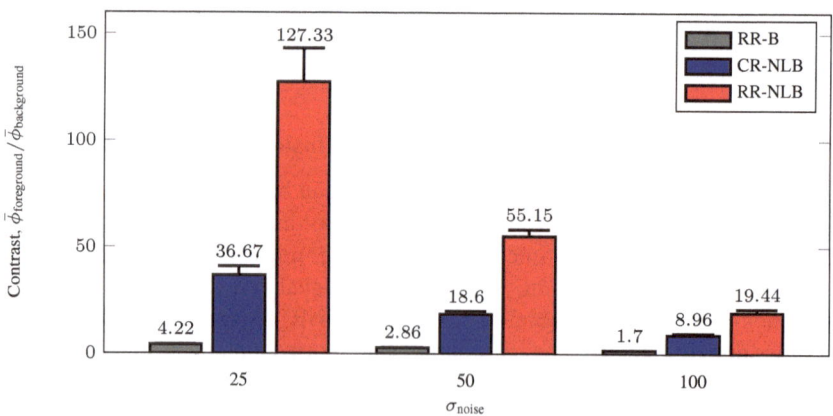

Fig. 2. Contrast. The average foreground-background contrast based on the ϕ-values. The error bars (some barely visible due to insignificant variability) indicate the standard deviations.

3   Experimental Results

We evaluated the effectiveness of the proposed bootstrap strategies (CR-NLB and RR-NLB) using *in silico* and *in vivo* diffusion MRI data. The conventional residual-resampling bootstrap (RR-B) [2], with spherical harmonics as the model [15], was used as comparison baseline. Unless otherwise stated, the neighborhood block radius was set to 2, giving a block of size $2(2) + 1 = 5$ in each dimension and a predictor vector $\mathbf{x}$ of size $d_X = 5^3|\mathcal{G}| = 125|\mathcal{G}|$. $B = 1,000$ bootstrap samples were generated for all cases. The bandwidth $\mathbf{H}$ was determined based on the data noise level, as described previously.

3.1   In Silico Data

We used diffusion tensors and their mixtures to generate a phantom of size 56×56 for evaluation [see Fig. 1(a)]. One group of tensors were oriented in the horizontal direction and another group in the vertical direction. At locations where these two groups cross, a mixture of two tensors with equal volume fraction was used to model the crossings. The tensor parameters were $\lambda_1 = 8 \times 10^{-4}\,\mathrm{mm^2/s}$, $\lambda_2 = \lambda_3 = 1.5 \times 10^{-4}\,\mathrm{mm^2/s}$, and $b = 1,000\,\mathrm{s/mm^2}$. The baseline signal was $S_0 = 1,000$. The background isotropic signal was generated using an isotropic tensor with $\lambda = 1.5 \times 10^{-3}\,\mathrm{mm^2/s}$ and $S_0 = 500$. The (42) gradient directions were taken from the *in vivo* dataset (see next section). Note that these diffusion parameters were carefully chosen to mimic the *in vivo* data.

To evaluate the effectiveness of the proposed bootstrap strategies, we evaluated whether they result in correct inference of the anisotropy of the diffusion signal. To achieve this, we evaluated whether the high-order spherical harmonic coefficients are significant in the presence of noise. That is, we were interested whether the statistic

$$T = \sum_{l=2,4,6} \sum_{m=-l,-l+1,\ldots,l} c_{l,m}^2 \tag{14}$$

was significant. Coefficient $c_{l,m}$ is real-valued and is associated with the spherical harmonic function of order l and degree m. Only even orders were used because of the antipodal symmetric assumption associated with the diffusion signal. The more significant the coefficients associated with the higher order spherical harmonic functions ($l > 0$), i.e., the anisotropic energy, the greater the possibility that the diffusion signal is anisotropic. The coefficient for $l = 0$ is associated with isotropic diffusion. To gauge the significance, we determined the variability of T with respect to noise, i.e., the standard error of T, using CR-NLB, RR-NLB, and RR-B. An indicator of the significance of the observed anisotropic energy T_{observed} is given by measure

$$\phi = \frac{T_{\text{observed}}}{\hat{\mathrm{se}}_B}, \tag{15}$$

where $\hat{\mathrm{se}}_B$ is the bootstrap estimate of the standard error using B bootstrap samples. A large value for ϕ indicates high significance; a small value indicates otherwise.

For RR-B, the spherical harmonic coefficients estimated by fitting the spherical harmonic functions to the diffusion signal were used to compute T_{observed} as given by (14).

The standard error of the statistic was then estimated using the bootstrap replicates computed from the bootstrap samples that were generated via resampling of the residuals, as done in standard practice [2, 12]. For CR-NLB and RR-NLB, $T_{observed}$ was computed by spherical harmonics fitted to $\hat{m}_{\mathbf{H}}(\mathbf{x})$ and the respective standard errors were estimated based on the resampling schemes described in Section 2.2. A goal common to these methods is the attempt to determine the variability of some form of regression function.

For evaluation, various levels ($\sigma_{noise} = 25, 50, 100$) of Rician noise was added to the synthesized diffusion signal. Noise level $\sigma_{noise} = 100$ corresponds to that of the *in vivo* data. We computed the Rician noise corrupted signal $\tilde{S}$ as

$$\tilde{S} = \sqrt{(S + n_1)^2 + (n_2)^2} \tag{16}$$

where n_1 and n_2 are sampled from normal distributions with zero mean and variance σ_{noise}^2. Each value for $\tilde{S}$ is a sample from a Rician distribution with parameters S and σ_{noise}.

We computed ϕ with 10 noisy realizations of the phantom and the average ϕ-images for the case of $\sigma_{noise} = 100$ are shown in Fig. 1. Note that ideally the ϕ-value should be high for the (anisotropic) foreground and low for the (isotropic) background. RR-B [Fig. 1(C)] is apparently less capable in differentiating between isotropic and anisotropic voxels in severely noisy conditions. CR-NLB [Fig. 1(D)] and RR-NLB [Fig. 1(E)] yield much better contrast between the foreground and the background. Fig. 1(B) shows that, due to noise, the contrast of the (generalized) anisotropy between the anisotropic and isotropic regions is low. Despite the heavy amount of noise, the results indicate that the anisotropy of the original data [Fig. 1(A)] can still be inferred quite accurately using CR-NLB and RR-NLB. For quantitative evaluation, we computed the contrast between the foreground and the background, i.e., the ratio of the ϕ-value averages: $\bar{\phi}_{foreground}/\bar{\phi}_{background}$. The results for all tested noise levels, shown in Fig. 2, again validate that CR-NLB and RR-NLB give much improved contrast over RR-B.

3.2   In Vivo Data

A set of high-resolution $(1mm)^3$ diffusion-weighted images were acquired using a Siemens 3T TIM Trio MR scanner with the acquisition technique reported in [22]. Diffusion gradients were applied in 42 non-collinear directions with diffusion weighting $b = 1,000\,s/mm^2$. The imaging matrix was 192×192 with a field of view of $192 \times 192\,mm^2$. The slice thickness was 1 mm. The low SNR of this dataset, due to the small voxel volume, makes it ideal for testing the various bootstrap strategies.

It is a well-accepted fact that the anisotropy of the white matter (WM) is high owing to diffusion anisotropy resulting from restricted diffusion. On the other hand, the diffusion signal captured from the gray matter (GM) and the cerebrospinal fluid (CSF) should be very close to isotropic. We expect to see similar patterns for results given by the different bootstrap methods.

The same evaluation, as performed on the synthetic data, was performed on this *in vivo* data. The results, shown in Fig. 3, indicate that CR-NLB and RR-NLB correctly yield high ϕ-values for WM regions and low ϕ-values for GM and CSF regions. RR-B

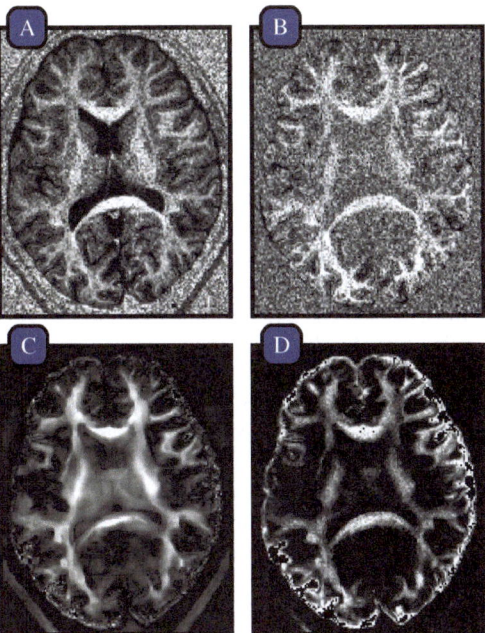

Fig. 3. Real Data. The ϕ-images as indicator of anisotropy. (A) The anisotropy image of the DWI data. The results given by (B) RR-B, (C) CR-NLB, and (D) RR-NLB.

shows a much reduced contrast between these regions, indicating low differentiability between them. As was done for the synthetic data, we computed the contrast between the anisotropic WM regions and the isotropic GM and CSF regions. We obtained results similar to those of the synthetic data: 1.68 for RR-B, 2.51 for CR-NLB, and 2.26 for RR-NLB. These values indicate that CR-NLB and RR-NLB are significantly more likely than RR-B to result in correct inferences of the anisotropy in the presence of noise.

4   Conclusion

We have presented two novel bootstrap strategies that show that bootstrapping can be performed within a regression framework that pulls together non-local information coming from the whole image. To the best of our knowledge, this is the first work that marries non-local estimation, non-parametric kernel regression, and the bootstrap in a single unified framework. Recasting non-local means as a regression problem allows us to further refine non-local means by studying different kernel estimators, by performing bias analysis [10], and by incorporating other more advanced techniques such as adaptive kernel regression [25] and local polynomial regression [7]. Our results indicate that both case-resampling and residual-resampling non-local bootstrap approaches yield results that are markedly better than the commonly used residual bootstrap. Future directions entail applying these bootstrap strategies to evaluating the variability of local fiber orientations, fiber trajectories, and connectivity between brain regions.

Acknowledgment. This work was supported in part by a UNC start-up fund and NIH grants (EB006733, EB008374, EB009634, MH088520, AG041721, and MH100217).

References

1. Buades, A., Coll, B., Morel, J.M.: A review of image denoising algorithms, with a new one. Multiscale Modeling and Simulation 4(2), 490–530 (2005)
2. Chung, S., Lu, Y., Henry, R.G.: Comparison of bootstrap approaches for estimation of uncertainties of DTI parameters. NeuroImage 33(2), 531–541 (2006)
3. Coupé, P., Yger, P., Prima, S., Hellier, P., Kervrann, C., Barillot, C.: An optimized blockwise nonlocal means denoising filter for 3-D magnetic resonance images. IEEE Transaction on Medical Imaging 27, 425–441 (2008)
4. Dabov, K., Foi, A., Katkovnik, V., Egiazarian, K.: Image denoising by sparse 3D transform-domain collaborative filtering. IEEE Transactions on Image Processing 16(8), 2080–2095 (2007)
5. Davison, A., Hinkley, D.: Bootstrap Methods and their Application. Cambridge Series in Statistical and Probabilistic Mathematics. Cambridge University Press (1997)
6. Efron, B., Tibshirani, R.J.: An Introduction to the Bootstrap. Monographs on Statistics and Applied Probablilty. Chapman and Hall (1994)
7. Fan, J., Gijbels, I.: Local Polynomial Modelling and Its Applications. Monographs on Statistics and Applied Probablilty. Chapman and Hall (1996)
8. Friman, O., Farnebäck, G., Westin, C.F.: A Bayesian approach for stochastic white matter tractography. IEEE Transactions on Medical Imaging 25, 965–977 (2006)
9. Härdle, W.: Applied Nonparametric Regression. Cambridge University Press (1992)
10. Härdle, W., Bowman, A.W.: Bootstrapping in nonparametric regression: Local adaptive smoothing and confidence bands. Journal of the American Statistical Association 83(401), 102–110 (1988)
11. Härdle, W., Müller, M.: Multivariate and semiparametric kernel regression. In: Schimek, M.G. (ed.) Smoothing and Regression: Approaches, Computation, and Application. Wiley & Sons, Inc., Hoboken (2000)
12. Haroon, H.A., Morris, D.M., Embleton, K.V., Alexander, D.C., Parker, G.J.M.: Using the model-based residual bootstrap to quantify uncertainty in fiber orientations from Q-ball analysis. IEEE Transaction on Medical Imaging 28(4), 535–550 (2009)
13. Jbabdi, S., Woolrich, M., Andersson, J., Behrens, T.: A Bayesian framework for global tractography. NeuroImage 37(1), 116–129 (2007)
14. Jeurissen, B., Leemans, A., Tournier, J.D., Sijbers, J.: Can residual bootstrap reliably estimate uncertainty in fiber orientation obtained by spherical deconvolution from diffusion-weighted MRI? In: Proceedings 14th Annual Meeting of the Organization of Human Brain Mapping (2008)
15. Jeurissen, B., Leemans, A., Jones, D.K., Tournier, J.D., Sijbers, J.: Probabilistic fiber tracking using the residual bootstrap with constrained spherical deconvolution. Human Brain Mapping 32(3), 461–479 (2011)
16. Johansen-Berg, H., Behrens, T.E. (eds.): Diffusion MRI — From Quantitative Measurement to In-Vivo Neuroanatomy. Elsevier (2009)
17. Jones, D.: Determining and visualizing uncertainty in estimates of fiber orientation from diffusion tensor MRI. Magnetic Resonance in Medicine 49(1), 7–12 (2003)
18. Lazar, M., Alexander, A.L.: Bootstrap white matter tractography (BOOT-TRAC). NeuroImage 24(2), 524–532 (2005)

19. Manjón, J., Carbonell-Caballero, J., Lull, J., García-Martí, G., Martí-Bonmatí, L., Robles, M.: MRI denoising using non-local means. Medical Image Analysis 12(4), 514–523 (2008)

20. Manjón, J., Coupé, P., Martí-Bonmatí, L., Collins, D., Robles, M.: Adaptive non-local means denoising of MR images with spatially varying noise levels. Journal of Magnetic Resonance Imaging 31(1), 192–203 (2010)

21. Nadaraya, E.: On estimating regression. Theory of Probability and its Applications 9(1), 141–142 (1964)

22. Porter, D.A., Heidemann, R.M.: High resolution diffusion-weighted imaging using readout-segmented echo-planar imaging, parallel imaging and a two-dimensional navigator-based reacquisition. Magnetic Resonance in Medicine 62(2), 468–475 (2009)

23. Ruppert, D., Wand, M.: Multivariate locally weighted least squares regression. The Annals of Statistics 22(3), 1346–1370 (1994)

24. Shi, F., Yap, P.T., Gao, W., Lin, W., Gilmore, J., Shen, D.: Altered structural connectivity in neonates at genetic risk for schizophrenia: A combined study using morphological and white matter networks. NeuroImage 62(3), 1622–1633 (2012)

25. Silverman, B.: Density Estimation for Statistics and Data Analysis. Monographs on Statistics and Applied Probablilty. Chapman and Hall (1998)

26. Watson, G.: Smooth regression analysis. Sankhyā: The Indian Journal of Statistics Series A 26(4), 359–372 (1964)

27. Wee, C.Y., Yap, P.T., Li, W., Denny, K., Browndyke, J.N., Potter, G.G., Welsh-Bohmer, K.A., Wang, L., Shen, D.: Enriched white matter connectivity networks for accurate identification of MCI patients. NeuroImage 54(3), 1812–1822 (2010)

28. Wee, C.Y., Yap, P.T., Zhang, D., Denny, K., Browndyke, J.N., Potter, G.G., Welsh-Bohmer, K.A., Wang, L., Shen, D.: Identification of MCI individuals using structural and functional connectivity networks. NeuroImage 59(3), 2045–2056 (2012)

29. Yap, P.T., Fan, Y., Chen, Y., Gilmore, J., Lin, W., Shen, D.: Development trends of white matter connectivity in the first years of life. PLoS ONE 6(9), e24678 (2011)

30. Yap, P.T., Wu, G., Shen, D.: Human brain connectomics: Networks, techniques, and applications. IEEE Signal Processing Magazine 27(4), 131–134 (2010)

Beyond Crossing Fibers: Tractography Exploiting Sub-voxel Fibre Dispersion and Neighbourhood Structure

Matthew Rowe, Hui Gary Zhang, Neil Oxtoby, and Daniel C. Alexander

Centre for Medical Image Computing, Department of Computer Science,
University College London, UK
matthew.rowe.09@ucl.ac.uk

Abstract. In this paper we propose a novel algorithm which leverages models of white matter fibre dispersion to improve tractography. Tractography methods exploit directional information from diffusion weighted magnetic resonance (DW-MR) imaging to infer connectivity between different brain regions. Most tractography methods use a single direction (e.g. the principal eigenvector of the diffusion tensor) or a small set of discrete directions (e.g. from the peaks of an orientation distribution function) to guide streamline propagation. This strategy ignores the effects of within-bundle orientation dispersion, which arises from fanning or bending at the sub-voxel scale, and can lead to missing connections. Various recent DW-MR imaging techniques estimate the fibre dispersion in each bundle directly and model it as a continuous distribution. Here we introduce an algorithm to exploit this information to improve tractography. The algorithm further uses a particle filter to probe local neighbourhood structure during streamline propagation. Using information gathered from neighbourhood structure enables the algorithm to resolve ambiguities between converging and diverging fanning structures, which cannot be distinguished from isolated orientation distribution functions. We demonstrate the advantages of the new approach in synthetic experiments and *in vivo* data. Synthetic experiments demonstrate the effectiveness of the particle filter in gathering and exploiting neighbourhood information in recovering various canonical fibre configurations and experiments with *in vivo* brain data demonstrate the advantages of utilising dispersion in tractography, providing benefits in practical situations.

1 Introduction

Tractography is a powerful tool to probe the geometric structure of white matter in vivo from non-invasive DW-MR imaging, allowing us to infer the anatomical connectivity of the separate functional regions of the brain. Information gained from tractography has great potential to advance our understanding of neurological function and disease.

Tractography algorithms infer connectivity by propagating streamlines between locations in the brain using directional information derived from DW-MR

J.C. Gee et al. (Eds.): IPMI 2013, LNCS 7917, pp. 402–413, 2013.

images. Early techniques were deterministic and followed a single direction per voxel, taken from the principal eigenvector of the diffusion tensor. The simplest method involves nearest neighbour interpolation FACT (Fiber Assignment by Continuous Tracking) [1], others involve trilinear interpolation [2, 3]. As the local fibre orientation estimates are prone to errors and uncertainty, probabilistic techniques were developed which assume a variance on the dominant fibre orientation and propagate a large collection of streamlines from each seed location using monte-carlo sampling of each fibre orientation estimate, thus inferring an index of connection probability between separate locations related to the number of streamlines which connect them [4, 5]. Multi-fibre techniques addressed the potential existence of multiple fibre populations traversing a voxel [6–9]. The majority of these techniques make use of a discrete set of fibre orientation estimates in each voxel (e.g. from the peaks of a fibre orientation distribution function). They assume that the uncertainty in the peak directions captures orientation dispersion due to noise and underlying fibre dispersion [10], while some [11] sample a fibre orientation distribution function (fODF) directly via a rejection sampling scheme for streamline propagation. While these methods provide good solutions to the crossing fibre problem, they do not account for other sub-voxel fibre configurations such as fanning and bending. This can lead to false negative connections in regions where such fibre architecture exists such as the corona radiata.

Global tractography methods [12–14] pose a potential solution to these limitations of local tractography. These methods search for the set of all streamlines which best explain the entire DW-MR data set. In theory, this approach handles complex sub-voxel fibre architectures such as fanning and crossing since the distribution of orientations formed by the candidate streamlines passing through each voxel is required to support the DW-MR signal in each voxel. Also local ambiguities such as fanning vs. crossing and fanning polarity could also be resolved in theory, since the streamlines are continuous and must reflect the diffusion weighted data globally, hence data from multiple voxels supports or opposes the existence of any particular candidate streamline. Sherbondy [15] demonstrates that by combining such a global technique with microstructure modelling can resolve classic confounding fibre architectures such as kissing vs. crossing. However, the major drawback of global tractography is the computational cost. The search space is very high-dimensional so globally optimal solutions are impossible to find in practical timescales with current technology. Recent work [16] has questioned whether these suboptimal solutions offer any real advantage over local tractography in real brain data.

Recent DW-MR modelling and imaging techniques [17–20] use parametric models of the fODF to recover estimates of within-voxel dispersion. These techniques avoid the instability with non-parametric fODFs such as those from standard spherical deconvolution and have been shown to match well fODFs measured from histology [21]. Preliminary investigations have demonstrated that tractography techniques sampling these fODFs in full for streamline propagation can reduce false negatives in regions of high anatomical fibre dispersion such as the the corona radiata [22]. However, Jeurissen *et al.* [10] show that making use of the full fODF for sampling propagation directions renders tractography more susceptible to false positives due to ambiguities about the underlying anatomical basis of the orientation dispersion.

To resolve ambiguities in the local voxel model of fibre orientation, we can make use of information from local neighbourhood voxels in the vicinity of the region which a streamline is traversing in addition to the local model. Savadjiev *et al.* [23] demonstrate that information from a voxels neighbourhood can be used to disambiguate sub-voxel fibre architectures such as curving and fanning. Using helical curves projected into the neighbourhood of a voxel, Savadjiev derives markers distinguishing and quantifying fanning and crossing fibres and fanning polarity within each voxel and parameterises the set of streamline selections enabling evaluation of those which are most consistent with forthcoming local structure. These methods demonstrate nicely the potential of leveraging voxel neighbourhood information for disambiguating fibre architecture at the subvoxel level. These methods however do not make use of a parameterised local model of dispersion and carry a computational expense due to the complexity of the helical model of streamlines, which would be costly to apply in a probabilistic tractography framework.

In this paper we present a new tractography method which combines local models of sub-voxel fibre dispersion with voxel neighbourhood exploration via a particle filter. Particle filter methods have been used previously in tractography [24–26] to estimate global connectivity in DW-MR images. In contrast to these methods we use the particle filter over a short range at each step of the streamline propagation to sample the set of possible future trajectories suggested by the local dispersion model and probe their compatibility with the neighbouring image structure. The particle filter informs the next single step selected from the local model, after which we repeat the whole procedure. Each step is stochastic and so, therefore, is the final resulting streamline. Thus the full algorithm repeats the whole process, as in traditional probabilistic tractography, to establish a collection of candidate streamlines from which we can derive probabilistic indices of connectivity in the usual way [4, 5]. We demonstrate the behaviour of the particle filter in gathering information on neighbourhood geometry in common fibre configurations on synthetic data and demonstrate the advantages of using dispersion in tractography on *in vivo* brain data tracking through the corona radiata.

2   Methods

In this section we describe our tracking algorithm that exploits local fibre dispersion and neighbourhood structure via a particle filter. Section 2.1 explains the details of the local model and Section 2.2 presents the technique to create a directional distribution informed by both local and neighbourhood information.

2.1   Locally-Estimated Dispersion ODF

To capture dispersion at each voxel locally, we model the fODF as a Bingham distribution. The Bingham distribution is a function on the sphere with a mean direction μ and two concentration parameters κ_1 and κ_2 which control the degree of dispersion along the two axes orthogonal to the mean direction μ_1 and μ_2 respectively:

$$f(\mathbf{n}) = F_1\left(\frac{1}{2}, \frac{3}{2}, \kappa_1, \kappa_2\right)^{-1} \exp\left[\kappa_1(\mu_1 \cdot \mathbf{n})^2 + \kappa_2(\mu_2 \cdot \mathbf{n})^2\right], \qquad (1)$$

where F_1 is the hypergeometric function (note: $F_1(1/2, 3/2, \kappa_1, \kappa_2)$ is a number, not a function).

The Bingham distribution has been used to model fibre dispersion in [17, 19]. For this work, we make use of the NODDI technique for fitting fibre dispersion models. The NODDI technique fits the cylindrically symmetric Watson distribution and introduces an imaging protocol better able to support the estimation of fibre dispersion. Here we use an extension of the NODDI technique to fit a Bingham distribution to the DW data. The Bingham distribution captures cylindrically asymmetric dispersion, which can better represent planar dispersion, representative of fanning white matter fibre structure [19].

Although such a local model of dispersion can improve exploration of sub-voxel fibre trajectories, it exhibits a number of ambiguities which cannot be resolved by examining each voxel in isolation. Due to the symmetrical nature of DW-MR measurements, the resulting distributions are symmetric, meaning there is an ambiguity between sub-voxel curving and fanning, and also fanning polarity. To address these ambiguities, it is necessary to gather information from voxels in the neighbourhood of the subject voxel to inform on the treatment of the local model for streamline propagation. For this purpose we use a particle filter framework explained in Section 2.2.

2.2   Voxel Neighbourhood-Informed Dispersion ODF

In this section, we describe a technique that creates a neighbourhood-informed fODF from the local dispersion estimates by fusing the information from the neighbourhood structure of the dominant fibre orientation. We draw candidate directions from the local dispersion fODF and propagate these directions into the local neighbourhood. By examining the coherence of each projected streamline with neighbourhood structure we can then weight each of these candidate directions according to the coherence of the respective projected streamline with the neighbourhood structure. This process is illustrated in Figure 1 for various canonical neighbourhood structures. The streamlines which are misaligned with neighbourhood structure are downweighted (coloured in blue) and the streamlines which align with the neighbourhood structure have their weights increased (coloured in red). This shows that fanning polarity and curvature can be distinguished. In the case of a diverging neighbourhood structure, the streamlines propagated from the dispersed candidate directions drawn from the fODF in the subject voxel find good alignment with the neighbourhood structure and are therefore evenly weighted. In contrast, in the presence of a convergent neighbourhood structure, the streamlines propagated from the peripheral candidate directions drawn from the local fODF misalign with neighbourhood structure and are downweighted. In the case of a curving structure, the candidate directions propagating against the curve are downweighted.

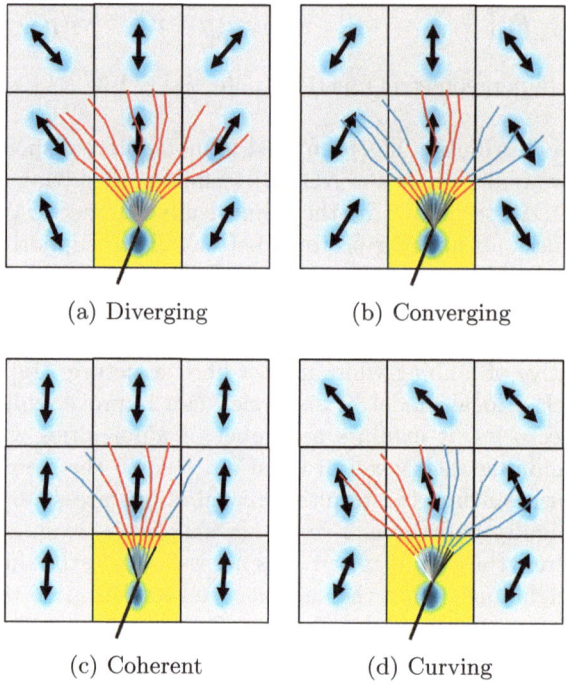

(a) Diverging   (b) Converging

(c) Coherent   (d) Curving

Fig. 1. Illustration of neighbourhood exploration in the case of of diverging (a), converging (b), coherent (c) and curving (d) neighbourhood structure in the tracking direction. Red streamlines are highly weighted, blue are low weighted.

This neighbourhood exploration scheme falls naturally into a particle filter framework. The particle filter is a simulation based model estimation technique used in non-linear, non-Gaussian dynamical systems. Through a process of prediction and update, the particle filter provides a discrete approximation of a posterior disribution $p(x_k|y_{0:k})$ on a time-varying parameter x_k at timestep k given the observations $y_{0:k}$ for timesteps $0, 1, 2, ..., k$ and the initial state distribution $p(x_0)$. At each timestep k, N particles are propagated by sampling from an importance density $\pi(x_k^{(i)}|x_{0:k-1}^{(i)}, y_{0:k})$, then assigned importance weights $w_k^{*(i)}$ which depend on a likelihood model $p(y_k|x_k^{(i)})$. Subsequently the discrete approximation to the posterior distribution $p(x_k|y_{0:k})$, denoted by $\tilde{w}_k^{(i)}$, is computed by normalising $w_k^{*(i)}$. This operation of a particle filter is summarised in Algorithm 1. Futher details on particle filtering can be found in [27].

State initialization, sample x_0 from $p(x_0)$;
Initialise importance weights
for $i = 1, ..., N$, **do**
$\quad | \quad w_0^{*(i)} = \frac{1}{N}$
end
for *times* $k = 1, 2, ..., K$ **do**
$\quad$ **for** $i = 1, ..., N$, **do**
$\quad\quad | \quad$ sample $x_k^{(i)}$ from $\pi(x_k | x_{0:k-1}^{(i)}, y_{0:k})$
$\quad$ **end**
$\quad$ calculate weight up to normalisation factor:
$\quad$ **for** $i = 1, ..., N$, **do**
$\quad\quad | \quad w_k^{*(i)} = w_{k-1}^{*(i)} p(y_k | x_k^{(i)})$
$\quad$ **end**
$\quad$ normalise the importance weights:
$\quad$ **for** $i = 1, ..., N$, **do**
$\quad\quad | \quad \tilde{w}_k^{(i)} = \frac{w_k^{*(i)}}{\sum_{j=1}^N w_k^{*(i)}}$
$\quad$ **end**
end

Algorithm 1. Sequential importance sampling

In this implementation, the importance density $\pi(x_k^{(i)} | x_{0:k-1}^{(i)}, y_{0:k})$ is chosen as a Watson distribution and the initial state distribution $p(x_0)$ is the Bingham distribution (described in Section 2.1) from the current voxel. A cloud of N particles defines a set of N streamlines defined by a string of vectors of fixed length connected end to end. At each timestep k each streamline is propagated one step from its previous location $u_{k-1}^{(i)}$ with a direction vector $v_k^{(i)}$ sampled from the importance density by a step length d such that $u_k^{(i)} = u_{k-1}^{(i)} + d v_k^{(i)}$. The state of a particle at timestep k $x_k^{(i)}$ is defined by its location $u_k^{(i)}$ and direction vector $v_k^{(i)}$. At each step the particle weights $w_k^{*(i)} = w_{k-1}^{*(i)} p(y_k | x_k^{(i)})$ are calculated to reflect their alignment with neighbourhood structure and the process is repeated for K steps. The likelihood $p(y_k | x_k^{(i)}) = (v_k \cdot D(u_k))^\gamma$ where $D(u_k)$ is the interpolated direction of the vector field D, defined by the mean directions of the Bingham distributions in each voxel, at the point location u_k. The stages of the particle filter scheme from streamline propagation to the selection of tract propagation direction is illustrated in Figure 2.

3   Experiments and Results

3.1   Synthetic Experiments

We use simulated data to examine the behaviour of the neighbourhood exploration by the particle filter. We simulate vector fields to mimic neighbourhood

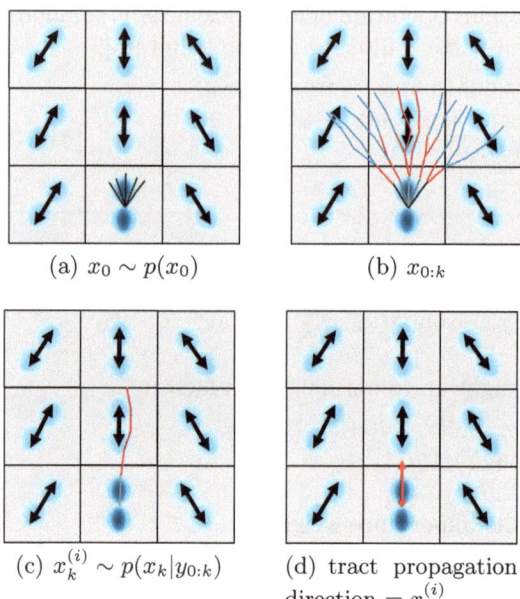

(a) $x_0 \sim p(x_0)$ (b) $x_{0:k}$

(c) $x_k^{(i)} \sim p(x_k|y_{0:k})$ (d) tract propagation
direction $= x_0^{(i)}$

Fig. 2. Illustration of the stages of neighbourhood exploration: initialisation from the local Bingham distribution (a), particle update and weighting (b), particle selection (c) and tract propagation direction selection (d).

structures which can arise in conjunction with dispersive local fODFs which are not distinguishable from the information from an isolated voxel. Figure 3 shows the behaviour of the particle filter in regions of diverging 3(a), converging 3(b), coherent 3(c), and curving 3(d) neighbourhood structure. The figure shows the particle weights at their final iteration step K.

Figure 4 shows a demonstration of the proposed tracking algorithm over 100 repetitions in diverging and converging local structure.

3.2 *in vivo* Experiments

We apply the algorithm on *in vivo* brain data. DW-MR images of a healthy male were acquired on a clinical 3T Philips system with isotropic voxels of 2mm, TE=78ms, TR=12.5ms, with one 30 direction shell and one 60 direction shell with b-values of 1000 s/mm^2 and 2000 s/mm^2, respectively. This dataset is the same as that used in [20]. Tracking experiments were performed from a single seed in the midbody of the corpus callosum (CC) at the mid-sagittal position, using the proposed algorithm and diffusion tensor (DT) PICo [4]. 5000 repetitions were used and results are shown in Figure 5. Tractography is also performed on 4 major white matter pathways: the inferior longitudinal fasciculus, the superior longitudinal fasciculus, the cingulum and the occipito-frontal fasciculus, for validation of expected performance in standard tracts. All *in vivo* results are displayed as maximum connection probability maps with a threshold of 1%.

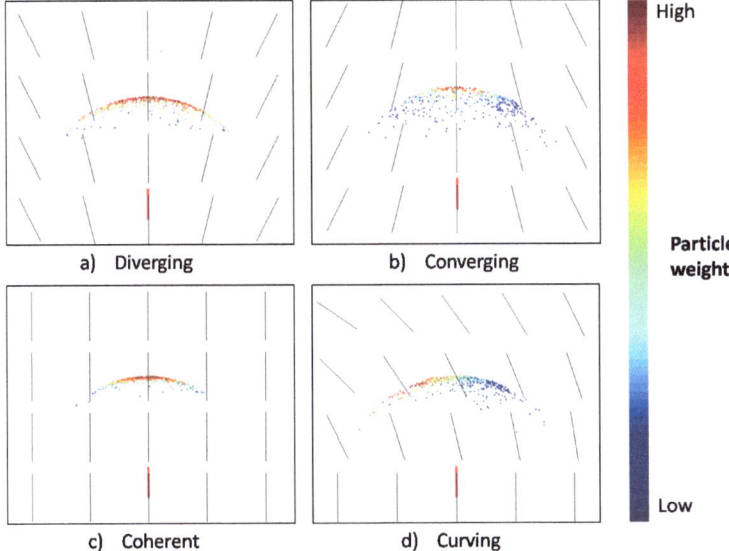

Fig. 3. Demonstration of particle filter behaviour in regions of diverging (a), converging (b), coherent (c) and curving (d) neighbourhood structure in the tracking direction. Colour denotes particle weight, blue is low through to red, which is high, yellow is intermediate.

4   Discussion and Conclusions

We have presented a tractography algorithm that combines information from both a local model of fibre orientation, which captures sub-voxel fibre dispersion with information drawn from the structural information available in the voxels in the immediate neighbourhood of the current tracking location. The simulations in Figure 3 demonstrate that the neighbourhood exploration particle filter behaves in practice like the conceptual illustration in Figure 1. In the case of divergent structure in the tracking direction (Figure 3(a)), the particles have an evenly spread distribution of weights, allowing full exploration of the orientations from the local model. In the case of convergent neighbourhood structure in the tracking direction (Figure 3(b)), the high particle weights are concentrated in the middle, limiting the selection of directions to align with forthcoming structure. Figure 4 shows the result of multiple iterations of the tractography algorithm in converging and diverging structure. In Figures 4(a) and 4(c) neighbourhood exploration is used, while in 4(b) and 4(d) neighbourhood exploration is not used, a curvature prior is used instead. The dispersion of streamline trajectories is exploited in the diverging case while the dispersion is restrained in the converging case over multiple repetitions. These simulations show that combining information from the voxel neighbourhood with information from the local fODF, we can resolve some of the remaining structural ambiguities of the

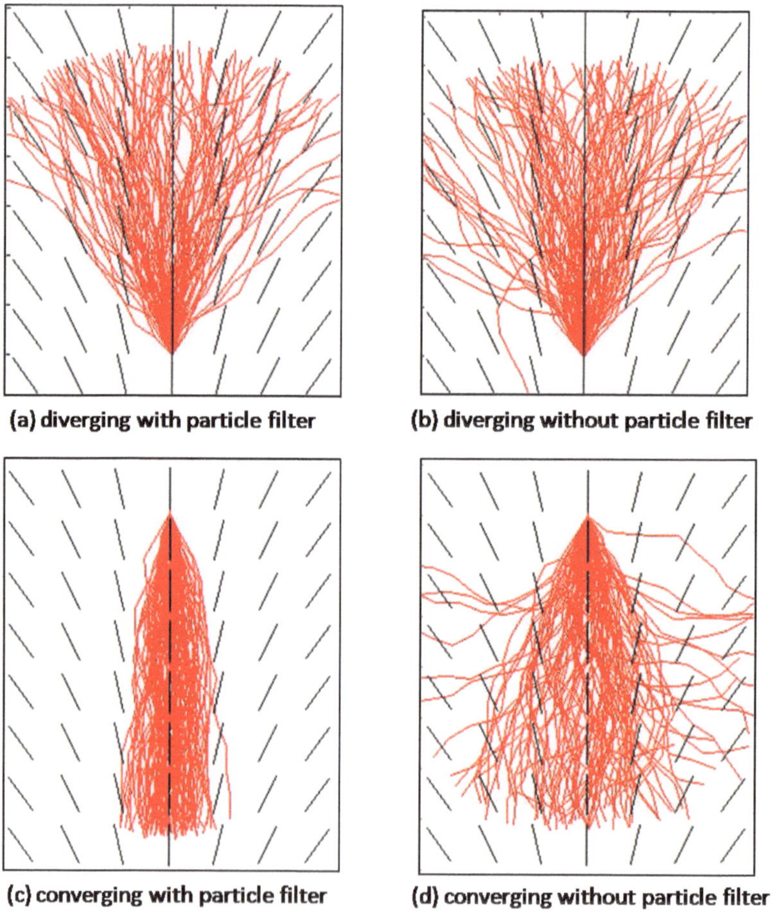

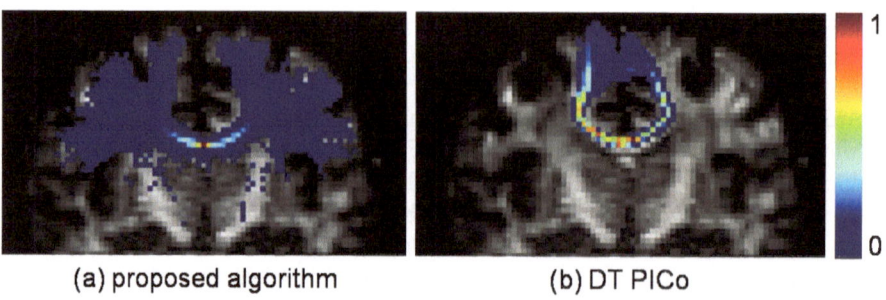

Fig. 4. 100 repetitions of the tracking algorithm in regions of diverging (a), (b) and converging (c) and (d) neighbourhood structure in the tracking direction. In (a) and (c), particle filter neighbourhood exploration is used, while in (b) and (d) only a curvature prior is used.

Fig. 5. Tracking from a single seed in the corpus callosum

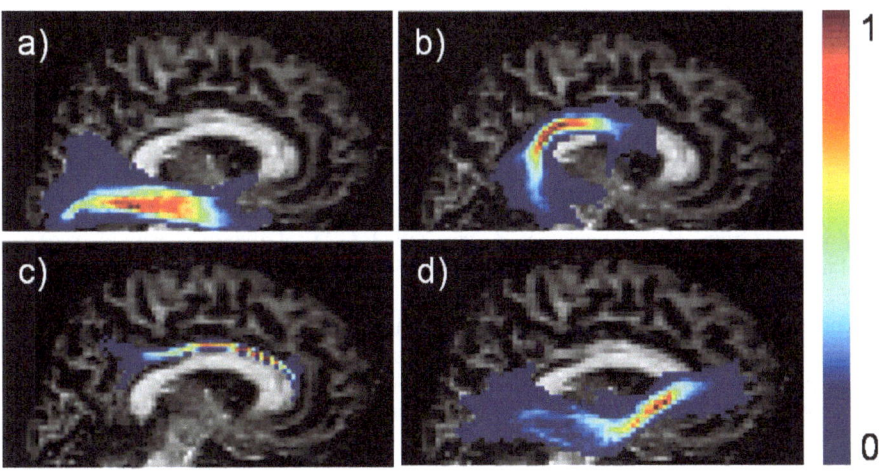

Fig. 6. Tracking of major white matter structures using proposed algorithm. a) inferior longitudinal fasciculus, b) superior longitudinal fasciculus, c) cingulum, d) cccipito-frontal fasciculus.

local model such as fanning polarity, which cannot be resolved from the voxel information in isolation.

Figure 5(a) shows the advantages of using dispersion in tractography in *in vivo* data. Tracking from a single seed in the corpus callosum, we can recover a wide range of connectivity to areas of the peripheral cortex. Both lateral and vertical connections are covered evenly with the oblique connections between. These streamlines traverse the corona radiata, which is a brain region known from anatomy to exhibit dispersing white matter structure. Figure 5(b) shows tracking from the same seed with PICo tractography based on the diffusion tensor (DT), which only uses a single discrete direction per voxel. DT PICo only recovers the vertical connections from the CC to the cortex as it does not exploit the dispersion in the corona radiata.

Figure 6 shows validation of the algorithm in tracking major white matter pathways, for which standard tractography algorithms work well, showing that the algorithm performs as expected in these structures.

Using a hybrid method utilising local fODFs modelling dispersion and neighbourhood exploration, we can capture complex dispersing subvoxel fibre architectures and include information from multiple voxels to resolve ambiguities of the local model and improve connectivity estimation. The synthetic experiments demonstrate the ability of the neighbourhood exploration to resolve ambiguities of local dispersive fODF such as fanning polarity and curvature, while the *in vivo* experiments show the advantages of exploiting fibre dispersion in tractography.

This technique represents a middle ground between local and global tractography, making use of the global tractography paradigm of pooling information from multiple voxels to overcome the limitations of condisering each voxel individually, while not inflating the problem to computationally intractible proportions. In future work we can explore other areas of this middle ground with larger neighbourhood exploration regions and using alternative fODFs such as those derived from spherical deconvolution.

References

1. Mori, S., Crain, B.J., Chacko, V.P., van Zijl, P.C.M.: Three dimensional tracking of axonal projections in the brain by magnetic resonance imaging. Ann. Neurol. 45, 265–269 (1999)
2. Conturo, T.E., Lori, N.F., Cull, T.S., Akbudak, E., Snyder, A.Z., Shimony, J.S., McKinstry, R.C., Burton, H., Raichle, M.E.: Tracking neuronal fiber pathways in the living human brain. Proc. Natl. Acad. Sci. U.S.A. 96, 10422–10427 (1999)
3. Basser, P.J., Pajevic, S., Pierpaoli, C., Duda, J., Aldroubi, A.: In vitro fiber tractography using DT-MRI data. Magn. Reson. Med. 44, 625–632 (2000)
4. Parker, G.J., Alexander, D.C.: Probabilistic Monte Carlo based mapping of cerebral connections utilising whole-brain crossing fibre information. In: Taylor, C.J., Noble, J.A. (eds.) IPMI 2003. LNCS, vol. 2732, pp. 684–695. Springer, Heidelberg (2003)
5. Behrens, T.E.J., Johansen-Berg, H., Woolrich, M.W., Smith, S.M., Wheeler-Kingshott, C.A.M., Boulby, P.A., Barker, G.J., Sillery, E.L., Sheehan, K., Cicarelli, O., Thompson, A.J., Brady, J.M., Matthews, P.M.: Characterization and propagation of uncertainty in diffusion-weighted MR imaging. Magn. Reson. Med. 50, 1077–1088 (2003)
6. Parker, G.J., Alexander, D.C.: Probabilistic anatomical connectivity derived from the microscopic persistent angular structure of cerebral tissue. Philosophical Transactions of the Royal Society B: Biological Sciences 360, 893–902 (2005)
7. Behrens, T.E.J., Johansen-Berg, H., Jbabdi, S., Rushworth, M.F.S., Woolrich, M.W.: Probabilistic diffusion tractography with multiple fibre orientations: What can we gain? NeuroImage 34, 144–155 (2007)
8. Tournier, J., Calamante, F., Connelly, A.: Robust determination of the fibre orientation distribution in diffusion mri: non-negativity constrained super-resolved spherical deconvolution. NeuroImage 35, 1459–1472 (2007)
9. Jeurissen, B., Leemans, A., Tournier, J.D., Sijbers, J.: Estimation of uncertainty in constrained spherical deconvolution fiber orientations. In: IEEE International Symposium on Biomedical Imaging: Macro to Nano, pp. 907–910 (2008)
10. Jeurissen, B., Leemans, A., Jones, D.K., Tournier, J.D., Sijbers, J.: Probabilistic fiber tracking using the residual bootstrap with constrained spherical deconvolution. Human Brain Mapping 32, 461–479 (2011)
11. Tournier, J.D., Calamante, F., Gadian, D.G., Connelly, A.: Probabilistic fibre tracking through regions containing crossing fibres. In: Proc. Intl. Soc. Mag. Reson. Med., vol. 13, p. 1343 (2005)
12. Sherbondy, A.J., Dougherty, R.F., Ananthanarayanan, R., Modha, D.S., Wandell, B.A.: Think Global, Act Local; Projectome Estimation with Bluematter. In: Yang, G.-Z., Hawkes, D., Rueckert, D., Noble, A., Taylor, C. (eds.) MICCAI 2009, Part I. LNCS, vol. 5761, pp. 861–868. Springer, Heidelberg (2009)
13. Fillard, P., Poupon, C., Mangin, J.-F.: A Novel Global Tractography Algorithm Based on an Adaptive Spin Glass Model. In: Yang, G.-Z., Hawkes, D., Rueckert, D., Noble, A., Taylor, C. (eds.) MICCAI 2009, Part I. LNCS, vol. 5761, pp. 927–934. Springer, Heidelberg (2009)

14. Kreher, B.W., Mader, I., Kiselev, V.G.: Gibbs Tracking: A Novel Approach for the Reconstruction of Neuronal Pathways. Magnetic Resonance in Medicine 60, 953–963 (2008)

15. Sherbondy, A.J., Rowe, M.C., Alexander, D.C.: MicroTrack: an algorithm for concurrent projectome and microstructure estimation. In: Jiang, T., Navab, N., Pluim, J.P.W., Viergever, M.A. (eds.) MICCAI 2010, Part I. LNCS, vol. 6361, pp. 183–190. Springer, Heidelberg (2010)

16. Li, L., Rilling, J.K., Preuss, T.M., Glasser, M.F., Damen, F.W., Hu, X.: Quantitative assessment of a framework for creating anatomical brain networks via global tractography. NeuroImage 61, 1017–1030 (2012)

17. Kaden, E., Knosche, T.R., Anwander, A.: Parametric spherical deconvolution: Inferring anatomical connectivity using diffusion MR imaging. NeuroImage 37, 474–488 (2007)

18. Zhang, H., Hubbard, P.L., Parker, G.J.M., Alexander, D.C.: Axon diameter mapping in the presence of orientation dispersion with diffusion MRI. NeuroImage 56, 1301–1315 (2011)

19. Sotiropoulos, S.N., Behrens, T.E.J., Jbabdi, S.: Ball and rackets: Inferring fiber fanning from diffusion-weighted MRI. NeuroImage 60, 1412–1425 (2012)

20. Zhang, H., Shneider, T., Wheeler-Kingshott, C., Alexander, D.C.: NODDI: Practical in vivo neurite orientation dispersion and density imaging of the human brain. NeuroImage 61, 1000–1016 (2012)

21. Jespersen, S.N., Leigland, L.A., Cornea, A., Kroenke, C.D.: Determination of axonal and dendritic orientation distributions within the developing cerebral cortex by diffusion tensor imaging. IEEE Trans. Med. Imaging 31, 16–32 (2012)

22. Rowe, M., Zhang, H., Alexander, D.C.: Utilising measures of fiber dispersion in white matter tractography. In: MICCAI CDMRI Workshop (2012)

23. Savadjiev, P., Campbell, J.S.W., Descoteaux, M., Deriche, R., Pike, G.B., Siddiqi, K.: Labeling of ambiguous subvoxel fibre bundle configurations in high angular resolution diffusion MRI. NeuroImage 41, 58–68 (2008)

24. Zhang, F., Hancock, E.R., Goodlett, C., Gerig, G.: White matter tractography using sequential importance sampling. In: Proc. ISMRM Annual Meeting, vol. 10 (2002)

25. Zhang, F., Hancock, E.R., Goodlett, C., Gerig, G.: Probabilistic white matter fiber tracking using particle filtering and von Mises-Fisher sampling. Med. Image Anal. 13, 5–18 (2009)

26. Pontabry, J., Rousseau, F.: Probabilistic tractography using Q-ball modeling and particle filtering. In: Fichtinger, G., Martel, A., Peters, T. (eds.) MICCAI 2011, Part II. LNCS, vol. 6892, pp. 209–216. Springer, Heidelberg (2011)

27. Doucet, A., Godsill, S., Andrieu, C.: On sequential Monte Carlo sampling methods for Bayesian filtering. Stat. and Comput. 10, 197–208 (2000)

Learning from M/EEG Data
with Variable Brain Activation Delays

Wojciech Zaremba[1,2], M. Pawan Kumar[1,2,3],
Alexandre Gramfort[4,5], and Matthew B. Blaschko[1,2,3]

[1] Center for Visual Computing, École Centrale Paris, Châtenay-Malabry France
[2] INRIA Saclay–Île-de-France
[3] Université Paris-Est, LIGM (UMR CNRS), École des Ponts ParisTech, France
[4] Institut Mines-Télécom, Télécom ParisTech, CNRS LTCI, Paris, France
[5] CEA/Neurospin bât 145, 91191 Gif-Sur-Yvette

Abstract. Magneto- and electroencephalography (M/EEG) measure the electromagnetic signals produced by brain activity. In order to address the issue of limited signal-to-noise ratio (SNR) with raw data, acquisitions consist of multiple repetitions of the same experiment. An important challenge arising from such data is the variability of brain activations over the repetitions. It hinders statistical analysis such as prediction performance in a supervised learning setup. One such confounding variability is the time offset of the peak of the activation, which varies across repetitions. We propose to address this misalignment issue by explicitly modeling time shifts of different brain responses in a classification setup. To this end, we use the latent support vector machine (LSVM) formulation, where the latent shifts are inferred while learning the classifier parameters. The inferred shifts are further used to improve the SNR of the M/EEG data, and to infer the chronometry and the sequence of activations across the brain regions that are involved in the experimental task. Results are validated on a long term memory retrieval task, showing significant improvement using the proposed latent discriminative method.

Keywords: magnetoencephalography (MEG), electroencephalograpy (EEG), Latent SVM, classification, independant component analysis (ICA), functional connectivity, single-trial variability.

1 Introduction

Magnetoencephalography and electroencephalography (M/EEG) measure the electromagnetic fields induced by brain activity. Typically, when collecting M/EEG data in neurosciences, the same task is repeated several times, resulting in hundreds of trials. Given such data, a classical way to distinguish between two tasks (also called experimental conditions) is to average all the trials for each condition and compare the difference between the averages. The main issue with such an approach is that the latency and amplitudes of the responses of each individual activated brain region can vary across the trials. For example

J.C. Gee et al. (Eds.): IPMI 2013, LNCS 7917, pp. 414–425, 2013.

the measured P300 wave, often used for brain computer interface (BCI) systems, is a mix of P3a and P3b waves which are almost concomitant with the P2 wave [16]. Each wave can suffer from different variabilities. The reasons for such variabilities are many fold: fatigue, habituation or changes in attention to name but a few. This makes the process of averaging prone to modeling errors. An alternative approach is to cast the statistical test of distinguishing two tasks as a classification problem. This is similar to a BCI system, which predicts a behavioral variable from raw M/EEG recordings. When using such a supervised learning approach, repeated trials increase the amount of training data, which could in theory lead to better prediction. However, even in this setting, the prediction accuracy is inevitably affected by the variability between trials.

The above argument suggests that it is important to explicitly model the variabilities in brain responses in order to improve classification accuracy. To this end, we propose to use a supervised learning algorithm with latent variables. Specifically, we introduce latent variables for each trial, which represent its variability. This allows us to learn a classifier using the latent support vector machine (LSVM) framework, which iteratively estimates the value of the latent variables such that the training error is reduced. Our experiments show that this approach can provide a significant improvement in the prediction accuracy over a baseline method that does not explicitly model the sample transformation (Section 5.1). Moreover, the imputed latent variables allows us to improve the quality of the brain sources visualization (Section 5.2). Finally, as explained in Section 5.3, the latencies of the brain source responses offers the possibility to investigate the chronometry in functional networks at a millisecond time scale. Code of this implementation is available online.[1]

2   Related Work

This work explores use of latent support vector machines (LSVM) in M/EEG studies to improve prediction and discover brain functional connectivity. The problem of prediction using M/EEG signals has been extensively studied in the context of mind reading [6]. Recent works in this field mostly use classifiers like SVM or LDA, which cannot explicitly model the variability over trials. To overcome this deficiency, we employ the latent support vector machine (LSVM) classifier, whose ability to handle latent variables has been successfully exploited in other fields of research such as bioinformatics [20] and computer vision [9]. Note that, in contrast to previous latent models used in brain imaging that are purely unsupervised [11], LSVM is a supervised learning approach (that is, it makes use of the knowledge of the experimental conditions for various trials while estimating the latent variables).

The topic of brain functional connectivity has also received considerable attention in the literature [5]. Recent works in this field mostly use non-stationary time-frequency transforms for feature selection [4]. In contrast to previous work, our features are based on activation peak misalignment (where the misalignments

---

[1] `https://github.com/wojzaremba/active-delays`

can be estimated using any set of features using our LSVM formulation). While the latency in brain signals has been studied since at least the late 1960s [19], to the best of our knowledge, it has not been previously considered in the context of brain functional connectivity.

3   Latent SVM for M/EEG Data

In this section, we will describe how the latent support vector machine (LSVM) [20] framework can be used to classify M/EEG data in the presence of significant variability among trials. Furthermore, we will describe how LSVM can be used to improve the visualization of brain sources and to estimate the brain functional connectivity. We begin with a brief description of the general LSVM framework.

LSVM is an extension of the well-known support vector machine (SVM) [8] classifier, which allows for missing information in the training samples. Formally, let $x \in \mathcal{X}$ denote an input that needs to be assigned a classification label $y \in \mathcal{Y} \equiv \{-1, +1\}$. In the present case corresponds to one or multiple time series. The latent variable $h \in \mathcal{H}$ represents any missing information that can aid the classification process. Note that, by definition, the value of the latent variable is unknown while the domain, $\mathcal{H}$, is a modeling choice. We represent the joint feature vector of the input x and the latent variable h by $\phi(x, h)$. Given a training dataset $D = \{(x_i, y_i), i = 1, \cdots, n\}$, the parameters w of the LSVM are learned by solving the following optimization problem:

$$\min_{w \in \mathbb{R}^d, \xi \in \mathbb{R}^n} \frac{1}{2}\|w\|^2 + C \sum_i \xi_i \tag{1}$$

$$\text{s.t. } \max_{h \in \mathcal{H}} y_i w^\top \phi(x_i, h) - \max_{\hat{h} \in \mathcal{H}}(-y_i) w^\top \phi(x_i, \hat{h}) \geq 1 - \xi_i, \tag{2}$$

$$\xi_i \geq 0, \forall i. \tag{3}$$

The regularization term $\|w\|^2$ in the objective function helps to avoid over-fitting. In addition, the objective function also minimizes the sum of the slack variables ξ_i, one for each sample (x_i, y_i). A small value of the slack variable results in the correct classification of a training sample. The constraints in problem (1) encourage the best latent variable for the correct output to have a score that is greater than all other possible latent variable assignments for the incorrect output. The number of constraints (2) is large. They consist of all possible assignments of $\hat{h}$ for every sample (precisely $|H| \times |X|$ constraints). However, the cutting plane algorithm [13] enables this optimization procedure in an efficient way regardless of the number of constraints.

In other words, the values of the latent variables are estimated such that the classification performance is maximized over the training set. Note that, for simplicity, we have restricted our description to a binary LSVM. However, we note that more general structured output LSVMs have also been proposed in the literature [20].

Algorithm 1. The CCCP method for learning the parameters of LSVM

Input: Training set $\mathcal{D} = \{(x_i, y_i), i = 1, \cdots, n\}$, initial parameters w_0, tolerance ϵ.
  Initialize $w = w_0$. Set $t = 0$.
  repeat
    Estimate the latent variables as $h_i \leftarrow \arg\max_{h \in \mathcal{H}} y_i w_t^\top \phi(x_i, h)$, for all i.
    Update the parameters by solving the following convex optimization problem:

$$w_{t+1} = \underset{w \in \mathbb{R}^d, \xi \in \mathbb{R}^n}{\arg\min} \quad \frac{1}{2}\|w\|^2 + C \sum_i \xi_i \tag{4}$$

$$\text{s.t.} \quad y_i w^\top \phi(x_i, h_i) - \max_{\hat{h} \in \mathcal{H}}(-y_i) w^\top \phi(x_i, \hat{h}) \geq 1 - \xi_i, \xi_i \geq 0, \forall i.$$

    Set $t \leftarrow t + 1$.
  until The decrease in the objective function of problem (1) is below tolerance ϵ.

While problem (1) is not convex, it was shown to have the special form of a difference-of-convex program [20]. This observation leads to an approximate algorithm based on the concave-convex procedure (CCCP) [21] as outlined in Algorithm 1. The CCCP method iterates over two main steps: (i) the latent variable values are imputed using the current set of parameters; and (ii) the parameters are updated while keeping the imputed latent variables fixed, which is equivalent to optimizing the convex problem (4). In our work, we used the 1-slack reformulation based cutting plane algorithm [13] to solve problem (4). Each iteration of CCCP decreases the objective function of problem (1) until we reach a local minimum or saddle point solution [17].

3.1   Classification of M/EEG Data

We now describe how the above LSVM framework can be adapted for the classification of M/EEG data. The input x corresponds to an M/EEG recording where data was collected from a single subject. The output y denotes the outcome. The unknown latent variables model the variation of a sample. The latent variable represents the possible transformations that M/EEG data may undergo. Such transformations are a result of the variability of the brain responses over trials. The latent space $\mathcal{H}$ can vary from a simple translation of the signal to multiple translations for different signal components (as determined by ICA).

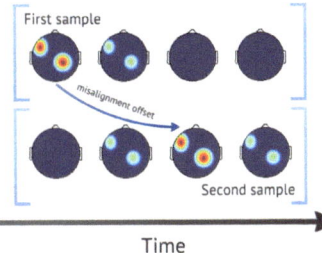

Fig. 1. In this work, we primarily consider variations in the data due to offsets in the time domain. By appropriately modeling such offsets, we are able to register the data samples with respect to each other and to enable the use of non-shift-invariant function classes. Additionally, the values of the latent variables are informative to quantify variations in brain responses.

We consider a simple distortion model where samples are shifted with respect to each other. We model this distortion using latent variables that represent the putative offset of the misalignment as shown in Figure 1. The latent space $\mathcal{H}$ contains a finite set of translations.

In more detail, we consider an input x that consists of c channels and multiple samples collected from the single subject. Each channel consists of m observed values:

$$x = x^{(1)}, \ldots, x^{(c)} \tag{5}$$
$$x^k = (a_1^k, a_2^k, \cdots, a_m^k)^\top \tag{6}$$

In the absence of misalignment between the trials, we use the elements in the range $(s, s + l)$ for each of the c channels to perform classification. However, as mentioned earlier, the prediction performance can be considerably improved by explicitly modeling the misalignment using a variable $h \in \mathcal{H}$. In such a setting, we define the joint feature vector $\phi(x, h)$ as follows:

$$\phi(x, h) = (\phi(x^{(1)}, h)^\top, \ldots \phi(x^{(c)}, h)^\top)^\top \tag{7}$$
$$\phi(x^{(k)}, h) = (a_{s+h}^{(k)}, a_{s+1+h}^{(k)}, \cdots, a_{s+l+h}^{(k)})^\top, \tag{8}$$
$$1 \leq s + h \leq s + l + h \leq m. \tag{9}$$

The joint feature vector consists of elements in the range $(s + h, s + l + h)$ for all the c channels. Note that when the latent space $\mathcal{H} = \{\gamma\}$ for any constant γ, the resulting LSVM simplifies to the standard SVM formulation.

In our experiments, x consist of data on the basis of channels as in the experiment described in Section 5.1 (c indexes channels), or on the basis of ICA components as in the experiments described in Sections 5.2 and 5.3 (c indexes components).

3.2   Component Quality Measure

ICA components are often considered as a proxy to brain sources [7], and in this studies we perform experiments on ICA components. A common approach in visualization studies is to average data coming from multiple samples in order to improve the signal-to-noise ratio. However, the averaging of slightly misaligned time-series often manifests itself in the elimination of high frequency components of the signal (Figure 2). By using the imputed values of the latent variables, we can correct for this loss and greatly improve the quality of M/EEG signals. In order to quantify this improvement, we propose a quality measure. We would like such a measure to favor sharpness (that is, the presence of high frequency components) over smoothness (that is, a lack of high frequency components). To this end, we propose to use the H^1 norm [1], which is defined as follows:

$$\|u\|_{H^1} = \left(\|u(x)\|_{L^2}^2 + \|Du(x)\|_{L^2}^2\right)^{\frac{1}{2}} \tag{10}$$

For a function of two variables, the H^1 norm tends to infinity if a function has a discontinuity over a 1-dimensional curve. The H^1 norm assigns high values to functions of M/EEG recordings that have sharp transitions spatially and over short time spans. This therefore favors functions that are spatially and temporally well-localized within the brain. In our experiments, we will calculate the H^1 norm of time series that are 2D flattened topographies arising as the difference of means of samples belonging to individual classes.

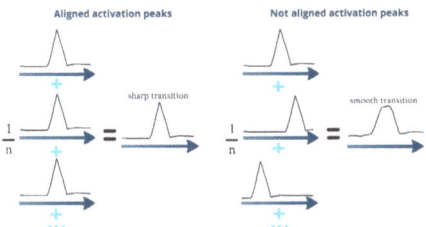

Fig. 2. Averaging over aligned data results in sharp peaks (n is a number of samples). In contrast, averaging over misaligned samples tends to smooth the data. Sharpness and smoothness can be quantified with the H^1 norm that takes a high value for sharp peaks and a low value for smooth time series.

3.3   Inferring Brain Functional Connectivity from the Latent Variables

The brain is a distributed system with cognitive processes involving multiple brain regions that are recruited sequentially or simultaneously. In order to understand brain processes, one has to find which parts of brain are associated with a particular cognitive task, but also the chronometry of information flow between each of these regions. Here we propose a method to infer statistical dependence and brain functional connectivity. To investigate couplings and interaction between sources we propose to use the estimates of the latent variables that encode the trial-to-trial variability of the response of each source. Intuitively if two sources have similar variability, here delays, it means they have a statistical dependency that could originate from a common node in the brain communication network, or that one of them interacts directly with the another. Delays to a common ancestor might cause a delay in all its descendants (e.g. the visual cortex can process data as soon as it receives a signal from retina, but not before).

Imputed offsets are not easy to compare directly between components. Firstly, as all offsets can be shifted by a constant value, the resulting offsets give the same relative misplacement. Secondly, M/EEG data is noisy and some samples might be aligned incorrectly or only approximately. Even comparing imputed offsets from two perfectly dependent components can be difficult. Rather than compare the resulting offsets from separate LSVM setups (each for different components), we propose to use a single LSVM with a shared latent variable between components. We use obtained offsets to align components and then measure the quality of the result by calculating its H^1 norm as described in Section 3.2. A high value of the H^1 norm indicates correct alignment, as misalignment removes high frequency components of the signal. As each pair of components optimized with a shared latent variable gives us two measures (one for each component), we combine them by multiplication. Multiplication is chosen over addition to ensure a high value of this score only if the resulting functions are sharp for both components, and not just one.

4   Data Collection and Experimental Paradigm

The considered dataset explores the process of long term memory (LTM) retrieval. The goal of the experiment is to elucidate the dynamics of long term memory encoding. The dataset is publicly available.[2] Details of data acquisition can be found in [2]. The task includes visual presentation, and the subject has to determine whether an abstract visual pattern corresponds to a presented natural object. The discriminative task to be solved with the LSVM is a binary classification problem (green color recall vs. red color recall). In these studies we have considered a single subject (number 8).

The long term memory retrieval experiment involves performing a complex, high level task by participants. The outcome of this kind of task is dependent on the subject's mental state, such as the level of concentration, vigilance, or familiarly with the experimental setting. We hypothesize that these factors cause the brain to respond with different temporal delays. While earlier visual processing may additionally have variable delays, high level cognitive functions, which are particularly challenging and interesting to study, are more susceptible to this form of variability due to the longer time frames involved, and the recruitment of multiple brain regions. For this reason, the LTM dataset considered in this study is particularly suited to the form of statistical modeling proposed here.

For further analysis, we have processed the dataset by dropping 10% of trials with the highest variance. 69 trials were removed out of 681 by this process. We reduced the data dimensionality with PCA to 60 dimensions and whitened the data. Finally, we applied InfoMax ICA with full rank [3]. We have applied PCA in conjunction with ICA in line with standard practice [12].

5   Results

To test the efficacy of LSVM, we performed a binary color prediction task on the LTM dataset. We first evaluated the prediction performance quantitatively, and subsequently visualized the ICA components after discriminative alignment with the LSVM. Finally, we used the learned offsets of the ICA components to infer a graph indicating likely functional connectivity between components.

5.1   LSVM Using All Channels

Here, we used data before the application of ICA, i.e. the dataset has been cleaned by dropping malicious samples and further whitened with PCA, however we have not applied ICA as the learned decision function will linearly transform the data. This experiment does not treat individual components differently, but instead learns a single offset parameter for the entire trial.

We considered a distortion model where the latent space H consists of a finite number of translations. Figure 3 presents the accuracy results for

---

[2] http://www.biomag2012.org/content/data-analysis-competition

various sizes of the latent space. The dataset was balanced with a chance
level at 50%. The point denoted by 10ms in the x-axis denotes the experiment where the putative translation is restricted to lie in the interval
$[-10\text{ms}, 10\text{ms}]$. For computational efficiency, we discretized the space of putative translations into 7 equally spaced values, resulting in the latent space
$H = \{-10\text{ms}, -6.7\text{ms}, -3.3\text{ms}, 0\text{ms}, 3.3\text{ms}, 6.6\text{ms}, 10\text{ms}\}$ (the data acquisition
rate is 300Hz). For the sake of brevity, we refer to the LSVM setup with max-
imum misalignment N ms as $MisAlign_N$. Particularly, for $N = 0$, $MisAlign_0$
simplifies to a classical SVM setup, where no misalignment is considered.

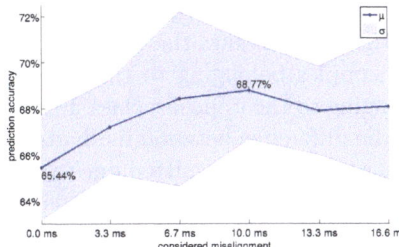

Fig. 3. Results of a LSVM for the long
term memory dataset where the latent
variable models misalignment. A paired t-
test indicates with p-value smaller than 5%
that, LSVM for misalignment up to 10ms
performs statistically significantly better
than a classical SVM.

Based on a preliminary analysis accuracy results obtained for very high C
parameter where indistinguishable from results for cross validated C. In this
and all further experiments we consider only a hard margin SVM (equivalent
to setting C to infinity). The results presented in Figure 3 are averaged over
5-folds. The accuracy obtained for $MisAlign_{10}$ is 3.33% higher compared to the
accuracy obtained by a standard SVM. The accuracy peaks when we consider
the latent variable to lie in the interval $[-10\text{ms}, 10\text{ms}]$ and it slowly decays for
larger values of misalignment. Our experiments indicate that the misalignment of
most of the samples is up to 10ms and considering higher values gives too much
capacity to the learning algorithm (for the majority of samples, higher values do
not correspond to actual data misalignment). A paired t-test indicates that the
accuracy of $MisAlign_{10}$ is significantly improved over the accuracy distribution
obtained for a standard SVM, and rejects the null hypothesis with p-value equal
to 4.36%. Note that we are able to achieve higher classification performance with
statistical significance which is a strong evidence that the use of latent variables
for discriminative alignment is an appropriate modeling choice for this class of
data.

5.2   LSVM on ICA Components

Over the course of this experiment, we consider single ICA components computed
from 200ms long time slices. We regard a single component as a proxy to a
brain source [14]. We visualize components by averaging them over trials. We
may consider such averaging with or without first aligning the trials using the
offsets learned by the LSVM. We considered 60 components and 3 time intervals
(0-200ms, 200ms-400ms, 400ms-600ms). We have used each of these component-
interval pairs in separate prediction tasks, and we focus on the four pairs with

highest prediction accuracy. Moreover, we focus only on component-interval pairs that give at least 1% improvement in $MisAlign_{10}$ over a classical SVM. In this way, we examine only components that carry an informative signal (high accuracy), and substantially suffering from misalignment.

To compare the discriminative alignments learned from the LSVM to the previous state of the art, we compare to the continuous profile model (CPM) [15], an unsupervised method. In total, we present three visualizations: (i) the unaligned ICA component, (ii) the ICA component aligned by the application of CPM, and (iii) the ICA component after aligning samples according to the learned offset from LSVM. In order to visualize a single component, first we mapped the data back to the channel space. Next, we took a single time slice and computed the mean for each prediction class separately. Figure 4 presents the absolute value of results. Red indicates that the mean of samples belonging to the one class highly differs from the mean of samples belonging to the opposite class. Figure 4 presents three time slices that demonstrate the difference between methods (additional results do not show a qualitative difference and are omitted due to space restrictions). The visualization obtained after alignment with LSVM is significantly sharper, while the other two visualizations are diffuse and the underlying structure is not visible.

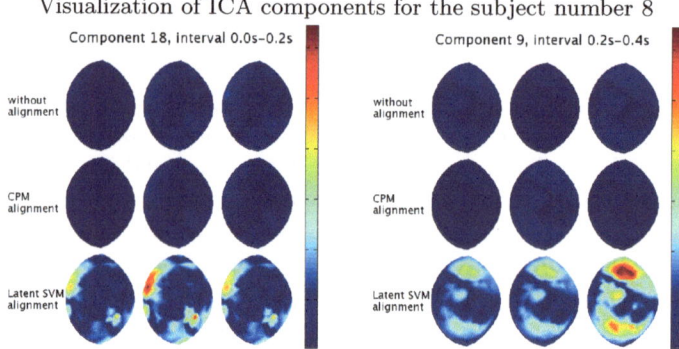

Fig. 4. Visualization of two ICA components with various alignment techniques. The figure presents the absolute value of the difference between the target class means. A difference between samples corresponding to the first outcome of a mental state and the second outcome (in this case mean of samples of green color recall minus mean of samples of red color recall). Red on this figure indicates regions that discriminate between classes. All methods make use of the same color palette to facilitate the comparison between subfigures.

Table 1 presents the H_1 norm for four different components and four different alignment methods. Images are first normalized by setting their mean to zero (centering) and standard deviation to one. The score obtained for data aligned according to the LSVM is much higher than for data without any alignment and for data aligned with the continuous profile model method [15]. Moreover, we evaluated the stability of the H^1 norm over randomly aligned images.

Table 1. The H^1 norm over normalized difference of means of samples belonging to individual classes. Results are computed for different methods of alignment. For every component LSVM achieves significantly higher values of the H^1 norm. The H^1 norm measures the spatio-temporal sharpness of a time series that are 2d flattened topographies.

		(component; time interval)			
		(18; 0s–0.2ms)	(58; 0s–0.2ms)	(9; 0.2s–0.4s)	(2; 0.4s–0.6s)
method	none	2.44	5.17	2.26	1.61
	random	2.51 ± 0.08	5.07 ± 0.31	2.18 ± 0.05	1.54 ± 0.08
	CPM	3.49	4.71	1.65	1.20
	LSVM	10.28	17.52	7.19	8.02

We randomly generated alignment offsets and shifted images with respect to them. For the resulting randomly aligned images we calculated the H^1 norm. The second row of Table 1, results for random alignment, presents the mean and standard deviation achieved over 5-folds. Values in this row are not substantially different from values in the first row, where none of the alignment methods have been applied. The relatively small standard deviation indicates that the H^1 norm is very stable in our setting.

5.3   Inference of Brain Functional Connectivity with LSVM

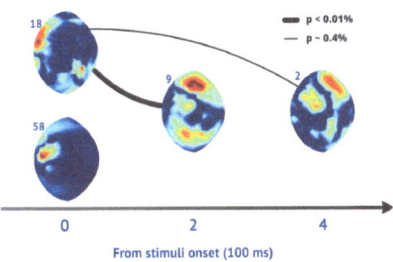

Fig. 5. Components giving similar misalignment offsets. An edge indicates that aligning components according to a common latency results in a high product of H^1 norms (c.f. Section 3.3). Statistical significance was verified with a permutation test. Edges are annotated by their p-values.

As described in Section 5.2, we focus on four components in these experiments. For each of the $\binom{4}{2}$ pairs of components and three subintervals of length 200ms, we have computed the product of their H^1 norms resulting from latent alignments estimated by joint discriminative training. Considering this score as a statistic, we verify if it is significantly larger than chance by computing permutation tests. Under the null hypothesis (H0) that there is no delay dependency between components across trials, we generated permuted data by shuffling the trials for one component leaving the other one unchanged. For each resulting permuted data we computed the same statistic to assemble a histogram generated under H0. The original statistic value is then positioned in the histogram to derive a p-value. Component 18 over interval 0.0s–0.2s and component 9 over interval 0.2s–0.4s achieved significant statistical scores using 10000 permutations (Figure 5). We observe 4 topographies, the 2 on the left exhibit dipolar patterns located at the back on the helmet above the occipital cortex that contains the visual cortex. Component 9 is statistically related to component 18 over the interval 0.0s–0.2s ($p < 0.01\%$) and shows a relative symmetric pattern that could correspond to a deep subcortical source involved in long term memory. Component 2 reflects an activation over interval 0.4s–0.6s ($p < 0.4\%$ with component 18) on the left side of the helmet over more frontal sensors which could correspond to higher level cognitive processing that naturally appears later in time after the stimulus onset.

6   Discussion

By modeling and estimating parameters of variations on single trial M/EEG data, LSVM has demonstrated a significant improvement with respect to a standard SVM, which has been previously used in neurosciences and for BCI applications [18]. The proper modeling of brain response variabilities via latent variables allowed us to estimate in a supervised way the parameters reflecting the changes in brain activations due for example to fatigue or subject habituation.

Exploiting the ability of ICA to exhibit components that are plausible brain sources according to the physics of the measurement system (high activations spatially localized with spatial smoothness and dipolar field patterns), we then run LSVM on ICA components to investigate the dynamics and chronometry of different brain source configurations. Results from Section 5.3 show the potential of this approach for functional connectivity studies as it offers a way to elucidate delays in brain responses from single trial data. Indeed, from correlated delays between sources one can for example infer if a source activation precedes another one or have a common cause that could be a deep subcortical source.

Future directions for this work is to investigate recovery of brain functionality graph for large number of components. Finally a next step is the localization of the ICA components in the brain by solving the M/EEG inverse problem [10].

Acknowledgements. This work is partially funded by the European Research Council under the Seventh Framework Programme (FP7/2007-2013)/ERC Grant 259112.

References

1. Adams, R., Fournier, J.: Sobolev Spaces: Pure and Applied Mathematics. Academic Press (2003)
2. Backus, A., Jensen, O., Meeuwissen, E., van Gerven, M., Dumoulin, S.: Investigating the temporal dynamics of long term memory representation retrieval using multivariate pattern analyses on magnetoencephalography data. MSc thesis (2011)
3. Bell, A.J., Sejnowski, T.J.: An information-maximization approach to blind separation and blind deconvolution. Neural Computation 7, 1129–1159 (1995)

4. Bénar, C., Clerc, M., Papadopoulo, T.: Adaptive time-frequency models for single-trial M/EEG analysis. In: Karssemeijer, N., Lelieveldt, B. (eds.) IPMI 2007. LNCS, vol. 4584, pp. 458–469. Springer, Heidelberg (2007)
5. Biswal, B., Yetkin, F.Z., Haughton, V.M., Hyde, J.S.: Functional connectivity in the motor cortex of resting human brain using echo-planar MRI. Magnetic Resonance in Medicine 34(4), 537–541 (1995)
6. Blankertz, B., Muller, K., Curio, G., Vaughan, T., Schalk, G., Wolpaw, J., Schlogl, A., Neuper, C., Pfurtscheller, G., Hinterberger, T., et al.: The bci competition 2003: progress and perspectives in detection and discrimination of eeg single trials. IEEE Transactions on Biomedical Engineering 51(6), 1044–1051 (2004)
7. Chen, Y., Akutagawa, M., Katayama, M., Zhang, Q., Kinouchi, Y.: Ica based multiple brain sources localization. In: Conf. Proc. IEEE Eng. Med. Biol. Soc. 2008, pp. 1879–1882 (2008)
8. Cortes, C., Vapnik, V.: Support-vector networks. Machine Learning, 273–297 (1995)
9. Felzenszwalb, P.F., Girshick, R.B., McAllester, D., Ramanan, D.: Object detection with discriminatively trained part-based models. IEEE Transactions on Pattern Analysis and Machine Intelligence 32(9), 1627–1645 (2010)
10. Gramfort, A., Strohmeier, D., Haueisen, J., Hamalainen, M., Kowalski, M.: Functional brain imaging with m/eeg using structured sparsity in time-frequency dictionaries. In: Székely, G., Hahn, H.K. (eds.) IPMI 2011. LNCS, vol. 6801, pp. 600–611. Springer, Heidelberg (2011)
11. Held, K., Kops, E., Krause, B., Wells III, W., Kikinis, R., Muller-Gartner, H.: Markov random field segmentation of brain MR images. IEEE Transactions on Medical Imaging 16(6), 878–886 (1997)
12. Hyvärinen, A., Karhunen, J., Oja, E.: Independent Component Analysis. Wiley-Interscience (2001)
13. Joachims, T., Finley, T., Yu, C.N.J.: Cutting-plane training of structural svms. Machine Learning 77(1), 27–59 (2009)
14. Jung, T., Makeig, S., Mckeown, M.J., Bell, A.J., won Lee, T., Sejnowski, T.J.: Imaging brain dynamics using independent component analysis. Proceedings of the IEEE 89, 1107–1122 (2001)
15. Listgarten, J., Neal, R.M., Roweis, S.T., Emili, A.: Multiple alignment of continuous time series. In: Advances in Neural Information Processing Systems, pp. 817–824. MIT Press (2005)
16. Polich, J.: Updating p300: An integrative theory of P3a and P3b. Clinical Neurophysiology 118(10), 2128 (2007)
17. Sriperumbudur, B., Lanckriet, G.: On the convergence of the concave-convex procedure. In: Bengio, Y., Schuurmans, D., Lafferty, J., Williams, C.K.I., Culotta, A. (eds.) Advances in Neural Information Processing Systems, vol. 22, pp. 1759–1767 (2009)
18. Thulasidas, M., Guan, C., Wu, J.: Robust classification of EEG signal for brain-computer interface. IEEE Transactions on Neural Systems and Rehabilitation Engineering 14(1), 24–29 (2006)
19. Woody, C.: Characterization of an adaptive filter for the analysis of variable latency neuroelectrical signals. Medical and Biological Engineering 5, 539–553 (1967)
20. Yu, C.N.J., Joachims, T.: Learning structural SVMs with latent variables. In: Proceedings of the International Conference on Machine Learning, ICML (2009)
21. Yuille, A.L., Rangarajan, A.: The concave-convex procedure. Neural Computation 15(4), 915–936 (2003)

Unsupervised Learning of Functional Network Dynamics in Resting State fMRI

Harini Eavani[1], Theodore D. Satterthwaite[2], Raquel E. Gur[2],
Ruben C. Gur[2], and Christos Davatzikos[1]

[1] Section of Biomedical Image Analysis, Department of Radiology,
University of Pennsylvania
[2] Brain Behavior Laboratory, Department of Psychiatry, University of Pennsylvania

Abstract. Research in recent years has provided some evidence of temporal non-stationarity of functional connectivity in resting state fMRI. In this paper, we present a novel methodology that can decode connectivity dynamics into a temporal sequence of hidden network "states" for each subject, using a Hidden Markov Modeling (HMM) framework. Each state is characterized by a unique covariance matrix or whole-brain network. Our model generates these covariance matrices from a common but unknown set of sparse basis networks, which capture the range of functional activity co-variations of regions of interest (ROIs). Distinct hidden states arise due to a variation in the strengths of these basis networks. Thus, our generative model combines a HMM framework with sparse basis learning of positive definite matrices. Results on simulated fMRI data show that our method can effectively recover underlying basis networks as well as hidden states. We apply this method on a normative dataset of resting state fMRI scans. Results indicate that the functional activity of a subject at any point during the scan is composed of combinations of overlapping task-positive/negative pairs of networks as revealed by our basis. Distinct hidden temporal states are produced due to a different set of basis networks dominating the covariance pattern in each state.

Keywords: resting state fMRI, functional connectivity, temporal network dynamics.

1 Introduction

Resting state fMRI[1] has emerged as a powerful tool in understanding the effect of mental illnesses on brain function[2]. Functional connectivity or strength of synchronous activity between regions of interest is an important measure that could reveal disease-related changes in brain physiology. Correlation values are widely used as a measure of connectivity but estimation is restricted to a single value obtained from the entire duration of the scan. This could lead to loss of potentially valuable information, since recent exploratory work seems to indicate significant temporal variation in the correlation between regions [3–5]. Using a sliding window framework, the authors reported the presence of repetitive patterns of whole-brain network activity. However sampling the correlation values

J.C. Gee et al. (Eds.): IPMI 2013, LNCS 7917, pp. 426–437, 2013.
© Springer-Verlag Berlin Heidelberg 2013

may not be very reliable due to high estimation error from the smaller windows. Hence, in this paper, we propose modeling the fMRI time-series directly, avoiding explicit sampling of the correlation values.

In this paper, we present a novel method that uses a HMM framework to discretize the temporal variation into a temporal sequence of hidden states. These hidden states could be cognitive processes like introspection, memory consolidation or arising due to unknown external or internal triggers or stimuli[6]. Within each state, the fMRI time-series data is modeled as observations sampled from a multi-variate Gaussian. Each state is characterized by a mean vector value and a unique covariance matrix or whole-brain network. We assume a relatively small number of underlying regions or processes drive the variation in the fMRI signals, introducing subtle changes in the covariance matrices, from which these hidden states can be identified. We model these underlying co-varying regions as a set of sparse rank-one basis matrices, such that non-negative combinations of these basis matrices act as priors for each of the HMM covariance matrices. These basis matrices are unknown and are learned from the data. Thus, our method is a joint framework that solves for the basis vectors as well as the hidden states simultaneously.

The rest of the paper is organized as follows. In section 2 we discuss our generative model in detail. In section 3 we describe the performance of our method on a simulated dataset. We apply our algorithm to resting state fMRI data, and the results are described in section 4. We wrap up with our conclusions and future work in section 5.

2   Approach

2.1   Hidden Markov Model

We begin by describing the first-order HMM framework. Let $\mathbf{Y}^s = [\mathbf{y}_1^s, \mathbf{y}_2^s, \ldots, \mathbf{y}_T^s]$, $\mathbf{y}_t^s \in \mathbf{R}^p$ be the fMRI time-series of a subject s, where p is the number of ROIs and T is the total number of time-points per subject. The superscript s denotes subject index, and the subscript t denotes time-index. Since resting state fMRI is acquired without any control over the subject's stimulus or environment, it is reasonable to assume that the subject wanders in and out of various cognitive states during the duration of the scan. Hence, we will assume that every time-point belongs to one of a finite number N of states. Each state is associated with an occurrence probability δ_i, and every pair of states i, j is associated with a transition probability Π_{ij} of moving from state i to state j. We are interested in describing these states quantitatively, as well finding the optimal sequence of states for each subject. A schematic diagram of an HMM with $N = 3$ states is shown in Fig 1.

We model the "emission" probabilities by a Gaussian distribution. Let $S_t^s \in \{1, 2, \ldots, N\}$ be a random variable denoting the state assignment for subject s at time t. Then, given the state assignment $S_t^s = i$, we let $\mathbf{y}_t^s \sim \mathcal{N}(\mu_i, \mathbf{\Sigma}_i)$, i.e.,

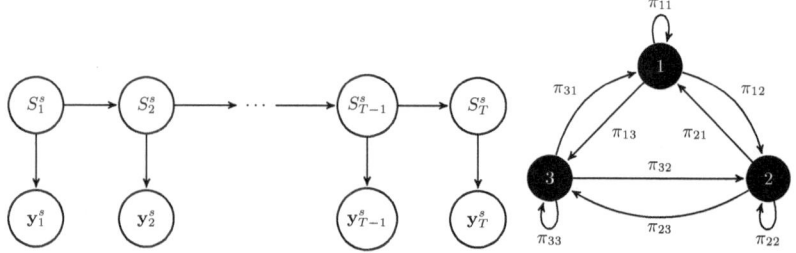

Fig. 1. Schematic of an HMM with $N = 3$. Left shows the temporal sequence $S_1^s, S_2^s, \ldots, S_T^s$ associated with a subject s. Each S_t^s could be one of N states (right).

$$p(\mathbf{y}_t^s | S_t^s = i, \mu_i, \mathbf{\Sigma}_i) = \frac{1}{(2\pi)^{p/2} |\mathbf{\Sigma}_i|^{1/2}} \exp\left\{ -\frac{1}{2} (\mathbf{y}_t^s - \mu_i)^T (\mathbf{\Sigma}_i)^{-1} (\mathbf{y}_t^s - \mu_i) \right\} \tag{1}$$

where $|\cdot|$ denotes determinant. The log-likelihood of the data as a function of the variables is

$$l_1 \left(\{\mu_i\}_1^N, \{\mathbf{\Sigma}_i\}_1^N \right) = \sum_{i=1}^N N_i \left\{ \log \det \mathbf{\Sigma}_i^{-1} - \text{tr} \left(\mathbf{S}_i \mathbf{\Sigma}_i^{-1} \right) \right\} \tag{2}$$

where N_i is the number of time-points that exist in state i, and $\mathbf{S}_i$ is the sample covariance matrix computed using all the time-points assigned to state i.

2.2 Sparse Dictionary Learning for Positive Definite Matrices

We hypothesize that a relatively small number of ROIs change their co-variance pattern from state to state. Similar to the basis learning formulation proposed in [7, 8], let $\mathbf{B} = [\mathbf{b}_1, \mathbf{b}_2, \ldots, \mathbf{b}_K]$, $-1 \preceq \mathbf{b}_k \preceq 1$, $\mathbf{b}_k \in \mathbf{R}^p$ be a set of K basis vectors such that each vector $\mathbf{b}_k$ reflects the membership of the ROIs to the basis network k. If $|\mathbf{b}_k(i)| > 0$, ROI i belongs to the basis vector k, and if $\mathbf{b}_k(i) = 0$ it does not. If two ROIs in $\mathbf{b}_k$ have the same sign, then they are positively correlated and opposing sign reflects that they are anti-correlated. Therefore, the rank-one matrix $\mathbf{b}_k \mathbf{b}_k^T$ reflects the covariance behavior of basis k. In addition, we constrain these basis networks to be much smaller than the whole-brain network by restricting their l_1-norm to a constant value λ.

We would like to approximate the matrices $\{\mathbf{\Sigma}_i\}_{i=1}^N$ representing the HMM states by a non-negative combination of a these basis networks. Thus, we want

$$\mathbf{\Sigma}_i \approx \sum_{k=1}^K c_i(k) \mathbf{b}_k \mathbf{b}_k^T = \mathbf{B} \, \text{diag}(\mathbf{c}_i) \, \mathbf{B}^T \triangleq \hat{\mathbf{\Sigma}}_i$$

$$||\mathbf{b}_k||_1 \leq \lambda, \quad -1 \preceq \mathbf{b}_k \preceq 1, \quad \mathbf{c}_i \geq 0 \tag{3}$$

where diag($\mathbf{c}_i$) denotes a diagonal matrix with values $\mathbf{c}_i$ along the diagonal. In practice, another term $\alpha\mathbf{I}_p$ is added to the $\hat{\boldsymbol{\Sigma}}_i$ matrix to make it positive definite. Here $\mathbf{I}_p$ is the identity matrix of size $p \times p$, and α is a small, fixed ($= 0.1$) value.

We quantify the approximation between $\boldsymbol{\Sigma}_i$ and $\hat{\boldsymbol{\Sigma}}_i$ using the Kullback-Liebler divergence:

$$\mathrm{KL}(\hat{\boldsymbol{\Sigma}}_i \,\|\, \boldsymbol{\Sigma}_i) = \mathrm{tr}(\hat{\boldsymbol{\Sigma}}_i\boldsymbol{\Sigma}_i^{-1}) - \log\det(\hat{\boldsymbol{\Sigma}}_i\boldsymbol{\Sigma}_i^{-1}) \tag{4}$$

The KL divergence described above quantifies the amount of information *lost* when a Gaussian distribution with covariance matrix $\hat{\boldsymbol{\Sigma}}_i$ is instead modeled by covariance matrix $\boldsymbol{\Sigma}_i$. A low value of $\mathrm{KL}(\hat{\boldsymbol{\Sigma}}_i\|\boldsymbol{\Sigma}_i)$ indicates a good approximation between the two matrices. Therefore, we are interested in minimizing the KL-divergence for all the pairs $(\hat{\boldsymbol{\Sigma}}_i, \boldsymbol{\Sigma}_i)$. This amounts to maximizing the function

$$l_2(\mathbf{B}, \mathbf{C}) = \sum_{i=1}^{N} N_i \left\{ \log\det(\hat{\boldsymbol{\Sigma}}_i\boldsymbol{\Sigma}_i^{-1}) - \mathrm{tr}(\hat{\boldsymbol{\Sigma}}_i\boldsymbol{\Sigma}_i^{-1}) \right\} \tag{5}$$

where $\mathbf{C} = [\mathbf{c}_1, \mathbf{c}_2, \ldots, \mathbf{c}_N]$ and N_i is defined as before in equation 2.

We are interested in finding HMM states that are distinct primarily due to differences in their covariance matrices $\boldsymbol{\Sigma}_i$. Clustering data solely based on co-variances is a challenging problem. However, if we assume that the matrices are generated from a common underlying basis $\mathbf{B}$ (as described above), we may be able to separate the clusters by forcing the coefficients $\mathbf{c}_i$ to be distinct, or equivalently, requiring that the inner product $\langle \mathbf{c}_i, \mathbf{c}_j \rangle$, $i \neq j$ be small. This constraint can be imposed by making the term $C^T C$ resemble the identity matrix. Thus, we would like to maximize

$$l_3(\mathbf{C}) = -\left(\sum_{i=1}^{N} N_i\right) \mathrm{KL}(C^T C \,\|\, \mathbf{I}_N) = \left(\sum_{i=1}^{N} N_i\right) \left\{ \log\det(C^T C) - \mathrm{tr}(C^T C) \right\} \tag{6}$$

where $\mathbf{I}_N$ is the identity matrix of size $N \times N$.

2.3 Joint Framework: HMM + Sparse Dictionary Learning

As mentioned earlier, a joint framework causes the HMM to converge to hidden states with distinct covariance matrices. Combining the three objectives in equations 2, 5 and 6 amounts to imposing a prior on the covariance matrices $\boldsymbol{\Sigma}_i$ with prior variables $\mathbf{B}$ and $\mathbf{C}$. We would like to maximize the joint log-likelihood

$$l\left(\{\mu_i\}_1^N, \{\boldsymbol{\Sigma}_i\}_1^N, \mathbf{B}, \mathbf{C}\right) = l_1\left(\{\mu_i\}, \{\boldsymbol{\Sigma}_i\}\right) + v_1\, l_2(\mathbf{B}, \mathbf{C}) + v_2\, l_3(\mathbf{C}) \tag{7}$$

where v_1 and v_2 are user-defined scalar parameters that control the amount of coupling between the HMM and priors. The constraints on the variables are given by

$$\boldsymbol{\Sigma}_i \succ 0, \quad \|\mathbf{b}_k\|_1 \leq \lambda, \quad -1 \preceq \mathbf{b}_k \preceq 1, \quad \mathbf{c}_i \succeq 0, \quad i = 1, 2, \ldots, N, \quad k = 1, 2, \ldots, K \tag{8}$$

Algorithm 1. Optimization strategy for maximizing log-likelihood in Eqn. 7

Input: Data $\mathbf{Y}$, Parameters v_1, v_2, λ, K, N
Initialize: Π, δ, $\mathbf{B}$, $\mathbf{C}$, $\{\mu_i\}_1^N$, $\{\Sigma_i\}_1^N$
   while Log-likelihood in Eqn. 7 is increasing **do**
   E-step
      Compute weights $q_1(S_t^s = i)$ and $q_2(S_t^s = i, S_{t-1}^s = j)$ using Baum-Welch[9]
   M-step:
      Update $\{\mathbf{S}_i\}_1^N$, $\{\mu_i\}_1^N$ and $\{\Sigma_i\}_1^N$ using Equations 9 and 10
      Solve for $\mathbf{B}$ and $\mathbf{C}$ using SPG solver, similar to [10]
      Update Π and δ using standard HMM update formulae[11]
   end while
   Compute optimal state sequences using Viterbi algorithm [12]

2.4   Joint Optimization Strategy

We use Expectation-Maximization[11] to obtain a local maximum. In the Expectation step the posterior marginals $q_1(S_t^s = i) = p(S_t^s = i|\mathbf{Y})$ and $q_2(S_t^s = i, S_{t-1}^s = j) = p(S_t^s = i, S_{t-1}^s = j|\mathbf{Y})$ are efficiently computed using the Baum-Welch[9] algorithm. These values are used as weights for the log-likelihood function. In the Maximization step the weighted log-likelihood function maximized with respect to each of the variables.

The joint log-likelihood is jointly non-concave, but individually concave w.r.t the variables $\{\Sigma_i^{-1}\}_1^N$, $\mathbf{B}$ and $\mathbf{C}$. Hence we will adopt a block optimization strategy that repeatedly solves for one variable (e.g. $\mathbf{B}$) while holding the others fixed (e.g. $\mathbf{C}$ and $\{\Sigma_i^{-1}\}_1^N$) until a local optimum is reached.

The optimal values for $\{\mu_i\}_1^N$ and $\{\Sigma_i\}_1^N$ have closed form expressions given by

$$\mu_i = \frac{\sum_{s,t} q_1(S_t^s = i)\, \mathbf{y}_t^s}{N_i}, \qquad \Sigma_i = \frac{1}{v_1 + 1}\, \mathbf{S}_i + \frac{v_1}{v_1 + 1}\, \hat{\Sigma}_i \qquad (9)$$

where

$$N_i = \sum_{s,t} q_1(S_t^s = i), \quad \mathbf{S}_i = \frac{1}{N_i} \sum_{s,t} q_1(S_t^s = i)(\mathbf{y}_t^s - \mu_i)(\mathbf{y}_t^s - \mu_i)^T, \quad i = 1, \dots, N \tag{10}$$

The optimization w.r.t the variables $\mathbf{B}$ and $\mathbf{C}$ is a constrained maximization problem without closed form solutions. We use the spectral projected gradient (SPG) solver with an efficient projection method, similar to the algorithm proposed in [10] to solve for $\mathbf{B}$ and $\mathbf{C}$ separately.

Matrices $\mathbf{B}$ and $\mathbf{C}$ are initialized randomly. The state transition matrix Π and occurrence probabilities δ are initialized as $\Pi_{ii} = 0.5$, $\Pi_{ij} = 0.5 * (N - 1), i \neq j$, $\delta_i = 1/N$ for $i, j = 1, 2, \dots, N$. Mean vectors μ_i and covariance matrices Σ_i are initialized by using random selection of data points. After the local optima for the unknowns are found using EM, the optimal state sequence for each subject

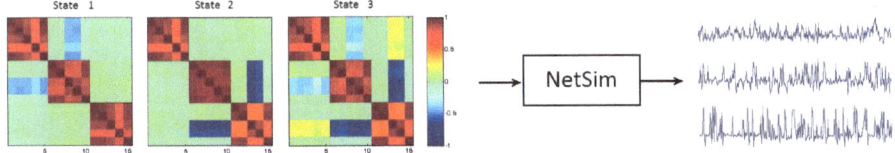

Fig. 2. Simulated data: Ground truth correlation matrices (left) and 50 randomly generated temporal state sequences was input to NetSim [13]. The resulting time-series form the input to our method.

can be found using the Viterbi algorithm [12]. The overall strategy is summarized in Algorithm 1.

2.5   Choice of Free Parameters

Parameters v_1 and v_2 control the effect of the prior variables $\mathbf{B}$ and $\mathbf{C}$ on the model. $v_1 = v_2 = 0$ reduces the model to a standard HMM. Observe from Equation 9 that the optimal value of $\mathbf{\Sigma}_i$ at every M-step is a weighted average of the sample covariance matrix $\mathbf{S}_i$ and the approximation $\hat{\mathbf{\Sigma}}_i$. The weight is controlled by the free parameter v_1. The v_2 parameter controls the orthogonality constraint on the coefficient vectors $\mathbf{c}_i$. For all our experiments in this paper, we set $v_1 = v_2 = 1$. Parameter λ controls the amount of sparsity in the basis vectors and can be set based on known clinical information, for e.g., the average size of a sub-network, like the default mode network(DMN) or the fronto-parietal network.

The number of basis vectors K and the number of HMM states N can be chosen based on how the estimated values for $\mathbf{\Sigma}_i$, $\mathbf{B}$ and $\mathbf{C}$ generalize. To assess generalizability, we will resort to Monte-Carlo split-sample cross-validation. All the other parameters being held fixed, for every value of K and N, the dataset is split into two halves. The model is trained on one half, and using the parameters $\mathbf{\Sigma}_i$, $\mathbf{B}$, $\mathbf{C}$ computed from this half, the weights $q_t^s(i)$ are computed for the second half. This procedure is repeated multiple times and the average cross-validated log-likelihood is computed. The optimal choice of the parameters is considered to be the value at which the average log-likelihood does not significantly change. In this paper we will only examine the case when $K = N$.

3   Validation Using Simulated Data

3.1   Data

We used NetSim [13] to generate time-series data in order to evaluate our method. This software takes as input the underlying network configuration(s) and temporal state sequences. It returns realistic BOLD time series while incorporating neural lag (50 ms), variability in Hemodynamic Response Function (0.5 s) and thermal noise(1% of signal power).

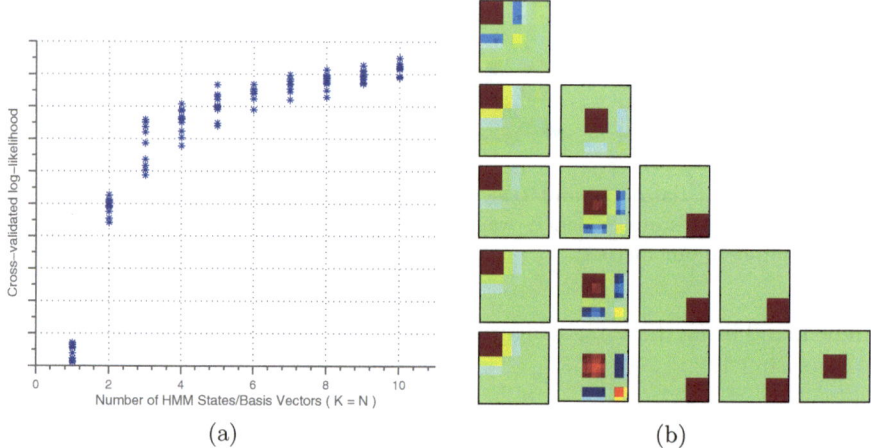

(a)   (b)

Fig. 3. (a) Monte-Carlo cross-validation log-likelihood for simulated data (b) Basis vectors for $K \in \{1, 2, 3, 4, 5\}$. Each row corresponds to a fixed value for K.

At any point in time and in any subject, the data is generated from one of the three network configurations, characterized by the covariance matrices shown in Figure 2. Our simulation consists of 15 nodes arranged in three subnetworks, which are positively correlated within each other (color scale red shown in Figure 2). The between-network connections vary with time - they are either zero (green), or negative (blue). Fifty temporal state sequences are used as input - the mean duration for each state was 40s (~13 TRs). The data was generated by applying Gaussian noise with mean zero as the stimulus at nodes 1,6 and 11. This ensures that the resulting data has mean value close to zero for all the nodes. The basis networks and the temporal state sequences was input to NetSim. This resulted in BOLD time series data for 50 "subjects", with TR=3 s and 120 time-points each.

3.2   Results on Simulated Data

Figure 3a shows the results of the Monte-Carlo cross-validation procedure on the simulated data as N is varied. The average cross-validated log-likelihood with increases with increasing $K = N$, showing that the HMM clusters generalize well. The other parameters are fixed at $v_1 = v_2 = 1$ and $\lambda = 0.2$. The gain in generalizability is reduced after $K \sim 3$ or 4.

The rank-one basis matrices $\mathbf{b}_k \mathbf{b}_k^T$, $k = 1, 2, \ldots, K$ computed for $K \in \{1, 2, 3, 4, 5\}$ are shown in Figure 3b. Each row corresponds to a fixed value for K. The values of the other parameters were fixed at $v_1 = v_2 = 1$ and $\lambda = 0.2$. It is evident that our algorithm effectively recovers the network basis. Our basis clearly identifies the clustering of the nodes into sub-networks and the anti-correlated relationship between them. Also, observe that each time K is increased by one, the method incrementally adds to the previous basis.

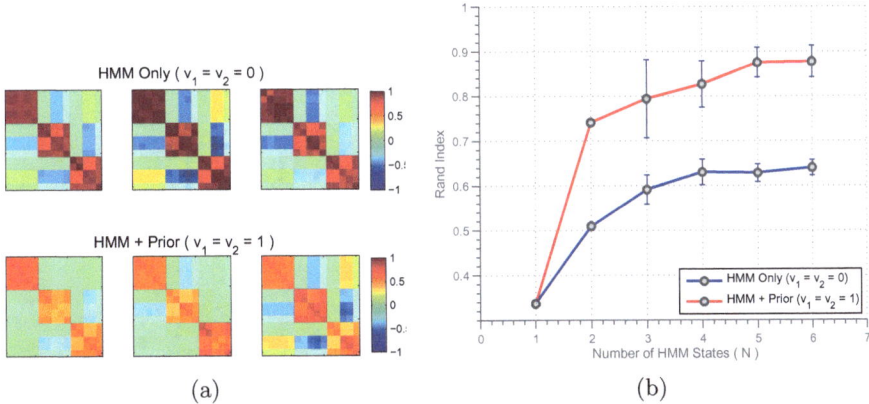

Fig. 4. (a) Covariance matrices Σ_i for HMM only (top) and our method (bottom) (b) Cross-validated Rand Index vs. N for both cases

The comparison between the performance of our method with the HMM alone is shown in Figure 4 . Figure 4a shows the estimated covariance matrices $\{\Sigma_i\}_{i=1}^{N}$ for $N = K = 3$, when only the HMM is used (top) and with the priors (bottom). Clearly, our method accurately estimates the underlying covariance matrices for all three states. Due to the lack of a significant difference in the mean vectors, the HMM alone performs poorly, with little or no difference between the three states. The optimal state-paths output by the Viterbi algorithm are also compared with the ground truth for both cases using the Rand Index (Figure 4b). Our method is able to achieve close to 90% clustering accuracy, while the HMM alone fails.

4   Application to Resting State fMRI Data

4.1   Data

BOLD fMRI was acquired with a Siemens 3 Tesla system using a whole-brain, gradient-echo echo planar sequence with TR/TE = 3000/32 ms, voxel resolution = 3x3x3 mm and number of time-points = 120. We used data from 420 normal participants, with age range 15.9 ± 3 years.

Pre-processing. Functional images were motion corrected, spatially smoothed (6mm FWHM) and temporally altered to retain frequencies 0.01-0.1 Hz. Several sources of confounding variance, including six motion parameters and mean whole-brain, WM, CSF time-courses were regressed out. The residual time course for each subject was transformed to standard MNI anatomical space. We used 160 regions of interest (ROIs) described by Dosenbach et al. [14], which were derived from a meta-analysis of a large sample of task-based fMRI studies. Each ROI was a non-overlapping 10mm diameter sphere, and was categorized by Dosenbach et al. as belonging to one of six networks, including: default-mode, cingulo-opercular, fronto-parietal, sensorimotor, occipital or cerebellar. The mean time-series of each ROI is

434   H. Eavani et al.

extracted from the registered fMRI image. The time-series is demeaned and scaled to have an average variance value of unity.

4.2 Results on fMRI Data

Fig. 5. Monte-Carlo cross-validation log-likelihood for fMRI data. The log-likelihood is greatest for $K = N \in \{2, 3, 4, 5\}$. The generalizability is variable for $N \in \{6, 7\}$ and begins to fall after $N = 7$, showing that our model begins to over-fit the data after this value. Thus, from the given data, we are able to obtain $N = 6$ distinct HMM states.

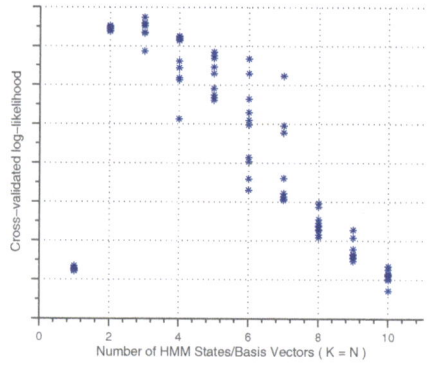

Figure 6 shows the six rank-one basis matrices obtained from our method. The ROIs are sorted according to their Dosenbach[14] network labels. It is easy to observe that our method is fairly accurate in identifying the general clustering

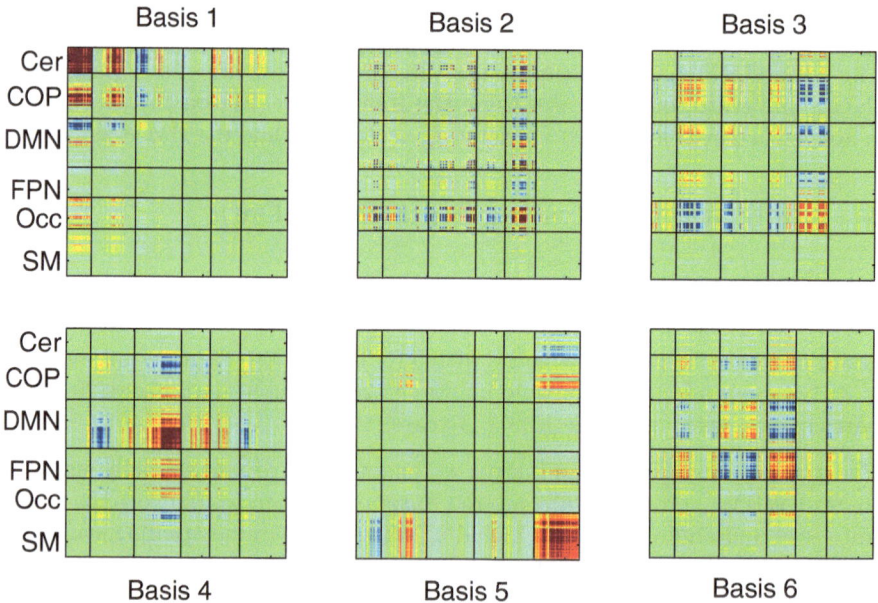

Fig. 6. Rank-one basis matrices for fMRI data. The Dosenbach [14] labels are given on the left. Abbreviations Cer: Cerebellum, COP: Cingulo-opercular network, DMN: Default-mode network, FPN: Fronto-Parietal network, Occ: Occipital network, SM: Sensori-motor network.

of the ROIs, since most ROIs belonging to a basis network are assigned the same Dosenbach labels. For example, all the ROIs belonging to the cerebellum are clustered in basis 1. Same is the case with occipital cortex (basis 3), default mode (basis 4), sensori-motor (basis 5) and fronto-parietal (basis 6).

We looked at two sub-networks in particular - the fronto-parietal network ("dorsal attentional network") and the cingulo-opercular network ("ventral attentional network"). Both are task-positive networks that activate when the subject is in an "extrospective" state, and it is well-established that activation of either of these networks causes the default mode network (DMN) to deactivate [1]. This behavior is captured in basis 6, which shows the anti-correlated nature of the fronto-parietal network and default mode. The anti-correlation between the cingulo-opercular network (COP) and the DMN is captured across multiple basis networks (1, 4 and 6).

We also note that the most amount of overlap between the basis networks occurs at the COP, with different aspects of it positively correlating with the cerebellum, sensori-motor and fronto-parietal networks(in basis 1, 5 and 6 respectively) and negatively correlating with the default mode and occipital

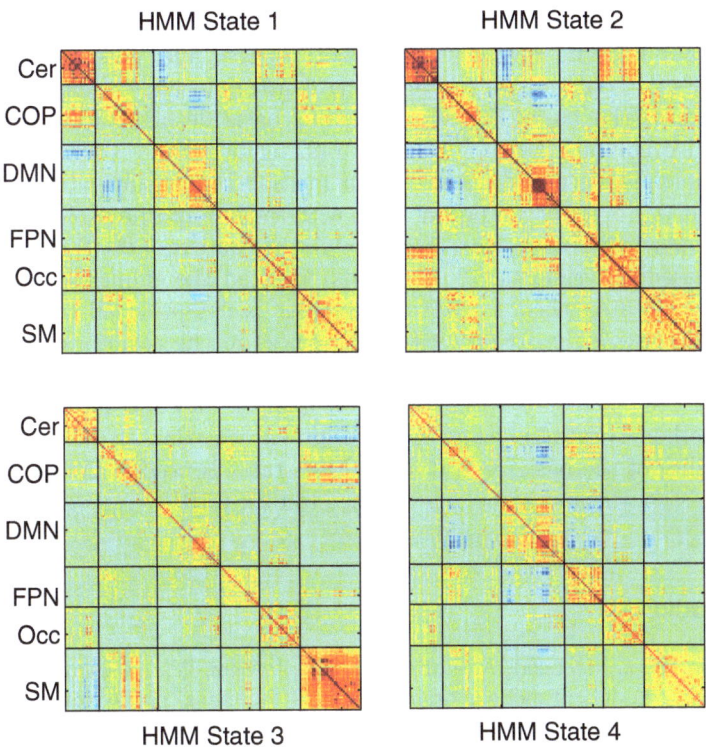

Fig. 7. Four HMM States obtained from resting state fMRI data. Abbreviations Cer: Cerebellum, COP: Cingulo-opercular network, DMN: Default-mode network, FPN: Fronto-Parietal network, Occ: Occipital network, SM: Sensori-motor network.

networks (in basis 1 and 3). The fact that these correlation/anti-correlation relationships are split amongst the basis networks suggests that they have different temporal behavior.

The covariance matrices Σ_i are shown in Figure 7. Due to the page limit only the four of the six covariance matrices are shown. It is clear that the states are separated based on the dominant basis networks. The cingulo-opercular network is most active in states 1 and 2, positively correlating with the cerebellum and negatively correlating with the DMN. State 2 shows greater activity in the occipital network. The sensori-motor network is active in state 3. State 4 is dominated by the anti-correlated pair of the fronto-parietal network and the DMN. The average duration the subjects existed in each of these states was between 12 and 20 time-points.

5   Conclusion

To our knowledge, this is the first attempt at resolving functional connectivity in resting state fMRI data into discrete temporal states, each associated with a distinct connectivity pattern. Each subject is assigned a sequence of states, which can then be used for group comparisons.

Our basis learning formulation provides sparse and possibly overlapping components without having to use strong constraints like orthogonality or independence of the basis. Further more, our basis decomposition only allows non-negative combinations of basis vectors, making the resulting basis more interpretable. These properties make our method better suited than spatial or temporal ICA [15] for decomposing brain activity into interpretable components.

Hidden Markov Models have been used in the context of fMRI, but primarily for task-based experiments [16][17]. In our method the emphasis is on finding hidden brain-states when an external stimulus is not provided to the subject. The HMM is strongly driven by the differences in the covariance matrices of these hidden brain states.

As a part of our future work, we hope to analyze the effect of model selection on our method is greater detail. A thorough examination of the functional interpretability of the basis vectors and HMM states is needed. As an additional validation step, this method can be applied to task-fMRI to recover the stimulus sequence.

References

1. Raichle, M.E., MacLeod, A.M., Snyder, A.Z., Powers, W.J., Gusnard, D.A., Shulman, G.L.: A default mode of brain function. Proceedings of the National Academy of Sciences 98(2), 676–682 (2001)
2. Broyd, S.J., Demanuele, C., Debener, S., Helps, S.K., James, C.J., Sonuga-Barke, E.J.S., et al.: Default-mode brain dysfunction in mental disorders: a systematic review. Neuroscience and Biobehavioral Reviews 33(3), 279 (2009)
3. Chang, C., Glover, G.H.: Time-frequency dynamics of resting-state brain connectivity measured with fMRI. Neuroimage 50(1), 81–98 (2010)

4. Majeed, W., Magnuson, M., Hasenkamp, W., Schwarb, H., Schumacher, E.H., Barsalou, L., Keilholz, S.D.: Spatiotemporal dynamics of low frequency bold fluctuations in rats and humans. Neuroimage 54(2), 1140–1150 (2011)
5. Hutchison, R.M., Womelsdorf, T., Gati, J.S., Everling, S., Menon, R.S.: Resting-state networks show dynamic functional connectivity in awake humans and anesthetized macaques. Human Brain Mapping (2012)
6. Buckner, R.L., Vincent, J.L., et al.: Unrest at rest: default activity and spontaneous network correlations. Neuroimage 37(4), 1091–1096 (2007)
7. Sra, S., Cherian, A.: Generalized dictionary learning for symmetric positive definite matrices with application to nearest neighbor retrieval. In: Gunopulos, D., Hofmann, T., Malerba, D., Vazirgiannis, M. (eds.) ECML PKDD 2011, Part III. LNCS (LNAI), vol. 6913, pp. 318–332. Springer, Heidelberg (2011)
8. Sivalingam, R., Boley, D., Morellas, V., Papanikolopoulos, N.: Positive definite dictionary learning for region covariances. In: 2011 IEEE International Conference on Computer Vision (ICCV), pp. 1013–1019. IEEE (2011)
9. Baum, L.E., Petrie, T., Soules, G., Weiss, N.: A maximization technique occurring in the statistical analysis of probabilistic functions of markov chains. The Annals of Mathematical Statistics, 164–171 (1970)
10. Batmanghelich, N.K., Taskar, B., Davatzikos, C.: Generative-discriminative basis learning for medical imaging. IEEE Transactions on Medical Imaging 31(1), 51–69 (2012)
11. Bishop, C.M., et al.: Pattern recognition and machine learning, vol. 4. Springer, New York (2006)
12. Viterbi, A.: Error bounds for convolutional codes and an asymptotically optimum decoding algorithm. IEEE Transactions on Information Theory 13(2), 260–269 (1967)
13. Smith, S.M., Miller, K.L., Salimi-Khorshidi, G., Webster, M., Beckmann, C.F., Nichols, T.E., Ramsey, J.D., Woolrich, M.W.: Network modelling methods for fmri. Neuroimage 54(2), 875–891 (2011)
14. Dosenbach, N.U.F., Fair, D.A., Miezin, F.M., Cohen, A.L., et al.: Distinct brain networks for adaptive and stable task control in humans. Proceedings of the National Academy of Sciences 104(26), 11073 (2007)
15. Smith, S.M., Miller, K.L., Moeller, S., Xu, J., Auerbach, E.J., Woolrich, M.W., Beckmann, C.F., Jenkinson, M., Andersson, J., Glasser, M.F., et al.: Temporally-independent functional modes of spontaneous brain activity. Proceedings of the National Academy of Sciences 109(8), 3131–3136 (2012)
16. Faisan, S., Thoraval, L., Armspach, J.P., Heitz, F.: Hidden markov multiple event sequence models: A paradigm for the spatio-temporal analysis of fmri data. Medical Image Analysis 11(1), 1 (2007)
17. Janoos, F., Machiraju, R., Singh, S., Morocz, I.Á.: Spatio-temporal models of mental processes from fmri. Neuroimage 57(2), 362–377 (2011)

Cohort-Level Brain Mapping:
Learning Cognitive Atoms
to Single Out Specialized Regions

Gaël Varoquaux[1,2,3], Yannick Schwartz[1,2], Philippe Pinel[2,3],
and Bertrand Thirion[1,2]

[1] INRIA, Parietal Team, Saclay, France
[2] NeuroSpin, CEA Saclay, Bat. 145, 91191 Gif-sur-Yvette, cedex France
[3] INSERM U992 Cognitive Neuroimaging Unit, France

Abstract. Functional Magnetic Resonance Imaging (fMRI) studies map
the human brain by testing the response of groups of individuals to
carefully-crafted and contrasted tasks in order to delineate specialized
brain regions and networks. The number of functional networks extracted
is limited by the number of subject-level contrasts and does not grow with
the cohort. Here, we introduce a new group-level brain mapping strategy to differentiate many regions reflecting the variety of brain network
configurations observed in the population. Based on the principle of functional segregation, our approach singles out functionally-specialized brain
regions by learning group-level functional profiles on which the response
of brain regions can be represented sparsely. We use a dictionary-learning
formulation that can be solved efficiently with on-line algorithms, scaling to arbitrary large datasets. Importantly, we model inter-subject correspondence as structure imposed in the estimated functional profiles,
integrating a structure-inducing regularization with no additional computational cost. On a large multi-subject study, our approach extracts a
large number of brain networks with meaningful functional profiles.

1 Introduction

Using fMRI, the systematic study of which areas of the brain are recruited
during various experiments has led to accumulation of activation maps related
to specific tasks or cognitive concepts in an ever growing literature. Mapping a
given population requires careful crafting of a set of tasks that are contrasted to
reveal networks. These networks form a natural representation of brain function
and are of particular interest to study its variability in a population, for instance
to correlate it to pathologies or genetic information. However, each subject can
only perform a small number of tasks in a scanner; particularly so for disabled
subjects. As a result, in a given study the number of networks that is identified by
standard task-activation mapping is small and limited by the number of contrasts
of the study. On the other hand, it is not uncommon to scan a large number of
subjects. Indeed, clinical studies must often resort to larger sample sizes due to
the intrinsic variability of pathologies. Massive cohorts can be acquired, *e.g.* to
learn diagnosis markers for Alzheimer's disease [10], or in neuroimaging-genetics.

J.C. Gee et al. (Eds.): IPMI 2013, LNCS 7917, pp. 438–449, 2013.

In large cohorts, a small set of contrasts reveals effects throughout the whole brain [16]. This observation suggests that more information can be extracted at the cohort level. In this paper, we address precisely this challenge by decomposing brain activity and experimental conditions at the group level to assign a specific cognitive function to each voxel. For this purpose, inter-subject variability is a blessing as functional variability reveals *functional degeneracy*, *i.e.* that different networks sustain the same cognitive function across individuals [9]. However, this variability is also a curse when it arises from spatial realignment error.

Compressed spatial representations were put forward for group studies by Thirion *et al.* [15] using clustering of the activation maps. This early work did not address the functional specificity of the clusters. Conversely, Lashkari *et al.* [7] discard spatial information and focus on extracting common functional profiles across subject, removing the need for spatial normalization. Following this idea of functional correspondence across subject, although not leading to the definition of regions, Sabuncu *et al.* [12] use this correspondence for inter-subject alignment. Linear models such as independent component analysis (ICA) have been used to extract modes of brain function across subjects [2] before clustering approaches. Laird *et al.* [6] have recently shown that the modes that it extracts from task-activation data capture meaningful structure in the space of cognitive processes. Beyond ICA, Varoquaux *et al.* [18] use dictionary learning to segment a functional parcellation from resting-state. Very interesting preliminary work by Chen *et al.* [3] integrates spatial normalization with dictionary learning to estimate jointly an inter-subject warping and functional regions.

The present paper combines ideas from this prior art in a new inter-subject model with an associated computationally-scalable estimation algorithm. Our contributions are *i)* a joint model of the position and functional tuning of brain networks, *ii)* explicit separation of the variance into intra-subject and inter-subject components, *iii)* a fast and scalable algorithm that can impose this particular variance structure. We show with simple simulations that controlling inter-subject variance is crucial, as unsupervised learning approaches such as dictionary learning or clustering will fit this variance and extract modes reflecting inter-subject variability. The paper is organized as followed. We start by giving a multi-subject model combining random effects (RFX) with functional segregation hypothesis. In section 3, we introduce an on-line and computationally-efficient algorithm to estimate this model. In section 4, we present a simulation study, and in section 5 results on an fMRI dataset comprising 150 subjects.

2   A Multi-subject Sparse-Coding Model of Brain Response

Sparse coding brain response. Our model is based on two basic neuroscience principles: *i) functional segregation* which states that brain territories are formed of elementary, functionally-specific units [17] and *ii) functional degeneracy* which states that a particular function may recruit different networks across subjects [9]. We combine these principles at the subject and group level to learn the correct basis to describe the macroscopic level of brain organization.

Experimental stimuli and contrasts do not correspond simply to elementary cognitive processes. For instance to isolate brain regions involved in a calculation tasks, instructions to perform arithmetics will be given to a subject, however these instructions are given via a modality: auditory or visual, and will induce a word-comprehension task in addition to the calculation. Investigators use *contrast maps* to cancel out secondary effects and focus on *word – calculations*, but these contrasts can carry also some auditory, visual, or language effects as the stimuli content in the different tasks are not perfectly matched.

A typical fMRI experiment thus yields a set of task-specific contrast maps: for each subject s, $\boldsymbol{X}^s \in \mathbb{R}^{t \times n}$, where t is the number of tasks and n the number of voxels. Based on the principles of functional specialization, we stipulate that the tasks used are formed of elementary cognitive processes associated with a set of corresponding sparse neural substrates: there exist combinations of tasks $\boldsymbol{D} = \{\boldsymbol{d}_j\}$ such that each $\boldsymbol{d}_j$ is expressed on a small number of brain regions:

$$\boldsymbol{X}^s = \boldsymbol{D}\boldsymbol{A}^{s\top}, \qquad \text{where } \boldsymbol{A}^s \text{ is sparse.} \qquad (1)$$

We are interested in learning a dictionary of k functional profiles $\boldsymbol{D} \in \mathbb{R}^{t \times k}$ and the associated sparse spatial code $\boldsymbol{A}^s \in \mathbb{R}^{n \times k}$, that we call *functional networks*. The number of atomic cognitive functions recruited by the tasks explored in an fMRI experiment is most likely much larger than the number of experimental conditions t. Drawing from a large number of subjects can help to estimate more functional profiles, as subjects will resort to different *cognitive strategies*, engaging differently atomic cognitive functions. To give a clichéd image, right-handed and left-handed subjects could rely on different visuo-spatial representations to perform a hand motion task. In practice, variability in cognitive strategy is often very subtle and can be related to variability in attention, engagement to the task, background processes, rather than high-level strategies [9]. Modeling this inter-subject variability should improve the quantification of population-level estimates and enable the separation of atoms of brain function.

Multi-subject modeling. We introduce subject-specific expressions of the functional profiles:

$$\boldsymbol{F}^s = (\boldsymbol{I} + \boldsymbol{\Delta}^s)\boldsymbol{D}, \qquad \text{where } \boldsymbol{\Delta}^s \sim \mathcal{N}(0, \sigma^2 \boldsymbol{I}_t), \quad \boldsymbol{\Delta}^s \in \mathbb{R}^{t \times t}, \quad \boldsymbol{F}^s \in \mathbb{R}^{t \times k} \qquad (2)$$

An approach commonly used when dealing with such unsupervised learning problem on multi-subject fMRI data is to concatenate the data spatially [2,15], learning an augmented dictionary,

$$\overline{\boldsymbol{F}} = \left[\boldsymbol{F}^{1\top} \ldots \boldsymbol{F}^{s\top}\right]^\top = \left[(\boldsymbol{I} + \boldsymbol{\Delta}^1)^\top, \ldots (\boldsymbol{I} + \boldsymbol{\Delta}^s)^\top\right]^\top \boldsymbol{D} \in \mathbb{R}^{st \times k}. \qquad (3)$$

The multi-subject model resulting from (1) and (2) can then be written as a standard dictionary-learning problem: $\overline{\boldsymbol{X}} = \overline{\boldsymbol{F}}\boldsymbol{A}^\top$, with $\overline{\boldsymbol{X}} \in \mathbb{R}^{st \times n}$ the spatial concatenation of the data and $\boldsymbol{A}$ functional networks independent of the subject. By learning a dictionary spanning multiple datasets, it can estimate inter-subject loadings that reveal the different cognitive strategies, drawing from the *spatial correspondence* of the coding of the information. However, estimating high-dimensional dictionaries has two major drawbacks: *i)* it is more challenging from the statistical standpoint because the residuals implicit in eq. 3 are non white and *ii)* this approach is fragile to errors in inter-subject correspondence.

To remove the need for spatial matching, Lashkari *et al.* [7] cluster the activity profiles, grouping voxels that respond similarly to the tasks across subjects. This *functional correspondence* hypothesis leads to a functional concatenation of the data: $\underline{\boldsymbol{X}} = [\boldsymbol{X}^1_\cdot \dots \boldsymbol{X}^{s\mathsf{T}}]^\mathsf{T} \in \mathbb{R}^{t \times sn}$. The multi-subject model is then written $\underline{\boldsymbol{X}} = \boldsymbol{D}\underline{\boldsymbol{A}}^\mathsf{T}$ with $\underline{\boldsymbol{A}} = [(\boldsymbol{I}_k + \boldsymbol{\Delta}^1)\boldsymbol{A}^1_\cdot \dots (\boldsymbol{I}_k + \boldsymbol{\Delta}^s)\boldsymbol{A}^{s\mathsf{T}}]^\mathsf{T} \in \mathbb{R}^{k \times sn}$, which amounts to learning a dictionary common to all subjects and different spatial maps.

Modeling Random effects. Both spatial and functional concatenation approaches lead to a simple formulation in terms of learning a dictionary of functional profiles and spatial code. However a naive resolution of these dictionary learning problems neglects that both spatial code and functional profiles share information across subjects. In functional neuroimaging data analysis, the standard way to model both common effects and variability across datasets relies on hierarchical linear models, often mixed- or random-effects (RFX) models that assume that the effect has two components of variance: inter-subject and intra-subject [19]. We can adapt this model to enhance the spatial correspondence approach by constraining the ratio of the intra- and inter-subject variance of the functional profiles in the augmented dictionary $\overline{\boldsymbol{F}}$. For this purpose, we introduce a *common effect matrix* made of s $k \times k$ identity matrices concatenated: $\boldsymbol{C} = \frac{1}{s}[\boldsymbol{I}_k, \dots \boldsymbol{I}_k]^\mathsf{T} \in \mathbb{R}^{k \times sk}$ and the *differential effects matrix* $\boldsymbol{C}_\perp \in \mathbb{R}^{(s-1)k \times sk}$, which is an orthogonal completion of $\boldsymbol{C}$. To impose an RFX structure on the dictionary, we present in section 3 an algorithm controlling $\|\overline{\boldsymbol{f}}_i\boldsymbol{C}\|_2^2 / \|\overline{\boldsymbol{f}}_i\boldsymbol{C}_\perp\|_2^2$, where $i \in [1, t]$ is the index of a dictionary element.

Proposition 1. $\boldsymbol{C}$ *and* $\boldsymbol{C}_\perp$ *isolate* i) *group-level profiles:* $\mathbb{E}[\overline{\boldsymbol{f}}_i\boldsymbol{C}] = \boldsymbol{d}_i$,

ii) *intra-subject variance:* $\mathbb{E}[\|\overline{\boldsymbol{f}}_i\boldsymbol{C}\|_2^2] = (1 + \frac{\sigma^2}{s})\|\boldsymbol{d}_i\|_2^2 \sim \|\boldsymbol{d}_i\|_2^2$,

iii) *inter-subject variance:* $\mathbb{E}[\|\overline{\boldsymbol{f}}_i\boldsymbol{C}_\perp\|_2^2] = (\sigma^2 - \frac{\sigma^2}{s})\|\boldsymbol{d}_i\|_2^2 \sim \sigma^2\|\boldsymbol{d}_i\|_2^2$.

The first and the second equalities stem from Eq. (3), while the last one follows from the fact that $\|\overline{\boldsymbol{f}}_j\|_2^2 = \|\overline{\boldsymbol{f}}_j\boldsymbol{C}\|_2^2 + \|\overline{\boldsymbol{f}}_j\boldsymbol{C}_\perp\|_2^2$, as $[\boldsymbol{C}^\mathsf{T}, \boldsymbol{C}_\perp^\mathsf{T}]$ forms a basis of $\mathbb{R}^{sk}$.

3   Efficient Learning of RFX-Structured Dictionaries

State-of-the-art dictionary learning algorithm. A general approach to learn dictionaries for sparse coding is to optimize the dictionary so that is leads to a sparse regression on train data, using an ℓ_1 penalty on the code [8]:

$$\hat{\boldsymbol{D}} = \underset{\boldsymbol{A}, \boldsymbol{D}, \, \boldsymbol{D} \in \mathcal{C}}{\operatorname{argmin}} \; \|\boldsymbol{X} - \boldsymbol{D}\boldsymbol{A}^\mathsf{T}\|_2^2 - \lambda\|\boldsymbol{A}\|_1, \tag{4}$$

where $\boldsymbol{X}, \boldsymbol{D}, \boldsymbol{A}$ should be replaced by $\overline{\boldsymbol{X}}, \overline{\boldsymbol{F}}, \boldsymbol{A}$ or $\underline{\boldsymbol{X}}, \boldsymbol{D}, \underline{\boldsymbol{A}}$ depending on the choice of correspondence. Note that the dictionary $\boldsymbol{D}$ is constrained to a convex set $\mathcal{C}$, typically by bounding the ℓ_2 norm of its atoms: $\|d_i\|_2 \leq 1$. This constraint is technical, as without it the penalty on A could be made arbitrarily small by scaling up D and down A and thus keeping the data-fit term constant. Let us rewrite the optimization problem:

$$\hat{D} = \underset{D,\ D \in \mathcal{C}}{\operatorname{argmin}} \sum_v \min_{a_v} \left(\|x_v - Da_v^{\mathsf{T}}\|_2^2 + \lambda \|a_v\|_1 \right). \tag{5}$$

This new expression highlights that, when learning the dictionary, the objective function is the sum over a large number of different realizations of the same problem, here sparse coding a simple voxel activation profile x_v. The optimization problem can thus be tackled using stochastic gradient descent with on-line or mini-batch strategies [8]: small numbers of voxels randomly drawn from the data are successively considered and a corresponding sparse code a_v is learned by solving a Lasso-type problem. The dictionary can then be updated to minimize the data-fit error given the code. The algorithm iterates over small batches of voxels (hundreds) to incrementally improve the dictionary. When the number of voxels is large, such an approach can be orders of magnitude faster than the alternate optimization strategies used by [18,3], because these require solving brain-wide sparse regression for each update of the dictionary.

Szabo *et al.* [14] extend this approach to structured dictionaries by replacing the ℓ_1 norm on α_v with a structure-inducing norm, such as the ℓ_{21} norm used in the group lasso. However, the corresponding algorithms to learn the sparse code a_v are much more costly as they rely in general on optimizing augmented problems over auxiliary variables [14]. On the opposite, efficient algorithms to solve the ℓ_1 problem benefit from the sparsity of the solution and can be much less costly than a least-square estimate for very sparse problems [4].

Imposing RFX-structured dictionaries. We introduce a simple modification to the on-line algorithm [8] to impose an RFX structure on the dictionary. Our approach is based on spatial correspondence to learn an augmented dictionary $\overline{F}$ and sets different intra and inter-subject variance using proposition 1: controlling the ratio of the norm of $\overline{F}C$ and $\overline{F}C_\perp$. For this purpose, we use a careful choice of constraint set $\mathcal{C}$ on the dictionary; namely, we impose on each atom

$$\Omega(\overline{f}_i) \leq 1, \qquad \text{with } \Omega(\overline{f}_i) = \max(\|\overline{f}_i C\|_2^2, \ \mu \|\overline{f}_i C_\perp\|_2^2), \tag{6}$$

where μ controls the ratio of intra to inter subject variance. Because of the penalty on A, it is highly likely that the constraint will be saturated. This constraint is an ℓ_∞ norm, which tends to enforce equality when saturated[1]: $\|\overline{f}_i C\|_2^2 = \mu \|\overline{f}_i C_\perp\|_2^2$.

In the on-line dictionary learning algorithm, this constraint is enforced by an Euclidean projection (see algorithm 2 of [8]): at each iteration

$$d_{n+1} \leftarrow \underset{d}{\operatorname{argmin}} \|d_n - d\|_2^2 \quad \text{subject to } \Omega(d) \leq 1. \tag{7}$$

---

[1] Indeed, combined with an ℓ_2 loss, an ℓ_∞ constraint tends to saturate at its *kinks* enforcing equality between variables, as an ℓ_1 constraint enforces sparsity.

The *max* operator in Ω imposes that $\|\overline{f_i}C\|_2^2 \leq 1$ and $\|\overline{f_i}C_\perp\|_2^2 \leq \frac{1}{\mu}$. As C and $C_\perp$ span orthogonal subspaces, the Euclidean distance decomposes in two independent optimization problems on those subspaces: the projection on a ball of radius 1 (resp. $\frac{1}{\mu}$), $c_{n+1} \leftarrow c_n / \|c_n\|_2$, where c is the restriction of d to the subspace spanned by C (resp. $C_\perp$). In practice, to implement this projection, we apply the dictionary-update algorithm after rotating the dictionary and the code to express them in the basis of $\mathbb{R}^{sk}$ formed by $[C^\mathsf{T}, C_\perp^\mathsf{T}]$, and for the sparse-coding step, we rotate back the dictionary to the basis that leads to sparse codes. With this strategy, the Euclidean projection Eq. (7) has the same computational cost with norm Ω than with the standard ℓ_2 norm proposed in [8]. As the computational cost of the dictionary update step is already quadratic in the length of the atoms, this strategy to impose an RFX structure on the dictionary does not change the overall algorithmic complexity of dictionary learning, neither asymptotically nor for small dictionaries.

Parameter choice and initialization. Our algorithm has two parameters: λ, that controls the sparsity of the spatial maps, and μ that controls the ratio of intra-subject to inter-subject variance. We set that ratio to 10. Typically in fMRI study, inter-subject variance is 4 to 9 times larger than intra-subject variance [19], thus we are over-penalizing. However, in statistics, over-penalization is considered as preferable to under-penalization, as the former leads to bias, here to a common effect, while the later can easily lead to an explosion of variance. With regards to λ, the natural scaling factor is $\lambda \propto \frac{1}{\sqrt{p}}\varepsilon$ where p is the size of the atoms, and ε^2 the variance of the residuals [1]. We assume that $\varepsilon^2 \propto \mathrm{std}\, X$ and use the simple choice $\lambda \propto \frac{1}{\sqrt{p}}\mathrm{std}\, X$. Similar scalings are suggested in [8]. They lead to having a number of non-zero constant on average in the code A. In other words, each voxel is coded on the same number of maps, independently of the size of the problem (number of maps extracted, number of contrasts).

The dictionary learning problem is not convex. The starting point is important because a good choice can significantly speed up the convergence, and also determine the final results. We use spatially-constrained clustering on spatially-concatenated data [15] to learn an initial parcellation and associated dictionary.

4   Results on Simulated Data

Synthetic data generation. We generate a simple and well-understood synthetic dataset to illustrate how the different approaches work, as well as the impact of spatial variability. We study the scenario in which two observed contrasts are generated from three functional networks, each one of them made of a single blob (Fig. 1, top left). Group-level loadings are generated from a uniform $[0, 1]$ distribution, and for each subject one cognitive strategy out of two, corresponding to a variation in 20% of the weights, is affected randomly. Finally, Gaussian-distributed noise is added with a variance of 0.1. We generate images of size 50×50 for 32 subjects. Optionally, we add spatial variability across subjects with Gaussian noise of 3 pixel standard deviation on the positions of the blobs.

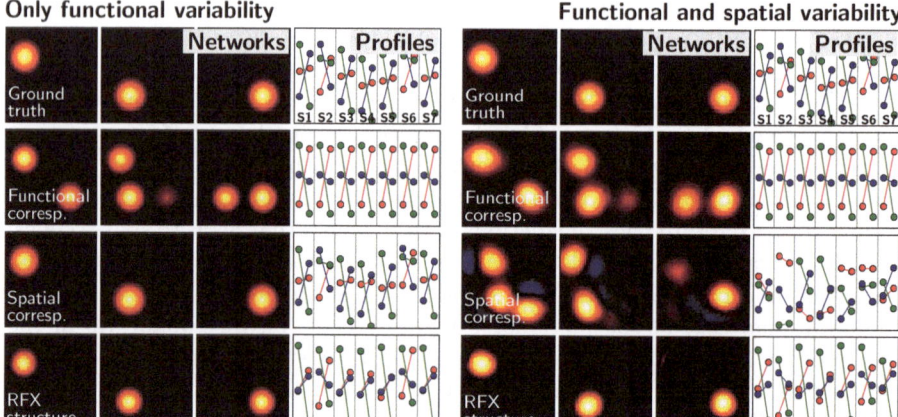

Fig. 1. Simulations: functional networks and subject-level profiles as estimated by different dictionary learning strategies – right column: with only functional variability – left column: with spatial variability. On the ground-truth profile plot the second cognitive strategy can be seen from the red loadings in the second and sixth subjects.

Results. Without spatial variability, spatial correspondence and RFX-structure are very successful at singling out the blobs, however the functional correspondence strategy is less so (see Fig. 1). This is not surprising, as in the functional correspondence case, the dictionary learning task amounts to separating out 3 vectors (functional profiles) in a 2-dimensional space, which corresponds to an under-determined source separation problem. The under-determined problem is much harder than the over-determined problem, as in the spatial correspondence approach. Indeed, learning an augmented dictionary across subjects can benefit from inter-subject functional variability to tease out networks. However, in the presence of spatial variability, the simple spatial correspondence fits this variability and the estimated maps exhibit *adjustment* modes, combining different networks with negative regions that correspond to network spatial derivatives. Indeed, the loadings show little consistency across subjects, as the spatial maps learning are combined to compensate for spatial fluctuations. The RFX structure prevents such a combination to happen via a shrinkage to common factors. As a result the spatial maps are more faithful to the true networks. Note that the inter-subject profiles are overly shrunk. This an expected consequence of strong regularization: suppressing the variance comes to the cost of a bias. However this bias is not detrimental to the mean profile or the spatial maps.

5 Learning a Cognitive Brain Atlas from fMRI

Functional localizer dataset. We use a functional localizer that targets a wide spectrum of cognitive processes, namely visual, auditory and sensorimotor processes, as well as reading, language comprehension and mental calculation.

This protocol [11] lasts only 5 minutes, in order to be performed routinely on top of other protocols. We use 151 subjects that were acquired on the same 3T SIEMENS Trio scanner. 6 contrast maps best represent the brain activity for the cognitive processes recruited in this protocol. The contrast maps are both a combination of several conditions (e.g., sentence reading, calculation), and a difference of those conditions (e.g., right click versus left click) to draw out the effect of interest. For instance, the map "calculation - words" aims to isolate the effect of calculation by canceling out the modality of the stimulus (auditory or visual), and the residual effect of the comprehension of the stimulus (reading or listening). The effect of words is then encoded by negative loadings.

Networks and profiles extracted. Fig. 2 shows some functional networks and profiles extracted using $k = 50$. The profiles are represented by their loadings on the contrasts of the original experiment, that oppose one type of brain function to another. Some networks extracted correspond across methods: for instance the network corresponding to a left click (a1, b1 and c1), for which the spatial map highlights the hand area of the motor cortex and the functional profiles are concentrated on the motor and left contrasts. As finger movement gives very strong activations, this network is reliable across subjects: standard errors on contrast loadings are small and the inter-subject functional profiles (Fig. 3) are similar across subjects even without enforcing structure. Note that a similar right-click network is also extracted (not shown). Extracting such a network is no surprise, as it maps well to a task performed in the study. More interestingly, networks corresponding to higher-level cognition are also extracted, *e.g.* the language network (a2, b2 and c2) and the dorsal-attentional network (a3, a4 and, b3 and c3), or a salience network (a4) [13]. We report a qualitative comparison of all the networks extracted for the different multi-subject approaches. As in the simulations, some maps learned by spatial correspondence have loadings that are not reproducible across subjects (b4 on Fig. 2 –note the large error bars– and on Fig. 3). Functional correspondence tends to mix well-known networks and produce degenerate maps. For instance, it extracts for the dorsal-attentional attentional network two components (a3 and a4) that are not well differentiated and include other regions. Indeed, the dorsal-attentional network is made of the intra-parietal sulci and the frontal eye fields and is well known for high-level visuo-spatial tasks, for instance during eye saccades. Maps a4 and a3 also outline the visual area MT (V5) and the dorsal ACC, part of respectively the visual system and the salience network. The corresponding functional profiles indeed stray away from the accepted functions of this network: a3 does not present any visual loading, while a4 shows right motor clicks and a preference for horizontal checkerboards. On the opposite, the RFX-structure approach selects only the frontal eye field and the intra-parietal sulci on the spatial map. The cognitive loadings are limited to visual and calculation tasks. While it may seem surprising to find calculation in a visuo-spatial network, this specific network has recently been reported as recruited in mental arithmetics [5]. Finally, we find that all the networks extracted by the RFX-structure approach outline known structure and have sensible cognitive loadings.

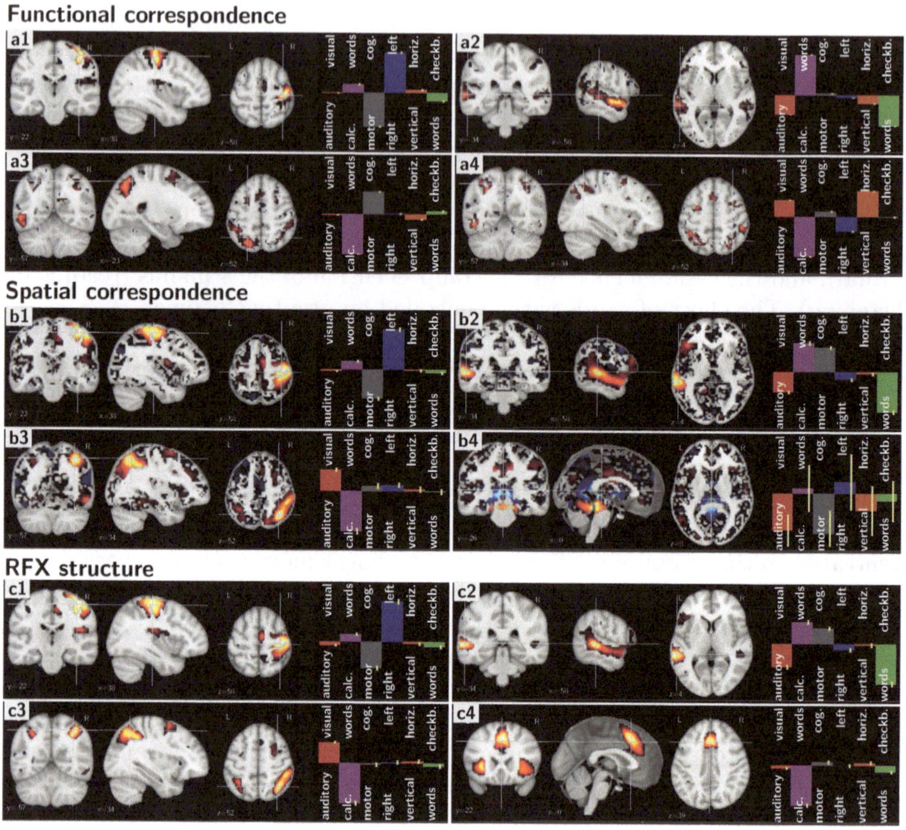

Functional correspondence

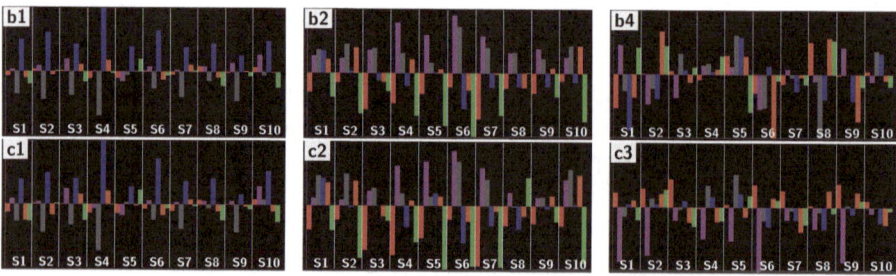

Spatial correspondence

RFX structure

Fig. 2. Networks learned on the localizer dataset with different strategies. Each box represents the functional network and the group-level profile as loadings on the contrasts of the study: auditory - visual, calculation - word, motor - cognition, right click - left click, vertical checkerboard - horizontal checkerboard, and words - checkerboard. The standard error across the group is displayed as a yellow bar for each loading. **a1**, **b1** and **c1** correspond to the left hand region of the motor cortex, **a2**, **b2** and **c2** to the language network, **a3**, **a4**, **b3**, **c3** to the dorsal-attentional network, and **c4** to a salience network. **b4** is likely a noise pattern.

Fig. 3. Inter-subject functional profiles $\underline{D}$ for the first 10 subjects, for spatial correspondence –top row– and RFX structure –bottom row. A white line separates subjects.

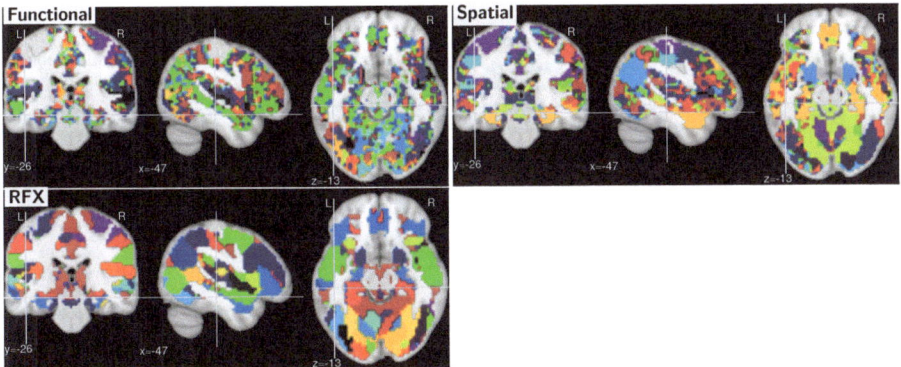

Fig. 4. Parcellations for the different strategies. The colors are random.

Towards a cognitive brain atlas. To evaluate the overall spatial layout of the networks extracted we turn the decomposition in a hard assignment: we assign each voxel to the component for which it has the highest value in the spatial map. This procedure retrieves a cognitive label for each voxel and thus establishes a cognitively-informed brain parcellation. The maps extracted by functional correspondence often lack spatial structure and segment redundant regions across the different components (as with a3 and a4), as a result the corresponding parcellation appears noisy (see Fig. 4). The parcellations for spatial correspondence show more regularity, and even more so for the RFX-structured approach. The later gives sensible divisions of well-known parts of the cortex, such as the motor cortex, or the ventral visual stream.

Functional richness of the profiles. The corresponding functional profiles are summarized by computing the t-value (mean effect divided by standard error) per network and contrast, across subjects. These values, clipped to [-10, 10], are presented in Fig. 5(left), which shows that the RFX model achieves an intermediate level of sensitivity between spatial correspondence, that yields smaller t values, and functional correspondence that exhibits high t-values.

A way of assessing the functional significance of these decompositions is to quantify how specific the encoding of functional profiles into networks is. To do so, we label each network as showing negative, none or positive activation, by thresholding the t values, and compute the entropy of the resulting assignment. Fig 5 (right) presents the results for a standard range of thresholds, obtained through 100 bootstrap replications of the t values and entropy computation. In a range of values that is usable in practice (t values between 2. and 4.) the RFX model yields a more efficient encoding than the other decompositions; the spatial decomposition dominates for very low t-values while the functional decomposition outperforms the others for extremely high t values. Altogether, this suggests that the RFX model encodes efficiently the possible functional profiles, while the spatial model is more sensitive to between-subject variability and the

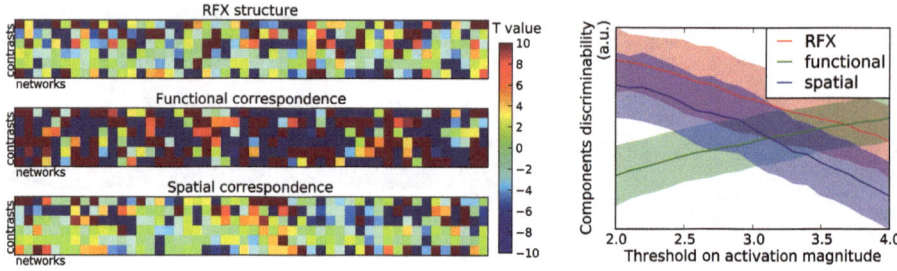

Fig. 5. Extracted functional profiles. (Left) These profiles summarize the functional activation per network (columns) and contrast (lines) of interest through a t-value per network and contrast, across subjects. The contrasts are identical to those in Fig. 2. The color scale, clipped to [-10, 10], shows that the RFX model achieves an intermediate level of sensitivity. (right) The specificity of the encoding of cognitive contrasts into networks is summarized by the entropy of an assignment to negative, none or positive activation: for most thresholds the RFX model yields the most efficient encoding.

functional model underestimates the group-level variance and thus overestimates the functional specificity of brain networks.

6   Conclusion

We have introduced a multi-subject model for task-induced fMRI activations that combines the principles of functional segregation and inter-subject degeneracy in a structured sparse coding problem. Technically, a major contribution of our formulation is to bound the ratio of inter-subject to intra-subject variance as it prevents extracting maps from non-reproducible variability. On a mid-sized cohort (150 subject, 6 contrasts) our model extracts a large number brain networks that are meaningful both in terms of cognitive content and of spatial maps. Applying this approach to larger studies should reveal richer and more specific effects. For larger cohorts, it can easily be extended to multi-level model specification, for instance in multi-centric studies, adding a center effect. An exciting direction of future research is to use this possibility to combine multiple studies in a meta analysis. Importantly, our approach is very computationally efficient: it is $\mathcal{O}\left(n^2\right)$ in the number of subjects, and the analysis presented in this paper runs in 10 mn on a single CPU, compared to several hours for non on-line learning. It is thus applicable to mining of massive datasets. Altogether, our results provide the basis of a framework to derive a synthetic and optimized representation of large amount of multi-subject fMRI data in terms of specialized brain regions.

This work was supported by the ANR grants BrainPedia ANR-10-JCJC 1408-01 and IRMGroup ANR-10-BLAN-0126-02.

References

1. Bickel, P., Ritov, Y., Tsybakov, A.: Simultaneous analysis of lasso and dantzig selector. The Annals of Statistics 37, 1705 (2009)
2. Calhoun, V.D., Adali, T., Pearlson, G.D., Pekar, J.J.: A method for making group inferences from fMRI data using independent component analysis. Hum. Brain Mapp. 14, 140 (2001)
3. Chen, G.H., Fedorenko, E.G., Kanwisher, N.G., Golland, P.: Deformation-invariant sparse coding for modeling spatial variability of functional patterns in the brain. In: Langs, G., Rish, I., Grosse-Wentrup, M., Murphy, B. (eds.) MLINI 2011. LNCS (LNAI), vol. 7263, pp. 68–75. Springer, Heidelberg (2012)
4. Efron, B., Hastie, T., Johnstone, I., Tibshirani, R.: Least angle regression. Ann. Statist. 32, 407 (2004)
5. Knops, A., Thirion, B., Hubbard, E., Michel, V., Dehaene, S.: Recruitment of an area involved in eye movements during mental arithmetic. Science 324, 1583 (2009)
6. Laird, A., Fox, P., Eickhoff, S., et al.: Behavioral interpretations of intrinsic connectivity networks. J. Cog. Neurosci. 23, 4022 (2011)
7. Lashkari, D., Golland, P.: Exploratory fMRI analysis without spatial normalization. In: Prince, J.L., Pham, D.L., Myers, K.J. (eds.) IPMI 2009. LNCS, vol. 5636, pp. 398–410. Springer, Heidelberg (2009)
8. Mairal, J., Bach, F., Ponce, J., Sapiro, G.: Online learning for matrix factorization and sparse coding. Journal of Machine Learning Research 11, 19 (2010)
9. Noppeney, U., Friston, K., Price, C.: Degenerate neuronal systems sustaining cognitive functions. J. Anat. 205, 433 (2004)
10. Petersen, R., Aisen, P., Beckett, L., et al.: Alzheimer's disease neuroimaging initiative (ADNI) clinical characterization. Neurology 74, 201 (2010)
11. Pinel, P., Thirion, B., Meriaux, S., Jobert, A., Serres, J., Le Bihan, D., Poline, J., Dehaene, S.: Fast reproducible identification and large-scale databasing of individual functional cognitive networks. BMC Neuroscience 8, 91 (2007)
12. Sabuncu, M., Singer, B., Conroy, B., Bryan, R., Ramadge, P., Haxby, J.: Function-based intersubject alignment of human cortical anatomy. Cereb. Cortex 20, 130 (2010)
13. Seeley, W., Menon, V., Schatzberg, A., Keller, J., Glover, G., Kenna, H., Reiss, A., Greicius, M.: Dissociable intrinsic connectivity networks for salience processing and executive control. J. Neurosci. 27, 2349 (2007)
14. Szabó, Z., Póczos, B., Lorincz, A.: Online group-structured dictionary learning. In: CVPR, p. 2865 (2011)
15. Thirion, B., Flandin, G., Pinel, P., Roche, A., Ciuciu, P., Poline, J.: Dealing with the shortcomings of spatial normalization: Multi-subject parcellation of fMRI datasets. Hum. Brain Map. 27, 678 (2006)
16. Thyreau, B., Schwartz, Y., Thirion, B., et al.: Very large fMRI study using the imagen database: Sensitivity–specificity and population effect modeling in relation to the underlying anatomy. NeuroImage 61, 295 (2012)
17. Tononi, G., McIntosh, A., Russell, D., Edelman, G.: Functional clustering: Identifying strongly interactive brain regions in neuroimaging data. Neuroimage 7, 133 (1998)
18. Varoquaux, G., Gramfort, A., Pedregosa, F., Michel, V., Thirion, B.: Multi-subject dictionary learning to segment an atlas of brain spontaneous activity. In: Székely, G., Hahn, H.K. (eds.) IPMI 2011. LNCS, vol. 6801, pp. 562–573. Springer, Heidelberg (2011)
19. Worsley, K., Liao, C., Aston, J., Petre, V., Duncan, G., Morales, F., Evans, A.: A general statistical analysis for fMRI data. NeuroImage 15, 1 (2002)

Rapid Multi-organ Segmentation Using Context Integration and Discriminative Models

Nathan Lay, Neil Birkbeck, Jingdan Zhang, and S. Kevin Zhou

Siemens Corporate Technology, 755 College Road East, Princeton NJ
{nathan.lay,neil.birkbeck,jingdan.zhang,shaohua.zhou}@siemens.com

Abstract. We propose a novel framework for rapid and accurate segmentation of a cohort of organs. First, it integrates *local and global image context* through a product rule to *simultaneously* detect multiple landmarks on the target organs. The global posterior integrates evidence over all volume patches, while the local image context is modeled with a local discriminative classifier. Through non-parametric modeling of the global posterior, it exploits sparsity in the global context for efficient detection. The complete surface of the target organs is then inferred by robust alignment of a shape model to the resulting landmarks and finally deformed using discriminative boundary detectors. Using our approach, we demonstrate efficient detection and accurate segmentation of liver, kidneys, heart, and lungs in challenging low-resolution MR data in *less than one second*, and of prostate, bladder, rectum, and femoral heads in CT scans, in *roughly one to three seconds* and in both cases with accuracy *fairly close to inter-user variability*.

Keywords: Local & global context, context integration, multi-landmark detection, discriminative learning, multi-organ segmentation.

1 Introduction

Algorithms for segmenting anatomical structures in medical imaging are often targeted to individual structures [1–4]. Instead, when the problem is posed as the joint segmentation of multiple organs, constraints can be formulated between the organs, e.g., non-overlapping, and the combined formulation allows for a richer prior model on the joint shape of the multiple structures of interest. Such multi-organ segmentation is often posed with atlas-based or level-set based formulation due to the ease at which geometric constraints can be modeled [5, 6].

However, level set methods are computationally demanding, and still require a decent initialization so as to not fall into a local minimum. Discriminative learning-based methods are often an alternative approach to initializing such segmentations (e.g., [5]), but, again, these methods often treat the initialization of each organ as an independent problem. While solving the single organ segmentation problem with learning-based methods can be fast (e.g., [2]), in order to achieve efficient multi-object segmentation, often a tree-like search structure has to be imposed on the detection order of the structures [7, 8].

J.C. Gee et al. (Eds.): IPMI 2013, LNCS 7917, pp. 450–462, 2013.
© Springer-Verlag Berlin Heidelberg 2013

The sequential ordering is used to avoid evaluating local classifiers everywhere in the image. However, as shapes of adjacent structures are often correlated, the appearance of neighboring image patches are often consistent, meaning image patterns commonly associated with one organ, say the liver, are likely to appear next to the right kidney. Instead of modeling dependency among structures at the algorithm level, e.g., with generative models [7], the correlation between such *global image context* and the shapes can be learned directly (e.g., [4, 9, 10]).

One method to utilize global contextual cues is to regress the position of the organ bounding boxes from each voxel location in the image [4, 9, 10]. Others suggested that this global information alone may not be accurate enough, and further improved the accuracy using a cascade of locally trained regressors [11].

In this work, we propose a novel integration of both local and global discriminative information for efficient multiple organ segmentation. Unlike other learning-based approaches, we do not rely on a tree-like dependency structure of organ detections to obtain an efficient detection algorithm. Instead, our global image context is only sparsely sampled, allowing us to derive an efficient detection algorithm: global context is used to hypothesize locations that need to be evaluated with the local discriminative classifier. Our non-parametric representation of global image context models correlations in the target shape, allowing us to jointly localize landmarks on multiple target organs. We impose a constraint on the distribution of allowable shapes, enabling us to initialize a likley shape from only a few landmarks per organ. The initialized shape is then deformed using learned discriminative boundary detector to better fit image appearance. We demonstrate that the combination of local and global image context outperforms either local and global context alone, and illustrate the use of the proposed joint landmark detection, robust shape initialization, and discriminative boundary deformation to segment up to 6 organs in either CT or MR data in *roughly one to three seconds* with segmentation in MR data taking *less than one second*. The segmentation accuracy is *fairly close to inter-user variability*.

2   Method

We aim to segment C organ shapes, $\mathbf{S} = [\mathbf{S}_1, ..., \mathbf{S}_C]$, given a volumetric image $\mathbf{I}$. We denote the set of all voxels in the image $\mathbf{I}$ by Ω and its size by $|\Omega|$. We assume that there exists a set of D corresponding landmarks, $\mathbf{X} = [\mathbf{x}_1, ..., \mathbf{x}_D]$, on the multiple shapes $\mathbf{S}$ and decompose the problem into estimating (i) the landmarks given the image using the posterior $P(\mathbf{X}|\mathbf{I})$ defined in §2.1 and (ii) the shapes given the landmarks and the image using energy minimization in §2.2. We use the notation $[\mathbf{x}, ..., \mathbf{x}]_D$ to represent repeating $\mathbf{x}$ in D times.

2.1   Joint Landmark Detection Using Context Integration

To jointly detect the landmarks, we integrate both local and global image context using a product rule into one posterior probability $P(\mathbf{X}|\mathbf{I})$:

$$P(\mathbf{X}|\mathbf{I}) = P^L(\mathbf{X}|\mathbf{I})P^G(\mathbf{X}|\mathbf{I}), \tag{1}$$

where $P^L(\mathbf{X}|\mathbf{I})$ and $P^G(\mathbf{X}|\mathbf{I})$ are local and global context posteriors, respectively.

Local Context Posterior. Though not necessarily true, we assume that the landmarks are *locally independent*:

$$P^L(\mathbf{X}|\mathbf{I}) = \prod_{i=1}^{D} P^L(\mathbf{x}_i|\mathbf{I}). \tag{2}$$

For modeling $P^L(\mathbf{x}_i|\mathbf{I})$, we exploit the local image context to learn a discriminative detector for landmark $\mathbf{x}_i$ (using *e.g.* PBT [12]), that is,

$$P^L(\mathbf{x}_i|\mathbf{I}) = \frac{1}{Z_i}\omega_i^L(+1|\mathbf{I}[\mathbf{x}_i]), \tag{3}$$

with $\mathbf{I}[\mathbf{x}_i]$ being the local image patch centered at $\mathbf{x}_i$, $\omega_i^L(+1|\cdot)$ the local context detector for landmark $\mathbf{x}_i$ and $Z_i = \sum_{\mathbf{x}\in\Omega}\omega_i^L(+1|\mathbf{I}[\mathbf{x}_i])$ is a normalizing constant.

Global Context Posterior. We integrate global evidence from all voxels in Ω.

$$P^G(\mathbf{X}|\mathbf{I}) = \sum_{\mathbf{y}\in\Omega} P^G(\mathbf{X}|\mathbf{I},\mathbf{y})P(\mathbf{y}|\mathbf{I}) = |\Omega|^{-1}\sum_{\mathbf{y}\in\Omega} P^G(\mathbf{X}|\mathbf{I}[\mathbf{y}]). \tag{4}$$

In (4), we assume a uniform prior probability $P(\mathbf{y}|\mathbf{I}) = |\Omega|^{-1}$ and $P^G(\mathbf{X}|\mathbf{I}[\mathbf{y}])$ is the probability of the landmarks at $\mathbf{X}$ when observing the image patch $\mathbf{I}[\mathbf{y}]$ at a location $\mathbf{y}$.

To learn $P^G(\mathbf{X}|\mathbf{I}[\mathbf{y}])$, we leverage annotated datasets and a 'randomized' K-nearest neighbor (NN) approach [13]. For a complete set of training images with annotated landmarks, we randomly form K subsets. From each subset of images with corresponding landmarks, we construct a training database $\{(\mathbf{J}_n, d\mathbf{X}_n)\}_{n=1}^{N}$ consisting of N pairs of image patch $\mathbf{J}$ and relative shift $d\mathbf{X}$ in an iterative fashion.

> **for** *n=1,...,N* **do**
> | Randomly sample in the subset an image say $\tilde{\mathbf{J}}$ with landmarks $\tilde{\mathbf{X}}$;
> | Randomly sample a voxel location, say $\mathbf{z}$, from Ω;
> | Set the image patch $\mathbf{J}_n = \tilde{\mathbf{J}}[\mathbf{z}]$;
> | Set the relative shift $d\mathbf{X}_n = \tilde{\mathbf{X}} - [\mathbf{z},...,\mathbf{z}]_D$.
> **end**

For a test image patch $\mathbf{I}[\mathbf{y}]$, we first find its NN $\hat{\mathbf{J}}_k$ from each subset; this way we find its K neighbors $\{\hat{\mathbf{J}}_1,...,\hat{\mathbf{J}}_K\}$ along with their corresponding shift vectors $\{d\hat{\mathbf{X}}_1[\mathbf{y}],...,d\hat{\mathbf{X}}_K[\mathbf{y}]\}$. How to efficiently find the NN for each subset is elaborated later. We then simply approximate $P^G(\mathbf{X}|\mathbf{I}[\mathbf{y}])$ as

$$P^G(\mathbf{X}|\mathbf{I}[\mathbf{y}]) = K^{-1}\sum_{k=1}^{K}\delta(\mathbf{X} - [\mathbf{y},...,\mathbf{y}]_D - d\hat{\mathbf{X}}_k[\mathbf{y}]). \tag{5}$$

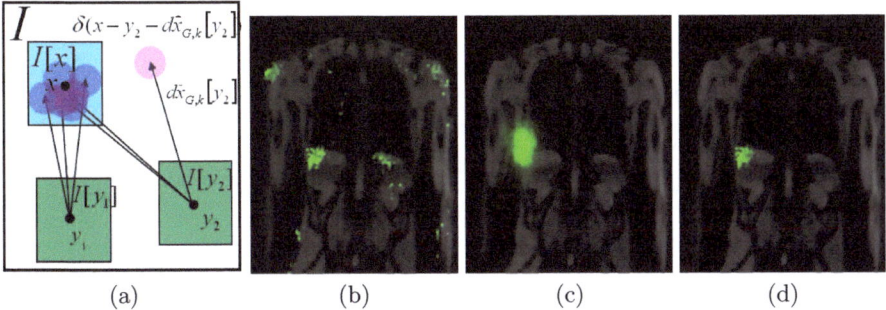

(a)   (b)   (c)   (d)

Fig. 1. (a) An illustration of how image patches (green) predict the landmark location using global context and Eq. (5) and then these predictions are combined with local context at (blue) **x**. (b) Detection scores for a landmark on the top left of the liver in a low resolution MR FastView 3D volume, where local context gives spurious responses. (c) Global context gives a coarse localization. (d) The integration of local and global detection gives a fine scale density.

Figure 1 graphically illustrates how the approach works. It also gives an example of the local, global and joint posteriors. Even though the local detector may be inaccurate, it is only being applied at locations predicted from the global context, meaning it is possible to get a highly peaked posterior when integrating evidence from local and global context.

MMSE and MAP Estimate for Landmark Location. The expected landmark location $\bar{\mathbf{X}}$, also the minimum mean square error (MMSE) estimate, is computed as

$$\bar{\mathbf{X}} = \sum_{\mathbf{X}} \mathbf{X} \, P(\mathbf{X}|\mathbf{I}) = \sum_{\mathbf{X}} \mathbf{X} \, P^L(\mathbf{X}|\mathbf{I}) P^G(\mathbf{X}|\mathbf{I}) \tag{6}$$

$$= \frac{1}{K|\Omega|} \sum_{\mathbf{X}} \sum_{\mathbf{y}\in\Omega} \sum_{k=1}^{K} \mathbf{X} \prod_{i=1}^{D} \frac{1}{Z_i} \omega_i^L(+1|\mathbf{I}[\mathbf{x}_i]) \delta(\mathbf{X} - [\mathbf{y},...,\mathbf{y}]_D - d\hat{\mathbf{X}}_k[\mathbf{y}]).$$

where $Z_i = \sum_{\mathbf{x}} \omega_i^L(+1|\mathbf{I}[\mathbf{x}_i])$ is a normalizing constant. Using the local independence and vector decomposition, it can be shown that the expected location $\bar{\mathbf{x}}_i$ for a single landmark is computed as

$$\bar{\mathbf{x}}_i = Z^{-1}K^{-1}|\Omega|^{-1} \sum_{\mathbf{y}\in\Omega} \sum_{k=1}^{K} (\mathbf{y} + d\hat{\mathbf{x}}_{k,i}[\mathbf{y}]) \omega_i^L(+1|\mathbf{I}[\mathbf{y} + d\hat{\mathbf{x}}_{k,i}[\mathbf{y}]]). \tag{7}$$

where $Z = \sum_{\mathbf{y}\in\Omega} \sum_{k=1}^{K} \omega_i^L(+1|\mathbf{I}[\mathbf{y} + d\hat{\mathbf{x}}_{k,i}[\mathbf{y}]])$ is a normalizing constant. Eq. (7) implies an efficient scheme – evaluating the local detector only for the locations predicted from the global context posterior instead of the whole image! Since the predicted locations are highly clustered around the true location, this brings the first significant reduction in computation.

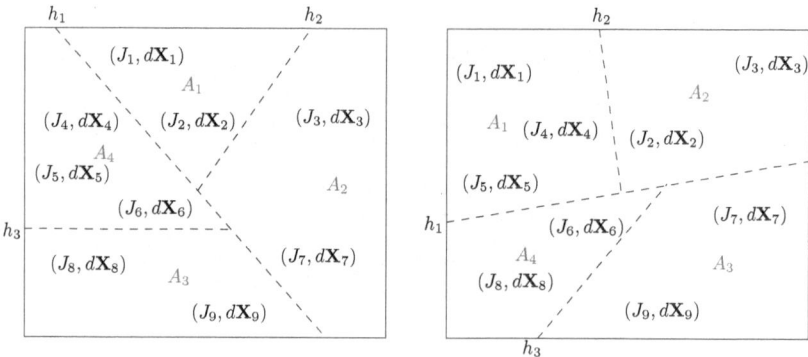

Fig. 2. Two BSP trees for different subsets of the training data are used to partition the space into convex regions (e.g., the leafs), A_j, using a set of hyperplanes h_i. Instead of searching over all entries within a leaf of the tree to find an exact NN, we simply store the average relative offset vector for the training samples that fell into the leaf.

Similarly, the maximum a posterior (MAP) estimate $\hat{\mathbf{x}}_i$ can be derived as

$$\hat{\mathbf{x}}_i = \arg\max_{\mathbf{x}} \omega_i^L(+1|\mathbf{I}[\mathbf{x}]) \sum_{\mathbf{y}\in\Omega} \sum_{k=1}^{K} \delta(\mathbf{x} - \mathbf{y} - d\hat{\mathbf{x}}_{k,i}[\mathbf{y}]). \qquad (8)$$

Sparsity in Global Context. The global context from all voxels is highly redundant as neighboring patches tend to predict nearby landmark locations. Therefore, we can 'sparsify' the global context by constructing the subset Ω_ℓ from the full voxel set Ω; for example, we can skip every other l voxels. This brings the second significant reduction in computation complexity by $O(l^3)$!

Efficient Approximate NN Search. Computing the expected landmark location in (7) relies on the ability to compute the NN from the training database of $\{\mathbf{J}_n, d\mathbf{X}_n\}_{n=1}^N$ for one subset of training images. The time and space efficiency of this operation is influenced by two factors: the size of the database, N, and the dimension of the points, D, in the database. With, for example 100 training volumes of dimension 128^3, we have a potential database size of $N = 128^3 \times 100 > 209$ million. Furthermore, in order to have enough contextual information, an image patch J_n, with size up to 32^3 voxels, is used, meaning that the NN query must be performed in a high dimensional space of up to $D = 32768$.

For efficiency, we relax the requirement of finding the exact nearest Euclidean neighbor to that of finding an approximate NN. We then take a similar approach as local sensitive hashing [14] and build multiple hash indexes on the data (Fig. 2). However, instead of using a hash function, we construct a random Binary Space Partition (BSP) tree that is similar to a random projection tree [15]. At each node of our BSP tree, we choose a random hyperplane to split the data. Unlike random projection trees, which choose the split hyperplane uniformly random on a D-dimensional hypersphere, we restrict the hyperplanes to be Haar wavelets. We have two reasons for doing this: 1) Haar wavelets provide a class of features often used to discriminate appearance in classification problems, and 2) any Haar feature can be instantaneously evaluated using an integral image. Further, instead of storing all training sample patches in their respective leaf nodes within the tree, we choose a single representative relative shift vector–this way the space requirements are dependent on the size of the tree instead of $O(ND)$.

In our experiments, we typically form $K = 10$ subsets and hence train 10 BSP-trees with each tree built up to depth 10. This means that an approximate NN match for a single tree is computed using at most 10 Haar wavelet evaluations, and all $K = 10$ approximate neighbors can be found in as little as 100 Haar wavelet evaluations.

2.2   Shape Initialization Using Robust Model Alignment

An initial segmentation for each organ is then aligned to the sparse detected landmarks through the use of a statistical model of shape variation. Here we use a point distribution model, where each organ shape is represented as a mean shape or mesh with M mesh nodes, $\bar{\mathbf{V}} = [\bar{\mathbf{v}}_1, \bar{\mathbf{v}}_2, \ldots, \bar{\mathbf{v}}_M]$, plus a linear combination of a set of N eigenmodes, $\mathbf{U}_n = [\mathbf{u}_{1,n}, \mathbf{u}_{2,n}, \cdots \mathbf{u}_{M,n}]$, with $1 \leq n \leq N$.

As a complete organ shape is characterized by only a few coefficients that modulate the eigenmodes, the point distribution model can be used to infer a shape from a sparse set of landmark points. Given a set of detected landmarks, $\{\mathbf{x}_i\}$, the best fitting instance of the complete shape is found by minimizing the following robust energy function:

$$(\beta, \{a_n\}) = \operatorname{argmin}_{\beta, \{a_n\}} \sum_i \psi \left(\|\mathbf{x}_i - T_\beta\{\bar{\mathbf{v}}_{\pi(i)} + \sum_{n=1}^{N} a_n \mathbf{u}_{\pi(i),n}\}\|^2 \right) + \sum_{n=1}^{N} a_n^2 / \lambda_n \tag{9}$$

where the function $\pi(i)$ maps the landmark $\mathbf{x}_i$ to the corresponding mesh index in $\bar{\mathbf{V}}$, the function $T_\beta\{\cdot\}$ is a 9D similarity transform parameterized by the vector $\beta = [t_x, t_y, t_z, \theta_x, \theta_y, \theta_z, s_x, s_y, s_z]$, and λ_n are the corresponding eigenvalues. The first term measures the difference between a predicted shape point under a hypothesis transformation from the detected landmark, and the second term is a prior keeping the eigenmodes responsible for smaller variation closer to zero. As we typically only have a few landmarks, and have a PCA model for a larger number of vertices, using no prior term gives rise to an ill-posed problem. Finally, ψ is a robust norm, reducing the effect of outliers. We use $\psi(s^2) = s$.

2.3   Discriminative Boundary Refinement

Using the initialization from §2.2, a fine refinement of the points on the surface mesh is obtained by iteratively displacing each vertex along its surface normal, $\mathbf{v}_i \leftarrow \mathbf{v}_i + \mathbf{n}_i \hat{r}_i$. The best displacement for each point is obtained by maximizing the output of a discriminative classifier [3]:

Table 1. Accuracy (measured in mm) and timing results for the landmark detection using local, global, and local + global context posterior

	Global		Local		Local + Global	
Spacing	Time	Median	Time	Median	Time	Median
1 (5mm)	2.76s	**25.0 ± 17.4**	1.91s	16.4 ± 10.6	-	-
5 (25mm)	0.92s	39.9 ± 33.4	-	-	2.11s	**12.9 ± 7.52**
7 (35mm)	0.91s	54.1 ± 54.1	-	-	0.91s	13.0 ± 7.56
15 (75mm)	**0.89s**	79.0 ± 85.6	-	-	**0.23s**	14.1 ± 8.25

$$\hat{\tau}_i = \mathrm{argmax}_{\tau_i} \omega^B(+1|\mathbf{v}_i + \mathbf{n}_i \tau_i). \tag{10}$$

Here, $\omega^B(+1|\cdot)$ is the boundary detector that scores whether the point, $\mathbf{v}_i + \mathbf{n}_i \tau_i$, is on the boundary of the organ being segmented. Regularity is incorporated in the previously independent estimated displacements by projecting the resulting mesh onto the linear subspace spanned by the linear shape model, as in the active shape model [16].

3   Results

Our system was implemented in C++ using OpenMP and compiled using Visual Studio 2008. In the experiments below, timing results are reported for an Intel Xeon 64-bit machine running Windows Server 2008 and using 16 threads. We illustrate the results on segmenting 6 organs in MR scans (§3.1) and 5 organs in CT (§3.2).

3.1   Lungs, Heart, Liver, and Kidneys in MR Localizer Scans

We tested our approach on a challenging set of MR localizer scans acquired using a fast continuously moving table technique (syngo TimCT FastView, Siemens). Such scans are often used for MR examination planning to increase scan reproducibility and operator efficiency. A total of 185 volumes having 5mm isotropic spacing were split into a training set of 135 and test set of 50. This data is challenging due to the low resolution, weak boundaries, inhomogeneous intensity within scan, and varying image contrast across scans. For this example, we used $K = 10$ NN. The local detectors were also trained on 5mm resolution using a PBT [12] and a combination of Haar and image gradient features. A total of 33 landmarks were selected on the 6 organs, with 6 landmarks each on the liver and the lungs, and 5 landmarks each on the kidneys and heart.

First, we demonstrate the effectiveness of integrating local and global context with respect to accuracy and evaluation time. Table 1 illustrates median errors for all landmark positions averaged over the testing set. For the local context detector and local+global posterior, we used the MMSE estimate. While it is

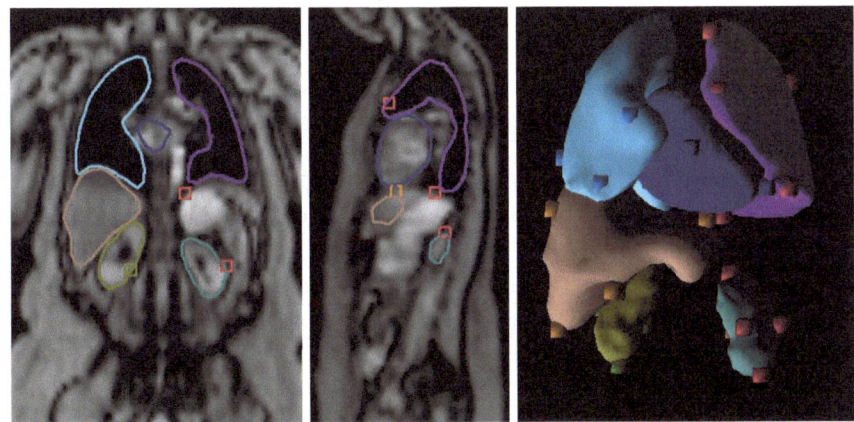

Fig. 3. An illustration of the landmarks in 3D and automatic segmentation results. Our method is robust to a few failed landmarks.

possible to get better speed-up with a sparse sampling of the global context when computing the expected value, we noticed that the MAP estimate gave better results as we reported in the table. Obtaining the MAP estimate requires populating a probability image and scanning through the image to get the MAP estimate (this is proportional to the number of landmarks, which is why no speedup is reported in the table). Besides, the accuracy of the global context posterior suffers from sparse sampling, and even with dense sampling it still performs worse than the local + global method. On the other hand, it is evident that a sparser sampling of the volume has little impact on the accuracy of the local+global method. The local classifier is computed using a constrained search over the volume (e.g., using bounds for the landmark positions relative to the image [2]), but achieves worse accuracy and is still slower than our combined local+global posterior modeling.

The shape landmarks are used to infer the shape of all the organs (see Fig. 3). We compare the resulting segmentation results at several phases to a state-of-the-art hierarchical detection using marginal space learning (MSL) [2] that is known as both fast and accurate. For the MSL setup, the kidneys were predicted from the liver bounding box, meaning the kidney search range was more localized allowing the detection to be faster (the lungs were predicted relative to the heart in a similar manner). Table 2 illustrates the timing and accuracy results for the 50 unseen test cases using both MSL and our method. The accuracy is gauged by symmetric surface-to-surface distance. Figure 4 illustrates two qualitative results.

The fast landmark detection and robust shape initialization can provide an approximate shape in as little as 0.33s (for spacing of 75mm, e.g., 15 voxels). The improvement of our initialization on the liver and lungs over the MSL approach is likely due to our use of more landmarks to capture more variations associated with complex anatomies than MSL that fits shapes of varying complexities into a rigid bounding box. On the other hand, for both kidneys with less variations

Table 2. Accuracy (measured in mm) and timing for segmentation results using our approach compared to the state-of-the-art MSL model on the MR FastView data

	Skip (mm)	Time	Liver	R. Kidney	L. Kidney	R.Lung	Heart	L. Lung
	Detection & Shape initialization							
MSL	-	5.50s	9.21 ± 1.82	**3.44 ± 1.16**	**3.08 ± 1.21**	7.29 ± 1.64	5.98 ± 1.59	7.42 ± 1.71
Local+Global	25mm	2.21	**7.41±1.91**	4.10±1.34	4.31±1.81	**6.60±1.74**	**5.64±1.41**	**6.72±1.55**
	35mm	1.01	7.43±1.95	4.18±1.39	4.39±1.89	6.67±1.79	5.69±1.40	6.78±1.53
	50mm	0.55	7.55±2.03	4.36±1.43	4.57±1.93	6.77±1.86	5.78±1.48	6.83±1.64
	60mm	0.39	7.63±1.95	4.59±1.52	4.70±1.98	6.86±1.91	5.92±1.53	6.91±1.68
	75mm	**0.33**	7.94±2.21	5.13±1.77	5.38±2.90	6.97±1.95	5.98±1.57	6.88±1.75
	With boundary refinement							
MSL	-	6.36s	4.87 ± 1.46	**2.26 ± 0.61**	**2.12 ± 0.68**	3.67 ± 0.95	**3.99 ± 1.36**	3.55 ± 0.97
(BSP)	25mm	2.89	**4.07±0.99**	2.33±0.68	2.41±1.61	**3.56±0.96**	4.02±1.50	**3.35±0.83**
	35mm	1.60	4.08±0.99	2.37±0.69	2.47±1.72	3.57±0.98	4.02±1.52	**3.35±0.83**
	50mm	1.13	4.09±1.01	2.37±0.73	2.48±1.66	3.57±0.95	4.06±1.62	3.36±0.83
	60mm	0.97	4.08±1.00	2.42±0.79	2.42±1.57	3.57±0.97	4.07±1.63	3.35±0.84
	75mm	**0.89**	4.17±1.14	2.51±1.00	2.84±2.51	3.57±0.95	4.11±1.64	3.37±0.83
Inter-user variability			4.07±0.93	1.96±0.43	2.10±0.51	3.79±0.36	4.54±0.88	3.52±0.63

in the shape but more in the appearance, MSL performs better as it considers kidney as a whole. The discriminative boundary deformation significantly improves the segmentation accuracy for both approaches, which yield comparable overall accuracy for all organs. Our approach is more efficient, e.g., over 5 times faster if we skip every 12th voxel (65mm) in the global context. With a skipping factor of 75mm, we achieved segmentation of 6 organs *within one second* and with accuracy almost as good as the best quality! Both methods perform fairly close to inter-user variability[1].

One potential concern with relying on far away global context information is that the reliability of the detection and segmentation may degrade or vary when given a subvolume. To investigate this, we evaluated the lung, liver, and heart segmentation accuracy on the same subset of unseen volumes, but this time we cropped the volumes 10cm below the lung and heart, meaning that the kidneys and liver are not present. In these cropped volumes, using a spacing factor of 50mm, we find the accuracy of our local+global method to be consistent with that in Table 2, where right lung accuracy was 3.57 ± 1.32, heart accuracy was slightly worse at 4.53 ± 2.39, and the left lung was 3.22 ± 1.02. Although the global model may predict instances of missing organs (e.g., the kidney and liver), these detections can be pruned by thresholding the local classifier scores or by identifying missing organs as those with a low average boundary detector score.

3.2 Prostate, Bladder, Rectum, Femoral Heads in CT Scans

In this second data set, we detect the prostate, bladder, rectum, and femoral heads in CT scans. The detection and segmentation of these structures is useful

---

[1] The inter-user variability was measured over 10 randomly selected unseen test cases.

Table 3. Accuracy and timing for segmentation results using our model compared to the state of the art MSL model on CT prostate, bladder, rectum and femoral heads

	Detection, shape initialization, & boundary refinement						
	Skip(mm)	Time	Prostate	Bladder	Rectum	R.Fem	L.Fem
MSL	-	9.67s	3.57±2.01	**2.59±1.70**	4.36±1.70	1.89±0.99	2.05±1.27
BSP	10 (30mm)	1.76s	**3.35±1.40**	3.08±2.25	**3.97±1.43**	**1.88±0.78**	**1.90±1.18**
	12 (36mm)	1.36s	3.48±1.53	3.17±2.28	3.98±1.49	1.93±1.00	2.23±1.76
	15 (45mm)	1.09s	3.70±1.64	3.28±2.42	4.03±1.48	2.04±1.18	2.25±2.04
	Inter-user variability		3.03±1.15	2.03±0.11	2.93±1.10	1.29 ± 0.12	1.16±0.21

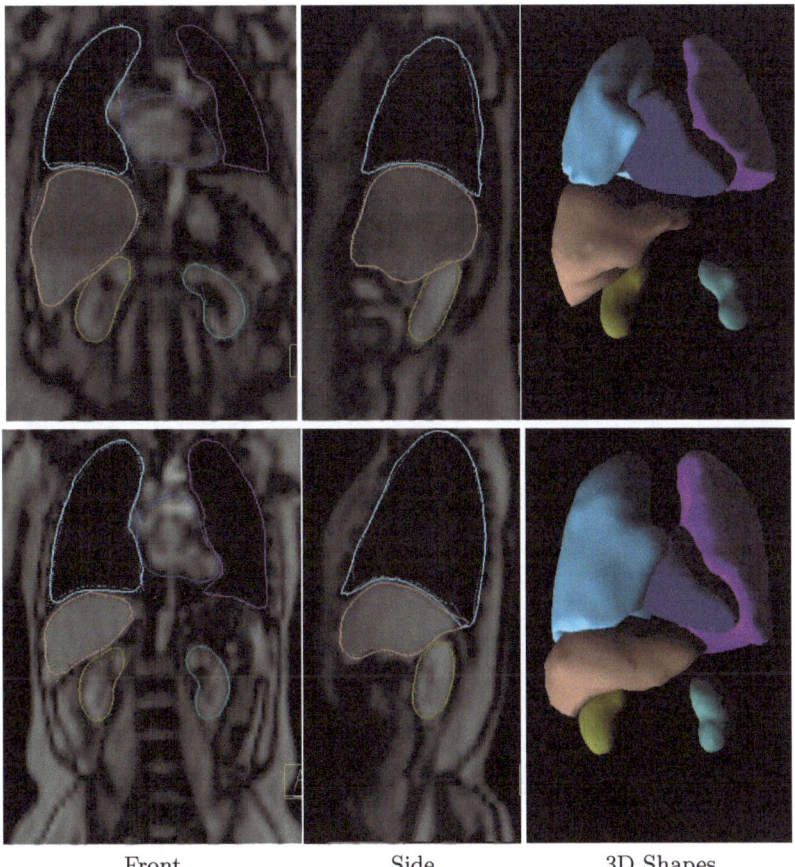

Front   Side   3D Shapes

Fig. 4. Qualitative results of the MR FastView segmentation (solid) on unseen cases with ground truth (dotted)

for radiation therapy planning. This data exhibits challenges in weak boundaries between soft tissues, complex shapes in rectum and femoral head, large scale variation in bladder, etc. A total of 145 cases were used, with 100 randomly selected for training and the remaining 45 used in testing. The volumes were isotropically resampled to have a resolution of 3mm. Six manually selected landmarks were identified on each of the objects, with the exception of the bladder which used 7 as it had large variability. And a similar configuration as described in the previous section was used to train the local and global context models.

Table 3 shows the timing and accuracy results for the final segmentation compared to an MSL pipeline. Even with a spacing factor of 36mm, our local+global model behaves similarly to or better than MSL on all organs except for the bladder while giving an overall speedup of 6 times over MSL. MSL seems to better handle the large scale variability observed in the bladder. Our approach significantly outperforms MSL for rectum, possibly because of the aforementioned reason – the rectum shape varies a lot and landmark-based shape initialization is better. Both approaches achieved accuracy fairly close to the inter-user

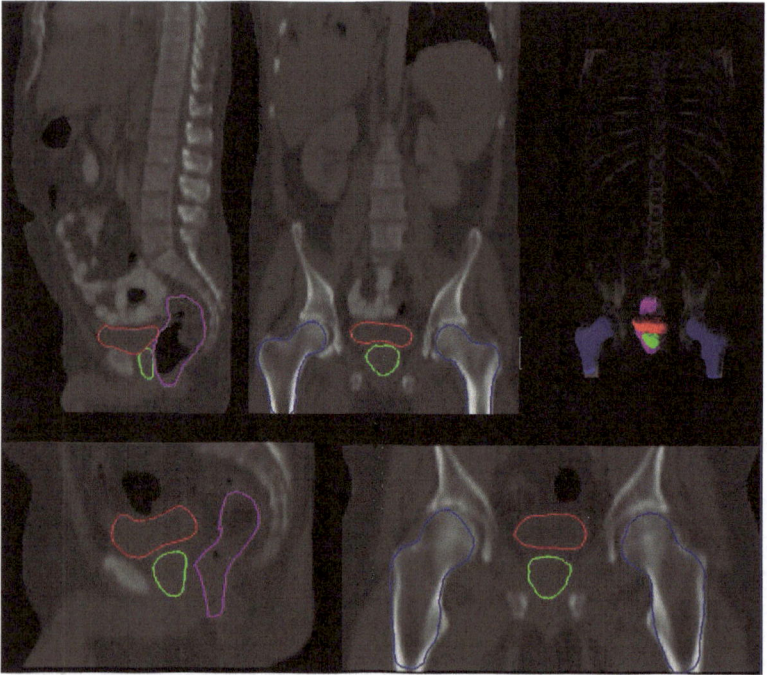

Fig. 5. An illustration of the segmentation results on two of the CT prostate data sets. The data has wildy varying dimensions, some being full body scans, and others localized near the prostate. Our method works well across this variation and handles large variability in shape and appearance of the organs, such as drastic changes in appearance in the rectum.

variability except the rectum[2]. We achieved a speed of just over one second by skipping every 16th voxel with decent accuracy. Figure 5 illustrates two of the automatic CT segmentations on unseen images. The femoral accuracy of the femoral head is limited by the low resolution of our mesh and due to using a 3mm isotropic resolution. However, this serves as a good initialization for voxel-based refinement using graph cut or random walker.

4   Conclusion

In this work we proposed a fusion of local and global context, coupled with discriminative models, for rapid multi-organ segmentation. Exploiting sparsity of the non-parametric global context led to a fast algorithm: the global context is only evaluated at sparse regions and is used to predict hypotheses for all landmarks simultaneously. By robustly fitting statistical shape model to these landmarks and deforming the fitted shape using learned boundary detector, we achieved segmentation accuracy comparable to inter-user variability.

Although our approach is already efficient, we feel that there is still room for improvement. Specifically, the local detectors often get evaluated on the same voxel multiple times; a simple caching of classifier results could be used to improve efficiency. Along a similar line, if results are cached, there may also be benefit in having a multi-class classifier be used to model the local posterior. We will also investigate how to further improve the segmentation accuracy for organs with simple shape but large variability in appearance like kidney or in scale like bladder.

References

1. Yang, J., Duncan, J.S.: 3D image segmentation of deformable objects with joint shape-intensity prior models using level sets. Medical Image Analysis 8(3), 285–294 (2004)
2. Zheng, Y., Georgescu, B., Ling, H., Zhou, S.K., Scheuering, M., Comaniciu, D.: Constrained marginal space learning for efficient 3D anatomical structure detection in medical images. In: CVPR, pp. 194–201. IEEE (2009)
3. Ling, H., Zhou, S.K., Zheng, Y., Georgescu, B., Suehling, M., Comaniciu, D.: Hierarchical, learning-based automatic liver segmentation. In: CVPR (2008)
4. Zhou, S.K.: Shape regression machine and efficient segmentation of left ventricle endocardium from 2D b-mode echocardiogram. Medical Image Analysis 14(4), 563–581 (2010)
5. Kohlberger, T., Sofka, M., Zhang, J., Birkbeck, N., Wetzl, J., Kaftan, J., Declerck, J., Zhou, S.K.: Automatic multi-organ segmentation using learning-based segmentation and level set optimization. In: Fichtinger, G., Martel, A., Peters, T. (eds.) MICCAI 2011, Part III. LNCS, vol. 6893, pp. 338–345. Springer, Heidelberg (2011)
6. Shimizu, A., Ohno, R., Ikegami, T., Kobatake, H., Nawano, S., Smutek, D.: Segmentation of multiple organs in non-contrast 3D abdominal CT images. International Journal of Computer Assisted Radiology and Surgery 2, 135–142 (2007)

---

[2] The inter-user variability was measured over 5 randomly selected unseen test cases.

7. Sofka, M., Zhang, J., Zhou, S.K., Comaniciu, D.: Multiple object detection by sequential Monte Carlo and hierarchical detection network. In: CVPR, June 13-18 (2010)
8. Liu, D., Zhou, S.K., Bernhardt, D., Comaniciu, D.: Search strategies for multiple landmark detection by submodular maximization. In: CVPR. IEEE (2010)
9. Criminisi, A., Shotton, J., Bucciarelli, S.: Decision forests with long-range spatial context for organ localization in ct volumes. In: MICCAI-PMMIA Workshop (2009)
10. Criminisi, A., Shotton, J., Robertson, D., Konukoglu, E.: Regression forests for efficient anatomy detection and localization in CT studies. In: Menze, B., Langs, G., Tu, Z., Criminisi, A. (eds.) MICCAI 2010 Workshop MVC. LNCS, vol. 6533, pp. 106–117. Springer, Heidelberg (2011)
11. Cuingnet, R., Prevost, R., Lesage, D., Cohen, L.D., Mory, B., Ardon, R.: Automatic detection and segmentation of kidneys in 3D CT images using random forests. In: Ayache, N., Delingette, H., Golland, P., Mori, K. (eds.) MICCAI 2012, Part III. LNCS, vol. 7512, pp. 66–74. Springer, Heidelberg (2012)
12. Tu, Z.: Probabilistic boosting-tree: Learning discriminative models for classification, recognition, and clustering. In: ICCV, pp. 1589–1596 (2005)
13. Friedman, J., Hastie, T., Tibshirani, R.: The elements of statistical learning. Springer Series in Statistics, vol. 1 (2001)
14. Datar, M., Indyk, P.: Locality-sensitive hashing scheme based on p-stable distributions. In: SCG 2004: Proceedings of the Twentieth Annual Symposium on Computational Geometry, pp. 253–262. ACM Press (2004)
15. Dasgupta, S., Freund, Y.: Random projection trees and low dimensional manifolds. In: Proceedings of the 40th Annual ACM Symposium on Theory of Computing, STOC 2008, pp. 537–546. ACM, New York (2008)
16. Cootes, T.F., Taylor, C.J., Cooper, D.H., Graham, J.: Active shape models their training and application. Comput. Vis. Image Underst. 61, 38–59 (1995)

Edge- and Detail-Preserving Sparse Image Representations for Deformable Registration of Chest MRI and CT Volumes

Mattias P. Heinrich[1,2,*], Mark Jenkinson[2], Bartlomiej W. Papież[1],
Fergus V. Glesson[3], Sir Michael Brady[4], and Julia A. Schnabel[1]

[1] Institute of Biomedical Engineering, University of Oxford, UK
[2] Oxford University Centre for Functional MRI of the Brain, UK
[3] Department of Radiology Churchill Hospital, Oxford, UK
[4] Department of Oncology, University of Oxford, UK
mattias.heinrich@eng.ox.ac.uk
http://users.ox.ac.uk/~shil3388

Abstract. Deformable medical image registration requires the optimisation of a function with a large number of degrees of freedom. Commonly-used approaches to reduce the computational complexity, such as uniform B-splines and Gaussian image pyramids, introduce translation-invariant homogeneous smoothing, and may lead to less accurate registration in particular for motion fields with discontinuities. This paper introduces the concept of sparse image representation based on supervoxels, which are edge-preserving and therefore enable accurate modelling of sliding organ motions frequently seen in respiratory and cardiac scans. Previous shortcomings of using supervoxels in motion estimation, in particular inconsistent clustering in ambiguous regions, are overcome by employing multiple layers of supervoxels. Furthermore, we propose a new similarity criterion based on a binary shape representation of supervoxels, which improves the accuracy of single-modal registration and enables multi-modal registration. We validate our findings based on the registration of two challenging clinical applications of volumetric deformable registration: motion estimation between inhale and exhale phase of CT scans for radiotherapy planning, and deformable multi-modal registration of diagnostic MRI and CT chest scans. The experiments demonstrate state-of-the-art registration accuracy, and require no additional anatomical knowledge with greatly reduced computational complexity.

Keywords: supervoxels, sliding motion, multi-modal fusion, pulmonary.

1 Introduction

Registering medical images of three (or more) dimensions with high spatial image resolution results in a highly complex optimisation problem, which is usually

---

* We thank EPSRC and Cancer Research UK for funding this work in the Oxford Cancer Imaging Centre.

J.C. Gee et al. (Eds.): IPMI 2013, LNCS 7917, pp. 463–474, 2013.

impractical to solve directly. A common approach to address this is the use of coarse-to-fine optimisation schemes. Representing the images by a Gaussian or spline pyramid [13], in which the spatial resolution is decreased by a certain factor between pyramid levels, is a popular strategy to tackle the challenges involved with high resolution data. It involves first solving a relaxed problem using a low-dimensional data representation and then refining the solution at a finer scale. A disadvantage of such multi-resolution approaches is the loss of detail at lower resolutions, which can and does lead to errors that cannot be compensated for at a finer scale. In addition, most approaches are limited by the use of a Cartesian grid representation and restricted spatially uniform subsampling. Furthermore, multi-resolution schemes do not preserve image boundaries and edges, which has a negative influence when estimating complex motion (with discontinuities).

In this work, we discuss the use of an alternative, low parametric, image representation, namely supervoxels. The motivation for the use of supervoxels is their ability to group voxels, which are close both **spatially and visually** into perceptually meaningful clusters. The locations of cluster centres do not have to lie on a regular grid, making them more versatile than traditional parametric image representations such as B-splines (with the exception of the recent work on sparse free-form deformations [12]). Supervoxels are not restricted to be uniformly shaped, enabling a better preservation of image edges. Figure 1 shows an example over-segmentation of an axial slice of a CT scan using 250 superpixels and the image reconstruction, obtained by assigning the mean intensity value of each cluster to each pixel within a superpixel. Note, that although only 2D superpixels are shown all steps in our implementation use 3D supervoxels. The advantages of preserving image edges and small anatomical detail is shown in comparison to a low-parametric B-spline representation. The disadvantage is that because superpixel segmentation relies on a piecewise constant image model, it shows poor performance in homogeneous or gradually changing image regions, resulting in inconsistent clustering. This reason has largely restricted the use of superpixels to image segmentation or classification tasks. These shortcoming will be addressed in this paper.

2   Related Work Using Supervoxels

Motion estimation or tracking using supervoxels relies on the assumption that all pixels contained in a cluster have the same (translational) motion. This precondition improves the robustness against image noise, reduces the ambiguity in homogeneous regions, and substantially reduces the complexity of the optimisation problem, in turn simplifying global regularisation of the motion field. Another advantage of this piecewise constant motion model is that it enables the preservation of motion discontinuities, so long as they coincide with intensity steps. In [9], stereo depth estimation is performed based on an over-segmentation of one of the two views. Employing a segmentation in only one view does not reduce the space of the potential motion vectors, hence extending this approach to higher dimensional problems substantially increases the complexity. An alternative approach, which is used in this work, is to perform supervoxel clustering

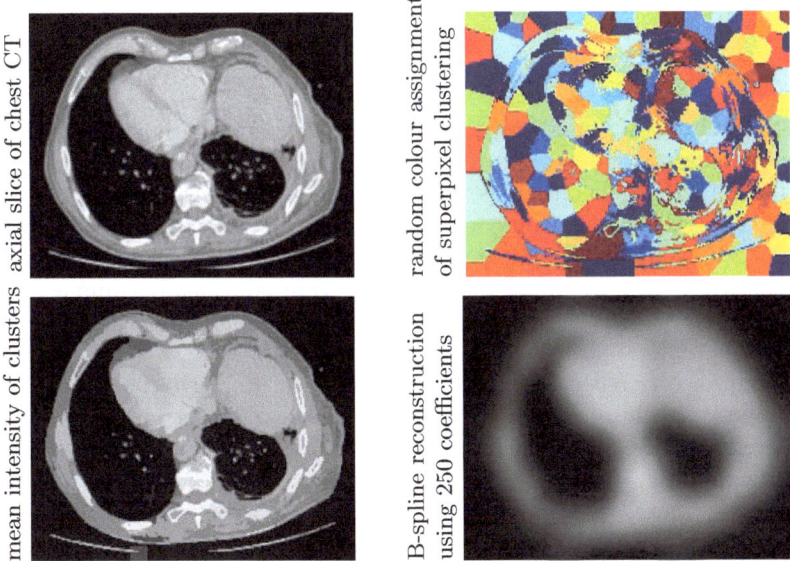

Fig. 1. Examples of sparse image representations. Image representation using 250 superpixels is able to preserve image edges and small-scale structures. While a reconstruction using 250 equally spaced coefficients [13] loses most fine details.

in both images and restrict the motion to corresponding cluster centres, thus directly matching segments across images. The main challenge here is the inconsistency of supervoxel clustering across images. [17] attempts to address this challenge by alternating steps of segmentation and matching to obtain a final segmentation, which is consistent across images.

The concept we introduce in this paper overcomes the disadvantages of previous approaches by using multiple layers of supervoxels. Sections 3.1 and 3.2 describe how two volumes (to be registered) are clustered into layers of supervoxels, which enable a better image representation in ambiguous (homogeneous or gradually changing intensity) regions, while at the same time preserving important details and edges. Sec. 3.2 shows that these complementary (not hierarchical) 3D layers of supervoxels form a low-parametric image representation with similar qualities as the popular joint bilateral filter [8] with very low computational complexity. We make further use of the clustering by introducing a new similarity criterion between single- and multi-modal scans, using a binary representation of the shape of the supervoxel (see Sec. 3.3). Section 3.4 describes the graph based optimisation, which uses a discretised, sparse displacement space. For each 3D layer, a separate graph connects supervoxels of the reference image, which are close both spatially and based on intensity. A combined energy term (Eq. 7) consisting of a diffusion regularisation term and similarity criterion is optimised using belief propagation [3] to obtain piecewise smooth transformations. The optimal transformations for all layers are then finally combined voxelwise in the original image domain (see Sec. 3.5).

3   Methods

3.1   Supervoxel Clustering

Supervoxel clustering performs an over-segmentation of an image that respects image boundaries. Supervoxels remove the redundant intensity information of voxels within homogeneous areas, which are likely to belong to the same object. Supervoxels enable a more compact image representation with little loss of detail. Due to their flexibility they are also more adaptive to the local shape of the images. Because they significantly reduce the computationally complexity, they have attracted a lot of attention in a range of image analysis tasks like stereo matching [9], optical flow [17], and segmentation [10].

We adapt a very recent algorithm, "simple linear iterative clustering" (SLIC) [1] for supervoxel clustering. Its complexity is linear w.r.t. the number of pixels N and therefore easily applicable to large datasets. It clusters voxels based on their grayscale similarity and spatial Euclidean distance. The algorithm is designed to create approximately K equally-sized supervoxels $\mathbf{S} = \{S_1, S_2, \ldots, S_k\}$. It starts from a set of equally spaced seed cluster centres with distance $s \approx \sqrt[3]{N/K}$. The distance d_{ik} between a voxel $p_i = [l_i, x_i, y_i, z_i]^T$ (where l is intensity value) and a cluster centre $S_k = [l_k, x_k, y_k, z_k]^T$ is given by Eq. 1.

$$d_{ik}^v = |l_k - l_i| , \quad d_{ik}^{xyz} = \sqrt{(x_k - x_i)^2 + (y_k - y_i)^2 + (z_k - z_i)^2}$$
$$d_{ik} = d_{ik}^v + \frac{m}{s} d_{ik}^{xyz} \tag{1}$$

The weighting m determines the compactness of the clusters, where higher values result in more regularly shaped supervoxels. It is assumed that the spatial extent of a supervoxel lies within a compact search region R of spatial extent $3s$ x $3s$ x $3s$. Therefore each voxel p_i has to be compared only to all centres which are within R and is afterwards assigned to the closest cluster (see Eq. 3.1):

$$S(p_i) = \arg\min_{S_j \in R} d_{ij} \tag{2}$$

After one pass over all pixels, the cluster centres are recomputed. This process is iterated until the clusters no longer change, or a fixed iteration number is reached. The algorithm does not guarantee connectedness within clusters, thus a simple connectivity enforcing step could be performed afterwards to eliminate stray labels. This method achieves substantial improvements in computation time compared to state-of-the-art methods, while yielding similar or better segmentation accuracy [1]. An example output of the method is displayed in Fig. 1, in which we compare the representation of an axial CT slice with the same number (250) of free parameters, using the supervoxels clustering and then a cubic B-spline basis function. It can be seen that the supervoxels better preserve image details and edges.

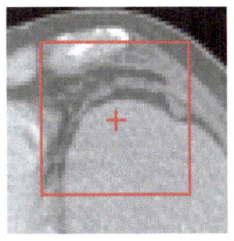 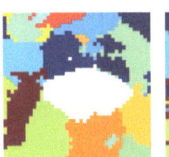 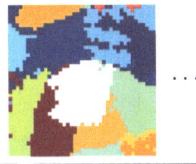 . . .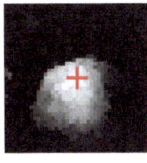

CT scan detail of liver   multiple layers of supervoxels   spatial weight of 20 layers

Fig. 2. Concept of layers of supervoxels for particular region (anterior part of liver) in axial CT plane, with central voxel p_c marked with red cross. Multiple clusterings **S** are obtained using different seeds. Shape of supervoxels is used as similarity criterion (see Sec. 3.3). Linear combination of all clusters of which p_c is part of, results in a spatial weighting similar to the bilateral filter.

3.2   Multiple Layers of Supervoxels

A disadvantage of supervoxel clustering is its inconsistent clustering in homogeneous or gradually changing image regions. In the context of motion estimation this is a major limitation, because it is important which correspondence within a homogeneous region is selected. One of the main contributions of this work is to use multiple layers of supervoxels to obtain a piecewise smooth motion model for accurate deformable registration.

To create multiple layers of supervoxels, the clustering algorithm of Sec. 3.1 is run several times with slightly different initialisation (random offset of seed locations with maximum magnitude $s/2$). Image regions with sufficient structural content (e.g. edges) are not affected by this disturbance and the clustering is therefore very similar for all layers. Homogeneous or gradually changing areas do not provide sufficient guidance for the supervoxel, resulting in arbitrarily different clusters for each layer. This means that when a separate optimisation is performed for each layer of supervoxels, the combination of these transformation is a smooth average in homogeneous regions, but adheres to discontinuities at image boundaries. Figure 2 demonstrates this concept. Two different layers of supervoxels of an axial CT slice are shown. The linear combination of the spatial layout of supervoxels of different layers for one particular voxel is shown. The close relation to the joint bilateral filter [8], and the ability to model smooth regions and at the same time preserve edges can be clearly seen. Furthermore, the supervoxel based approach enables a low parametric representation for each layer, which is beneficial for the optimisation, and the complexity of the clustering is independent of the number or size of the clusters.

3.3   Shape of Supervoxel as Similarity Criterion

The spatial context of a voxel's intensity has been used in many applications as it provides a good descriptor of local geometric and anatomical structure [5].

The census transform [16] uses a binary representation $\mathbf{B}$ of local shape. For each voxel p_i in an image, $\mathbf{B}$ is obtained by comparing its intensity l_i to the intensities l_n of all voxels in a certain spatial neighbourhood $\mathcal{I}$ and setting $B(p_i, p_n) = 1$ if $l_n < l_i$ and $B(p_i, p_n) = 0$ if $l_n \geq l_i$ for all $p_n \in \mathcal{I}$. It has been shown that these representations are well suited to define similarity across images, because they are sensitive to edges, local orientation and invariant to monotonic grayscale transformations. However, it cannot be employed for multi-modal images where gradients of corresponding anatomies might be reversed. We therefore propose to use the shape of supervoxels as a multi-modal similarity criterion. Given a supervoxel clustering $\mathbf{S}$, the binary vector $\mathbf{B}_i$ for a voxel p_i is defined as:

$$B(p_i, p_n) = \begin{cases} 1, & \text{if } S(p_i) = S(p_n) \\ 0, & \text{if } S(p_i) \neq S(p_n) \end{cases} \text{ for all } p_n \in \mathcal{I} \qquad (3)$$

We show examples of this binary shape representation in Fig. 2. We define the neighbourhood $\mathcal{I}$ to be the subset of the 320 closest points p_n (multiples of 64 are well suited for computation) based on the distance $|d_{in}^{xyz} - r|$ of p_n to the surface of a sphere centred at p_i with radius of $r = \frac{1}{2}s\sqrt[3]{6/\pi}$. The binary representation has the advantage that the L_1 distance between two vectors $|\mathbf{B}_i - \mathbf{B}_j|$ can be efficiently evaluated by the Hamming weight (bit count of all pair-wise unequal binary values [16]). The computation for a vector of size 64 takes less time than calculating a single absolute difference of two intensities.

3.4   MRF-Based Optimisation

Discrete optimisation methods have become very popular for deformable registration, due to their flexibility, computational efficiency and guarantees of optimality [4]. Our aim is to find the best correspondence for each supervoxel $S_p \in \mathbf{S}$ of the reference scan, in terms of similarity and subject to a global regularisation. This optimisation problem is solved independently for each 3D layer in the reference scan. The combination of several optimal transformations and the reverse mapping into the voxelwise image domain is detailed in Sec. 3.5. The set of potential displacement labels $\mathbf{f}_p = \{f_p^1, f_p^2, \ldots\}$ is defined for a supervoxel S_i as the sparse set of all supervoxel locations within a rectangular search window W (centred around $\mathbf{x}_p$) in any layer of the moving image (see Fig. 3 for a visual example). Each label f_p^j corresponds to a spatial displacement $\Delta\mathbf{x}(f_p^j) = \mathbf{x}_p - \mathbf{x}_j$ between reference and moving scan. The similarity cost of a label f_p based on the intensities I and I' (normalised to $[0,1]$) of reference and moving scan respectively is then defined as:

$$D(f_p) = |I(\mathbf{x}_i) - I'(\mathbf{x}_i + \Delta\mathbf{x}(f_p))| \qquad (4)$$

Likewise, the similarity criterion based on the local shape of supervoxels, which was introduced in Sec. 3.3, can now be defined for a certain label f_p:

$$\bar{D}(f_p) = \sum_{n \in \mathcal{I}} |B(\mathbf{x}_p, n) - B'(\mathbf{x}_p + \Delta\mathbf{x}(f_p), n)| \qquad (5)$$

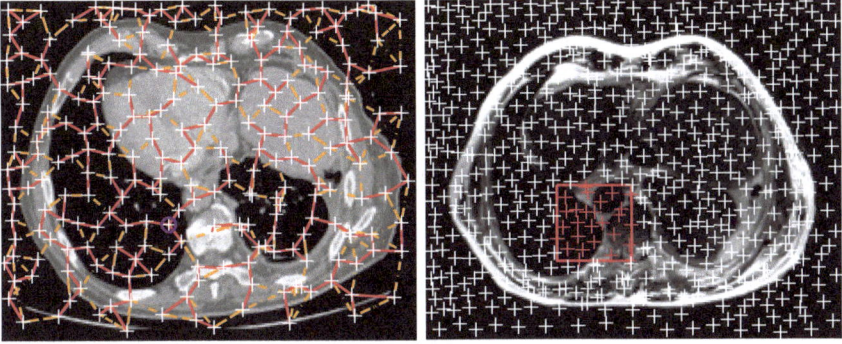

Fig. 3. Concept of supervoxel matching across scans. Cluster centres are denoted by white crosses. Left: Edges of kNN spanning graph in the reference image are shown with yellow dashed lines, edges which are also part of the Euclidean minimum spanning tree (EMST) with red lines. The possible displacements for a voxel of interest (purple circle) within a rectangular window in moving image are shown in red. Note that all 3D layers of the the moving image are considered simultaneously, resulting in more cluster centres.

In order to enforce spatial regularity of the displacements of all supervoxels, a graph is introduced, which connects all clusters that are close both spatially and in intensity. A diffusion regularisation term $R(f_p, f_q)$ is defined between two displacements f_p and f_q of two clusters, which penalises the squared Euclidean distance of displacements divided by the distance of the supervoxels (see Eq. 1):

$$R(f_p, f_q) = \frac{||\Delta\mathbf{x}(f_p) - \Delta\mathbf{x}(f_q)||^2}{\frac{s}{m}|l_p - l_q| + ||\mathbf{x}_p - \mathbf{x}_q||} \qquad (6)$$

Notice that the regularisation between clusters with different appearances is reduced. This enables the preservation of discontinuities, which are likely to coincide with image boundaries. Since the cluster centres are non-uniformly distributed across the image grid, conventional neighbourhood connections do not apply. We employ two steps to obtain a suitable graph representation. First, a k-nearest neighbour (kNN) graph with edges $\mathcal{E}$ is extracted based on the supervoxel cluster distances (see Eq. 1). The value of k is incrementally increased until a spanning graph (connecting all supervoxels in the reference image) is found. For large numbers of supervoxels K the naïve nearest neighbour search with K^2 complexity would be impractical, so we employ an accelerated ($\sim$50x) search using the vantage-point tree (see [15] for details).

The global energy term to be minimised is a weighted combination of intensity similarity D, shape similarity $\bar{D}$ and a diffusion regularisation term:

$$E(f) = \underbrace{(1 - \alpha) \sum_{p \in \mathbf{S}} D(f_p)}_{\text{intensity similarity}} + \underbrace{\alpha \sum_{p \in \mathbf{S}} \bar{D}(f_p)}_{\text{shape similarity}} + \underbrace{\lambda \sum_{(p,q) \in \mathcal{E}} R(f_p, f_q)}_{\text{diffusion regularisation}} \qquad (7)$$

Using the kNN graph, this energy can be minimised with a number of discrete optimisation methods (see [7] for an overview). Similar to [6], we make a further approximation to employ belief propagation on a tree (BP-T), which guarantees a global optimum of the energy on this relaxed graph. By iteratively removing edges with highest distance between clusters (and therefore smallest influence on the regularisation) we find a Euclidean minimum-spanning-tree, which is shown with red lines in Fig. 3.

3.5   Linear Combination of Optimal Transformations

Once the optimal transformation is found for each 3D layer in the reference image, the final deformation field can be obtained as a linear combination of all transformations. For each voxel p_i the resulting displacement is found by averaging over all displacement vectors of the particular supervoxel of which p_i is part in the respective 3D layer. This results in a spatial weighting of displacement vectors, which is similar to the bilateral filter, as displayed in Fig. 2. The advantage is that this linear combination can both preserve discontinuities in the motion field and model gradually changing motion magnitudes.

4   Experiments

We perform experiments on two clinical 3D datasets to demonstrate the suitability of our contributions. First, the benefits of using multiple layers of supervoxels to model piecewise smooth, edge-preserving deformations is evaluated on 4D-CT scans. Second, the similarity criterion based on the shape of supervoxels is applied successfully to the multi-modal fusion of chest CT and MRI scans.

4.1   Inhale-Exhale Volumetric CT Registration

Sliding motion is a particular challenge when estimating motion of lung CT scans acquired at different phases of the breathing cycle, which is clinically useful for radiotherapy of lung cancer and the assessment of breathing disorders. Most approaches to this problem have used a manual or automatically detected segmentation of the thoracic cage [11], [14]. Our approach relies solely on the over-segmentation from the supervoxel clustering to preserve motion boundaries and requires no further manual interaction. We perform our experiments on the extreme phases (inhale and exhale) of 4D respiratory CT scans of 5 lung cancer patients. The dataset has been made publicly available by the DIR-lab, University of Texas, manually annotated with 300 landmark per scan pair [2]. We use the most challenging cases #6-10, which have a very large diaphragm displacement and particularly strong sliding motion at the lung/rib cage interface.

  With a slice thickness of 2.5 mm, the volumes have strongly anisotropic voxel-sizes, so the axial resolution was resampled to 1.5 mm. The scans were slightly cropped to exclude regions outside the body. We found that around 15000 supervoxels are sufficient to represent the details of these images, which yields

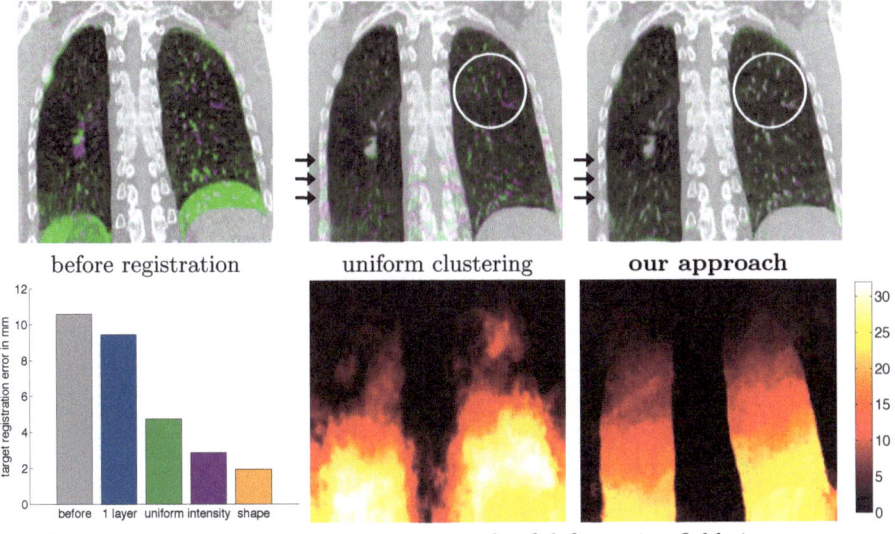

before registration   uniform clustering   **our approach**

quantitative registration error   magnitude of deformation fields in mm

Fig. 4. Example of deformable registration of an inhale-exhale CT scan pair. Overlay before and after registration is shown in green (inhale phase) and magenta (exhale phase). Uniform clustering approximates the traditional coarse-scale representation. Our approach using layers of supervoxels outperforms this for the matching of small vessels (see white circle) and the preservation of sliding motion (see black arrows). The quantitative evaluation shows a significantly lower registration error of our method using absolute intensity differences and a further improvement when employing the binary shape similarity criterion.

an average distance of 5 voxels between cluster centres. The supervoxel compactness parameter m is chosen empirically as 20 (for an intensity range of $[0, 255]$ and similar to [1]). We restrict the spatial extent of the (sparsely sampled) displacement space to ± 9 voxels in the axial plane and ± 15 voxels in proximal-distal direction (to cover the expected respiratory motion). For each 3D layer of supervoxels the computation takes roughly 5 sec. for the clustering, 1 sec. for similarity evaluation and graph extraction and 4 sec. for the BP-T optimisation using a C++ implementation on a quad-core CPU. We used 20 layers of super-voxels, tuned all parameters on a single scan pair and found their setting to be relatively insensitive. For the regularisation parameter $\lambda = \frac{1}{8}$ is chosen, but doubling or halving the value leads to a deviation of less than 10% in accuracy. The registration quality was examined visually and evaluated quantitatively using 300 manually annotated landmarks per scan pair.

Four different variations of our proposed method were tested to assess the individual influence of our contributions. The initial average landmark displacement was **10.6±7.5 mm**. First, our method was applied using only a **single layer** of supervoxels, similar to previous work on supervoxel matching. It yielded unsatisfactory results, as only the outer lung boundaries are aligned. Second, multiple layers were used and the image-adaptivity of the supervoxels was substantially

axial plane   sagittal plane

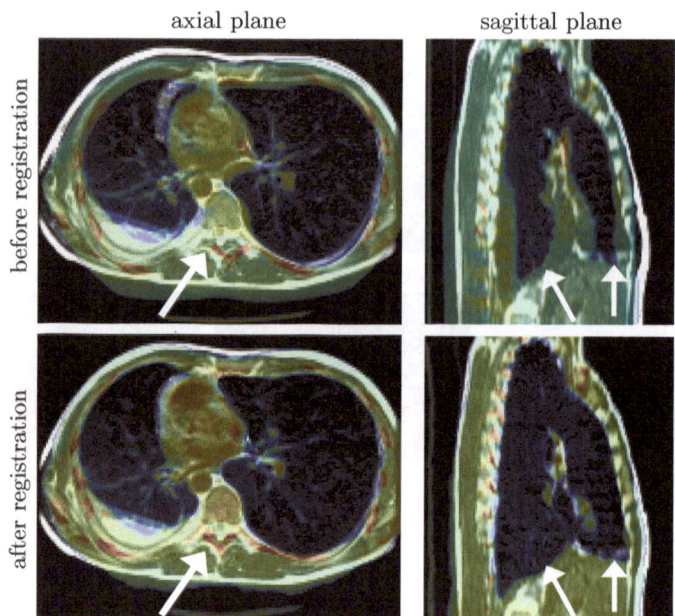

before registration

after registration

Fig. 5. Example of multi-modal fusion using the presented method. The sagittal and axial planes of a CT/MRI scan pair are shown. The MRI scan is displayed with greyscale intensities, while the CT scan is shown in pseudo-colours (red indicates high intensities and blue low intensities). A clearly improved alignment can be seen after deforming the CT scan with the estimated deformation field.

reduced ($m = 2000$) resulting in a very **uniform clustering** and a target registration error (TRE) of **4.72±3.5 mm**. Figure 4 demonstrates the main problem of this approach, which is similar to a traditional coarse-scale image representation. The motion field is smooth across the interface at which discontinuous sliding motion occurs (see black arrows). Additionally small details (lung vessels) are lost due to uniform smoothing, resulting in an inaccurate alignment of them (see white circle). Third, our approach was tested using only **intensity-based similarity** ($\alpha = 0$ in Eq. 7), achieving a significant improvement and a TRE of **2.87±1.9 mm**. Finally, the **shape similarity** $\bar{D}$ was included with a weighting of $\alpha = \frac{4}{5}$. Adding this structural image information, with negligible computational complexity, has clear advantages to match fine image details and further reduces the registration error to **1.94±1.3 mm**. Figure 4 demonstrates the accurate alignment of our approach and the well-preserved sliding motion at the thoracic cage.

4.2   Multi-modal Fusion of MRI and CT Chest Scans

Additionally, we applied our method to five pairs of longitudinal diagnostic MRI and CT scans from patients with lung diseases. The additional challenges here are lower scan quality in the MRI, large slice thicknesses of up to 8 mm, and pathological changes. The volumes have been manually cropped to a similar field of view (compensating global translation) and resampled to form isotropic voxels of 2x2x2 mm^3. The parameter settings were kept the same as before, except now only the shape similarity criterion was used $\alpha = 1$, since there is no direct relation of intensities between CT and MRI. The number of supervoxels was set to 15000 as before, which resulted in a spacing of 7 voxels. The search space is defined to be ±10 voxels in all dimensions. Figure 5 shows a successful multi-modal fusion of MRI in greyscale with the deformed CT as pseudo-colour overlay. A small number of anatomical landmarks (12 per scan) has been manually annotated by a radiologist, this tasks, however, is very difficult and resulted in a large intra-observer error ($\geq$ 5mm). The landmark distance could be reduced significantly (p =0.028) from **10.43±7.1 mm** to **7.33±4.3 mm** for this challenging fusion.

5   Conclusion

We have presented a novel concept for sparse image representation with application to deformable registration and fusion. Using multiple layers of supervoxels, each representing the grouped voxels with one constant intensity and motion vector, enables a very efficient piecewise smooth transformation model with very low computational complexity. We have demonstrated that our approach is able to deal well with complex lung motion containing both smooth deformations and discontinuities. Our resulting TRE of **1.94 mm** for the registration of inhale-exhale CT compares favourable with the published results of [11] and [14], which specifically address the challenge of sliding motion using a segmentation mask, and achieve a TRE of **2.68 mm** and **2.09 mm** for these particularly challenging scan pairs (#6-10 of [2]). It is worth noting that they found similar results (TRE 4.27 and 4.23 mm) when not using a lung segmentation compared to our uniform clustering variant, which confirms the advantages of the presented image-adaptive supervoxel clustering. Our second contribution, the formulation of a binary shape representation based on the clusters as a similarity criterion, improves accuracy of single-modal registration and enables multi-modal fusion.

While our results already demonstrate state-of-the-art performance for the given tasks, further improvements are possible (e.g. by employing twice as many layers of supervoxels, the TRE of the 4DCT registration is reduced to 1.75 mm – at the cost of higher computational complexity). Making use of the symmetry of the registration problem by enforcing inverse consistency would further improve the robustness. The use of an optimisation strategy, which can include a larger set of edges (e.g. loopy BP [3]) is likely to perform better. Rather than resampling the scans to avoid large anisotropy of voxel-sizes, isotropic supervoxels could be calculated directly using world instead of voxel coordinates. Finally, this concept has potential use in many other image analysis tasks, such as probabilistic segmentation and parameter map estimation.

474 M.P. Heinrich et al.

References

1. Achanta, R., Shaji, A., Smith, K., Lucchi, A., Fua, P., Süsstrunk, S.: SLIC superpixels compared to state-of-the-art superpixel methods. IEEE Trans. Pattern Anal. Mach. Intell. 34(11), 2274–2282 (2012)
2. Castillo, E., Castillo, R., Martinez, J., Shenoy, M., Guerrero, T.: Four-dimensional deformable image registration using trajectory modeling. Phys. Med. Biol. 55(1), 305 (2009)
3. Felzenszwalb, P., Huttenlocher, D.: Efficient Belief Propagation for Early Vision. Int. J. Comp. Vis. 70(1), 41–54 (2006)
4. Glocker, B., Komodakis, N., Tziritas, G., Navab, N., Paragios, N.: Dense image registrations through MRFs and efficient linear programming. Med. Imag. Anal. 12(6), 731–741 (2008)
5. Heinrich, M.P., Jenkinson, M., Bhushan, M., Matin, T., Gleeson, F.V., Brady, M., Schnabel, J.A.: MIND: Modality independent neighbourhood descriptor for multimodal deformable registration. Med. Imag. Anal. 16(7), 1423–1435 (2012)
6. Heinrich, M., Jenkinson, M., Brady, M., Schnabel, J.: MRF-based deformable registration and ventilation estimation of lung CT. IEEE Trans. Med. Imag. (2013)
7. Kolmogorov, V., Rother, C.: Minimizing nonsubmodular functions with graph cuts - a review. IEEE Trans. Pattern Anal. Mach. Intell. 29(7), 1274–1279 (2007)
8. Kopf, J., Cohen, M.F., Lischinski, D., Uyttendaele, M.: Joint bilateral upsampling. ACM Trans. Graph. 26(3), 96 (2007)
9. Lei, C., Selzer, J., Yang, Y.H.: Region-tree based stereo using dynamic programming optimization. In: CVPR, pp. 2378–2385. IEEE (2006)
10. Lucchi, A., Smith, K., Achanta, R., Knott, G., Fua, P.: Supervoxel-based segmentation of mitochondria in EM image stacks with learned shape features. IEEE Trans. Med. Imag. 31(2), 474–486 (2012)
11. Schmidt-Richberg, A., Werner, R., Handels, H., Ehrhardt, J.: Estimation of slipping organ motion by registration with direction-dependent regularization. Med. Imag. Anal. 16(1), 150–159 (2012)
12. Shi, W., Zhuang, X., Pizarro, L., Bai, W., Wang, H., Tung, K.P., Edwards, P., Rueckert, D.: Registration using sparse free-form deformations. In: Ayache, N., Delingette, H., Golland, P., Mori, K. (eds.) MICCAI 2012, Part II. LNCS, vol. 7511, pp. 659–666. Springer, Heidelberg (2012)
13. Unser, M.A., Aldroubi, A., Gerfen, C.R.: Multiresolution image registration procedure using spline pyramids. In: Int. Symp. on Optics, Imaging, and Instrumentation, SPIE, pp. 160–170 (1993)
14. Vandemeulebroucke, J., Bernard, O., Rit, S., Kybic, J., Clarysse, P., Sarrut, D.: Automated segmentation of a motion mask to preserve sliding motion in deformable registration of thoracic CT. Med. Phys. 39, 1006 (2012)
15. Yianilos, P.N.: Data structures and algorithms for nearest neighbor search in general metric spaces. In: ACM-SIAM Symp. on Discrete Algorithms, pp. 311–321 (1993)
16. Zabih, R., Woodfill, J.: Non-parametric local transforms for computing visual correspondence. In: Eklundh, J.-O. (ed.) ECCV 1994. LNCS, vol. 801, pp. 151–158. Springer, Heidelberg (1994)
17. Zitnick, C.W., Jojic, N., Kang, S.B.: Consistent segmentation for optical flow estimation. In: ICCV, pp. 1308–1315. IEEE (2005)

Multimodal Surface Matching: Fast and Generalisable Cortical Registration Using Discrete Optimisation

Emma C. Robinson[1], Saad Jbabdi[1], Jesper Andersson[1], Stephen Smith[1],
Matthew F. Glasser[2], David C. Van Essen[2], Greg Burgess[2],
Michael P. Harms[3], Deanna M. Barch[4], and Mark Jenkinson[1]

[1] FMRIB, Nuffield Department of Clinical Neurosciences, University of Oxford, UK
[2] Department of Anatomy and Neurobiology, Washington University School
of Medicine, St Louis, MO, USA
[3] Department of Psychiatry, Washington University School of Medicine, St Louis,
MO, USA
[4] Department of Psychology, Washington University, St Louis, MO, USA

Abstract. Group neuroimaging studies of the cerebral cortex benefit
from accurate, surface-based, cross-subject alignment for investigating
brain architecture, function and connectivity. There is an increasing
amount of high quality data available. However, establishing how different modalities correlate across groups remains an open research question.
One reason for this is that the current methods for registration, based on
cortical folding, provide sub-optimal alignment of some functional sub-
regions of the brain. A more flexible framework is needed that will allow
robust alignment of multiple modalities. We adapt the Fast Primal-Dual
(Fast-PD) approach for discrete Markov Random Field (MRF) optimisation to spherical registration by reframing the deformation labels as a
discrete set of rotations and propose a novel regularisation term, derived
from the geodesic distance between rotation matrices. This formulation
allows significant flexibility in the choice of similarity metric. To this end
we propose a new multivariate cost function based on the discretisation
of a graph-based mutual information measure. Results are presented for
alignment driven by scalar metrics of curvature and myelination, and
multivariate features derived from functional task performance. These
experiments demonstrate the potential of this approach for improving
the integration of complementary brain data sets in the future.

1 Introduction

Automated and accurate registration of the cortical sheet is an increasingly important topic of neuroimaging methods research. However, the use of volumetric
registration approaches in functional studies is sub-optimal, since functional areas are often spaced much further apart across the two-dimensional surface than
is represented in volumetric space, because of the cortical folds.

Spherical registration algorithms [1,2] simplify the cortical matching problem
by inflating the surface to a two dimensional sphere. Current approaches pre-
dominantly use measures of sulcal depth or mean curvature (folding) to perform

J.C. Gee et al. (Eds.): IPMI 2013, LNCS 7917, pp. 475–486, 2013.
© Springer-Verlag Berlin Heidelberg 2013

the cross-surface matching. This leads to a reasonable first approximation of brain alignment, but is limited by the fact that significant variability in cortical folding manifests across populations [3].

A more fundamental caveat of morphologically driven alignment is that cortical folding imperfectly reflects functional sub-divisions[3]. The fundus of a sulcus does not generally align with the boundary between two functional regions. Since the ultimate goal of inter-subject registration is to match functional regions across subjects, matching anatomies yields only an approximation.

Connectivity-based alignment [4] has been proposed as an additional means for driving registration. Connections may be a more direct correlate of brain function than local morphology. However, it is unclear how well we can estimate connections that are relevant to drive registration. Another alternative is to use functional (task) activation data to drive registration, though at the cost of increasing data requirements and incomplete brain coverage.

It is unlikely that any single measure of brain structure or function will be sufficient for consistent, whole brain, and functionally accurate inter-subject registration. A multimodal approach is likely to yield significant improvements, but requires a more flexible registration framework that is adaptable to multivariate correlates of functional, structural and connectional brain data.

Discrete optimisation approaches to image registration constitute such a flexible framework. They were first proposed by Glocker et al [5] who converted a B-spline free-form deformation model [6] into a discrete setting. Discrete sets of deformation labels were assigned to the control points of the B-spline model, and the problem was re-formulated using graph cuts [7]. Alternative approaches that do not tie the framework to use of the free-form deformation model have also been proposed by [8,9].

Discrete methods in general offer advantages in terms of reduced sensitivity to local minima combined with a fast and efficient optimisation approach that provides flexibility by not restricting the choice of similarity measure. Here, we introduce a multivariate mutual-information measure derived from entropic graphs [10,11]. These measures were first proposed for use in volumetric registration by [10] in order to allow fast estimation of multivariate mutual information without the need for costly estimations of high dimensional histograms. To our knowledge, ours is the first application of multivariate matching within the discrete optimisation framework.

One restriction of the MRF-based optimisation framework is that the regularisation term must be reformulated in terms of pair-wise edge potentials between neighbouring vertices. This can limit the choice of regulariser to measures derived from the first order derivatives of the deformation warp, which are not invariant to scaling or rotations. Alternative methods have been proposed in [12,13]. Here we propose a new regularisation potential based on the geodesic distance between rotation matrices. This is not a metric and therefore we benefit from applying Fast-PD optimisation of the MRF, proposed in [14,15] and first used for registration by Glocker et al in [5].

In the next section we provide an overview of the new Multimodal Surface Matching (MSM) approach and its reformulation to fit the spherical coordinate system. Results are presented using simulated data, univariate measures of sulcal depth and curvature, and finally multivariate features derived from functional task performance.

2   MRF-Based Optimisation for Spherical Registration

2.1   Discrete Optimisation and Fast-PD

Discrete registration methods redefine the image as a weighted graph $G(P, E, \omega)$ formed from control point nodes (P), edges (E), and weights (ω), and solve the optimisation in the form of a Markov Random Field labelling. This approach limits the movement of any vertex point p to a set of discrete displacements $\mathbf{d}^{l_p}$ determined by a predefined label set $L = \{a, b.....\}$. For spherical registration these displacements may be governed by a finite set of rotations (Fig . 1).

The optimal deformation can be found by minimising the following energy function:

$$COST = \sum_{p \in P} \mathbf{c}_p(l_p) + \sum_{(p,q) \in E} \omega_{pq} V(l_p, l_q) \tag{1}$$

This is formed from a similarity term $\mathbf{c}_p(l_p)$ and a weighted ω_{pq} penalisation term $V(l_p, l_q)$, which limits the extent to which neighbouring vertices (p, q) can be assigned different displacement labels (l_p, l_q). The penalisation term controls regularisation of the deformation. The key advantage of the MRF formulation is that any similarity metric may be used.

Volumetric methods, such as [5,8] propose using a low-resolution control point grids or regular sampling of the image space to define the nodes in G. In this way image similarity, for each label a, is approximated by factorizing the expression for whole image similarity into cliques, as:

$$\sum_{p \in P} \mathbf{c}_p(l_p) = \sum_{p \in P} \sum_{i \in N} \hat{n}(\mathbf{x}_i - \mathbf{x}_p)(sim(F(\mathbf{x}_i), M((\mathbf{x}_i + \mathbf{d}^a)))) \tag{2}$$

This sums over pair-wise similarities between points in the moving mesh $M((\mathbf{x}_i + \mathbf{d}^a)$ (transformed by the proposed deformation $\mathbf{d}^a$) and their neighbours within the fixed/target image $F(\mathbf{x}_i)$, for all data points in the neighbourhood of control point p. The $\hat{n}(\mathbf{x}_i - \mathbf{x}_p)$ is a weighting term controlling the zone of influence of each control point. In this instance, $\hat{n}(\mathbf{x}_i - \mathbf{x}_p)$ is either 0 or 1.

There are several methods for solving the MRF problem, amongst which are the well-known graph cut [7] and max-flow min-cut algorithms, used often in computer vision for image restoration and segmentation. In [5] the authors use the Fast-PD algorithm, proposed by Komodakis et al [14,15] which takes advantage of the primal-dual schema of linear programing to derive an efficient approximation. For full comprehensive details of the algorithm we refer to [14,15]. However, the main advantages is that it generates fast solutions that can be shown to be close to the global optimum even for pair-wise potential terms which are not metrics. That is, potentials can be used that do not have to satisfy the conditions $V(a, b) = 0 \; \forall a = b$; $V(a, b) = V(b, a) \geq 0$ and $V(a, b) = V(b, a) \leq V(a, c) + V(c, b)$.

2.2   Deformation Labels and the Control Point Grid

In this framework, spherical registration is driven using a series multi-resolution control point grids. Currently three regular icosahedrons of order 3-5 (161, 642 and 2542 vertices) are used, with respective mean vertex distances (MVD) of 26.7mm, 13.8mm and 6.9mm. Similarity is estimated by dividing all vertices of the original mesh into sets of cliques as for eq. 2. Interpolation of the control point warp to the original surface mesh is performed using spline-based interpolation.

Image data is downsampled to a 10,000 vertex regular mesh $(MVD = 3.5mm)$ to speed up the sampling of the image space. In general, this is a reasonable approximation as the original volumetric image data will typically be of a resolution between 1mm for structural data and 3mm for functional data. Downsampling is performed using Gaussian interpolation, which enables simultaneous smoothing of the data. Note, although higher resolution control point and image grids can be used with minimal additional computational overhead, these were not found to improve the results of the data in this paper.

Deformation labels are defined via a simple and approximate solution to sampling on the sphere: a higher resolution icosahedron grid is projected below each control point and used to define the sampling grid (see Fig. 1). MRF labels are represented as discrete rotations between the control point and the vertices of the higher resolution sampling grid. For a sampling grid formed from an icosahedron 2 orders higher than the control point grid, there is typically between 10 and 20 labels per control point. The spacing between labels at the highest resolution level is roughly 1mm.

At each level the maximum sampling distances, and thus biggest possible control point deformation, is set to $0.4 * MVD$. This ensures diffeomorphic warps by forcibly preventing mesh folding. However, this also means that it is not guaranteed that optimal alignment can be reached within one cycle of labelling. Therefore, the algorithm iterates over several cycles of labelling at each resolution. As the MRF will be optimised for the label set after each cycle, the label set iterates between using the vertices and barycentres of the faces of the sampling grid to prevent the registration getting trapped in local minima. After each stage the deformation is projected to the image grid and the control point grid is reset.

2.3   Regularisation

Regularisation in discrete optimisation methods has conventionally been imposed by pair-wise potentials calculated from the distance between the deformations assigned to neighbouring points: $V(l_p, l_q) = \lambda(|d^{l_p} - d^{l_q}|)$. However, in methods such as this where registration iterates over several cycles of MRF optimisation, symmetric pairwise potentials are unsuited as they cannot capture

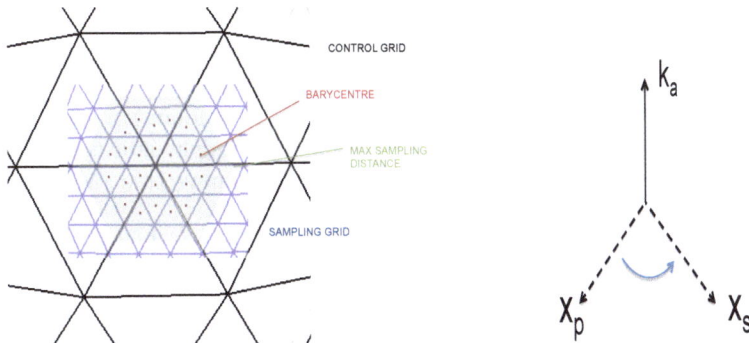

Fig. 1. The sampling (blue) and control point grids (black). Sampling points vary between the vertices and the barycentres (red points) of the high res grid. Max sampling distance is 0.4 times the control point spacing. Rotation matrices, estimated between the control point and each of the sampling points, are used to define the deformation labels.

the properties of the previous warps. Estimates of the deformation from previous iterations (R_p, R_q) can be used to provide a full regularisation over time as: $V(l_p, l_q) = \lambda(|\mathbf{R}_p d^{l_p} - \mathbf{R}_q d^{l_q}|)$ [5]. Nevertheless, this automatically renders any distance non-metric as the penalisation need no longer be same for points assigned the same label: $V(l_p, l_q) \neq 0 \; if \; l_p = l_q$.

In the spherical registration format, it is no longer desirable to project deformations as Cartesian deformation vectors, as the deformation is constrained to the spherical surface, and thus the space is not Euclidean. Instead we choose to represent the deformation labels as rotation matrices defined using the Rodrigues rotation formula:

$$\mathbf{R}_p^{l_p} = I + sin\theta_{l_p}[\mathbf{k}_{l_p}]_\times + (1 - cos\theta_{l_p})(\mathbf{k}_{l_p}\mathbf{k}_{l_p}^T - I) , \tag{3}$$

where, the axis $\mathbf{k}_{l_p} = \mathbf{x}_p \times \mathbf{x}_s$ and angle θ_{l_p} of rotation for label l_p are estimated using the initial $\mathbf{x}_p$ and final point of the rotation $\mathbf{x}_s$ (Fig. 1). $[\mathbf{k}_{l_p}]_\times$ is the cross product matrix.

This form is also conveniently linked to the definition of a geodesic distance between rotation matrices: $d_g(\mathbf{A}, \mathbf{B}) := ||log(\mathbf{A}^T\mathbf{B})||_F = ||[\mathbf{k}_{ab}]_\times \theta_{ab}||_F$, where $||.||_F$ represents the Frobenius norm and $d_g(A, B)$ is proportional to the angle of difference (θ_{ab}) between the rotation matrices. This allows warps from previous iterations to contribute to the estimation of the pairwise potential. As the control point grid is reset each time, the past deformation of each control point p is estimated from the warped imaged data, and summarised by rotation matrix $\mathbf{R}_p$. The full rotation matrix for the combined deformation can then be estimated as $\mathbf{A} = \mathbf{R}_p^{l_p}\mathbf{R}_p$, and compared against the full deformation of its neighbour $\mathbf{B} = \mathbf{R}_q^{l_q}\mathbf{R}_p$.

3   Multivariate Similarity Measures

A significant advantage of the flexibility of the MRF framework is that it is straightforward to replace scalar similarity terms with a multivariate measure.

Therefore, our framework can incorporate a multivariate measure such as the estimate of mutual information known as α-entropy, derived by [10] from entropic graphs. Rényi, or α-entropy is a generalisation of Shannon's entropy of the form: $H_\alpha(z) = \frac{1}{1-\alpha}log(\sum_{i=1}^n p_i^\alpha)$, where z is a random variable. Entropic graphs are any graph whose normalised total edge weight is a consistent estimator of α-entropy. These include the minimal spanning tree (MST) and the k-nearest neighbour (kNN) graph.

The basic principle is as follows: if each point in the fixed image is described by a multivariate feature vector $\mathbf{z}^f(\mathbf{x}_i) = [z_1^f(\mathbf{x}_i)...z_d^f((\mathbf{x}_i)]$ of dimension d, and the equivalent point in the moving image is $\mathbf{z}^m(\mathbf{x}_i + \mathbf{d}^a)$, then a graph-based measure of mutual information may be calculated from the kNN graph as:

$$\alpha - \hat{M}I(Z_f, Z_m, Z_{fm}) = \frac{1}{\alpha - 1}log\frac{1}{N^\alpha}\sum_{i=1}^{N_f}\left(\frac{\Gamma_i^{fm}}{\sqrt{\Gamma_i^f\Gamma_i^m}}\right)^\gamma \quad (4)$$

For:

$$\Gamma_i^f = \sum_{n=1}^k ||\mathbf{z}^f(\mathbf{x}_i) - \mathbf{z}^f(\mathbf{x}_{in})|| \quad (5)$$

$$\Gamma_i^m = \sum_{n=1}^k ||\mathbf{z}^m(\mathbf{x}_i + \mathbf{d}^a) - \mathbf{z}^m(\mathbf{x}_{in} + \mathbf{d}^a)|| \quad (6)$$

$$\Gamma_i^{fm} = \sum_{n=1}^k ||\mathbf{z}^{fm}(\mathbf{x}_i, \mathbf{x}_i + \mathbf{d}^a) - \mathbf{z}^{fm}(\mathbf{x}_p, \mathbf{x}_{in} + \mathbf{d}^a)|| \quad (7)$$

Here, $\mathbf{z}^{fm}$ is the result of concatenating the feature vectors from the fixed and moving image at the transformed position $(\mathbf{x}_i + \mathbf{d}^a)$. Z_f, Z_m, and Z_{fm} represent the set of feature vectors for each kNN graph, $\gamma = d(1 - \alpha)$ and α are user defined tuning parameters, and Euclidean distances are estimated between feature vectors. Currently each feature is given a equal weighting when estimating the cost. However, given that the end goal is to combine complementary data sets, each of which are shown to be consistent across subjects in different areas, this term could be replaced by a weighted sum of squares.

Approximate k-nearest neighbours are calculated using [16]. This method has been shown to lead to a significant boost in speed in solving for k, provided a small error in the graph estimation is tolerable. For this purpose approximate neighbours are sufficient as the principal goal of using the α-MI measure to drive the registration is to ensure that the spatial distribution of image features is the same for source and target meshes.

4   Validation

In this section we test the algorithm on scalar image data and use a simulation to show the algorithm performs as well as the state of the art in this respect.

Table 1. Comparing the new Multimodal Surface Matching method against the state of the art. Performance is judged in terms of Dice overlap results for simulated data, and run times for real data (averaged over 14 test sessions).

	FreeSurfer	Spherical Demons	MSM
Dice Overlap	N/A	0.892 ± 0.002	0.922 ±0.002
Speed	> 1hr	2 min	4 min

We test the performance of the algorithm against FreeSurfer [1] and Spherical Demons (SD) [2], measuring success in terms of speed and generalisability to new data sets. Given that curvature metrics have been shown to be highly variable across the population, and in the absence of any better neurological marker of ground truth, we use a simulated test case to quantify alignment. We then extend the comparison to standard measures of sulcal depth and curvature, as well as a new data set composed of estimates of cortical myelination [17] to provide more concrete evidence that the algorithm performs well on real data.

4.1 Simulated Deformations

A test case (Fig. 2 a), with colour patches each representing a different scalar value, was created and then transformed by applying a known deformation, in order to generate a target (Fig. 2 b). The deformation was obtained through registration of real image data to the fsaverage template using the FreeSurfer algorithm. The discrete optimisation approach was run for three resolution levels, with 5 internal iterations at each level. At each internal iteration the algorithm reset the control point grid and recalculated the label set as described in section 2.2. The data cost term was estimated using cross correlation. We found the framework largely insensitive to the choice of regularisation parameter. The results of the registration (fig. 2 c) were compared with those obtained from applying Spherical Demons (fig. 2 d), run using the default parameters. FreeSurfer was not used as it could not be adapted to accept non-curvature data.

The accuracy of each approach was assessed using the mean Dice overlap of the sampling patches (Table 1 top row). In general, although both approaches estimate the affine component of the registration correctly, Spherical Demons fails to capture the majority of the non-linear deformation fig. 2 d). Some investigation showed this to be linked to the regularisation; controlled by modifying the number of times a smoothing kernel is applied to the deformation warp in the second step of the Demons algorithm. Setting the number of smoothing iterations to one managed to capture some, but not all, of the remaining non-linear warp.

4.2 Experiments on Real Data

For the next experiment we used 10 subjects (four with repeat sessions) acquired as pilot data for the WU-Minn Human Connectome Project (HCP). The HCP (http://humanconnectome.org) is collecting a large and comprehensive database

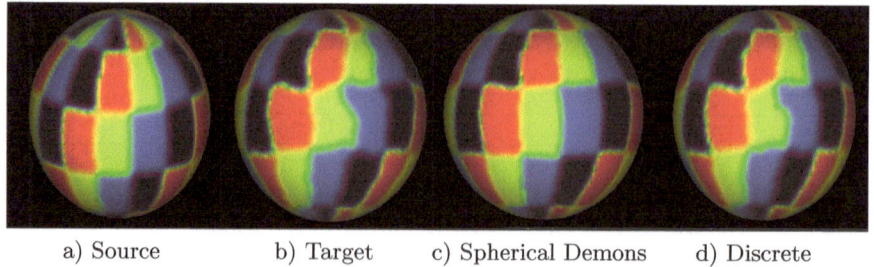

a) Source   b) Target   c) Spherical Demons   d) Discrete

Fig. 2. Simulation. Colours represent scalar values in the range 0-4 with borders showing partial volume values

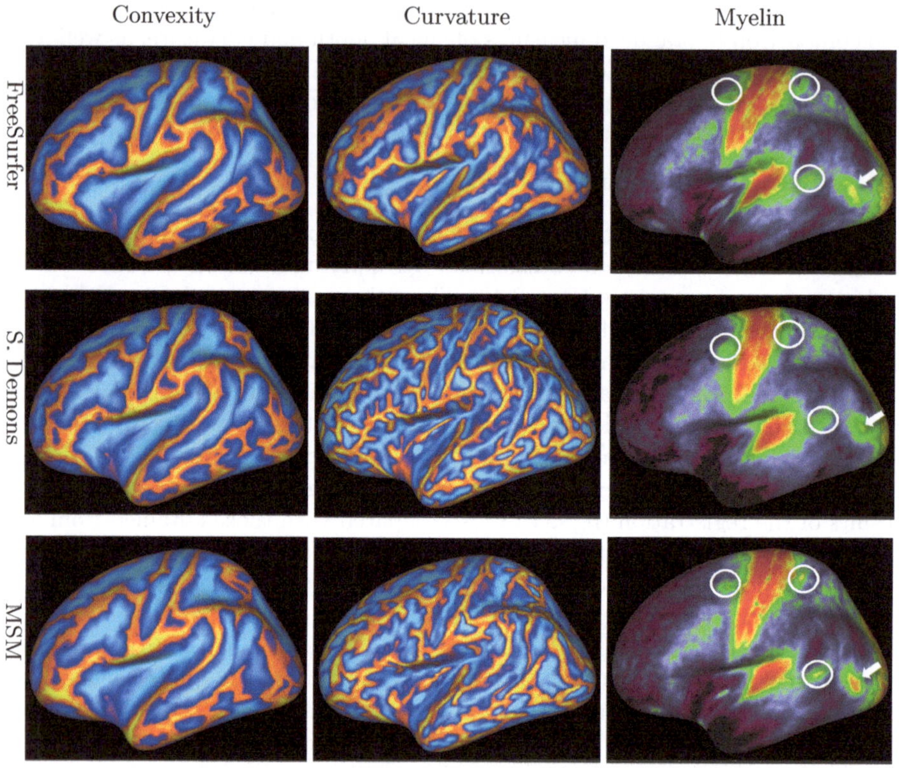

<table>
<tr><td></td><td>Convexity</td><td>Curvature</td><td>Myelin</td></tr>
<tr><td>FreeSurfer</td><td></td><td></td><td></td></tr>
<tr><td>S. Demons</td><td></td><td></td><td></td></tr>
<tr><td>MSM</td><td></td><td></td><td></td></tr>
</table>

Fig. 3. Results of univariate registration. Top row: cross-subject mean atlases generated by convexity-driven FreeSurfer alignment. Centre row: averaged results after driving Spherical Demons using (from left to right) convexity, curvature and myelin data. Bottom row: results of registration using MSM. MSM driven myelin alignment pulls out structures (circled) that are not present after convexity-driven FreeSurfer or myelin-driven Spherical Demons alignment. The MT+ region is much stronger after myelin driven MSM (white arrow).

of neuroimaging data, including high resolution diffusion, task and resting state functional MRI. For each subject MRI scans were obtained over 3 sessions. Pilot data used here includes structural MRI and five task FMRI (tfMRI) scans (working memory, motor, biological motion, language, and social cognition), acquired using multiband acquisition at 2mm isotropic.

The bottom row of Table 1 displays the speed of the different algorithms. Unlike MSM and Spherical Demons, which use multi-resolution control-point grids, FreeSurfer estimates a dense displacement field for every vertex in the high resolution mesh ($\sim$ 160K vertices). Thus it is much slower. FreeSurfer is also limited to registration of sulcal-depth measures as this is seen to be less sensitive to inter-subject variability in folds.

The top row of Fig. 3 shows group-average maps of sulcal depth (yellow = gyral, near the exterior of the brain; blue = buried cortex), curvature (yellow = gyral folds; blue = sulcal fundi), and myelin maps (ratio of T1- and T2-weighted scans) after registration to FreeSurfers fsaverage surface. In contrast to the sulcal depth and curvature maps, which only reflect cortical shape, the myelin maps [19] highlight regions of functional significance, including the primary sensory areas and the motion sensitive area MT+.

Fig. 3 also shows results from univariate registration using Spherical Demons (middle row) and MSM (bottom row; parametrised as for section 4.1) driven by the three different data sets (sulcal depth/curvature/myelin). In each case, registration is initialised by affine alignment of the subjects' native sulcal depth surfaces to the fsaverage template. The results of the non-linear component of the convexity (left column) and curvature (middle column) driven alignment compare well to the FreeSurfer averages. However, myelin-driven MSM produces a much sharper average than can be achieved through sulcal depth-driven FreeSurfer registration, or myelin-driven Spherical Demons alignment.

5   Multimodal Surface Matching

We now test the performance of the algorithm on multivariate data and present results using a novel dataset derived from functional task performance. The

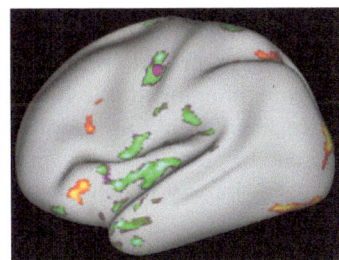
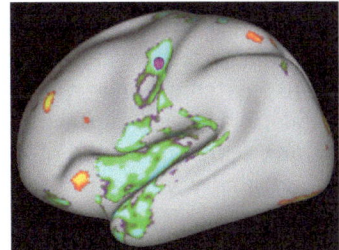

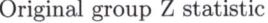

Original group Z statistic   Group Z statistic after MSM

Fig. 4. Group Z statistic images for the working memory task, before and after registration. After MSM, cluster size grows and absolute value of the peak statistic (pink circle) increase from 4.49 to 5.54.

full set of five tasks collected in the pilot HCP protocol was used. tfMRI data were corrected for volumetric image distortions, registered to standard structural space, mapped to the cortical surface, and regularized by surface-constrained smoothing (2mm FWHM). Statistical analysis was performed using the FEAT tool from FSL [18] whereby task time courses were regressed against the vertex-wise time series using a general linear model (GLM). Z statistic images estimated for the parameters of interest of each task (in this instance 37 correlates of mean activity) were concatenated into one feature vector for each vertex. Z values were squared to downweight the contribution of low intensity, noisy variations when estimating of the image similarity.

A registration target was chosen at random from the dataset in the absence of a suitable average target. Registration was initialised using convexity-driven affine alignment and then driven using the task features over 3 resolution levels, again with 5 iterations at each level. At each level the α-entropy measure was estimated using gamma of 1 as recommended in [10]. The k-nearest neighbour graphs were estimated for 10 neighbours at each level and a 10% error in the neighbour calculation was allowed.

Following tfMRI-constrained registration, a group level general linear model (GLM) was used to look for improvements in alignment across the group. Fig. 4 shows good improvements in the size and peak statistics of the clusters for the working memory task after MSM. Fig. 5 shows results for myelin maps (top row) transformed using the warp estimated for the task data. The source myelin map is initially not well aligned to the target myelin map (see white reference contour), but becomes better aligned, especially in occipital cortex (left on the surface), after registration. The transformed tfMRI activation for the social task (Fig. bottom row) is also better aligned in occipital cortex even though this particular tfMRI activation differs markedly between the source and target individuals. Further work will explore the potential for using independent components derived from resting state fMRI analyses.

6   Discussion

The advent of large data collection projects such as the HCP and UK Biobank means that it has never been more important to provide schemes for fast and accurate matching of a wide range of brain imaging data. However, current methods for cortical surface matching are insufficient, as they are limited to matching scalar measures of cortical shape. In this paper we propose a new, fast and highly generalisable surface registration approach based on discrete optimisation.

The use of discrete optimisation offers significant flexibility to choice of similarity measure, and through the fast-PD framework it is possible to incorporate non-metric regularisation penalties. To this end we have proposed a new smoothness penalty for spherical registration based on penalising the geodesic distance between the rotation matrices that define the deformation labels. We find this generates remarkably smooth warps. Nevertheless, regularisation based on first

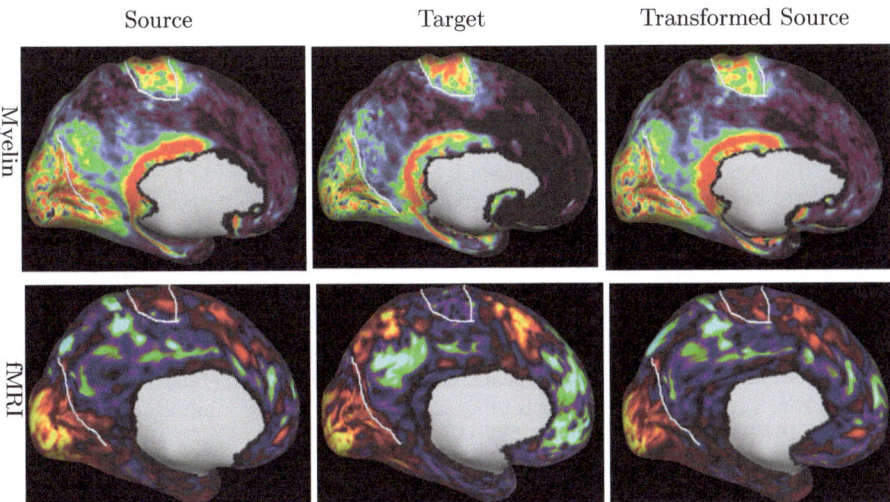

Fig. 5. The results of transforming myelin data using task-driven registration. White dots show the boundaries of structures in the target myelin map. Bottom row: the social task fMRI features before and after registration.

order smoothness penalties, as used here and in [5] are limited as they penalise linear transformations [13]. Therefore future work will explore the potential for higher order smoothness terms as proposed in [13].

To our knowledge this is the first discrete registration method that has used multivariate features. Our preliminary analysis suggests that alignment can be improved using features from a battery of functional tasks, and that it has potential both for increasing the statistical power of functional experiments and improving alignment of other functionally correlated datasets.

Further improvements should be attainable by harnessing complementary information from multiple modalities. Myelin maps have features which are consistent across subjects in regions that are highly variable in cortical folding. In addition, neuronal fibres provide the structure which underpins functional communication. Thus combined estimates of structural (via diffusion tractography) and functional connectivity (via resting-state fMRI) also have significant potential.

References

1. Fischl, B., Sereno, M.I., Tootell, R.B.H., Dale, A.M.: High-resolution intersubject averaging and a coordinate system for the cortical surface. Human Brain Mapping 8(4), 272–284 (1999)
2. Yeo, T., Sabuncu, M., Vercauteren, T., Ayache, N., Fischl, B., Golland, P.: Spherical demons: fast diffeomorphic landmark free surface registration. IEEE Transaction on Medicial Imaging 29(3), 650–668 (2010)

3. Fischl, B., Rajendran, R., Busa, E., Augustinack, J., Hinds, O., Yeo, B.T.T., Mohlberg, H., Amunts, K., Zilles, K.: Cortical folding patterns and predicting cytoarchitecture. Cerebral Cortex 18, 1973–1983 (2008)
4. Petrović, A., Smith, S.M., Menke, R.A., Jenkinson, M.: Methods for tractography-driven surface registration of brain structures. In: Yang, G.-Z., Hawkes, D., Rueckert, D., Noble, A., Taylor, C. (eds.) MICCAI 2009, Part I. LNCS, vol. 5761, pp. 705–712. Springer, Heidelberg (2009)
5. Glocker, B., Komodakis, N., Paragios, N., Navab, N.: Dense image registration through MRFs and efficient linear programming. Medical Image Analysis 12, 731–741 (2008)
6. Rueckert, D., Sonoda, L.I., Hayes, C., Hill, D.L.G., Leach, M.O., Hawkes, D.J.: Nonrigid registration using free-form deformations: Application to breast MR images. IEEE Transaction on Medical Imaging 18(8), 712–721 (1999)
7. Boykov, Y., Veksler, O., Sabik, R.: Fast approximate energy minimization via graph cuts. IEEE PAMI 23(11), 1–17 (2001)
8. Heinrich, M.P., Jenkinson, M., Brady, M., Schnabel, J.A.: Globally optimal deformable registration on a minimum spanning tree using dense displacement sampling. In: Ayache, N., Delingette, H., Golland, P., Mori, K. (eds.) MICCAI 2012, Part III. LNCS, vol. 7512, pp. 115–122. Springer, Heidelberg (2012)
9. Cobzas, D., Sen, A.: Random walks for deformable image registration. In: Fichtinger, G., Martel, A., Peters, T. (eds.) MICCAI 2011, Part II. LNCS, vol. 6892, pp. 557–565. Springer, Heidelberg (2011)
10. Neemuchwala, H.F.: Entropic graphs for image registration. PhD thesis, University of Michigan (2005)
11. Staring, M., van der Heide, U.A., Klein, S., Viergever, M.A., Pluim, J.P.W.: Registration of cervical mri using multifeature mutual information. IEEE Transactions on Medical Imaging 28(9), 1412–1421 (2009)
12. Glocker, B., Komodakis, N., Paragios, N., Navab, N.: Approximated curvature penalty in non-rigid registration using pairwise MRFs. In: Bebis, G., et al. (eds.) ISVC 2009, Part I. LNCS, vol. 5875, pp. 1101–1109. Springer, Heidelberg (2009)
13. Kwon, D., Lee, K.J., Yun, I.D., Lee, S.U.: Nonrigid image registration using dynamic higher-order MRF model. In: Forsyth, D., Torr, P., Zisserman, A. (eds.) ECCV 2008, Part I. LNCS, vol. 5302, pp. 373–386. Springer, Heidelberg (2008)
14. Komodakis, N., Tziritas, G.: Approximate labeling via graph cuts based on linear programming. PAMI 29(8) (2007)
15. Komodakis, N., Tziritas, G.: Performance vs computational efficiency for optimizing single and dynamic MRFs: Setting the state of the art with primal dual strategies. Computer Vision and Image Understanding 112(1), 14–29 (2008)
16. Arya, S., Mount, D., Netanyahu, N., Silverman, R., Wu, A.: An optimal algorithm for approximate nearest neighbor searching fixed dimensions. J. ACM 45(6), 891–923 (1998)
17. Glasser, M.F., Van Essen, D.C.: Mapping human cortical areas in vivo based on myelin content as revealed by T1- and T2-weighted MRI. J. Neuroscience 31(32), 11597–11616 (2011)
18. Jenkinson, M., Beckmann, C.F., Behrens, T.E., Woolrich, M.W., Smith, S.M.: FSL. NeuroImage 62(2), 782–790 (2012)

Globally Optimal Cortical Surface Matching with Exact Landmark Correspondence

Alex Tsui[1,3], Devin Fenton[2,3], Phong Vuong[1,3], Joel Hass[2], Patrice Koehl[1],
Nina Amenta[1], David Coeurjolly[4], Charles DeCarli[3], and Owen Carmichael[1,3]

[1] Computer Science Department, University of California, Davis, USA
[2] Mathematics Department, University of California, Davis, USA
[3] Neurology Department, University of California, Davis, USA
[4] LIRIS, Université de Lyon, CNRS, France

Abstract. We present a method for establishing correspondences between human cortical surfaces that exactly matches the positions of given point landmarks, while attaining the global minimum of an objective function that quantifies how far the mapping deviates from conformality. On each surface, a conformal transformation is applied to the Euclidean distance metric, resulting in a hyperbolic metric with isolated *cone point* singularities at the landmarks. Equivalently, each surface is mapped to a hyperbolic *orbifold*: a pillow-like surface with each point landmark corresponding to a pillow corner. An initial surface-to-surface mapping exactly aligns the landmarks, and gradient descent is used to find the single, global minimum of the Dirichlet energy of the remainder of the mapping. Using a population of real MRI-based cortical surfaces with manually labeled sulcus endpoints as landmarks, we evaluate the approach by how much it distorts surfaces and by its biological plausibility: how well it aligns previously-unseen anatomical landmarks and by how well it promotes expected associations between cortical thickness and age. We show that, compared to a painstakingly-tuned approach that balances a tradeoff between minimizing landmark mismatch and Dirichlet energy, our method has similar biological plausibility, superior surface distortion, a better theoretical foundation, and fewer arbitrary parameters to tune. We also compare to conformal mapper in the spherical domain to show that sacrificing exact conformality of the mapping does not cause noticeable reductions in biological plausibility.

1 Introduction

Cortical surface matching– establishing point-wise correspondences between cerebral cortex surfaces– is a crucial step in MRI-based studies of brain morphology. Algorithms typically aim to induce a surface-to-surface mapping that minimally distorts morphological features. It is also desirable to use information provided by experts to guide the mapping. This information can consist of landmarks, labeled as points or curves on the surfaces, that are required to correspond to each other. Our goal is a cortical surface matching method that exactly matches point landmarks while insuring that the mapping minimizes distortion.

J.C. Gee et al. (Eds.): IPMI 2013, LNCS 7917, pp. 487–498, 2013.
© Springer-Verlag Berlin Heidelberg 2013

We quantify surface distortion in terms of *conformality*, or angle preservation. Conformal maps have been studied intensely due to their ability to preserve key shape properties of biological specimens [9], and because conformal maps from any genus-zero surface to the sphere, and from any higher-genus surface to a surface of constant curvature, provably exist regardless of surface morphology [2] [21]. However, point landmarks are difficult to incorporate into conformal maps. A conformal map to the sphere, for example, is uniquely determined by the mapping of exactly three surface points; matching more than three requires sacrificing either conformality or exact landmark matching. For this reason, we seek maps that minimally deviate from conformality, using the Dirichlet energy of the mapping to quantify this deviation. Specifically, we conformally map each cortical surface to a hyperbolic orbifold, and find Dirichlet energy minimizing maps between the orbifolds that exactly align an arbitrary number of point landmarks. We show that the Dirichlet energy has exactly one, unique, global minimum over the relevant set of orbifold-to-orbifold maps, making it computationally robust.

Our approach is summarized in Figure 1. Given two triangulated cortical surfaces, we first alter the distance metrics on the two surfaces using conformal transformations [19]. This results in hyperbolic metrics on both surfaces with singularities at a finite number of isolated cone points, near which the metric behaves as though the surface is shaped locally like the vertex of a cone. One such cone point is located at each of the point landmarks. We then calculate an initial mapping from one surface to the other that exactly aligns the corresponding point landmarks. There is exactly one deformation of the initial map that maintains these point landmark matches while obtaining a minimum of the Dirichlet energy among the set of maps reachable by continuous deformation, *i.e.* within the homotopy class of the initial map. Given the uniminimal nature of the Dirichlet energy landscape, finding the energy minimizing mapping within the homotopy class is straightforward using gradient descent.

Using brains from a large epidemiological study [4] with manual point landmarks, we assessed whether exact landmark matching (versus approximate *e.g.*, [15]) results in greater surface distortion, and less utility in practical situations, that counterbalance the theoretical advantage of guaranteed globally-optimal mapping. We also assessed whether abandoning truly conformal mapping for Dirichlet energy minimizing mapping results in noteworthy practical disadvantages. To do this we compared our method (`OrbifoldExact`) to two competing methods that minimized landmark mismatch in a least-squares sense. An *orbifold least squares* method (`OrbifoldLS`), inspired by earlier work [15], balanced a tradeoff between Dirichlet energy minimization and landmark mismatch in a least squares sense. A *conformal least squares* method (`ConformalLS`) found the conformal map in the spherical domain that minimized landmark mismatch [15]. We compared the methods in terms of point landmark mismatch, surface distortion, mismatch of novel (*i.e.,* not used to define the mapping) point landmarks, and ability to re-capitulate known population-level associations between cortical thickness and age [16]. Finally, we assessed whether the behavior of `OrbifoldLS` is stable with respect to critical but difficult-to-set operating parameters.

2   Prior Work

Prior landmark-based cortical surface matching methods begin by finding harmonic energy minimizing mappings to spherical [15] or Euclidean [1] canonical domains as an initial step, or finding initial conformal maps to canonical Euclidean annuli [24] or hyperbolic "pairs of pants" [23]. One such canonical domain is then mapped onto the other in a way that encourages landmark matching. Using a Mobius transformation for this mapping [15] insures conformality but it is restricted to either exactly match only 3 points, or inexactly match a larger number. Harmonic maps are more flexible, but guarantee neither conformality nor exact landmark matching [1]. Quasi-conformal maps have bounded angle distortion, but the practical utility of recent implementations is not clear [25]. Methods that cut the brain surface and map the cut to the boundary of a canonical domain have the additional limitation that conformality is lost along the cut [24], and there is an arbitrary decision about how exactly to map out the cut to the boundary. Note that while we specify paths between point landmarks that are similar to cuts, these instead constitute a *marking*, i.e. a landmark ordering convention that insures that the eventual mapping comes from a natural homotopy class, i.e. that the mapping can be connected to the desired optimal mapping by some deformation.

Building on earlier work on mapping cortical surfaces to the hyperbolic disc for visualization [9], we leverage an earlier observation that there is a single globally optimal map between hyperbolic discs that minimizes the Dirichlet energy [12], and model the landmarks as cone points in the hyperbolic metric to insure exact matching. Such cone point singularities have been considered previously to reduce area and length distortions during flattening to the plane, for applications such as texture mapping [22]. Other discrete conformal mapping methods [10] [19] incorporate cone point singularities into their conformal transformation of the surface distance metric without cutting.

3   Method

We begin with a pair of triangulated surfaces whose topology is spherical; in our experiments, each of these is the outer pial surface of a human cerebral cortex hemisphere output by commonly available software. Each surface has been annotated by an expert with a set of k point landmarks that are known to be in correspondence across surfaces. There are four key steps to our approach. The first, **orbifold mapping**, calculates conformally equivalent hyperbolic metrics on the surfaces, or equivalently, conformally maps the surface to a k pointed orbifold such that landmark points map to its cone points. Next, **marking** allows us to constrain the surface-to-surface mapping to a natual homotopy class of mappings: those that preclude reflections, complex surface folding, twisting, etc, in between exact point matches. For this step we define a tree that connects the landmark points analogously across surfaces. An **initial mapping** is constructed that maps the first tree to the second one, and extends that mapping continuously across the rest of the surfaces; this mapping belongs to the natural homotopy class. Finally, **energy minimization** is used to adjust this mapping so that it arrives at the unique Dirichlet energy minimizing map within this homotopy class that leaves the landmark matches fixed.

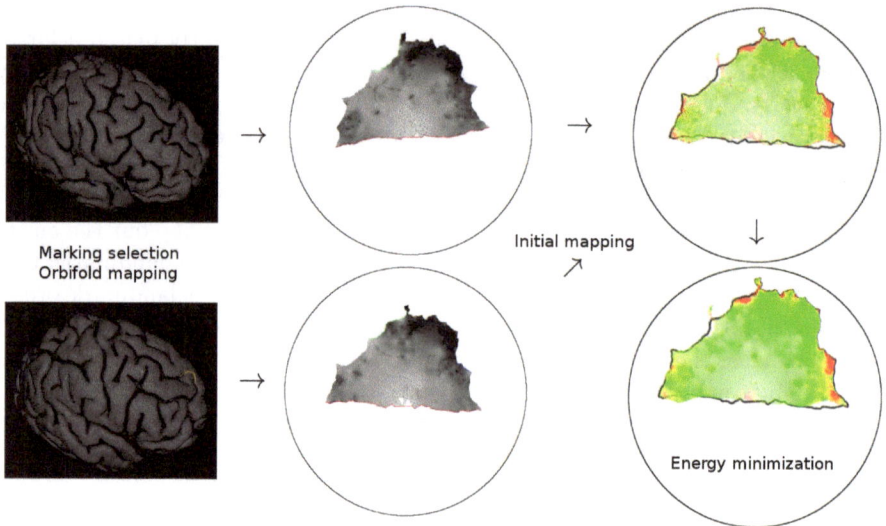

Fig. 1. Overview of surface-to-surface mapping algorithm. Given two brain hemisphere surfaces (left), orbifold mapping constructs hyperbolic metrics on each surface. Then, marking selection identifies a natural homotopy class of mappings to optimize over. These steps allow us to map the surfaces to the hyperbolic plane (middle: sulci shown as colored boundary curves). Next, an initial curface-to-surface mapping is constructed in the hyperbolic plane (top right). This mapping introduces surface distortions in the form of dilatations (redder colors suggest greater distortion). Dirichlet energy minimization in hyperbolic space adjusts the mapping to obtain the global minimum of such distortions over the homotopy class (bottom right).

3.1   Orbifold Mapping

We use a conformal factors-based method [3] to calculate a conformal transformation of the surface distance metric. Briefly, a surface triangulation T is a set of vertices V, edges E, and faces F, and a discrete metric $l : V \to \mathbb{R}$ assigns lengths to each edge such that the triangle inequality at each face is satisfied. Two combinatorially equivalent triangulations, one with a Euclidean metric l and the other with hyperbolic metric $\tilde{l}$, are discretely conformally equivalent if their respective metrics l and $\tilde{l}$ are related by

$$\sinh \frac{\tilde{l}_{ij}}{2} = e^{\frac{1}{2}(u_i + u_j)} l_{ij} \tag{1}$$

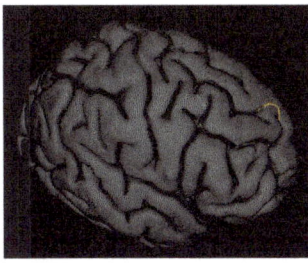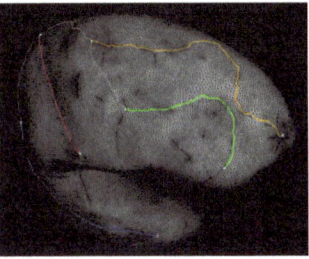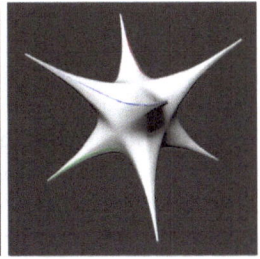

Fig. 2. Identifying a cortical surface (left) with a hyperbolic orbifold (right). Landmark points (white dots) are selected and connected by a set of paths to form a marking tree (colored curves, shown on an inflated cortical mesh, center). The point-to-point distance metric on the mesh can be conformally transformed into a hyperbolic metric by imposing an angle constraint at each landmark point, effectively identifying the brain with the hyperbolic orbifold.

where $u : V \to \mathbb{R}$ is an assignment of conformal factors to each vertex. This is an equivalence relation, and the set of discrete metrics in the same equivalence class is called a discrete conformal class. In this way, the conformal factors u define a conformal transformation of the Euclidean metric into a hyperbolic one.

Starting with a triangulation and the Euclidean metric (T, l), we seek a discretely conformally equivalent triangulation with hyperbolic metric, such that the metric treats the k provided landmark points as cone points. One way to formulate this requirement is to consider the angle sum of vertex $v_i \in V$: this is the sum, over all mesh triangles that include v_i, of angles with v_i as the vertex. An angle sum of 2π means that the surface is locally flat at v_i, while angle sums less than 2π mean that the surface in the neighborhood of v_i more resembles the vertex of a cone. As described previously [3], we solve for conformal factors u such that the above equation is satisfied and each vertex is constrained to have a certain angle sum: for all point landmarks, the required sum is π to treat them as cone points; for all other points, the required sum is 2π to treat them as locally flat. For a genus zero surface to have a hyperbolic orbifold metric with cone point singularities, the sum of the angle defects (2π - angle sum) across all vertices must be greater than 4π. With an angle sum of π at the cone points and 2π everywhere else, this means we must have at least five cone points to insure that the resulting metric is hyperbolic. We use a trust region Newton's method [13] to minimize an energy function [3] to compute the conformal factors.

3.2 Marking Selection

Once the hyperbolic metric is defined on both surfaces, we impose an ordering on the set of landmarks that constrains the surface-to-surface mapping to be simple and well-behaved, *i.e.* to map corresponding points onto each other exactly while inducing no gross foldings or twists to the rest of the mapping. To do so, we first draw vertex-constrained paths that connect one sulcal endpoint to the opposite endpoint. We then insert additional paths connecting endpoints across sulci until all endpoints are connected in a tree, called the *marking tree* (see Figure 2 middle). Note that paths must not intersect with themselves or other paths, but otherwise any tree of paths will suffice.

The purpose of the marking tree is to specify the homotopy class of the mapping ie. it allows us to specify an initial mapping such that one tree is mapped onto the other in a natural way, and the tree-to-tree mapping is extrapolated continuously over the rest of the surfaces. Optimization is then constrained such that the mapping remains within the same homotopy class. Thus, this step effectively allows us to rule out unnatural mappings. Together with the fact that under hyperbolic space, there exists a unique harmonic map that minimizes Dirichlet energy in each homotopy class, the mapping can be refined to obtain the globally unique map in the sense of minimum Dirichlet energy.

3.3   Initial Mapping

Because there is a single, unique global minimum for Dirichlet energy within each homotopy class, the initial mapping that is optimized to minimize Dirichlet energy is arbitrary– the only requirement is that it belong to the homotopy class of mappings that map one surface onto the other in a simple, reasonable way (*i.e.*, with no complex folding or twisting of the surface in between landmarks). We parameterize this initial mapping in the Euclidean disc to make use of existing computational methods [12] that insure the mapping is in the correct homotopy class, but we note that the optimization itself is governed by the hyperbolic metric induced upon the surface as described above. The initial mapping is constructed by assigning each edge of the marking tree to a side of a regular polygon in the Euclidean disc and filling in the remainder of the mapping by minimizing harmonic energy. One such parameterization is performed for each surface; the overlay of the two Euclidean polygons provides the initial surface-to-surface mapping. The corners of the polygon are identified with the landmark points in the order that they appear in a traversal of the marking tree, and thus one marking tree maps to the other in a simple way while filling in the remainder of the mapping in a smooth, reasonable manner. We emphasize that while this approach effectively cuts the spherical-topology surface open along the marking tree, resulting in a topological disc in 3D that is then flattened into a disc contained in the plane as in prior work [12], this is solely for the purpose of establishing an approximate initial mapping that is then optimized based on the hyperbolic metrics described above; the optimized mapping does not contain discontinuities or other distorting artifacts along the marking tree edges. We also emphasize that this initial mapping is arbitrary: other methods may be applied without impact to the optimality of the final mapping.

3.4   Energy Minimization

Suppose one surface contains edges e_{ij} that connect vertices v_i to v_j, w_{ij} are the cotangent weights $w_{ij} = 0.5(\cot \alpha + \cot \beta)$, where α and β are the two angles opposite the edge e_{ij}, and the other surface lies in the hyperbolic plane. The initial mapping f maps the points of this surface onto the other surface such that point landmarks are kept in correspondence. The Dirichlet energy of f under the hyperbolic metric can be approximated as follows:

$$E(f) = \frac{1}{2} \sum_{e_{ij}} w_{ij}(f(v_j) - f(v_i))^2 \tag{2}$$

Given hyperbolic orbifold structures defined on each surface and an initial map between them, the theorems of Eells and Sampson [5] and of Hartman [8] imply that there is a unique harmonic map that minimizes Dirichlet energy in the homotopy class of maps that can be realized by deforming the original map.

To compute the Dirichlet energy minimizing map, we re-parameterize the the initial 2D polygon-to-polygon mapping in the Euclidean disc to the hyperbolic disc (specifically the Poincare disc). We use steepest descent to minimize the Dirichlet energy: this amounts to adjusting surface vertex positions in the Poincare disc but constraining the vertices corresponding to landmark points to stay fixed and in correspondence. To overcome numerical issues, we follow a prior approach by [12] optimizing the mapping of each surface vertex one at a time: this point and its surrounding one-ring of mesh faces (its local "chart") is translated to the Poincare disc origin, where the hyperbolic metric is well approximated by a corresponding Euclidean metric. The position of that point is then adjusted to minimize the Dirichlet energy and translated back to its original position. See [20] for implementation of local charts.

4   Experiments

4.1   Data

We obtained brain MRI of 50 healthy elderly subjects from a prior study [4], identified gray matter voxels [6], used BrainVisa to convert each hemisphere's cortical gray matter mask into matching inner and outer pial surface meshes [14], from which we removed small or slivery mesh triangles [7]. Cortical thickness was estimated at each outer pial surface vertex using a "normal-average" approach [11]. A set of 16 sulcal endpoints were annotated on each outer pial hemisphere by an expert rater using a validated protocol [18].

4.2   Competing Methods

Experiments compared the method described above, termed `OrbifoldExact`, to two competing methods that strike a different balance between landmark matching and surface distortion. One competitor, `OrbifoldLS`, is identical to `OrbifoldExact` except that point landmarks are not constrained to be fixed during energy minimization, and the energy function balances a tradeoff between landmark mismatch and Dirichlet energy:

$$E(f) = (1 - \lambda)\frac{1}{2}\sum_{e_{ij}} w_{ij}(f(v_j) - f(v_i))^2 + \lambda \sum_{v_i \in L_1}(f(v_i) - L_2(v_i))^2 \quad (3)$$

where L_1 is the set of landmark points on the source surface and $L_2(v_i)$ is the landmark point on the target surface corresponding to landmark point v_i on the source surface.

The other competitor, ConformalLS, first conformally maps each triangular mesh onto the unit sphere [19], then solves for a Möbius transformation (*i.e.*, a conformal mapping of the first sphere to the second one) that minimizes point landmark mismatch in the same least squares sense as in OrbifoldLS.

4.3   Performance Measures

Surface Distortion. OrbifoldLS and OrbifoldExact, are able to induce surface distortions in the form of *dilatations*– stretches that transform local circles to local ellipses under the mapping– while ConformalLS precludes such dilatations by construction. For the former, we compute a discrete approximation of dilatation [17] at every mesh triangle and report summaries of dilatation over all vertices. We also show brain surfaces color-coded by dilatation under various mappings.

Landmark Mismatch. OrbifoldLS and ConformalLS allow imperfect matching of point landmarks, while OrbifoldExact requires exact landmark matches by construction. We report the mean Euclidean distance between corresponding landmark points under the mapping for the former two approaches.

Strength of Expected Associations. We selected one of the 50 left outer pial surfaces as a canonical brain surface and used each of the three techniques to map the remaining 49 surfaces onto it. The mappings allowed us to transfer cortical thicknesses from the 49 surfaces onto the canonical one, and interpolate the thicknesses to the positions of canonical mesh points. This resulted in 50 cortical thicknesses (one per subject) at each canonical mesh point. We calculated a linear regression model at each mesh point to assess the strength of association between that point's local cortical thickness and the age of the corresponding subjects. The p values for these regressions were corrected for multiple comparisons [26], and the p values at the vertices were interpolated across intervening mesh faces. The surface area that had $p < .05$ was then calculated. Numerous studies (*e.g.*, [16]), agree that the thickness of the cortical mantle reduce with age, so we seek mapping methods that give rise to a statistically significant relationship with age across the largest possible cortical area.

4.4   Experimental Settings

Comparison of 3 Methods. Given 16 point landmarks on a hemisphere surface, we consider two experimental settings. In the first, we use the full set of landmarks to define the mappings, and evaluate surface distortion, landmark mismatch, and strength of expected associations on appropriate methods. In the second, we cross-validate: we use 14 of the 16 landmarks to define the mapping and evaluate landmark mismatch for the remaining two.

Practical Limitations of OrbifoldLS. OrbifoldLS includes two operating parameters that are difficult for a user to know how to set optimally: the marking tree and λ. We assessed whether settings of these parameters impact landmark mismatch and surface distortion by running OrbifoldLS over a range of settings for both and assessing variability in both performance characteristics.

5 Results

Landmark mismatch for OrbifoldLS and ConformalLS is in Table 1. Mismatch is substantial for each method, averaging greater than 5 mm for most sulci (note that mean mesh edge length is 0.55 mm). This motivates exact landmark matching as in our method: the mapping problem is difficult enough that least squares methods do not readily find a solution that matches landmarks closely. Dilatation for OrbifoldLS and OrbifoldExact are in Table 2, and anecdotal dilatation maps are in Figure 3. As expected, OrbifoldExact gives rise to dramatic maximum dilatations, which occur at the isolated point landmarks where the orbifold construction has dramatically changed the surface distance metric. But large dilatations do not broadly affect large surface regions (see Figure 3 and mean dilatations in Table 2), suggesting that requiring exact landmark matches does not preclude broadly well-behaved mappings.

Table 1. Average landmark mismatches, in mm, for sulcal endpoints across 50 subjects. Note that landmark mismatch for OrbifoldExact is zero by construction.

Sulcus	ConformalLS	OrbifoldLS, $\lambda = 0.1$	OrbifoldLS, $\lambda = 0.5$
Central	19.95	7.62	6.29
Precentral	20.01	7.80	6.33
Postcentral	21.42	9.56	7.40
Cingulate	26.61	7.16	6.11
Intraparietal	25.54	8.66	7.25
Superior Temporal	29.40	8.16	6.46
Superior Frontal	24.12	6.45	5.28
Inferior Frontal	24.31	5.90	4.90

Table 3 shows landmark mismatch for the left-out landmark in cross-validation. OrbifoldLS conferred no notable benefit over OrbifoldExact, again suggesting that requiring exact landmark matches draws no appreciable cost in terms of practical performance. ConformalLS provides superior matching of the left-out point for approximately half of the landmarks, but matching is similar to OrbifoldExact

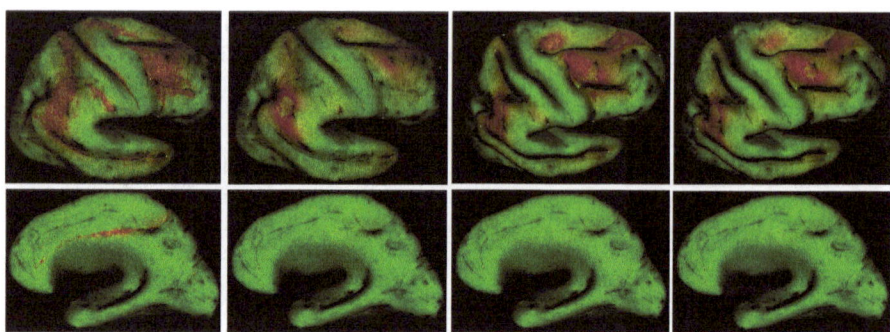

Fig. 3. Mesh face dilations for one example pair of surfaces (greener/redder indicates lesser/greater dilatation). Recall that dilatation is exactly one for `ConformalLS`. Left to right, columns show dilatation of the initial mapping, `OrbifoldExact`, `OrbifoldLS` with $\lambda = 0.5$, and `OrbifoldLS` with $\lambda = 0.1$. White dots indicate landmark points.

Table 2. Left: Mean, median, and maximum distortion from conformality (dilatation) across all mesh faces on all 50 surfaces, for three competing methods. Note that dilatation of 1 is realized in an isometry and by construction is 1 everywhere for `ConformalLS`. **Right:** Total area (mm^2) of cortex showing statistically significant evidence of a linear relationship with cortical thickness.

Method	Mean	Median	Max
`OrbifoldExact`	1.489	1.300	2089
`OrbifoldLS`, $\lambda = 0.1$	1.452	1.283	320
`OrbifoldLS`, $\lambda = 0.5$	1.503	1.288	732

Method	Age
`ConformalLS`	450.0
`OrbifoldExact`	3885.8
`OrbifoldLS`, $\lambda = 0.1$	4020.8

or worse for the other half. This suggests that `ConformalLS` offers no obvious performance advantage over `OrbifoldLS` in terms of matching previously-unseen landmarks, and the landmarks used to define the mapping again exhibit substantial mismatch.

Table 2 summarizes the cortical surface area significantly associated with age. `OrbifoldExact` and `OrbifoldLS` are highly similar in this regard, while `ConformalLS` lags far behind. This suggests that `OrbifoldLS` and `ConformalLS` holds no obvious practical advantage in terms of relevant applications that might compensate for their other theoretical or computational limitations.

Variability in landmark mismatch for `OrbifoldLS` is shown in Table 4. Landmark matching varies with respect to marking tree and λ, although users cannot know *a priori* what setting is favorable. So while matching of `OrbifoldLS` and `OrbifoldExact` are similar, variability due to arbitrary parameter settings reduces the robustness of `OrbifoldLS`. Indeed, this demonstrates the difficulty in least squares approaches as optimizing an energy function with local minima is subject to initial conditions.

In conclusion, our method provides a surface-to-surface mapping that exactly matches point landmarks and arrives at the global minimum of a particular

Table 3. Mean sulcal endpoint deviations in mm of the left-out sulcus using a map created by applying the given method. Numbers in parentheses indicate the landmark deviation (mm) averaged over the remaining seven sulci.

Sulcus	ConformalLS	OrbifoldLS, $\lambda = 0.1$	OrbifoldLS, $\lambda = 0.5$	OrbifoldExact
Central	12.49 (20.90)	25.59 (7.22)	25.61 (6.53)	25.18
Cingulate	28.96 (21.23)	26.65 (6.93)	26.65 (6.27)	25.20
Inferior Frontal	24.31 (21.11)	24.57 (6.87)	24.56 (6.03)	22.82
Intraparietal	30.44 (21.21)	31.37 (7.08)	31.35 (6.18)	30.39
Postcentral	21.62 (20.28)	28.92 (7.01)	28.92 (6.20)	30.93
Precentral	17.04 (21.05)	25.84 (6.83)	25.85 (6.01)	26.12
Superior Frontal	23.86 (20.77)	36.75 (5.79)	35.89 (4.95)	35.90
Superior Temporal	39.57 (23.52)	33.84 (7.69)	33.85 (6.81)	31.16

Table 4. Mean landmark deviations with respect to marking tree and λ. Experiment was conducted with eight point landmarks. We set $\lambda = 0.1$ when varying the marking tree, and we fix marking tree A when varying λ. Tree A is the same as shown in Figure 2. Trees B and C connect the landmarks instead in a single path.

Marking tree	Deviation (mm)	λ	Deviation (mm)
A	2.05	0.1	2.05
B	0.23	0.5	0.24
C	0.53	0.8	0.027

surface distortion energy. Experiments suggest that neither requiring exact landmark matches, nor failing to require conformality, reduce the practical performance of the method, suggesting usefulness in practice.

Acknowledgements. This work was supported by NSF grant IIS-1117663 and NIH grants AG010129, AG030514.

References

1. Auzias, G., Lefèvre, J., Le Troter, A., Fischer, C., Perrot, M., Régis, J., Coulon, O.: Model-driven harmonic parameterization of the cortical surface. In: Fichtinger, G., Martel, A., Peters, T. (eds.) MICCAI 2011, Part II. LNCS, vol. 6892, pp. 310–317. Springer, Heidelberg (2011)
2. Bers, L.: Uniformization, moduli, and kleinian groups. Bull. London Math. Soc. 4, 257–300 (1972)
3. Bobenko, A., Pinkall, U., Springborn, B.: Discrete conformal maps and ideal hyperbolic polyhedra, pp. 1–49 (2010)
4. Debette, S., Beiser, A., DeCarli, C., Au, R., Himali, J.J., Kelly-Hayes, M., Romero, J.R., Kase, C.S., Wolf, P.A., Seshadri, S.: Association of MRI markers of vascular brain injury with incident stroke, mild cognitive impairment, dementia, and mortality the framingham offspring study. Stroke 41(4), 600–606 (2010)
5. Eells, J., Sampson, J.H.: Harmonic mappings of riemannian manifolds. American Journal of Mathematics 86, 109–160 (1964)
6. Fletcher, E., Singh, B., Harvey, D., Carmichael, O., DeCarli, C.: Adaptive image segmentation for robust measurement of longitudinal brain tissue change. In: EMBC, pp. 5319–5322. IEEE (2012)

7. Fuhrmann, S., Ackermann, J., Kalbe, T., Goesele, M.: Direct Resampling for Isotropic Surface Remeshing. In: VMV, pp. 9–16 (2010)
8. Hartman, P.: On homotopic harmonic maps. Canadian Journal of Mathematics 19, 673–687 (1967)
9. Hurdal, M.K., Stephenson, K.: Discrete conformal methods for cortical brain flattening. NeuroImage 45, S86–S98 (2009)
10. Kharevych, L., Springborn, B., Schröder, P.: Discrete conformal mappings via circle patterns. ACM Trans. Graph. 25, 412–438 (2006)
11. Kochunov, P., Rogers, W., Mangin, J.-F., Lancaster, J.: A library of cortical morphology analysis tools to study development, aging and genetics of cerebral cortex. Neuroinformatics 10, 81–96 (2012)
12. Li, X., Bao, Y., Guo, X., Jin, M., Gu, X., Qin, H.: Globally optimal surface mapping for surfaces with arbitrary topology. IEEE Trans. Vis. Comput. Graphics 14, 805–819 (2008)
13. Lin, C., Moré, J.: Newton's method for large bound-constrained optimization problems. SIAM Journal on Optimization 9, 1100–1127 (1999)
14. Mangin, J.F., Frouin, V., Bloch, I., Régis, J., López-Krahe, J.: From 3d magnetic resonance images to structural representations of the cortex topography using topology preserving deformations. Journal of Mathematical Imaging and Vision 5(4), 297–318 (1995)
15. Ming, L., Wang, Y., Chan, T.F., Thompson, P.: Landmark constrained genus zero surface conformal mapping and its application to brain mapping research. Appl. Numer. Math. 57, 847–858 (2007)
16. Salat, D.H., Buckner, R.L., Snyder, A.Z., Greve, D.N., Desikan, R.S.R., Busa, E., Morris, J.C., Dale, A.M., Fischl, B.: Thinning of the cerebral cortex in aging. Cerebral Cortex 14(7), 721–730 (2004)
17. Sander, P.V., Snyder, J., Gortler, S.J., Hoppe, H.: Texture mapping progressive meshes. In: SIGGRAPH, pp. 409–416 (2001)
18. Sowell, E.R., Thompson, P.M., Rex, D., Kornsand, D., Tessner, K.D., Jernigan, T.L., Toga, A.W.: Mapping sulcal pattern asymmetry and local cortical surface gray matter distribution in vivo: maturation in perisylvian cortices. Cerebral Cortex 12, 17–26 (2002)
19. Springborn, B., Schröder, P., Pinkall, U.: Conformal equivalence of triangle meshes. ACM Trans. Graph. 27, 1–11 (2008)
20. Surazhsky, V., Gotsman, C.: Explicit surface remeshing. In: SGP, pp. 20–30 (2003)
21. Thurston, W.P.: Three dimensional manifolds, kleinian groups and hyperbolic geometry. Bull. Amer. Math. Soc. 6, 357–382 (1982)
22. Tong, Y., Alliez, P., Cohen-Steiner, D., Desbrun, M.: Designing quadrangulations with discrete harmonic forms. In: SGP, pp. 201–210 (2006)
23. Wang, Y., Dai, W., Chou, Y.-Y., Gu, X., Chan, T.F., Toga, A.W., Thompson, P.M.: Studying brain morphometry using conformal equivalence class. In: ICCV, pp. 2365–2372 (2009)
24. Wang, Y., Gu, X., Chan, T.F., Thompson, P.M., Yau, S.-T.: Conformal slit mapping and its applications to brain surface parameterization. In: Metaxas, D., Axel, L., Fichtinger, G., Székely, G. (eds.) MICCAI 2008, Part I. LNCS, vol. 5241, pp. 585–593. Springer, Heidelberg (2008)
25. Weber, O., Myles, A., Zorin, D.: Computing extremal quasiconformal maps. Computer Graphics Forum 31, 1679–1689 (2012)
26. Worsley, K.J., Marrett, S., Neelin, P., Vandal, A.C., Friston, K.J., Evans, A.C., et al.: A unified statistical approach for determining significant signals in images of cerebral activation. Human Brain Mapping 4(1), 58–73 (1996)

Joint Learning of Appearance and Transformation for Predicting Brain MR Image Registration

Qian Wang[1,2], Minjeong Kim[1], Guorong Wu[1], and Dinggang Shen[1]

[1] Department of Radiology and BRIC, [2] Department of Computer Science
University of North Carolina at Chapel Hill, US
qianwang@cs.unc.edu, {mjkim,grwu,dgshen}@med.unc.edu

Abstract. We propose a new approach to register the subject image with the template by leveraging a set of training images that are pre-aligned to the template. We argue that, if voxels in the subject and the training images share similar local appearances and transformations, they may have common correspondence in the template. In this way, we learn the sparse representation of certain subject voxel to reveal several similar candidate voxels in the training images. Each selected training candidate can bridge the correspondence from the subject voxel to the template space, thus predicting the transformation associated with the subject voxel at the confidence level that relates to the learned sparse coefficient. Following this strategy, we first *predict* transformations at selected key points, and retain multiple predictions on each key point (instead of allowing a single correspondence only). Then, by utilizing all key points and their predictions with varying confidences, we adaptively *reconstruct* the dense transformation field that warps the subject to the template. For robustness and computation speed, we embed the *prediction-reconstruction* protocol above into a multi-resolution hierarchy. In the final, we efficiently refine our estimated transformation field via existing registration method. We apply our method to registering brain MR images, and conclude that the proposed method is competent to improve registration performances in terms of time cost as well as accuracy.

1 Introduction

Image registration has been intensively investigated and widely applied in medical image analysis during past decades. By normalizing individual images into the same space, researchers are able to conduct population-based analysis. A typical setting in processing brain MR images, for instance, often involves selecting template and then aligns each subject image to the template via pairwise registration. After registering all subject images, qualitative and quantitative analyses can be performed in the template space, e.g., to infer the population atlas or to measure group difference.

Pairwise registration between individual subject and the template is usually formulated as an optimization problem [1], with the objective function evaluating both the subject-template *similarity* and the *smoothness* of the non-rigid transformation field. However, this straightforward optimization scheme may suffer when applied to subject images that have significant anatomical differences to the template. Further, the independent registration can hardly take advantages of intrinsic similarity of subject

J.C. Gee et al. (Eds.): IPMI 2013, LNCS 7917, pp. 499–510, 2013.

images, although similar subjects share similar transformations to the template and can potentially help each other in registration.

In fact, performances of image registration can be greatly improved if information from other images in the population is well incorporated. For example, recent studies show very promising alignment of images in the groupwise manner [2]. Although it is difficult to directly warp a significantly different subject to the template in pairwise registration, the problem could become much easier when using other intermediate images as bridges [3-5]. That is, the input subject can deform first towards its nearby intermediate image, and then towards the template by borrowing the already established pathway from the intermediate to the template.

We here propose a novel approach to predict the transformation between a new *subject* image and the *template* by leveraging a set of images that are pre-registered with the template. Specifically, the prediction is achieved by joint learning of patch-based image appearances and transformations, which significantly differs from existing methods. For clarity, we term the images to help estimate the subject-template transformation as *training* images, and denote the transformation in the Lagrangian framework. In particular, we aim to estimate the field $\phi(\cdot)$ that warps the subject (as well as any training image) to the template. That is, for the grid point x in the template, $\phi(x)$ maps it to the subject space. Reversely, $\phi^{-1}(\cdot)$ projects from subject to template. The template voxel x and the subject voxel $\phi(x)$ are regarded as *correspondences* to each other.

The transformation associated with certain subject voxel can be predicted by proper candidate voxels in the training images, if they are correspondences. Fig. 1(a) shows an intuitive example, where voxels from the template, a training image, and the subject are enumerated in red boxes, respectively. For y in the training image, we locate its template correspondence at $x = \phi_{tr}^{-1}(y)$. Further, supposing $\hat{x}$ in the subject to be the correspondence of y (i.e., with similar local appearances in red circles), $\hat{x}$ should locate its template correspondence at $x = \phi_s^{-1}(\hat{x})$ as well. The established correspondence between the template voxel x and the subject voxel $\hat{x}$, bridged by the training voxel y, implies that $\phi_s^{-1}(\hat{x})$ can be predicted by the training field $\phi_{tr}^{-1}(y)$.

We will develop the **Prediction-Reconstruction** (P-R) protocol to directly estimate $\phi_s(\cdot)$ instead of its inverse $\phi_s^{-1}(\cdot)$, and further apply it to registering brain MR images. For given subject voxel, we identify its correspondences in training images to bridge the subject-template correspondence. To this end, we learn the sparse representation of the patch-based appearance of the subject voxel by all possible correspondence candidate voxels in training images. The sparse learning reveals several training candidates, each of which predicts the local transformation at the confidence relating to the learned sparse coefficient. Therefore, we can *predict* multiple transformations on a set of selected key points, and adaptively *reconstruct* the dense transformation field by considering the confidence of each prediction. For the sake of robustness and computation speed, the P-R protocol is embedded in a multi-resolution hierarchy. Moreover, since the tentative transformation field conveys important voxel descriptions other than appearances, it also participates into the sparse learning to better predict transformations. In the end, we can refine our estimated transformation field via existing registration method efficiently (i.e., with limited iterations of optimization).

The major contributions of this work include:

1. We investigate the appearance-transformation relationship to derive the hierarchy for predicting the transformation field in registration;
2. We apply sparse representation to local appearance/transformation and then propagate the sparse learning to update predictions of the transformation field;
3. We introduce an adaptive way to reconstruct the dense transformation field based on key points and their associated multiple predictions with varying confidences.

We will detail the proposed method in Section 2 and demonstrate its performances in Section 3. We will conclude this work with discussions in Section 4.

2   Method

We introduce the **Prediction-Reconstruction** protocol in Section 2.1, which predicts transformations at selected key points and then reconstructs the dense field accordingly. The protocol is embedded into a hierarchical framework in Section 2.2, and specifically applied to brain MR image registration. In order to predict the transformation of each key point, we apply sparse representation for joint learning of appearances and transformations in Section 2.3. Finally, in Section 2.4, we show details on adaptive reconstruction of the dense transformation field.

2.1   The P-R Protocol

We aim to estimate the transformation field $\phi_s(\cdot)$ that warps the subject image to the template in the P-R protocol. For the template voxel x, we can predict its correspondence $\phi_s(x)$ in the subject by utilizing the correspondence between x in the template and $\phi_{tr}(x)$ in the training image. In Fig. 1(b), we assume the subject voxel $\hat{x}$ and the training voxel y to be a pair of correspondences. Then, the offset from $\phi_s(x)$ to $\hat{x}$ in the subject image should equal the offset from $\phi_{tr}(x)$ to y in the training image

$$\phi_s(x) - \hat{x} = \phi_{tr}(x) - y. \tag{1}$$

The relation above, proved in the appendix, implies that the subject transformation $\phi_s(x)$ and the training transformation $\phi_{tr}(x)$ are closely related if $\hat{x}$ and y are correspondences in terms of their similar appearances. Based on (1), we can *predict* transformations on selected key points in the template, and then adaptively *reconstruct* the dense transformation field $\phi_s(\cdot)$.

Predicting $\phi_s(x)$ in (1) requires several inputs that are addressed in the following. Specifically, we convert (1) to an incremental refinement model by letting $\hat{x} = \phi_s^{\tau_{l-1}}(x)$ that reflects the tentatively deformed location of the template voxel x at time τ_{l-1}. Then, the prediction at time τ_l, later than τ_{l-1}, is updated by

$$\phi_s^{\tau_l}(x) = \phi_s^{\tau_{l-1}}(x) + \phi_{tr}^{\tau_l}(x) - y, 0 \le \tau_{l-1} \le \tau_l. \tag{2}$$

This incremental refinement is also illustrated in Fig. 1(c), where blue and red dashed arrows denote transformations at τ_{l-1} and τ_l, respectively.

After fixing $\hat{x} = \phi_s^{\tau_{l-1}}(x)$, we further select the training image with $\phi_{tr}^{\tau_l}(\cdot)$ and determine the training voxel y as the correspondence to $\hat{x}$ for predicting $\phi_s^{\tau_l}(x)$. Multiple predictions usually exist for a single template voxel x. Given the two training images in Fig. 1(c), for instance, two predictions on $\phi_s^{\tau_l}(x)$ are available by choosing y_1 from the first training image and y_2 from the second. Moreover, the number of predictions on $\phi_s^{\tau_l}(x)$ can be much higher, since multiple correspondence candidates to $\phi_s^{\tau_{l-1}}(x)$ may emerge from even a single training image. To acquire only reliable predictions on $\phi_s^{\tau_l}(x)$, we apply sparse representation to qualify both transformation $\phi_{tr}^{\tau_l}(x)$ and candidates of y in the training images, with details provided in Section 2.3. The sparse learning also computes the confidence for each specific prediction attempted by an arbitrary combination of $\phi_{tr}^{\tau_l}(x)$ and y.

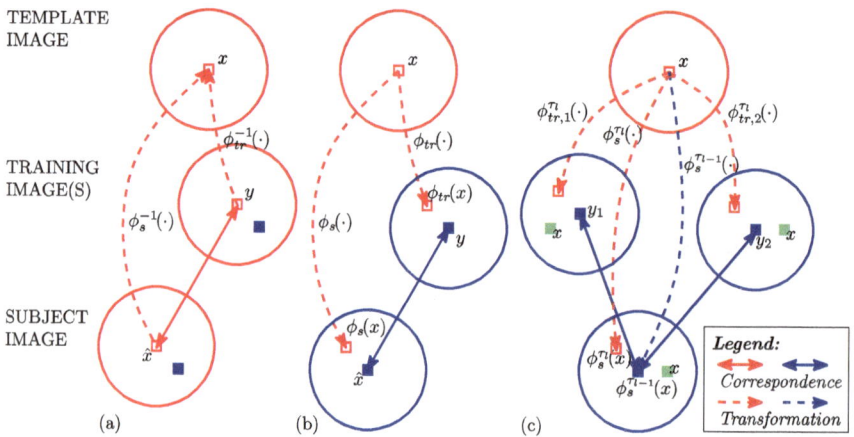

Fig. 1. Illustration of the predictable transformation: (a) The correspondence between the subject voxel $\hat{x}$ and the template voxel x is established due to the correspondence from $\hat{x}$ to y in the training image and from y to x as $x = \phi_{tr}^{-1}(y)$; (b) The template voxel x deforms to $\phi_s(x)$ in the subject, if $\hat{x}$ is the correspondence to y and the offset from $\phi_s(x)$ to $\hat{x}$ equals the offset from $\phi_{tr}(x)$ to y; (c) Multiple predictions are available given several candidates of y, and the prediction fits an incremental refinement model if $\hat{x}$ is assigned according to the tentative transformation.

The prediction is further applied to a set of key points that are automatically selected in the template space. Then, utilizing all key points scattered in the template space and their associated predictions, we are able to reconstruct the dense transformation field $\phi_s^{\tau_l}(\cdot)$ that warps the subject to the template. Note that the reconstruction is adaptive in order to account for multiple predictions (with varying confidences) of each key point, as detailed in Section 2.4.

2.2   The P-R Hierarchy in Brain MR Image Registration

We further embed the P-R protocol above into a hierarchical framework and apply it to registering bran MR images in this work. The hierarchy accounts for evolving resolutions, with the goal to provide better robustness. The transformation field output by the previous level works as initialization to the next level at higher resolution. In particular, after denoting the l-th level to finish at τ_l, the P-R hierarchy is as follows

```
Select a set of template key points X;
FOR each level l
  Select a subset of key points X_l ⊆ X;
  FOR each key point x ∈ X_l
    Predict φ_s^{τ_l}(x) following the rule in (2);
  END FOR
  Reconstruct the dense field φ_s^{τ_l}(·);
END FOR
```

The hierarchy above functions in the way similar to typical multi-resolution image registration methods. In particular, we use HAMMER [6] to align all training images to the template with recommended configurations (i.e., low-middle-high resolutions). The transformation fields of training images are then utilized at each level of our P-R hierarchy. The key points in the template are mostly sampled near the transitions of different brain tissues (i.e., white matter, grey matter, and cerebrospinal fluid), following the same strategy with [6]. The key points are abundant in contexture information and crucial to accurate alignment of neuroanatomical structures. Locations of all key points are available as part of the training data, thus resulting in no additional computation for a new subject. The subset of key points X_l in the l-th level is randomly sampled from X, while the size of X_l enlarges when the level increases (i.e., 1.0e4 for the size of X_1, 4.0e4 for X_2, and 1.6e5 for X_3 in the end). After exhausting all levels, the P-R hierarchy estimates the dense transformation field that registers the subject with the template. We can further refine the estimated transformation field efficiently, i.e., by feeding the field as initialization and running HAMMER with limited number of iterations at the high resolution only.

2.3   Predict Transformations via Joint Learning

The rule in (2) requires specific $\phi_{tr}^{\tau_l}(x)$ and y when attempting to predict $\phi_s^{\tau_l}(x)$. The selection of the two inputs determines the confidence of the resulted prediction. To this end, we evaluate the respective confidences of $\phi_{tr}^{\tau_l}(x)$ and y in predicting $\phi_s^{\tau_l}(x)$, and then define their product as the overall confidence of the resulted prediction. In particular, we *first* select several training images and assign specific confidences to their fields. *Then*, from those selected training images, we locate candidates of y that are correspondences to $\phi_s^{\tau_{l-1}}(x)$ in terms of local image appearances. The combination of certain $\phi_{tr}^{\tau_l}(x)$ and the candidate of y yields a prediction on $\phi_s^{\tau_l}(x)$, along with the respective confidence.

Confidence of $\phi_{tr}^{\tau_l}(x)$

The correspondence detected in brain MR images is meaningful only if restricted within a limited range such that $\|\phi_s^{\tau_{l-1}}(x) - y\|$ is small. The latent intimacy between $\phi_s^{\tau_{l-1}}(x)$ and y encourages us to select the training image with the field $\phi_{tr}^{\tau_l}(x)$ highly resembling $\phi_s^{\tau_l}(x)$ according to (2). The importance in selecting $\phi_{tr}^{\tau_l}(\cdot)$ can also be observed in Fig. 1(c). The two candidates y_1 and y_2, from two respective training images, yield the same predictions for $\phi_s^{\tau_l}(x)$. However, the training field $\phi_{tr,2}^{\tau_l}(x)$ in the right is more similar to $\phi_s^{\tau_l}(x)$ than the left field $\phi_{tr,1}^{\tau_l}(x)$, in reference to the coordinate of x in green. The correspondence between $\phi_s^{\tau_{l-1}}(x)$ and y_1 thus can only be detected by searching in a much wider area, with more computation, as $\|\phi_s^{\tau_{l-1}}(x) - y_1\| > \|\phi_s^{\tau_{l-1}}(x) - y_2\|$. Therefore, we conclude that $\phi_{tr,2}(x)$ is superior to $\phi_{tr,1}(x)$ in predicting $\phi_s^{\tau_l}(x)$ due to the relatively high similarity between $\phi_{tr,2}(x)$ and $\phi_s(x)$. Consequently, we relate the confidence of $\phi_{tr}^{\tau_l}(x)$ in predicting $\phi_s^{\tau_l}(x)$ as their in-between similarity, since more similar $\phi_{tr}^{\tau_l}(x)$ can better approximate $\phi_s^{\tau_l}(x)$ in (2).

In order to determine the confidence of $\phi_{tr}^{\tau_l}(x)$ from individual training image, we investigate the sparse representation of $\phi_s^{\tau_l}(x)$ in terms of all possible training fields at x. The coefficient in representing $\phi_s^{\tau_l}(x)$ indicates the similarity between $\phi_s^{\tau_l}(x)$ and $\phi_{tr}^{\tau_l}(x)$ from a specific training image [7], thus capturing the confidence of $\phi_{tr}^{\tau_l}(x)$ in predicting $\phi_s^{\tau_l}(x)$. The confidence of $\phi_{tr}^{\tau_l}(x)$, however, can hardly be estimated directly since $\phi_s^{\tau_l}(x)$ is not yet predicted. To this end, we evaluate the similarity of $\phi_{tr}^{\tau_{l-1}}(x)$ and $\phi_s^{\tau_{l-1}}(x)$ as an alternative, by assuming that the transformation fields at different levels are mildly changing. To facilitate sparse representation [7] for the evaluation of the confidence of each training field, we denote the set of training images as $\{I_{tr,i} | i = 1, \cdots M\}$ and their transformations as $\{\phi_{tr,i}^{\tau_l}(\cdot) | i = 1, \cdots M\}$. The local patch of the transformation field ϕ centered at x is then vectorized to the column vector ψ. The patch for the subject transformation ψ_s can thus be represented as $\psi_s = \Psi_{tr} \mathbf{u}$ by solving

$$\mathbf{u} = \arg \min_{\mathbf{u}} \|\psi_s - \Psi_{tr}\mathbf{u}\|^2 + \alpha \|\mathbf{u}\|_1, \tag{3}$$

where $\mathbf{u} = [u_1, \cdots, u_i, \cdots, u_M]^T$, $\Psi_{tr} = [\psi_{tr,1} \cdots, \psi_{tr,i}, \cdots \psi_{tr,M}]$, and $\forall u_i \geq 0$. The matrix Ψ_{tr} is the dictionary wrapping up all patches of training fields. The vector $\mathbf{u}$ records the coefficients to linearly represent $\phi_s(x)$, where the superscript τ_{l-1} indicating the level is intentionally omitted for short. The non-negative scalar α imposes the sparseness of $\mathbf{u}$ by penalizing its L_1-norm $\|\mathbf{u}\|_1$. The derived u_i, measuring the *similarity* of $\psi_{tr,i}$ and ψ_s [7], indicates the *confidence* to predict $\phi_s(x)$ by $\phi_{tr,i}(x)$.

Confidence of y

Given the i-th training image with the field $\phi_{tr,i}^{\tau_l}(\cdot)$, we aim to locate candidate voxels of y that are correspondences of $\phi_s^{\tau_{l-1}}(x)$. The search for y can be conducted as typical *correspondence detection*, by evaluating the appearance similarity between $\phi_s^{\tau_{l-1}}(x)$ and the candidate of y in the nearby. Higher similarity measure indicates better reliability of the detected correspondence, thus implying higher confidence of the prediction. To this end, we learn the sparse representation of the patch-based appearance of $\phi_s^{\tau_{l-1}}(x)$ based on candidates of y from all training images. The coefficients computed in sparse learning, also measuring the similarities between $\phi_s^{\tau_{l-1}}(x)$ and individual training candidates [7], tell the confidences in predicting $\phi_s^{\tau_l}(x)$ according to different candidates of y.

We denote y_{ij} for the j-th candidate of y from the i-th training image. All candidates y_{ij} for y, which satisfy $\|\phi_s^{\tau_{l-1}}(x) - y_{ij}\| \le \rho_l$ with ρ_l the maximal magnitude of a reasonable correspondence, are enumerated. We then denote $\boldsymbol{\theta}_s$ for the intensity patch centered at $\phi_s^{\tau_{l-1}}(x)$ and $\boldsymbol{\theta}_{ij}$ for the patch at y_{ij}. All training patches are concatenated in the dictionary $\boldsymbol{\Theta}_{tr} = \left[\cdots, \boldsymbol{\theta}_{1j}, \cdots, \boldsymbol{\theta}_{ij}, \cdots, \boldsymbol{\theta}_{Mj}, \cdots\right]$. Consequently, the coefficient vector $\mathbf{v}$ to represent $\boldsymbol{\theta}_s$ based on the dictionary matrix $\boldsymbol{\Theta}_{tr}$ can be obtained by solving

$$\mathbf{v} = \arg\min_{\mathbf{v}} \|\boldsymbol{\theta}_s - \boldsymbol{\Theta}_{tr}\mathbf{v}\|^2 + \beta\|\mathbf{v}\|_1,$$

$$\text{s.t.} \quad \mathbf{v} = \left[\cdots, v_{1j}, \cdots, v_{ij}, \cdots, v_{Mj}, \cdots\right]^T, \forall v_{ij} \ge 0. \tag{4}$$

The non-negative constant β, similar to α in (3), encourages deriving $\boldsymbol{\theta}_s$ by a sparse linear representation of column basis in $\boldsymbol{\Theta}_{tr}$. Note that the training candidate $\boldsymbol{\theta}_{ij}$ can be automatically excluded from $\boldsymbol{\Theta}_{tr}$ if the confidence of $\phi_{tr,i}^{\tau_l}(x)$, or u_i obtained in the step above, happens to be zero. That is, the previous sparse learning upon training fields helps reduce the size of $\boldsymbol{\Theta}_{tr}$, thus the optimization in (4) can be expedited significantly.

Any arbitrary combination of $\phi_{tr,i}^{\tau_l}(x)$ and y_{ij} yields an attempt to predict $\phi_s^{\tau_l}(x)$. In particular, we define the confidence w_{ij} for the attempt as the product of confidences of $\phi_{tr,i}^{\tau_l}(x)$ and y_{ij}, or $w_{ij} = u_i v_{ij}$. The sparsity enforced in selecting $\phi_{tr}^{\tau_l}(x)$ and y results in multiple, but limited number of, predictions with non-zero confidences. In this way, we **1)** avoid local minima if only acquiring a single but incorrect prediction for the key point; **2)** suppress a majority of predictions of low reliability. We further normalize the confidences of each key point by $w_{ij} \leftarrow w_{ij}/\sum\|w_{ij}\|$, to impose equal priors of all key points.

2.4   Reconstruct Dense Transformation Field

In the next, we reconstruct the dense transformation field to fit the multiple predictions of all key points. We turn to radial basis function (RBF) to represent the field. Suppose the RBF kernel function is $G(\cdot)$ and γ_x the RBF coefficient vector for the key point $x \in \mathbb{X}$, the dense field at the arbitrary location x' is then computed by

$$\phi(x') = \sum_{x \in \mathbb{X}} G(\|x' - x\|)\gamma_x. \tag{5}$$

We further define the kernel matrix $\mathbf{G}$, in which the entry at the m-th row and the n-th column is calculated by feeding the distance between the m-th and the n-th key points to the kernel function $G(\cdot)$. If only a single prediction was ever attempted for each key point, the residuals for the dense field to fit the predicted transformations of all key points could be easily computed as $\|\mathbf{\Phi} - \mathbf{G\Gamma}\|^2$, while the predicted transformation (in row vector form) of the m-th key point is recorded in the m-th row of $\mathbf{\Phi}$ and its RBF coefficient in the m-th row of $\mathbf{\Gamma}$ accordingly.

Due to multiple predictions of each key point, we further expand $\mathbf{\Phi}$ and introduce the confidence matrix $\mathbf{W}$ to fitting. Suppose the p-th row of $\mathbf{\Phi}$ records the prediction for the m-th key point with the confidence w_{ij}, we set the entry of $\mathbf{W}$ at the p-th row and the m-th column as w_{ij} and set all other entries in the p-th row as zero. The overall residuals then become $\|\mathbf{\Phi} - \mathbf{WG\Gamma}\|^2$.

Smoothness regularization is essentially important to the reconstruction of the dense field. To this end, the kernel functions $G(\cdot)$ is usually designed as low-pass filter [8]. Further, if $\mathbf{G}$ is positive definite, the regularization can be attained by solving $\mathbf{\Gamma} = \arg\min_{\mathbf{\Gamma}} \|\mathbf{\Phi} - \mathbf{WG\Gamma}\|^2 + \lambda \text{tr}(\mathbf{\Gamma}^T \mathbf{G\Gamma})$ [9], where λ controls the strength of the smoothness constraint. To generate the dense transformation field, the RBF coefficients in $\mathbf{\Gamma}$ are solvable in the following

$$(\mathbf{G} + \lambda(\mathbf{W}^T\mathbf{W})^{-1})\mathbf{\Gamma} = (\mathbf{W}^T\mathbf{W})^{-1}\mathbf{W}^T\mathbf{\Phi}. \tag{6}$$

Here, $\mathbf{W}^T\mathbf{W}$ is a diagonal matrix, where the m-th diagonal entry equals the sum of squares of the confidences for all predictions upon the m-th key point.

The kernel $G(\cdot)$ is designed such that $\mathbf{G}$ is positive definite and $G(\cdot)$ has low-pass response. Abundant choices of RBF kernels are available, i.e., the thin plate splines (TPS) [10, 11] with polynomial decay in frequency domain. Most RBF kernels, however, are globally supported, leading to dense matrix $\mathbf{G}$ and suffering from numerical instability. As a remedy, we use the compactly supported kernel [12] in this work

$$G(\|x' - x\|) = \left(1 - \frac{\|x' - x\|}{c}\right)^2 \cdot \exp\left(-\frac{\|x' - x\|^2}{2\sigma^2}\right), \forall \|x' - x\| \le c. \tag{7}$$

The kernel function $G(\cdot)$ cuts to zero if beyond the compact support, or $\|x' - x\| > c$. The resulted matrix $\mathbf{G}$ is thus sparse and further benefits solving (6).

To tackle the concern on the optimal scale of the kernel, we apply multi-kernel strategy to recursively reconstruct the transformation field [13]. In particular, we fix σ in (7) and adjust c to derive a set of RBF kernels $\{G_h\}$. The size of the compact support for G_h, or c_h, satisfies to $c_{h-1} = 2c_h$. We start reconstruction by applying G_1 to (6). The residuals after G_{h-1} are further reconstructed by G_h. The recursion iterates until that the overall residual, or $\|\mathbf{\Phi} - \mathbf{WG\Gamma}\|^2$, is tiny enough.

3   Experimental Results

We apply the proposed P-R hierarchy to NIREP datasets to verify its time cost and accuracy in estimating the transformation fields. The NIREP datasets contain 16 images, each of which is labeled by 32 ROIs. All images are resampled to the isotropic size of 256×256×256 and pre-processed (including bias correction, skull-stripping, etc.). We then randomly select one image (i.e., the fourth image) as the template and align all other images to the template in affine registration (i.e., using FLIRT). The estimation of the rest non-rigid transformation between each subject and the template is the focus of our study. All experiments are performed on a machine with an Intel Core i5 CPU (3.1GHz, single thread only) and 8G RAM.

We apply HAMMER to carefully register all images to the template, in order to acquire transformation fields as training data. The code of HAMMER is freely available through NITRC[1]. We follow the recommended settings for HAMMER and specify 50 iterations to each of the low, middle, and high resolutions. The outputs of HAMMER are comparable to [14], assuring the quality of the training data.

Time Cost

In order to predict the transformation for a certain subject image by our method, we utilize all other 14 images and their transformations from HAMMER for training. A leave-one-out cross validation is conducted for each subject image. The predicted transformation usually needs further refinement (i.e., applying HAMMER for a limited number of iterations at the high resolution only). In particular, we designate 0 (Setting 1), 10 (Setting 2), and 50 (Setting 3) iterations of refinement, respectively, for the proposed method. Note that Setting 1 produces results with no refinement via registration, while refinement in Setting 3 is the same with the high resolution of standard HAMMER. The time cost for each setting, compared with HAMMER, is summarized in Table 1.

We observe that the proposed method can efficiently predict the dense transformation field in 5.0min by average (Setting 1). With 10 iterations of refinement in Setting 2, the overall time cost rises to 8.6min, which is still significant lower (64.5% less) than direct registration via HAMMER (24.2min in average). With 50 iterations of refinement (Setting 3), which is equal to the high-resolution setting of HAMMER, our method costs comparable time (22.1min in average). Since our method also achieves reasonable accuracy in estimating the transformation field as shown in the next, we conclude that the proposed method can potentially save computation time in deforming the subject to the template.

Table 1. Average time costs of HAMMER and different settings of the proposed method (unit: minute). The number in parenthesis counts iterations of registration.

		Stages of prediction/registration				Overall
		Low level	Mid level	High level	Refinement	time cost
HAMMER		1.7 (50)	5.3 (50)	17.2 (50)	NA	**24.2**
Proposed Method	Setting 1	0.2	0.9	3.9	NA	**5.0**
	Setting 2				3.6 (10)	**8.6**
	Setting 3				17.1 (50)	**22.1**

[1] http://www.nitrc.org/projects/hammerwml/

Accuracy of Estimated Transformation

The accuracy of the estimated transformation is evaluated in terms of the spatial alignment of neuroanatomical structures. To this end, after warping the ROIs of the subject image to the template, we calculate the Dice overlap ratio between all pairs of corresponding ROIs. We further compute the average Dice ratio, as well as the standard deviation, associated with each ROI and plot the results in Fig. 2. The left panel of Fig. 2 shows the Dice ratios for 16 ROIs in the left hemisphere, while the right panel is for the other 16 ROIs in the right hemisphere.

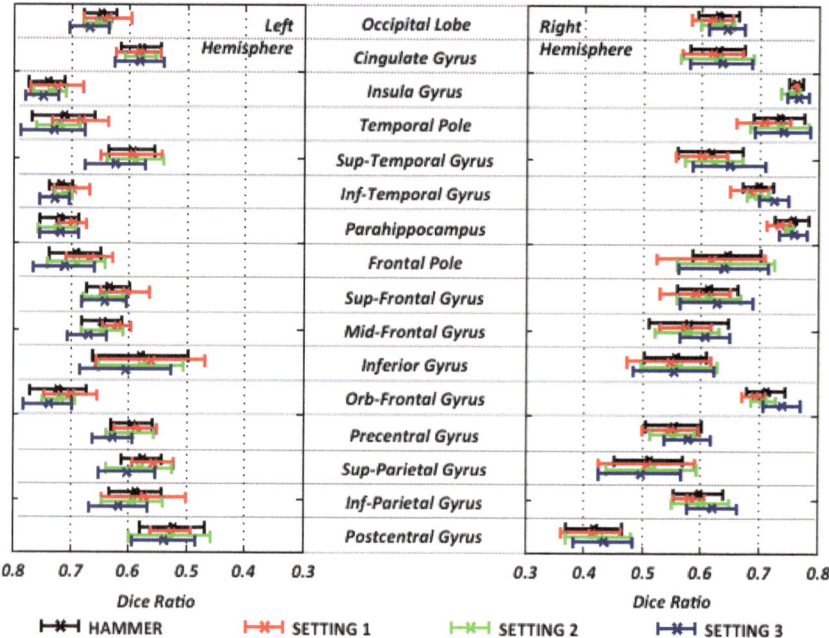

Fig. 2. The average Dice overlap ratios, as well as standard deviations, associated with 32 ROIs in NIREP datasets yield by HAMMER and the three different settings of the proposed method. The left panel shows scores for 16 ROIs in the left hemisphere, while the right panel is for the other ROIs in the right hemisphere.

Without any refinement to the proposed method (Setting 1, red bars in Fig. 2), the predicted transformation leads to an overall Dice ratio 2.01% lower than HAMMER (black bars). However, compared to the output of the middle resolution of HAMMER, our method yields 2.65% higher Dice ratio. The predicted transformation thus provides better initialization to the high-resolution refinement. Moreover, the Dice ratio can be rapidly improved by using only 10 iterations of refinement as in Setting 2 (green bars), which scores only 0.03% lower than HAMMER in the final. Considering the time cost of Setting 2, we conclude that *the proposed method is superior as it can achieve comparable accuracy in registration more efficiently.*

The accuracy in estimating transformations can be further enhanced in Setting 3, which utilizes 50 iterations of refinement. In particular, the average Dice ratio for Setting 3 is 1.87% higher than HAMMER, while its time cost is close to (or slightly less than) the counterpart. We further compute the Dice ratios of white matter and grey matter, as Setting 3 scores 4.05% and 4.28% higher than HAMMER, respectively. As the result, we claim that *our method achieves more accurate transformation fields given computation resources comparable to conventional registration method.*

4   Discussion

We have proposed an efficient approach to predict the transformation field for registering a new subject to the template. The prediction relies on the high correlation between image appearances and transformations. Thus, the sparse learning upon appearances can propagate to the prediction of transformations. After predicting transformations for selected landmarks, the dense field can be reconstructed adaptively. Compared with conventional registration method, the proposed method convincingly improves both time cost and accuracy of the estimated transformation field.

When predicting the transformation for a certain key point, we first select training images via sparse learning of transformations, and then locate correspondence candidate voxels from selected training images only. This sequential solution effectively lowers the number of training candidates involved in correspondence detection. Moreover, with even more training images, the speed performance of our method is not expected to deteriorate, as the learning on transformations is fast and it regulates the complexity of the learning on appearances.

The P-R hierarchy provides a robust way to estimate the final dense transformation field. As level increases, more key points predict their transformations and the reconstructed field is obviously more accurate. Due to initialized transformation field at high levels, the search range in correspondence detection can gradually reduce compared with low levels. As the result, the size of the appearance dictionary matrix Θ_{tr} decreases, thus obtaining better speed performance for the proposed method.

5   Appendix – The Rule in Predicting Transformations

Fig. 1(b) explains the rule in predicting transformations. Following the transformation field $\phi_{tr}(\cdot)$ that deforms a certain training image to the template, the template voxel x identifies its correspondence $\phi_{tr}(x)$ in the training image. Then, our task is to determine $\phi_s(\cdot)$ that assigns x to its correspondence $\phi_s(x)$ in the subject. We define the perturbation δx for x in the template and specifically let $\phi_s(x + \delta x) = \hat{x}$. We presume that voxels $\hat{x}$ in the subject and y in the training image form a pair of correspondences. The correspondence between $(x + \delta x)$ in the template and y in the training image, bridged by $\hat{x}$ in the subject, can immediately be established as $\phi_{tr}(x + \delta x) = y$. By expanding both transformations in their Taylor series, we have

$$\hat{x} = \phi_s(x + \delta x) = \phi_s(x) + \nabla\phi_s(x)\delta x + \mathcal{O}(\delta x^T \delta x),$$
$$y = \phi_{tr}(x + \delta x) = \phi_{tr}(x) + \nabla\phi_{tr}(x)\delta x + \mathcal{O}(\delta x^T \delta x). \tag{8}$$

An obvious solution of $\phi_s(x)$ to the equations above is

$$\phi_s(x + \delta x) = \phi_{tr}(x + \delta x) + \hat{x} - y, \forall \delta x, \tag{9}$$

such that $\nabla^z \phi_s(x) \equiv \nabla^z \phi_{tr}(x)$ for any $z \in \mathbb{Z}^+$. It leads to (1) when δx vanishes.

Acknowledgement. This paper was supported in part by NIH grants (EB006733, EB008374, EB009634, MH088520, AG041721, and MH100217).

References

1. Rueckert, D., Schnabel, J.A.: Medical Image Registration. In: Deserno, T.M. (ed.) Biomedical Image Processing, pp. 131–154. Springer, Heidelberg (2011)
2. Wu, G., Jia, H., Wang, Q., Shi, F., Yap, P.-T., Shen, D.: Emergence of Groupwise Registration in MR Brain Study. In: Liang, H., Bronzino, J.D., Peterson, D.R. (eds.) Biosignal Processing: Principles and Practices (2012)
3. Jia, H., Yap, P.T., Shen, D.: Iterative multi-atlas-based multi-image segmentation with tree-based registration. NeuroImage 59, 422–430 (2012)
4. Kim, M., Wu, G., Yap, P.-T., Shen, D.: A General Fast Registration Framework by Learning Deformation-Appearance Correlation. IEEE Transactions on Image Processing 21, 1823–1833 (2012)
5. Wolz, R., Aljabar, P., Hajnal, J.V., Hammers, A., Rueckert, D.: LEAP: Learning embeddings for atlas propagation. NeuroImage 49, 1316–1325 (2010)
6. Shen, D., Davatzikos, C.: HAMMER: hierarchical attribute matching mechanism for elastic registration. IEEE Transactions on Medical Imaging 21, 1421–1439 (2002)
7. Wright, J., Ma, Y., Mairal, J., Sapiro, G., Huang, T.S., Yan, S.: Sparse Representation for Computer Vision and Pattern Recognition. Proceedings of the IEEE 98, 1031–1044 (2010)
8. Myronenko, A., Song, X.: Point Set Registration: Coherent Point Drift. IEEE Transactions on Pattern Analysis and Machine Intelligence 32, 2262–2275 (2010)
9. Girosi, F., Jones, M., Poggio, T.: Regularization Theory and Neural Networks Architectures. Neural Computation 7, 219–269 (1995)
10. Bookstein, F.L.: Principal warps: thin-plate splines and the decomposition of deformations. IEEE Transactions on Pattern Analysis and Machine Intelligence 11, 567–585 (1989)
11. Chui, H., Rangarajan, A.: A new point matching algorithm for non-rigid registration. Computer Vision and Image Understanding 89, 114–141 (2003)
12. Genton, M.G.: Classes of kernels for machine learning: a statistics perspective. The Journal of Machine Learning Research 2, 299–312 (2002)
13. Floater, M.S., Iske, A.: Multistep scattered data interpolation using compactly supported radial basis functions. Journal of Computational and Applied Mathematics 73, 65–78 (1996)
14. Klein, A., Andersson, J., Ardekani, B.A., Ashburner, J., Avants, B., Chiang, M.C., Christensen, G.E., Collins, D.L., Gee, J., Hellier, P., Song, J.H., Jenkinson, M., Lepage, C., Rueckert, D., Thompson, P., Vercauteren, T., Woods, R.P., Mann, J.J., Parsey, R.V.: Evaluation of 14 nonlinear deformation algorithms applied to human brain MRI registration. NeuroImage 46, 786–802 (2009)

Automatic Prostate MR Image Segmentation with Sparse Label Propagation and Domain-Specific Manifold Regularization

Shu Liao[1], Yaozong Gao[1], Yinghuan Shi[1], Ambereen Yousuf[2],
Ibrahim Karademir[2], Aytekin Oto[2], and Dinggang Shen[1]

[1] Department of Radiology and BRIC, University of North Carolina at Chapel Hill,
`dgshen@med.unc.edu`
[2] Department of Radiology, Section of Urology, University of Chicago

Abstract. Automatic prostate segmentation in MR images plays an important role in prostate cancer diagnosis. However, there are two main challenges: (1) Large inter-subject prostate shape variations; (2) Inhomogeneous prostate appearance. To address these challenges, we propose a new hierarchical prostate MR segmentation method, with the main contributions lying in the following aspects: First, the most salient features are learnt from atlases based on a subclass discriminant analysis (SDA) method, which aims to find a discriminant feature subspace by simultaneously maximizing the inter-class distance and minimizing the intra-class variations. The projected features, instead of only voxel-wise intensity, will be served as anatomical signature of each voxel. Second, based on the projected features, a new multi-atlases sparse label fusion framework is proposed to estimate the prostate likelihood of each voxel in the target image from the coarse level. Third, a domain-specific semi-supervised manifold regularization method is proposed to incorporate the most reliable patient-specific information identified by the prostate likelihood map to refine the segmentation result from the fine level. Our method is evaluated on a T2 weighted prostate MR image dataset consisting of 66 patients and compared with two state-of-the-art segmentation methods. Experimental results show that our method consistently achieves the highest segmentation accuracies than other methods under comparison.

1 Introduction

Prostate cancer is the second leading cause of cancer death for American males. It is estimated by the American Cancer Society that in year 2012, around 241,740 new cases of of prostate cancer will be diagnosed, and around 28,170 men will die because of prostate cancer. Image guided radiation therapy (IGRT), as a non-invasive approach, is one of the major treatment methods for prostate cancer, and accurate prostate segmentation is a critical step in IGRT.

The T2 weighted magnetic resonance image (MRI) is one of the most commonly used prostate image modalities to perform treatment planning in IGRT due to its superior soft tissue contrast. There are many novel prostate MR image

J.C. Gee et al. (Eds.): IPMI 2013, LNCS 7917, pp. 511–523, 2013.
© Springer-Verlag Berlin Heidelberg 2013

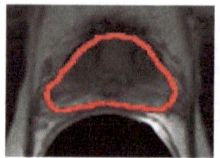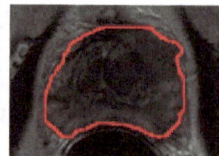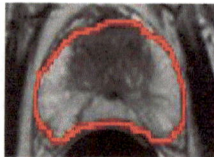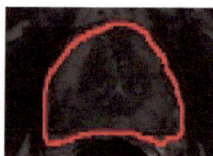

Fig. 1. Illustrations of large inter-subject shape and appearance variations of prostate in MR images, where the manual segmentation groundtruths are highlighted by the red contours. Note also the large inhomogeneous image appearances within the prostate region.

segmentation algorithms proposed in the literature, and they can be broadly classified into two main categories, namely multi-atlases based segmentation methods [1,2] and deformable model based segmentation methods [3,4]. Multi-atlases based segmentation methods generally have two main steps. First, atlases (i.e., training images with segmentation groundtruths) are registered to the target image. Second, label fusion is performed with the registered atlases to obtain the final segmentation result of the target image. The most commonly used label fusion techniques include majority voting (MV), STAPLE based methods [5,6], the SIMPLE algorithm [7], and the non-local mean based label propagation [8,9]. Deformable model based methods first construct a shape prior from available training images. Then, the prostate in the target image is segmented by fitting the deformable model onto the prostate boundary with both shape and appearance constraints. Representative deformable model based methods include the active appearance model (AAM) based methods [3] and probabilistic spatial constrained deformable model based methods [4].

Although many prostate MR image segmentation methods have been proposed, there are still two existing main challenges. The first challenge exists in all prostate image modalities, which is the large inter-subject prostate shape variation. It brings difficulty for multi-atlases based and deformable model based methods to accurately segment the prostate if prostate shape in the target image is significantly different from prostate shapes in the atlases. The second challenge is that the image appearance inside the prostate can have very large variations, which brings difficulty in learning effective image appearance features to capture all the anatomical properties of the prostate. These two challenges are also illustrated by Figure 1.

Therefore, we are motivated to propose a new prostate MR image segmentation method to address the two main challenges mentioned above. Specifically, the most salient anatomical features to aid segmentation are learnt by subclass discriminant analysis (SDA), which is a discriminant subspace learning method. SDA simultaneously maximizes the inter-class distances and minimizes the intra-class variations of the learnt features. Based on the learnt features, a hierarchical segmentation framework is proposed. In the coarse level, a multi-atlases based sparse label propagation method is proposed to estimate the prostate likelihood of each voxel in the target image, which provides a rough labeling of prostate

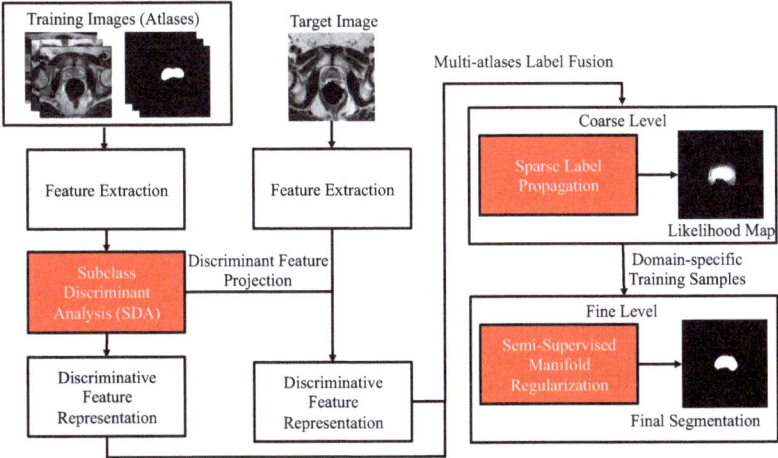

Fig. 2. Flow chart of our method, where all rectangles highlighted in red denote the main contributions of the proposed method

and non-prostate voxels. Then, voxels with high segmentation confidence can be determined based on the likelihood map. In the fine level, voxels with high segmentation confidence in the target image are served as labeled domain-specific samples, while voxels with low segmentation confidence are served as unlabeled domain-specific samples. These labeled and unlabeled domain-specific samples reflect the prostate anatomical properties in the target image more precisely than those from atlases, and thus they can be used as input for the semi-supervised manifold regularization method to refine the final segmentation result. A prostate MR image dataset consisting of 66 patients is used to evaluate our method, and further compare it with the two state-of-the-art prostate segmentation methods. Experimental results show that our method consistently achieves the highest segmentation accuracies than other methods under comparison.

2   Method

The proposed method can be summarized by Figure 2. Details of each component in Figure 2 is explained below.

2.1   Discriminant Feature Learning with SDA

As illustrated in Figure 1, using voxel intensity alone is insufficient to distinguish voxels belonging to the prostate and non-prostate regions. Therefore, it is of essential importance for designing highly discriminant voxel signatures. In the ideal case, discriminant voxel signatures should exhibit large inter-class distances and small intra-class variations for different tissue types, which is also known as the linear discriminant analysis (LDA) [10]. LDA aims to project the original

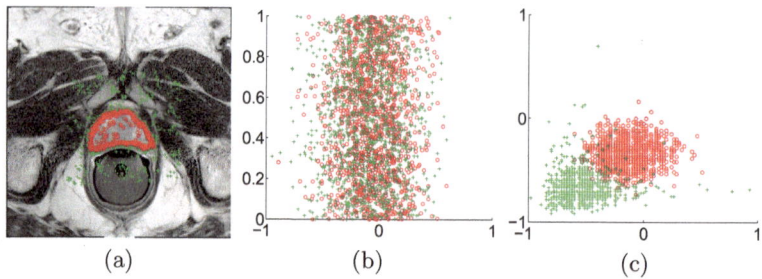

Fig. 3. (a) A typical example of sampling voxels drawn from a training image. Samples belonging to the prostate and non-prostate regions are highlighted by small red circles and green crosses, respectively. (b) shows the scatter plot of 1D discriminant feature learnt by LDA, where the horizontal axis represents the projected value of the features. For easy visualization, the projected data points are uniformly distributed along the vertical axis. (c) shows the scatter plot of the top two most discriminant feature learnt by the SDA algorithm.

signature to a feature subspace such that the projected features can maximize the separation of different classes measured by the Fisher-Rao's separation criterion.

In this paper, the Gabor wavelet function was used to extract the original feature signature. Specifically, given N training images I_i $(i = 1, ..., N)$, each image I_i is convolved with 50 Gabor wavelet kernels ψ^j $(j = 1, ..., 50)$, to obtain the resulting feature maps F_i^j. In each feature map, the multi-resolution patch-based representation [9] with patch sizes $K_1 = 5, K_2 = 9$, and $K_3 = 13$ are used as signature for each voxel x, denoted as $f(x)$.

Note that the original signature $f(x)$ may contain many redundant and noisy features. We aim to project the original signature to a discriminant subspace such that the projected features can maximize the inter-class distances and minimize the intra-class variations. Specifically, P voxels are drawn from the training images (e.g., Figure 3 (a)), denoted as $x_1,...,x_P$. Each voxel x_k $(k = 1, ..., P)$ has an anatomical label l_k, with $l_k = 1$ if x_k belongs to the prostate and $l_k = 0$ otherwise. We can learn the most discriminant features based on LDA [10] by finding projection vectors w which can maximize the Fisher-Rao's criterion:

$$J(w) = \frac{w^T S_B w}{w^T S_W w},$$ (1)

where S_B and S_W denote the between class scatter matrix and the within class scatter matrix defined by Equations 2 and 3, respectively.

$$S_B = \sum_{i=1}^{C} (\mu_i - \mu)(\mu_i - \mu)^T,$$ (2)

where C denotes the number of classes (i.e., $C = 2$ in our prostate segmentation problem), μ_i denotes the sample mean of class i, and μ denotes the global mean of all the samples.

$$\mathbf{S}_W = \sum_{i=1}^{C} \sum_{\boldsymbol{x}_k \in \zeta_i} (\boldsymbol{f}(\boldsymbol{x}_k) - \boldsymbol{\mu}_i)(\boldsymbol{f}(\boldsymbol{x}_k) - \boldsymbol{\mu}_i)^T, \tag{3}$$

where ζ_i denotes the set of voxels belonging to class i, and $\boldsymbol{f}(\boldsymbol{x}_k)$ is the multi-resolution patch signature of voxel $\boldsymbol{x}_k$.

The most discriminant direction $\boldsymbol{w}$ to project the original features can be obtained by selecting the eigenvectors with the largest eigenvalues of $(\mathbf{S}_W)^{-1}\mathbf{S}_B$.

The basic assumption of LDA in defining $\mathbf{S}_B$ by Equation 2 is that samples belonging to the same class are generated from a unimodal Gaussian distribution. This assumption generally does not hold for voxels belonging to the prostate and non-prostate regions due to the complex anatomical structure composition in MR images (e.g., in peripheral zones, central zones, rectum, and bladder). In this case, voxels belonging to the same class may exhibit significantly different distributions in the feature space and LDA is no longer applicable. Another limitation of LDA is that it can only project the original feature to a subspace with at most $C - 1$ dimensions since the rank of $\mathbf{S}_B$ can be at most $C - 1$. In binary medical image segmentation problems (i.e., $C = 2$ in our problem), LDA can only derive 1-dimensional feature, which is unlikely to well separate voxels belonging to different regions. Figure 3 (b) shows the projected 1D feature with LDA on the drawn samples shown in Figure 3 (a), and it can be observed that samples belonging to the prostate and non-prostate regions cannot be satisfactorily separated.

Therefore, we assume that samples belonging to the same class can belong to different clusters in the feature space. Specifically, for voxels belonging to class i (i.e., only two classes in binary segmentation problem), they can be further partitioned into H_i clusters (i.e., subclasses). Following this assumption, we propose the usage of subclass discriminant analysis (SDA) [12] to learn the most discriminant features. Specifically, we redefine $\mathbf{S}_B$ by Equation 4

$$\mathbf{S}_B = \sum_{i=1}^{C-1} \sum_{j=1}^{H_i} \sum_{k=i+1}^{C} \sum_{l=1}^{H_k} p_{ij}p_{kl}(\boldsymbol{\mu}_{ij} - \boldsymbol{\mu}_{kl})(\boldsymbol{\mu}_{ij} - \boldsymbol{\mu}_{kl})^T, \tag{4}$$

where $p_{ij} = P_{ij}/Q$ denotes the weight of the jth subclass of class i, with P_{ij} denoting the number of samples of the jth subclass in class i and Q denoting the total number of samples. $\boldsymbol{\mu}_{ij}$ is the sample mean of the jth subclass in class i. H_i denotes the number of subclasses in class i. Equation 4 aims to maximize the separability of subclasses belonging to different classes. Also, in Equation 4, $rank(\mathbf{S}_B) \leq \min(\sum_{i=1}^{C} H_i - 1, rank(\mathbf{S}_W))$, which resolves the rank deficiency problem. The number of subclasses H_i of each class i is automatically determined by affinity propagation clustering [13] on samples belonging to each class i.

The SDA discriminant feature extraction procedure can be summarized by Algorithm 1. The dimension of the final features extracted by SDA is determined as the least subset of eigenvectors which occupy more than 95% of the variance similar to [10]. Figure 3 (c) shows the scatter plot of the first two dimensions of the projected features with respect to the drawn voxel samples shown in Figure 3

Algorithm 1. Discriminant Feature Extraction by SDA

Input: Drawn training voxel samples $x_1, ..., x_P$, with their multi-resolution patch signature $f(x_i)$ $(i = 1, ..., P)$ and anatomical label l_i.

Output: Projected signature $\hat{f}(x_i)$ $(i = 1, ..., P)$, and projection matrix $\mathbf{M}$.

1. Compute the within class scatter matrix $\mathbf{S}_W$ by Equation 3.
2. Perform affinity propagation to cluster voxel samples belonging to the prostate region into H_1 subclasses and voxel samples belonging to the non-prostate region into H_2 subclasses.
3. Compute the between class scatter matrix $\mathbf{S}_B$ by Equation 4.
4. Perform eigen-analysis on $(\mathbf{S}_W)^{-1}\mathbf{S}_B$ to obtain its most significant eigenvectors forming matrix $\mathbf{V}$, and diagonal matrix $\mathbf{\Lambda}$ containing the largest eigenvalues.
5. Let $\mathbf{M} = \mathbf{\Lambda}^{-1/2}\mathbf{V}^T$.
6. Calculate the projected feature signature $\hat{f}(x_i) = \mathbf{M}f(x_i)$ $(i = 1, ..., P)$.
7. Return $\hat{f}(x_i)$ $(i = 1, ..., P)$, and $\mathbf{M}$.

(a) by SDA. It can be visually observed that SDA can separate voxels belonging to the prostate and non-prostate regions more effectively than LDA.

2.2 Coarse Level: Multi-atlases Based Sparse Label Propagation

After learning the feature projection matrix $\mathbf{M}$ by Algorithm 1, we can calculate the signature $\hat{f}(x)$ of each voxel x in the target image I_{new} as $\hat{f}(x) = \mathbf{M}f(x)$, where $f(x)$ is the original feature signature of x. The extracted features are then integrated with a multi-atlases based sparse label propagation framework to roughly estimate the prostate likelihood map in the target image.

Given N aligned training images (i.e., atlases) $\check{I}_i$ $(i = 1, ..., N)$ with I_{new} and their segmentation groundtruths $\check{S}_i$, the principle of label propagation [8,9] can be illustrated by Figure 4. For each voxel $x \in I_{new}$, its prostate likelihood is estimated by the voxels $y \in \check{I}_i$ around the neighborhood of x, namely the candidate voxels. The contribution of each $y \in \check{I}_i$ is represented by a graph weight $w_i(x, y)$, and its corresponding label $\check{S}_i(y)$ in $\check{S}_i$ can be propagated to voxel x with weight $w_i(x, y)$. In this paper, the multi-resolution fast free-form deformation (FFD) with the localized mutual information (LMI) registration algorithm [2] was used. Then, the prostate likelihood $S_{new}(x)$ in I_{new} can be estimated by label propagation [9] as defined in Equation 5:

$$S_{new}(x) = \frac{\sum_{i=1}^{N} \sum_{y \in \mathcal{N}_i(x)} w_i(x, y)\check{S}_i(y)}{\sum_{i=1}^{N} \sum_{y \in \mathcal{N}_i(x)} w_i(x, y)}, \qquad (5)$$

where $\mathcal{N}_i(x)$ denotes the set of neighboring voxels of x in image $\check{I}_i$, and it is defined as a $W \times W \times W$ window centered at voxel x. $\check{S}_i(y) = 1$ if voxel y belongs to the prostate region in $\check{I}_i$, and $\check{S}_i(y) = 0$ otherwise.

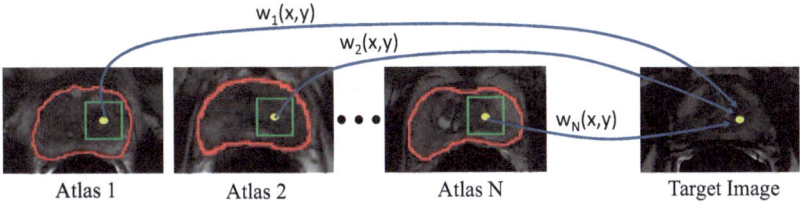

Fig. 4. The schematic illustration of multi-atlases label propagation. In this example, N atlases with their segmentation groundtruths highlighted by red contours are available. For the reference voxel highlighted by the yellow dot in the target image, its prostate likelihood can be estimated by comparing its feature signature with those of the neighboring candidate voxels within the green squares in the atlases. The contribution of each candidate voxel y in the ith atlas during label propagation is determined by the graph weight $w_i(x, y)$.

The most straightforward way to determine $w_i(x, y)$ is to directly compute the Euclidean distance between the feature signatures of x and y as similar to [9]. However, the graph weight $w_i(x, y)$ determined in this way may be sensitive to outliers and may not be able to effectively identify the most appropriate candidate voxels for label propagation. Therefore, we are motivated to estimate the graph weight $w_i(x, y)$ based on a group sparse representation framework. Specifically, signatures $\hat{f}(y)$ of voxels $y \in \mathcal{N}_i$ are reshaped into column vectors and organized into a matrix $\mathbf{A} = [\mathbf{A}_1^1, \mathbf{A}_1^2, ..., \mathbf{A}_i^1, \mathbf{A}_i^2, ..., \mathbf{A}_N^1, \mathbf{A}_N^2]$, where $\mathbf{A}_i^1$ and $\mathbf{A}_i^2$ ($i = 1, ..., N$) are matrices with candidate voxels belonging to the prostate and non-prostate regions in the ith training image, respectively. We aim to reconstruct the signature $\hat{f}(x)$ of each voxel $x \in I_{new}$ by the group sparse representation of columns of $\mathbf{A}$. The sparse coefficient vector β_x associated with x is organized as $\beta_x = \left[(\beta_x^{1,1})^T, (\beta_x^{1,2})^T, ..., (\beta_x^{i,1})^T, (\beta_x^{i,2})^T, ..., (\beta_x^{N,1})^T, (\beta_x^{N,2})^T\right]^T$, where $(\beta_x^{i,1})^T$, $(\beta_x^{i,2})^T$ is the coefficient vector corresponding to $\mathbf{A}_i^1$, $\mathbf{A}_i^2$. The graph weight $w_i(x, y)$ is set to the corresponding element in β_x^{opt} for voxel $y \in \check{I}_i$, where β_x^{opt} denotes the optimal solution for minimizing Equation 6:

$$E(\beta_x) = \frac{1}{2}||\hat{f}(x) - \mathbf{A}\beta_x||_2^2 + \lambda||\beta_x||_1 + \sum_{i=1}^{N}\sum_{k=1}^{2}||\beta_x^{i,k}||_2, \quad \beta_x \geq 0, \quad (6)$$

where $|| \cdot ||_1$ denotes the L_1 norm, and λ is the parameter controlling the global sparsity. Equation 6 can be optimized by using Nesterov's method [14].

The group sparsity constraint (third term) enforced in Equation 6 plays the role of atlas selection, as it tends to give more emphasis to candidate voxels from atlases similar to the target image, and effectively excludes outlier candidate voxels from atlases which are significantly different from the target image. On the other hand, the sparsity constraint (second term) further assigns more weights to the candidate voxels from atlases with similar feature signatures to the reference voxel in the target image.

Note that the estimated prostate likelihood map may still not be able to accurately delineate the prostate boundary as illustrated by a challenging

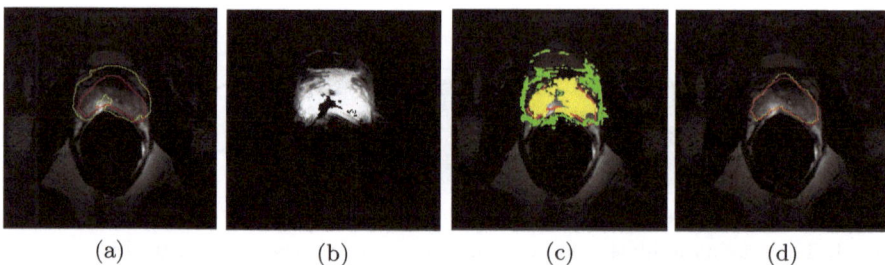

(a)	(b)	(c)	(d)

Fig. 5. Demonstration on how our method works on a challenging example. (a) shows the estimated prostate boundary (yellow contour) by using sparse label propagation in the coarse level, with the groundtruth prostate boundary overlayed (red contour), and (b) is the corresponding prostate likelihood map. Voxels highlighted with yellow in (c) are determined as domain-specific prostate samples, and voxels highlighted with green in (c) are determined as domain-specific non-prostate samples. (d) shows the estimated prostate boundary (yellow contour) by applying the fine level domain-specific manifold regularization, with the groundtruth prostate boundary overlayed (red contour).

example shown in Figure 5. The main reason is that the population information alone cannot fully reflect the anatomical details of the underlying patient. On the other hand, voxels with the highest segmentation confidence (i.e,. with high or low prostate likelihood values) can generally be classified correctly as shown in Figure 5 (c), which can be actually served as additional training samples to reflect the domain-specific knowledge of the target image. In this paper, voxels with prostate likelihood value $S_{new}(\boldsymbol{x}) \geq 0.85$ are determined as domain-specific prostate samples, while voxels with prostate likelihood value $0 < S_{new}(\boldsymbol{x}) \leq 0.15$ are used as domain-specific non-prostate samples. Other voxels in the target image can be used to serve as unlabeled domain-specific samples.

2.3   Fine Level: Semi-supervised Manifold Regularization

As described in Section 2.2, if the prostate shape and appearance information in the target image is significantly different from those in atlases, the segmentation result can be inaccurate. The origin of this problem is that population information from atlases alone is insufficient to represent the anatomical properties in the target image. Figure 5 (a) shows an example of the poor segmentation result obtained by the coarse level sparse label propagation.

Although the likelihood map estimated in the coarse level may not be able to accurately locate the prostate boundary, voxels with the highest segmentation confidences can be reliably identified and served as labeled domain-specific samples as described in Section 2.2 and shown in Figure 5 (c). Other voxels in the target image can be served as unlabeled domain-specific samples to encode the manifold configuration information in the feature space. These voxels provide more relevant and direct anatomical information to guide the segmentation process than voxels from atlases. In this paper, semi-supervised manifold regularization method based on the Laplacian Regularized Least Squares (LapRLS) [15] is used to integrate such information.

Specifically, given t labeled domain-specific training voxels z_i^L $(i = 1, ..., t)$, with anatomical label $v_i = 1$ if z_i^L is determined as prostate samples and $v_i = 0$ otherwise, and also h unlabeled domain-specific training voxels z_j^U $(j = 1, ..., h)$, LapRLS can be formulated as the optimization problem in Equation 7:

$$\min_{\Phi \in \mathcal{H}_K} \frac{1}{t} \sum_{i=1}^{t} (v_i - \Phi(\hat{f}(z_i^L)))^2 + \gamma_A ||\Phi||_K^2 + \frac{\gamma_I}{(t+h)^2} q^T L q, \qquad (7)$$

where $\hat{f}(z_i^L)$ denotes the discriminant feature representation of voxel z_i^L. $\mathcal{H}_K$ denotes the reproducing kernel Hilbert spaces (RKHS), and Φ is a mapping function in $\mathcal{H}_K$ to map a discriminant feature representation to a prostate likelihood value. $q = \left[\Phi(\hat{f}(z_1^L)), ..., \Phi(\hat{f}(z_t^L)), \Phi(\hat{f}(z_1^U)), ..., \Phi(\hat{f}(z_h^U)) \right]^T$, and L is the graph Laplacian of all the training samples computed based on the heat kernel [15]. γ_A and γ_I are weighting parameters of the second and third terms.

Based on the Representer Theorem [15], Φ can be represented as an expansion of kernel functions over both the labeled and unlabeled samples:

$$\Phi(\hat{f}(z)) = \sum_{i=1}^{t} \alpha_i K(\hat{f}(z), \hat{f}(z_i^L)) + \sum_{j=1}^{h} \alpha_{t+j} K(\hat{f}(z), \hat{f}(z_j^U)). \qquad (8)$$

Once the kernel function K is determined, the optimal parameters α_i $(i = 1, ..., t + h)$ in Equation 8 which yield the optimal mapping function Φ^{opt} to minimize Equation 7 can be obtained by Equation 9:

$$\alpha^* = (JK + \gamma_A tI + \frac{\gamma_I t}{(t+h)^2} LK)^{-1} Y, \qquad (9)$$

where $J = diag(1, ..., 1, 0, ..., 0)$ is a $(t + h) \times (t + h)$ diagonal matrix with the first t diagonal entries as 1 and the rest as 0. K is the $(t + h) \times (t + h)$ Gram matrix with $K_{ij} = K(\hat{f}(z_i), \hat{f}(z_j))$. Y is a $(t+h)$ dimensional label vector with $Y = [v_1, ..., v_t, 0, ..., 0]$, and $\alpha^* = [\alpha_1, ..., \alpha_{t+h}]$.

After estimating α^*, the optimal mapping function Φ^{opt} can be obtained by Equation 8. The final segmentation result can be obtained by applying Φ^{opt} to the feature signature $\hat{f}(z)$ of each voxel z in the target image, and classified it to the prostate region if $\Phi(\hat{f}(z)) \geq 0.5$, and classified to the non-prostate region otherwise. Figure 5 (d) shows the estimated prostate boundary refined by the fine level semi-supervised manifold regularization, and it can be observed that the prostate boundary has been accurately located, which implies the importance of incorporating domain-specific appearance information for classification.

3   Experimental Results

Our method was evaluated on a prostate T2 weighted MR image dataset consisting of 66 images taken from 66 different patients in the University of Chicago Hospital, and 9 prostate MR images taken from 9 different patients other than

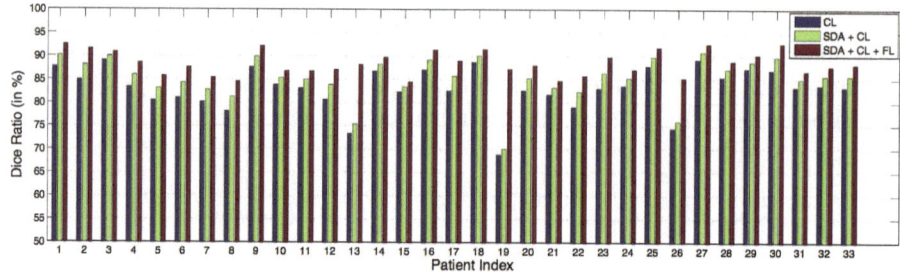

Fig. 6. Dice ratio between the estimated prostate volume and the groundtruth of the first 33 patients by using coarse level (CL) segmentation only, SDA derived feature with CL, and finally integrated with the fine level (FL) segmentation.

Table 1. The comparison of different methods with different evaluation metrics. The last three rows show the segmentation accuracy of our method with coarse level (CL) sparse label propagation only, CL based on the features derived by SDA, and finally integrated with domain-specific manifold regularization in the fine level (FL), respectively. The best results are bolded.

Method	Mean Dice + SD (in %)	Min Dice (in %)	Mean Hausdorff + SD (in mm)	Mean ASD + SD (in mm)
Klein *et al.* [2]	81.8 ± 4.3	47.3	11.7 ± 3.2	2.8 ± 1.2
Coupe *et al.* [9]	78.4 ± 3.6	34.2	15.8 ± 3.6	4.1 ± 1.5
CL	82.6 ± 4.8	51.4	10.6 ± 3.3	2.6 ± 1.4
SDA+CL	85.1 ± 4.1	63.2	9.6 ± 2.7	2.4 ± 1.2
SDA+CL+FL	$\mathbf{88.3 \pm 2.6}$	$\mathbf{84.6}$	$\mathbf{7.7 \pm 2.1}$	$\mathbf{1.8 \pm 0.9}$

those 66 patients were used as atlases. All MR images were also taken from different MR scanners. For each image, its manual segmentation groundtruth is provided by a clinical expert. The parameters of our method were set as follows by cross validation: $W = 15$, $\lambda = 10^{-4}$, $\gamma_A = 10^{-6}$, and $\gamma_I = 10^{-7}$. The Gaussian RBF kernel $K(\hat{f}(z_1), \hat{f}(z_2)) = \exp(-\tau||\hat{f}(z_1) - \hat{f}(z_2)||^2)$ was used in the fine level, with kernel parameter $\tau = \frac{1}{128}$.

The following preprocessing procedure was performed: The N3 bias correction algorithm [16] was first performed, followed by the histogram equalization procedure. Three different evaluation measures are used: Dice ratio, Hausdorff distance, and the average surface distance (ASD). Our method was also compared with the two state-of-the-art multi-atlases based segmentation methods proposed by Klein *et al.* [2] and Coupe *et al.* [9].

Table 1 lists the average Dice ratio, minimum Dice ratio, mean Hausdorff distance, and mean ASD, along with respective standard deviations (SD), across all the patients for different approaches.

It can be observed from Table 1 that by using the coarse level (CL) only, the segmentation accuracy of our method is slightly higher than Klein's method. By integrating CL with the salient features extracted by SDA, the segmenta-

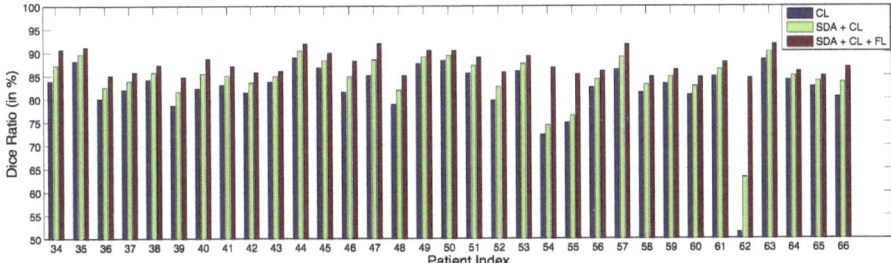

Fig. 7. Dice ratio between the estimated prostate volume and the groundtruth of the rest of the 33 patients by using coarse level (CL) segmentation only, SDA derived feature with CL, and finally integrated with the fine level (FL) segmentation

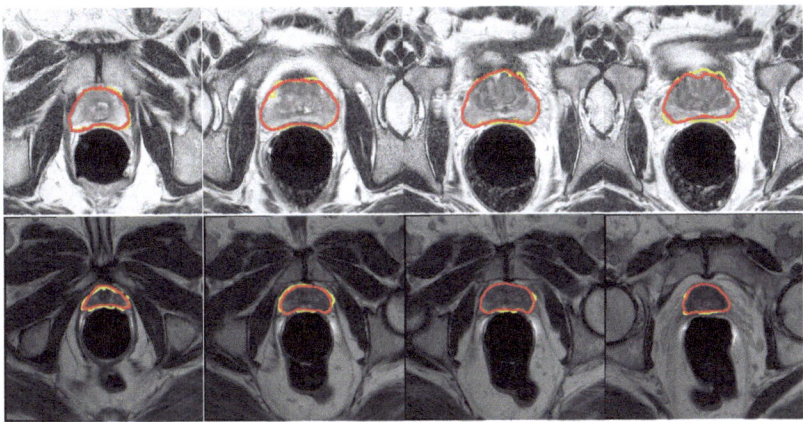

Fig. 8. Exemplar segmentation results obtained by the proposed method, where each row represents the segmentation results of a particular patient. Here, the estimated prostate boundary is highlighted in yellow, and the groundtruth prostate boundary is highlighted in red.

tion accuracy can be further improved, which reflects the contribution of SDA. Finally, by incorporating the fine level (FL) semi-supervised manifold regularization framework, the segmentation accuracy can be significantly boosted up, which is particularly reflected by the minimum Dice ratio.

Figures 6 and 7 show the Dice ratio between the estimated prostate volume and the segmentation groundtruth of each patient with our method by using the CL only, SDA derived features with CL, and further integrated with FL. It can be observed that the segmentation accuracies consistently and progressively increase for all the patients, which illustrates the contribution of each component.

Figure 8 shows some typical segmentation results by our method, and it can be observed that the estimated prostate boundaries by the proposed method are very close to the groundtruth, which implies the effectiveness of our method.

The proposed method takes around 2.9 mins on average to segment a 3D prostate MR image. All the experiments were conducted on an Intel Xeon 2.66-GHz CPU computer with MATLAB implementation.

4   Conclusion

In this paper, we propose a new prostate MR image segmentation method. The most discriminant feature signatures for each voxel are learnt by the subclass discriminant analysis (SDA) to aid segmentation. SDA aims to find a discriminant feature subspace which simultaneously maximizes the inter-class distance and minimizes the intra-class variations. The learnt features are integrated with a hierarchical segmentation framework. In the coarse level, a sparse label propagation method is proposed to propagate the population information from atlases to the target image. The estimated prostate likelihood map can reliably identify voxels with the highest segmentation confidences to serve as labeled domain-specific samples of the target image, and voxels with low segmentation confidences are served as unlabeled domain-specific samples to describe the underlying manifold configuration in the feature space. A semi-supervised manifold regularization method is proposed to construct the domain-specific classifier, and it is used to refine the final segmentation result in the fine level. Our method has been evaluated on a prostate MR image dataset consisting of 66 patients and compared with two state-of-the-art multi-atlases based segmentation methods. Experimental results demonstrate that our method consistently achieves the highest segmentation accuracy among the methods under comparison.

References

1. Chandra, S., Dowling, J., Shen, K., Raniga, P., Pluim, J., Greer, P., Salvado, O., Fripp, J.: Patient specific prostate segmentation in 3D magnetic resonance images. TMI 31, 1955–1964 (2012)
2. Klein, S., Heide, U., Lips, I., Vulpen, M., Staring, M., Pluim, J.: Automatic segmentation of the prostate in 3D MR images by atlas matching using localized mutual information. Medical Physics 35, 1407–1417 (2008)
3. Toth, R., Madabhushi, A.: Multi-feature landmark-free active appearance models: Application to prostate MRI segmentation. TMI 31, 1638–1650 (2012)
4. Martin, S., Troccaz, J., Daanen, V.: Automated segmentation of the prostate in 3D MR images using a probabilistic atlas and a spatially constrained deformable model. Medical Physics 37, 1579–1590 (2010)
5. Warfield, S., Zou, K., Wells, W.: Simultaneous truth and performance level estimation (STAPLE): An algorithm for the validation of image segmentation. TMI 23, 903–921 (2004)
6. Asman, A.J., Landman, B.A.: Characterizing spatially varying performance to improve multi-atlas multi-label segmentation. In: Székely, G., Hahn, H.K. (eds.) IPMI 2011. LNCS, vol. 6801, pp. 85–96. Springer, Heidelberg (2011)
7. Langerak, T., van der Heide, U., Kotte, A., Viergever, M., van Vulpen, M., Pluim, J.: Label fusion in atlas-based segmentation using a selective and iterative method for performance level estimation (simple). TMI 29, 2000–2008 (2010)
8. Rousseau, F., Habas, P., Studholme, C.: A supervised patch-based approach for human brain labeling. TMI 30, 1852–1862 (2011)
9. Coupe, P., Manjon, J., Fonov, V., Pruessner, J., Robles, M., Collins, D.: Patch-based segmentation using expert priors: application to hippocampus and ventricle segmentation. NeuroImage 54, 940–954 (2011)

10. Belhumeur, P., Hespanha, J., Kriegman, D.: Eigenfaces vs. fisherfaces: Recognition using class specific linear projection. PAMI 19(7), 711–720 (1997)
11. Li, W., Liao, S., Feng, Q., Chen, W., Shen, D.: Learning image context for segmentation of prostate in CT-guided radiotherapy. In: Fichtinger, G., Martel, A., Peters, T. (eds.) MICCAI 2011, Part III. LNCS, vol. 6893, pp. 570–578. Springer, Heidelberg (2011)
12. Zhu, M., Martinez, A.: Subclass discriminant analysis. PAMI 28(8), 1274–1286 (2006)
13. Frey, B., Dueck, D.: Clustering by passing messages between data points. Science 315, 972–976 (2007)
14. Nesterov, Y.: Introductory Lectures on Convex Optimization: A Basic Course. Kluwer Academic Publishers (2004)
15. Belkin, M., Niyogi, P., Sindhwani, V.: Manifold regularization: A geometric framework for learning from labeled and unlabeled examples. Journal of Machine Learning Research 7, 2399–2434 (2006)
16. Sled, J., Zijdenbos, A., Evans, A.: A nonparametric method for automatic correction of intensity nonuniformity in MRI data. TMI 17, 87–97 (1998)

Moving Frames for Heart Fiber Geometry

Emmanuel Piuze[1], Jon Sporring[2,1], and Kaleem Siddiqi[1]

[1] School of Computer Science & Centre for Intelligent Machines, McGill University
[2] eScience Center, Department of Computer Science, University of Copenhagen

Abstract. Elongated cardiac muscle cells named cardiomyocytes are densely packed in an intercellular collagen matrix and are aligned to helical segments in a manner which facilitates pumping via alternate contraction and relaxation. Characterizing the geometrical variation of their groupings as cardiac fibers is central to our understanding of normal heart function. Motivated by a recent abstraction by Savadjiev et al. of heart wall fibers into generalized helicoid minimal surfaces, this paper develops an extension based on differential forms. The key idea is to use Maurer-Cartan's method of moving frames to study the rotations of a frame field attached to the local fiber direction. This approach provides a new set of parameters that are complimentary to those of Savadjiev et al. and offers a framework for developing new models of the cardiac fiber architecture. This framework is used to compute the generalized helicoid parameters directly, without the need to formulate an optimization problem. The framework admits a straightforward numerical implementation that provides statistical measurements consistent with those previously reported. Using Diffusion MRI we demonstrate that one such specialization, the homeoid, constrains fibers to lie locally within ellipsoidal shells and yields improved fits in the rat, the dog and the human to those obtained using generalized helicoids.

Keywords: Heart Myofibers, Differential Geometry, Connection Forms, Moving Frames, Diffusion MRI, Generalized Helicoids.

1   Introduction

Cardiac myofibers are densely packed in the heart wall and are locally aligned to helical curves [1]. Helices act as geodesics between points in the myocardium and mathematical analyses by Peskin [2] and Horowitz et. al [3] support the view that this alignment is mechanically optimal. As a result, geometric descriptions of cardiac fibers using the helix angle, taken to be the projected angle between the fiber direction and the short-axis plane (see Fig. 1a), are popular in the literature. Several accounts from both small-scale histology and voxel-scale studies based on Diffusion MRI (dMRI) report that along a transmural penetration line from the heart's outer to inner wall, the helix angle varies smoothly and regularly undergoing a total change in orientation of about 120° [1, 4–7]. The range of the transverse angle, which is the angle formed by a fiber moving away from a plane perpendicular to the transmural direction, is much smaller, about ±10° [4, 8], and is therefore often ignored in the literature.

J.C. Gee et al. (Eds.): IPMI 2013, LNCS 7917, pp. 524–535, 2013.
© Springer-Verlag Berlin Heidelberg 2013

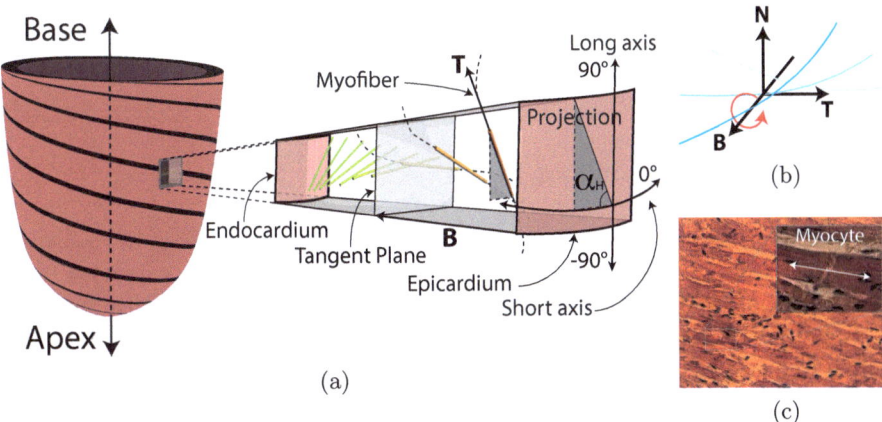

Fig. 1. (1a) The helix angle α_H is defined as the angle between the short axis of the heart and the projected myofiber orientation in a plane orthogonal to the transmural direction. (1b) The transmural change in the helix angle in the direction $\boldsymbol{B}$, orthogonal to the heart wall tangent plane. (1c) A histological slice of cardiac tissue showing individual elongated cardiomyocytes and their nuclei (dark) in the intercellular collagen network (*adapted from Wikimedia Commons*).

The analysis of myofibers from histological slices is cumbersome and their invasiveness does not easily admit an association with the original intact three-dimensional geometry. Thus, many modern analysis methods work with cardiac fiber orientation data derived from dMRI measurements [4–6, 9, 10]. However, the scale at which current dMRI measurements are made is at least one order of magnitude larger than the length of individual cardiomyocytes [8]. The measured signal therefore reflects the composite behaviour of large groups of cardiac muscle cells within the collagen matrix (Fig. 1c). Savadjiev et al. [12] have recently obtained a promising characterization of the collective geometrical variation of cardiac fibers, using a method derived from texture flow analysis [11]. They arrived at the conclusion that the cardiac fiber directions across three mammalian species – the rat, the canine and the human – are locally described by a particular minimal surface, the generalized helicoid model (GHM).

A limitation of the GHM is that its streamlines lie on a planar manifold in spite that the heart wall is curved (Fig. 1a). The GHM thus captures the variability of cardiac fibers in a plane tangent to the local cardiac wall but not orthogonally to it. Moreover, experimental results have shown that the GHM is only accurate in the immediate neighborhood of a voxel, with fitting errors growing rapidly as the neighborhood in which the fits are applied is increased [12]. Motivated by these observations, this paper develops an extension by attaching a local frame field to the fiber and transmural directions and studying the full differential geometry of this moving frame through the Maurer-Cartan connection one-forms. We show that locally the GHM can in fact be measured directly using a combination of connection forms. We then introduce a sub-class of differential form-based models for which the streamlines lie on ellipsoidal shells or *homeoids* (Section 3.4). Using the same database examined by Savadjiev et al. in [12] we demonstrate that local measurements on homeoids give lower fitting errors than generalized helicoids. We begin by introducing the Maurer-Cartan form in Section 2.

2   The Maurer-Cartan Form

We characterize the differential geometry of fibers in the heart wall by measuring the manner in which they turn locally. For this purpose, we construct a frame field $F_1, F_2, F_3 \in \mathbb{R}^3$, $F_i \cdot F_j = \delta_{ij}$, where δ_{ij} is the Kronecker delta, in such a manner that the turning of the frame field characterizes the turning of the fibers. The frame field is expressed as a rotation of the cartesian frame $\begin{bmatrix} e_1 & e_2 & e_3 \end{bmatrix}^T$,

$$\begin{bmatrix} F_1 & F_2 & F_3 \end{bmatrix}^T = A \begin{bmatrix} e_1, e_2, e_3 \end{bmatrix}^T, \tag{1}$$

where the attitude matrix $A \in \mathrm{SO}(3)$ is a smoothly varying orthonormal matrix, and where the basis vectors e_j are treated as symbols such that $F_i = \sum_j a_{ij} e_j$.

The differential geometry of the fibers is now directly characterized by the attitude transformation. Its differential structure is found to be [13]

$$\mathrm{d} \begin{bmatrix} F_1 \\ F_2 \\ F_3 \end{bmatrix} = \begin{bmatrix} \mathrm{d}F_1 \\ \mathrm{d}F_2 \\ \mathrm{d}F_3 \end{bmatrix} = (\mathrm{d}A) \begin{bmatrix} e_x \\ e_y \\ e_z \end{bmatrix} = (\mathrm{d}A) A^{-1} \begin{bmatrix} F_1 \\ F_2 \\ F_3 \end{bmatrix} = C \begin{bmatrix} F_1 \\ F_2 \\ F_3 \end{bmatrix}, \tag{2}$$

where d is the differential operator, $A^{-1} = A^T$, $C = (\mathrm{d}A) A^{-1}$ is the Maurer-Cartan form, and where for simplicity the notation $\mathrm{d}F_i = \sum_j c_{ij} F_j$ is used. The Maurer-Cartan matrix is skew symmetric, i.e., $C = -C^T$. Hence it has at most 3 independent, non-zero elements: c_{12}, c_{13}, and c_{23}. Each c_{ij} is a one-form in $\mathbb{R}^3$ that can be contracted on a vector $v = \begin{bmatrix} v_1, v_2, v_3 \end{bmatrix}^T \in \mathbb{R}^3$ to yield the initial rate of turn of F_i towards F_j when moving in the direction of v. We denote this contraction $c_{ij}\langle v \rangle$, which is found to be $c_{ij}\langle v \rangle = \nabla_v F_i \cdot F_j|_x$, where $x \in \mathbb{R}^3$ is a point in the fiber field and $\nabla_v F_i$ is the covariant derivative of F_i in the direction v. Thus,

$$c_{ij}\langle v \rangle = \begin{bmatrix} F_{j1} & F_{j2} & F_{j3} \end{bmatrix} \begin{bmatrix} \partial_x F_{i1} & \partial_y F_{i1} & \partial_z F_{i1} \\ \partial_x F_{i2} & \partial_y F_{i2} & \partial_z F_{i2} \\ \partial_x F_{i3} & \partial_y F_{i3} & \partial_z F_{i3} \end{bmatrix} \begin{bmatrix} v_1 \\ v_2 \\ v_3 \end{bmatrix}, \tag{3}$$

where the components of the frame vectors are enumerated as $F_i = \begin{bmatrix} F_{i1}, F_{i2}, F_{i3} \end{bmatrix}^T$ and where $\partial_x \equiv \frac{\partial}{\partial x}$ is used to denote partial derivatives. Since we are interested in studying the change of the frame field in the direction of its basis vectors we study the contractions $c_{ijk} \equiv c_{ij}\langle F_k \rangle$. Note that the frame field F_1, F_2, F_3 has 3 degrees of freedom. Since this field roams a 3-dimensional space, a linear model of the spatial change of the frame field must have 9 degrees of freedom, which are embodied in e_{ijk}.

The abstraction and the comprehensiveness in the one-form description of the geometrical behavior of a frame field can be harnessed to develop models that are descriptive of the variability of cardiac fiber orientations across multiple species. The next section introduces a class of fiber models based on one-forms and reintroduces the GHM of [12] as a planar approximation to the complete one-form parameterization.

3 Measures on a Discrete Fiber Frame Field

We analyze hearts represented as diffusion MRI volumes embedded in 3D rectangular lattices with coordinates $x = xe_1 + ye_2 + ze_3 = [x, y, z]^T \in \mathbb{Z}^3$. A tangent vector T is identified as the principal eigenvector of the diffusion tensor field. Consistency in T amongst voxel neighbours is enforced by adopting an adaptive cylindrical coordinate system. The centroid c_z of the chamber within each short-axis slice s_z is first determined. $T(x)$ is then made to turn clockwise with respect to that centroid as follows:

$$T(x) \rightarrow \text{sign}\big((T \times (x - c_z)) \cdot l(s_z) \big) \, T(x), \tag{4}$$

where $l(s_z)$ is the local approximation of the heart's long-axis. For all the hearts that we consider, $l(s_z)$ approximately coincides with the world's z axis. In the spirit of [12], the heart transmural direction $\hat{B}$ is estimated as the gradient vector of a distance transform produced as follows: a) the binary image (mask) of the heart is closed using mathematical morphological operations, b) the closest distance to the heart wall is evaluated at every point, c) the gradient of the distance transform is computed, and finally d) the skeletal points of colliding fronts are removed and interpolated by thresholding the magnitude of the gradient vectors. The normals $\hat{B}$ are then aligned to point from outer to inner wall. With T and $\hat{B}$ we specify a local frame

$$F_1 = \frac{T}{\|T\|}, \quad F_2 = N = F_3 \times F_1, \quad F_3 = B = \frac{\big(\hat{B} - (\hat{B} \cdot T)T\big)}{\|\hat{B} - (\hat{B} \cdot T)T\|}, \tag{5}$$

where B is the part of $\hat{B}$ orthogonal to T. From here on, we will use the symbols T, N, and B interchangeably with the corresponding symbols F_j. We will also refer to the local plane spanned by T and N as the *tangent plane*.

3.1 One-Form Intuition

One-form contractions c_{ijk} can be interpreted as the amount of turning of F_i towards F_j in the direction F_k. For example, c_{TNB} describes a transmural rotation of T towards N, as shown in Fig. 1b. c_{ijk} were computed at each voxel from the discrete fiber frame field combined with (3). Histograms for three species (rat, canine, human) are shown in Fig. 2 and illustrate statistics on the local turning of the frame field. The rotations of T towards N, $c_{TN}\langle F_k \rangle$, are

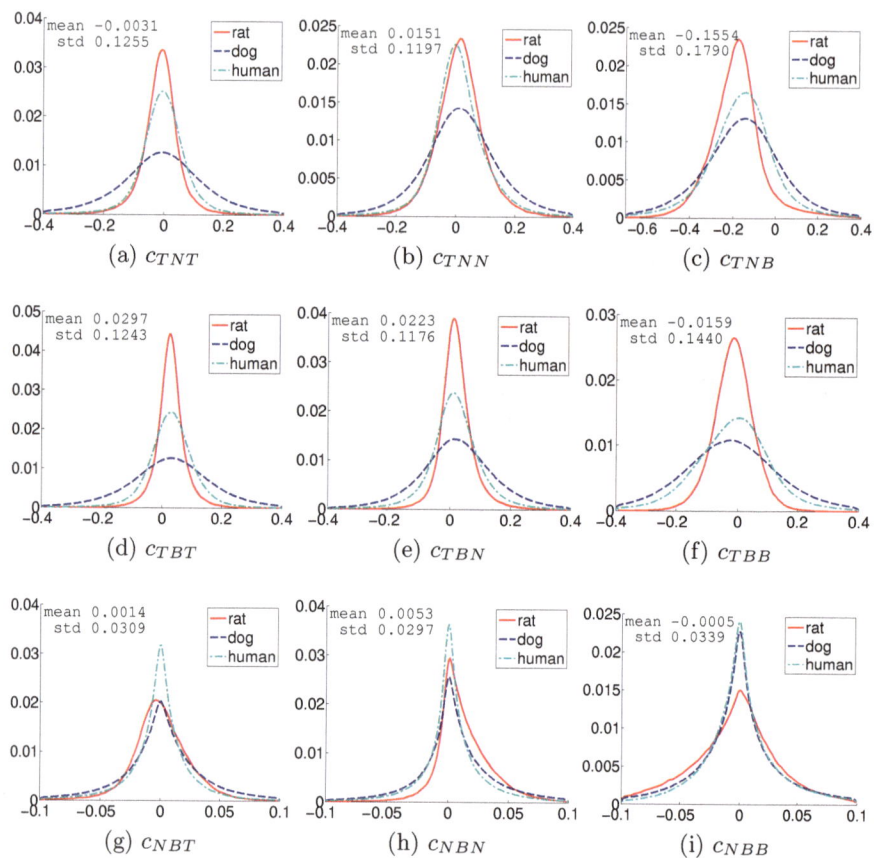

Fig. 2. Histogram of $c_{ijk} \equiv c_{ij}\langle F_k \rangle$ for 3 species: rat, human, dog. All measures have been normalized such that the horizontal axis is in mm.

intimately linked to the curvature parameters of the GHM in [12]. These rotations intuitively describe the manner in which fibers turn in the tangent plane of the heart: c_{TNT}, shown in Fig. 2a, describes their tangential curvature, c_{TNN}, shown in Fig. 2b, their fanning in the tangent plane, and c_{TNB}, shown in Fig. 1b, their transmural turning or equivalently the rate of change of the *helix angle*. This is arguably the most salient variation of the cardiac fibers. The rotations of T towards B, $c_{TB}\langle F_k \rangle$, express the turning of the fibers towards the inner wall: c_{TBT} effectively measures the first the local curvature of the heart, c_{TBN} describes a twisting of the tangent plane and the rate of change of the *transverse angle*, and c_{TBB} measures a fanning or thickening of the local fiber population away from the tangent plane, towards the inner wall. As shown in Fig. 2g–2i, the remaining rotations of N towards B, $c_{NB}\langle F_k \rangle$, are an order of magnitude smaller in all 3 directions which indicate that the frame field axis N is constrained within the local tangent plane. c_{NBT} measures a twisting of the tangent plane, c_{NBN} the second curvature of the heart wall, and c_{NBB} a transmural fanning or thickening.

3.2   The One-Form Model

The Maurer-Cartan form extrapolates the local shape to first order as

$$\tilde{T}_h = T + c_{TN}\langle h \rangle N + c_{TB}\langle h \rangle B \tag{6}$$

$$= T + (c_{TNT}\, h \cdot T + c_{TNN}\, h \cdot N + c_{TNB}\, h \cdot B)\, N \tag{7}$$

$$+ (c_{TBT}\, h \cdot T + c_{TBN}\, h \cdot N + c_{TBB}\, h \cdot B)\, B,$$

where h is an offset from the point at which the frame is expressed and $\tilde{T}_h$ represents the predicted direction of this neighbor by the one-form extrapolation to first-order approximation. As in [12], we construct an error measure by computing the average angular difference between the measured and predicted directions in an isotropic neighborhood $\mathcal{N}_i$,

$$e(\mathcal{N}_i) = \frac{1}{|\mathcal{N}_i|} \sum_{h \in \mathcal{N}_i} \arccos \left(T_h \cdot \frac{\tilde{T}_h}{\|\tilde{T}_h\|} \right), \tag{8}$$

where $|\mathcal{N}_i| = i^3$ for odd $i \in \mathbb{Z}$ and T_h is the true neighbor's measured direction. The associated errors of fit for different species are shown in Fig. 3. Diffusion MRI noise and resolution, heart size, and underlying fiber geometry are factors that account for the error disparity across different species. We delay further analysis of these errors to Section 4, where they will be compared against those of the other models we will introduce next.

3.3   The Generalized Helicoid as a Subset of the One-Form Model

The generalized helicoid model of Savadjiev et al. [12] expresses the local fiber direction in a plane tangent to the heart wall. Within the local coordinate frame, the fiber direction at a point $x = x_T T + x_N N + x_B B \in \mathbb{R}^3$ is given as the angle

$$\theta(x, K_T, K_N, K_B) = \arctan \left(\frac{K_T x_T + K_N x_N}{1 + K_N x_T - K_T x_N} \right) + K_B x_B, \tag{9}$$

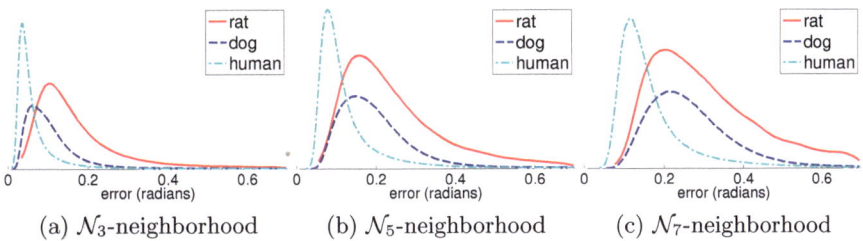

(a) $\mathcal{N}_3$-neighborhood   (b) $\mathcal{N}_5$-neighborhood   (c) $\mathcal{N}_7$-neighborhood

Fig. 3. One-form extrapolation error for neighborhoods of size $|\mathcal{N}_i| = 3^3, 5^3, 7^3$

where $K_* \in \mathbb{R}$ are the GHM curvature parameters. Direct calculations show that a frame field spanned by $\boldsymbol{T}(\theta)$, $\boldsymbol{N}(\theta)$, $\boldsymbol{B}(\theta)$ has instantaneous turning given by $c_{TN}\langle \boldsymbol{T}(\theta)\rangle = K_T$, $c_{TN}\langle \boldsymbol{N}(\theta)\rangle = K_N$, $c_{TN}\langle \boldsymbol{B}(\theta)\rangle = K_B$, with the remaining one-forms all being zero. The GHM parameters can thus be estimated directly using (3) and the GHM model may be evaluated directly using (7) and central differences as an alternative to the generative model (9). To compare these 2 representations, the parameter vector $\boldsymbol{K} = (K_T, K_N, K_B)$ of the GHM was estimated at each voxel using a standard Nelder-Mead optimization scheme. The problem was formulated as the selection of the parameters $\boldsymbol{K}$ which minimize an extension of (8), where $\tilde{\boldsymbol{T}}_h \longrightarrow \tilde{\boldsymbol{T}}_h(\boldsymbol{K}) = (\cos\theta, \sin\theta, 0)$ and $\theta = \theta(\boldsymbol{K})$ as given by (9). Results for the fitting error and a comparison with the one-forms are shown in Fig. 4. The results indicate that the one-form model is able to capture the GHM's parameterization accurately and that it consistently yields lower errors. Note that in addition to an improved fitting method – continuous rather than discrete – we estimate heart wall normals slightly differently than is done in the original work [12]. Consequently, our GHM parameters estimates are more precise and still support the overall shape distribution reported. From here on, we will therefore consider the GHM using its one-form approximation, which we refer to as the *ghm-form*.

The following section introduces a differential model, the *homeoid*, that can also be expressed using a subset of the one-forms, and has the advantage that it is intuitively connected to the large-scale structure of the heart by enforcing the ellipsoidal topology of the local tangent plane.

3.4 The Generalized Helicoid on an Ellipsoid is a Homeoid

The calculations of the previous section can be applied to model fibers with smoothly varying fiber orientations, such that the differential operations are well defined. Motivated by evidence that fibers wind around the heart wall while remaining approximately parallel to the tangent plane to the wall at each location [1,5,9], we now consider a specialization to the case where the fibers lie locally on *thin homeoids*, which are shells composed of two concentric and similar ellipsoids.

As introduced in Section 2, the Maurer-Cartan form has only 3 independent one-forms: $c_{TN}\langle\cdot\rangle$, $c_{TB}\langle\cdot\rangle$, and $c_{NB}\langle\cdot\rangle$ with 3 associated spatial degrees of freedom, for a total of 9 possible combinations. Working with the intuition given in Section 3.2 of each c_{ijk}, this is a convenient space to develop models of fiber geometry. For example, in Section 3.3 we showed that for the GHM only $c_{TN}\langle\boldsymbol{T}\rangle$, $c_{TN}\langle\boldsymbol{N}\rangle$, and $c_{TN}\langle\boldsymbol{B}\rangle$ are non-zero. Based on a general description of the cardiac fiber architecture as collections of fibers that i) vary smoothly and ii) are locally constrained to the tangent space of smooth and orthogonal surfaces to the heart wall, the following contractions of 1-forms must occur:

$$c_{TN}\langle\boldsymbol{T}\rangle = \alpha, c_{TN}\langle\boldsymbol{N}\rangle = \beta, c_{TN}\langle\boldsymbol{B}\rangle = \gamma, c_{TB}\langle\boldsymbol{B}\rangle \approx 0, c_{NB}\langle\boldsymbol{B}\rangle \approx 0. \quad (10)$$

Locally, these fibers lie in the tangent plane of a thin homeoid. The parameter fields α, β, and γ are introduced as the curvature parameters of the fibers. c_{NBB}

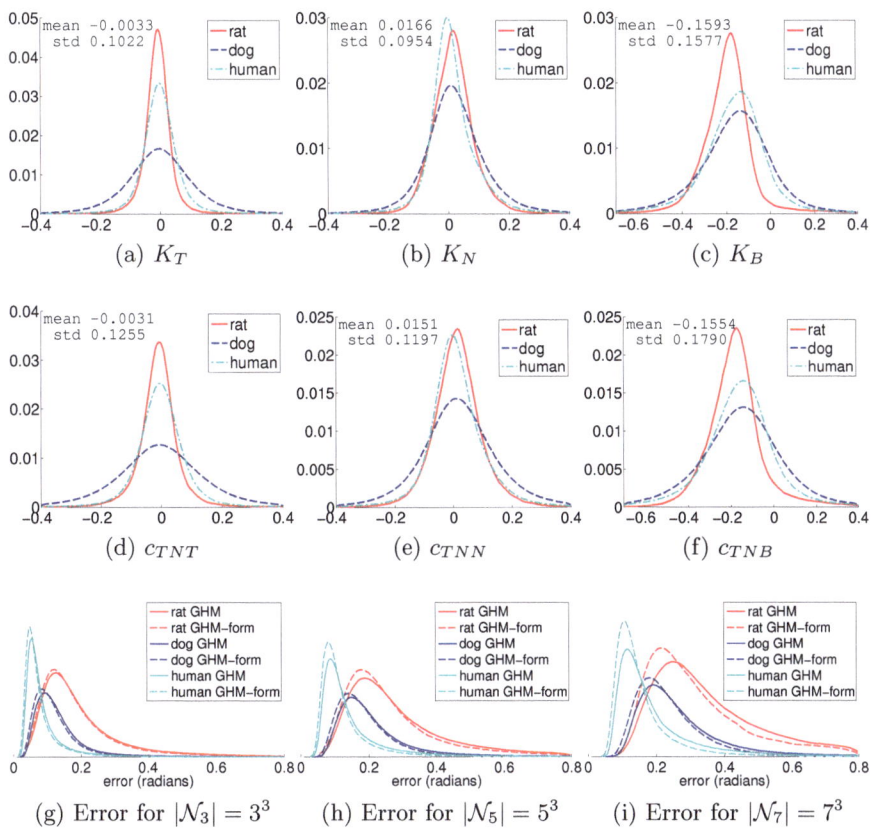

Fig. 4. Rows 1 and 2 compare the one-form approximation to the GHM for the neighborhood $\mathcal{N}_3$. Horizontal axes are given in radians/mm. Row 3 compares the error of each model as a function of $\mathcal{N}_i$.

must be zero otherwise fibers could move in and out of the local tangent plane and our hypothesis ii) would not be satisfied. The remaining contractions specify the shape of the homeoid and we have

$$c_{TB}\langle \boldsymbol{T} \rangle = \frac{1}{\rho_1}, c_{NB}\langle \boldsymbol{N} \rangle = \frac{1}{\rho_2}, c_{TB}\langle \boldsymbol{N} \rangle = 0, c_{NB}\langle \boldsymbol{T} \rangle = 0, \qquad (11)$$

where ρ_1 and ρ_2 are the radii fields of the osculating ellipsoid. Using (7), the model can be employed to extrapolate the orientation of fibers in the neighborhood of a point $\boldsymbol{x}$. Constraints given by (10) and (11) are satisfied by enforcing the nullity of c_{TBN} and c_{TBB} such that we obtain

$$\tilde{\boldsymbol{T}}_h = \boldsymbol{T} + c_{TN}\langle \boldsymbol{h} \rangle \boldsymbol{N} + (c_{TBT}\, \boldsymbol{h} \cdot \boldsymbol{T})\boldsymbol{B}. \qquad (12)$$

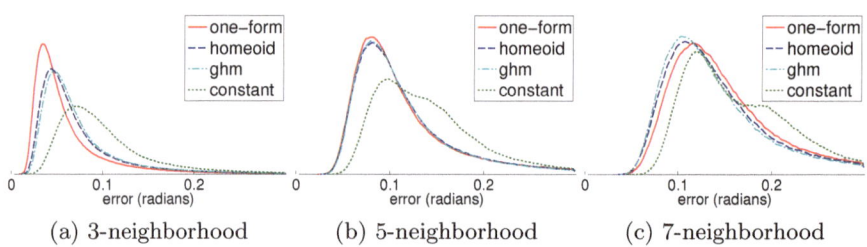

Fig. 5. Human error of fit for the different models analyzed in this paper. Results are shown for isotropic voxel neighbourhoods of size 3^3, 5^3, and 7^3.

4 Model Space Comparison

The analytical models of fiber geometry described so far vary in their parametric complexity. The one-form, homeoid and generalized helicoid models respectively have 9, 5, and 3 parameters. We introduce the *constant* model which will serve as a base-line to which the remaining models can be compared. This parameter-free model simply assumes $\tilde{\boldsymbol{T}}_h = \boldsymbol{T}$ in (7). To compare the different models in terms of their fitting accuracy, we have evaluated each c_{ijk} on the human data set using first-order central differences on 3^3 neighbors. We then used these one-forms to extrapolate each model using (7) and (8) in isotropic neighborhoods $\mathcal{N}_i$ where $|\mathcal{N}_i| = i^3$ for $i = 3, 5, 7, 9$. Fig. 5 shows a distribution of the error of fit in the human dataset for the different models across increasingly large voxel neighborhoods. Error generally increases with neighborhood size but the relative performance of each model is difficult to assess. We therefore fitted a log-normal distribution to each error plot and show the resulting log-normal mode $e^{\mu - \sigma^2}$ and mean $e^{\mu + \frac{1}{2}\sigma^2}$ as a function of neighborhood size in Fig. 6. As expected, the constant model provides an upper bound on the error of fit and is a measure of the smoothness in the data. The one-form model has the lowest error of fit when the neighborhood size reflects the scale at which central differences were computed but behaves poorly for larger neighborhood sizes, which we attribute to local overfitting. On the other hand, the ghm-form and the homeoid models are well-behaved for all neighborhood sizes and differ only slightly from one another. In Section 3.4 we showed that their extrapolated $\tilde{\boldsymbol{T}}_h$ axis only differs by the c_{TBT} one-form which is a measure of the curvature of the heart wall. For the human, this value is small and therefore the two models should be very similar. The rat hearts is smaller in size and therefore has larger per voxel curvature. In this case Table 1 shows that the homeoid is a better fit.

A moving frame in $\mathbb{R}^3$ has 3 degrees of freedom of which 2 are captured by the error vector $\boldsymbol{T} - \tilde{\boldsymbol{T}}_h$: the angular difference $e(\mathcal{N})$ between dMRI orientations and extrapolations specified by (8), and a rotation ϕ about $\boldsymbol{T}$. The third DOF is the rotation ψ of $\boldsymbol{N}$ about $\boldsymbol{T}$. ψ strongly depends on the calculations of $\hat{\boldsymbol{B}}$ and much less on the direct measurements. In contrast to the GHM, the homeoid

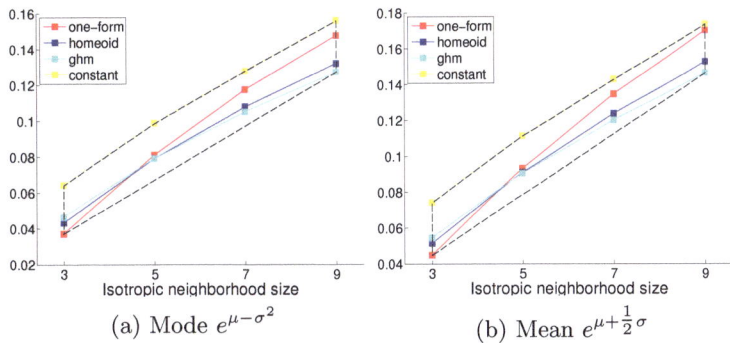

(a) Mode $e^{\mu - \sigma^2}$

(b) Mean $e^{\mu + \frac{1}{2}\sigma}$

Fig. 6. Log-normal fits of the human heart extrapolation error. The mode and mean describe the precision of the fit and the skewness of the distribution.

model considers this angle. However, since we focus on the direct measurement of the fiber geometry given by T, we leave further investigation of ψ as future work. ϕ can be obtained by projecting $T - \tilde{T}_h$ onto the local NB plane and measuring its angle with respect to the frame axis N: $\phi = \arctan \frac{(T - \tilde{T}_h) \cdot B}{(T - \tilde{T}_h) \cdot N}$, i.e., values of $\phi = (0, \pi)$ and $(\frac{\pi}{2}, \frac{3\pi}{2})$ respectively indicate alignment with the frame vectors N and B. Fig. 5 showed the marginal distributions of $e(\boldsymbol{x}, \mathcal{N})$ for various neighborhoods sizes and Fig. 7 shows the marginal distributions of ϕ. In Fig. 8 we show the joint histogram of these marginal distributions for the human heart and for the 4 different models in a 3^3 extrapolation neighborhood. Note that the error along ϕ is negligible when e is small. The spread of ϕ measures the rotation of the local NB plane, which for the one-form model results in overfitting for larger neighborhood sizes.

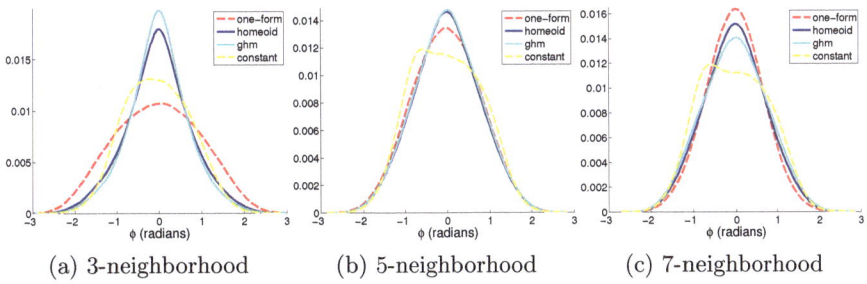

(a) 3-neighborhood   (b) 5-neighborhood   (c) 7-neighborhood

Fig. 7. Rotational angle ϕ of the different models analyzed in this paper for the human heart in isotropic voxel neighbourhoods of size 3^3, 5^3, and 7^3

Table 1. Extrapolation error in radians for each species, differential model, and neighborhood $\mathcal{N}_i$ from the mode $e^{\mu-\sigma^2}$ and the mean $e^{\mu+(1/2)\sigma^2}$ of log-normal fits. The model with the best performance is selected as the one that minimizes the mode (and the mean to resolve multiplicity), and is highlighted for each $\mathcal{N}_i$.

$|\mathcal{N}_i|$		Rat (mode, mean)	Dog (mode, mean)	Human (mode, mean)
3^3	one-form	**0.093, 0.113**	**0.076, 0.092**	**0.039, 0.054**
	homeoid	0.094, 0.115	0.085, 0.102	0.046, 0.063
	ghm-form	0.099, 0.118	0.089, 0.106	0.050, 0.066
	constant	0.163, 0.181	0.110, 0.128	0.070, 0.090
5^3	one-form	0.146, 0.175	0.157, 0.181	0.085, 0.112
	homeoid	**0.145, 0.173**	0.152, 0.176	0.085, 0.112
	ghm-form	0.150, 0.175	**0.147, 0.171**	**0.085, 0.111**
	constant	0.271, 0.286	0.156, 0.178	0.109, 0.135
7^3	one-form	0.202, 0.239	0.220, 0.251	0.124, 0.161
	homeoid	**0.200, 0.234**	0.202, 0.235	0.117, 0.152
	ghm-form	0.206, 0.237	0.189, 0.221	**0.114, 0.147**
	constant	0.389, 0.402	**0.189, 0.215**	0.141, 0.172

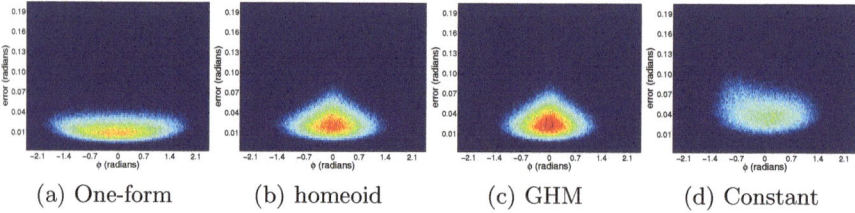

(a) One-form   (b) homeoid   (c) GHM   (d) Constant

Fig. 8. Joint histogram of the angular errors e and ϕ in the human heart for different models. Results are shown for an isotropic 3^3 neighborhood with minimum values colored in dark blue and maximum values in dark red.

In summary, we have shown that the one-form model yields the lowest fitting error for small neighborhoods and that the homeoid model is as accurate as or better than the GHM depending on the per-voxel curvature of the heart wall.

5   Conclusion

We have presented a framework for analyzing cardiac fiber geometry based on the method of Maurer-Cartan's moving frames. Using this framework we were able to make predictions of the differential geometry of fibers that corroborate previously reported values. We proposed the homeoid as an extension to the GHM for characterizing cardiac geometry. We demonstrated that this model a) lowers the error of fit across multiple species, b) offers a trade-off between the geometrical comprehensiveness of the complete one-form model and the minimality of the GHM, and finally c) incorporates two important parameters, $\rho_1 = c_{TBT}^{-1}$

and $\rho_2 = c_{TBN}^{-1}$ which measure the curvature of the local tangent plane. Our framework provides intuitive tools for reasoning about the differential geometry of cardiac muscle and opens up many possibilities. Further work includes exploring the behavior of cardiac fibers in their one-form description, possibly across a greater number of species, for assessing the existence of cardiac sheets and uncovering descriptors of heart pathology and fiber remodeling. Future work also includes the consideration of higher-order and scale-space approaches to differentiation, the study of different cardiac frame fields, and a study of the relative information content stored in individual one-forms.

References

1. Streeter, D.D.: Gross morphology and fiber geometry of the heart. In: Berne, R.M., Sperelakis, N. (eds.) Handbook of Physiology, Section 2. The Heart, pp. 61–112. Williams and Wilkins, New York (1979)
2. Peskin, C.S.: Mathematical aspects of heart physiology. Technical report, Courant Institute of Math. Sciences, New York University, New York, NY, USA (1975)
3. Horowitz, A., Perl, M., Sideman, S.: Geodesics as a mechanically optimal fiber geometry for the left ventricle. Basic. Res. Cardiol. 88(suppl. 2), 67–74 (1993)
4. Geerts, L., Bovendeerd, P., Nicolay, K., Arts, T.: Characterization of the normal cardiac myofiber field in goat measured with mr-diffusion tensor imaging. Am. J. Physiol.: Heart and Circ. Physiol. 283, H139–H145 (2002)
5. Beg, M.F., Helm, P.A., McVeigh, E.M., Miller, M.I., Winslow, R.L.: Computational cardiac anatomy using mri. Magn. Reson. Med. 52, 1167–1174 (2004)
6. Chen, J., Liu, W., Zhang, H., Lacy, L., Yang, X., Song, S.K., Wickline, W.A., Yu, X.: Regional ventricular wall thickening reflects changes in cardiac fiber and sheet structure during contraction: quantification with diffusion tensor mri. Am. J. Physiol.: Heart and Circ. Physiol. 289, H1898–H1907 (2005)
7. Streeter, D., Bassett, D.: An engineering analysis of myocardial fiber orientation in pig's left ventricle in systole. The Anatomical Record 155(4), 503–511 (2005)
8. LeGrice, I.J., Smaill, B.H., Chai, L.Z., Edgar, S.G., Gavin, J.B., Hunter, P.J.: Ventricular myocyte arrangement and connective tissue architecture in the dog. Am. J. Physiol.: Heart and Circ. Physiol. 269 (1995)
9. Rohmer, D., Sitek, A., Gullberg, G.T.: Reconstruction and visualization of fiber and laminar structure in the normal human heart from ex vivo diffusion tensor magnetic resonance imaging (dtmri) data. Invest. Radiol. 42(11), 777–789 (2007)
10. Lombaert, H., Peyrat, J.-M., Croisille, P., Rapacchi, S., Fanton, L., Clarysse, P., Delingette, H., Ayache, N.: Statistical analysis of the human cardiac fiber architecture from DT-MRI. In: Metaxas, D.N., Axel, L. (eds.) FIMH 2011. LNCS, vol. 6666, pp. 171–179. Springer, Heidelberg (2011)
11. Ben-Shahar, O., Zucker, S.W.: The perceptual organization of texture flow: A contextual inference approach. IEEE TPAMI 25(4) (2003)
12. Savadjiev, P., Strijkers, G.J., Bakermans, A.J., Piuze, E., Zucker, S.W., Siddiqi, K.: Heart wall myofibers are arranged in minimal surfaces to optimize organ function. Proc. Natl. Acad. Sci. USA 109(24), 9248–9253 (2012)
13. Koenderink, J.: Solid shape, vol. 2. Cambridge Univ. Press (1990)

Structural Brain Network Constrained Neuroimaging Marker Identification for Predicting Cognitive Functions

De Wang[1], Feiping Nie[1], Heng Huang[1,*], Jingwen Yan[2], Shannon L. Risacher[2], Andrew J. Saykin[2], Li Shen[2,*], and for the Alzheimer's Disease Neuroimaging Initiative[**]

[1] Computer Science and Engineering, University of Texas at Arlington, Arlington, TX, USA
{wangdelp,feipingnie}@gmail.com,heng@uta.edu
[2] Department of Radiology and Imaging Sciences, Indiana University School of Medicine, Indianapolis, IN, USA
jingyan@umail.iu.edu,{srisache,asaykin,shenli}@iu.edu

Abstract. Neuroimaging markers have been widely used to predict the cognitive functions relevant to the progression of Alzheimer's disease (AD). Most previous studies identify the imaging markers without considering the brain structural correlations between neuroimaging measures. However, many neuroimaging markers interrelate and work together to reveal the cognitive functions, such that these relevant markers should be selected together as the phenotypic markers. To solve this problem, in this paper, we propose a novel network constrained feature selection (NCFS) model to identify the neuroimaging markers guided by the structural brain network, which is constructed by the sparse representation method such that the interrelations between neuroimaging features are encoded into probabilities. Our new methods are evaluated by the MRI and AV45-PET data from ADNI-GO and ADNI-2 (Alzheimer's Disease Neuroimaging Initiative). In all cognitive function prediction tasks, our new NCFS method outperforms other state-of-the-art regression approaches. Meanwhile, we show that the new method can select the correlated imaging markers, which are ignored by the competing approaches.

Keywords: Neuroimaging Marker Identification, Brain Network Based Feature Selection, Correlated Marker Selection, Imaging Genetics.

---

[*] Corresponding author.
[**] Data used in preparation of this article were obtained from the Alzheimer's Disease Neuroimaging Initiative (ADNI) database (adni.loni.ucla.edu). As such, the investigators within the ADNI contributed to the design and implementation of ADNI and/or provided data but did not participate in analysis or writing of this report. A complete listing of ADNI investigators can be found at: http://adni.loni.ucla.edu/wp-content/uploads/how_to_apply/ADNI_Acknowledgement_List.pdf .

J.C. Gee et al. (Eds.): IPMI 2013, LNCS 7917, pp. 536–547, 2013.
© Springer-Verlag Berlin Heidelberg 2013

1   Introduction

Alzheimer's disease (AD) is the most common dementia that has acquired tremendous research attention due to its wide range of effects and mysterious underlying mechanisms. AD is a neurodegenerative disorder characterized by progressive impairment of cognitive functions, and thus it is crucial to understand how structural and functional changes in brain can influence cognitve performance. As a powerful tool for capturing neurodegenerative process in AD progression, neuroimaging data have been widely studied for classification of disease status [9,3] and more recently for prediction of disease-relevant cognitive scores [13,10].

Regression analyses were commonly used to predict cognitive scores from imaging measures. In [13], stepwise regression was performed in a pairwise way to associate the Magnetic Resonance Imaging (MRI) and FDG-PET (Positron Emission Tomography) measures to memory scores. Because the univariate model was used in this study, their results neglected the interrelated structures within both imaging and clinical data. As a special case of a sparse linear model, the relevance vector regression method was applied to relate the Voxel-Based Morphometry (VBM) features to selected clinical scores [10]. This approach was connected to the combination of Bayesian model and least absolute shrinkage and selection operator (LASSO) model [12]. Another study [14] used the structured sparsity-inducing norm, $\ell_{2,1}$-norm, to select neuroimaging markers that are important to most prediction tasks. Later work [15,16] presented joint sparse multitask models to identify the imaging markers related to both cognitive scores and outcomes. In most recent work, we introduced the high-order low-rank sparse learning models to select the longitudinal neuroimaging markers associated to genetic basis [17] or cognitive scores [18].

Most existing studies selected the neuroimaging features totally based on their influences on the prediction results, *i.e.* in a model-driven way. However, from the functional brain circuitry point of view, many neuroimaging markers interrelate with each other and work together to reveal the brain cognitive functions. Thus, it is desired to explore and utilize such interrelation structures and select these important and structurally correlated features together.

In this paper, we propose a new brain network constrained feature selection (NCFS) method to naturally integrate the structural brain network into cognitive function prediction model. As a result, our selected imaging markers not only have prediction power, but also indicate the feature interrelations in structural brain network. We apply the new method to analyze the MRI, AV45-PET and cognitive data from the Alzheimer's Disease Neuroimaging Initiative (ADNI) database. The neuroimaging markers are identified to predict the cognitive scores from five sets of different neuropsychological tests.

2   Structural Brain Network Construction Using A New Sparse Representation Model

To understand and characterize the underlying architectures of complex brain networks, previous neuroscience studies utilized the Pearson correlation coefficients of cortical thickness measurements from MRI to create the network of anatomical connections [2,6]. Thus, given the neuroimaging measures, we can create the structural brain network using their correlation coefficients. In this constructed brain network, each vertex represents one neuroimaging feature and each edge between two vertices encodes their correlation. However, this simple correlation analysis may not effectively construct the brain anatomical structure. To solve this problem, we propose a new sparse representation model to construct an effective structural brain network among neuroimaging measures.

Denote the neuroimaging features are $F = [f_1, f_2, \cdots, f_d] \in \Re^{n \times d}$, where n is the number of subject and d is the number of features. Our goal is to construct a connectivity matrix A, in which $A_{i,j}$ encodes the correlation between features f_i and f_j. A popular method to compute A is using the Gaussian kernel function. The major disadvantage of this method is that the hyper-parameter σ in the Gaussian kernel function is very sensitive and is difficult to tune in practice.

Recently, as an approximate formulation for Gaussian graphical modeling [7], the sparse coding method was applied to compute the similarity matrix A. The similarity vector α_i includes the similarities between the i-th feature and the rest features, and is calculated by the sparse representation as follows:

$$\min_{\alpha_i} ||F^{-i}\alpha_i - f_i||_2^2 + \lambda||\alpha_i||_1, \tag{1}$$

where $F^{-i} = [f_1, \cdots, f_{i-1}, f_{i+1}, \cdots, f_d] \in \Re^{n \times (d-1)}$. However, the above model is not shift-invariant. We propose to impose two new constraints: $\alpha_i^T 1 = 1$ and $\alpha_i \geq 0$, such that $||(F^{-i} + t1^T)\alpha_i - (f_i + t)||_2^2 = ||F^{-i}\alpha_i - x_i||_2^2$. More important, based on these two new constraints, the learned similarities in α_i can be interpreted as probabilities. Interestingly, the new constraints make the second term be constant. So the sparse representation model is to solve:

$$\min_{\alpha_i \geq 0, \alpha_i^T 1 = 1} ||F^{-i}\alpha_i - f_i||_2^2. \tag{2}$$

Because the parameter λ is canceled, our new model doesn't require any parameter tuning and is suitable for practical applications. Our new objective is a non-smooth convex problem. We use the accelerated projected gradient method to solve this problem.

3   Structural Brain Network Constrained Neuroimaging Feature Learning

To identify biologically meaningful markers, we integrate the structural brain network into cognitive function prediction model. The structural brain network can constrain and guide the machine learning model to identify important and correlated biomarkers, which potentially play the key roles in memory and cognition circuitry. To predict cognitive scores, we use regression methods, but it is challenging to incorporate the network connectivity matrix A into a regression model. To solve this problem, we introduce a novel structural brain network constrained feature selection (NCFS) method with new optimization algorithm.

To select the correlated features, in the regression model, if the i-th and j-th features have high similarity in A, their coefficient vectors w^i and w^j ($w^i \in \Re^{c \times 1}$ is the transpose of the i-th row of parameter matrix W) should be both large or both small, $i.e.$, similar to each other. Because the similarity vector α_i encodes the similarity between the i-th feature and other features, the coefficient vector w^i and the rest coefficient vectors $W^{-i} = [w^1, ..., w^{i-1}, w^{i+1}, ..., w^d] \in \Re^{c \times (d-1)}$ should also have similar sparse representation with α_i. Thus, we should minimize:

$$\sum_{i=1}^{d} ||W^{-i}\alpha_i - w^i||^2 = Tr(W^T(I - A)(I - A)^T W), \tag{3}$$

where $A = [\tilde{\alpha}_1, ..., \tilde{\alpha}_d] \in \Re^{d \times d}$, in which $\tilde{\alpha}_i \in \Re^{d \times 1}$ is an augmented $\alpha_i \in \Re^{(d-1) \times 1}$ with the i-th element as 0.

Denoting $L = (I - A)^T(I - A)$, our new NCFS objective is to solve:

$$\min_{W,b} ||X^T W + 1b^T - Y||_F^2 + \gamma_1 Tr(W^T LW) + \gamma_2 ||W||_{2,1}. \tag{4}$$

In our new objective, the first regularization term imposes the structural brain network constraint, and the second regularization term is the structured sparse mixed norm to select features which are important to all prediction tasks. Thus, the features identified by our NCFS model are important to all cognitive functions prediction and also correlated in the structural brain network.

Taking the derivative w.r.t. b and setting to zero, we have $b = \frac{1}{n}Y^T 1 - \frac{1}{n}W^T X1$. Thus, our objective becomes:

$$\min_{W} ||CX^T W - CY||_F^2 + \gamma_1 Tr(W^T LW) + \gamma_2 ||W||_{2,1}, \tag{5}$$

where $C = I - \frac{1}{n}11^T$ is the centering matrix. This new objective is a non-smooth convex problem with two regularization terms. We will derive an efficient algorithm to optimize the new objective.

3.1   New Optimization Algorithm to Solve Problem (5)

By taking the derivative of Eq. (5) w.r.t. W and setting to zero, we have:

$$XCX^T W - XCY + (\gamma_1 L + \gamma_2 P)W = 0, \tag{6}$$

where P is a diagonal matrix, the i-th diagonal element is $\frac{1}{2||w^i||_2}$. Eq. (6) leads to the solution W as:

$$W = (XCX^T + \gamma_1 L + \gamma_2 P)^{-1}XCY. \tag{7}$$

Note that P is not a constant and depends on the unknown W. We propose an iterative algorithm to solve W based on Eq. (7). As initialization, we guess a

Initialize $W \in \Re^{d \times c}$
repeat
    1. Calculate diagonal matrix P, the i-th diagonal element is $\frac{1}{2||w^i||_2}$.
    2. Update W by $W = (XCX^T + \gamma_1 L + \gamma_2 P)^{-1} XCY$
until *Converges*

Algorithm 1. Optimization algorithm to solve problem (5)

solution W, then we calculate P with current W and update W with Eq. (7). The detailed algorithm is summarized in Algorithm 1.

If Algorithm 1 converges, then the converged solution W satisfies Eq. (6). Since problem (5) is convex, the converged solution W is the global optimal solution to problem (5). In next subsection, we will prove that Algorithm 1 indeed converges.

3.2 Convergence Analysis on Our New Algorithm

For the Algorithm 1, we have the following theorem:

Theorem 1. *In each iteration, Algorithm 1 will decrease the objective value of problem (5) till the algorithm converges.*

Proof: In the Step 2 of Algorithm 1, we denote the updated solution W as $\tilde{W}$. According to Step 2, we have

$$\tilde{W} = \arg\min_{W} ||CX^T W - CY||_F^2 + Tr(W^T(\gamma_1 L + \gamma_2 P)W). \qquad (8)$$

Since $\tilde{W}$ is the optimal solution in Eq. (8), we have

$$||CX^T\tilde{W} - CY||_F^2 + Tr(\tilde{W}^T(\gamma_1 L + \gamma_2 P)\tilde{W}) \le ||CX^T W - CY||_F^2 + Tr(W^T(\gamma_1 L + \gamma_2 P)W)$$

According to the definition of P in Step 1 of Algorithm 1, we have

$$\begin{aligned} ||CX^T\tilde{W} - CY||_F^2 + \gamma_1 Tr(\tilde{W}^T L\tilde{W}) + \gamma_2 \sum_{i=1}^{d} \frac{||\tilde{w}^i||_2^2}{2||w^i||_2} \\ \le ||CX^T W - CY||_F^2 + \gamma_1 Tr(W^T LW) + \gamma_2 \sum_{i=1}^{d} \frac{||w^i||_2^2}{2||w^i||_2} \end{aligned} \qquad (9)$$

Based on a inequality $||\tilde{w}||_2 - \frac{||\tilde{w}||_2^2}{2||w||_2} \le ||w||_2 - \frac{||w||_2^2}{2||w||_2}$ for any vectors w and $\tilde{w}$, we have

$$\gamma_2 \sum_{i=1}^{d} ||\tilde{w}^i||_2 - \gamma_2 \sum_{i=1}^{d} \frac{||\tilde{w}^i||_2^2}{2||w^i||_2} \le \gamma_2 \sum_{i=1}^{d} ||w^i||_2 - \gamma_2 \sum_{i=1}^{d} \frac{||w^i||_2^2}{2||w^i||_2} \qquad (10)$$

Summing over Eq. (9) and Eq. (10) on both sides, we arrive at

$$\begin{aligned} ||CX^T\tilde{W} - CY||_F^2 + \gamma_1 Tr(\tilde{W}^T L\tilde{W}) + \gamma_2||\tilde{W}||_{2,1} \\ \le ||CX^T W - CY||_F^2 + \gamma_1 Tr(W^T LW) + \gamma_2||W||_{2,1}. \end{aligned} \qquad (11)$$

Table 1. Participant characteristics

Category	HC	MCI	AD
Number	105	237	18
Gender(M/F)	53/52	137/100	11/7
Handness(R/L)	98/7	208/29	16/2
Baseline age (mean±std)	74.2±5.7	71.1±7.5	76.2±11.0
Education (mean±std)	16.4±2.6	16.2±2.6	15.3±2.7

Thus, our algorithm will decrease the objective value of problem (5) in each iteration till it converges.   □

Because the objective value of problem (5) has a lower bound 0, the algorithm will converge. As mentioned before, the algorithm will converge to the global optimal solution of problem (5).

4   Experimental Results and Discussions

4.1   Neuroimaging and Cognition Data Descriptions

We have applied and evaluated the proposed new models on the neuroimaging and cognitive data downloaded from the ADNI database (adni.loni.ucla.edu). One goal of ADNI has been to test whether serial MRI, PET, other biological markers, and clinical and neuropsychological assessment can be combined to measure the progression of mild cognitive impairment (MCI) and early AD. For up-to-date information, see www.adni-info.org.

We downloaded corrected 3T structural MRI scans [4], pre-processed AV-45 PET scans [5], and cognitive data from the ADNI website. Our analysis focused on the baseline MRI, AV45-PET and cognitive data at the ADNI-GO/2 phase. All the participants with a baseline diagnosis were involved in the study, including 105 health control (HC), 237 MCI and 18 AD participants (Table 1).

VBM in SPM8 [1] was applied to preprocess structural MRI scans, as previously described [8]. Briefly, scans were aligned to a T1-weighted template image, segmented into gray matter (GM), white matter (WM) and cerebrospinal fluid (CSF) maps, normalized to MNI space, and smoothed with an 8mm FWHM kernel. Besides, all scans were also processed through automated segmentation and parcellation using Freesurfer version 5.1.

AV-45 PET scans were pre-processed using techniques identical to the previous techniques for processing ADNI PiB PET scans [5]. Standardized uptake value ratio (SUVR) AV-45 PET images were created by intensity normalizing to a mean cerebellar GM region of interest (ROI). Downloaded scans were co-registered to the structural MRI scan from the corresponding visit and normalized to MNI space using SPM8, as described in [11]. Mean AV-45 measures were calculated for ten ROIs, including frontal lobe, parietal lobe, temporal lobe,Limbic lobe, occipital lobe, anterior cingulate, poster cingulate, precuneus, and cerebellum. In addition, a summarized measure were calculated based on the ROIs that best differentiate AD and HC in previous experiment.

Table 2. Comparisons of cognitive score prediction performance of five methods using the average RMSEs (mean+std)

		FLU	ADAS	TRAILS	RAVLT	MMSE
VBM	NCFS	**5.0772±0.6240**	**6.2277±0.5672**	**41.8300±2.7196**	**5.4153±0.2972**	1.8822±0.0821
	$\ell_{2,1}$	5.0819±0.6452	6.3236±0.6508	43.3156±2.9257	5.4931±0.3308	1.8657±0.112
	Lasso	5.0820±0.6452	6.3239±0.6505	42.5423±2.2569	5.4760±0.3057	1.8657±0.1112
	Ridge	5.1109±0.6410	6.2382±0.5833	42.1515±2.8509	5.4517±0.2611	**1.8437±0.0743**
	MVLR	5.8757±0.6087	7.0166±0.5415	48.6541±3.9337	6.2138±0.3610	2.1477±0.0920
FS	NCFS	**4.7605±0.5210**	**5.8323±0.3874**	**40.3119±3.3601**	**5.2145±0.3722**	**1.7694±0.1230**
	$\ell_{2,1}$	4.7608±0.4870	5.8441±0.4006	40.9824±3.3570	5.2553±0.33593	1.7719±0.1261
	Lasso	4.7611±0.4869	5.8443±0.4007	40.9353±3.6106	5.2530±0.3814	1.7719±0.1262
	Ridge	4.8796±0.5050	5.8887±0.4198	40.7526±3.0069	5.2245±0.3180	1.7830±0.1017
	MVLR	5.6263±0.3744	6.6088±0.2690	49.0891±2.9285	6.0465±0.4743	2.0364±0.1004
AV45	NCFS	**5.0983±0.5416**	**6.5406±0.2506**	**41.0382±3.2921**	**5.6701±0.5030**	**1.8664±0.1170**
	$\ell_{2,1}$	5.1015±0.5557	6.5554±0.2456	41.9643±3.1609	5.7316±0.6920	1.8673±0.1241
	Lasso	5.1015±0.5557	6.5554±0.2456	41.8831±3.2199	5.7454±0.6409	1.8673±0.1241
	Ridge	5.1448±0.5889	6.5491±0.2529	42.0099±3.2689	5.8452±0.6344	1.8776±0.1291
	MVLR	5.1907±0.6372	6.5793±0.2652	42.9643±3.3477	5.9513±0.7656	1.9226±0.1679

Overall, we had 90 VBM measures, 95 Freesurfer measures, and eleven AV45 measures for each subject. Based on these imaging measures, we performed different regression models to predict five types of cognitive scores: (1) Alzheimer's Disease Assessment Scale-Cognitive test (ADAS); (2) Rey Auditory Verbal Learning Test (RAVLT); (3) FLUENCY; (4) Mini-Mental State Examination (MMSE); and (5) Trail Making Test (TRAILS).

4.2   Experimental Setting

We compared our new method (NCFS) with several competing regression models: multivariate linear regression (MVLR), ridge regression, structured sparsity-inducing norm regularized regression [14] (denoted as $\ell_{2,1}$), and Lasso regularized regression. The evaluation metric used was the standard root mean square error (RMSE), which has been widely used in performance evaluation of regression analysis. For each method, five-fold cross-validation was performed to obtain the average RMSE. In each of five trials, an internal five-fold cross-validation was done to tune the parameters using grid search for different methods. The range of each parameter varied from 10^{-5} to 10^5. The reported results were the best results of each method with the optimal parameter.

4.3   Cognitive Functions Prediction Performance Comparisons

The cognitive scores prediction results were reported in Table 2. The proposed method NCFS consistently outperformed other methods by predicting five cognitive scores more accurately with lower RMSEs. The key difference between NCFS and other methods was that the NCFS method utilized the correlation between features by incorporating the structural brain network as the regularization term, whereas other methods tended to select individual feature and ignored other less important but correlated features. Thus, NCFS had a

Table 3. Average correlation values of top ranked features in structural brain network (mean+std) constructed by the sparse representation model

		Top 5	Top 10	Top 20			Top 2
VBM	NCFS	**0.0508±0.0472**	**0.0282±0.0179**	**0.0200±0.0070**			**0.1980±0.1182**
	$\ell_{2,1}$	0.0227±0.0078	0.0119±0.0097	0.0126±0.0037			0.1342±0.1225
	Lasso	0.0240±0.0083	0.0142±0.0074	0.0131±0.0039	AV45		0.1342±0.1225
	Ridge	0.0491±0.0298	0.0277±0.0146	0.0161±0.0047			0.1533±0.1453
	MVLR	0.0196±0.0200	0.0156±0.0093	0.0157±0.0032			0.1395±0.1278
FS	NCFS	**0.0625±0.0332**	**0.0334±0.0165**	0.0196±0.0057			
	$\ell_{2,1}$	0.0299±0.0359	0.0237±0.0112	0.0153±0.0060			
	Lasso	0.0269±0.0311	0.0227±0.0113	0.0131±0.0039	–		–
	Ridge	0.0395±0.0331	0.0258±0.0147	**0.0217±0.0080**			
	MVLR	0.0278±0.0316	0.0207±0.0132	0.0162±0.0044			

built-in mechanism to select structural correlated features which acted together to impact human cognitive functions. MVLR had the largest RMSEs than all other methods, because it was prone to overfit the training data. Table 2 also indicated that FreeSurfer measures were more powerful for predicting cognitive performance than VBM and AV45 measures.

We also evaluated the average correlation values of top ranked features in all methods. For each method, we extracted top 5, 10 and 20 features for FreeSurfer and VBM measures. Because AV45 only had 11 features, we selected top 2 features (*i.e.* top 20% of all features) for each method. The correlation of features was computed from the structural brain network obtained by the sparse representation model, which reflected the similarity between features. Table 3 showed the average correlations of top ranked features by different methods. In most case, top ranked features by NCFS method were more correlated than that of other methods. The correlations of top ranked features in $\ell_{2,1}$ and Lasso approaches were relatively low because they tended to select a single feature from a group of correlated features. NCFS selected more (correlated) features in structural brain network, which helped achieve better prediction performance.

4.4   Imaging Markers Analysis and Discussions

Figure 1 visualized the resulting structural brain network of 95 FreeSurfer measures as a connectivity matrix. Indices 1-7 corresponded to seven unilateral measures, which were listed in blue (from BrainStem to CSF) on the x axis of Figures 2. Indices 8-51 (52-95) corresponded to 44 bilateral measures on the left (right) hemisphere, which were listed in black (from AccumVol to TransvTemporal) on the x axis of Figures 2. The white lines separated the unilateral and bilateral measures as well as left and right measures. It was obvious that the left and right hemispheres demonstrated a very similar pattern.

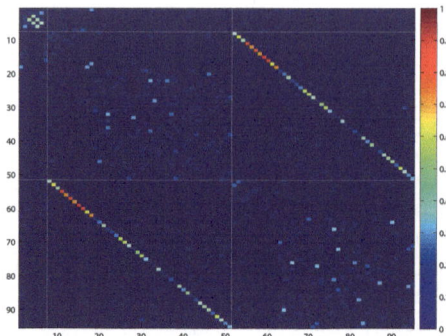

Fig. 1. The resulting structural brain network of 95 freesurfer measures is shown as a connectivity matrix. Indices 1-7 correspond to seven unilateral measures, which are listed in blue (from BrainStem to CSF) on the x axis of Figure 2. Indices 8-51 (52-95) correspond to 44 bilateral measures on the left (right) hemisphere, which are listed in black (from AccumVol to TransvTemporal) on the x axis of Figure 2.

The results of linear regression and ridge regression were not sparse, making it difficult for biomarker identification. Thus, here we only compared the feature selection results between NCFS and $\ell_{2,1}$. Both NCFS and $\ell_{2,1}$ were sparse models that were able to identify a compact set of relevant imaging markers and to explain the underlying brain structural changes related to cognitive status. Shown in Figure 2 were the maps of regression weights for predicting various cognitive scores (from top to bottom: Fluency, ADAS, TRAIL, RAVLT and MMSE) using the FreeSurfer measures. Average regression weights of 5-fold cross-validation trials were plotted for NCFS (the even panels) and $\ell_{2,1}$ (the odd panels). In each panel, the odd (even) rows showed the weights from left (right) hemisphere. Note that the first seven measures (from BrainStem to CSF, colored in blue) were unilateral, and thus their left and right measures were set to be the same. Blue indicated negative correlation, while red indicated positive correlation. The bigger the magnitude of a coefficient was, the more important its imaging measure was in predicting the corresponding cognitive score.

Clearly, $\ell_{2,1}$ yielded more sparse patterns than NCFS. However, for highly correlated features, $\ell_{2,1}$ tended to identify one and ignore the others. This was inadequate for yielding a biologically meaningful interpretation. In contrast, NCFS did seem to work in terms of structuring the identified patterns. For example, the hippocampal volume and amygdala volume were correlated (Fig. 1). They were selected together by NCFS for predicting ADAS and RAVLT scores, while $\ell_{2,1}$ only selected hippocampal volume in this case. In addition, bilateral measures of the same structure were often highly correlated. The NCFS yielded a more symmetric pattern than $\ell_{2,1}$ in many cases.

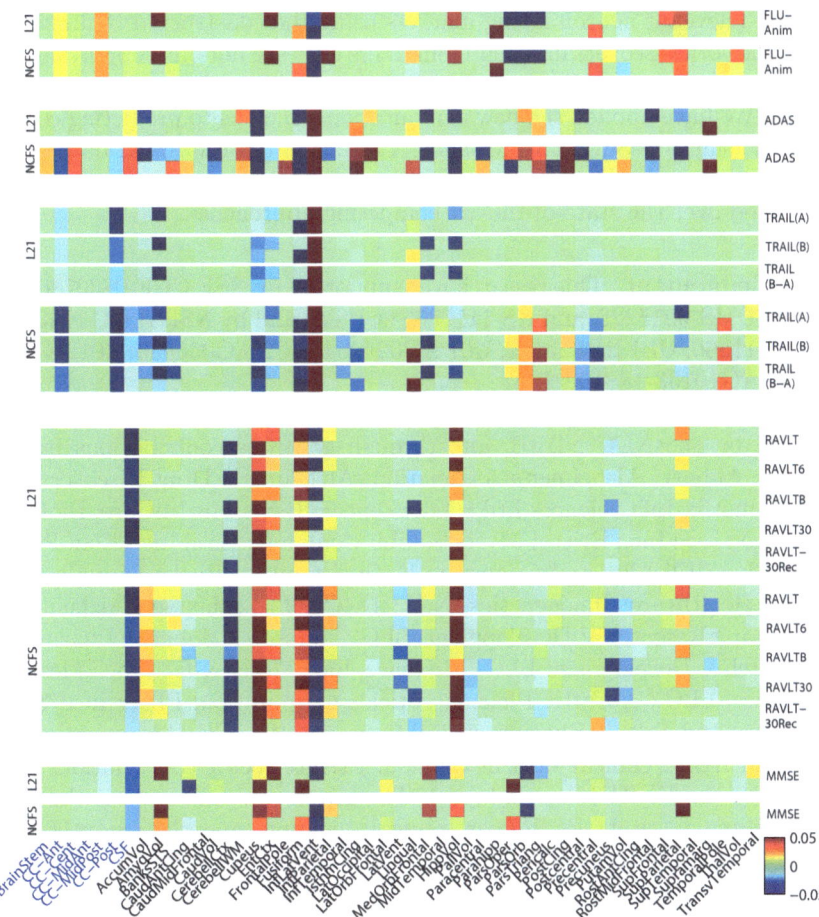

Fig. 2. Heat maps of regression weights for predicting cognitive scores (from top to bottom: Fluency, ADAS, TRAIL, RAVLT and MMSE) from FreeSurfer measures using NCFS (the even panels) and $\ell_{2,1}$ (the odd panels) methods. In each panel, the odd (even) rows show the weights from left (right) hemisphere. Note that the first seven measures (from BrainStem to CSF, colored in blue) are unilateral, and thus their left and right measures are set to be the same. Blue indicates negative correlation, while red indicates positive correlation.

Finally, the identified patterns were in fact expected based on our prior knowledge. For example, RAVLT measured verbal learning memory; and the identified regions included hippocampus, fusiform, entorhinal cortex, and other regions relevant to learning and memory.

5   Conclusions

In this paper, we have proposed two new machine learning models, one for constructing a structural brain network and the other for identifying cognition-releveant neuroimaging markers using the constructed brain network. This framework discovers imaging biomarkers that are not only important to the cognitive outcomes but also interrelating with each other in the structural brain network. We have applied the new computational models to predicting cognitive outcomes using FreeSurfer, VBM, and AV45 data from the ADNI database. All the empirical results have demonstrated consistently improved performance of our method over the state-of-the-art competing approaches.

Acknowledgement. This research was supported by NSF CCF-0830780, CCF-0917274, DMS-0915228, and IIS-1117965 at UTA; and by NSF IIS-1117335, NIH R01 LM011360, UL1 RR025761, U01 AG024904, RC2 AG036535, R01 AG19771, and P30 AG10133-18S1 at IU.

Data used for this project was funded by the ADNI (U01AG024904). ADNI is funded by the NIA, NIBIB, and through generous contributions from the following: Abbott; Alzheimer's Association; Alzheimer's Drug Discovery Foundation; Amorfix Life Sciences Ltd.; AstraZeneca; Bayer HealthCare; BioClinica, Inc.; Biogen Idec Inc.; Bristol-Myers Squibb Company; Eisai Inc.; Elan Pharmaceuticals Inc.; Eli Lilly and Company; F. Hoffmann-La Roche Ltd; Genentech, Inc.; GE Healthcare; Innogenetics, N.V.; IXICO Ltd.; Janssen Alzheimer Immunotherapy Research & Development, LLC.; Johnson & Johnson Pharmaceutical Research & Development LLC.; Medpace, Inc.; Merck & Co., Inc.; Meso Scale Diagnostics, LLC.; Novartis Pharmaceuticals Corporation; Pfizer Inc.; Servier; Synarc Inc.; and Takeda Pharmaceutical Company. The CIHR is providing funds to support ADNI clinical sites in Canada. Private sector contributions are facilitated by the FNIH (www.fnih.org). The grantee organization is the Northern California Institute for Research and Education, and the study is coordinated by the Alzheimer's Disease Cooperative Study at UCSD. ADNI data are disseminated by LONI at UCLA.

References

1. Ashburner, J., Friston, K.: Voxel-based morphometry–the methods. Neuroimage 11(6), 805–821 (2000)
2. Chen, Z.J., He, Y., Rosa-Neto, P., Germann, J., Evans, A.C.: Revealing modular architecture of human brain structural networks by using cortical thickness from mri. Cerebral Cortex 18, 2374–2381 (2008)
3. Hinrichs, C., Singh, V., et al.: Spatially augmented LPboosting for AD classification with evaluations on the ADNI dataset. Neuroimage 48(1), 138–149 (2009)
4. Jack Jr., C.R., Bernstein, M.A., Borowski, B.J., Gunter, J.L., Fox, N.C., Thompson, P.M., Schuff, N., Krueger, G., Killiany, R.J., Decarli, C.S., Dale, A.M., Carmichael, O.W., Tosun, D., Weiner, M.W.: Update on the magnetic resonance imaging core of the alzheimer's disease neuroimaging initiative. Alzheimers Dement 6(3), 212–220 (2010)
5. Jagust, W.J., Bandy, D., Chen, K., Foster, N.L., Landau, S.M., Mathis, C.A., Price, J.C., Reiman, E.M., Skovronsky, D., Koeppe, R.A.: The alzheimer's disease neuroimaging initiative positron emission tomography core. Alzheimers Dement 6(3), 221–229 (2010)

6. Khundrakpam, B.S., Reid, A., Brauer, J., et al.: Developmental changes in organization of structural brain networks. Cerebral Cortex (2012)
7. Meinshausen, N., Bühlmann, P.: High-dimensional graphs and variable selection with the Lasso. The Annals of Statistics 34(3), 1436–1462 (2006)
8. Risacher, S.L., Saykin, A.J., West, J.D., Shen, L., Firpi, H.A., McDonald, B.C.: Baseline mri predictors of conversion from mci to probable ad in the adni cohort. Curr. Alzheimer Res. 6(4), 347–361 (2009)
9. Shen, L., Qi, Y., Kim, S., Nho, K., Wan, J., Risacher, S.L., Saykin, A.J., ADNI: Sparse bayesian learning for identifying imaging biomarkers in AD prediction. In: Jiang, T., Navab, N., Pluim, J.P.W., Viergever, M.A. (eds.) MICCAI 2010, Part III. LNCS, vol. 6363, pp. 611–618. Springer, Heidelberg (2010)
10. Stonnington, C.M., Chu, C., et al.: Predicting clinical scores from magnetic resonance scans in alzheimer's disease. Neuroimage 51(4), 1405–1413 (2010)
11. Swaminathan, S., Shen, L., Risacher, S.L., Yoder, K.K., West, J.D., Kim, S., Nho, K., Foroud, T., Inlow, M., Potkin, S.G., Huentelman, M.J., Craig, D.W., Jagust, W.J., Koeppe, R.A., Mathis, C.A., Jack Jr., C.R., Weiner, M.W., Saykin, A.J.: Amyloid pathway-based candidate gene analysis of [(11)c]pib-pet in the Alzheimer's disease neuroimaging initiative (adni) cohort. Brain Imaging Behav. 6(1), 1–15 (2012)
12. Tibshirani, R.: Regression shrinkage and selection via the LASSO. J. Royal. Statist. Soc. B 58, 267–288 (1996)
13. Walhovd, K., Fjell, A., et al.: Multi-modal imaging predicts memory performance in normal aging and cognitive decline. Neurobiol. Aging 31(7), 1107–1121 (2010)
14. Wang, H., Nie, F., Huang, H., Risacher, S.L., Ding, C., Saykin, A.J., Shen, L.: Sparse multi-task regression and feature selection to identify brain imaging predictors for memory performance. In: IEEE Conference on Computer Vision, pp. 557–562 (2011)
15. Wang, H., Nie, F., Huang, H., Risacher, S., Saykin, A.J., Shen, L., ADNI: Identifying AD-sensitive and cognition-relevant imaging biomarkers via joint classification and regression. In: Fichtinger, G., Martel, A., Peters, T. (eds.) MICCAI 2011, Part III. LNCS, vol. 6893, pp. 115–123. Springer, Heidelberg (2011)
16. Wang, H., Nie, F., Huang, H., Risacher, S.L., Saykin, A.J., Shen, L., ADNI: Identifying disease sensitive and quantitative trait relevant biomarkers from multi-dimensional heterogeneous imaging genetics data via sparse multi-modal multi-task learning. In: 20th Annual International Conference on Intelligent Systems for Molecular Biology (ISMB), vol. 28, pp. i127–i136 (2012)
17. Wang, H., Nie, F., Huang, H., Yan, J., Kim, S., Nho, K., Risacher, S.L., Saykin, A.J., Shen, L.: From Phenotype to Genotype: An Association Study of Candidate Phenotypic Markers to Alzheimer's Disease Relevant SNPs. Bioinformatics 28, i619–i625 (2012)
18. Wang, H., Nie, F., Huang, H., Yan, J., Kim, S., Nho, K., Risacher, S., Saykin, A., Shen, L.: High-Order Multi-Task Feature Learning to Identify Longitudinal Phenotypic Markers for Alzheimer Disease Progression Prediction. In: Advances in Neural Information Processing Systems, NIPS (2012)

Multi-atlas Segmentation with Robust Label Transfer and Label Fusion

Hongzhi Wang[1], Alison Pouch[2], Manabu Takabe[2], Benjamin Jackson[3],
Joseph Gorman[3], Robert Gorman[3], and Paul A. Yushkevich[1,*]

[1] Department of Radiology, [2] Department of Bioengineering, [3] Department of Surgery
University of Pennsylvania

Abstract. Multi-atlas segmentation has been widely applied in medical image analysis. This technique relies on image registration to transfer segmentation labels from pre-labeled atlases to a novel target image and applies label fusion to reduce errors produced by registration-based label transfer. To improve the performance of registration-based label transfer against registration errors, our first contribution is to propose a label transfer scheme that generates multiple warped versions of each atlas to one target image through registration paths obtained by composing inter-atlas registrations and atlas-target registrations. The problem of decreasing quality of warped atlases caused by accumulative errors in composing multiple registrations is properly addressed by an atlas selection method that is guided by atlas segmentations. To improve the performance of label fusion against registration errors, our second contribution is to integrate the probabilistic correspondence model employed by the non-local mean approach with the joint label fusion technique, both of which have shown excellent performance for label fusion. Experiments on mitral-valve segmentation in 3D transesophageal echocardiography (TEE) show the effectiveness of the proposed techniques.

1 Introduction

Label fusion based multi-atlas segmentation has been widely applied in medical image analysis. This technique applies deformable image registration to establish one-to-one correspondence between each pre-labeled training image, called an atlas, and a novel target image. Then, the segmentation label is transferred to the target image by warping each atlas based on the correspondence. Each warped atlas provides one candidate segmentation for the target image. To reduce segmentation errors produced by registration-based label transfer, label fusion is applied to combine all candidate segmentations into a consensus segmentation.

As empirical studies [1,13] have shown, the performance of multi-atlas segmentation usually can be improved when the number of applied atlases increases. However, generating atlases with high quality segmentation is time consuming and labor intensive. Hence, atlases that can be applied in practice are often

* Grant support: NIH AG037376, EB014346, HL63954, HL73021, and HL103723.

J.C. Gee et al. (Eds.): IPMI 2013, LNCS 7917, pp. 548–559, 2013.

very limited. Under such circumstances, how to effectively apply limited atlases for optimal segmentation performance is an important problem. To address this problem, our main contribution is to propose techniques that allow more effective label transfer and more accurate label fusion.

Most existing multi-atlas segmentation techniques register and warp each atlas to a target image only once. If the registration fails, the information provided by the atlas for segmenting the target image may be completely wasted. Since any single registration may be unreliable, one natural solution to make the solution more robust to registration failures is to generate multiple registrations and warps for each atlas.

To address this problem, [7] proposed an atlas propagation approach that warps each atlas to a novel target image through other novel target images. To generate multiple warped versions of each atlas for a target image, multiple registration paths obtained by composing registrations between different novel target images are applied. Although this approach significantly improves single atlas segmentation performance [7], the requirement for inter-target registrations makes it computationally expensive.

To make the idea of atlas propagation through various registration paths more practical and more effective, our first contribution is to propose warping each atlas to a target image through registration paths obtained from composing inter-atlas registrations. This approach has two key advantages: 1) Since inter-atlas registrations can be computed off-line, this approach does not increase on-line registration burden. 2) Since the manual segmentation of each atlas is known, it allows an atlas segmentation guided atlas selection method, which can reliably detect and remove poor quality warps obtained through composing inter-atlas registrations.

To fuse the warped atlases, we apply local weighted voting with the joint label fusion technique [17]. Unlike most other label fusion techniques, which rely on the assumption of independence between atlases, joint label fusion explicitly incorporate correlations between atlases in label fusion. As shown in [17], joint label fusion performed better than label fusion with independent voting weight estimation. To further improve the performance of joint label fusion against registration errors, our second contribution is to integrate the probabilistic correspondence model employed by the non-local mean approach, which has proven to be highly effective for addressing image registration related uncertainties [5,2], into the joint label fusion approach.

For validation, we apply our method to mitral valve segmentation in 3D transesophageal echocardiography (TEE) and compare with the original joint label fusion approach. We show that our atlas propagation approach and the enhanced joint label fusion approach produce significant improvements.

2   A Bayesian View for Multi-atlas Segmentation

First, we give a brief overview for multi-atlas segmentation. Let $\mathcal{A} = \{A^1 = (A_F^1, A_S^1), ..., A^n = (A_F^n, A_S^n)\}$ be n independently constructed atlases, where A_F^i

is an atlas image and A_S^i is the atlas segmentation. For a target image T_F, its segmentation, T_S, can be estimated using the atlases as follows:

$$p(T_S|T_F, \mathcal{A}) = \int_D p(T_S|T_F, D)p(D|T_F, \mathcal{A})dD \tag{1}$$

where $D = (D_F, D_S)$ is one feasible warp of the atlases into the native space of T_F. D_F and D_S denote the warped atlas image and the corresponding warped atlas segmentation, obtained by performing deformable image registration between one atlas to the target image. $p(D|T_F, \mathcal{A})$ is the probability of observing the warped atlas D given the target image T_F and the atlas set $\mathcal{A}$. One common way to estimate this probability is based on image similarity between the warped atlas image and the target image over local patches, under the assumption that high similarities indicate high probabilities of observing the warps.

Due to the uncertainty in image registration, each atlas may generate multiple feasible warps for one target image. However, most work only produces one warp for each atlas, where the warped atlas is often generated by a maximum a posterior (MAP) registration result produced by some registration algorithm. Under the assumption that the posterior distribution of feasible warps produced by one atlas is narrowly peaked around its maximum, this approach usually can give reasonable solutions when the registration algorithms can reliably find the MAP solution. However, when the assumption is invalid or the registration algorithm works poorly, only using the MAP registration warp produced by one registration algorithm may be inadequate.

By contrast, since the Bayesian approach requires to marginalize over all feasible warped atlases, it is more robust against any single registration failures. This advantage can be crucial for applications such as mitral valve segmentation in ultrasound images addressed in this paper, where reliable image registrations are hard to generate due to poor image quality and large motion induced deformations. Although computing all feasible warped atlases is intractable, it is still beneficial if multiple feasible warps can be generated for each atlas. In the next section, we discuss some possible solutions to address this problem.

3   Sampling Strategies for Registration-Based Label Transfer

3.1   Sampling with Different Registrations

One way to generate additional independently warped atlases using a fixed atlas set is by applying different registration algorithms with different parameter settings to compute the registrations for warping each atlas. The main limitation of this approach is that the computational cost for image registration increases linearly with the number of warped atlases. Given the fact that multi-atlas segmentation is already one of the most computationally expensive segmentation techniques due to the requirement for one registration between each atlas and a target image, further increasing registration costs will make this technique less practical.

3.2 Atlas Propagation through Various Registration Paths Obtained from Composing Registrations

As discussed in the introduction, warping one atlas to a target image through various registration paths constructed by composing registrations is an efficient approach for generating multiple warps for each atlas because each registration can be utilized in multiple registration paths for generating new warps. [7] first applied this idea through composing inter-target registrations and showed its effectiveness. To make the idea more practical and more effective, we propose to generate multiple warps through composing inter-atlas registrations.

Let $\phi_{i \to T}$ be the diffeomorphic map between atlas i and a target image computed by some registration algorithm. We call warped atlases obtained from such single registrations *first-order warps*. Let $\phi_{i \to j}$ be the estimated diffeomorphic map from atlas i to atlas j. Then the composed diffeomorphic map $\phi_{i \to j \to T} = \phi_{i \to j} \circ \phi_{j \to T}$ gives a correspondence map from atlas i to T as well. We call the warped atlases obtained from composing two independent registrations *second-order warps*. Similarly, higher-order warps can be produced from composing lower-order warps, e.g. $\phi_{i \to j \to k \to T} = \phi_{i \to j} \circ \phi_{j \to k \to T}$ for $i \neq j \neq k \neq i$.

Advantages. Since pairwise registrations among the atlases can be computed offline, one advantage is that it can significantly increase the number of warped atlases without substantially increasing the online computational burden, as only the registrations from each atlas to the target image are required. Furthermore, in some cases, high-order warps may improve the accuracy of the warped atlas. Typically, image registration can be more reliably done when the deformations between two images are small. When the deformations are large, registration is more likely to fail. One approach to address this problem is to decompose a large deformation into a series of small deformations [8]. As shown in [18,4,12], high-order atlas propagation is one way to achieve this goal. When each of the first-order registrations required for warping one atlas to a target image can be reliably estimated, high-order warps obtained by composing these first-order registrations may produce a more accurate warp than the one obtained from directly registering the atlas to the target image (see Fig. 1 for one example).

Limitations. Since generating high-order warps requires composing multiple independently estimated registrations, errors produced in estimating these registrations will accumulate in the composed solution. Hence, it is reasonable to expect that high-order warps should overall produce less accurate candidate segmentations than low-order warps.

For demonstration, we conducted an empirical study to quantitatively measure the segmentation accuracy produced by first and second-order atlas warping. We used one set of 10 atlases used in our mitral valve segmentation experiments (data description in section 5). We computed pairwise deformable image registration between each pair of the atlases, from which each atlas was warped to each of the remaining 9 atlases through first-order and second-order warping. Fig. 2(a) shows the distribution of segmentation accuracy produced by first-order

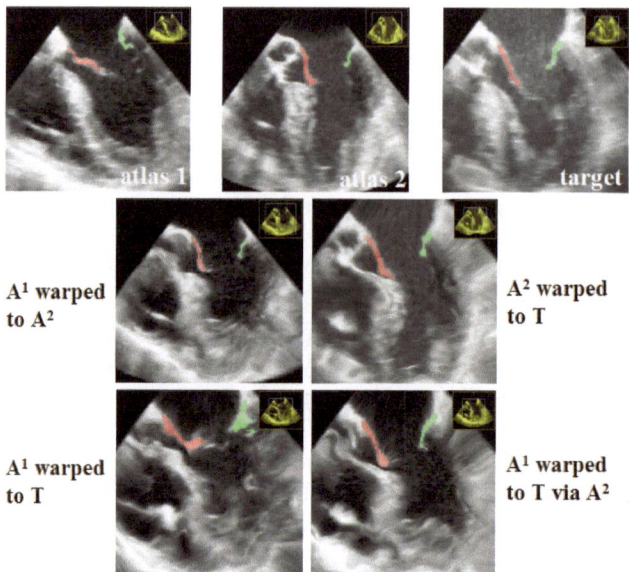

Fig. 1. Atlas warping through inter-atlas registration for mitral valve segmentation in 3D transesophageal echocardiography, shown in the septolateral plane of the valve. The anterior and posterior leaflets are in red and green, respectively. Directly registering atlas A^1 to the target image produces a low quality warp due to large deformations. However, since the registration between A^1 and A^2 and the registration between A^2 and T can be done more accurately, warping A^1 to T through A^2 produces a more accurate warp than directly warping A^1 to T.

and second-order warping, respectively. It clearly shows that second-order warping produces less accurate segmentations than first-order warping.

Atlas selection guided by atlas segmentations. To make label fusion more reliable with high-order warps, we propose an atlas selection technique that is capable of removing most of the low quality warped atlases. Since the ground truth segmentation of the target image is unknown, it is difficult to quantitatively estimate the registration accuracy in the final warped atlases. However, since the manual segmentation of each intermediate atlas is known, it is possible to quantitatively evaluate the quality of intermediately warped atlases. For instance, let atlas j be the last propagating atlas before warping atlas i to a target image. Let $D_S^{i \to j}$ be the segmentation obtained from propagating atlas i's segmentation to atlas j. Note that $D_S^{i \to j}$ may or may not be obtained through high-order warping. Under the assumption that the segmentation of atlas i and atlas j are different only due to random effects in producing manual segmentation, the overlap between the manual segmentation of atlas A^j and $D_S^{i \to j}$ is a good indicator of accumulative errors for propagating atlas i to atlas j. We measure the Dice similarity coefficient (DSC) [6] for each label between $D_S^{i \to j}$ and A_S^j and compute the average DSC over all labels. Then a threshold can be applied to remove those atlases

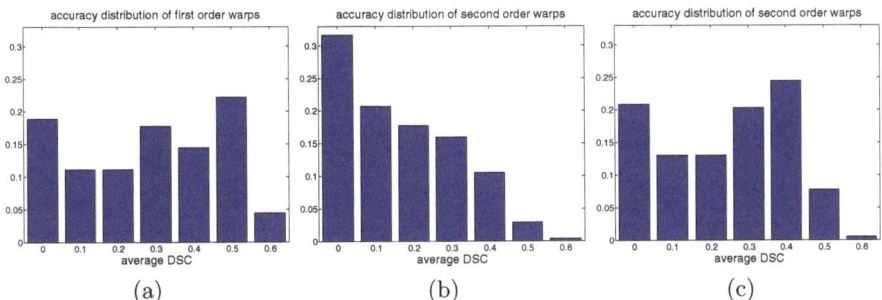

Fig. 2. Distribution of segmentation accuracy produced by first-order atlas warping (a) and second-order atlas warping (b) for the mitral valve segmentation problem. (c) shows the results of second-order warping with atlas segmentation guided atlas selection with a threshold of average Dice similarity coefficient (DSC)=0.5 (see text in section 3 for more detail). For this mitral valve segmentation problem, reliable image registrations are hard to generate. The average DSC produced by first-order warping is 0.328. The average DSC produced by second-order warping without/with atlas selection is 0.209/0.285, respectively. Atlas segmentation guided atlas selection significantly improves the overall quality of the warped atlases produced by second-order warping.

that propagate poorly. Fig. 2 shows that this approach can significantly improve the overall quality of high-order atlas warps.

4   Label Fusion

We apply local weighted voting with the joint label fusion algorithm [17] to fuse warped atlases. Comparing to other label fusion methods, the key advantage of joint label fusion is that it explicitly considers atlas correlations to reduce bias in the atlas set. To improve the performance of joint label fusion against registration errors, we adopt the probabilistic correspondence model employed by the non-local mean approach to improve the estimation accuracy of atlas correlations. For self completeness, we briefly summarize the joint label fusion approach below.

4.1   Joint Label Fusion

Joint label fusion models segmentation errors produced by each warped atlas as $T_{S,l}(x) = D_{S,l}^i(x) + \delta^i(x)$. $T_{S,l}(x), D_{S,l}^i(x) \in \{0, 1\}$ are the observed votes for label l produced by the target image and the ith warped atlas, respectively. Hence, $\delta^i(x) \in \{-1, 0, 1\}$ is the observed label difference. The correlation between the segmentation errors produced by any two atlases at location x are captured by a dependency matrix M_x, with $M_x(i, j) = p(\delta^i(x)\delta^j(x) = 1 \mid T_F, D_F^i, D_F^j)$ measuring the probability that atlas i and j produce the same label error for the target image. The expected label difference between the consensus solution obtained from weighted voting and the target segmentation is:

$$E_{\delta^1(x),\ldots,\delta^n(x)}\left[(T_{S,l}(x)-\sum_{i=1}^{n}w_x^i D_{S,l}^i(x))^2 \mid T_F, D_F^1, \ldots, D_F^n\right] = \mathbf{w}_x^t M_x \mathbf{w}_x \quad (2)$$

where w_x^i is the voting weight for atlas i at location x and t stands for transpose. To minimize the expected label difference, the optimal voting weights can be solved by $\mathbf{w}_x = \frac{M_x^{-1}1_n}{1_n^t M_x^{-1}1_n}$, where n is the number of warped atlases and $1_n = [1;1;\ldots;1]$ is a vector of size n.

4.2   Robust Estimation of Pairwise Atlas Correlations

To estimate the pairwise atlas dependency matrix M_x, [17] applies an image similarity based model over local patches as follows:

$$M_x(i,j) \sim \langle|D_F^i(\mathcal{N}(x)) - T_F(\mathcal{N}(x))|, |D_F^j(\mathcal{N}(x)) - T_F(\mathcal{N}(x))|\rangle^\beta \quad (3)$$

where $|D_F^i(\mathcal{N}(x)) - T_F(\mathcal{N}(x))|$ is the vector of absolute intensity difference between a warped atlas and the target image over a local patch $\mathcal{N}(x)$ centered at x and $\langle\cdot,\cdot\rangle$ is the dot product. β is a model parameter.

To make the estimation more robust against registration errors, [17] applies a local search algorithm to find the patch from each warped atlas within a small neighborhood $\mathcal{N}_s(x)$ that is the most similar to the target patch in the target image. Under the assumption that more similar patches are more likely to be correct correspondences, instead of the original corresponding patches in the warped atlases, the searched patches are applied for label fusion. However, since image similarities over local patches are not always reliable indicators of registration errors, the searched most similar patch may still give an incorrect correspondence. To address the unreliability in choosing any single candidate corresponding patch for label fusion, we propose to consider all feasible corresponding patches. We achieve this goal by integrating the non-local mean patch-based label fusion technique [5,2], which is shown to be effective for handling the unreliability in determining the correct correspondence, into the above atlas correlation estimation method (3).

First, a probability model is applied to represent the correspondence between each warped atlas and a target image. For each voxel x in the target image, the probability that a voxel x^i in the warped atlas i is the correct corresponding voxel is estimated by:

$$p(x^i|x, D_F^i, T_F) = \begin{cases} \frac{1}{Z_x^i}e^{-\frac{\|D_F^i(\mathcal{N}(x^i))-T_F(\mathcal{N}(x)))\|_2^2}{\sigma}} & \text{if } x^i \in \mathcal{N}_s(x); \\ 0 & \text{otherwise,} \end{cases} \quad (4)$$

where a Gaussian model is applied to transfer image similarity into a probability measure. In our experiments, we normalize the intensity vector obtained from each local image intensity patch, such that the normalized vector has zero mean and a constant norm and σ is fixed to be 0.1. Z_x^i is a normalization factor.

Combining this probability correspondence representation model and the patch-based atlas correlation model in (3), we estimate the probability that two atlases produce the same segmentation error for the target image by:

$$M_x(i,j) \sim \sum_{x^i \in \mathcal{N}_s(x)} \sum_{x^j \in \mathcal{N}_s(x)} p(x^i|x, D_F^i, T_F) p(x^j|x, D_F^j, T_F)$$

$$\langle |D_F^i(\mathcal{N}(x^i)) - T_F(\mathcal{N}(x))|, |D_F^j(\mathcal{N}(x^j)) - T_F(\mathcal{N}(x))| \rangle^\beta \quad (5)$$

In comparison to the local search algorithm, the key difference in (5) is that each patch within the searching area are considered as a potential match, but weighted by the estimated probability of being the correct match. Hence, it is more robust to the errors produced by the hard decision made by selecting the correspondence based on local image similarities.

5   Experiments

We apply our approach to segment the mitral valve in 3D transesophageal echocardiography (3D TEE). The mitral valve supports physiologically normal cardiac function by maintaining unidirectional blood flow across the left heart. Common valve diseases, such as ischemic and degenerative mitral regurgitation, are associated with pathological alterations in mitral leaflet and annular morphology. 3D examination of these morphological abnormalities, which vary substantially between individuals, is critical to the diagnosis and personalized surgical treatment of mitral valve disease. 3D TEE is the most practical imaging modality for 3D mitral valve assessment in the operating room and has been effectively used in both research and clinical settings to visualize and quantify mitral leaflet and annular geometry in vivo [11,15,16]. Segmentation of the mitral valve from 3D TEE is crucial for quantitative assessment.

Three new methods are proposed in this paper, which include atlas propagation through composing inter-atlas registrations (AP), atlas segmentation guided atlas selection (AS) and non-local mean based robust atlas correlation estimation (NL). To evaluate the performance of each proposed method, in addition to the overall performance produced by combining the three components, we also evaluated the effectiveness of each component. The tested methods include LWJoint-NL, LWJoint-AP, LWJoint-AP-AS, LWJoint-AP-AS-NL, where the method's name shows how different methods are combined. In our experiments, we only included first and second-order warps for AP. For atlas segmentation guided atlas selection, since the empirical study on atlases in Fig. 2.(c) shows that a threshold 0.5 average DSC can effectively remove most poor quality warped atlases, we fixed the threshold to be 0.5 average DSC.

Data Acquisition and Manual Segmentation. Twenty patients undergoing cardiac surgery were imaged pre-operatively using real-time 3D TEE. This cohort included 6 subjects with normal mitral valve anatomy and function, and 14 subjects with mild to severe mitral valve disease. All studies were performed after induction of general anesthesia and before initiation of cardiopulmonary bypass. Electrocardiographically gated full-volume images were acquired with the iE33 platform (Philips Medical Systems, Andover, MA) using a 2 to 7 MHz transesophageal matrix-array transducer over four consecutive cardiac cycles. The frame rate was 17 to 30 Hz, and the imaging depth was 12 to 16 cm. From each subject's data series, 3D TEE images of the mitral valve at mid-diastole were selected for analysis. These 3D TEE images were exported in Cartesian format (224×208×208 voxels), with an approximate isotropic resolution of 0.6 to 0.8 mm. The 20 images selected for analysis were uploaded to ITK-SNAP [19], an open source software package for medical image segmentation. An expert observer manually segmented the anterior and posterior leaflets in their entirety, associating the two leaflets with separate labels.

Experimental Setup. For cross-validation evaluation, we randomly selected 10 images to be the atlases and the other 10 images for testing. Each atlas was registered to each test image, as well as to each other atlas. Global registration was performed using the FSL FLIRT tool [14] with 12 degrees of freedom and using the default parameters (normalized mutual information similarity metric; search range from -5 to 5 in x, y and z). Deformable registration was performed using the ANTS Symmetric Normalization (SyN) algorithm [3], with the cross-correlation similarity metric (with radius 2) and a Gaussian regularizer with $\sigma = 3$. The cross-validation experiment was repeated 10 times. In each experiment, a different set of atlases and test images were randomly selected. The results reported below are averaged over the 10 experiments.

The baseline performance is produced by joint label fusion (LWJoint) without high-order warps. As described in section 4, LWJoint has three free parameters: r, the radius of the local appearance window $\mathcal{N}$ used in similarity-based M_x estimation; r_s, the radius of the local searching window $\mathcal{N}_s$; and β, the parameter used for estimating atlas correlation in (3). For each cross-validation experiment, the parameters are optimized by exhaustive search among a range of values in each parameter ($r \in \{1, 2, 3\}$; $r_s \in \{0, 1, 2, 3\}$; $\beta \in \{0.5, 0.75, ..., 2\}$) using the atlases in a leave-one-out strategy. We measure the average DSC between the automatic segmentation of each atlas obtained via the remaining atlases and the manual segmentation of that atlas, and find the optimal parameters that maximize this average DSC. For the 10 cross-validation experiments, the most frequently selected parameters are $(r, r_s, \beta)=(2,3,1)$. The same parameters selected for LWJoint were also applied for other LWJoint-based methods.

For more comprehensive comparison, we also produced results by majority voting (MV), image similarity based local weighted voting with the inverse weighting model $w_x^i = \frac{1}{Z(x)} exp \left(-\sum_{y \in \mathcal{N}(x)} \left[D_F^i(y) - T_F(y) \right]^2 /\sigma \right)$ (LWInverse) [1,10] and the Gaussian weighting model $w_x^i = \frac{1}{Z(x)} \left(\sum_{y \in \mathcal{N}(x)} \left[D_F^i(y) - T_F(y) \right]^2 \right)^{-\beta}$ (LW-Gaussian) [13]. The weighting model parameters, σ and β, are optimized along with r and r_s using the atlases through the leave-one-out strategy as well.

Table 1. The performance of mitral valve segmentation in terms of Dice similarity coefficient produced by each method

method	anterior leaflets	posterior leaflets
MV	0.348±0.229	0.250±0.187
LWInverse	0.573±0.144	0.422±0.172
LWGaussian	0.576±0.159	0.411±0.183
LWJoint	0.609±0.157	0.453±0.179
LWJoint-NL	0.616±0.150	0.464±0.174
LWJoint-AP	0.615±0.150	0.468±0.176
LWJoint-AP-AS	0.619±0.131	0.482±0.164
LWJoint-AP-AS-NL	0.623±0.126	0.490±0.158

Results. Table 1 summarizes the performance of each automatic segmentation method. The results are given in DSC between manual segmentation and automatic segmentation. Due to the large mitral valve deformations across different subjects and high noises in the TEE images, most warped atlases produced by image registration are in low qualities. Hence, the results produced by MV have low accuracy. Image similarity based local weighted voting produced significantly better segmentation accuracy than MV. Among the three baseline local weighted voting methods, LWJoint produced the best results.

Overall, each of the three methods proposed in this paper produced prominent improvements. The non-local mean based robust atlas correlation estimation technique consistently improved the accuracy of LWJoint with/without high-order atlas warps. The overall improvements produced by combining the three methods, i.e. LWJoint-AP-AS-NL, over LWJoint are statistically significant, with $p<0.05$ on the paired Students t-test. Fig. 3 shows some results produced by LWJoint and the full proposed method.

To report the mean surface distance between manual and automatic segmentation, for each voxel on one segmentation surface, we search for the closest voxel on the other segmentation surface and calculate the Euclidean distance between them. To make the measurement symmetric, the point-to-surface distance is calculated in two directions, from the automatic segmentation to manual segmentation surfaces and vice versa, and the average distance is taken as the final measurement for surface distance. When the mitral valve segmentation is evaluated as a whole, the average surface distances produced by MV, LWInverse, LGaussian, LWJoint and LWJoint-AP-AS-NL are 3.84 mm, 2.07 mm, 1.86 mm, 1.66 mm and 1.52 mm, respectively.

In the literature, [9] is the only existing work addressing fully automatic mitral valve segmentation. This work is based on discriminative learning and model fitting and was evaluated through a three-fold cross-validation on a set of 1516 TEE volumes. The mean point-to-surface distance between reference segmentation and automatic segmentation is 1.54 mm, which is comparable to that produced by our full method. However, we only used 10 training images, which is significantly fewer than those used in [9].

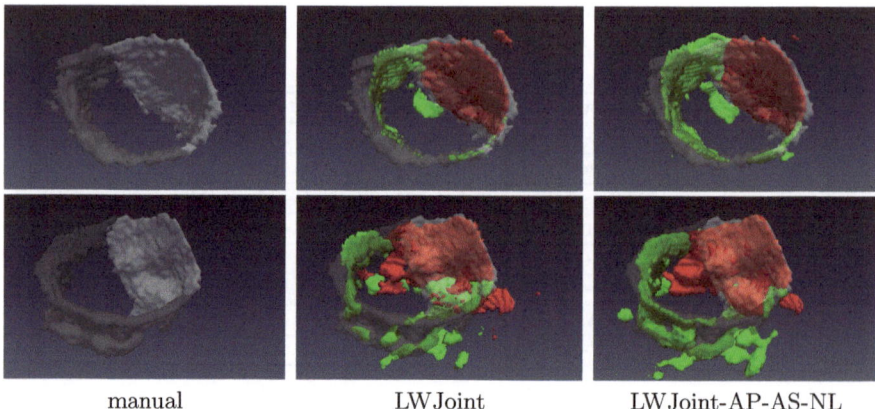

| manual | LWJoint | LWJoint-AP-AS-NL |

Fig. 3. Mitral valve segmentation. The anterior and posterior leaflets are shown in red(bright) and green(gray) in automatic(manual) segmentation, respectively.

6   Conclusions and Discussion

To improve the performance of label fusion based multi-atlas segmentation, we proposed a robust label transfer technique that can efficiently generates multiple warps for each atlas through registration paths obtained from composing inter-atlas registrations. To address the potential risk caused by accumulative errors in composing multiple registrations, we also proposed an atlas selection method that is guided by atlas segmentations to remove poorly warped atlases. To improve the performance of joint label fusion, we proposed a new technique for robust estimation of atlas correlations. The proposed methods were validated in a mitral valve segmentation problem using 3D transesophageal echocardiography and produced significant improvements over the state of the art label fusion algorithm. Using significantly fewer manually labeled images for training, our mitral valve segmentation accuracy is also comparable to previous fully automatic mitral valve segmentation work.

In our current experiments, we only included second-order atlas warps for label fusion and we used a fixed threshold for atlas segmentation guided atlas selection. In future work, higher-order warps will be included. A study on the impact of the threshold choice on the performance will be studied as well.

References

1. Artaechevarria, X., Munoz-Barrutia, A., de Solorzano, C.O.: Combination strategies in multi-atlas image segmentation: Application to brain MR data. IEEE TMI 28(8), 1266–1277 (2009)
2. Asman, A.J., Landman, B.A.: Non-local STAPLE: An intensity-driven multi-atlas rater model. In: Ayache, N., Delingette, H., Golland, P., Mori, K. (eds.) MICCAI 2012, Part III. LNCS, vol. 7512, pp. 426–434. Springer, Heidelberg (2012)

3. Avants, B., Epstein, C., Grossman, M., Gee, J.: Symmetric diffeomorphic image registration with cross-correlation: Evaluating automated labeling of elderly and neurodegenerative brain. Medical Image Analysis 12(1), 26–41 (2008)
4. Cardoso, M.J., Wolz, R., Modat, M., Fox, N.C., Rueckert, D., Ourselin, S.: Geodesic information flows. In: Ayache, N., Delingette, H., Golland, P., Mori, K. (eds.) MICCAI 2012, Part II. LNCS, vol. 7511, pp. 262–270. Springer, Heidelberg (2012)
5. Coupe, P., Manjon, J., Fonov, V., Pruessner, J., Robles, N., Collins, D.: Patch-based segmentation using expert priors: Application to hippocampus and ventricle segmentation. NeuroImage 54(2), 940–954 (2011)
6. Dice, L.: Measure of the amount of ecological association between species. Ecology 26, 297–302 (1945)
7. Gass, T., Székely, G., Goksel, O.: Semi-supervised segmentation using multiple segmentation hypotheses from a single atlas. In: Menze, B.H., Langs, G., Lu, L., Montillo, A., Tu, Z., Criminisi, A. (eds.) MCV 2012. LNCS, vol. 7766, pp. 29–37. Springer, Heidelberg (2013)
8. Hamm, J., Ye, D., Verma, R., Davatzikos, C.: Gram: A framework for geodesic registration on anatomical manifolds. MedIA 14(5), 633–642 (2010)
9. Ionasec, R., Voigt, I., Georgescu, B., Wang, Y., Houle, H., Vega-Higuera, F., Navab, N., Comaniciu, D.: Patient-specific modeling and quantification of the aortic and mitral valves from 4-d cardiac ct and tee. IEEE Transactions on Medical Imaging 29(9), 1636–1651 (2010)
10. Isgum, I., Staring, M., Rutten, A., Prokop, M., Viergever, M., van Ginneken, B.: Multi-atlas-based segmentation with local decision fusion–application to cardiac and aortic segmentation in CT scans. IEEE Trans. on MI 28(7), 1000–1010 (2009)
11. Grewal, J., Mankad, S., Freeman, W., Click, R., Suri, R., Abel, M., Oh, J., Pellikka, P., Nesbitt, G., Syed, I., Mulvagh, S., Miller, F.: Real-time three-dimensional transesophageal echocardiography in the intraoperative assessment of mitral valve disease. J. Am. Soc. Echocardiogr. 22(1), 34–41 (2009)
12. Jia, H., Yap, P., Shen, D.: Iterative multi-atlas-based multi-image segmentation with tree-based registration. Neuroimage 59(1), 422–430 (2012)
13. Sabuncu, M., Yeo, B., Leemput, K.V., Fischl, B., Golland, P.: A generative model for image segmentation based on label fusion. IEEE TMI 29(10), 1714–1720 (2010)
14. Smith, S., Jenkinson, M., Woolrich, M., Beckmann, C., Behrens, T., Johansen-Berg, H., Bannister, P., Luca, M., Drobnjak, I., Flitney, D., Niazy, R., Saunders, J., Vickers, J., Zhang, Y., Stefano, N., Brady, J., Matthews, P.: Advances in functional and structural MR image analysis and implementation as FSL. Neuroimage 23(suppl. 1), 208–219 (2004)
15. Sugeng, L., Shernan, S., Salgo, I.S., Weinert, L., Shook, D., Raman, J., Jeevanandam, V., Dupont, F., Settlemier, S., Savord, B., Fox, J., Mor-Avi, V., Lang, R.: Live 3-dimensional transesophageal echocardiography initial experience using the fully-sampled matrix array probe. J. Am. Coll. Cardiol. 52(6), 446–449 (2008)
16. Vergnat, M., Jassar, A., Jackson, B., Ryan, L., Eperjesi, T., Pouch, A., Weiss, S., Cheung, A., Acker, M., Gorman, J., Gorman, R.: Ischemic mitral regurgitation: a quantitative three-dimensional echocardiographic analysis. Ann. Thorac. Surg. 91(1), 157–164 (2011)
17. Wang, H., Suh, J.W., Das, S., Pluta, J., Craige, C., Yushkevich, P.: Multi-atlas segmentation with joint label fusion. IEEE Trans. on PAMI 35(3), 611–623 (2013)
18. Wolz, R., Aljabar, P., Hajnal, J., Hammers, A., Rueckert, D.: Leap: Learning embeddings for atlas propagation. NeuroImage 49(2), 1316–1325 (2010)
19. Yushkevich, P., Piven, J., Hazlett, H., Smith, R., Ho, S., Gee, J., Gerig, G.: User-guided 3D active contour segmentation of anatomical structures: significantly improved efficiency and reliability. NeuroImage 31(3), 1116–1128 (2006)

A Hierarchical Geodesic Model
for Diffeomorphic Longitudinal Shape Analysis

Nikhil Singh, Jacob Hinkle, Sarang Joshi, and P. Thomas Fletcher

Scientific Computing and Imaging Institute, University of Utah, Salt Lake City, Utah

Abstract. Hierarchical linear models (HLMs) are a standard approach for analyzing data where individuals are measured repeatedly over time. However, such models are only applicable to longitudinal studies of Euclidean data. In this paper, we propose a novel hierarchical geodesic model (HGM), which generalizes HLMs to the manifold setting. Our proposed model explains the longitudinal trends in shapes represented as elements of the group of diffeomorphisms. The individual level geodesics represent the trajectory of shape changes within individuals. The group level geodesic represents the average trajectory of shape changes for the population. We derive the solution of HGMs on diffeomorphisms to estimate individual level geodesics, the group geodesic, and the residual geodesics. We demonstrate the effectiveness of HGMs for longitudinal analysis of synthetically generated shapes and 3D MRI brain scans.

Keywords: Diffeomorphisms, Longitudinal, Hierarchical Model.

1   Introduction

A longitudinal study of neuroanatomical aging, development and disease progression necessitates modeling anatomical changes over time. A convenient representation of anatomical variability is via maps of diffeomorphisms, which are topology-preserving smooth and invertible transformations of a template image. Recently proposed methods, such as *geodesic regression* [5,10,11], effectively represent smooth trajectories of changes in anatomy. However, regression is not an appropriate model of longitudinal data.

Related work [3,4,7] estimate the group trajectory by averaging individual trajectories in the diffeomorphic setting. Durrleman et. al [3] estimates a spatiotemporal piecewise geodesic atlas. Although this method estimates a continuous evolution of spatial change, it does not guarantee smoothness of the resulting average estimate across the time span. The average shape trajectory estimates by Fishbaugh et. al [4] are also not guaranteed to be smooth in time. The approach based on stationary velocity fields presented in [7] does not model *distances* between trajectories, which makes it difficult to compare the differences in trends for statistical analysis.

Another important shortcoming of the contemporary methods of averaging trajectories is that they do not apply when the time ranges of measurements of individuals are staggered. For instance, [3] and [4] both require extrapolation

J.C. Gee et al. (Eds.): IPMI 2013, LNCS 7917, pp. 560–571, 2013.

and resampling for each individual trajectory estimates outside their time-range before an average evolution of the population can be computed. Muralidharan et. al [9] address these problems and estimate smooth geodesic representations for individual and group trends for a population of staggered individual measurements. They utilize a Sasaki metric on the tangent bundle of the manifold of finite-dimensional shapes to compare geodesic trends. However, their methods are difficult to apply to the infinite-dimensional space of diffeomorphic transformations, due to the need for curvature computations of the underlying manifold.

In this paper, we present a hierarchical geodesic model (HGM) on diffeomorphisms that generalizes classical hierarchical linear models (HLMs) on Euclidean spaces. HGMs utilize the metric on the space of diffeomorphisms to define the group geodesic given a population of geodesics. It applies to commonly occurring unbalanced designs in medical imaging data where measurements are staggered, i.e., not every individual is measured at the same time points. The consequence of this modeling is an estimate of a smooth "average geodesic" and a common reference coordinate system to represent longitudinal trends of multiple individuals for longitudinal studies.

2   Hierarchical Geodesic Models

We begin by defining HGMs in the simplest scenario in which the data lie in a Euclidean space. In this case, the geodesic models of longitudinal trends reduce to straight lines, and we give a procedure for estimation of model parameters defining the group level trend in a hierarchical fashion. We later present the generalization of this model and its estimation to diffeomorphisms.

2.1   Hierarchical Geodesic Models in Euclidean Space

Consider the univariate longitudinal case with independent time variable, t, and dependent response variable, y. Say we are given a population of N individuals with M_i measurements for the ith individual. The design can be unbalanced, meaning there are potentially a different number of measurements for each individual. Denote y_{ij} as the jth measurement of the ith individual at time t_{ij}. Motivated by classical hierarchical linear models [6] for repeated measurements, this is modeled in two levels as

$$
\begin{aligned}
&\textit{Group Level:} && \textit{Individual Level:} \\
&a_i \sim \mathcal{N}(\alpha + \beta t_{i0}, \sigma_I^2) && y_{ij} \sim \mathcal{N}(a_i + b_i(t_{ij} - t_{i0}), \sigma_i^2) \\
&b_i \sim \mathcal{N}(\beta, \sigma_S^2)
\end{aligned}
$$

The estimation of the parameters for this model proceeds in two stages. First, the individual level parameters a_i and b_i are estimated. These estimates are then used to estimate α and β at the group level. The solution to this model thus corresponds to minimizing the negative log-likelihood at individual and group levels, respectively, where

$$-\log(p(y_{ij}|a_i,b_i)) = \frac{1}{2\sigma_i^2}\sum_{j=1}^{M_i}[y_{ij}-(a_i+b_i(t_{ij}-t_{i0}))]^2 \tag{1}$$

$$-\log(p(a_i,b_i|\alpha,\beta)) = \frac{1}{2\sigma_I^2}\sum_{i=1}^{N}[(\alpha+\beta t_{i0})-a_i]^2 + \frac{1}{2\sigma_S^2}\sum_{i=1}^{N}[\beta-b_i]^2 \tag{2}$$

Individual level: The solution for the slope-intercept pair, a_i, b_i, in the individual level that minimize (1) is given by the standard ordinary least-squares regression solution. An equivalent solution more directly generalizable to the diffeomorphic case is to solve this problem as an optimal control, as detailed in [10]. This is done by adding Lagrange multipliers to constrain the curves to be straight lines and derive the system of equation termed the *adjoint equations*.

Group level: The maximum likelihood group estimate represents an "average line", $\alpha(t)$, that best matches the individual lines, (a_i, b_i), in least-squares sense. From an optimal control viewpoint, we add Lagrange multipliers to constrain the curve $\alpha(t)$ to be a straight line. This is done by introducing time-dependent adjoint variables, λ^α and λ^β, in the log-likelihood in (2), giving

$$\mathcal{E}(\alpha,\beta) = \int_0^{t_N}(\lambda^\alpha(\dot{\alpha}-\beta)+\lambda^\beta\dot{\beta})dt + \frac{1}{2}\sum_{i=1}^{N}(\frac{1}{\sigma_I^2}(\alpha(t_i)-a_i)^2 + \frac{1}{\sigma_S^2}(\beta(t_i)-b_i)^2)$$

The gradients of this functional are $\delta_{\alpha(0)}\mathcal{E} = -\lambda^\alpha(0^-)$ and $\delta_{\beta(0)}\mathcal{E} = -\lambda^\beta(0^-)$. These are evaluated by integrating backwards the adjoint equations, $-\dot{\lambda}^\alpha = 0$, and $\dot{\lambda}^\beta = -\lambda^\alpha$, subject to the following boundary and jump conditions:

$$\lambda^\alpha(t_N) = -\frac{1}{\sigma_I^2}(\alpha(t_N)-a_N) \qquad\qquad \lambda^\beta(t_N) = -\frac{1}{\sigma_S^2}(\beta(t_N)-b_N)$$

$$\lambda^\beta(t_k^+)-\lambda^\beta(t_k^-) = \frac{1}{\sigma_S^2}(\beta(t_i)-b_i) \qquad\qquad \lambda^\alpha(t_k^+)-\lambda^\alpha(t_k^-) = \frac{1}{\sigma_I^2}(\alpha(t_i)-a_i)$$

Notice that unlike least squares regression, the velocity term in the group log-likelihood at group level also influences the group estimate. In particular, the jumps in integrating λ^β are interpreted as the forces by the initial velocities pulling the group geodesic. The solution for $\alpha(0)$ and $\beta(0)$ in this Euclidean case corresponds to the solution of the linear system $Ax = b$, where:

$$A = \begin{pmatrix} N\frac{1}{\sigma_I^2} & \frac{1}{\sigma_I^2}\sum_{i=0}^{N}t_i \\ \frac{1}{\sigma_I^2}\sum_{i=0}^{N}t_i & N\frac{1}{\sigma_S^2}+\frac{1}{\sigma_I^2}\sum_{i=0}^{N}t_i^2 \end{pmatrix}, \quad b = \begin{pmatrix} \frac{1}{\sigma_I^2}\sum_{i=0}^{N}a_i \\ \frac{1}{\sigma_I^2}\sum_{i=0}^{N}a_it_i+\frac{1}{\sigma_S^2}\sum_{i=0}^{N}b_i \end{pmatrix}$$

Notice that if there is no slope term in the energy functional, i.e., as $\sigma_S^2 \to \infty$, this reduces to the standard ordinary least squares solution for linear regression. An example of synthetically generated longitudinal data is shown in Figure 1. This example illustrates the importance of modeling correlations within each individual by including individual slope terms in the likelihood function. Ignoring

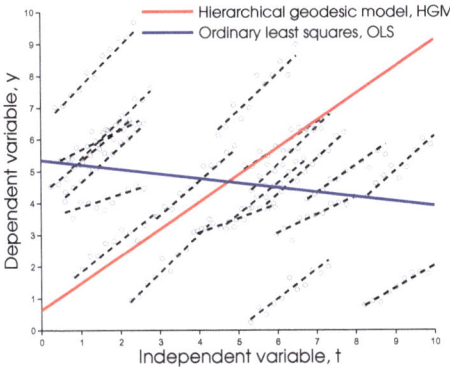

Fig. 1. Comparing HGM and OLS in Euclidean space

these correlations leaves us with a simple linear regression fit to the data, which does not reflect the longitudinal trends that individuals experience. In contrast, the group trend, $\alpha(t)$, estimated in the hierarchical model by including slope terms, better summarizes the average behavior of the individual trends.

2.2 Background on Diffeomorphisms

We follow the well-established framework of large deformation diffeomorphic metric mapping (LDDMM) [2,12]. Before introducing our longitudinal model on manifold of anatomical shape changes, we briefly review some necessary background of the mathematical framework of diffeomorphisms.

Diffeomorphisms: Let Ω be the coordinate space of the image, I. A diffeomorphism, $\phi(t)$, is constructed by the integration of an ordinary differential equations (ODE) on Ω defined via a smooth, time-indexed velocity field, $v(t)$. The deformation of an image I by ϕ is defined as the action of the diffeomorphism, given by $\phi \cdot I = I \circ \phi^{-1}$. The choice of a self-adjoint differential operator, L determines the right-invariant Riemannian structure on the collection of velocity fields with the norm defined as, $\|v\|^2 = \int_{\Omega} (Lv(x), v(x)) dx$.

Deformation Momenta and EPDiff Evolution: The tangent space at identity, $V = T_{\mathrm{Id}}\mathrm{Diff}(\Omega)$ consists of all vector fields with finite norm. Its dual space, $V^* = T_{\mathrm{Id}}^*\mathrm{Diff}(\Omega)$ consists of vector-valued distributions over Ω. The velocity, $v \in V$, maps to its dual deformation momenta, $m \in V^*$, via the operator L such that $m = Lv$ and $v = Km$. The operator $K : V^* \to V$ denotes the inverse of L. Note that constraining ϕ to be a geodesic with initial momentum, $m(0)$ implies that ϕ, m, and I all evolve in a way entirely determined by the metric L, and that the deformation is determined entirely by the initial deformation momenta, $m(0)$. Given the initial velocity, $v(0) \in V$, or equivalently, the initial momentum, $m(0) \in V^*$, the geodesic path $\phi(t)$ is constructed as per the following EPDiff equations [1,8]:

$$\partial_t m = -\mathrm{ad}_v^* m = -(Dv)^T m - Dmv - (\mathrm{div}\, v)m \qquad (3)$$

where D denotes the Jacobian matrix, and the operator ad^* is the dual of the negative Jacobi-Lie bracket of vector fields [1,8,12] such that, $\text{ad}_v w = -[v, w] = Dvw - Dwv$. The deformed image $I(t) = I(0) \circ \phi^{-1}(t)$, evolves via: $\partial_t I = -v \cdot \nabla I$.

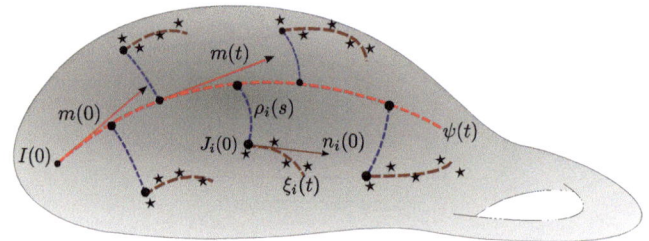

Fig. 2. Hierarchical geodesic modeling in diffeomorphisms

2.3 Hierarchical Geodesic Models for Diffeomorphisms

Similar to the setup discussed for Euclidean data, we are given a population of N individuals with M_i measurements for the ith individual. There can be a variable number of measurements for each individual. Denote H_{ij} as the jth measured image of the ith individual at time t_{ij}.

Figure 2 shows a schematic of the HGM. We model geodesic trend for an individual with a diffeomorphism, $\xi_i(t)$ (brown). The initial image, or intercept, $J_i(0)$, and the initial momenta, or slope, $n_i(0)$, fully parameterize the trajectory for the ith individual. At the group level, we model the group geodesic trend with the diffeomorphism, $\psi(t)$, (red) starting at identity, parameterized by initial momenta, $m(0)$. Let ϕ_i denote the diffeomorphism that matches individual baseline $J_i(0)$ from identity and ρ_i denote the residual geodesic between $\psi(t_i)$ and ϕ_i: $\rho_i = \phi_i \circ \psi^{-1}(t_i)$. The initial momenta, $p_i(0)$, parameterize residual, ρ_i.

We now present the hierarchical geodesic estimation procedure on diffeomorphisms in two stages. For the first stage, we note that estimates at individual level amounts to solving N geodesic regression problems for each individual as proposed in [10,11]. We briefly review it here under the vectorized deformation momenta formulation (details in [11]). In the second stage at the group level, we address the more interesting question of averaging the individual geodesics in the space of diffeomorphisms.

Individual level: Given M_i observed images H_{ij} at time points t_{ij} for an individual such that $j = 1, \ldots, M_i$, the geodesic that passes closest, in the least squares sense, to the data minimizes the energy functional:

$$\mathcal{E}(J_i(0), n_i(0)) = \frac{1}{2}\|n_i(0)\|_K^2 + \frac{1}{2\sigma_i^2} \sum_{j=1}^{M_i} \|J_i(t_{ij}) - H_{ij}\|_{L^2}^2$$

where $J_i(0)$ and $m_i(0)$ are the initial "intercept" and "slope" to be estimated that completely parameterize the geodesic for the ith individual. Here, $J_i(t) = \xi_i(t) \cdot J_i(0)$ and $\|.\|_K$ is the norm defined by the kernel, K, in the dual space of momenta, as per the metric induced by Sobolev operator, L, on velocity fields. This is done by adding time-dependent Lagrange multipliers,$\hat{n}_i, \hat{J}_i$, and $\hat{w}_i$, to constrain $\xi_i(t)$ to be along the EPDiff geodesic path:

$$\tilde{\mathcal{E}}(J_i(0), n_i(0)) = \mathcal{E} + \int_0^1 \langle \hat{n}_i, \dot{n}_i + \text{ad}_{w_i}^* n_i \rangle_{L^2} dt$$
$$+ \int_0^1 \langle \hat{J}_i, \dot{J}_i + \nabla J_i \cdot w_i \rangle_{L^2} dt + \int_0^1 \langle \hat{w}_i, n_i - Lw_i \rangle_{L^2} dt.$$

The variation of $\tilde{\mathcal{E}}$ with respect to the initial momenta is

$$\delta_{n_i(0)}\tilde{\mathcal{E}} = K \star n_i(0) - \hat{n}_i(0) \tag{4}$$

The optimality conditions for n_i and J_i result in the time-dependent *adjoint* system of ODEs which are integrated backward in time to obtain $\hat{n}_i(0)$ to compute gradient update in (4). The variation of $\tilde{\mathcal{E}}$ with respect to the initial image, $\delta_{J_i(0)}\tilde{\mathcal{E}}$, can be directly computed from the energy functional, $\tilde{\mathcal{E}}$. Since $J_i(t) = \xi_i(t) \cdot J_i(0) = J_i(0) \circ \xi_i^{-1}(t)$, a change of variables for ξ_i, followed by taking the derivative with respect to $J_i(0)$, results in the closed form solution for optimum initial image, $J_i(0)$, as

$$J_i(0) = \frac{\sum_{j=1}^{M_i} H_{ij} \circ \xi_i(t_{ij}) |D\xi_i(t_{ij})|}{\sum_{j=1}^{M_i} |D\xi_i(t_{ij})|}.$$

Note that the solution to the geodesic regression problem presented in [10] is based on optimization over scalar deformation momentum. In our formulation, the evolution of the geodesic and adjoint system is decoupled from the template image resulting in a closed-form for image update. In the discussion that follows, for clarity and ease of notation, we will use $J_i = J_i(0)$ to denote the initial "intercept" and $n_i = n_i(0)$ to denote initial "slope" for an individual.

Group level: At the group level (Figure 2), the idea is to estimate the average geodesic, $\psi(t)$, that is a representative of the population of geodesic trends denoted by the initial intercept-slope pair, (J_i, n_i), for N individuals, $i = 1, \ldots, N$. The required estimate for $\psi(t)$ must span the entire range of time along which the measurements are made for the population and must minimize residual diffeomorphisms ρ_i from $\psi(t)$.

Analogous to the Euclidean case, we propose a formulation that includes influences from forces by initial velocities along with initial intercepts from each individual. The following energy functional generalizes the log-likelihood presented for the group estimate in the Euclidean case:

$$\mathcal{E}(\psi, \rho_i, I(t_i)) = \frac{1}{2}\mathrm{d}(e, \psi(1))^2 + \frac{1}{2\sigma_I^2}\sum_{i=1}^{N}\left(\mathrm{d}(e, \rho_i)^2 + \|\rho_i \cdot I(t_i) - J_i\|_{L^2}^2\right)$$

$$+ \frac{1}{2\sigma_S^2}\sum_{i=1}^{N}\|\rho_i \cdot m(t_i) - n_i\|_K^2,$$

where d is the distance metric on diffeomorphisms, which corresponds to the norm of initial momentum under unit-time parameterization of the geodesic. The energy, $\mathcal{E}$, is to be minimized subject to geodesic constraints on $\psi(t)$ and ρ_i for $i = 1, \ldots, N$. Here, σ_I^2 and σ_S^2 represent the variances corresponding to the likelihood for the intercept and slope terms respectively. Also, $\rho_i \cdot I(t_i)$ is the group action of the residual diffeomorphism ρ_i on the image, $I(t_i)$, and $\rho_i \cdot m(t_i)$ is its group action on the momenta, $m(t_i)$. This group action on momenta also coincides with the co-adjoint transport in the group of diffeomorphisms.

The above energy functional is written in terms of initial conditions of the group geodesic as:

$$\mathcal{E}(\psi, \rho_i, m(0), p_i(0), I(0)) = \frac{1}{2}\|m(0)\|_K^2$$

$$+ \frac{1}{2\sigma_I^2}\sum_{i=1}^{N}(\|p(0)_i\|_K^2 + \|\rho_i \cdot \psi(t_i) \cdot I(0) - J_i\|_{L^2}^2)$$

$$+ \frac{1}{2\sigma_S^2}\sum_{i=1}^{N}\|\rho_i \cdot \psi(t_i) \cdot m(0) - n_i\|_K^2.$$

This optimization problem corresponds to jointly estimating the group geodesic flow, ψ, and residual geodesic flows, ρ_i, and the group baseline template, $I(0)$.

Evaluating Gradients of $\mathcal{E}$: We introduce the time-dependent Lagrange multipliers, $\hat{m}, \hat{I}, \hat{v}$ to constrain the group trend, ψ, to be a geodesic and $\hat{p}_i, \hat{\rho}_i, \hat{u}_i$ to constrain the residuals, ρ_i, to be geodesics. We write the augmented energy as:

$$\tilde{\mathcal{E}} = \mathcal{E} +$$

$$\int_0^1 \langle \hat{m}, \dot{m} + \mathrm{ad}_v^* m\rangle_{L^2}dt + \int_0^1 \langle \hat{I}, \dot{I} + \nabla I \cdot v\rangle_{L^2}dt + \int_0^1 \langle \hat{v}, m - Lv\rangle_{L^2}dt +$$

$$\sum_{i=1}^{N}\int_0^1 \langle \hat{p}_i, \dot{p}_i + \mathrm{ad}_{u_i}^* p_i\rangle_{L^2}ds + \int_0^1 \langle \hat{u}_i, p_i - Lu_i\rangle_{L^2}ds + \int_0^1 \langle \hat{\rho}_i, \dot{\rho}_i \circ \rho_i^{-1} - u_i\rangle_{L^2}ds.$$

The variation of the energy functional $\tilde{\mathcal{E}}$ with respect to all time dependent variables results in ODEs in the form of dependent adjoint equations with boundary conditions and added jump conditions. For clarity we report derivatives first for the residual geodesics followed by that for the group geodesic.

For the residual geodesics, ρ_i parameterized by s: The resulting adjoint systems for the residual geodesics for $i = 1, \dots, N$ are:

$$\left.\begin{aligned}
\hat{u}_i - \dot{\hat{p}}_i + \mathrm{ad}_{u_i}\hat{p}_i &= 0\\
\hat{p}_i - L\hat{u}_i - \mathrm{ad}^*_{\hat{p}_i}p_i &= 0\\
-\dot{\hat{\rho}}_i - \mathrm{ad}^*_{u_i}\hat{\rho}_i &= 0
\end{aligned}\right\} \tag{5}$$

with boundary conditions:

$$\left.\begin{aligned}
\hat{p}_i(1) = 0, \text{ and } \hat{\rho}_i(1) = &-\frac{1}{\sigma_I^2}\left[(I(t_i) \circ \rho_i^{-1} - J_i)\right]\nabla(I(t_i) \circ \rho_i^{-1})\\
&-\frac{1}{\sigma_S^2}\left(\mathrm{ad}^*_{K\star[\mathrm{Ad}^*_{\rho_i^{-1}}m(t_i)-n_i]}\mathrm{Ad}^*_{\rho_i^{-1}}m(t_i)\right)
\end{aligned}\right\} \tag{6}$$

The gradients for update of initial momenta, p_i for residual diffeomorphisms are:

$$\delta_{p_i(0)}\tilde{\mathcal{E}} = \frac{1}{\sigma_I^2}K\star p_i(0) - \hat{p}_i(0). \tag{7}$$

The initial momenta, $p_i(0)$, for each individual is updated via gradient descent, using the gradient in (7), by first evaluating $\hat{p}_i(0)$ via backward integration of N adjoint systems in (5) starting from initial conditions in (6) for each individual. It is important to note that the residual diffeomorphisms, ρ_i, are not estimated using the usual image matching solution. Rather, this estimate maximizes the combined matching of both the base image J_i with $I(t_i)$ under the group action on images, and the momentum n_i with $m(t_i)$ under the co-adjoint transport, jointly over all the individuals.

For the group geodesic parameterized by t: The resulting adjoint system for the group geodesic:

$$\left.\begin{aligned}
-\dot{\hat{m}} + \mathrm{ad}_v\hat{m} + \hat{v} &= 0\\
-\dot{\hat{I}} - \nabla \cdot (\hat{I}v) &= 0\\
-\mathrm{ad}^*_{\hat{m}}m + \hat{I}\nabla I - L\hat{v} &= 0
\end{aligned}\right\} \tag{8}$$

with boundary conditions:

$$\hat{I}(1) = 0, \text{ and } \hat{m}(1) = 0, \tag{9}$$

with added jumps at measurements, t_i, such that,

$$\left.\begin{aligned}
\hat{I}(t^{i+}) - \hat{I}(t^{i-}) &= \frac{1}{\sigma_I^2}|D\rho_i|(I(t_i) \circ \rho_i^{-1} - J_i) \circ \rho_i\\
\hat{m}(t^{i+}) - \hat{m}(t^{i-}) &= \frac{1}{\sigma_S^2}\mathrm{Ad}_{\rho_i^{-1}}\left(K\star(\mathrm{Ad}^*_{\rho_i^{-1}}m(t_i) - n_i)\right)
\end{aligned}\right\} \tag{10}$$

Finally, the gradients for update of the initial group momentum is:

$$\delta_{m(0)}\tilde{\mathcal{E}} = K\star m(0) - \hat{m}(0) \tag{11}$$

The variation of $\tilde{\mathcal{E}}$ with respect to the group initial image, $\delta_{I_0}\tilde{\mathcal{E}}$, can be directly computed from the energy functional, $\tilde{\mathcal{E}}$. Since, $\rho_i \cdot \psi(t_i) \cdot I(0) = I(0) \circ \psi^{-1}(t_i) \circ \rho_i^{-1}(1) = I(0) \circ \phi^{-1}$, a change of variable for ϕ_i followed by taking the derivative with respect to $I(0)$ results in the closed form solution for optimum initial image, $I(0)$, for the group geodesic as:

$$I(0) = \frac{\sum_{i=1}^{N} J^i \circ \phi_i |D\phi_i|}{\sum_{i=1}^{N} |D\phi_i|} \tag{12}$$

During the joint optimization for computing group geodesic, the initial momenta, $m(0)$, is updated via gradient descent, using the gradient in (11), by first evaluating $\hat{m}(0)$ via backward integration of the adjoint system for the group in (8) starting from initial conditions in (9) with added jumps in (10). This can be interpreted as forces influencing the group geodesic by the individual initial images, J_i, and the momenta, n_i, that parameterize the individual trends. Thus, in effect, such a formulation incorporates the pull arising from the "differences" in the individual trajectories with the group trajectories and not just their base images. The energy functional at the group level is jointly minimized such that the group estimates, $I(0), m(0)$, and all the N residual estimates, $\rho_i(1), p_i(0)$, are updated at each iteration of gradient descent according to (7), (11) and (12).

3 Results

We evaluate our proposed model using synthetic and 3D-structural MRI data. Our focus in these experiments is to evaluate our primary proposed contribution, i.e., the estimation of group level trajectory given a population of trajectories. In our experiments, the kernel K corresponds to the invertible and self-adjoint fluid operator, $L = -a\nabla^2 - b\nabla(\nabla \cdot) + c$, with $a = 0.01$, $b = 0.01$, and $c = 0.001$.

Experiments with Synthetic Data: To test the group estimation in HGM, we generated the synthetic data using the forward model. We first generated a ground truth group geodesic in diffeomorphisms by solving the image matching problem to give initial conditions, $I(0)$, and $m(0)$. The image, $I(t)$, and momenta, $m(t)$, can be generated along the group geodesic via the EPDiff evolution equations. Figure 3 (first row) visualizes the trajectory of this group trend in terms of sampled shapes along this geodesic: plus to flower.

To generate the individual, random perturbations from the group trend were computed. This was done by generating initial conditions: images, $J_i(0)$, and momenta, $n_i(0)$, for the ith individual at time, t_i. In particular, the $J_i(0)$ are constructed by shooting the image $I(t_i)$ along the group geodesic at time, t_i, with a randomly generate momenta that consequently also defines a residual geodesic diffeomorphism ρ_i for this individual. Correspondingly, the initial individual momenta, $n_i(0)$, are generated by co-adjoint transport of $m(t_i)$ along the diffeomorphisms, ρ_i. In Figure 3 (second row), we visualize one such individual's own EPDiff geodesic evolution for which the initial conditions are generated at

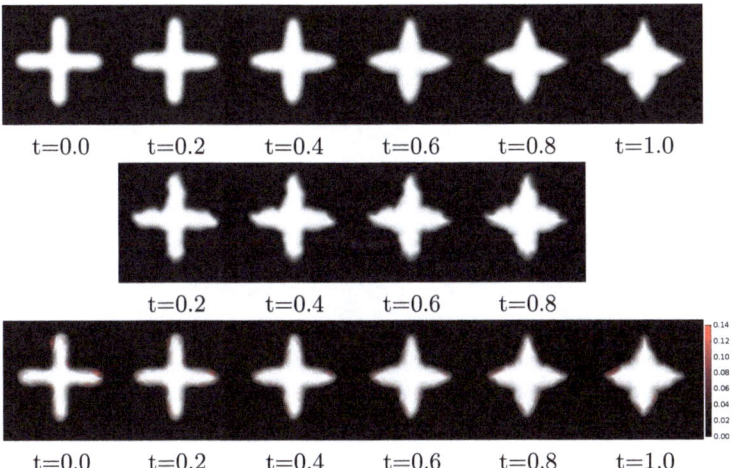

$t=0.0$ $t=0.2$ $t=0.4$ $t=0.6$ $t=0.8$ $t=1.0$

$t=0.2$ $t=0.4$ $t=0.6$ $t=0.8$

$t=0.0$ $t=0.2$ $t=0.4$ $t=0.6$ $t=0.8$ $t=1.0$

Fig. 3. First row: Synthetically generated ground truth group shape geodesic. Second Row: An example of a perturbed individual starting at t=0.2. Twenty four randomly perturbed individuals along the span of the geodesics were generated. Only the initial conditions of the perturbed individuals were used in the group trend estimation. Third Row: Recovered ground truth geodesic by HGM overlaid with difference in intensities relative to ground truth (in red).

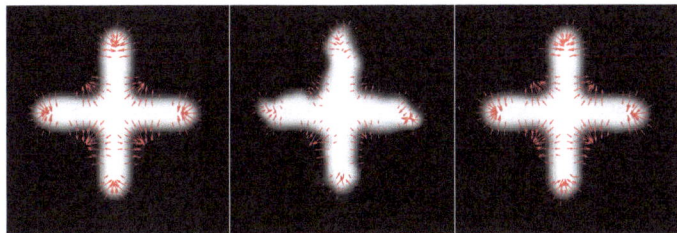

Fig. 4. Left: Initial conditions, intercept image and slope for ground truth group geodesic. Center: Example of the initial conditions for one perturbed individual from the group trend. Right: Recovered initial conditions for the group geodesic from randomly perturbed initial conditions using 24 individuals.

time $t = 0.2$. Using this procedure, we generate 24 such randomly perturbed trends from the group trend. The HGM algorithm only uses the initial conditions of the individual geodesics as input, i.e., images, $J_i(0)$, and initial momenta, $n_i(0)$, for all individuals, $i = 1, \ldots, 24$ for estimation of the group geodesics initial conditions, $m(0)$, and $I(0)$. The resulting estimated group trend closely match the ground truth geodesic, Figure 3 (third row). Head-to-head comparison of the initial conditions between estimated and ground truth are depicted in Figure 4, together with an example of one of the individual's perturbed initial conditions.

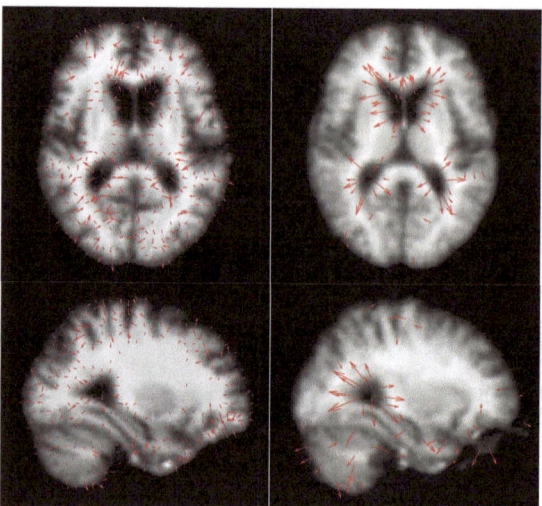

Fig. 5. Estimated group geodesics initial conditions for 3D MRI using HGM. Left column: $\sigma_S \gg \sigma_I$, does not represent average trend. Right column: $\sigma_I = 0.1, \sigma_S = 0.1$, better representative of the average trend. For fair comparison same cut-off was used for visualization of deformation momenta on both the runs.

Experiments with Brain Images from OASIS: We performed HGM analysis on longitudinal 3D-MRI sequences for seven individuals diagnosed with Alzheimer's disease with maximum scan range of 5 years. At the individual level of HGM, seven geodesic regressions are performed independently on the time-series of scans. At the group level, the initial conditions of the average geodesic are estimated based on the estimated initial conditions of seven individuals at individual level. The naive serial implementation of this algorithm took 7.5 hours to run 500 iterations of gradient descent for optimization on this dataset. Figure 5 reports the estimated initial conditions for the group geodesic at age=66 for different level of noise variance in intercept and slope terms.

We observe that forcing both the image and momenta to match the corresponding initial conditions of individual geodesics results in a different estimate of initial conditions for the group geodesic when compared to ignoring the momenta and forcing the image matching alone. For higher variance on the momenta matching term ($\sigma_S^2 \rightarrow \infty$), the resulting deformation directions exhibit patterns of deformation across the whole brain (Figure 5, Left). This is because variability across the subjects is very high. These deformations are capturing variability in brain shape across the population more than representing an average trajectory within an individual and hence is not a representative of the longitudinal trend in the population.

On the other hand, lowering the variance in the momenta matching term ($\sigma_S = 0.1, \sigma_I = 0.1$, Figure 5, Right) results in deformation patterns around regions expected to be changing for an individual as time progresses. In particular, the information about individual trajectories are taken into account in the averaging process more than inter-subject variability information, thus resulting in an average shape change that represents the longitudinal trend in the population. This is in accordance with the simple Euclidean case presented earlier (Figure 1), where ignoring the velocity matching results in an average line that does not represent the longitudinal variability in the population and hence fail to represent an average trajectory of changes in the dependent variable.

Acknowledgments. This research was supported by NIH grants 5R01EB007688, U01 AG024904, R01 MH084795 and P41 RR023953, and NSF CAREER Grant 1054057.

References

1. Arnol'd, V.I.: Sur la géométrie différentielle des groupes de Lie de dimension infinie et ses applications à l'hydrodynamique des fluides parfaits. Ann. Inst. Fourier 16, 319–361 (1966)
2. Beg, M., Miller, M., Trouvé, A., Younes, L.: Computing large deformation metric mappings via geodesic flows of diffeomorphisms. IJCV 61(2), 139–157 (2005)
3. Durrleman, S., Pennec, X., Trouvé, A., Gerig, G., Ayache, N.: Spatiotemporal atlas estimation for developmental delay detection in longitudinal datasets. In: Yang, G.-Z., Hawkes, D., Rueckert, D., Noble, A., Taylor, C. (eds.) MICCAI 2009, Part I. LNCS, vol. 5761, pp. 297–304. Springer, Heidelberg (2009)
4. Fishbaugh, J., Prastawa, M., Durrleman, S., Piven, J., Gerig, G.: Analysis of longitudinal shape variability via subject specific growth modeling. In: Ayache, N., Delingette, H., Golland, P., Mori, K. (eds.) MICCAI 2012, Part I. LNCS, vol. 7510, pp. 731–738. Springer, Heidelberg (2012)
5. Fletcher, P.T.: Geodesic regression on Riemannian manifolds. In: MICCAI Workshop on Mathematical Foundations of Computational Anatomy, pp. 75–86 (2011)
6. Laird, N.M., Ware, J.H.: Random-effects models for longitudinal data. Biometrics 38(4), 963–974 (1982)
7. Lorenzi, M., Ayache, N., Frisoni, G.B., Pennec, X., The Alzheimer's Disease Neuroimaging Initiative: Mapping the Effects of $A\beta_{1-42}$ Levels on the Longitudinal Changes in Healthy Aging: Hierarchical Modeling Based on Stationary Velocity Fields. In: Fichtinger, G., Martel, A., Peters, T. (eds.) MICCAI 2011, Part II. LNCS, vol. 6892, pp. 663–670. Springer, Heidelberg (2011)
8. Miller, M.I., Trouvé, A., Younes, L.: Geodesic shooting for computational anatomy. Journal of Mathematical Imaging and Vision 24(2), 209–228 (2006)
9. Muralidharan, P., Fletcher, P.: Sasaki metrics for analysis of longitudinal data on manifolds. In: IEEE Conference on CVPR, pp. 1027–1034 (June 2012)
10. Niethammer, M., Huang, Y., Vialard, F.-X.: Geodesic regression for image timeseries. In: Fichtinger, G., Martel, A., Peters, T. (eds.) MICCAI 2011, Part II. LNCS, vol. 6892, pp. 655–662. Springer, Heidelberg (2011)
11. Singh, N., Hinkle, J., Joshi, S., Fletcher, P.T.: A vector momenta formulation of diffeomorphisms for improved geodesic regression and atlas construction. In: International Symposium on Biomedial Imaging (ISBI) (April 2013)
12. Younes, L., Arrate, F., Miller, M.I.: Evolution equations in computational anatomy. Neuroimage 45(1 suppl.), S40–S50 (2009)

Active Testing Search for Point Cloud Matching

Miguel Amável Pinheiro[1], Raphael Sznitman[2], Eduard Serradell[3], Jan Kybic[1], Francesc Moreno-Noguer[3], and Pascal Fua[2]

[1] Center for Machine Perception, Faculty of Electrical Engineering,
Czech Technical University in Prague, Czech Republic
amavemig@cmp.felk.cvut.cz
http://cmp.felk.cvut.cz/~amavemig
[2] Computer Vision Laboratory, École Polytechnique Fédérale de Lausanne (EPFL),
Lausanne, Switzerland
[3] Institut de Robòtica i Informàtica Industrial (CSIC-UPC), Barcelona, Spain

Abstract. We present a general approach for solving the point-cloud matching problem for the case of mildly nonlinear transformations. Our method quickly finds a coarse approximation of the solution by exploring a reduced set of partial matches using an approach to which we refer to as *Active Testing Search* (ATS). We apply the method to registration of graph structures by branching point matching. It is based solely on the geometric position of the points, no additional information is used nor the knowledge of an initial alignment. In the second stage, we use dynamic programming to refine the solution. We tested our algorithm on angiography, retinal fundus, and neuronal data gathered using electron and light microscopy. We show that our method solves cases not solved by most approaches, and is faster than the remaining ones.

Keywords: point cloud matching, graph matching, image registration, active search, dendrites.

1 Overview

In this manuscript we consider the problem of point-cloud to point-cloud (PTP) matching. The problem consists of finding correspondences between two populations of points, related by a geometrical transformation. The transformation is assumed to be non-linear but not far from affine. The correspondences can be partial. We do not require an initial alignment nor any additional information except the point coordinates. However, if such information is available (e.g. local appearance or connectivity), it can be incorporated to reduce the search problem.

The main difficulty of the PTP problem is the large set of possible matches. The major challenge lies in the ability to formulate a search procedure that is tractable and still provides an acceptable solution. This is particularly true when the transformation between the two populations is non-rigid.

We consider this problem in the context of medical image registration. Three important challenges lie in such registration tasks. First, the transformation

J.C. Gee et al. (Eds.): IPMI 2013, LNCS 7917, pp. 572–583, 2013.

between curvilinear structures is generally non-rigid, which induces complex solutions that are difficult to compute. Second, appearance based measures of similarity (e.g. key point descriptors) cannot be used in some cases due to the fact that registration may be between different modalities (e.g. Electron Microscopy (EM) and Light Microscopy (LM)) [1]. Finally, registration may be at different physical scales (e.g. nm and μm) and hence consists of registering one domain to a substructure of another much larger structure.

In our approach, *Active Testing Search* (ATS) we take a Bayesian point of view and consider the correspondences to be random. We use a *sensor*: a black box function, which scores the quality any set of partial or complete point correspondences. The probability of the correctness of the match given a sensor output is given by a *sensor model*, which we learn from data. We make observations sequentially and integrate information received from the sensor by computing the posterior probability of the correspondence correctness. We explore the space of possible potential correspondences by performing a priority search based on the information gain, adding one point match per step, similar to the *Twenty Questions* game with noisy outputs [2–5].

2   Related Work

The difficulty of registering medical images lies on the nonlinearity between structures and also high number of outliers, such as in the case of EM and LM images. These structures can be interpreted as point clouds or as graphs. In the first case, some authors have proposed transformation minimizations between the sets [6, 7], which however fails when the sets are not roughly aligned or when the number of outliers is too high. Another approach to this problem is to try to find the correct correspondence between the points [8–10].

Another popular approach is ICP (Iterative Closest Point) [11], which iteratively calculates the closest distance between points, assigns correspondences and calculates the rigid transformation between the sets until convergence. The method and its variants [12, 13] also require the initial position of the sets to be relatively close.

Local similarities such as geometric compatibilities and feature descriptors could also help establish correspondences between points [14, 15]. However, in the presence of shearing and nonrigid transformations, the approach proves to be sensitive.

Using graph information can provide further constraints in the problem, such as local connectivity and geodesic distance preservation [16, 1]. However, most of these approaches are either not robust enough to solve harder cases [17] or are not scalable [1].

3   Notation

Consider two sets of points $X^A = \{x_1^A, ..., x_N^A\}$ and $X^B = \{x_1^B, ..., x_M^B\}$ of size N and M respectively, with $x_i^A \in \mathbb{R}^{D_A}$ and $x_j^B \in \mathbb{R}^{D_B}$. We want to find a matching where each element x_i^A of X^A maps to at most one element of X^B, which is

Table 1. Summary of Notation

$X^A = \{x_1^A, ..., x_N^A\}$	Source point cloud
$X^B = \{x_1^B, ..., x_M^B\}$	Target point cloud
$Y = (Y_1, ..., Y_N)$	Correspondences for X^A
$Y^* = (Y_1^*, ..., Y_N^*)$	True correspondences
$\mathcal{Y}$	Space of feasible correspondences
$A = \{Y_1 = y_1, ..., Y_d = y_d\}$	Partial assignment
$\mathcal{A}_d$	Set of partial assignments of length d
$\psi(A)$	Sensor function
$(\boldsymbol{\theta}_1, \boldsymbol{\theta}_0)$	Sensor noise model parameters
γ	Minimum number of required assignments for ψ
S_A	Sensor response for set A
$r(S_A)$	Sensor likelihood ratio
K	Total number of iterations
π_k	Assignment to evaluate at iteration k
$\boldsymbol{\pi} = (\pi_1, ..., \pi_K)$	Sequence of observations to make
$\mathcal{C}_A$	Set of children of A

represented by an index $Y_i \in \{-1, 1, ..., M\}$ to X^B, with a virtual element of index -1 meaning no match (an outlier). We consider $Y = (Y_1, ..., Y_N) \in \mathcal{Y}$, where $\mathcal{Y}$ is the space of all possible solutions, to be a discrete random vector, with probability $P(Y) = P(Y_1, ..., Y_N)$. Note that the ordering of Y is important. Our objective is to find Y^*, the true correspondence between X^A and X^B.

A *partial assignment* is a vector $A = (Y_1 = y_1, ..., Y_d = y_d)$, where we require the correspondences to be determined in order. We denote $\mathcal{A}_d$ the set of all possible partial correspondences of d elements.

The sets $\mathcal{A}_d$ can be organized hierarchically into a tree, where children are formed from parents by adding one additional match. The children of A are $\mathcal{C}_A = \{A \cup \{Y_{|A|+1} = y\}\}$, with $y \in \{-1, 1, ..., M\}, y \notin A$.

A sensor is a task specific function $\psi : \mathcal{A} \to \mathbb{R}$ such that $S_A = \psi(A)$ evaluates a partial correspondence A for $|A| \geq \gamma$, where γ is the minimum number of matches required to calculate ψ. Let $\boldsymbol{\pi} = (\pi_1, ..., \pi_K)$ be the sequence of subsets observed throughout the algorithm, where $\pi_k \in \mathcal{A}$, is the kth set of partial assignments to observe.

4   Objective

Our objective is to estimate Y^* from some observation S_{π_k}. To do this, we consider solving the MAP,

$$Y^* = \arg\max_{y \in \mathcal{Y}} P(Y|S_{\pi_1}, ..., S_{\pi_K}) = \arg\max_{y \in \mathcal{Y}} \left\{ \frac{1}{Z} P(Y) P(S_{\pi_1}, ..., S_{\pi_K}|Y) \right\}$$

$$= \arg\max_{y \in \mathcal{Y}} \left\{ \frac{1}{Z} P(Y) \prod_{i=1}^{K} P(S_{\pi_k}|Y) \right\}, \quad (1)$$

where Z is a constant factor.

Clearly, considering all possible correspondences in $\boldsymbol{\pi}$ is intractable. RANSAC [8] and MLESAC [9] can been viewed as solving Eq. 1 when $\boldsymbol{\pi}$ contains only randomly chosen partial assignments of fixed size (i.e. $\forall k, |\pi_k| = $ const, depending on the number of degrees of freedom of the transformation).

In our approach, we differ from RANSAC and MLESAC in two important ways. First, π_k are selected sequentially and on the fly, based on the previous values observed from $\pi_1, \ldots, \pi_{k-1}$. This makes our selection process adaptive and fully data-driven. Second, to allow maximum flexibility with respect to the types of possible correspondences (i.e. non-rigid transformations), we let $|\pi_k|$ vary; it will typically increase as the transformation is refined and which is vital for estimating correspondences for non-rigid transformations..

5   Active Testing Search

Our method attempts to approximately solve the MAP of Eq. 1. To do this, we begin with a prior on Y, observe π_1 using our chosen sensor ψ, compute the posterior distribution of Y given the new information, S_{π_1}, and select the most promising new set π_2 to evaluate based on the posterior distribution. This process repeats K times and the best correspondence set, defined as the set with the highest number of inliers, is retained.

5.1   Sensor and Sensor Model

As described previously, our sensor is a function $\psi : \mathcal{A} \to \mathbb{R}$, with a random response $\psi(A) = S_A$. We assume the following model

$$P(S_A = s_A | Y) = \begin{cases} \xi(S_A = s_A; \boldsymbol{\theta}_1^d), & \text{if } A \subset Y^* \\ \xi(S_A = s_A; \boldsymbol{\theta}_0^d), & \text{if } A \not\subset Y^* \end{cases} \qquad (2)$$

where $d = |A|$, $\xi(S_A = s_A; \boldsymbol{\theta}_1^d)$ and $\xi(S_A = s_A; \boldsymbol{\theta}_0^d)$ are respectively the *positive* and *negative* distributions and $\boldsymbol{\theta}_1^d$ and $\boldsymbol{\theta}_0^d$ its parameters. We also define likelihood ratio

$$r(s_A) = \frac{\xi(S_A = s_A ; \boldsymbol{\theta}_1^d)}{\xi(S_A = s_A ; \boldsymbol{\theta}_0^d)}. \qquad (3)$$

The sensor score implicitly characterizes the expected geometrical transformations and depends directly on the number of assignments d in A. For simplicity, we will assume $\xi(\cdot; \boldsymbol{\theta}_1^d)$ and $\xi(\cdot; \boldsymbol{\theta}_0^d)$ to be Gaussian and we will describe in Sec. 7 how the parameters of these distributions can be obtained from training data. Using the Gaussian Processes non-linear regression (GPR) described in [1], we can estimate the position of a match of a point x_i^A in X^A, which we denote $\bar{x}_i^A$. The GPR models the geometrical transformation as affine with a small random nonlinear component, which is spatially correlated and its amplitude is controlled by a parameter σ_n^2. Note that the prediction is based on a partial assignment A. We have used GPR to generate the following two sensors:

Assigned Distance. We use the predictions from GPR to define the total cost of assigning the points $\{\bar{x}_i^A\}$ to X^B

$$S_A = \sum_{i=1}^{N} \sum_{j=1}^{M} H_{i,j} \cdot \text{dist}(\bar{x}_i^A, x_j^B), \tag{4}$$

where $\text{dist}(\bar{x}_i^A, x_j^B)$ is the Euclidean distance between $\bar{x}_i^A$ and x_j^B and H is the optimal assignment matrix computed by the Hungarian algorithm [18] so that S_A is minimal. We make use of an assignment so that we penalize situations where $\bar{x}_i^A$ is positioned solely around a subset of small size of X_B.

Number of inliers. We also calculate the relative number of points consistent with the GPR. This is calculated as the ratio over $|X^A|$ of the number of points in X^B which have some point $\{\bar{x}_i^A\}$ closer than σ_n^2,

$$S_A = \frac{|I|}{|X^A|}, \quad I = \left\{ x_j^B \in X^B \mid \exists \bar{x}_i^A, \text{dist}(x_j^B, \bar{x}_i^A) < \sigma_n^2 \right\}. \tag{5}$$

5.2 Hierarchical Search

In many datasets, we can select a smaller number of important points B^A from all points X^A to be matched, $B^A \ll X^A$. For example, in a dataset created by segmenting a dendritic tree, the branching points are structurally more important than points on the edges connecting the branching points.

Our strategy then is to use the sensor $S_A = \psi(A)$ from (4) only on the 'important' points B^A, for 'small' partial matches A where $|A| < \delta$. For partial matches bigger than δ, we switch to the sensor (5) evaluated on the full set of points X^A. This allows for a fast search at low depths of the search tree, which constitutes most of the evaluated proposals π_k, and a more discriminative selection at higher depths.

5.3 Computing Posterior Probability Distributions

In this setting, aggregating observations can be achieved by using a Bayesian formulation. We can compute the posterior distribution when π_k has been observed by

$$P(Y|S_{\pi_1}, \ldots, S_{\pi_k}) = \frac{1}{Z} \left[r(S_{\pi_k}) \mathbb{1}_{\pi_k \subset Y} + \mathbb{1}_{\pi_k \not\subset Y} \right] P(Y|S_{\pi_1}, \ldots, S_{\pi_{k-1}}), \tag{6}$$

where

$$Z = r(S_{\pi_k}) P(\pi_k) + 1 - P(\pi_k) \tag{7}$$

and $r(S_{\pi_k})$ is defined in Eq. 3. There are two important aspects of (6). First, it is recursive, allowing the posterior $P(Y \mid S_{\pi_1} \ldots S_{\pi_k})$ to be computed from the previous posterior. This allows online integration of new information. Second, the normalization factor Z is independent on Y and can therefore be ignored when comparing the likelihood of different hypotheses Y.

5.4   Implementation and Algorithm

The search method is given in Algorithm 1. The probabilities $P(Y|S_{\pi_1}, \ldots, S_{\pi_k})$ are stored in a priority queue Q (line 1). Initially, this queue will hold all the elements of the subspace $\mathcal{A}_\gamma$ with the same likelihood $\epsilon = 1/|\mathcal{A}_\gamma|$ of being contained in the true set of correspondences (i.e. uniform prior on Y). The priority queue is ordered by the likelihood ϵ that a partial assignment is correct.

Algorithm 1. Active Testing Search $(X^A, X^B; K, \psi, \boldsymbol{\theta}_1, \boldsymbol{\theta}_0, \gamma)$

1: Initialize Priority Queue: $Q \leftarrow Push(A, 1/|\mathcal{A}_\gamma|), \forall A \in \mathcal{A}_\gamma$
2: **for** $k = 1 \ldots K$ **do**
3:     $\{\pi_k, \epsilon_k\} = \text{pop}(Q)$; //choose the most likely π_k
4:     $S_{\pi_k} = \psi(\pi_k)$
5:     **for** $y \in \mathcal{C}_{\pi_k}$ **do**
6:         $Q \leftarrow Push(\pi_k \cup \{Y_{|\pi_k|+1} = y\}, \epsilon_k r(S_{\pi_k})/|\mathcal{C}_{\pi_k}|)$
7:     **end for**
8: **end for**
9: **return** $\pi^* = \arg\max_{\{\pi_1, \ldots, \pi_K\}} S_{\pi_k}$

For each iteration k, we select the partial assignment with the biggest likelihood ϵ_k. We use the sensor and compute the noisy score $S_{\pi_k} = \psi(\pi_k)$. At this point we must compute the posterior distribution given this new observation. To do this, we first generate children $\mathcal{C}_{\pi_k}$ of π_k and insert them into the queue using (6) (line 6). The queue maintains an unnormalized posterior distribution to avoid unnecessary computational costs. This process is repeated K times, at which point we return the assignment π^* which scored the highest. Our method does not perform a breadth-first, or depth-first search as in traditional search strategies. Rather, it is an adaptive strategy which allows constant backtracking and avoids hand-tune pruning of the search space.

6   Fine Alignment

Depending on the choice of K, Algorithm 1 will find only a subset of all inliers. A fine alignment can be added as a post-processing stage, to identify remaining inliers and if possibly slightly modifies the transformation. An algorithm such as the coherent point drift [7] is very well suited for this task. We use the approach described in [1], which locally finds assignment of the yet unassigned points by the Hungarian algorithm [18], using the already assigned points as constraints. The GPR transformation model is updated and the process is iterated until convergence.

7   Learning the Distributions

Given a specific sensor ψ, as described in Sec. 5.1, we need to learn the sensor model parameters. To reduce the number of degrees of freedom, we assume that

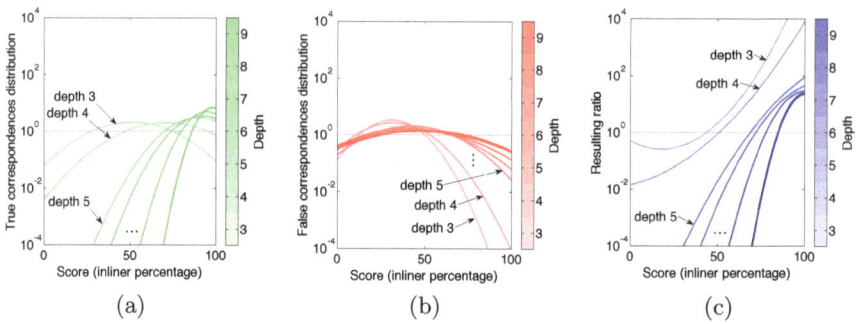

Fig. 1. Example for values of distributions taken from **(a)** true correspondences samples, **(b)** false correspondences and **(c)** ratio between the true and false distributions. The sensor used to compute this example was the number of inliers – described in Eq. 5.

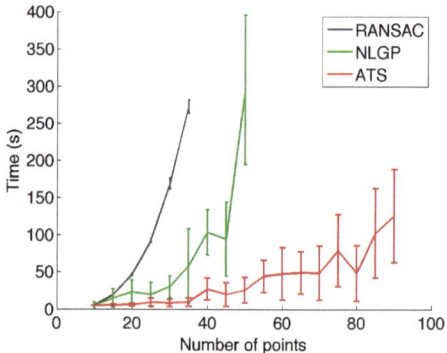

Fig. 2. Processing time required by RANSAC and NLGP in comparison to our method as a function of the number of points

it does not depend on the number of points M of X^B, at least when M is of the same order of magnitude as N.

In general, for a given sensor ψ, an outlier ratio R_O and a point set size N, we learn the parameters $\boldsymbol{\theta}_1^d$ and $\boldsymbol{\theta}_0^d$ as follows: we generate L point clouds X^A and L random affine transformations, together with a nonlinear deformation to each point from which we compute X^B and for which we know the correspondence Y^* – generating a set $\{\{X^A\}_l, \{X^B\}_l, Y_l^*\}_{l=1}^L$. Then, for $\gamma \leq d \leq N$, we sample assignments $A \in \mathcal{A}_d$ such that $A \in Y$ and compute S_A. Once all $N - \gamma$ scores on all L generated sets are computed, we estimate the Gaussian distribution parameters $\{\boldsymbol{\theta}^d\}_{d=\gamma}^N = \{\mu_d, \sigma_d\}_{d=\gamma}^N$. The learned probability densities can be seen in Fig. 1(a).

For the distribution of false correspondences we follow a similar sampling approach. However, especially for larger correspondences deeper in the tree, we

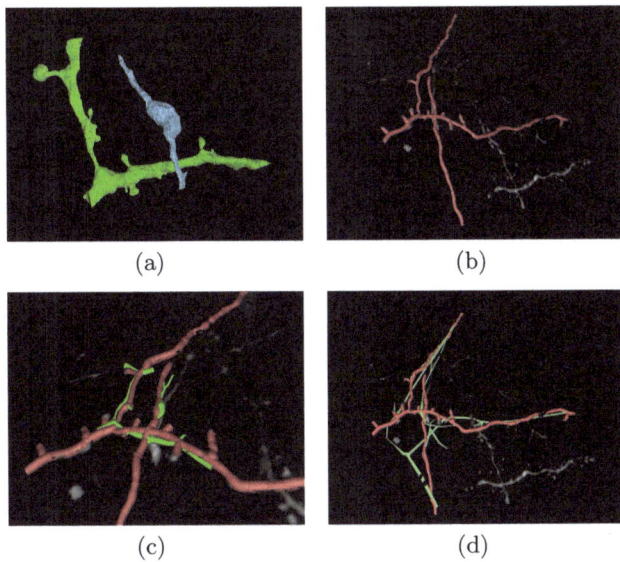

(a)   (b)

(c)   (d)

Fig. 3. Light and electron microscopy neuronal trees. **(a):** Segmented electron microscopy data. **(b):** Segmented light microscope data. **(c):** Registration of structures using ATS. **(d):** Registration using CPD.

will mostly encounter correspondences composed of mostly true correspondences, except for the last one. Therefore, we sample many random false correspondences at lower depths and false correspondences close to the true ones at higher depths. An example of such distribution can be seen in Fig. 1(b).

In Fig. 1(c), we can see the likelihood ratio between the distributions for true and false correspondences. This shows that the sensor gets more discriminative as the size of the partial correspondence being tested increases.

8   Experiments

We present a number of experiments to illustrate the performance of our method (Active Testing Search – ATS) against state of the art approaches in point matching, with or without additional structure information. We have tested: Non-Linear GP (NLGP) [1], Coherent Point Drift (CPD) [7], Iterative Closest Point [11] and RANSAC [8]. For RANSAC, we test affine transformations from the random branching points, applying the result on all the nodes.

8.1   Experiments on Synthetic Data

We generated random two dimensional point data sets with random affine transformation. For the NLGP that requires connection information, a Minimum Spanning Tree was found. Observe that the processing time (Fig. 2) increases much faster with both NLGP and RANSAC, while for ATS it stays manageable.

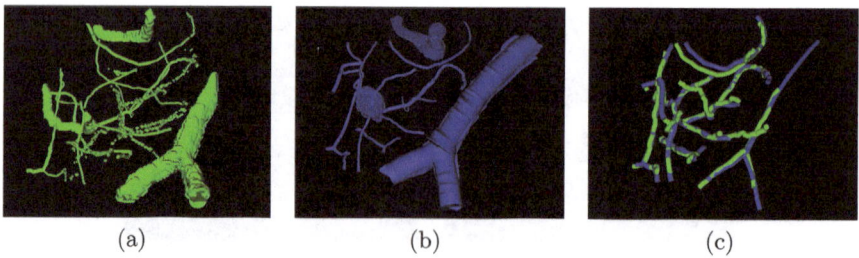

(a)   (b)   (c)

Fig. 4. Blood vessels in brain tissue. **(a):** Segmented two photon microscopy data. **(b):** Segmented bright-field optical microscopy data. **(c):** Registration of structures using Active Testing Search.

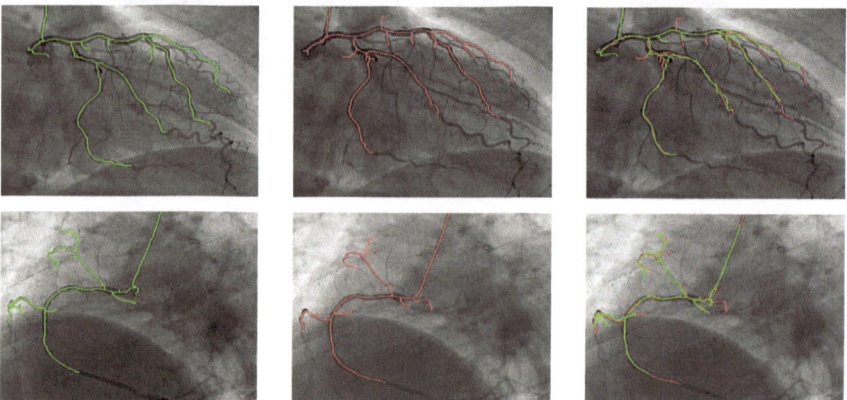

Fig. 5. Matching and registration of heart angiograms. **Left and center:** Original data. **Right:** Registration of structures using Active Testing Search.

8.2   Experiments on Real Data

A variety of datasets from medical imaging was collected. The graphs were extracted through a semi-automatic approach using the Fiji[1] platform and its plugins. In Tables 2 and 3, we can see the error obtained and times elapsed, respectively, for every method tested. The computed error is the mean distance of each point to its nearest neighbor in the original data to which the graph was matched. For ATS and NLGP, we show the coarse and fine alignment algorithm times separately.

Fig. 3 shows 3D neuronal structures from electron (EM) and light (LM) microscopy, where electron microscopy data is a nonlinearly deformed subset of the data light microscopy. The intended application is to automatically localize the EM volume in the LM volume. Only ATS and NLGP are able to correctly align the structures. CPD obtains a numerically small error, but as seen

---

[1] http://pacific.mpi-cbg.de

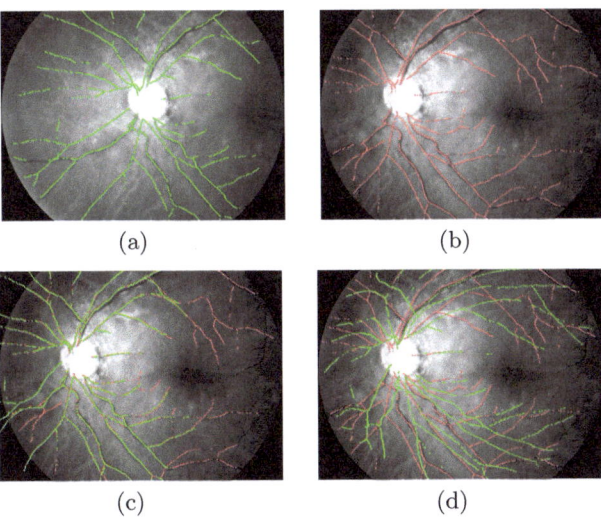

(a)   (b)

(c)   (d)

Fig. 6. Retinal fundus tree images. **(a) and (b):** Original data. **(c):** Registration of structures using Active Testing Search, **(d):** Registration using CPD.

in Fig. 3, the alignment is not correct and the resulting deformation is not realistic. The great advantage of ATS over NLGP is the much shorter elapsed time (Table 3).

In Fig. 4, a blood vessels network in brain tissue is imaged. One of the 3D image stacks is acquired using a two photon microscope and the other using bright-filed microscopy after excision and fixation.

In Fig. 5 and Fig. 6, we show 2D datasets of heart angiograms and retinal fundus images. The angiograms present a nonlinear transformation which is correctly recovered by the approach. The retinal fundus images present a high number of outliers in both images. Nonetheless, the algorithm correctly identifies the alignment. For the data from retinal fundus, the remaining methods do not recover correctly the alignment, although CPD and ICP present a small error (Table 2).

Table 2. Real data error for ATS and other state of the art methods. * Not correctly aligned (see Fig. 3(d) or Fig. 6(d) for example).

Error (pixels)					
Dataset (Fig.)	**ATS**	**NLGP**	**CPD**	**ICP**	**RANSAC**
Neuronal (3)	0.161	0.181	0.563*	2.995*	0.449*
Brain tissue (4)	0.159	0.171	0.164	0.851*	0.606*
Angio. (5 Top)	1.361	1.178	1.232	1.430	12.487*
Angio. (5 Bottom)	2.072	2.074	2.195	2.122	35.384*
Retina (6)	5.587	5.613	5.503*	6.524*	10.762*

582   M.A. Pinheiro et al.

Table 3. Processing time for each method and each dataset, in seconds

Dataset (Fig.)	ATS (coarse+fine)	NLGP (coarse+fine)	CPD	ICP	RANSAC
	Elapsed time (seconds)				
Neuronal (3)	42.4 + 15.8	116.1 + 18.2	22.2	28.2	606.9
Brain tissue (4)	593.7 + 55.5	15029.1 + 19.9	37.1	30.9	570.7
Angio. (5 Top)	307.8 + 129.4	1240.9 + 162.8	144.3	8.1	1608.1
Angio. (5 Bottom)	167.9 + 77.2	112.0 + 95.4	68.8	5.0	346.5
Retina (6)	1293.3 + 406.4	5998.9 + 336.8	580.2	24.3	8901.5

9 Conclusion

We presented a general approach for the exploration of a tree of possible correspondences between two sets of points, using partial assignments and a Bayesian model. We have shown how we can include graph constraints to reduce the number of points, allowing for a faster search. We have also shown that our method is able to correctly align biological structures that are nonlinearly transformed and extracted with different techniques. These structures need not to be pre-aligned. Our method finds the correct alignment for all considered datasets and is faster than NLGP and RANSAC. It allows a considerably faster exploration of correspondences over the method which correctly finds a solution for harder datasets.

Acknowledgments The authors would like to acknowledge the Fundação para a Ciência e Tecnologia (FCT) for the Ph.D. grant SFRH/BD/77134/2011. This work was also supported by the Czech Science Foundation under the project P202/11/0111, by the Grant Agency of the Czech Technical University in Prague under the grant SGS12/190/OHK3/3T/13, by the EU ERC project Micro-Nano, and also by the Spanish Ministry of Economy and Competitiveness under projects PAU+ DPI2011-27510 and MIPRCV Consolider Ingenio 2010 CSD2007-00018.

References

1. Serradell, E., Glowacki, P., Kybic, J., Moreno-Noguer, F., Fua, P.: Robust non-rigid registration of 2D and 3D graphs. In: IEEE CVPR, pp. 996–1003 (2012)
2. Geman, D., Jedynak, B.: An active testing model for tracking roads in satellite images. IEEE Trans. on Pattern Analysis and Machine Intelligence 18, 1–14 (1995)
3. Yuille, A., Coughlan, J.: Twenty questions, focus of attention, and A*: A theoretical comparison of optimization strategies. In: International Workshop on Energy Minimization Methods in CVPR, pp. 197–212 (1997)
4. Sznitman, R., Jedynak, B.: Active testing for face detection and localization. IEEE Trans. on Pattern Analysis and Machine Intelligence 32(10), 1914–1920 (2010)
5. Sznitman, R., Richa, R., Taylor, R.H., Jedynak, B., Hager, G.D.: Unified detection and tracking of instruments during retinal microsurgery. IEEE Trans. on Pattern Analysis and Machine Intelligence 99, 1 (2012)

6. Gold, S., Rangarajan, A., Lu, C.P., Mjolsness, E.: New algorithms for 2D and 3D point matching: Pose estimation and correspondence. Pattern Recognition 31, 957–964 (1997)
7. Myronenko, A., Song, X.: Point set registration: Coherent point drift. IEEE Trans. on Pattern Analysis and Machine Intelligence 32(12), 2262–2275 (2010)
8. Fischler, M.A., Bolles, R.C.: Random sample consensus: a paradigm for model fitting with applications to image analysis and automated cartography. Commun. ACM 24, 381–395 (1981)
9. Torr, P.H.S., Zisserman, A.: MLESAC: A new robust estimator with application to estimating image geometry. Computer Vision and Image Understanding 78, 138–156 (2000)
10. Chum, O., Matas, J.: Matching with PROSAC – progressive sample consensus. In: IEEE CVPR, pp. 220–226 (2005)
11. Besl, P.J., McKay, N.D.: A method for registration of 3-D shapes. IEEE Trans. on Pattern Analysis and Machine Intelligence 14(2), 239–256 (1992)
12. Pajdla, T., Van Gool, L.: Matching of 3-D curves using semi-differential invariants. In: IEEE ICCV, pp. 390–395 (1995)
13. Rusinkiewicz, S., Levoy, M.: Efficient variants of the icp algorithm. In: International Conference on 3-D Digital Imaging and Modeling, pp. 145–152 (2001)
14. Belongie, S., Malik, J., Puzicha, J.: Shape matching and object recognition using shape contexts. IEEE Trans. on Pattern Analysis and Machine Intelligence 24, 509–522 (2001)
15. Leordeanu, M., Hebert, M.: A Spectral Technique for Correspondence Problems Using Pairwise Constraints. In: IEEE ICCV, vol. 2, pp. 1482–1489 (2005)
16. Serradell, E., Moreno-Noguer, F., Kybic, J., Fua, P.: Robust elastic 2D/3D geometric graph matching. SPIE Medical Imaging 8314(1), 831408-1–831408-8 (2012)
17. Cour, T., Srinivasan, P., Shi, J.: Balanced graph matching. In: Neural Information Processing Systems, pp. 313–320 (2006)
18. Kuhn, H.W.: The Hungarian method for the assignment problem. Naval Research Logistics 2(1-2), 83–97 (1955)

Relating Fisher Information to Detectability of Changes in Nodule Characteristics with CT

Qin Li, Rongping Zeng, Kyle J. Myers, Berkman Sahiner, Marios A. Gavrielides, and Nicholas Petrick

Division of Imaging and Applied Mathematics, Office of Science and Engineering Laboratories, Center for Devices and Radiological Health, US Food and Drug Administration, Silver Spring, MD, USA

Abstract. Fisher information provides a bound on the variance of any unbiased estimate for estimation tasks involving nonrandom parameters. In addition, a Fisher information approximation for ideal-observer detectability has been derived. We adopt and generalize such an approximation to establish a method to assess a system's ability to detect small changes in lesion characteristics. By representing the lesion by a size parameter, the ability to detect small changes can be approximated by a function involving the size difference and the Fisher information. A concept, termed the approximated least required difference (ALRD), is introduced and evaluated as an upper bound for assessing a system's power in size discrimination. We present a simulation study for lung nodules as an example to illustrate such a framework, where the image model incorporates a simulated CT imaging system, a thorax background and parameterized nodules. The noise is assumed to be multivariate Gaussian and the noise power spectrum (NPS) method is used to estimate the covariance matrix for the Fisher information calculation. In addition to bounding performance, our results also provide insights into factors, including nodule characteristics and acquisition parameters, that influence ALRD performance. This framework can be extended to connect other discrimination and estimation tasks, facilitating objective assessment and optimization of quantitative imaging systems.

1 Introduction

Lung nodule growth or shrinkage is an important indicator of nodule malignancy, with growing nodules much more likely to be malignant. Likewise, tracking changes in nodule size as part of treatment monitoring allows patient response and treatment effectiveness to be monitored for individual patients. While early determination of small changes in nodules is desired, it is quite difficult due to the uncertainties associated with the imaging and size measurement processes. For instance, the standard RECIST criteria, which applies only for lesions of 10mm size or greater, only allows for determination of progressive disease when a 20% growth in longest diameter is observed [1]. There is a clear need for improved image acquisition and analysis methods that enable the detection of smaller changes in nodule size, and the quantification of such changes accurately, so they can be reliably applied to smaller nodules.

J.C. Gee et al. (Eds.): IPMI 2013, LNCS 7917, pp. 584–593, 2013.

Modern multi-detector row CT (MDCT) systems can now scan the whole lung within a single breath hold with a thin reconstructed slice thickness, facilitating 3D nodule volume estimation. However, efforts are still needed to quantitatively assess the bias and variance of volumetric measurements, which depend on a number of factors including scan acquisition and reconstruction parameters, nodule characteristics, and estimation methods [2]. In [3, 4], phantom studies were conducted to quantify the magnitude of such effects. Phantom studies provide a framework with known truth, enabling the determination of performance estimates under well-controlled conditions. It would also be useful to derive theoretical bounds on performance for this lung nodule volume estimation task and evaluate them by means of simulation studies, where we are not constrained to a limited set of nodule phantoms and imaging conditions.

Fisher information is a common construct in parameter estimation problems. It is well known that for estimation of nonrandom parameters, a lower bound of the variance of an unbiased estimator is given by the Cramer-Rao inequality, which is directly related to the Fisher information matrix. On the other hand, Fisher information also enters into the figure of merit for performance of classification tasks [5]. Intuitively, the performance of a classification task depends on how well the distributions of the classes are separated. Therefore, Fisher information must be tied with classification problems since it is also known as a metric to measure the informational difference between two probability distributions in information geometry [6].

The receiver operating characteristic (ROC) curve is a plot of the relationship between the true positive fraction and the false positive fraction for a decision-maker in a binary classification task, which is becoming increasingly widely used in the medical community [7]. Shen and Clarkson [8, 9] investigated the relation between Fisher information and area under the ROC curve (AUC), a figure of merit for binary classification problems. They derived a simple approximation relating the Fisher information to the detectability of a small change in the parameter of the probability distribution function (PDF) that governs the statistics of the data. In particular, the square of the detectability can be approximated to the second order as a product involving the parameter difference and the Fisher information.

Inspired by such a connection, we are proposing a method to assess the ability of a system to detect lesion size changes, particularly for the problem of lung nodule size change detection in CT images. Instead of looking at the signal size estimation task directly, we evaluate the difference that ensures size change detection at a certain level of detectability. By using the connection between Fisher information and AUC, we tie together estimation and detection tasks for this application.

2   Fisher Information and Detectability of Small Changes

We consider signals $\mathbf{f}(\mathbf{a})$ in physical space, parameterized by a nonrandom parameter vector $\mathbf{a}$. We denote the observed data as vector $\mathbf{g}$. For an estimation task, we wish to estimate parameter vector $\mathbf{a}$ from $\mathbf{g}$. Let $\hat{\mathbf{a}}(\mathbf{g})$ be an unbiased estimate, and ϵ_i be the ith component of the estimation error $\hat{\mathbf{a}}(\mathbf{g}) - \mathbf{a}$; then its variance satisfies

$$\sigma_{\epsilon_i}^2 \triangleq \mathrm{Var}\left(\hat{a}_i(\mathbf{g}) - a_i\right) \geq \left(F_{ii}(\mathbf{a})\right)^{-1} , \tag{1}$$

where the Fisher information matrix $\mathbf{F}(\mathbf{a}) = (F_{ij}(\mathbf{a}))$,

$$F_{ij}(\mathbf{a}) = \mathrm{E}\left\{\frac{\partial \ln pr(\mathbf{g}|\mathbf{a})}{\partial a_i} \cdot \frac{\partial \ln pr(\mathbf{g}|\mathbf{a})}{\partial a_j}\right\} , \tag{2}$$

assuming that the first and second derivative of $\ln pr(\mathbf{g}|\mathbf{a})$ exist [5], where $pr(\mathbf{g}|\mathbf{a})$ is the probability density of $\mathbf{g}$ conditioned on $\mathbf{a}$.

Instead of estimating $\mathbf{a}$, we are interested in detecting changes in $\mathbf{a}$. Assume there are two classes H_0 and H_1 of which the signal parameter vector has value $\mathbf{a}_0$ and $\mathbf{a}_1$ respectively. The question we address is determining which signal, $\mathbf{f}(\mathbf{a}_0)$ or $\mathbf{f}(\mathbf{a}_1)$, is present based on $\mathbf{g}$. The ideal-observer decides in favor of one or the other hypothesis by comparing the likelihood ratio Λ to a threshold, where

$$\Lambda = \frac{pr(\mathbf{g}|H_1)}{pr(\mathbf{g}|H_0)} , \text{ or alternatively, } \Lambda = \frac{pr(\mathbf{g}|\mathbf{a}_1)}{pr(\mathbf{g}|\mathbf{a}_0)} . \tag{3}$$

The ideal-observer utilizes all statistical information about the data, and as a result maximizes the AUC. Let $\Delta \mathbf{a} = \mathbf{a}_1 - \mathbf{a}_0$. Following [8, 9], we define $d_A(\mathbf{a}_0, \Delta\mathbf{a})$ as an index on the ability to differentiate between $\mathbf{f}(\mathbf{a}_0)$ and $\mathbf{f}(\mathbf{a}_1)$. The AUC and this index are related by

$$\mathrm{AUC} = \frac{1}{2} + \frac{1}{2}\mathrm{erf}\left(\frac{1}{2} d_A(\mathbf{a}_0, \Delta\mathbf{a})\right). \tag{4}$$

When $\Delta\mathbf{a}$ is small, by expanding $d_A^2(\mathbf{a}_0, \Delta\mathbf{a})$ at $\mathbf{a}_0$, a second order approximation is obtained as in [8]

$$d_A^2(\mathbf{a}_0, \Delta\mathbf{a}) \approx \Delta\mathbf{a}^T \cdot \mathbf{F}(\mathbf{a}_0) \cdot \Delta\mathbf{a} . \tag{5}$$

Hence, a firmer mathematical connection between the detection and estimation tasks is given by:

$$\mathrm{AUC} \approx \frac{1}{2} + \frac{1}{2}\mathrm{erf}\left(\frac{1}{2}\sqrt{\Delta\mathbf{a}^T \cdot \mathbf{F}(\mathbf{a}_0) \cdot \Delta\mathbf{a}}\right). \tag{6}$$

In [8], several examples for detecting weak signals were presented, showing high agreement between the approximation and the exact calculation of detection performance. In the remainder of this paper, we adopt and generalize this technique to our particular nodule size estimation task. To be more specific, we later introduce and evaluate ALRD, the approximated least required difference for differentiating spherical nodules of two different size estimates from reconstructed images. Compared to the formulation in previous studies where $\mathbf{f}(\cdot)$ was always linear in $\mathbf{a}$, $\mathbf{f}(\cdot)$ will be nonlinear in $\mathbf{a}$ in our work.

3   Image Model and Formulation of Fisher information

Let the imaging system be represented by

$$\mathbf{g}(\mathbf{x}; \mathbf{a}) = \mathcal{H} \circ \left(\mathbf{b}_{phy}(\mathbf{x}) + \mu\mathbf{f}(\mathbf{x}; \mathbf{a})\right) + \mathbf{n} , \tag{7}$$

where $\mathcal{H}$ represents a general imaging operator, linear or nonlinear, mapping the objects and background from physical space to image (reconstruction) space, $\mathbf{b}_{\mathrm{phy}}(\mathbf{x}) \in \mathbb{R}^3$ is the background in physical space, $\mathbf{f}(\mathbf{x}; \mathbf{a}) \in \mathbb{R}^3$ is the signal parameterized by a $m \times 1$ vector $\mathbf{a}$, μ is the density and $\mathbf{n}$ is the noise. Details of each component will be specified later. Let us emphasize that in the current formulation there are two sources of randomness in $\mathbf{g}$: the background and noise. For notational simplicity, we denote the noise-free image of the signal $\mathcal{H} \circ \mu \mathbf{f}(\mathbf{x}; \mathbf{a})$ as $\mathbf{s}(\mathbf{a})$ and the noise-free image $\mathcal{H} \circ \left(\mathbf{b}_{\mathrm{phy}}(\mathbf{x}) + \mu \mathbf{f}(\mathbf{x}; \mathbf{a}) \right)$ as $\bar{\mathbf{g}}$. Then the noise-free background image $\mathbf{b} \in \mathrm{B}$ is defined as $\mathbf{b} = \bar{\mathbf{g}} - \mathbf{s}(\mathbf{a})$. We further assume that $\mathbf{b}$ and $\mathbf{a}$ are independent. Now we derive the Fisher information at $\mathbf{a}_0$ by first manipulating $pr(\mathbf{g}|\mathbf{a})$. Let $\mathrm{L}(\mathbf{g}|\bar{\mathbf{g}}) = \ln pr(\mathbf{g}|\mathbf{b}, \mathbf{a})$,

$$\frac{\partial \ln pr(\mathbf{g}|\mathbf{a})}{\partial \mathbf{a}} = \frac{1}{pr(\mathbf{g}|\mathbf{a})} \int_{\mathrm{B}} \frac{\partial pr(\mathbf{g}|\mathbf{b}, \mathbf{a})}{\partial \mathbf{a}} pr(\mathbf{b}) d\mathbf{b}$$

$$\text{(chain rule)} \quad = \frac{1}{pr(\mathbf{g}|\mathbf{a})} \int_{\mathrm{B}} \frac{\partial pr(\mathbf{g}|\mathbf{b}, \mathbf{a})}{\partial \mathbf{s}(\mathbf{a})} \frac{\partial \mathbf{s}(\mathbf{a})}{\partial \mathbf{a}} pr(\mathbf{b}) d\mathbf{b}$$

$$= \left(\int_{\mathrm{B}} \frac{\partial \ln pr(\mathbf{g}|\mathbf{b}, \mathbf{a})}{\partial \mathbf{s}(\mathbf{a})} \frac{pr(\mathbf{g}|\mathbf{b}, \mathbf{a}) pr(\mathbf{b})}{pr(\mathbf{g}|\mathbf{a})} d\mathbf{b} \right) \frac{\partial \mathbf{s}(\mathbf{a})}{\partial \mathbf{a}}$$

$$\text{(Byes's rule)} \quad = \left(\int_{\mathrm{B}} \frac{\partial \mathrm{L}(\mathbf{g}|\bar{\mathbf{g}})}{\partial \mathbf{s}(\mathbf{a})} pr(\mathbf{b}|\mathbf{g}, \mathbf{a}) d\mathbf{b} \right) \frac{\partial \mathbf{s}(\mathbf{a})}{\partial \mathbf{a}} = \mathbf{G}(\mathbf{a}). \tag{8}$$

By definition, $\mathbf{F}(\mathbf{a}_0)$ is the mean of $\mathbf{G}(\mathbf{a}_0)^T \mathbf{G}(\mathbf{a}_0)$ over the ensemble of noisy $\mathbf{g}$ from class H_0, thus

$$\mathbf{F}(\mathbf{a}_0) = E\{\mathbf{G}(\mathbf{a}_0)^T \mathbf{G}(\mathbf{a}_0)\} . \tag{9}$$

Assume that the noise follows a multivariate Gaussian with zero mean and covariance matrix $\mathbf{K}$, then

$$pr(\mathbf{g}|\mathbf{b}, \mathbf{a}) = \frac{1}{(2\pi)^{m/2}|\mathbf{K}|^{1/2}} exp \left(-\frac{1}{2} (\mathbf{g} - \bar{\mathbf{g}})^T \mathbf{K}^{-1} (\mathbf{g} - \bar{\mathbf{g}}) \right) \tag{10}$$

and the derivative of the log likelihood function $\frac{\partial \mathrm{L}(\mathbf{g}|\bar{\mathbf{g}})}{\partial \mathbf{s}(\mathbf{a})} = (\mathbf{g} - \bar{\mathbf{g}})^T \mathbf{K}^{-1}$. Then $\mathbf{G}(\mathbf{a})$ becomes,

$$\mathbf{G}(\mathbf{a}) = \left(\mathbf{g} - \mathbf{s}(\mathbf{a}) - \int_{\mathrm{B}} \mathbf{b} pr(\mathbf{b}|\mathbf{g}, \mathbf{a}) \, d\mathbf{b} \right)^{\mathrm{T}} \mathbf{K}^{-1} \left(\frac{\partial \mathbf{s}(\mathbf{a})}{\partial \mathbf{a}} \right) \tag{11}$$

If the $\mathbf{b}$ is fixed, according to the definition of $\mathbf{K}$,

$$\mathbf{F}(\mathbf{a}) = \left(\frac{\partial \mathbf{s}(\mathbf{a})}{\partial \mathbf{a}} \right)^{\mathrm{T}} \mathbf{K}^{-1} \left(\frac{\partial \mathbf{s}(\mathbf{a})}{\partial \mathbf{a}} \right) . \tag{12}$$

When $\mathbf{a}$ is a scalar, $\mathbf{F}(\mathbf{a})$ reduces to a scalar as well.

4   Simulations and Implementation

We simulated a helical multi-detector row CT scanner (MDCT). Our imaging operator $\mathcal{H}$ maps an object from the object space to the image space, including the forward projection and reconstruction process. The projection views of the virtual helical MDCT were generated by ray-tracing continuous objects that were analytically described by their parameters and then contaminated by the Poisson distribution. The reconstruction was obtained using the FBP-based helical CT image reconstruction algorithm [10]. Note that when the photo count I_0 is sufficiently large, the noise in the CT scans can be modeled reasonably well as a Gaussian distribution, ensured by the central limit theorem [11]. The reader may refer to [11] for more details about the MDCT simulation. The signal $\mathbf{f}(\mathbf{x}; \mathbf{a})$ were modeled as location-known solid spheres parameterized by a single parameter, the diameter a.

Unlike some other medical images, such as mammography images, which feature a more complex textured background, the lung area background for a CT acquisition is relatively uniform when vessels and air pathway structures are not considered. Therefore, we have considered the background to be deterministic in this study. More realistic and complex backgrounds which increase the complexity of calculating the posterior mean in Eq. (11) will be studied in our future work. For now, we simulated a simplified thorax which contained large structures including the lung, heart, and spine (Fig.1a). The thorax, organs and other internal structures were modeled as analytical shapes, allowing the imaging process to be defined as a continuous-to-discrete mapping. The thorax (as illustrated in Fig. 1a) was modeled as an elliptical cylinder ($[r_x, r_y, l_z] = [17,10,35]$cm, $\mu = 40$HU); the two lungs were modeled as ellipsoids ($[r_x, r_y, r_z] = [7,5,15]$cm, $\mu = -850$HU); the heart was modeled as a sphere ($r = 3.5$cm, $\mu = 65$HU); the spine was modeled as two concentric cylinders ($[r_{out}, r_{in}, l_z] = [1.75,1.5,35]$cm, $[\mu_{out}, \mu_{in}] = [1000,200]$HU).

In general, the noise in CT is location dependent. However, within a small region, the noise properties vary slowly and can be viewed as locally stationary. Therefore, we used the noise power spectrum (NPS)-based approximation method to estimate the covariance matrix $\mathbf{K}$, operating under the assumption of stationary noise [12]. With the stationarity assumption, K can be diagonalized by the Fourier transform as $\mathbf{K} = \mathbf{A}^T \mathbf{W} \mathbf{A}$, where $\mathbf{A}$ is the Fourier transform matrix and $\mathbf{W}$ is a diagonal matrix, given by the NPS. The NPS can be empirically estimated by averaging the spectrum of the Fourier transforms of many realizations of noise. Since we were interested in small nodules, the NPS only needed to be calculated for a region of interest (ROI) around the nodule. In our simulations, the size of the ROI was chosen to be $15 \times 15 \times 7$ voxels around the nodule. For this ROI size, only around 30 noisy realizations were needed to produce a stable estimate of NPS [10]. Based on Eq. (14) and method of NPS, the Fisher information was then calculated as

$$F(a) = (\mathbf{A}\mathbf{s}'(a))^T \mathbf{W}^{-1}(\mathbf{A}\mathbf{s}'(a)), \tag{13}$$

where $\mathbf{s}'(a)$ was numerically approximated using a finite difference technique since it was difficult to obtain an explicit expression for the first derivative of our signal.

Simulated images from the phantom and imaging model described above are shown in Fig.1. Fig.1a shows the central slice of the simple thorax with five 4mm (in diameter), -630HU spherical nodules centered at different locations within the xy-plane (all with the same z-direction position). Four are placed close to the boundary of the lung, in each of the four compass directions, and one in the center of the lung. The central slice of reconstruction passes through the nodule center. Note that although this image shows all five nodules, we only included a single nodule at one of these locations in the lung field for each realization to examine the location factor. We also included two cases where the nodules had the same xy-plane center as Location 1 but with a shift in z of 1mm (1/3 slice) and 1.5mm (1/2 slice), respectively. These situations were labeled as Location 6 and Location 7 (not shown in Fig.1a). The acquisition and reconstruction parameters were set as follows: $I_0 = 10^5$ (approximately equivalent to 100mAs), voxel size in x-, y- and z-dimensions were 0.78, 0.78 and 3mm respectively, targeted reconstruction ROI size was $15 \times 15 \times 7$ voxels around the nodule, reconstruction slice interval was 3mm with no overlap, the number of views was 300. Each NPS for a certain location was a $15 \times 15 \times 7$ matrix estimated from 30 noisy scans generated for each case. Fig. 1b shows images of the central slice of the 3D NPS for each location and Fig.1c shows the NPS for Location 2 as an example.

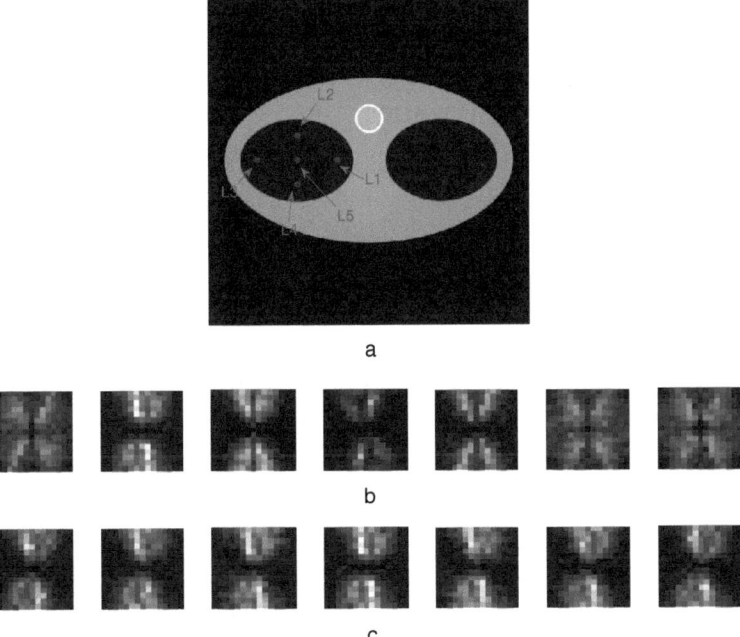

Fig. 1. a. Central slice of scan of the simplified thorax and nodule of Location 1-5. b. Examples of NPS (central slice) for the seven different nodule locations (Location 1-7 respectively). c. 3D NPS for a nodule centered at Location 2.

5   Approximated Least Required Difference (ARLD)

In practice, we often encounter the problem of determining whether or not a nodule size changes based on two estimates that are obtained at different time points without knowing the ground truth. To answer this question, we introduce the concept ALRD, the difference that ensures changes, at a given level of performance. First, let us define γ such that $|\Delta a| = \gamma a$. For a given nodule location l and γ, the approximated detectability is a function of a according to Eq. (5). We define the Fisher information approximation curve for a nodule at Location l as

$$C_l(\gamma; a) = \gamma a \sqrt{F(a)} . \tag{14}$$

Given l and γ, we assume that $C_l(\gamma; a)$ increases monotonically with a, i.e., the larger the nodule size is, the easier the detection of the same percentage for change. Therefore, there is a one-to-one relationship between any value of a and a particular C_l. For any desired level of detectability D for a change in nodule size, we can determine the associated nodule size parameter that gives that detectability value. We call the size parameter the critical size $a_{\gamma,D}^*$ such that $C_l(\gamma; a_{\gamma,D}^*) = D$. As we stated earlier, the detectability $d_A(a, \gamma a)$ (approximated by $C_l(\gamma, a)$) characterizes how well the ideal observer can differentiate nodules of size a and $(1 \pm \gamma)a$ after the objects are subjected to the imaging process. Thus, each D represents how well the distribution of the ideal observer test statistic for a nodule of size $a_{\gamma,D}^*$ can be separated from that for a nodule of size $(1 \pm \gamma)a_{\gamma,D}^*$. The larger D is, the less likely an estimate $\hat{a} = (1 + \gamma)a_{\gamma,D}^*$ ($\hat{a} = (1 - \gamma)a_{\gamma,D}^*$) is from the distribution of nodules with ground truth size smaller (larger) than $a_{\gamma,D}^*$. Let $\hat{a}_1, \hat{a}_2$ be two independent estimates with mean $a_{\gamma,D}^*$. If $\hat{a}_1 > (1 + \frac{2\gamma}{1-\gamma})\hat{a}_2$ (equivalently, $\hat{a}_1 > (1 + \gamma)a_{\gamma,D}^*, \hat{a}_2 < (1 - \gamma)a_{\gamma,D}^*$), then we say their underlying truth has the relation $a_{true,1} > a_{true,2}$ with confidence level D and call $\rho(a_{\gamma,D}^*) = \frac{2\gamma}{1-\gamma}$ the ARLD to tell a size change between nodules of two estimates around $a_{\gamma,D}^*$ at confidence level D. ALRD by definition is then a function of baseline nodule size and certainty of belief. ARLD would be expected to hold not only for $a_{\gamma,D}^*$ but for any $a > a_{\gamma,D}^*$ because of the monotonicity of $C_l(\gamma; a)$. We suggest that ρ can be used as an overall figure of merit for assuring real change from size estimates for nodules that are subjected to an imaging process.

6   Results and Discussion

Fig. 2 shows the Fisher information approximation curves $C_l(\gamma; a)$ evaluated for $\gamma = 1\%$, Locations $l = 1, 2, ..., 7$ and $a = 3, 4, ..., 8mm$. For a fixed location, $C_l(\gamma; a)$ monotonically increases with increasing nodule diameter a, as we would expect. We see that $C_l(\gamma; a)$ varies with location, with nodule locations closer to more attenuating areas resulting in reduced detectability. We also observe that Locations 6 and 7, which are offset, also have impact on detectability. The right plot of Fig. 2 gives an example of $a_{\gamma,D}^* = 5$ for Location 2, where $D = 4.35$ (or $AUC = 0.999$) and $\gamma = 2.42\%$ ($\rho = 4.95\%$). This value of ALRD corresponds to roughly a 15% volume

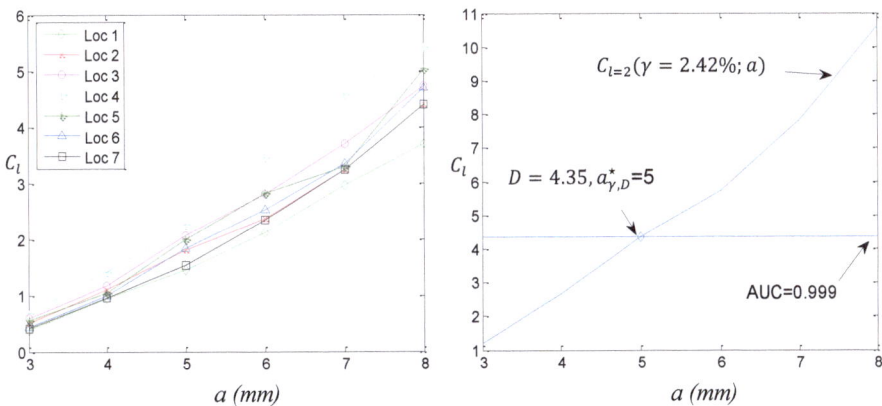

Fig. 2. Left: Plots of $C_l(1\%, a)$, the approximation to d_A, for locations $l = 1$ to 7. Right: Plot of $C_l(2.42\%, a)$ for Location 2 and the line $D = 4.35$ which corresponds to a 0.999 AUC. The intersection of these curves corresponds to a critical size of 5 mm.

difference in the spheres. Table 1 gives the ALRD for two D levels and different critical sizes, averaged among the seven locations. These results quantify the difficulty in determining the small changes in nodule size, especially for small nodules.

Table 1. ALRD (%) for different D(AUC) and critical sizes. Two quantities are given: the mean ALRD averaged across the seven locations and its standard deviation.

$a^\star_{\gamma,D}$ D	3mm	4mm	5mm	6mm	7mm	8mm
4.35	19.8	8.49	4.94	3.45	2.58	1.93
(0.999)	(4.56)	(1.20)	(0.81)	(0.54)	(0.34)	(0.24)
2.33	10.13	4.45	2.61	1.83	1.37	1.02
(0.95)	(2.23)	(0.62)	(0.42)	(0.29)	(0.18)	(0.13)

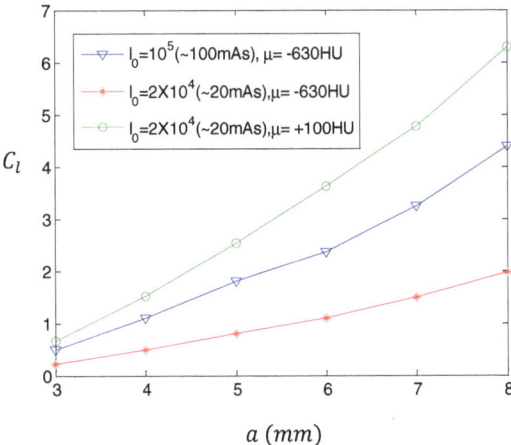

Fig. 3. Plots of curves $C_l(1\%, a)$ of Location 2 for three cases: (blue) -630HU nodule, $I_0 = 10^5$; (red) -630HU nodule, $I_0 = 2 \times 10^4$; (green) +100HU nodule, $I_0 = 2 \times 10^4$

Two more simulations were performed with a different simulated x-ray exposure I_0, one of which also involved a higher density object that resulted in higher contrast. Notice that the magnitude of the image of the object $\mathbf{s}(a)$, which is equal to $\mathcal{H} \circ \mu \mathbf{f}(\mathbf{x}; a)$, is directly proportional to μ. The NPS $\mathbf{W}$ for different doses (values of I_0) have similar shape but with magnitudes inversely proportional to I_0. Therefore, according to the formula for Fisher information (Eq. (13)), $\sqrt{F}$ should be directly proportional to μ and $\sqrt{I_0}$. Our numerical results given in Fig. 3 agree with this expectation: the d_A values of the blue curve are about $\sqrt{5} \times$ that of the red curve; the d_A values of the green curve are about $3\times$ that of the red curve (the attenuation coefficient of $+100\mathrm{HU}/-630\mathrm{HU}$ is equivalent to $1.1\mu_{water}/0.37\mu_{water}$).

7   Conclusions and Future Work

In this work we establish a method to facilitate the quantitative assessment of imaging systems, especially by further relating detection tasks to estimation performance. To this point, we have provided insights into factors, including nodule characteristics (size and density) and acquisition parameters (dose and reconstruction slice center relative to nodule center), that influence ALRD performance. In particular, the results show that ALRD for detecting nodule change decreases when the true nodule size increases. ALRD was also found to be location dependent, and affected by factors such as CT dose and lesion contrast.

Questions remain regarding the quality of the approximations. The approximation formula was obtained by expanding d_A^2 by Taylor expansion. Therefore, the approximation is good when higher order terms have reasonable values [7]. Now consider the efficient estimator of a nonrandom parameter, i.e., one that is unbiased with a variance that achieves the Cramer-Rao lower bound. When an efficient estimator exists, this observer achieves maximal AUC. Assuming that the data $\mathbf{g}$ are normally distributed, one can show that the approximation is good as long as Δa is sufficiently small, and is exact when the signal is linear in a and the covariance matrices are the same for the two classes. In the situation where the parameter influences the data in a highly nonlinear manner, the Fisher information will not provide a tight bound for estimator performance.

In future work, we plan to explore the appropriateness of the approximations and especially how the derived bound compares with experimental results and how this work can be applied to clinical practice. The current formulation is general but the application here has some restrictions: the parameter is a scalar, and the background is deterministic. Thus, further studies are needed to evaluate the effectiveness of our method in more complicated problems (e.g., multi-parameter, random background). In addition, we plan to investigate the impact of additional CT imaging parameters, reconstruction algorithms, and complex nodules (irregular shape, mixed density) through the expansion of the model of the imaging process and the signals. The presented framework can be extended to connect other discrimination and estimation tasks as well. For instance, estimates of lesion shape features, such as sphericity, could be related to shape discrimination in a quantitative way. We hope this framework will eventually help facilitate objective assessment and optimization of quantitative imaging systems.

References

1. Eisenhauer, E.A., Therasse, P., Bogaerts, J., Schwartz, L.H., Sargent, D., Ford, R., Dancey, J., Arbuck, S., Gwyther, S., Mooney, M., Rubinstein, L., Shankar, L., Dodd, L., Kaplan, R., Lacombe, D., Verweij, J.: New response evaluation criteria in solid tumors: revised RECIST guideline (version 1.1). European Journal of Cancer 45(2), 228–247 (2009)
2. Gavrielides, M.A., Kinnard, L.M., Myers, K.J., Petrick, N.: Noncalcified lung nodules: Volumetric Assessment with thoracic CT. Radiology 251(1), 26–37 (2009)
3. Gavrielides, M.A., Zeng, R., Kinnard, L.M., Myers, K.J., Petrick, N.: Information-theoretic approach for analyzing bias and variance in lung nodule size estimation. IEEE Trans. on Med. Imag. 29, 1795–1807 (2010)
4. Gavrielides, M.A., Kinnard, L.M., Myers, K.J., Peregoy, J., Pritchard, W.F., Zeng, R., Esparza, J., Karanian, J., Petrick, N.: A resource for the assessment of lung nodule size estimation methods: database of thoracic CT scans of an anthropomorphic phantom. Optics Express 18, 15244–15255 (2010)
5. Van Trees, H.L.: Detection, Estimation, and Modulation Theory, Part I. Wiley (1968)
6. Amari, S.I.: Differential geometrical theory of statistics. Springer (1985)
7. Barret, H.H., Myers, K.J.: Foundations of Image Science. Wiley (2004)
8. Shen, F., Clarkson, E.: Using fisher information to approximate ideal-observer performance on detection tasks for lumpy-background images. JOSA A 23(10), 2406–2414 (2006)
9. Clarkson, E., Shen, F.: Fisher information and surrogate figures of merit for the task-based assessment of image quality. JOSA A 27(10), 2313–2326 (2010)
10. Hsieh, J.: Computed Tomography: Principles, Design, Artifacts and Recent Advances. SPIE Press, Bellingham (2003)
11. Zeng, R., Petrick, N., Gavrielides, M.A., Myers, K.J.: Approximations of noise covariance in multi-slice helical CT scans: impact on lung nodule size estimation. Med. Phys. 56, 6223–6242 (2011)
12. Siewerdsen, J.H., Cunningham, I.A., Jaffray, D.A.: A framework for noise-power spectrum analysis of multidimensional images. Med. Phys. 29, 2655–2671 (2002)

Adaptive Multi-modal Particle Filtering for Probabilistic White Matter Tractography

Aymeric Stamm[1],[*], Olivier Commowick[1], Christian Barillot[1], and Patrick Pérez[2]

[1] VISAGES: INSERM U746 - CNRS UMR6074 - INRIA - Univ. of Rennes I, France
[2] Technicolor, Rennes, France
Aymeric.Stamm@irisa.fr

Abstract. Particle filtering has recently been introduced to perform probabilistic tractography in conjunction with DTI and Q-Ball models to estimate the diffusion information. Particle filters are particularly well adapted to the tractography problem as they offer a way to approximate a probability distribution over all paths originated from a specified voxel, given the diffusion information. In practice however, they often fail at consistently capturing the multi-modality of the target distribution. For brain white matter tractography, this means that multiple fiber pathways are unlikely to be tracked over extended volumes.

We propose to remedy this issue by formulating the filtering distribution as an adaptive M-component non-parametric mixture model. Such a formulation preserves all the properties of a classical particle filter while improving multi-modality capture. We apply this multi-modal particle filter to both DTI and Q-Ball models and propose to estimate dynamically the number of modes of the filtering distribution. We show on synthetic and real data how this algorithm outperforms the previous versions proposed in the literature.

1 Introduction

The advent of MRI technology has provided the medical community with a large amount of data that help clinicians in making decisions on a daily basis. Diffusion MRI is the sequence of choice for the study and analysis of the brain white matter (WM) neural network [16]. Yet, the **tractography** problem of inferring the WM neural system from noisy diffusion-weighted images is very challenging. It requires (i) an appropriate **diffusion model** that retrieves the diffusion information (e.g., diffusion orientations, diffusivities, anisotropies) and (ii) a **tracking algorithm** that generates pathways from the diffusion information.

Many diffusion models have been devised in the literature [3]. The very first proposed diffusion model in the literature is diffusion tensor imaging (DTI) [7], which can be viewed as the solution of the modified Bloch-Torrey equation for anisotropic media [24]. Despite its good performance in homogeneous regions of the brain, its robustness to noise and its low computational cost, DTI has

---

[*] Corresponding author.

J.C. Gee et al. (Eds.): IPMI 2013, LNCS 7917, pp. 594–606, 2013.

shortcomings: since it summarizes the diffusion in a second-order tensor, it characterizes well uni-oriented anisotropic media but fails to describe multi-oriented ones, which occurs in approximately a third of the voxels in the brain [9]. Solutions to the intra-voxel fiber heterogeneity problem rely on higher-order tensors [19], mixture models [26,8,2,23] or non-parametric models such as the Q-Ball model [25]. The latter is especially appealing since its estimation is linear (and thus fast) and directly provides the orientation information.

The second ingredient for tractography is the tracking algorithm itself [15]. The tractography problem that we tackle here is the generation of possible fiber pathways from one seed voxel without constraining the other extremity of the paths. Existing algorithms that address this problem can be classified as *deterministic* or *probabilistic*. The first category generates a single fiber pathway either by following the estimated local orientations [6,18] or by fast marching front propagation [20,22]. Local deterministic algorithms suffer from a possible accumulation of errors during the tracking process. Fast marching methods partially address this issue by reconstructing the fiber pathway that minimizes these errors. On the other hand, probabilistic algorithms generate several weighted fiber pathways that quantify the relative connectivity of the arrival point to the seed voxel (e.g. [9,12]). Randomness is often introduced on the estimated local diffusion orientations to account for their uncertainty. The von Mises & Fisher distribution on the sphere [14] is particularly well adapted to perform this sampling and has been used within a particle filter in which fiber pathways are reconstructed as first order Markov chains [28,21].

The use of particle filters for WM tractography has been pioneered in [28], where the diffusion information is estimated through DTI. The particle filter is improved in [21] by using the Q-Ball model to account for multiple local fiber orientations. However, particle filters often fail at consistently capturing the multi-modality of the filtering distribution [27]. Multiple fiber pathways are thus unlikely to be tracked over extended volumes. We propose an adaptive multi-modal particle filter for WM tractography that improves the multi-modality capture. We apply it to both DTI and Q-Ball models (Section 2). We then design an experimental framework for validation of the proposed methods (Section 3) and show results on both synthetic data with an extensive comparison to their classic particle filter counterparts and real clinical data (Section 4). Another contribution is that the number of modes of the filtering distribution is dynamically estimated. We show that our proposed algorithm greatly improves WM tractography and, when the associated diffusion model accurately captures multiple fiber orientations, it is able to distinguish crossings from bifurcations.

2   Proposed Algorithm

2.1   Tractography as a Mixture Filtering Problem

Denote $\Omega \subseteq \mathbb{R}^3$ the image spatial domain. An image over this domain is a set $A = \{a_{\mathbf{x}}, \mathbf{x} \in \Omega\}$. Let then $\{S_i\}_{i=1}^n$ be a set of n raw gradient images, S_0 be one non-weighted diffusion image and Ψ one diffusion model image.

At step k, a fiber pathway is a sequence $X^k = [(\mathbf{x}_0, \mathbf{v}_{-1}), \ldots, (\mathbf{x}_k, \mathbf{v}_{k-1})] \in (\Omega, \mathbb{S}^2)^{k+1}$ of successive pairs of positions and arrival directions, related by $\mathbf{x}_{k+1} = \mathbf{x}_k + \rho \mathbf{v}_k$, where $\rho > 0$ is the step size, which is assumed to be constant. The state space at step k is the set of all possible fiber pathways X^k originated from a specified position $\mathbf{x}_0$ and a specified arrival direction $\mathbf{v}_{-1}$.

The filtering distribution at step k is the distribution of X^k, given the diffusion data $\mathcal{Y}_k(X^k) = \{y_{\mathbf{x}_0}, y_{\mathbf{x}_1}, \ldots, y_{\mathbf{x}_k}\}$ where $y_{\mathbf{x}_j} = \{s_{\mathbf{x}_j,i}, \psi_{\mathbf{x}_j,i}\}_{i=1}^n$, for all $j = 0, \ldots, k$. At each step k, this distribution is sequentially determined by successively computing the prediction distribution $p(X^k|\mathcal{Y}_{k-1}(X^{k-1}))$ out of the previous filtering distribution and then using Bayes' rule to obtain $p(X^k|\mathcal{Y}_k(X^k))$. These **prediction** and **update** stages require to specify respectively the evolution model $p(\mathbf{x}_{k+1}, \mathbf{v}_k|X^k)$ and the likelihood $p(\mathcal{Y}_{k+1}(X^{k+1})|X^{k+1})$.

We assume that fiber pathways are first order Markov chains. Consequently, the evolution model simplifies to $p(\mathbf{v}_k|\mathbf{x}_k, \mathbf{v}_{k-1})$. In the remainder of the article, according to [28,21], we use the following evolution model:

$$p(\mathbf{v}_k|\mathbf{x}_k, \mathbf{v}_{k-1}) = \text{vMF}(\mathbf{v}_k; \mathbf{v}_{k-1}, \kappa) = \frac{\kappa}{4\pi \sinh \kappa} \exp\{\kappa \mathbf{v}_{k-1}^T \mathbf{v}_k\}, \qquad (1)$$

where $\text{vMF}(\cdot; \mathbf{v}_{k-1}, \kappa)$ is the von Mises & Fisher distribution [14] on the 2-dimensional sphere with mean direction $\mathbf{v}_{k-1} \in \mathbb{S}^2$ and concentration parameter $\kappa \geq 0$. The concentration parameter κ of the evolution model controls the smoothness of the reconstructed fiber pathways. Assuming conditional independence of the observations given a pathway, the observation model reads:

$$p(\mathcal{Y}_{k+1}(X^{k+1})|X^{k+1}) = \prod_{j=0}^{k} p(y_{\mathbf{x}_{j+1}}|\mathbf{v}_j), \qquad (2)$$

where $p(y_{\mathbf{x}_{j+1}}|\mathbf{v}_j)$ depends on the diffusion model and will be defined in Section 2.4. In order to better capture multi-modality, we follow the idea of [27] and formulate the filtering distribution as a mixture of M_k components:

$$p(X^k|\mathcal{Y}_k(X^k)) = \sum_{m=1}^{M_k} \pi_{m,k} p_m(X^k|\mathcal{Y}_k(X^k)), \qquad (3)$$

where $\sum_{m=1}^{M_k} \pi_{m,k} = 1$. Such a formulation allows us to perform the filtering recursion for each component p_m individually, provided that each mixture weight is updated as the normalized weighted likelihood for the associated component.

2.2 Mixture Particle Filter

In general, there is no closed-form expressions for the filtering recursion equations. A popular strategy is to resort to particle filters. They approximate the filtering distribution by a set of samples that are properly weighted to represent the filtering distribution at each step. Using the notations in [27], let $\mathcal{P}_k = \{M_k, \Pi_k, \mathcal{X}_k, \mathcal{W}_k, \mathcal{C}_k\}$ be the particle representation of the filtering distribution where M_k is the number of components, $\Pi_k = \{\pi_{m,k}\}_{m=1}^{M_k}$ the set of mixture weights, $\mathcal{X}_k = \{\mathbf{x}_k^{(\ell)}\}_{\ell=1}^N$ the set of N particles, $\mathcal{W}_k = \{w_k^{(\ell)}\}_{\ell=1}^N$ the set of particle weights and $\mathcal{C}_k = \{c_k^{(\ell)}\}_{\ell=1}^N$ the set of component indicators (i.e., $c_k^{(\ell)} = m$ if particle ℓ belongs to component m). Given $\mathcal{P}_k$, the particle approximation with mixture filtering distribution proceeds to step $k+1$ in five stages:

Proposition of New Samples: New samples are generated according to a proposal density $q(\cdot|\mathbf{v}_{k-1}^{(\ell)}, y_{\mathbf{x}_k^{(\ell)}})$ which depends on the previous direction and the diffusion information at step k:

$$\mathbf{v}_k^{(\ell)} \sim q(\mathbf{v}_k|\mathbf{v}_{k-1}^{(\ell)}, y_{\mathbf{x}_k^{(\ell)}}) \text{ and } \mathbf{x}_{k+1}^{(\ell)} = \mathbf{x}_k^{(\ell)} + \rho \mathbf{v}_k^{(\ell)}. \tag{4}$$

Update of Particle Weights: The weights of the new particles are updated in order to be representative of the filtering distribution according to [11]:

$$\tilde{w}_{k+1}^{(\ell)} = \frac{w_k^{(\ell)} p(y_{\mathbf{x}_{k+1}^{(\ell)}}|\mathbf{v}_k^{(\ell)}) p(\mathbf{v}_k^{(\ell)}|\mathbf{v}_{k-1}^{(\ell)})}{q(\mathbf{v}_k^{(\ell)}|\mathbf{v}_{k-1}^{(\ell)}, y_{\mathbf{x}_k^{(\ell)}})}. \tag{5}$$

The normalization of these weights is performed within each component:

$$w_{k+1}^{(\ell)} = \frac{\tilde{w}_{k+1}^{(\ell)}}{\sum_{j \in \mathcal{I}_{m,k}} \tilde{w}_{k+1}^{(j)}}, \tag{6}$$

where $\mathcal{I}_{m,k} = \{\ell \in [\![1, N]\!] : c_k^{(\ell)} = m\}$ is the set of indices of the particles that belong to the m-th mixture component at step k.

Update of Mixture Weights: The mixture weights need to be updated properly to ensure that the filter still acts on each component individually:

$$\pi_{m,k+1} = \frac{\pi_{m,k} \tilde{w}_{m,k+1}}{\sum_{i=1}^M \pi_{i,k} \tilde{w}_{i,k+1}} \text{ with } \tilde{w}_{m,k+1} = \sum_{\ell \in \mathcal{I}_{m,k}} \tilde{w}_{k+1}^{(\ell)}. \tag{7}$$

Resampling within Each Component: To avoid the degeneracy of the particle weights, occasional resampling is necessary [11]. The resampling stage can be performed within each subset of particles associated to a mixture component independently, according to the component particle weights [27]: we compute the effective number of particles in a mixture component as:

$$\text{ESS}_m = \left(\sum_{\ell \in \mathcal{I}_{m,k}} \left(w_{k+1}^{(\ell)} \right)^2 \right)^{-1}, \tag{8}$$

and perform resampling according to the weights in Eq.(6), if ESS_m is below a threshold $\alpha |\mathcal{I}_{m,k}|$, where $|\cdot|$ denotes the set size operator.

Reclustering of the Particles within New Components: The number of components M_k in the mixture is not known. At the end of each step, it is dynamically estimated by merging and/or splitting some of the components: M_k, $\mathcal{C}_k$ and $\mathcal{I}_{m,k}$ are updated to M_{k+1}, $\mathcal{C}_{k+1}$ and $\mathcal{I}_{m,k+1}$ accordingly.

In Section 2.3, we describe how the reclustering of the mixture filtering distribution is performed. In Section 2.4, we define the proposal density and the likelihood for the DTI and Q-Ball models following respectively [28] and [21].

2.3 Reclustering of the Filtering Distribution

After the resampling stage, we characterize each mixture component by a vMF distribution with mean direction $\boldsymbol{\mu}_{m,k}$ and concentration $\kappa_{m,k}$. The parameters of the distribution are estimated using the following equations:

$$\mathbf{r}_{m,k} := \frac{\sum_{\ell \in \mathcal{I}_{m,k}} \mathbf{v}_k^{(\ell)}}{|\mathcal{I}_{m,k}|}, \quad \boldsymbol{\mu}_{m,k} = \frac{\mathbf{r}_{m,k}}{\|\mathbf{r}_{m,k}\|}, \quad \kappa_{m,k} = \frac{\|\mathbf{r}_{m,k}\|(3 - \|\mathbf{r}_{m,k}\|^2)}{1 - \|\mathbf{r}_{m,k}\|^2}. \quad (9)$$

These estimators have been proposed in [4] and have been introduced for diffusion MRI in [10] for their unbiasedness and robustness.

We first test the components pairwise for merging. We merge two components if the two following conditions are met:

1. the Euclidean distance between the mean positions $\overline{\mathbf{x}}_{m,k} := \frac{\sum_{\ell \in \mathcal{I}_{m,k}} \mathbf{x}_k^{(\ell)}}{|\mathcal{I}_{m,k}|}$ is below a threshold ξ_1, and
2. the distance between the two vMF distributions computed with Eq.(9) is below a threshold ξ_2.

We compute the distance between two vMF distributions as proposed in [17]:

$$d\left((\kappa_i, \boldsymbol{\mu}_i), (\kappa_j, \boldsymbol{\mu}_j)\right) = \sqrt{\log^2\left(\frac{\kappa_j}{\kappa_i}\right) + \arccos^2\left(\boldsymbol{\mu}_i^T \boldsymbol{\mu}_j\right)}. \quad (10)$$

We then test each component for splitting. We split a component if its concentration parameter $\kappa_{m,k}$ drops below a threshold ξ_3.

Finally, the number of mixture components is updated to M_{k+1}, the component indicators to $\mathcal{C}_{k+1}$ and the set of indices to $\mathcal{I}_{m,k+1}$. In order to maintain a properly weighted sample from the filtering distribution and thus to preserve the convergence properties of the particle filter, we perform the following update of mixture and particle weights [27]:

$$\pi^\star_{m,k+1} = \sum_{\ell \in \mathcal{I}_{m,k+1}} \pi_{c_k^{(\ell)},k+1} w_{k+1}^{(\ell)}, \quad w_{k+1}^{(\ell)\star} = \frac{\pi_{c_k^{(\ell)},k+1} w_{k+1}^{(\ell)}}{\pi^\star_{c_{k+1}^{(\ell)},k+1}}. \quad (11)$$

2.4 Diffusion Models: Associated Proposal Densities and Likelihoods

The DTI Model. It provides a 2nd order diffusion tensor represented by its eigensystem $\{\lambda_1, \lambda_2, \lambda_3, \mathbf{e}_1, \mathbf{e}_2, \mathbf{e}_3\}$, of which we extract the fractional anisotropy FA [5], the linear coefficient c_l defined as in [28], the mean diffusivity

$\bar{\lambda} = (\lambda_1 + \lambda_2 + \lambda_3)/3$, the perpendicular diffusivity $\lambda_\perp = (\lambda_2 + \lambda_3)/2$, the principal eigenvector $\mathbf{e}_1$ and the minor eigenvector $\mathbf{e}_3$. The likelihood is given by:

$$p(y_{\mathbf{x}_{k+1}}|\mathbf{v}_k) =$$

$$\begin{cases} \left[\prod_{i=1}^n \frac{s^\star_{\mathbf{x}_{k+1},i}}{\sigma_i \sqrt{2\pi}} \exp\left\{ -\frac{(s^\star_{\mathbf{x}_{k+1},i})^2 (\log s_{\mathbf{x}_{k+1},i} - \log s^\star_{\mathbf{x}_{k+1},i})^2}{2\sigma_i^2} \right\} \right]^{\frac{1}{n}}, & c_l > \tau, \\[2ex] \frac{1}{\sigma\sqrt{(2\pi)^3}} \exp\left\{ -\frac{(\arccos(\mathbf{v}_k^T \mathbf{e}_3) - \pi/2)^2}{2\sigma^2} \right\}, & c_l \le \tau, \end{cases} \quad (12)$$

where the diffusion tensor is estimated at position $\mathbf{x}_{k+1}$, σ_i and $\mathbf{g}_i$ are the standard deviation and the gradient direction of the i-th gradient image respectively, estimated by least square estimation and pseudo-residuals [13], σ is a user-defined standard deviation and $s^\star_{\mathbf{x}_{k+1},i} = s^\star_{\mathbf{x}_{k+1},0} \exp\{-b(\lambda_\perp + 3(\mathbf{v}_k^T \mathbf{g}_i)^2(\bar{\lambda} - \lambda_\perp))\}$ is the diffusion signal simulated from the diffusion tensor cylindrically constrained along the sampled direction $\mathbf{v}_k$. The proposal density is given by:

$$q(\mathbf{v}_k|\mathbf{v}_{k-1}, y_{\mathbf{x}_k}) = \begin{cases} \text{vMF}(\mathbf{v}_k; \mathbf{e}_{1,k}, \nu_k), & c_l > \tau, \\[1ex] p(\mathbf{v}_k|\mathbf{v}_{k-1}), & c_l \le \tau, \end{cases} \quad (13)$$

where the diffusion tensor is estimated at $\mathbf{x}_k$ and ν_k is a function of FA [28].

The Q-Ball model. It provides an orientation distribution function (ODF) of which we extract the set Λ of maxima $\boldsymbol{\mu}$, the value of the ODF at its maxima $\psi(\boldsymbol{\mu})$ and the mean curvature of the ODF at its maxima $H(\boldsymbol{\mu})$. Borrowing ideas from [21], we define the likelihood as follows:

$$p(y_{\mathbf{x}_{k+1}}|\mathbf{v}_k) = \left[\prod_{i=1}^n \frac{1}{\sigma_i \sqrt{2\pi}} \exp\left\{ -\frac{(s_{\mathbf{x}_{k+1},i} - s^\star_{\mathbf{x}_{k+1},i})^2}{2\sigma_i^2} \right\} \right]^{\frac{1}{n}}, \quad (14)$$

where the ODF is estimated at position $\mathbf{x}_{k+1}$ and $s^\star_{\mathbf{x}_{k+1},i}$ is the diffusion signal simulated according to [1] from the ODF that has been rotated to align the sampling direction to the sampled one. The proposal density is given by:

$$q(\mathbf{v}_k|\mathbf{v}_{k-1}, y_{\mathbf{x}_k}) = \begin{cases} \sum_{\boldsymbol{\mu} \in \Lambda} \omega_{\boldsymbol{\mu}} \text{vMF}(\mathbf{v}_k; \boldsymbol{\mu}, \kappa_{\boldsymbol{\mu}}), & \Lambda \ne \emptyset, \\[2ex] p(\mathbf{v}_k|\mathbf{v}_{k-1}), & \Lambda = \emptyset, \end{cases} \quad (15)$$

where the ODF is estimated at $\mathbf{x}_k$, $\omega_{\boldsymbol{\mu}} \propto \psi(\boldsymbol{\mu})$ (normalized) and $\kappa_{\boldsymbol{\mu}} \propto H(\boldsymbol{\mu})$.

3   Experimental Setup and Evaluation Metrics

3.1   Phantom Diffusion Weighted Data

Two synthetic diffusion weighted phantoms were created for validation and are illustrated in Fig. 1: a case of two crossing fibers at a $90°$ angle and a case of one fiber splitting into two fibers at a 60° angle. For both phantoms, one non-weighted diffusion image and 81 raw gradient images with a single b-value of 3000 s.mm^{-2} were simulated using an equally weighted multi-tensor model at each voxel. Rician noise was then added on the noise-free images with a relative standard deviation of 5%, to generate 50 samples of each phantom.

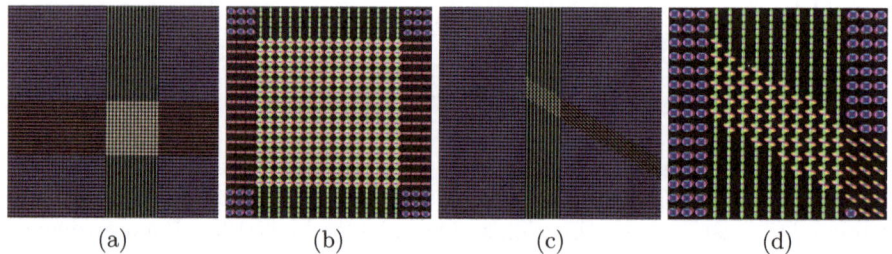

(a)   (b)   (c)   (d)

Fig. 1. Noise Free Diffusion Weighted Phantoms. ODF visualization of crossing fibers (a) with close-up view (b), and the bifurcating fibers (c) with close-up view (d).

3.2   Evaluation Measures for Phantom Data

Four methods were utilized: DTI-based "mono-modal" (i.e., without particle clustering mechanism) tractography (DTI mono), DTI-based multi-modal tractography (DTI multi), ODF-based mono-modal tractography (ODF mono) and ODF-based multi-modal tractography (ODF multi). For each phantom, a single seed voxel was placed in the upper branch. The initial direction of propagation was set towards the bottom. The following common parameters were used in all algorithms: resampling threshold $\alpha = 0.4$, number of particles $N = 1000$, step length $\rho = 1$ mm, prior concentration $\kappa = 30$, and merge and split thresholds $\xi_1 = 1$ mm, $\xi_2 = 1$ and $\xi_3 = 40$. Tensors were considered as oblate for $\tau = 0.25$. The output fiber pathways are the averaged of each cluster of particles (a single one in mono-modal versions).

The tractography results were evaluated visually and with 3 different quantitative measures: (i) the proportion of fibers branching from the main direction, which is an indicator of branching capacity (ii) the root-mean-square error between the end point (after $L_{\max}$ iterations of the particle filter) of each fiber following the main path and the expected arrival position (known in the phantoms), which gives an idea of how spread the fibers are around the true one and (iii) the local curvature along each branching fiber for the bifurcation phantom, which translates how each branch was created from the main direction (either by an uncertain turn or by a sharper local turn).

The expected arrival position in the bifurcation phantom is not obvious. In this phantom, fibers going straight follow the inaccurate diffusion orientations given by the diffusion model in the heterogeneous region and are thus expected to deviate exclusively towards the right border of the vertical band. Therefore, we have chosen the end position for the bifurcation phantom at the center of the segment joining the center of the vertical band and its right border.

3.3   Clinical Diffusion Acquisition

The 4 algorithms were also applied on real clinical scans, acquired on a Siemens 3T scanner with a matrix size of 128x128, 60 slices (voxel size 2x2x2 mm^3). The diffusion acquisition consisted of one non-weighted diffusion image and 30 gradient images with a b-value of 1000 $s.mm^{-2}$. Seed regions were placed by a radiologist at the basis of the left and right cortico-spinal tracts (CST) in the mesencephalon, with filtering regions in the posterior limb of the internal capsule to keep only the CST. The same parameters as for synthetic data were utilized for real data. A particle filter was initiated at each voxel of the seed regions and the fiber pathways are the averaged fibers of each cluster of particles.

4   Results

4.1   Experiments on Synthetic Data

We present a representative example of the results achieved by each method in Fig. 2. We clearly notice that the 2 mono-modal methods fail to capture the multi-modality of the bifurcation phantom and therefore follow only one of the two directions. On the contrary, the 2 multi-modal methods are visually well able to capture the two branching fiber tracts, thanks to the adaptive clustering based on the proposed directions. It may be noted that DTI multi tends to obtain more fanning fibers, because the observation model is wide for oblate tensors. These visual results are valid for both crossing and bifurcation phantoms. However, in the crossing, fibers are only expected to go straight since the crossing ones are

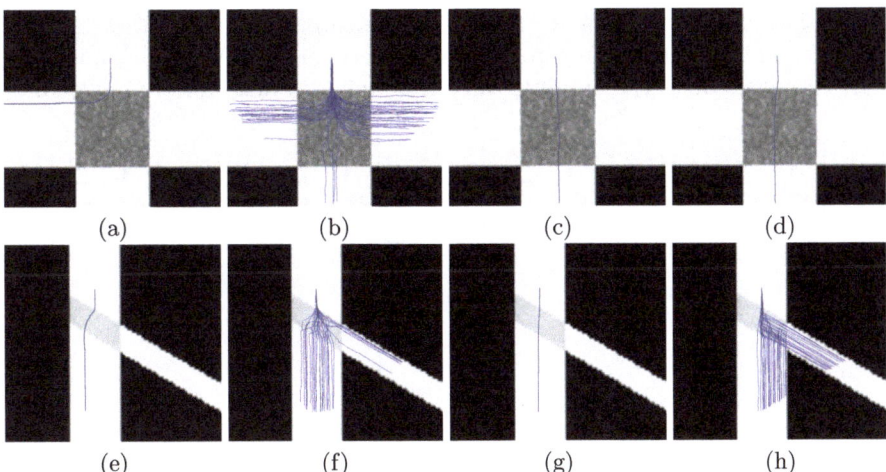

Fig. 2. Tractography Results on Phantom Data. First row: crossing phantom, Second row: bifurcation phantom. Methods used were DTI mono (a,e), DTI multi (b,f), ODF mono (c,g), ODF multi (d,h).

not part of the same pathway. Therefore, ODF mono and multi are performing well while DTI multi tends to capture too many branches.

We report in Table 1 the proportion of branching fibers for each phantom and each method. These quantitative results confirm the visual ones. When utilizing the mono-modal methods, only one of the two branches of each phantom is explored. On the contrary, multi-modal methods capture much better the 2 modes in the bifurcation phantom, with ODF multi being the closest to the half/half ground truth in each branch.

Table 1. Evaluation of Fibers on Phantom Data. Proportion of branching and straight fibers and Root Mean Squared error of fibers going straight with respect to true expected position, for each phantom.

	DTI mono	DTI multi	ODF mono	ODF multi
Crossing Phantom				
Fiber proportion straight (%)	0 ± 0	8.75 ± 3.06	100 ± 0	98.76 ± 6.14
Fiber proportion branch (%)	100 ± 0	91.25 ± 3.06	0 ± 0	1.24 ± 6.14
RMS (mm)	N/A	9.71 ± 3.71	2.09 ± 1.35	2.05 ± 1.15
Bifurcation Phantom				
Fiber proportion straight (%)	93.88 ± 24.22	66.53 ± 4.06	100 ± 0	56.63 ± 4.59
Fiber proportion branch (%)	6.12 ± 24.22	33.47 ± 4.06	0 ± 0	43.37 ± 4.59
RMS (mm)	20.16 ± 6.07	15.36 ± 1.28	12.94 ± 0.29	9.08 ± 0.41

In addition, Table 1 displays the RMS error towards the expected arrival point of the straight fibers only for those fibers which go in the straight branch of each phantom. For both phantoms, DTI mono and multi perform worse as DTI does not handle multiple directions. ODF multi outperforms the other methods, being able to better recover the final positions of the fibers.

The last metric, only for the bifurcation phantom, is the local curvature of each mean fiber that deviates from the main vertical path. We report one representative example of the obtained curves as well as a box-plot of inter-quantile

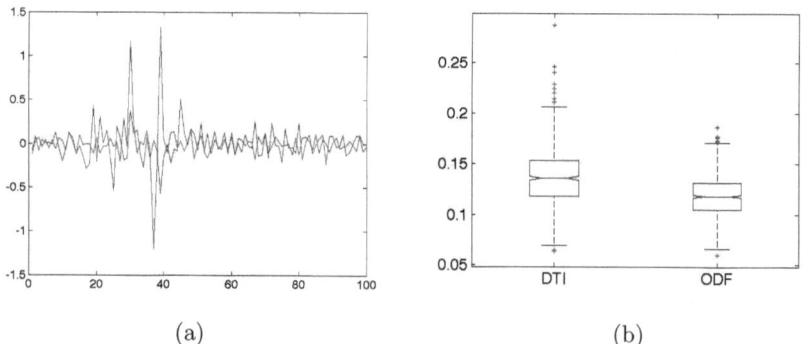

(a)   (b)

Fig. 3. Local Curvature of Branching Fibers. Evaluation of local curvature for the branching fibers of the splitting fibers phantom. (a): Local curvature on one single fiber (blue: DTI-based, multimodal, red: ODF-based, multimodal), (b): box-plot representation of inter-quantile range for DTI and ODF over all fibers and repetitions.

ranges of the curvatures along each mean fiber for all repetitions (Fig. 3). The curves of local curvatures clearly show a more peaked behavior for ODF multi (red curve), indicating that it branches more sharply. This was expected as the ODF model captures the 2 fiber orientations in the splitting region, whereas the DTI model inaccurately estimates the fiber orientations and thus the particle filter is mainly driven by the previous direction with a wide observation model. Also, a one-way ANOVA quantitatively shows a significant difference ($p \ll 10^{-3}$) between the standard deviations of the curvature of the 2 methods: away from the peaks, the curvature varies less with ODF multi than with DTI multi.

4.2   Experiments on Real Data

To illustrate the capacities of the proposed algorithms on real clinical datasets, we report in Fig. 4 the left and right cortico-spinal tracts (CST) obtained on

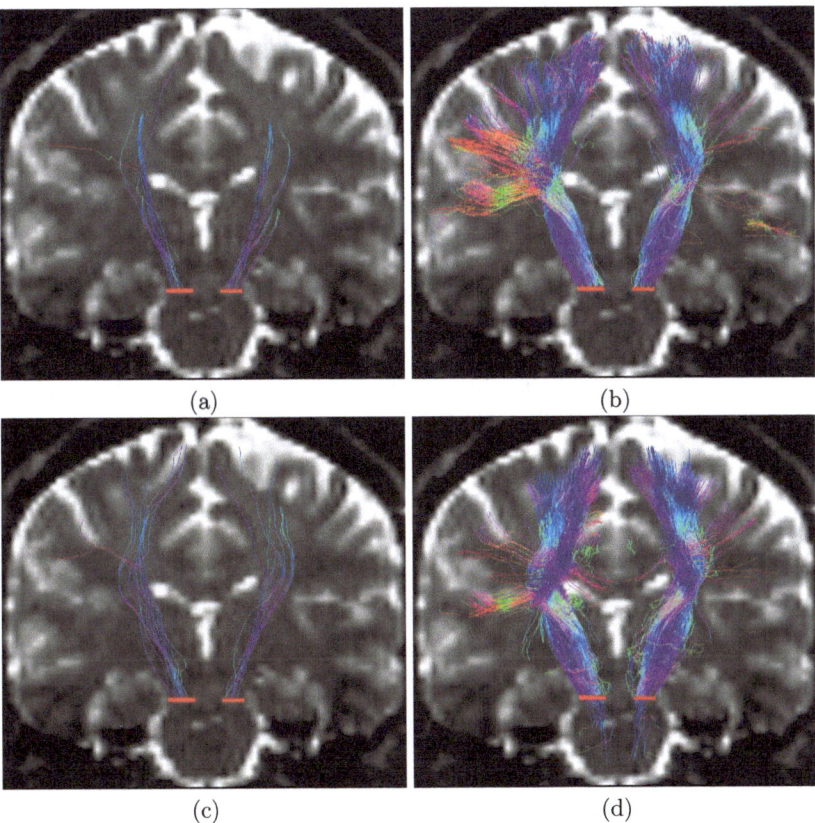

Fig. 4. Tractography of the Left and Right Corticospinal Tracts. Coronal view of both corticospinal tracts using the four proposed methods: (a): DTI mono, (b): DTI multi, (c): ODF mono, (d): ODF multi. Fiber tracts are overlaid on the T2-weighted volume from the diffusion acquisition, red bars indicate the seeding regions.

a normal control subject. The results obtained here are consistent with those obtained on synthetic data. While the mono-modal methods do not capture branchings to lateral parts of the CST, both DTI multi and ODF multi are able to capture branches to the hand area or even sometimes the face area. Interestingly, DTI multi seems a bit more able to capture branches than ODF multi especially on the right side of the brain (left in the images). Since the data was acquired with only 30 gradient directions and a single low b-value of 1000 s.mm^{-2}, it might indeed not be enough for the ODF model to identify accurately multiple orientations. However, ODF mono and multi seem overall able to capture more accurate directions of the main tract.

5   Discussion

We have presented a new adaptive multi-modal particle filter algorithm for diffusion MRI probabilistic tractography. It relies on the adaptive clustering of the filtering distribution through a new scheme for splitting and merging clusters based on the distribution of directions and positions among clusters. This strategy is applied after each step of the filtering recursion. We have implemented this algorithm with two different diffusion models: DTI and ODF on a spherical harmonics basis.

We have demonstrated through experiments on synthetic and real data that our proposed algorithms outperform more classical particle filtering approaches available in the literature, being more able to capture branching and crossing fibers. In addition, the ODF multi-modal algorithm produces more accurate branchings and differentiate crossing fibers from splitting fibers, thanks to the diffusion model that already accurately captures multiple orientations.

As noted in Section 4.2, it will be interesting in the near future to apply this algorithm using other diffusion models such as multi-compartment models [26,8,2,23], more adapted to data with a small number of gradient directions and a single low b-value. The proposed algorithm is very generic and can thus easily be extended to new diffusion models: only the proposal and the observation densities require to be modified to reflect the underlying diffusion model. Future work will also include evaluation on more real data cases, also with HARDI acquisitions, as well as an in-depth study of the usual parameters of a particle filter and their influence on the results.

References

1. Aganj, I., Lenglet, C., Sapiro, G., Yacoub, E., Ugurbil, K., Harel, N.: Reconstruction of the orientation distribution function in single- and multiple-shell q-ball imaging within constant solid angle. MRM 64(2), 554–566 (2010)
2. Assaf, Y., Basser, P.: Composite hindered and restricted model of diffusion (CHARMED) MR imaging of the human brain. NeuroImage 27(1), 48–58 (2005)
3. Assemlal, H., Tschumperlé, D., Brun, L., Siddiqi, K.: Recent advances in diffusion MRI modeling: Angular and radial reconstruction. MedIA (2011)

4. Banerjee, A., Dhillon, I., Ghosh, J., Sra, S.: Clustering on the unit hypersphere using von Mises-Fisher distributions. J. of Machine Learning 6, 1345–1382 (2006)
5. Basser, P., Pierpaoli, C.: Microstructural and physiological features of tissues elucidated by quantitative-diffusion-tensor MRI. J. Magn. Reson. 111(3), 209–219 (1996)
6. Basser, P.J., Pajevic, S., Pierpaoli, C., Duda, J., Aldroubi, A.: In vivo fiber tractography using DT-MRI data. MRM 44(4), 625–632 (2000)
7. Basser, P., Mattiello, J., Le Bihan, D.: MR diffusion tensor spectroscopy and imaging. Biophysical journal 66(1), 259–267 (1994)
8. Behrens, T., Woolrich, M., Jenkinson, M., Johansen-Berg, H., Nunes, R., Clare, S., Matthews, P., Brady, J., Smith, S.: Characterization and propagation of uncertainty in diffusion-weighted MR imaging. MRM 50(5), 1077–1088 (2003)
9. Behrens, T.E.J., Berg, H.J., Jbabdi, S., Rushworth, M.F.S., Woolrich, M.W.: Probabilistic diffusion tractography with multiple fibre orientations: What can we gain? NeuroImage 34(1), 144–155 (2007)
10. Bhalerao, A., Westin, C.-F.: Hyperspherical von Mises-Fisher Mixture (HvMF) Modelling of High Angular Resolution Diffusion MRI. In: Ayache, N., Ourselin, S., Maeder, A. (eds.) MICCAI 2007, Part I. LNCS, vol. 4791, pp. 236–243. Springer, Heidelberg (2007)
11. Doucet, A., Godsill, S., Andrieu, C.: On sequential Monte Carlo sampling methods for Bayesian filtering. Statistics and Computing 10(3), 197–208 (2000)
12. Friman, O., Farnebäck, G., Westin, C.: A Bayesian approach for stochastic white matter tractography. IEEE TMI 25(8), 965–978 (2006)
13. Gasser, T., Sroka, L., Jennen-Steinmetz, C.: Residual variance and residual pattern in nonlinear regression. Biometrika 73(3), 625–633 (1986)
14. Jupp, P., Mardia, K.: A unified view of the theory of directional statistics. International Statistical Review 57(3), 261–294 (1989)
15. Lazar, M.: Mapping brain anatomical connectivity using white matter tractography. NMR in Biomedicine 23(7), 821–835 (2010)
16. Le Bihan, D.: Looking into the functional architecture of the brain with diffusion MRI. Nature reviews. Neuroscience 4(6), 469–480 (2003)
17. McGraw, T., Vemuri, B.: Von Mises-Fisher mixture model of the diffusion ODF. In: IEEE ISBI, pp. 65–68 (2006)
18. Mori, S., Crain, B.J., Chacko, V.P., van Zijl, P.C.: Three-dimensional tracking of axonal projections in the brain by magnetic resonance imaging. Annals of Neurology 45(2), 265–269 (1999)
19. Ozarslan, E., Mareci, T.: Generalized diffusion tensor imaging and analytical relationships between diffusion tensor imaging and high angular resolution diffusion imaging. MRM 50(5), 955–965 (2003)
20. Parker, G., Wheeler-Kingshott, C., Barker, G.: Estimating distributed anatomical connectivity using fast marching methods and diffusion tensor imaging. IEEE TMI 21(5), 505–512 (2002)
21. Pontabry, J., Rousseau, F.: Probabilistic tractography using Q-ball modeling and particle filtering. In: Fichtinger, G., Martel, A., Peters, T. (eds.) MICCAI 2011, Part II. LNCS, vol. 6892, pp. 209–216. Springer, Heidelberg (2011)
22. Staempfli, P., Jaermann, T., Crelier, G.R., Kollias, S., Valavanis, A., Boesiger, P.: Resolving fiber crossing using advanced fast marching tractography based on diffusion tensor imaging. NeuroImage 30(1), 110–120 (2006)
23. Stamm, A., Pérez, P., Barillot, C.: A new multi-fiber model for low angular resolution diffusion MRI. In: IEEE ISBI, pp. 936–939 (2012)

24. Stejskal, E.O.: Use of spin echoes in a pulsed magneticfield gradient to study anisotropic, restricted diffusion and flow. J. Chem. Phys. 43, 3597 (1965)
25. Tuch, D.S.: Q-ball imaging. MRM 52(6), 1358–1372 (2004)
26. Tuch, D., Reese, T., Wiegell, M., Makris, N., Belliveau, J., Wedeen, V.: High angular resolution diffusion imaging reveals intravoxel white matter fiber heterogeneity. MRM 48(4), 577–582 (2002)
27. Vermaak, J., Doucet, A., Pérez, P.: Maintaining multimodality through mixture tracking. In: IEEE ICCV. vol. 2, pp. 1110–6 (2003)
28. Zhang, F., Hancock, E., Goodlett, C., Gerig, G.: Probabilistic white matter fiber tracking using particle filtering and von Mises-Fisher sampling. MedIA 13(1), 5–18 (2009)

Can T_2-Spectroscopy Resolve Submicrometer Axon Diameters?

Enrico Kaden* and Daniel C. Alexander

Centre for Medical Image Computing, Department of Computer Science,
University College London, Gower Street, London, WC1E 6BT, United Kingdom
e.kaden@ucl.ac.uk

Abstract. The microscopic geometry of white matter carries rich information about brain function in health and disease. A key challenge for medical imaging is to estimate microstructural features noninvasively. One important parameter is the axon diameter, which correlates with the conduction time delay of action potentials and is affected by various neurological disorders. Diffusion magnetic resonance (MR) experiments are the method of choice today when we aim to recover the axon diameter distribution, although the technique requires very high gradient strengths in order to assess nerve fibers with one micrometer or less in diameter. In practice *in-vivo* brain imaging is only sensitive to the largest axons, not least due to limitations in the human physiology which tolerates only moderate gradient strengths. This work studies, from a theoretical perspective, the feasibility of T_2-spectroscopy to resolve submicrometer tissue structures. Exploiting the surface relaxation effect, we formulate a plausible biophysical model relating the axon diameter distribution to the T_2-weighted signal, which is based on a surface-to-volume ratio approximation of the Bloch–Torrey equation. Under a certain regime of bulk and surface relaxation coefficients, our simulation results suggest that it might be possible to reveal axons smaller than one micrometer in diameter.

1 Introduction

The extrinsic connections, which link the cortical areas and subcortical nuclei distributed over the brain, are established by the axons. These cellular extensions of the neurons carry the neural signals over long distances of up to several centimeters, thereby leaving the gray matter and forming the white matter. We henceforth use the terms axons and (nerve) fibers interchangeably. An important aim of human brain research is to explore the wiring scheme of the long-range pathways, but also to characterize their biophysical properties such as the axon diameter. Most of the fibers in the central nervous system have a diameter between 0.2 and 20 μm. For instance, axons in the human corpus callosum larger than 1 μm, 3 μm, and 5 μm in diameter were found to represent about 20%, 0.1%, and 0.02% of the total axons counted (larger than 0.4 μm), respectively [1].

---

* Corresponding author.

J.C. Gee et al. (Eds.): IPMI 2013, LNCS 7917, pp. 607–618, 2013.

For other brain areas, however, the fiber density and the axon diameter distribution, especially their spatial variation and the differences between subjects, are less known. These parameters are crucial markers towards the understanding of brain function, since the conduction time delay of action potentials, hence the speed of information transmission between remote brain areas, is largely determined by the axon radius [2]. Moreover, the fiber microanatomy is affected by various neurological disorders. In multiple sclerosis it is well known that during the typical course of the disease the thin axons are preferentially damaged [3].

Nowadays diffusion MR experiments are the method of choice when we aim to recover the axon diameter distribution in brain white matter noninvasively. This technique allows us to encode the diffusion process of water molecules through the external application of time-dependent magnetic fields, which are under control of the experimenter. Considerable effort over the past few years [4] has gone into devising biophysical models or acquisition protocols for estimating the axon diameter from diffusion MR measurements. For instance, Stanisz *et al.* [5] proposed a tissue model that provides an estimate of the mean axon diameter and demonstrated their approach in bovine optic nerve. The AxCaliber framework describes the restricted diffusion process within the axons and the hindered water diffusion in the space between the nerve fibers [6,7]. The axon diameter distribution, which is parameterized by a Gamma density, was then estimated in excised nerve tissue and in the corpus callosum of living rat brain, respectively, thereby assuming parallel fibers with a single known orientation. The ActiveAx technique [8] allows orientationally invariant estimates of the axon diameter and shows the first *in-vivo* human maps of an index of axon diameter. This method still assumes that the nerve fibers in a voxel are parallel to each other. More recently, Zhang *et al.* [9] relaxed the assumption by allowing a Watson distribution of axon orientations to describe fiber dispersion known to exist even in the corpus callosum [10].

A key limitation of diffusion MR experiments is that the gradient strength places a lower bound on the measurable axon diameter [8,11]. The gradient systems available on human scanners are sensitive only to the largest nerve fibers. Moreover, the human physiology tolerates only moderate gradient strengths, suggesting that *in-vivo* diffusion imaging has fundamental limitations upon the resolution power. Even on dedicated animal systems we cannot distinguish diameters less than one or two micrometers where the bulk of the axon distribution resides. Also unduly long gradient durations are prohibitive because of the short T_2-relaxation time of white matter tissue. Here we consider, from a theoretical viewpoint, an alternative MR modality, T_2-spectroscopy, and its potential to resolve submicrometer axon diameters. Instead of the displacement of the diffusing water molecules, this method measures their interaction with the cellular boundaries, which may contain paramagnetic impurities that give rise to fluctuating microscopic fields. As a consequence, the water molecules close to the axonal membranes partially loose their phase coherence and thus the T_2-weighted signal attenuates faster. This surface relaxation effect is the contrast mechanism that gives the potential to measure axons with one micrometer or less in diameter. Intuitively, for a tissue sample of thin nerve fibers a large volume fraction of water molecules is located in the vicinity of the axonal membranes. Therefore, the transverse magnetization decays faster than for nerve fibers with a large radius because in the latter case only a small fraction of water molecules is influenced by the cellular boundaries.

This article lays the foundations for quantitative T_2-spectroscopy exploiting the surface relaxation in the underlying tissue material. The potential advantages over diffusion experiments are the possibility to map the full axon diameter distribution, including the nerve fibers with a submicrometer diameter, and independence from the directional tissue structure. In the following we start from the Bloch–Torrey equation for the description of the surface relaxation and present a general solution based on the eigenstructure of the pore geometry. Then a plausible biophysical model is developed for nervous tissue using a surface-to-volume ratio approximation. Under a certain regime of bulk and surface relaxivity parameters, our simulation results suggest that it might be possible to reveal axons smaller than one micrometer in diameter, even from spin-echo experiments achievable on clinical scanners. We conclude with a discussion of the proposed approach, including an outlook for future work.

2 Theory and Methods

2.1 Bloch–Torrey Equation

The Bloch equation [12] provides a phenomenological description for the evolution of the magnetization vector in a time-dependent magnetic field. We suppose that the repetition time is chosen much longer than the T_1-relaxation time, which means that the spin-lattice relaxation can be ignored. Let $m(x,t)$ be the magnetization perpendicular to the main magnetic field B_0 at position x and time t. Consider a large ensemble of water molecules undergoing Brownian motion with the (bulk) diffusion coefficient D in a region $\Omega \subseteq \mathbb{R}^d$ of dimension d. Torrey [13] proposed to modify the Bloch equation to include the signal decay due to the diffusion process. The transverse magnetization then obeys the partial differential equation

$$\left(\frac{\partial}{\partial t} - D\Delta + i\gamma B(x,t) + \frac{1}{T_{2,b}} \right) m(x,t) = 0 \quad \text{on } x \in \Omega, \, t \geq 0, \qquad (1)$$

where Δ denotes the Laplace operator describing the diffusive motion of the water molecules, γ is the gyromagnetic ratio of the hydrogen proton, and $B(x,t)$ represents the time-dependent magnetic field. Since for a plain spin-echo experiment [14] $B(x,t) = B_0$ is constant, the magnetic field encoding gives rise to a multiplicative factor $\exp(-i\gamma B_0 t)$ in the solution of Equation (1) and hence can be neglected. $T_{2,b}$ quantifies the bulk relaxation of water. The initial spin density $m(x,0) = m_0(x)$ of the water protons is assumed to be uniform over Ω. The observable MR signal at time t is the transverse magnetization $E(t) = \int_\Omega m(x,t) s(x) \, dx$ weighted by the sampling function $s(x)$ of the receiver coil, which is here uniform over the domain Ω. In the case of free (unrestricted) diffusion the solution of the Bloch–Torrey equation leads to the T_2-weighted signal $E(t) = E_0 \exp(-t/T_{2,b})$, where E_0 denotes the water proton density.

Since the diffusion process is confined in nervous tissue, we introduce appropriate boundary conditions. The Robin condition for the transverse magnetization at sufficiently smooth boundaries $\partial\Omega$ writes

$$\left(D\frac{\partial}{\partial n} + K \right) m(x,t) = 0 \quad \text{on } x \in \partial\Omega,\, t \geq 0, \tag{2}$$

where $\partial/\partial n$ denotes the outward normal derivative on $\partial\Omega$. The surface relaxivity $K \in [0, \infty]$ quantifies the influence of the cellular barriers on the phase coherence of the spin-bearing water molecules. This coefficient reflects the physicochemical properties of the boundary and we make the assumption that K is uniform over $\partial\Omega$. For a closed pore Ω the general solution of the Bloch–Torrey equation (1) under condition (2) yields the T_2-weighted MR signal [15]

$$E(t) = E_0 \sum_{m=0}^{\infty} v_m \exp(-(\lambda_m + 1/T_{2,b})\, t), \tag{3}$$

where λ_m denote the eigenvalues corresponding to the orthogonal eigenfunctions $u_m(x)$ of the eigenproblem $-D\Delta u_m(x) = \lambda_m u_m(x)$ on $x \in \Omega$ with the boundary condition $(D\partial/\partial n + K)u_m(x) = 0$ on $x \in \partial\Omega$. The initial density of the water protons is set to $m_0(x) = E_0/V$ and the sampling function reads $s(x) = 1$, where V denotes the volume of the pore. The coefficients v_m are given by $v_m = V^{-1}(\int_\Omega u_m(x)\,dx)^2/(\int_\Omega u_m(x)^2\,dx)$ and fulfill the relation $\sum_{m=0}^{\infty} v_m = 1$. In plain words, Ω gives the size and the shape of the pore (e.g., the axon diameter). The eigenvalues, which are sorted in increasing order $0 \leq \lambda_0 \leq \lambda_1 \leq \lambda_2 \leq \ldots$, depend on the geometry Ω, the bulk diffusion coefficient D, and the surface relaxivity K. As v_m may be zero for some indices m, the observable T_2-signal is controlled by a subset of the eigenmodes, which means that we are not able to reconstruct arbitrary shapes. The eigenspectrum for various simple geometries like the plane, the cylinder, or the sphere may be found in the literature [16].

From the general solution (3) of the Bloch–Torrey equation we can easily deduce the T_2-spectrum

$$\nu = E_0 \sum_{m=0}^{\infty} v_m \delta_{1/(\lambda_m + 1/T_{2,b})},$$

which is a discrete measure on $[0, \infty]$. ν is normalized with the spin density of the water protons $\nu([0, \infty]) = E_0$. The peaks can be found at $1/(\lambda_m + 1/T_{2,b})$, which are bounded from above by the bulk relaxation $T_{2,b}$ and are weighted by $E_0 v_m$. The (modified) Laplace transform of the spectrum, i.e., $E(t) = \int_0^\infty \exp(-t/\tau)\, d\nu(\tau)$, then yields the observable T_2-weighted MR data. For illustration purposes, Figure 1 exemplifies the discrete T_2-spectrum of an infinite cylinder with $1\,\mu\text{m}$ in diameter. In the left panel the magnetization of

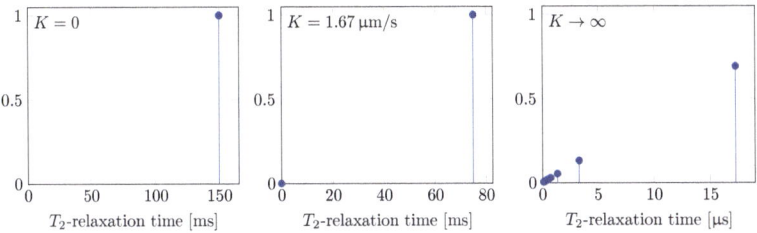

Fig. 1. Discrete T_2-spectrum for a cylinder with various surface relaxivities K. Its diameter is set to $1\,\mu m$, the bulk diffusion coefficient is fixed at $D = 2.5\,\mu m^2/ms$, the bulk relaxation time is $T_{2,b} = 150\,ms$, and the spin density reads $E_0 = 1$.

the nuclear spins does not alter during their interaction with the boundary (*i.e.*, $K = 0$), which gives rise to the Neumann boundary condition. The visible peak is due to the bulk relaxation, which is here set to $T_{2,b} = 150\,ms$, and thus the signal does not contain any information about the tissue geometry. The middle panel depicts the spectrum under the weak surface relaxation regime, which generally exhibits an infinite number of peaks that decay rapidly both in their intensity and the T_2-relaxation time. In practice it will be difficult to observe any other peaks than the one for the lowest eigenvalue. Therefore, Brownstein and Tarr [15,16] proposed a surface-to-volume ratio model

$$E(t) \approx E_0 \exp\left(-t\left(K\frac{S(\Omega)}{V(\Omega)} + \frac{1}{T_{2,b}}\right)\right) \qquad (4)$$

that approximates very closely the T_2-weighted signal for all closed pores Ω (not only the cylinder shown in the figure), where $S(\Omega)$ computes the surface area of Ω and $V(\Omega)$ the volume. The right panel depicts the eigenspectrum when the water molecules completely loose their transverse magnetization if they collide with the interface (*i.e.*, $K \to \infty$). Note that for the Dirichlet boundary regime we obtain very short T_2-relaxation times.

2.2   Biophysical Model of White Matter

In the following we develop a plausible biophysical model of white matter tissue based on the surface-to-volume ratio approximation of the Bloch–Torrey equation, which subsequently allows us to infer the fiber density and the axon diameter distribution. Although T_2-spectroscopy is not able to recover arbitrary shapes, the attenuation of the transverse magnetization can be still useful when we make some appropriate assumptions about the underlying tissue structure. The present work considers a two-compartment model similar to those used in diffusion MR techniques for axon diameter estimation (for a review see [4] and the references therein). Henceforth we assume that one signal component arises from the water pool inside the axons, while the other compartment comes from the extraaxonal space. The T_2-weighted signal may then be written as

$$E(t) = E_0 \exp(-t/T_{2,b})(P_1 E_{\text{intra}}(t) + (1 - P_1)E_{\text{extra}}(t)),$$

where $E(t)$ is the observable transverse magnetization after time t, E_0 quantifies the water proton density, $T_{2,b}$ denotes the bulk T_2-relaxation coefficient, $E_{intra}(t)$ is the surface relaxation signal from the intraaxonal compartment, $E_{extra}(t)$ the signal for the extraaxonal space, and $P_1 \in [0,1]$ quantifies the volume fraction occupied by the fiber population. Since the transverse relaxation encodes neither the intra-voxel position nor the orientation of a fiber segment, we do not need to consider the directional tissue architecture of white matter, for example, fiber dispersion and axon undulation.

First, we model the surface relaxation for the intraaxonal domain based on the surface-to-volume ratio approximation (4) under the weak surface relaxivity regime (compare left and middle panel of Figure 1). A key feature of the axon geometry is the radius, which exhibits multiple length scales in the brain white matter. This study adopts a statistical approach to describing the diversity of nerve fibers in terms of the axon diameter distribution μ, which is normalized with $\mu([0,\infty]) = 1$. The shape of an axon is approximated by a cylindrical tube with diameter ϕ. Integrating over the fiber population we obtain

$$E_{intra}(t) = \frac{\int_0^\infty V(\phi) \exp(-tKS(\phi)/V(\phi)) \, d\mu(\phi)}{\int_0^\infty V(\phi) \, d\mu(\phi)},$$

where $S(\phi) = \pi\phi$ quantifies the surface area of an axon and $V(\phi) = \pi\phi^2/4$ its volume in the two-dimensional plane perpendicular to the cylinder axis. In general the intraaxonal surface relaxation, which may be simplified to

$$E_{intra}(t) = \frac{\mathbb{E}_\mu[\phi^2 \exp(-4tK/\phi)]}{\mathbb{E}_\mu[\phi^2]},$$

exhibits a multiexponential decay, where $\mathbb{E}_\mu[\cdot]$ denotes the expectation with respect to the axon diameter measure μ.

Next, we describe the surface relaxation for the extraaxonal space. The particular placement of the axons within the domain has a negligible effect because under the weak surface relaxivity regime the observable signal largely depends on the surface-to-volume ratio, which is invariant with respect to the fiber configuration. In addition, we assume that the space between the nerve fibers is connected or, if not, that the various components of the extraaxonal space have a similar surface-to-volume ratio. The surface relaxation then takes the form

$$E_{extra}(t) = \exp\left(-tK \frac{\int_0^\infty S(\phi) \, d\mu(\phi)}{(1/P_1 - 1) \int_0^\infty V(\phi) \, d\mu(\phi)}\right),$$

where $S(\phi)$ and $V(\phi)$ quantify the surface area and the volume of a cylindrical axon with diameter ϕ, respectively, and P_1 denotes the volume fraction of the nerve fibers. The extraaxonal surface relaxation, which may be rewritten as

$$E_{extra}(t) = \exp\left(-\frac{4tK}{1/P_1 - 1} \frac{\mathbb{E}_\mu[\phi]}{\mathbb{E}_\mu[\phi^2]}\right),$$

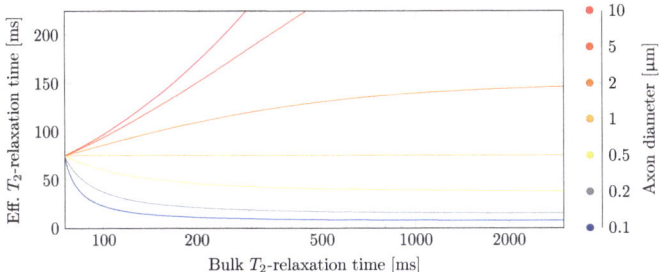

Fig. 2. The diagram plots the effective T_2-relaxation time for various bulk relaxation coefficients and different axon diameters. The surface relaxivity is chosen such that a nerve fiber with diameter of $1\,\mu m$ (neglecting the extraaxonal space) has an effective relaxation time of $75\,ms$.

has a monoexponential behavior. Note that the expectation functionals exist if a maximum radius can be given, which is always the case in brain white matter.

Finally, we provide two examples of specific diameter measures. In the case when all nerve fibers have the same diameter ϕ within a voxel, which means that the axon diameter distribution is described by a Dirac mass δ_ϕ, the signal writes

$$E(t) = E_0 \exp(-t/T_{2,b}) \left(P_1 \exp\left(-\frac{4tK}{\phi}\right) + (1 - P_1)\exp\left(-\frac{4tK}{(1/P_1 - 1)\phi}\right)\right).$$
(5)

Alternatively, as in [6] for a Gamma distribution model of μ, with the parameters α and β chosen such that $f_{\mathcal{G}a}(0; \alpha, \beta) = 0$ holds, the T_2-weighted signal takes the form

$$E(t) = E_0 \exp(-t/T_{2,b}) \left(P_1 \frac{2\left(\frac{4tK}{\beta}\right)^{\alpha/2+1}}{\Gamma(\alpha + 2)} K_{\alpha+2}\left(2\sqrt{\frac{4tK}{\beta}}\right)\right.$$

$$\left. + (1 - P_1)\exp\left(-\frac{4tK}{1/P_1 - 1}\frac{1}{(\alpha + 1)\beta}\right)\right),$$
(6)

where $K_{\alpha+2}(\cdot)$ denotes the modified Bessel function of the second kind with the order $\alpha + 2$. Other models for the axon diameter distribution, such as a scaled Beta density, also give closed form expressions for $E(t)$.

2.3   Bulk and Surface Relaxation Coefficients

The surface-to-volume ratio model (4) depends on the bulk relaxation coefficient $T_{2,b}$ and the surface relaxivity parameter K. Unfortunately, neither parameter is known for nervous tissue. Pure water has a relaxation time of about $3\,s$ [17], which is an upper bound. Ignoring any signal contributions from the extraaxonal space, let us assume that a fiber with diameter of $\phi = 1\,\mu m$ gives rise to an effective T_2-relaxation time $T_{2,\text{eff}} = 75\,\text{ms}$, which is defined by $T_{2,\text{eff}} = 1/(KS(\phi)/V(\phi) + 1/T_{2,b})$. This value is in the range of T_2-weighted signals we typically measure in brain white matter [17]. The surface relaxation coefficient can then be estimated from a given bulk relaxation time $T_{2,b}$. Figure 2 plots the effective T_2-relaxation time for various bulk relaxivities and different axon diameters. By definition we obtain a constant effective relaxation time for the fibers with $1\,\mu\text{m}$ in diameter. In the case of $T_{2,b} \to \infty$, the effective relaxation time of an axon is proportional to its diameter. If the bulk relaxation is decreased, the figure shows that the T_2-spectrum gets narrower. The literature [17] suggests that the spectrum is not very broad, which means that the bulk relaxation coefficient can only be slightly larger than $T_{2,\text{eff}} = 75\,\text{ms}$, but is much smaller than the T_2-relaxation time of pure water. This observation motivates our choice of these two parameters in the next section.

3   Experiments

For the following simulation study we set the bulk relaxation coefficient to $T_{2,b} = 150\,\text{ms}$. The surface relaxivity parameter $K = 1.67\,\mu\text{m/s}$ is chosen such that an axon of $1\,\mu\text{m}$ in diameter has an effective relaxation time of $75\,\text{ms}$. Note that all results, especially the resolution power of the axon diameter, depend on these two model parameters. We do not need to specify any diffusion coefficients. The T_2-weighted signal is sampled at 32 echo times ranging from 10 to $320\,\text{ms}$ with constant interecho spacing using a Carr-Purcell-Meiboom-Gill (CPMG) experiment. The phantom signals are disturbed by Gaussian noise. This report studies the statistical properties of the least-squares estimator which is used to infer the water proton density $E_0 > 0$, the intraaxonal volume fraction $P_1 \in [0, 1]$, and the fiber diameter distribution. The latter is constrained such that the density at an axon radius of zero vanishes, here $f_{\mathcal{G}a}(0; \alpha, \beta) = 0$. Thus, the estimated parameters are ensured to lie within a physically meaningful range. We run 5000 trials each to investigate the estimation error of the fiber density and the axon diameter (distribution) under various scenarios.

   The first case study generates a sample of different fiber populations where all axons have an identical radius, which means that the axon diameter distribution is described by a Dirac measure. Subsequently we try to recover the fiber density and the axon diameter from the simulated data. The top row of Figure 3 depicts the median of the estimates as well as their 0.05- and 0.95-quantiles for various signal-to-noise ratios E_0/σ, where E_0 denotes the water proton density and σ^2 is the Gaussian noise variance. The discontinuity in the quantiles is due to a second local optimum which gradually disappears as the signal-to-noise ratio increases. The bottom row shows the estimation results for simulated axon diameters ranging from 0.1 to $10\,\mu\text{m}$. For very thin fibers the T_2-signal vanishes at long echo times, which means that only few spin echoes contribute to the estimation of the biexponential decay. To reduce the higher estimation error, we would have to increase the temporal resolution of the CPMG sequence. In the opposite case of very thick axons the T_2-relaxation has a rather slow decay, which suggests sampling the transverse magnetization at longer echo times.

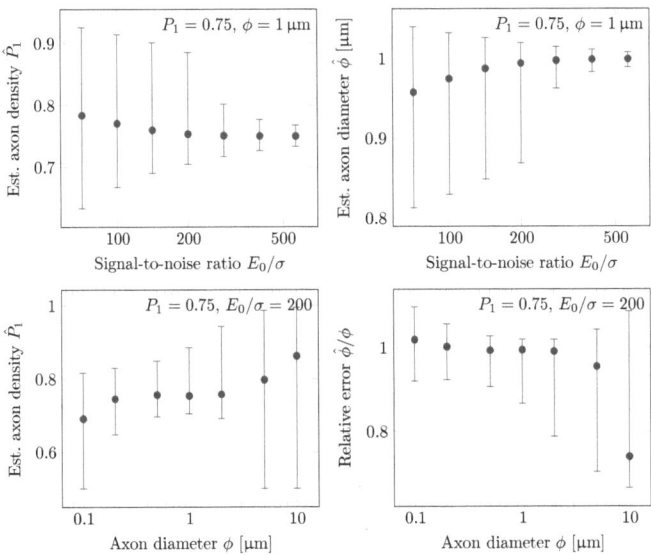

Fig. 3. Estimation accuracy for various tissue samples of white matter with a single axon diameter (Dirac measure). The four diagrams show the median of the least-squares estimates including their 0.05- and 0.95-quantiles for various signal-to-noise ratios and different axon diameters. The fixed model parameters are indicated in the upper right corner of these plots.

The next case study simulates tissue samples that consist of multiple axon diameters, which follow a Gamma density with the mean diameter $\bar{\phi} = 1\,\mu m$ and the variance $\mathrm{var}[\phi] = 0.5\,\mu m^2$. The intraaxonal volume fraction is set to 0.75 for all experiments. We estimate the axon density and the fiber diameter using the Dirac model (5) which assumes that the radii of the nerve fibers are constant. The upper row of Figure 4 shows the estimated tissue parameters for various levels of Gaussian noise. The variance decreases as expected when the signal-to-noise ratio is improved, but we observe a significant bias in the estimation of P_1 and $\bar{\phi}$ due to a model mismatch, which is particularly prominent for broad diameter distributions. In the lower row of this figure the estimation results are depicted when the variance of the axon diameter distribution is reduced, in which case the bias vanishes and the estimated parameters asymptotically converge towards their true values. Note that for a broad diameter distribution the T_2-signal decay can differ considerably from the magnetization attenuation of a narrow distribution even if the mean axon diameter is kept fixed. This signal behavior may explain the observed bias in the estimation of the tissue parameters. Nevertheless, the Dirac model can be used for the approximate estimation of the mean fiber radius, which, however, might be biased for broad diameter distributions.

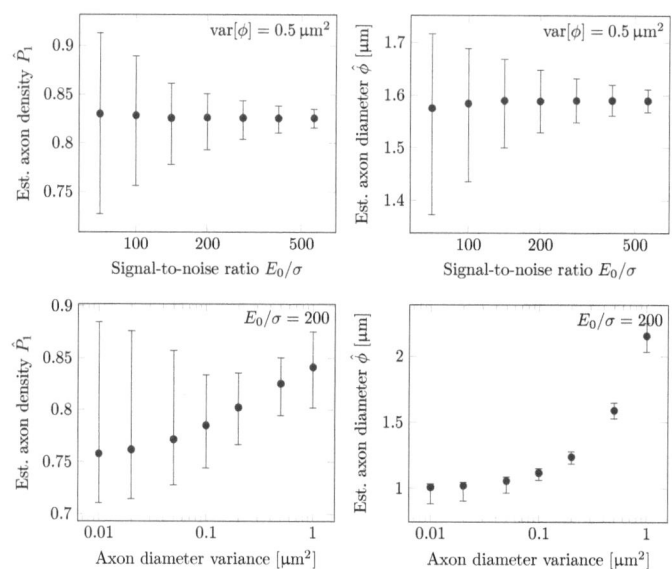

Fig. 4. Estimation accuracy of the axon density and the fiber diameter for tissue samples of white matter in which the axon diameter follows a Gamma distribution. The mean diameter of the nerve fibers is set to $1\,\mu m$ and the axon density is fixed at 0.75 for all experiments.

Provided that the intraaxonal volume fraction $P_1 = 0.75$ is known, Figure 5 demonstrates the parametric estimation of the fiber diameter distribution. In contrast to the previous experiment, there is no model misspecification here because we simulate and analyze the synthetic tissue samples using the same model of axon diameter distribution. More precisely, the multiple axon diameters are governed by a Gamma density with the mean $\bar{\phi} = 1\,\mu m$ and the variance $\text{var}[\phi] = 0.5\,\mu m^2$. The upper row shows the mean and variance estimates (right) and plots a sample of the estimated Gamma densities for the signal-to-noise ratio of $E_0/\sigma = 200$. The red square and the red line indicate the true value and density, respectively. The bottom row of Figure 5 depicts the median including the 0.05- and 0.95-quantiles of the mean axon diameter and the L_1-norm based distance between the estimated and the true density for various signal-to-noise ratios E_0/σ. The diagrams show that the variance of the mean diameter estimator decreases and the L_1-norm based error is reduced when the signal-to-noise ratio is improved. A noteworthy result is that there is no significant bias apparent in the mean axon diameter because the full diameter distribution is considered. Given the axon density, we should be able to recover the fiber diameter distribution, where its mean can be estimated in a quite robust manner. However, we expect considerable variance in the estimation of the shape of the parametric diameter density for realistic spin-echo experiments.

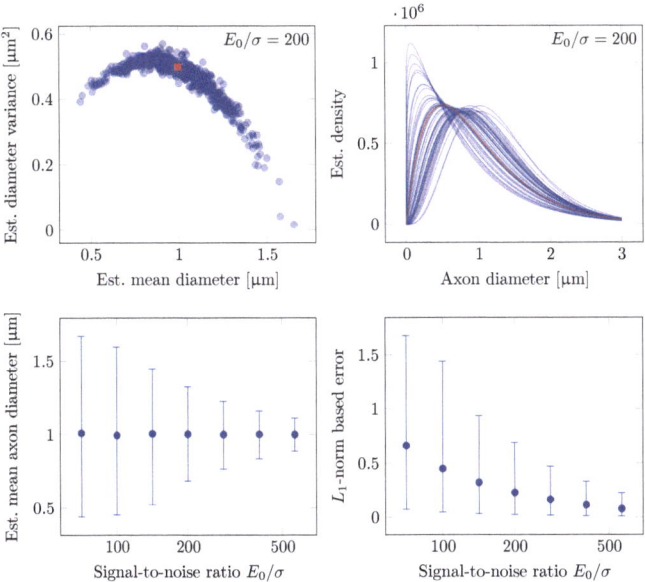

Fig. 5. Estimation accuracy of the axon diameter distribution parameterized by a Gamma density with the mean $\bar{\phi} = 1\,\mu\text{m}$ and the variance $\text{var}[\phi] = 0.5\,\mu\text{m}^2$, given the fiber density $P_1 = 0.75$ in the underlying substrate. See text for further details on this simulation study.

4   Discussion

In the present report we have proposed a novel strategy for assessing the axon diameter distribution including the fibers that have a diameter less than one micrometer. Our simulation results suggest that T_2-spectroscopy might be able to detect submicrometer axon diameters, depending on the temporal resolution of the CPMG experiment, the bulk and the surface relaxation coefficient. Figure 2 suggests that the bulk relaxivity parameter in nervous tissue is significantly lower than for pure water because otherwise the T_2-spectrum would be very broad. A possible explanation could be specific properties of the axoplasm or the cytoskeleton inside the nerve fibers (*e.g.*, neurofilaments and microtubules). The key question is whether the surface relaxation still dominates the bulk relaxation in the T_2-weighted signal. If not, we would not be able to recover the axon diameter distribution using the surface relaxation process. These theoretical results motivate work to evaluate the two relaxation coefficients. For example, we may estimate the two model parameters by conducting a calibration experiment using histological data. Knowing the fiber density and the axon diameter distribution for a small tissue sample, it should be possible to infer the bulk and surface relaxation coefficients from the measured MR data. Further advantages of T_2-spectroscopy are that the proposed method is independent of the tangential distribution of the axons within a voxel and that the CPMG experiments can be performed with a standard human scanner in a clinical environment. Future work may also consider the myelination of the axons, the presence of glial cells in white matter tissue, and exchange processes between different water pools.

Acknowledgment. The UK EPSRC supported this work with grant EP/E007748.

References

1. Aboitiz, F., Scheibel, A.B., Fisher, R.S., Zaidal, E.: Fiber composition of the human corpus callosum. Brain Research 598, 143–153 (1992)
2. Rushton, W.A.H.: A theory of the effects of fibre size in medullated nerve. Journal of Physiology 115, 101–122 (1951)
3. DeLuca, G.C., Ebers, G.C., Esiri, M.M.: Axonal loss in multiple sclerosis: a pathological survey of the corticospinal and sensory tracts. Brain 127, 1009–1018 (2004)
4. Panagiotaki, E., Schneider, T., Siow, B., Hall, M.G., Lythgoe, M.F., Alexander, D.C.: Compartment models of the diffusion MR signal in brain white matter: A taxonomy and comparison. NeuroImage 59, 2241–2254 (2012)
5. Stanisz, G.J., Szafer, A., Wright, G.A., Henkelman, R.M.: An analytical model of restricted diffusion in bovine optic nerve. Magnetic Resonance in Medicine 37, 103–111 (1997)
6. Assaf, Y., Blumenfeld-Katzir, T., Yovel, Y., Basser, P.J.: AxCaliber: A method for measuring axon diameter distribution from diffusion MRI. Magnetic Resonance in Medicine 59, 1347–1354 (2008)
7. Barazany, D., Basser, P.J., Assaf, Y.: *In vivo* measurement of axon diameter distribution in the corpus callosum of rat brain. Brain 132, 1210–1220 (2009)
8. Alexander, D.C., Hubbard, P.L., Hall, M.G., Moore, E.A., Ptito, M., Parker, G.J.M., Dyrby, T.B.: Orientationally invariant indices of axon diameter and density from diffusion MRI. NeuroImage 52, 1374–1389 (2010)
9. Zhang, H., Hubbard, P.L., Parker, G.J.M., Alexander, D.C.: Axon diameter mapping in the presence of orientation dispersion with diffusion MRI. NeuroImage 56, 1301–1315 (2011)
10. Axer, H., Axer, M., Krings, T., von Keyserlingk, D.G.: Quantitative estimation of 3-D fiber course in gross histological sections of the human brain using polarized light. Journal of Neuroscience Methods 105, 121–131 (2001)
11. Dyrby, T.B., Søgaard, L.V., Hall, M.G., Ptito, M., Alexander, D.C.: Contrast and Stability of the Axon Diameter Index from Microstructure Imaging with Diffusion MRI. Magnetic Resonance in Medicine (2012), http://dx.doi.org/10.1002/mrm.24501, doi:10.1002/mrm.24501
12. Bloch, F.: Nuclear induction. Physical Review 70, 460–474 (1946)
13. Torrey, H.C.: Bloch equations with diffusion terms. Physical Review 104, 563–565 (1956)
14. Hahn, E.L.: Spin echoes. Physical Review 80, 580–594 (1950)
15. Brownstein, K.R., Tarr, C.E.: Spin–lattice relaxation in a system governed by diffusion. Journal of Magnetic Resonance 26, 17–24 (1977)
16. Brownstein, K.R., Tarr, C.E.: Importance of classical diffusion in NMR studies of water in biological cells. Physical Review A 19, 2446–2453 (1979)
17. MacKay, A., Laule, C., Vavasour, I., Bjarnason, T., Kolind, S., Mädler, B.: Insights into brain microstructure from the T_2 distribution. Magnetic Resonance Imaging 24, 515–525 (2006)

Dictionary Learning on the Manifold of Square Root Densities and Application to Reconstruction of Diffusion Propagator Fields[*]

Jiaqi Sun[1], Yuchen Xie[2], Wenxing Ye[3], Jeffrey Ho[1], Alireza Entezari[1],
Stephen J. Blackband[4], and Baba C. Vemuri[1,**]

[1] CISE Department, University of Florida, Gainesville, FL 32611, USA
[2] Qualcomm Inc., San Diego, CA 92121, USA
[3] Google Inc., Mountain View, CA 94043, USA
[4] Department of Neuroscience, McKnight Brian Institute, University of Florida,
Gainesville, FL 32611, USA
vemuri@cise.ufl.edu

Abstract. In this paper, we present a novel dictionary learning framework for data lying on the manifold of square root densities and apply it to the reconstruction of diffusion propagator (DP) fields given a multi-shell diffusion MRI data set. Unlike most of the existing dictionary learning algorithms which rely on the assumption that the data points are vectors in some Euclidean space, our dictionary learning algorithm is designed to incorporate the intrinsic geometric structure of manifolds and performs better than traditional dictionary learning approaches when applied to data lying on the manifold of square root densities. Non-negativity as well as smoothness across the whole field of the reconstructed DPs is guaranteed in our approach. We demonstrate the advantage of our approach by comparing it with an existing dictionary based reconstruction method on synthetic and real multi-shell MRI data.

Keywords: Dictionary learning, Manifold, DW-MRI, Diffusion propagator reconstruction.

1 Introduction

Diffusion weighted MRI, as a non-invasive imaging technique, helps explore the complex micro-structure of fibrous tissues through sensing the Brownian motion of water molecules [1]. Water diffusion is fully characterized by the diffusion Probability Density Function (PDF) called the diffusion propagator (DP) [2]. Under the narrow pulse assumption, the diffusion propagator denoted by

---

[*] This research was in part funded by the NIH grant NS066340 to Baba C. Vemuri, and the following grants AFOSR FA9550-12-1-0304, ONR N000141210862, NSF CCF-1018149 to Alireza Entezari.

[**] Corresponding author.

J.C. Gee et al. (Eds.): IPMI 2013, LNCS 7917, pp. 619–631, 2013.

$P(\mathbf{r})$ and the diffusion signal attenuation $E(\mathbf{q})$ are related through the Fourier transform[2]:

$$P(\mathbf{r}) = \int E(\mathbf{q}) exp(-2\pi i \mathbf{q} \cdot \mathbf{r}) d\mathbf{q} \tag{1}$$

where $E(\mathbf{q}) = S(\mathbf{q})/S_0$, S_0 is the diffusion signal with zero diffusion gradient.

Given the diffusion MRI data, reconstructing the DP is one of the most important problems in the field. Numerous techniques have been proposed to this end [3–5]. For further reading, we refer the interested reader to a recent survey [6]. Most of these methods either assume a model in which case, the basis functions for reconstruction are predefined or in the case of model free approaches, they have to explicitly enforce the positivity constraints on the DP, which in some works was not done. In our work, we take a fresh approach to this problem namely a dictionary learning approach. This approach will move away from the requirement of pre-specifying the basis functions and instead learns it from the data and hence is data adaptive. This is a more flexible approach over fixing the basis. Further, by using the square root density representation of the DP, we make use of the intrinsic structure of the manifold of square root densities in the reconstruction process without having to resort to explicit enforcement of non-negativity constraint on DP reconstruction. In the following, we first present a brief review of relevant dictionary learning techniques and then present a review of state-of-the-art in DP reconstruction from multi-shell diffusion MRI.

1.1 Dictionary Learning on Riemannian Manifolds: Literature Review

Sparse coding which calls for modeling data as a linear combination of a small number of elements from a collection of atoms, i.e., the dictionary, has been proven very effective in many image processing tasks [7]. In these tasks, learning a dictionary that adapts well to the data is of great significance for a good performance of the sparse representation. Therefore, considering the geometric structure of the data space is critical to the success of dictionary learning. Most existing dictionary learning algorithms often assume that the data points and the atoms are vectors in a Euclidean space, and the dictionary is learned based on the vector space structure of the input data. However, the data involved in many image analysis tasks often reside on Riemannian manifolds such as the space of, symmetric positive definite (SPD) matrices [8] and square root densities. Therefore, the existing extrinsic approaches which overlook the potentially important intrinsic geometric structure of the data are inadequate in the context of such applications. Recently, this inadequacy was addressed by a few researchers [9] leading to the generalization of dictionary learning to manifolds, specifically, to the manifold of SPD matrices. However, most of these methods seek to transform the problem to a simpler space and solve it there, instead of respecting the geometric structure of the SPD matrix manifold. Needless to say, none of them truly incorporated the intrinsic geometry implied by the data as is done in this paper.

In general, dictionary learning in the Euclidean setting can be formulated as $\min_{c_1,\cdots,c_n,D} \sum_{i=1}^{n} \|s_i - Dc_i\|^2 + \mathbf{Sp}(c_i)$, where $s_1, \cdots, s_n$ is the given collection of data points, D is the matrix with columns composed of the atoms a_i, c_i the sparse coding coefficients and $\mathbf{Sp}(c_i)$ the sparsity promoting term. When generalizing it to a Riemannian manifold $\mathcal{M}$, one of the key difficulties that needs resolution is to make sure that the collection of atoms as well as the approximation of data points generated using the atoms still lie on the manifold. The reason being, in Euclidean space, it is the global linear structure that guarantees the data synthesized from the atoms is contained in the same space, whereas, on Riemannian manifolds the Riemannian geometry provides only local linear structures through the Riemannian exponential and logarithmic maps. Yet, by taking advantage of this diversity of linear structures it is possible to formulate the dictionary learning in a data specific way. Details regarding this formulation will be discussed in subsequent sections. It suffices to say that we employ the *log* and *exp* maps along with an affine constraint to achieve this goal.

1.2   DP Reconstruction from Multi-shell Acquisitions: Literature Review

We now present a brief review of DP reconstruction from multi-shell diffusion MRI data. Various techniques have been proposed to reconstruct the DP from multi-shell acquisitions of the diffusion signal[5, 10], which, compared to single shell acquisitions provide additional information about the radial signal decay. Most of them assume a particular model for the diffusion signal as in q-ball imaging (QBI) [11]. As an alternative, another category of methods place weak assumptions about the diffusion signal and therefore are capable of generating relatively unbiased reconstruction results, such as diffusion spectrum imaging (DSI) proposed in [12] and the tomographic reconstruction methods in [13–15]. These methods interpolate the spherical domain data samples onto a dense regular lattice and then reconstruct the DP using the Fourier transform relationship between $P(\mathbf{r})$ and $E(\mathbf{q})$. This idea is also adopted in our proposed method.

However, all of the aforementioned multi-shell methods solve the reconstruction problem in a voxel-wise manner, thereby always lead to a noisy reconstruction across the field. This gives us a strong motivation for applying dictionary learning to the reconstruction of DP fields, because the globally defined dictionary plays an implicit role in regularizing the reconstructions over the entire field. In recent years, a few dictionary learning based DP reconstruction methods have been proposed. In [16], Bilgic et al. applied adaptive dictionaries to accelerate the DSI method for estimating the DPs. In [17], Merlet et al. proposed a parametric dictionary learning framework obtaining a closed form DP and ODF modeling from diffusion MRI data. An over-complete dictionary based reconstruction of DP fields from single shell acquisition was presented in [18]. Nevertheless, due to the absence of explicit use of the geometric structure of the data space itself, none of these methods can guarantee the non-negativity of the reconstructed propagators, an intrinsic and basic property of the DP. Accordingly, these methods are prone to higher numerical errors.

Recently several approaches that guarantee the non-negativity of the reconstructed DP or ODF were proposed. For instance, in [19] authors used the Spherical Harmonic (SH) representation for ODF and enforced non-negativity on the continuous domain by enforcing the positive semi-definiteness of Toeplitz-like matrices constructed from the SH representation. Cheng et al. in [20] proposed to reconstruct ODFs (DPs) by estimating the square root of ODF (DP) called the wave-function directly from diffusion signals, ensuring non-negativity. The idea of taking advantage of the square root parameterization of DPs is also adopted in our proposed method. However, unlike dictionary based methods, the two methods discussed above are not guaranteed to yield a smooth reconstruction across the field and the reconstruction basis are pre-specified.

In this paper, we propose to apply the dictionary learning method generalized to the manifold of square root densities to the reconstruction of DP fields. As the nature of a globally learned dictionary indicates, our method will yield a smooth reconstruction which is desirable in real applications. By taking into consideration the intrinsic geometric structure of the manifold formed by the square root of DPs, our method performs better than the reconstruction techniques based on dictionary learning in a Euclidean setting. Furthermore, the non-negativity of the reconstructed DPs is naturally guaranteed due to the adoption of the square root representation and use of the intrinsic geometry of this space.

Rest of the paper is organized as follows. Section 2 contains brief background on Riemannian manifolds and the dictionary learning formulation. We present application to reconstruction of DP fields in section 3 and provide several examples in section 4. Finally section 5 contains conclusions.

2   Theory

2.1   Relevant Basics of Riemannian Manifolds

In this subsection, we briefly go over some fundamentals of Riemannian geometry, details of which can be found in [21]. A manifold $\mathcal{M}$ of dimension d is a topological space that is locally homeomorphic to open subsets of the Euclidean space $\mathbb{R}^d$ at each point. With a globally defined differential structure, manifold $\mathcal{M}$ becomes a differentiable manifold. The global differential structure allows one to define the globally differentiable tangent space. The tangent space at $p \in \mathcal{M}$ denoted by $T_p\mathcal{M}$ is a vector space that contains all the tangent vectors to $\mathcal{M}$ at point p. A Riemannian manifold is a differentiable manifold on which each tangent space $T_p\mathcal{M}$ at point p is equipped with a differentiable varying inner product $\langle \cdot, \cdot \rangle_p$. The family of the inner products is called a Riemannian metric. Let p_i, p_j be two points on manifold $\mathcal{M}$, the geodesic curve $\gamma : [0, 1] \rightarrow \mathcal{M}$ is a smooth curve with the minimum length connecting p_i and p_j. Let $v \in T_p\mathcal{M}$ be a tangent vector to the manifold at point p, there exists a unique geodesic γ_v satisfying $\gamma_v(0) = p$ with initial tangent vector v. The exponential map $exp_p : T_p\mathcal{M} \rightarrow \mathcal{M}$ of v is defined as $exp_p(v) = \gamma_v(1)$. Logarithmic map, as the inverse of the exponential map, is denoted as $log_p : \mathcal{M} \rightarrow T_p\mathcal{M}$. Given two points $p_i, p_j \in \mathcal{M}$, log_{p_i} maps point p_j to the unique tangent vector at p_i that is the initial velocity of the geodesic γ with $\gamma(0) = p_i$ and $\gamma(1) = p_j$. The geodesic distance between p_i and p_j is computed by $dist(p_i, p_j) = \|log_{p_i}(p_j)\|_{p_i}$.

2.2 Dictionary Learning on Riemannian Manifolds: Formulation

In the Euclidean setting, given a collection of signals $s_1, \ldots, s_n \in \mathbb{R}^d$, classical dictionary learning methods seek to find a dictionary $D \in \mathbb{R}^{d \times m}$ whose columns consist of m atoms such that each signal s_i can be approximated as a sparse linear combination of these atoms $s_i \approx D c_i$, where $c_i \in \mathbb{R}^m$ is the coefficient vector. Using l_1 regularization on c_i, the dictionary learning problem can be formulated as:

$$\min_{c_i, D} \sum_{i=1}^{n} \left(\|s_i - D c_i\|_2^2 + \lambda \|c_i\|_1 \right) \tag{2}$$

where λ is a regularization parameter.

In the Riemannian manifold setting, denote $s_1, \ldots, s_n \in \mathcal{M}$ as a collection of n data points on the manifold $\mathcal{M}$, and $a_1, \ldots, a_m \in \mathcal{M}$ as atoms of the learned dictionary $\mathcal{D} = \{a_1, \ldots, a_m\}$. Due to the local linear geometric structure of $\mathcal{M}$, it is improper to use the linear combination of atoms $\hat{s}_i = \sum_{j=1}^{m} c_{ij} a_j$ to approximate the data s_i, since there is no guarantee that $\hat{s}_i$ is on the manifold. Instead, by using the geodesic linear interpolation on $\mathcal{M}$, s_i can be estimated by $\hat{s}_i = \exp_{s_i} \left(\sum_{j=1}^{m} c_{ij} \log_{s_i}(a_j) \right)$ where, $\exp_{s_i}$ and $\log_{s_i}$ are exponential and logarithmic map at s_i respectively, and $c_{ij} \in \mathbb{R}$ are the coefficients. Intuitively, in order to approximate data point s_i, we project all the atoms in the dictionary to the tangent space at s_i and perform linear combination $v_i = \sum_{j=1}^{m} c_{ij} \log_{s_i}(a_j)$ on the tangent vector space $T_{s_i} \mathcal{M}$, then the approximation $\hat{s}_i$ is obtained by taking the exponential map of v_i at s_i.

Our goal is to build a dictionary that minimizes the sum of reconstruction error for each data point. Define

$$E_{\text{data}} = \sum_{i=1}^{n} dist(s_i, \hat{s}_i)^2 = \sum_{i=1}^{n} \|\log_{s_i}(\hat{s}_i)\|_{s_i}^2 = \sum_{i=1}^{n} \|\sum_{j=1}^{m} c_{ij} \log_{s_i}(a_j)\|_{s_i}^2. \tag{3}$$

By using the l_1 sparsity regularization, the dictionary learning problem on the manifold $\mathcal{M}$ can be formulated as the following optimization problem

$$\min_{C, \mathcal{D}} \sum_{i=1}^{n} \|\sum_{j=1}^{m} c_{ij} \log_{s_i}(a_j)\|_{s_i}^2 + \lambda \|C\|_1, s.t. \sum_{j=1}^{m} c_{ij} = 1, i = 1, \ldots, n \tag{4}$$

where $C \in \mathbb{R}^{n \times m}$ and the (i, j) entry of C is written as c_{ij}. A similar data term was used in [22] but the atoms were assumed fixed. The affine constraint implies that we are using affine subspaces to approximate the data instead of the usual subspaces, which are simply affine subspaces based at the origin. Generalizing from vector spaces to Riemannian manifolds, there is no corresponding notion of the origin that can be used to define subspaces, and this geometric fact requires the abandonment of the usual subspaces in favor of general affine subspaces. We can also introduce other regularizations in our framework instead of the l_1 norm but that will be a topic for future research. Similar to classical dictionary learning methods, we use the iterative method to solve this optimization problem:

1. **Sparse coding step:** fix the dictionary $\mathcal{D}$ and optimize with respect to the coefficients $\mathbf{C}$.
2. **Codebook optimization step:** fix $\mathbf{C}$ and optimize with respect to $\mathcal{D}$.

The first step is a regular sparse coding problem that can be easily solved by many existing fast algorithms. However the second subproblem is much more challenging, since the optimization methods in Euclidean space are not appropriate for atoms on manifolds.

We developed a line search based algorithm on Riemannian manifold to update the dictionary $\mathcal{D}$. Let the cost function to be minimized be denoted by $f(a_1, \ldots, a_m)$. First, we need to initialize the atoms in the dictionary. One possible choice of initialization is the m clusters of the data $s_1, \ldots, s_n$ generated by a K-means algorithm applied to all the data on $\mathcal{M}$. Then, a line search on the manifold is used to optimize $f(a_1, \ldots, a_m)$. Intuitively, the idea is to find a descent direction v on the tangent space, and then walk a step along the geodesic γ whose initial velocity is v. The details are listed in Algorithm 1. The convergence analysis of the line search method on manifold is discussed in [23].

Algorithm 1. Line search on Riemannian manifold

Input: A set of data $\mathcal{S} = \{s_1, \ldots, s_n\}$ on the manifold $\mathcal{M}$, coefficients $\mathbf{C} \in \mathbb{R}^{n \times m}$ and initial dictionary atoms $a_1^0, \ldots, a_m^0$.
Output: The optimal dictionary atoms $(a_1^*, \ldots, a_m^*)$ that minimize the cost function $f(a_1, \ldots, a_m)$.

1. Set scalars $\alpha > 0$, $\beta, \sigma \in (0, 1)$ and initialize $k = 0$.
2. Compute $\operatorname{grad} f(a_1^k, \ldots, a_m^k) = (\frac{\partial f(a_1^k)}{\partial a_1}, \ldots, \frac{\partial f(a_m^k)}{\partial a_m})$
3. Pick $\eta^k = (\eta_1^k, \ldots, \eta_m^k) = -\operatorname{grad} f$, where $\eta_i^k \in T_{a_i^k}\mathcal{M}$.
4. Find the smallest t such that

$$f(\exp_{a_1^k}(\alpha\beta^t\eta_1^k), \ldots, \exp_{a_m^k}(\alpha\beta^t\eta_m^k)) \leq f(a_1^k, \ldots, a_m^k) - \sum_{i=1}^{m} \sigma\alpha\beta^t \|\eta_i^k\|_{a_i^k}.$$

5. Set $a_i^{k+1} = \exp_{a_i^k}(\alpha\beta^t\eta_i^k)$, $i = 1, \ldots, m$.
6. Stop if f does not change much, otherwise set $k = k + 1$ and go back to step 2.

2.3   Manifold of Square Root Densities

In this section, without loss of generality we restrict the analysis to PDFs defined on the interval $[0, T]$ for simplicity: $\mathcal{P} = \{p : [0, T] \to \mathbb{R} | \forall s, p(s) \geq 0, \int_0^T p(s)ds = 1\}$.

In [24], the Fisher-Rao metric was introduced to study the Riemannian structure formed by the statistical manifold. For a PDF $p_i \in \mathcal{P}$, the Fisher-Rao metric is defined as $\langle v_j, v_k \rangle = \int_0^T v_j(s)v_k(s)\frac{1}{p_i(s)}ds$, where $v_j, v_k \in T_{p_i}\mathcal{P}$. The Fisher-Rao metric is invariant to reparameterizations of the functions. In order to facilitate easy computations when using Riemannian operations, the square root density representation $\psi = \sqrt{p}$ was used in [25]. The space of square root density functions is defined as $\Psi = \{\psi : [0,T] \to \mathbb{R} | \forall s, \psi(s) \geq 0, \int_0^T \psi^2(s)ds = 1\}$. As we can see, Ψ forms a convex subset of the unit sphere in a Hilbert space. Then the Fisher-Rao metric can be obtained as $\langle v_j, v_k \rangle = \int_0^T v_j(s)v_k(s)ds$, where $v_j, v_k \in T_{\psi_i}\Psi$ are tangent vectors. Given any two functions $\psi_i, \psi_j \in \Psi$, the geodesic distance between these two points is given in closed form by $\mathrm{dist}(\psi_i, \psi_j) = \cos^{-1}(\langle \psi_i, \psi_j \rangle)$, which is just the angle between ψ_i and ψ_j on the unit hypersphere. The geodesic at ψ_i with a direction $v \in T_{\psi_i}\Psi$ is defined as $\gamma(t) = \cos(t)\psi_i + \sin(t)\frac{v}{|v|}$. Then, the exponential map can be represented as $exp_{\psi_i}(v) = \cos(|v|)\psi_i + \sin(|v|)\frac{v}{|v|}$. To ensure the exponential map is a bijection, we restrict $|v| \in [0, \pi)$. The logarithmic map is then given by $log_{\psi_i}(\psi_j) = u \cos^{-1}(\langle \psi_i, \psi_j \rangle)/\sqrt{\langle u, u \rangle}$, where $u = \psi_j - \langle \psi_i, \psi_j \rangle \psi_i$.

Using the expressions for Ψ discussed above, we can perform the dictionary learning on square root density functions. Let $s_1, \ldots, s_n \in \Psi$ be a collection of square root density functions, and $a_i, \ldots, a_m \in \Psi$ be atoms in the dictionary $\mathcal{D}$. $\mathbf{C}$ is a $n \times m$ matrix. If we use l_1 regularization, our dictionary learning framework becomes

$$\min_{\mathbf{C},\mathcal{D}} \sum_{i=1}^n \| \sum_{j=1}^m c_{ij} \cos^{-1}(\langle s_i, a_j \rangle)\frac{u_{ij}}{|u_{ij}|} \|_{s_i}^2 + \lambda \|\mathbf{C}\|_1, s.t. \sum_{j=1}^m c_{ij} = 1, i = 1, \ldots, n.$$

(5)

where $u_{ij} = a_j - \langle s_i, a_j \rangle s_i$. Note that in this formulation, the normalization on atoms a_i is not needed. Because by incorporating the manifold structure of the square root densities, the atoms we learned are always on the hypersphere, while traditional dictionary learning (Equation (2)) needs the normalization to guarantee the unique solution. This optimization problem can be efficiently solved using the algorithm presented in section 2.2.

3   Application to Reconstruction of DP Fields

As mentioned in the introduction section, in the DP reconstruction problem, we aim to reconstruct a smooth field of DPs $P(\mathbf{r}, \mathbf{x})$ from a given field of multi-shell diffusion weighted MRI data $E(\mathbf{q}, \mathbf{x})$, where $\mathbf{x}$ represents the spatial locations. We propose to solve this problem in two steps. Briefly speaking, the first step is to acquire a rough estimation of the DP at each voxel through the Fourier transform relationship between the signal $E(\mathbf{q})$ and the DP, $P(\mathbf{r})$, specified in Equation (1). In the second step, in order to get a smooth reconstruction of the DPs over the entire field, we apply the proposed dictionary learning algorithm on the set of square root densities obtained by taking the square root of the DPs estimated from step 1. The implementation details are given below.

Despite the simple relationship between the diffusion signal and the DP described in Equation (1), it is often infeasible to reconstruct the DP from the diffusion signal directly through Fourier transform. The reason is that in practice, the diffusion signal is sampled in the $\mathbf{q}$ space following some pre-specified sampling scheme, which might not be uniform and regular. One solution is to define a regular lattice in $\mathbf{q}$ space and estimate the values on this lattice through interpolation. Inspired by the work of Ye et al.[15], we choose Body Centered Cubic (BCC) lattice to be our regular lattice for interpolation and apply Fourier transform to the interpolated values to get an estimate of the DPs. As demonstrated in [15], in 3-D, BCC lattice is the optimal lattice for $\mathbf{q}$ space sampling because its reciprocal lattice (i.e. the FCC lattice) is the densest sphere packing lattice.

Specifically, given N sample measurements $E(\mathbf{q}_n)$ on multiple spherical shells, the desired K values $E(\mathbf{x}_k)$ on the BCC lattice $\mathbf{x}_k \in \mathcal{L}$ can be estimated by solving the following linear system $E(\mathbf{q}_n) = \sum_{\mathbf{x}_k \in \mathcal{L}}^{1 \leq k \leq K} E(\mathbf{x}_k) sinc_{\mathcal{L}}(\mathbf{q}_n - \mathbf{x}_k), n = 1, \ldots, N$, where $sinc_{\mathcal{L}}(x)$ is the ideal interpolation function that depends on the sampling lattice $\mathcal{L}$. The $sinc_{\mathcal{L}}(x)$ for the BCC lattice is computed by Ye et. al in [15]. Once the K estimates $E(\mathbf{x}_k)$ on the lattice are obtained, we get a continuous representation of $E(\mathbf{q})$ as $E(\mathbf{q}) = \sum_{\mathbf{x}_k \in \mathcal{L}}^{1 \leq k \leq K} E(\mathbf{x}_k) sinc_{\mathcal{L}}(\mathbf{q} - \mathbf{x}_k)$. Taking Fourier transform on this equation, we get $P(\mathbf{r}) = box(\mathbf{r}) \sum_{\mathbf{x}_k \in \mathcal{L}}^{1 \leq k \leq K} E(\mathbf{x}_k) exp(-2\pi i \mathbf{x}_k \cdot \mathbf{r})$, where $box(\mathbf{r})$ is the Fourier transform of $sinc_{\mathcal{L}}(\mathbf{q})$.

According to the definition of DP, $P(\mathbf{r})$ is a PDF defined on a 3-D displacement $\mathbf{r}$ space. Therefore, by adopting the square root parameterization, we are able to map the estimated DPs from the space of PDFs to the manifold of square root densities. Let $\psi(\mathbf{r}) = \sqrt{P(\mathbf{r})}$ denote the square root of the DP at a single voxel, we apply the proposed dictionary learning algorithm on the set of $\psi(\mathbf{r})$ over the entire field. After solving for the globally defined dictionary $\mathcal{D}$ and the coefficient matrix $\mathbf{C}$ over the field, the reconstructed DPs can be obtained by solving a weighted mean problem on the hypersphere as described in section 2.2.

4   Experiments

In this section, we evaluate our reconstruction method by comparing it to a traditional dictionary learning based DP reconstruction method on both synthetic and real data sets.

4.1   Synthetic Data

We synthesized a 32×32 field of diffusion signals simulating two straight fibers crossing in the center. The signals were generated using a mixture of two Gaussian functions. The data was sampled on multiple $\mathbf{q}$ shells using the interlaced scheme described in [15]. Note that this sampling scheme is not a necessity for the application of our proposed method, we used it simply due to its high resolution in **q** space. Rician noise with level δ varying from 0.05 to 0.3 was added on the generated data.

Next we give the parameter settings in our reconstruction framework. In the first step, we chose a BCC lattice to interpolate the signals onto, which consists of two staggered Cartesian lattices of size $(11 \times 11 \times 11)$ and $(12 \times 12 \times 12)$ respectively. The $\|\mathbf{r}\|$ value to evaluate $P(\mathbf{r})$ on was set to be 18. Then in the process of dictionary learning on the square root density manifold, we set the dictionary size to be 100.

In order to demonstrate the advantage of incorporating the manifold structure into the reconstruction, we compared our method with the method in [18]. Since in [18] the authors adopted an adaptive kernel framework to model the signal in **q** space, which assumes a single b value in the signal acquisition, their framework can not handle data acquired on multiple **q** shells. Therefore, for the purpose of comparison we generalized it to make it applicable to multi-shell data, by using a tensor product of two 1-D splines in place of the 1-D spline in the Kernel they used. Also, we removed the NLM-based term in the cost function of [18] to achieve fair comparisons with our method.

We applied both methods to the synthetic data we generated with varying noise levels. The accuracy of the reconstruction was evaluated in terms of the average angular error over the entire field as well as within the crossing area. The angular error was computed based on the reconstructed $P(\mathbf{r})$ value at $\|\mathbf{r}\| = 18$. The quantitative comparisons of the two methods are given in Fig.1. The plot shows that our method has a higher accuracy in the reconstruction over the traditional dictionary learning based method. Note that the scales of the Average Angular Error axis are different in these two graphs. By comparing them we can see that the advantage of our scheme over the other one is more significant in the crossing area, where an accurate reconstruction is more difficult to achieve. This good performance is due to the incorporation of the intrinsic geometric structure of the Riemannian manifold in our reconstruction process.

In addition to the numerical comparison, a visual comparison is also shown above. The plots of the reconstructed $P(\mathbf{r})$ field from synthetic data with noise level $\delta = 0.25$ for the two methods are displayed side by side in Fig. 2. As is shown in the image, our method yields a smoother reconstruction over the entire field, especially in the crossing region. Furthermore, in our result(b), the fiber directions can be easily identified at each voxel in the crossing area whereas in the other one(a), the information is lost at some locations.

4.2   Real Data

In this section we present experimental results on real diffusion MRI data acquired from two different regions of a mouse brain: 1) a sagittal set through the midline and 2) a coronal set at the level of the corpus callosum. All magnetic resonance imaging was performed on a $600MHz$ Bruker imaging spectrometer, using a conventional diffusion weighted spin echo sequence. Parameters of the data acquisition for the two data sets are as follows. Dataset 1 was acquired with: $slicethickness = 0.35mm$, $1.8 \times 0.9cm^2$ field-of-view, 256×128 data matrix,

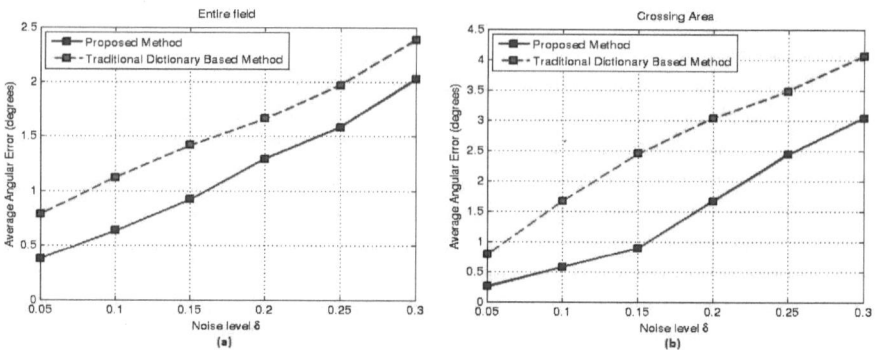

Fig. 1. The average angular error on the synthetic data set with varying noise levels. (a) Over the entire field. (b) Within the crossing area.

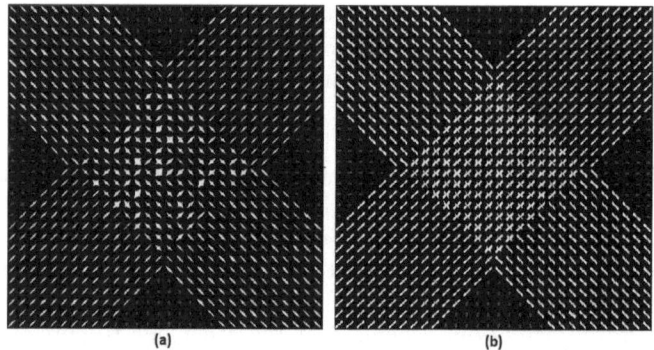

Fig. 2. Reconstruction of $P(\mathbf{r})$ on synthetic data set with noise level $\delta = 0.25$. (a) The traditional dictionary learning based method. (b) The proposed method.

and $70.3\mu m$ in-plane resolution. Diffusion parameters include: diffusion time, $\Delta = 12msec$, diffusion gradient duration, $\delta = 1msec$, and b-values of 187, 750, 1687 and $3000s/mm^2$. Dataset 2: $slicethickness = 0.3mm$, $1.2 \times 1.2cm^2$ field-of-view, 192×192 data matrix, and $62.5\mu m$ in-plane resolution, the diffusion parameters are identical to the ones in Dataset 1. The sampling scheme was the same as used in the synthetic experiments.

The $P(\mathbf{r})$ reconstruction results for both data sets are displayed in Fig.3. The images in the first row correspond to Dataset 1 while the second row Dataset 2. In each row, from left to right, the images are respectively the S0 image of the entire image plane including the ROI (the region in the red box), the reconstruction result using traditional dictionary learning based method and the one given by our proposed method. It is obvious from the visualization that our method performs better at smoothing out the noise from both data

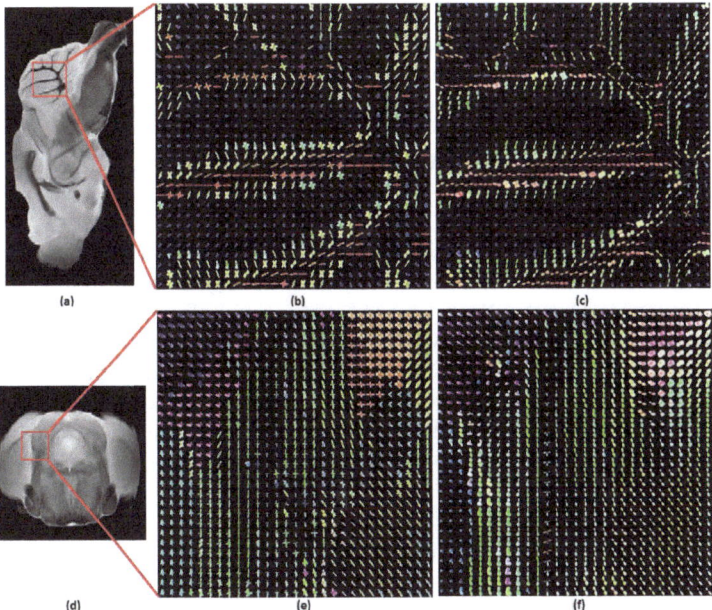

Fig. 3. Reconstruction results on real data. (a) The S0 image of the entire field of Dataset 1, where the ROI is indicated by the red box. (b) $P(\mathbf{r})$ Reconstruction using traditional dictionary learning based method on Dataset 1. (c) $P(\mathbf{r})$ Reconstruction using the proposed method on Dataset 1. (d)(e)(f) are the corresponding images for Dataset 2.

sets and therefore yields smoother DP fields. Furthermore, the fiber orientations estimated in our method are in accordance with expectations. As we can see in the ROI of Fig 3(a), which is part of the mouse cerebellum, the orientations of the DPs in the white matter (corresponding to the dark region in the S0 image) are more consistent in (c) than in (b).

5 Conclusions

In this paper, we generalized the traditional dictionary learning methods on Euclidean space to Riemannian manifolds. Specifically, we proposed a novel dictionary learning framework for data on the manifold of square root densities and applied it to the reconstruction of DP fields from multi-shell diffusion MRI data. Through multiple synthetic and real data experiments, we showed that our reconstruction method performs well in comparison to the traditional dictionary learning based DP reconstruction methods, hence, justifying the incorporation of the geometric structure of the data space (square root density Riemannian manifold in our case) into our reconstruction.

References

1. Basser, P., Mattiello, J., Lebihan, D.: Estimation of the effective self-diffusion tensor from the nmr spin echo. Journal of Magnetic Resonance (1994)
2. Callaghan, P.T.: Principles of nuclear magnetic resonance microscopy. Oxford University Press (1991)
3. Ozarslan, E., Shepherd, T.M., Vemuri, B.C., Blackband, S.J., Mareci, T.H.: Resolution of complex tissue microarchitecture using the diffusion orientation transform (DOT). Neuroimage (2006)
4. Jian, B., Vemuri, B.C., Ozarslan, E., Carney, P.R., Mareci, T.H.: A novel tensor distribution model for the diffusion-weighted MR signal. NeuroImage (2007)
5. Descoteaux, M., Deriche, R., Bihan, D.L., Mangin, J., Poupon, C.: Multiple q-shell diffusion propagator imaging. MIA (2011)
6. Assemlal, H., Tschumperle, D., Brun, L., Siddiqi, K.: Recent advances in diffusion MRI modeling: Angular and radial reconstruction. MIA (2011)
7. Aharon, M., Elad, M., Bruckstein, A.: K-svd: An algorithm for designing overcomplete dictionaries for sparse representation. IEEE Transactions on Signal Processing (2006)
8. Fletcher, P., Joshi, S.: Riemannian geometry for the statistical analysis of diffusion tensor data. Signal Processing (2007)
9. Sra, S., Cherian, A.: Generalized dictionary learning for symmetric positive definite matrices with application to nearest neighbor retrieval. In: Gunopulos, D., Hofmann, T., Malerba, D., Vazirgiannis, M. (eds.) ECML PKDD 2011, Part III. LNCS (LNAI), vol. 6913, pp. 318–332. Springer, Heidelberg (2011)
10. Caruyer, E., Deriche, R.: Diffusion MRI signal reconstruction with continuity constraint and optimal regularization. MIA (2012)
11. Tuch, D.S.: Q-ball imaging. MRM (2004)
12. Wedeen, V.J., Hagmann, P., Tseng, W.Y., Reese, T.G., Weisskoff, R.M.: Mapping complex tissue architecture with diffusion spectrum magnetic resonance imaging. MRM (2005)
13. Pickalov, V., Basser, P.: 3D tomographic reconstruction of the average propagator from MRI data. In: ISBI (2006)
14. Wu, Y., Alexander, A.: Hybrid diffusion imaging. NeuroImage (2007)
15. Ye, W., Portony, S., Entezari, A., Blackband, S.J., Vemuri, B.C.: An efficient interlaced multi-shell sampling scheme for reconstruction of diffusion propagators. IEEE TIP (2012)
16. Bilgic, B., Setsompop, K., Cohen-Adad, J., Wedeen, V., Wald, L.L., Adalsteinsson, E.: Accelerated diffusion spectrum imaging with compressed sensing using adaptive dictionaries. In: Ayache, N., Delingette, H., Golland, P., Mori, K. (eds.) MICCAI 2012, Part III. LNCS, vol. 7512, pp. 1–9. Springer, Heidelberg (2012)
17. Merlet, S., Caruyer, E., Deriche, R.: Parametric dictionary learning for modeling EAP and ODF in diffusion MRI. In: Ayache, N., Delingette, H., Golland, P., Mori, K. (eds.) MICCAI 2012, Part III. LNCS, vol. 7512, pp. 10–17. Springer, Heidelberg (2012)
18. Ye, W., Vemuri, B.C., Entezari, A.: An over-complete dictionary based regularized reconstruction of a field of ensemble average propagators. In: ISBI (2012)
19. Schwab, E., Afsari, B., Vidal, R.: Estimation of non-negative ODFs using the eigenvalue distribution of spherical functions. In: Ayache, N., Delingette, H., Golland, P., Mori, K. (eds.) MICCAI 2012, Part II. LNCS, vol. 7511, pp. 322–330. Springer, Heidelberg (2012)

20. Cheng, J., Jiang, T., Deriche, R.: Nonnegative definite EAP and ODF estimation via a unified multi-shell HARDI reconstruction. In: Ayache, N., Delingette, H., Golland, P., Mori, K. (eds.) MICCAI 2012, Part II. LNCS, vol. 7511, pp. 313–321. Springer, Heidelberg (2012)
21. Spivak, M.: A comprehensive introduction to differential geometry. Publish or Perish, Berkeley (1979)
22. Cetingul, H.E., Vidal, R.: Sparse Riemannian manifold clustering for HARDI segmentation. In: ISBI (2011)
23. Absil, P., Mahony, R., Sepulchre, R.: Optimization algorithms on matrix manifolds. Princeton University Press (2008)
24. Rao, C.R.: Information and accuracy attainable in the estimation of statitical parameters. Bull. Calcutta Math. Soc. (1945)
25. Srivastava, A., Jermyn, I., Joshi, S.: Riemannian analysis of probability density functions with applications in vision. In: CVPR (2007)

Diseased Region Detection
of Longitudinal Knee MRI Data

Chao Huang[1,3], Liang Shan[2], Cecil Charles[4], Marc Niethammer[2],
and Hongtu Zhu[3,*]

[1] Department of Mathematics, Southeast University, China
[2] Department of Computer Sciences and Biomedical Research Imaging Center,
University of North Carolina at Chapel Hill, USA
[3] Department of Biostatistics and Biomedical Research Imaging Center,
University of North Carolina at Chapel Hill, USA
[4] Department of Radiology, Duke University, USA
htzhu@email.unc.edu

Abstract. Statistical analysis of longitudinal cartilage changes in osteoarthritis (OA) is of great importance and still a challenge in knee MRI data analysis. A major challenge is to establish a reliable correspondence across subjects within the same latent subpopulations. We develop a novel Gaussian hidden Markov model (GHMM) to establish spatial correspondence of cartilage thinning across both time and subjects within the same latent subpopulations and make statistical inference on the detection of diseased regions in each OA patient. A hidden Markov random field (HMRF) is proposed to extract such latent subpopulation structure. The EM algorithm and pseudo-likelihood method are both considered in making statistical inference. The proposed model can effectively detect diseased regions and present a localized analysis of longitudinal cartilage thickness within each latent subpopulation. Simulation studies and diseased region detection on 2D thickness maps extracted from full 3D longitudinal knee MRI Data for Pfizer Longitudinal Dataset are performed, which show that our proposed model outperforms standard voxel-based analysis.

Keywords: Diseased regions detection, EM algorithm, Gaussian hidden Markov model, Longitudinal cartilage thickness, Pseudo-likelihood method.

1 Introduction

Osteoarthritis (OA) is the most common form of arthritis and a major cause of longterm disability in the US [18]. It is estimated that more than 16% of all adults 45 years or older suffer from symptomatic OA of the knee [5]. The OA symptoms include swelling, pain, discomfort and problems in mobility and are caused by the progressive loss of joint cartilage [5]. Fig. 1 shows the anatomy of the human knee and illustrates the cartilage loss.

---

* Corresponding author.

J.C. Gee et al. (Eds.): IPMI 2013, LNCS 7917, pp. 632–643, 2013.
© Springer-Verlag Berlin Heidelberg 2013

Cartilage loss [9] is believed to be the dominating factor in OA. Studying cartilage morphological changes will help understand OA progression and drug development. Magnetic resonance imaging (MRI) is a three-dimensional imaging technique able to directly measure cartilage volume and thickness and is thus sensitive to the detection of cartilage loss. Significant advances in MRI have resulted in the ability to quantify cartilage morphology [8]. Therefore, MRI is increasingly accepted as a primary method to evaluate progression of OA (see [6], [16]). Meanwhile, large image databases have been acquired for OA research. It would be of great value to fully analyze the MR images of the datasets such as the one form the osteoarthritis initiative to help understand the progression of OA.

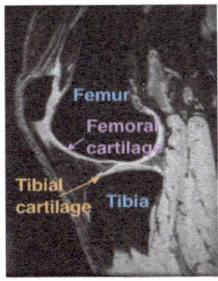 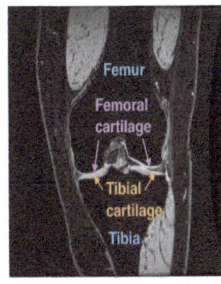 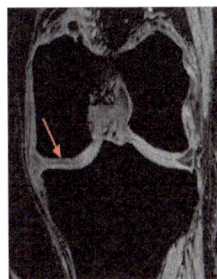

Fig. 1. Anatomy of human knee and illustration of cartilage loss. (*left*) A sagittal slice of a healthy knee. Bones are annotated in blue, femoral cartilage in purple and tibial cartilage in orange. (*middle*) A coronal slice of the same healthy knee. (*right*) A coronal slice of an OA knee with cartilage loss indicated by the red arrow.

Subregion-based analysis is one of the most popular approaches among existing statistical analysis methods (see [4], [17]). However, this approach can be problematic because changes within a specific subregion could happen only to a few subjects within a latent subpopulation whereas other subjects have strong progressions in different subregions and belong to different latent subpopulations. Local changes (that happen to a smaller region than the size of a subregion) are weakened by averaging over a particular subregion and are impossible to recover. So, statistical analysis of cartilage thickness changes is still a challenging problem. To fully understand the spatial pattern of OA progression, the analysis of localized cartilage thickness changes is necessary.

The aim of this paper is to develop a novel Gaussian hidden Markov model (GHMM) to establish spatial correspondence of cartilage thinning across time and subjects within the same subpopulation. A hidden Markov random field (HMRF) is developed to specifically discover the disease regions [2], [14]. The EM algorithm and pseudo-likelihood method are both considered in making statistical inference. The proposed model can can effectively detect diseased regions and presents a localized analysis of longitudinal cartilage thickness. Simulation studies and diseased regions detection of 2D thickness map extracted from full 3D

longitudinal knee MRI Data of the Pfizer Longitudinal Study (PLS-A9001140)
are performed, which shows that our proposed model outperforms the classical
linear mixed model.

The paper is organized as follows. Section 2 introduces GHMM and then the
related EM algorithm for the proposed model is derived. In Section 3, simulation
studies are performed to show the advantages of our proposed model in diseased
regions detection. Section 4 applies GHMM to the 2D thickness maps derived
from the 3D MRI data of the Pfizer Longitudinal Study (PLS-A9001140).

2   Background and Methods

2.1   Gaussian Hidden Markov Model

Suppose that we observe a longitudinal imaging data set with imaging data
$\{y_{ij}(s_k) : k = 1, \ldots, m\}$ measured at time t_j for $j = 1, \ldots, T_i$ and $i = 1, \ldots, n$,
where $S = \{s_1, \ldots, s_m\}$ is the set of pixels and T_i is the total number of time
points for the $i-$th subject. Let x_i represent disease status of osteo-arthritis
(OA) for each subject such that $x_i = 0$ and 1, respectively, represent normal
control and patient with OA. At each pixel s_k, we introduce an unobserved random effect $b_i(s_k)$ to label normal region R_{i0}, median diseased region R_{i1}, and
severely diseased region R_{i2} for each subject. For normal controls, both R_{i1} and
R_{i2} should be the empty set. Specifically, $b_i(s_k) \in L = \{0, 1, 2\}$ are label configurations of three nonoverlapping regions $\{R_{i0}, R_{i1}, R_{i2}\}$. Note that these three
unknown regions for each subject play a critical role in establishing spatial correspondences across subjects. Moreover, we introduce another unobserved random
effect $v_i(s_k)$ to characterize temporal correlations among repeated measures for
each subject.

Our Gaussian hidden Markov model consists of a a spatial random effect
model (SREM) and a Potts model. We first propose SREM to model the conditional distribution of the observed images given the random effects. Specifically,
given b_i and v_i, we propose a general spatial random effect model given by

$$y_{ij}(s_k) = \boldsymbol{w}_j^T \boldsymbol{\beta}(s_k) + c(x_i, \boldsymbol{w}_j, b_i(s_k), \bar{\boldsymbol{\beta}}) + \boldsymbol{w}_j^T \boldsymbol{v}_i(s_k) + \epsilon_{ij}(s_k), \qquad (1)$$

where $\boldsymbol{w}_j$ is a $q_w \times 1$ vector of covariates (e.g., time) and $\boldsymbol{\beta}(s_k)$ is a q_w dimensional
vector of regression coefficients representing the dynamic change of imaging in-
tensities at pixel s_k in normal controls. Moreover, $\bar{\boldsymbol{\beta}} = (\bar{\boldsymbol{\beta}}(1), \bar{\boldsymbol{\beta}}(2))^T$ is a $2q_w$
dimensional vector of coefficients to characterize the dynamic changes of imaging
intensities in the diseased region $R_{i1} \cup R_{i2}$. The function $c(x_i, \boldsymbol{w}_j, b_i(s_k), \bar{\boldsymbol{\beta}})$ is
defined as

$$c(x_i, \boldsymbol{w}_j, b_i(s_k), \bar{\boldsymbol{\beta}}) = \begin{cases} 0, & x_i = 0, \\ \displaystyle\sum_{l=1}^{2} \boldsymbol{w}_j^T \bar{\boldsymbol{\beta}}(l) \delta(b_i(s_k), l) & , x_i \neq 0. \end{cases} \qquad (2)$$

where $\delta(\cdot,\cdot)$ is the Kronecker function. Thus, $c(x_i, \boldsymbol{w}_j, b_i(s_k), \bar{\boldsymbol{\beta}})$ equals zero for all pixels for normal controls and the pixels with $b_i(s_k) = 0$ for OA patients. For OA patients, pixels in different diseased regions may have different dynamic changes of imaging intensities. Throughout the paper, we assume $\boldsymbol{w}_j = (1, t_j, t_j^2)^T$ and set $q_w = 3$. Moreover, $\epsilon_{ij}(s_k)$ are independent measurement errors across subjects, time, and pixels, while they follow $N(0, \sigma_{s_k}^2)$.

We model the random effects $\boldsymbol{b}_i$ and $\boldsymbol{v}_i$ as follows. First, it is assumed that $\boldsymbol{b}_i = (b_i(s_1), \ldots, b_i(s_m))^T$ and $\boldsymbol{v}_i = \{v_i(s_k) : k = 1, \ldots, m\}$ are mutually independent. Moreover, $\boldsymbol{v}_i(s_k)$ are mutually independent across pixels and $\boldsymbol{v}_i(s_k)$ follows $N(\boldsymbol{0}, \boldsymbol{\Sigma}_{v_{s_k}})$ at pixel s_k. It is assumed that $\boldsymbol{b}_i$ are independent across subjects and $\boldsymbol{b}_i$ follows a Potts model ([2], [14]), whose Gibbs form is given by

$$p(\boldsymbol{b}_i|\tau) = \exp\{-U(\boldsymbol{b}_i)\tau - \log C(\tau)\}, \tag{3}$$

where $U(\boldsymbol{b}_i) = -\sum_{s_k \sim s_l} \delta(b(s_k), b(s_l))$ and parameter τ, which introduces spatial consistency. $C(\tau)$ is the partition function such that $p(\boldsymbol{b}_i|\tau)$ is a probability function. The notation "$\sum_{s_i \sim s_j}$" means that s_i is a neighbor of s_j and each neighboring pair enters the summation only once. Throughout the paper, we only consider the closest neighbors for each pixel.

2.2 Estimation Procedure

Our primary problem of interest is to make inference on all unknown parameters, denoted as $\boldsymbol{\theta}$, and random effects. We decompose the parameter $\boldsymbol{\theta}$ into two parts: τ, introduced in (3), and all others, denoted as $\bar{\boldsymbol{\theta}}$. This is a standard incomplete-data problem. Since the Maximum likelihood estimation (MLE) of τ is generally difficult to compute due to the normalizing part of the probability function in (3), the MLE of $\bar{\boldsymbol{\theta}}$ can be calculated by using the EM algorithm [7], whereas τ can be estimated by using a pseudo-likelihood method [1], which is easy to compute.

Let $\boldsymbol{W}_i = (\boldsymbol{w}_1, \ldots, \boldsymbol{w}_{T_i})$, $\bar{c}(x_i, \boldsymbol{W}_i, b_i(s_k), \bar{\boldsymbol{\beta}}) = (c(x_i, \boldsymbol{w}_1, b_i(s_k), \bar{\boldsymbol{\beta}}), \ldots,$ $c(x_i, \boldsymbol{w}_{T_i}, b_i(s_k), \bar{\boldsymbol{\beta}}))^T$, and $\boldsymbol{\Sigma}_{s_k,i} = \{\kappa_{p,q}\}_{1 \leq p,q \leq T_i}$, where $\kappa_{p,q} = \sigma_{s_k}^2 \mathbf{1}(p=q)$, in which $\mathbf{1}(\cdot)$ is an indicator function. Thus, the distribution of $\boldsymbol{y}_i(s_k)$ conditional on random effects is given by $N(\boldsymbol{z}_i(s_k), \boldsymbol{\Sigma}_{s_k,i})$, where

$$\boldsymbol{z}_i(s_k) = \boldsymbol{y}_i(s_k) - \boldsymbol{W}_i^T \boldsymbol{\beta}(s_k) - \bar{c}(x_i, \boldsymbol{W}_i, b_i(s_k), \bar{\boldsymbol{\beta}}) - \boldsymbol{W}_i^T \boldsymbol{v}_i(s_k),$$

Thus, the complete-data log-likelihood function is given by

$$\log \tilde{L}(\boldsymbol{\theta}) \propto -\frac{1}{2}\sum_{i=1}^{n}\sum_{k=1}^{m}\log|\boldsymbol{\Sigma}_{s_k,i}| - \frac{1}{2}\sum_{i=1}^{n}\sum_{k=1}^{m}\boldsymbol{z}_i(s_k)^T\boldsymbol{\Sigma}_{s_k,i}^{-1}\boldsymbol{z}_i(s_k) - \sum_{i=1}^{n_0}U(\boldsymbol{b}_i)\tau$$

$$-n_0\log C(\tau) - \frac{n}{2}\sum_{k=1}^{m}\log|\boldsymbol{\Sigma}_{v_{s_k}}| - \frac{1}{2}\sum_{i=1}^{n}\sum_{k=1}^{m}\boldsymbol{v}_i^T(s_k)\boldsymbol{\Sigma}_{v_{s_k}}^{-1}\boldsymbol{v}_i(s_k), \tag{4}$$

where $n_0 = \#\{x_i : x_i \neq 0\}$ denotes the number of OA patients. Given the current estimate $\widetilde{\boldsymbol{\theta}}^{(r)}$ at iteration r, the value $\widetilde{\boldsymbol{\theta}}^{(r+1)}$ is obtained via maximizing the Q-function $E_{\widetilde{\boldsymbol{\theta}}^{(r)}}(\log \tilde{L}(\boldsymbol{\theta})|\boldsymbol{y}, \boldsymbol{x})$ with respect to $\bar{\boldsymbol{\theta}}$.

We consider the E-step and M-step of EM algorithm as follows.

E-step: In E-step, we need to calculate four conditional expectations

$$E\left[\boldsymbol{v}_i(s_k)\delta(b_i(s_k),l)\big|\boldsymbol{y}_i(s_k),\boldsymbol{x},\widetilde{\boldsymbol{\theta}}^{(r)}\right], E\left[\boldsymbol{v}_i(s_k)\boldsymbol{v}_i^T(s_k)\big|\boldsymbol{y}_i(s_k),\boldsymbol{x},\widetilde{\boldsymbol{\theta}}^{(r)}\right],$$

$$E\left[\boldsymbol{v}_i(s_k)\big|\boldsymbol{y}_i(s_k),\boldsymbol{x},\widetilde{\boldsymbol{\theta}}^{(r)}\right], E\left[\delta(b_i(s_k),l)\big|\boldsymbol{y}_i(s_k),\boldsymbol{x},\widetilde{\boldsymbol{\theta}}^{(r)}\right].$$

In order to calculate these conditional probability, the class labels $\boldsymbol{b}$ should be estimated first. The MRF-MAP estimation is adopted here. First, the conditional probability density function of $\boldsymbol{y}_i(s_k)$ given x_i and $\boldsymbol{b}_i(s_k)$ is derived as

$$f(\boldsymbol{y}_i(s_k)|x_i,b_i(s_k),\widetilde{\boldsymbol{\theta}}^{(r)}) \sim \mathcal{N}(\boldsymbol{\varpi}_i(s_k),\boldsymbol{W}_i^T\widetilde{\boldsymbol{\Sigma}}_{v_{s_k}}^{(r)}\boldsymbol{W}_i + \widetilde{\boldsymbol{\Sigma}}_{s_k,i}^{(r)}). \tag{5}$$

where $\boldsymbol{\varpi}_i(s_k) = \boldsymbol{W}_i^T\widetilde{\boldsymbol{\beta}}^{(r)}(s_k) + \bar{c}(x_i,\boldsymbol{W}_i,b_i(s_k),\widetilde{\boldsymbol{\beta}}^{(r)})$.

According to the MAP criterion, the estimate $\widetilde{\boldsymbol{b}}_i^{(r)}$ is defined as

$$\widetilde{\boldsymbol{b}}_i^{(r)} = \arg\max_{\boldsymbol{b}_i}\left\{\prod_{k=1}^{m} f(\boldsymbol{y}_i(s_k)|x_i,b_i(s_k),\widetilde{\boldsymbol{\theta}}^{(r)})p(\boldsymbol{b}_i|\widetilde{\tau}^{(r)})\right\}. \tag{6}$$

To obtain the optimal solution to (6), in this paper, we adopt the iterated conditional modes (ICM) algorithm proposed by [2]. As a result, the conditional expectation $E\left[\delta(b_i(s_k),l)\big|\boldsymbol{y}_i(s_k),\boldsymbol{x},\widetilde{\boldsymbol{\theta}}^{(r)}\right]$ can be calculated. Then, the desired expectations can be estimated respectively.

M-step: We find the updates of $\overline{\boldsymbol{\theta}}$ as follows. For $\boldsymbol{\beta}(s_k)$ and $\overline{\boldsymbol{\beta}}(l)$, we have

$$\widetilde{\boldsymbol{\beta}}^{(r+1)}(s_k) = [\sum_{i=1}^{n}\boldsymbol{W}_i\widetilde{\boldsymbol{\Sigma}}_{s_k,i}^{(r)-1}\boldsymbol{W}_i^T]^{-1}\sum_{i=1}^{n}\boldsymbol{W}_i\widetilde{\boldsymbol{\Sigma}}_{s_k,i}^{(r)-1}\left(\boldsymbol{y}_i(s_k) - \boldsymbol{W}_i^T E\left[\boldsymbol{v}_i(s_k)\big|\boldsymbol{y}_i(s_k),\right.\right.$$
$$\left.\left.\boldsymbol{x},\widetilde{\boldsymbol{\theta}}^{(r)}\right] - \delta(x_i,0)\boldsymbol{W}_i^T\sum_{l=1}^{M}\overline{\boldsymbol{\beta}}(l)E\left[\delta(b_i(s_k),l)\big|\boldsymbol{y}_i(s_k),\boldsymbol{x},\widetilde{\boldsymbol{\theta}}^{(r)}\right]\right), \tag{7}$$

$$\widetilde{\overline{\boldsymbol{\beta}}}^{(r+1)}(l) = \left[\sum_{i=1}^{n_0}\sum_{k=1}^{m}\boldsymbol{W}_i\widetilde{\boldsymbol{\Sigma}}_{s_k,i}^{(r)-1}\boldsymbol{W}_i^T E\left[\delta(b_i(s_k),l)\big|\boldsymbol{y}_i(s_k),\boldsymbol{x},\widetilde{\boldsymbol{\theta}}^{(r)}\right]\right]^{-1}\sum_{i=1}^{n_0}\sum_{k=1}^{m}\boldsymbol{W}_i\widetilde{\boldsymbol{\Sigma}}_{s_k,i}^{(r)-1}$$
$$\left\{\boldsymbol{y}_i(s_k) - \boldsymbol{W}_i^T\widetilde{\boldsymbol{\beta}}^{(r)}(s_k) - \boldsymbol{W}_i^T E\left[\boldsymbol{v}_i(s_k)\delta(b_i(s_k),l)\big|\boldsymbol{y}_i(s_k),\boldsymbol{x},\widetilde{\boldsymbol{\theta}}^{(r)}\right]\right\}. \tag{8}$$

For the covariance matrix $\boldsymbol{\Sigma}_{v_{s_k}}$, we have

$$\widetilde{\boldsymbol{\Sigma}}_{v_{s_k}}^{(r+1)} = \frac{1}{n}\sum_{i=1}^{n} E\left[\boldsymbol{v}_i(s_k)\boldsymbol{v}_i^T(s_k)\big|\boldsymbol{y}_i(s_k),\boldsymbol{x},\widetilde{\boldsymbol{\theta}}^{(r)}\right], \tag{9}$$

For $\sigma_{s_k}^2$ and ρ_{s_k}, we have

$$\widetilde{\sigma}_{s_k}^{2(r+1)} = \frac{1}{\sum_{i=1}^{n} T_i} \sum_{i=1}^{n} E\left[[\widetilde{L}_i^{(r)} z_i^{(r)}(s_k)]^T \widetilde{L}_i^{(r)} z_i^{(r)}(s_k) \Big| y_i(s_k), x, \widetilde{\theta}^{(r)}\right], \quad (10)$$

$$\widetilde{\rho}_{s_k}^{(r+1)} = \left[\sum_{i=1}^{n} E\left[[z_i^{(r)}(s_k)]^T K_i z_i^{(r)}(s_k) \Big| y_i(s_k), x, \widetilde{\theta}^{(r)}\right]\right]^{-1}$$

$$\sum_{i=1}^{n} E\left[[z_i^{(r)}(s_k)]^T R_i z_i^{(r)}(s_k) \Big| y_i(s_k), x, \widetilde{\theta}^{(r)}\right], \quad (11)$$

where $z_i^{(r)}(s_k) = y_i(s_k) - W_i^T \widetilde{\beta}^{(r)}(s_k) - \bar{c}(x_i, W_i, b_i(s_k), \widetilde{\widetilde{\beta}}^{(r)}) - W_i^T v_i(s_k)$, and $\widetilde{L}_i^{(r)}$, K_i and R_i are given by

$$\widetilde{L}_i^{(r)} = \begin{bmatrix} 1 & 0 & \cdots & 0 \\ -\widetilde{\rho}_{s_k}^{(r)} & 1 & \cdots & 0 \\ \vdots & \ddots & \ddots & \vdots \\ 0 & \cdots & -\widetilde{\rho}_{s_k}^{(r)} & 1 \end{bmatrix}_{T_i}, K_i = \begin{bmatrix} 1 & 0 & \cdots & 0 \\ 0 & \ddots & \cdots & 0 \\ \vdots & \ddots & 1 & \vdots \\ 0 & \cdots & 0 & 0 \end{bmatrix}_{T_i}, R_i = \begin{bmatrix} 0 & 0 & \cdots & 0 \\ 1 & \ddots & \cdots & 0 \\ \vdots & \ddots & \ddots & \vdots \\ 0 & \cdots & 1 & 0 \end{bmatrix}_{T_i}.$$

The parameter τ in MRF model (3) is estimated based on a pseudo-likelihood method. The pseudo-likelihood at the rth step is a simple product of the conditional likelihood

$$PL(\widetilde{b}^{(r)}) = \prod_{i=1}^{n_0} \prod_{s_k \in \mathcal{S} - \partial\mathcal{S}} PL(\widetilde{b}_i^{(r)}(s_k)|\widetilde{b}_i^{(r)}), \quad (12)$$

where $\partial\mathcal{S}$ denotes the set of points at the boundaries of $\mathcal{S}$. The pseudo-likelihood does not involve the partition function. Although the pseudo-likelihood is not the true likelihood function, the maximum pseudo-likelihood (MPL) estimate converges to the truth with probability one [10]. The logarithm pseudo-likelihood is given by

$$\ln PL(\widetilde{b}^{(r)}, \tau) = \sum_{i=1}^{n_0} \sum_{s_k \in \mathcal{S} - \partial\mathcal{S}} \ln\left[PL(\widetilde{b}_i^{(r)}(s_k)|\widetilde{b}_i^{(r)})\right], \quad (13)$$

Thus, the MPL estimate $\widetilde{\tau}^{(r+1)}$ can be obtained by solving

$$\frac{\partial \ln PL(\widetilde{b}^{(r)}, \tau)}{\partial \tau} = 0. \quad (14)$$

The E-step and M-step are alternately repeated until the difference between $\log L(\widetilde{\theta}^{(r+1)})$ and $\log L(\widetilde{\theta}^{(r)})$ is smaller than a desired small value (e.g., 0.0001).

3   Simulation Studies

We examine the finite sample performance of GHMM for diseased region detection. We chose the femoral cartilage thickness data of all the normal controls derived from the 3D MRI data of the Pfizer Longitudinal Study (PLS-A9001140) and fitted the model (1) to all MRI data obtained from normal controls. We set the obtained parameter estimators as the true values of parameters $\beta(s_k), \Sigma_{v_{s_k}}, \sigma^2_{s_k}$ and ρ_{s_k}. The related parameter $\overline{\beta}(l)$ are generated from $U(-0.1, 0.1)$ and $U(-0.5, 0.5)$ for $l = 1, 2$, respectively. The parameter τ was set as 0.5. The covariate W_i for each subject was generated according to the real dataset in Section 4. We generated 20 subjects from 3 groups with 7 subjects in group 1, 7 subjects in group 2, and 6 subjects in group 3. The location of the diseased region is predetermined and does not vary for subjects in the same group, whereas it varies across groups. These three kinds of the diseased regions are shown in Fig. 2.

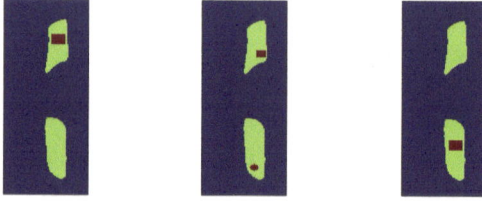

Fig. 2. Three kinds of the diseased regions: diseased region (*red*); normal region (*green*)

We applied GHMM to detect the diseased region in each subject. We randomly selected one subject from each group and presented its detection results in Fig. 3. For all selected subjects, the diseased regions can be successfully detected with few misclassifications in the results. To show the average detection performance among subjects in each group, the Dice metric [13], Rand index [15], adjusted Rand index, and Mirkin metric [11] were calculated to compare the detection results with the truth and the average of each index values were also calculated. For the first three indexes, a higher index value indicates a more accurate detection result, while it is the opposite case for the last index. Simulation results based on all the three groups are presented in Table 1. For all these groups, the average of the first three index values are larger than 88 percent, and the last index values are all less than 0.1. Fig. 3 and Table 1 indicate that GHMM performs very well in diseased region detection of cartilage MRI data.

4   Real Data Analysis

We consider the dataset of the Pfizer longitudinal study on osteoarthritis (PLS-A9001140). This dataset contains T1-weighted (3D SPGR) images for

Table 1. Average detection performance among subjects in different groups

	Dice metric	Rand index	Adjusted Rand index	Mirkin metric
Group 1	0.9818	0.9643	0.9008	0.0357
Group 2	0.9797	0.9602	0.8874	0.0398
Group 3	0.9688	0.9395	0.8802	0.0605

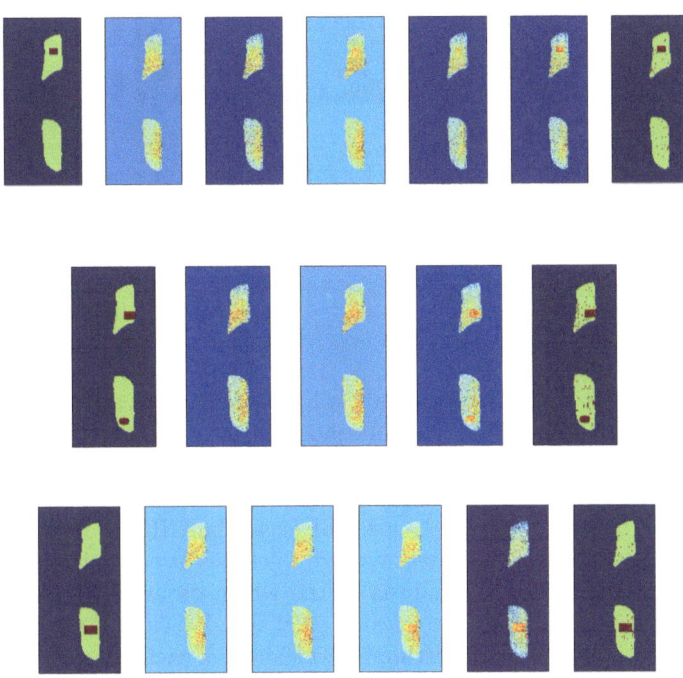

Fig. 3. Diseased region detection for subjects from three groups: subject with 5 time points in group 1 (*top*); subject with 3 time points in group 2 (*middle*); subject with 4 time point in group 3 (*bottom*). This is the simulated result and hence we have an imposed ground truth. In each group, the first image presents the true diseased region while the last image indicate the detection result, the remaining ones are the observations for the time points.

155 subjects, imaged at baseline, 3, 6, 12, and 24 months at a resolution of $1.00 \times 0.31 \times 0.31 mm^3$. Some subjects have missing scans and thus we have 706 MRIs in total. The Kellgren-Lawrence grades (KLG) [12] were determined for all subjects from the baseline scan, classifying 81 as normal control subjects (KLG0), 1 as KLG1 (mild OA), 40 as KLG2 (severe OA) and 33 as KLG3 (severe OA).

We applied a voxel-based analysis based on linear mixed models and GHMM to the OA data set. Moreover, the expert cartilage segmentations are available for all images in the native image space. The femoral cartilage segmentation was

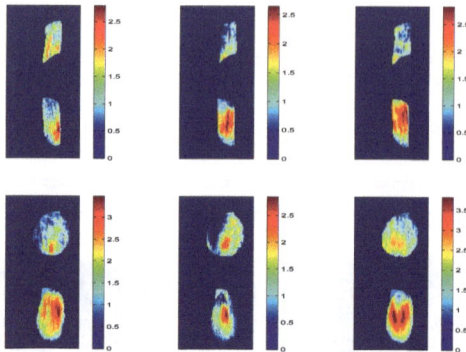

Fig. 4. Local cartilage thickness (mm) for subjects with expert segmentations at baseline with different KLG: (*left*) femoral cartilage thickness map(*top*) and tibial cartilage thickness map(*bottom*) for subject with KLG0; (*middle*) femoral cartilage thickness map(*top*) and tibial cartilage thickness map(*bottom*) for subject with KLG1; (*left*) femoral cartilage thickness map(*top*) and tibial cartilage thickness map(*bottom*) for subject with KLG3.

drawn only on the weight-bearing part, whereas the tibial cartilage segmentation covers the entire region. We randomly chose several subjects with different KLG from the dataset, and present the related cartilage segmentations for the chosen subjects at baseline in Fig. 4.

Firstly, we applied the voxel-based analysis to the MRI data from normal controls and calculated the estimated average thickness at each pixel site. Secondly, we applied the voxel-based analysis to the whole dataset and then calculated the estimated average thickness at each pixel site. We carried out a t test across pixels to identify whether the estimated thickness of each diseased patient is significantly different from the estimated average thickness obtained from normal controls. If the hypothesis is rejected at a pixel at a significance level 1%, then this pixel site is treated as the one from the disease region. Otherwise, it belongs to the normal region. Fig. 4 presents several randomly chosen subjects with KLG1 and KLG3, whereas Fig. 5 presents the related p-value at each pixel site. As a comparison, we applied GHMM to the whole dataset. The detection results of the two selected subjects are also plotted in Fig. 6, where the red area indicates the diseased region while the green one indicates the normal region. The probability that a pixel site comes from the diseased region can also be estimated. The empirical probability distribution of the diseased region based on GHMM and the voxel-based analysis are both presented in Fig. 7. From Fig. 5-Fig. 7, it follows that the p-value at most pixel sites is not significant and thus the voxel-based analysis fails to realize the diseased region detection. In contrast, for GHMM, the detected diseased regions probably locate in the center of the cartilage, which means that the cartilage loss in OA may not be uniform throughout the cartilage, but OA may affect certain regions (e.g. the center) more frequently than other regions [3]. Therefore, GHMM outperforms

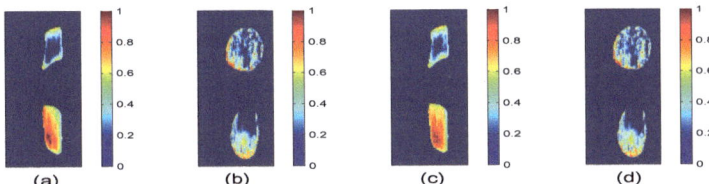

Fig. 5. P-value at each pixel site for subjects randomly chosen with different KLG: (*a*) p-value in femoral cartilage of subject with KLG1; (*b*) p-value in tibial cartilage of subject with KLG1; (*c*) p-value in femoral cartilage of subject with KLG3; (*d*) p-value in tibial cartilage of subject with KLG3.

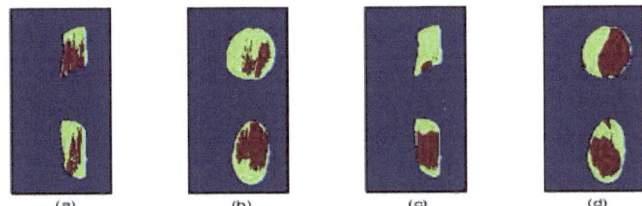

Fig. 6. Diseased region detection for subjects randomly chosen with different KLG: (*a*) diseased region (red) in femoral cartilage of subject with KLG1; (*b*) diseased region (red) in tibial cartilage of subject with KLG1; (*c*) diseased region (red) in femoral cartilage of subject with KLG3; (*d*) diseased region (red) in tibial cartilage of subject with KLG3.

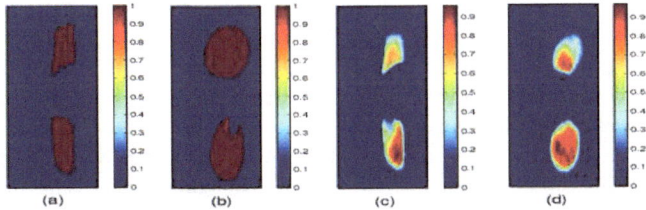

Fig. 7. Empirical probability distribution of the diseased region: (*a*) empirical probability distribution of the diseased region in femoral cartilage based on the voxel-based analysis; (*b*) empirical probability distribution of the diseased region in tibial cartilage based on voxel-based analysis; (*c*) empirical probability distribution of the diseased region in femoral cartilage based on GHMM; (*d*) empirical probability distribution of the diseased region in tibial cartilage based on GHMM.

the voxel-based analysis in localized analysis of longitudinal cartilage thickness and diseased region detection.

5   Concluding Remarks

We have developed a novel GHMM to establish spatial correspondence of cartilage thinning across time and subjects within the same latent subpopulation. A hidden Markov random field (HMRF) has been proposed to extract such latent subpopulation structure. Simulation studies and real data analysis demonstrate that GHMM can effectively realize diseased regions detection in localizing longitudinal cartilage thickness. However, one would like to estimate the continuous level of disease, i.e., from completely healthy to fully diseased. Thus, more research on this issue will be valuable and we believe this is an interesting direction for further exploration.

Acknowledgments. This work was supported in part by NIH grants R025747-01, CA142538-01, MH086633, B005149-01, R01 MH091645-01A1, R21 AR059890, and the Pfizer longitudinal study on osteoarthritis (PLS-A9001140).

References

1. Besag, J.E.: Statistical Analysis of Non-Lattice Data. Journal of Royal Statistical Society, Series D 24, 179–195 (1975)
2. Besag, J.E.: On the statistical analysis of dirty pictures (with discussion). Journal of Royal Statistical Society, Series B 48, 259–302 (1986)
3. Biswal, S., Hastie, T., Andriacchi, T.P., Bergman, G.A., Dillingham, M.F., Lang, P.: Risk factors and progressive cartilage loss in the knee: A longitudinal magnetic resonance imaging study in forty-three patients. Arthritis & Rheumatism 46, 2884–2892 (2002)
4. Buck, R.J., Wyman, B.T., Graverrand, M.P.L., Hudelmaier, M., Wirth, W., Eckstein, F.: Does the use of ordered values of subregional change in cartilage thickness improve the detection of disease progression in longitudinal studies of osteoarthritis? Arthritis and Rheumatism 61(7), 917–924 (2009)
5. Arthritis related statistics, Center of Disease Control, CDC (2008), http://www.cdc.gov/arthritis/data_statistics/arthritis_related_statistics.htm
6. Cicuttini, F., Hankin, J., Jones, G., Wluka, A.: Comparison of conventional standing knee radiographs and magnetic resonance imaging in assessing progression of tibiofemoral joint osteoarthritis. Oesteoarthritis Cartilage 13, 722–727 (2005)
7. Dempster, A.P., Laird, N.M., Rubin, D.B.: Maximum likelihood from incomplete data via the EM algorithm (with discussion). J. R. Stat. Soc. Series B 39(1), 1–38 (1977)
8. Eckstein, F., Cicuttini, F., Raynauld, J.P., Waterton, J.C., Peterfy, C.: Magnetic resonance imaging (MRI) of articular cartilage in knee osteoarthritis (OA): morphological assessment. Osteoarthritis and Cartilage 14, A46–A75 (2006)
9. Felson, D.T., Lawrence, R.C., Dieppe, P.A., Hirsch, R., Helmick, C.G., Jordan, J.M., Kington, R.S., Lane, N.E., Nevitt, M.C., Zhang, Y., Sowers, M., McAlindon, T., Spector, T.D., Poole, A.R., Yanovski, S.Z., Ateshian, G., Sharma, L., Buckwalter, J.A., Brandt, K.D., Fries, J.F.: Osteoarthritis: new insights, part 1: the disease and risk factors. Annals of Internal Medicine 133(8), 635–646 (2000)

10. Geman, S., Graffigne, C.: Markov random field image models and their applications to computer vision. In: Proceedings of the International Congress of Mathematicians: Berkeley, pp. 1496–1517 (1987)
11. Hubert, L., Arabie, P.: Comparing partitions. J. Classif. 2, 193–218 (1985)
12. Kellgren, J., Lawrence, J.: Radiological assessment of osteoarthritis. Annals of Rheumatic Diseases 16(4), 494–502 (1957)
13. Lynch, M., Ghita, O., Whelan, P.F.: Segmentation of the left ventricle of the heart in 3-D+t MRI data using an optimized nonrigid temporal model. IEEE Trans. Med. Imaging 27(2), 195–203 (2008)
14. Qian, W., Titterington, D.M.: Estimation of parameters in hidden Markov models. Philosophical Transactions of the Royal Society of London, Series A 337, 407–428 (1991)
15. Rand, W.M.: Objective criteria for the evaluation of clustering methods. J. Am. Stat. Assoc. 66, 846–850 (1971)
16. Raynauld, J.P.: Quantitative magnetic resonance imaging of articular cartilage in knee osteoarthritis. Current Opinions in Rheumatology 15(5), 647–650 (2003)
17. Wirth, W., Eckstein, F.: A technique for regional analysis of femorotibial cartilage thickness based on quantitative magenetic resonance imaging. IEEE Transactions on Medical Imaging 27(6), 737–744 (2008)
18. Woolf, A.D., Pfleger, B.: Burden of major musculoskeletal conditions. Bulletin of the World Health Organization 81, 646–656 (2003)
19. Zhang, Y., Brady, M., Smith, S.: Segmentation of brain MR images through a hidden Markov random field model and the expectation-maximization algorithm. IEEE Transactions on Medical Imaging 15, 45–57 (2001)

Model Selection and Estimation
of Multi-compartment Models
in Diffusion MRI with a Rician Noise Model

Xinghua Zhu[1], Yaniv Gur[2], Wenping Wang[1], and P. Thomas Fletcher[2]

[1] The University of Hong Kong, Department of Computer Science, Hong Kong
[2] University of Utah, School of Computing, Salt Lake City, UT 84112, USA

Abstract. Multi-compartment models in diffusion MRI (dMRI) are used to describe complex white matter fiber architecture of the brain. In this paper, we propose a novel multi-compartment estimation method based on the ball-and-stick model, which is composed of an isotropic diffusion compartment ("ball") as well as one or more perfectly linear diffusion compartments ("sticks"). To model the noise distribution intrinsic to dMRI measurements, we introduce a Rician likelihood term and estimate the model parameters by means of an Expectation Maximization (EM) algorithm. This paper also addresses the problem of selecting the number of fiber compartments that best fit the data, by introducing a sparsity prior on the volume mixing fractions. This term provides automatic model selection and enables us to discriminate different fiber populations. When applied to simulated data, our method provides accurate estimates of the fiber orientations, diffusivities, and number of compartments, even at low SNR, and outperforms similar methods that rely on a Gaussian noise distribution assumption. We also apply our method to *in vivo* brain data and show that it can successfully capture complex fiber structures that match the known anatomy.

1 Introduction

Diffusion Tensor Imaging (DTI) is a powerful technique that enables inferring white matter pathways of the brain from diffusion weighted (DW) MRI measurements. However, DTI can only describe one dominant diffusion direction per voxel, and therefore, cannot capture known complex fiber structures in the white matter in human brain. The limitation of DTI motivated the development of new imaging modalities that utilize higher angular resolution, as well as new methods to extract white matter structures from such data, including spherical deconvolution [1], Funk-Radon transform [2], multi-compartment models [3, 4], and higher-order tensors [5–7]. In this work, we consider a particular case of multi-compartment models, where the diffusivities in directions perpendicular to the white matter fiber are constrained to be zero. This model is known as the "ball-and-stick", where the "ball" stands for the isotropic diffusion compartment, and each "stick" corresponds to a perfectly linear diffusion compartment (white matter fiber).

J.C. Gee et al. (Eds.): IPMI 2013, LNCS 7917, pp. 644–655, 2013.

The ball-and-stick model was first proposed by Behrens et al. [8] as a constrained version of the multi-tensor model, which comprised only one ball and one stick compartment. A Bayesian framework for the ball-and-one-stick model estimation and tractography was also introduced in [8]. This framework was later elaborated in [9, 4], where multiple anisotropic compartments and model selection methods were proposed. In [9] Hosey et al. focused on the estimation of two-fiber models in a probabilistic manner under Rician noise assumption. They addressed the model selection problem by analyzing the probability density function (PDF) of the Bayes Factor of the one- and two- stick models. On the other hand, the method proposed in [4] did not limit the number of fiber compartments, and the estimation was done under Gaussian noise assumption. They adopted the automatic relevance determination (ARD) algorithm for model selection. However, the model selection methods in [9, 4] did not distinguish two-fiber models from more complicated ones, and no comprehensive evaluation of these methods was reported. More recently, Schultz et al. [11] proposed a spherical deconvolution operation to estimate the fiber orientations and volume fractions, which were refined by fitting a ball-and-stick model to the DW measurements. The number of fibers was selected at the spherical deconvolution level by directly thresholding the associated volume fractions. Similar to [4], this scheme did not account for the Rician noise in the DW measurements. Estimation of the more general two-tensor model, under Rician noise assumption, was presented in [10].

In this paper, the parameters of the ball-and-stick model are estimated by maximizing the log-likelihood function based on the Rician distribution. The maximization problem is solved using an EM algorithm, where the DW measurements with complex Gaussian noise represent the complete data. In addition, in order to find the number of compartments that best fit the data, we use a sparsity prior on the estimated volume fractions. The sparsity prior pushes to zero small volume fractions, and enables elimination of redundant terms that do not represent white matter fibers. In contrast to [9, 10], here we do not restrict our model to two stick compartments, and enable modeling of white matter structures in brain regions that contain up to three fiber populations. The results of the proposed model selection scheme provides a clear distinction between isotropic diffusion, and one, two, or three fiber populations.

The main contributions of this paper can be summarized as follows: 1) We solve the ball-and-stick estimation problem with multiple sticks, under the assumption of Rician noise distribution in the DW measurements. We use a Rician log-likelihood function which is maximized by a robust EM algorithm. 2) We assess the accuracy of our algorithm on simulated data at different b-values and low SNRs, and show that it introduces less bias in the model parameters compared to similar algorithms that rely on a Gaussian noise assumption. 3) We introduce an automatic model selection scheme, which is an integral part of our EM algorithm. This is done by introducing a sparsity prior on the volume fractions. 4) We evaluate the performance of the algorithm on in vivo brain data with deterministic tractography and show its ability to reproduce complex fiber structures matching the known anatomy.

2   Rician Likelihood and Expectation Maximization

In this paper, a parametric partial volume model is used to describe the local diffusion profile. The model we use is known as the "ball-and-sticks", which is composed of a mixture of an isotropic diffusion compartment ("ball"), and multiple directional anisotropic diffusion compartments ("sticks"). The "sticks" correspond to white matter fibers, and are represented by means of the unnormalized *Watson* distribution. That is, given a set of N diffusion weighted measurements, $\{\nu_i\}_{i=1}^N$, for each measurement in a gradient direction $\mathbf{g}_i$, we have

$$\nu_i = S_0 \left\{ w_0 \exp(-b\kappa_0) + \sum_{j=1}^{M} w_j \exp(-b\kappa_j (\mathbf{g}_i^T \mathbf{u_j})^2) \right\}, \quad (1)$$

where M is the number of anisotropic compartments, S_0 is the non-diffusion-weighted signal, and b represents the constant b-value. The model parameters are the white matter fiber orientations, $\mathbf{u}_1, \ldots, \mathbf{u}_M$, diffusion coefficients, $\kappa_0, \ldots, \kappa_M$, and volume fractions, $w_0, \ldots, w_M$, where $\sum_{j=0}^{M} w_j = 1, w_j \geq 0$.

In the rest of this paper, we will denote the set of model parameters by $\Theta = \{\mathbf{u}_1, \ldots, \mathbf{u}_M; w_0, \ldots, w_M; \kappa_0, \ldots, \kappa_M\}$. Also, we will use the notation $\nu_{i0}(\Theta) = S_0 \cdot w_0 \exp(-b\kappa_0)$ to represent the "ball" compartment in the i-th sampled direction, and $\nu_{ij}(\Theta) = S_0 \cdot w_j \exp(-b\kappa_j (\mathbf{g}_i^T \mathbf{u}_j)^2)$ for the j-th "stick" compartment in the i-th sampled direction. Using these notations, the expression for a "clean" signal in measurement direction $\mathbf{g}_i$ is given by the sum of the compartment signals, $\nu_i(\Theta) = \sum_{j=0}^{M} \nu_{ij}(\Theta)$.

2.1   Maximum Rician Likelihood

The MR signal in the complex domain is affected by Gaussian noise. However, the DW measurements are given as the magnitude of the complex MR signal, and, therefore, the noise distribution model becomes Rician. Thus, for a measured DW signal in the i-th gradient direction, S_i, we have $S_i \sim \mathrm{Ric}(\nu_i(\Theta), \sigma)$, given by the PDF

$$p(S_i|\Theta) = \frac{S_i}{\sigma^2} \exp\left(-\frac{S_i^2 + \nu_i(\Theta)^2}{2\sigma^2}\right) I_0\left(\frac{S_i \nu_i(\Theta)}{\sigma^2}\right). \quad (2)$$

We will use the notation $\mathbf{S}$ for the set of observed DW signals, i.e., $\mathbf{S} = \{S_i, i = 1, \ldots, N\}$. Assuming independent measurements in different gradient directions, the joint PDF for the signal $\mathbf{S}$ in each image voxel is given by $p(\mathbf{S}|\Theta) = \prod_{i=1}^{N} p(S_i|\Theta)$. We estimate the parameters Θ by maximization of the likelihood $l(\Theta|\mathbf{S}) = \log p(\mathbf{S}|\Theta)$, which is given by

$$l(\Theta|\mathbf{S}) = -2N \log(\sigma) + \sum_{i=1}^{N} \log(S_i) - \frac{S_i^2 + \nu_i(\Theta)^2}{2\sigma^2} + \log I_0\left(\frac{S_i \nu_i(\Theta)}{\sigma^2}\right). \quad (3)$$

2.2 Expectation Maximization Algorithm

One may apply a gradient ascent method to maximize the log-likelihood function. However, when directly maximizing $l(\Theta|\mathbf{S})$, the optimization parameters are variables of the modified Bessel function I_0. On the other hand, the proposed EM algorithm does not involve the computation of I_0 and its derivatives with respect to the optimization parameters. Therefore, maximizing the Q-function in the E-step is more stable numerically, and more tractable in terms of the analytical computations involved. Indeed, we have found that the proposed EM algorithm provides more accurate estimates of the model parameters.

Let us now consider a mixture model of one "ball" compartment and M different "stick" compartments. In the complex domain, the signal generated by the jth compartment in the ith sampled direction is corrupted by complex Gaussian noise, such that

$$Y_{ij} = \nu_{ij}(\Theta) + \epsilon, \quad \epsilon \sim \mathcal{CN}\left(0, \frac{2\sigma^2}{M+1}\right), \tag{4}$$

where $\mathcal{CN}$ denotes the circularly-symmetric complex normal distribution. Therefore, the PDF and log-likelihood of the complex signal, Y_{ij}, given Θ are

$$p(Y_{ij}|\Theta) = \frac{1}{2\pi\sigma^2/(M+1)} \exp\left(-\frac{\|Y_{ij} - \nu_{ij}(\Theta)\|^2}{2\sigma^2/(M+1)}\right), \tag{5}$$

$$l(\Theta|\{Y_{ij}\}) = \sum_{i=1}^{N}\sum_{j=0}^{M} -\log(2\pi\sigma^2/(M+1)) - \frac{\|Y_{ij} - \nu_{ij}(\Theta)\|^2}{2\sigma^2/(M+1)}. \tag{6}$$

Note that the complex signal, Y_{ij}, represent the complete data in our EM algorithm, whereas the observed incomplete data is the magnitude of a mixture of complex signals, that is $S_i = \left\|\sum_{j=0}^{M} Y_{ij}\right\|$, where $S_i \sim \text{Ric}\left(\nu_i(\Theta), \sigma^2\right)$ [12].

The E-step is derived by calculating the expected value of the log-likelihood with respect to the complete data $\mathbf{Y} = \{Y_{ij}, i = 1, \ldots, N, j = 0, \ldots, M\}$:

$$Q(\Theta|\Theta^{(k)}) = E\left[l(\Theta|\mathbf{Y})|\mathbf{S}, \Theta^{(k)}\right] = \int l(\Theta|\mathbf{Y})p(\mathbf{Y}|\mathbf{S}, \Theta^{(k)})d\mathbf{Y}. \tag{7}$$

Following some extensive derivations, which are too lengthy to be included in this paper, we arrive at the final expression for the Q-function:

$$Q(\Theta|\Theta^{(k)}) = \sum_{i,j} 2\nu_{ij}(\Theta)\left[\frac{S_i}{M+1}A\left(\frac{S_i\nu_i^{(k)}}{\sigma^2}\right) - \frac{\nu_i^{(k)}}{M+1} + \nu_{ij}^{(k)}\right] - \nu_{ij}(\Theta)^2,$$

where $A(x) = I_1(x)/I_0(x)$, $\nu_i^{(k)} = \nu_i(\Theta^{(k)})$, $\nu_{ij}^{(k)} = \nu_{ij}(\Theta^{(k)})$.

In the M-step, the model parameters Θ are updated to maximize Q via gradient ascent. The partial derivative of Q with respect to $\theta \in \Theta$ is given by

$$\frac{dQ}{d\theta} = 2\sum_{i,j}\left[\frac{S_i}{M+1}A\left(\frac{S_i\nu_i^{(k)}}{\sigma^2}\right) - \frac{\nu_i^{(k)}}{M+1} + \nu_{ij}^{(k)} - \nu_{ij}(\Theta)\right]\frac{d\nu_{ij}}{d\theta}. \tag{8}$$

The derivatives $d\nu_{ij}/d\mathbf{u}_j$ are computed in the tangent space of the real projective space, $\mathbb{RP}^2$, i.e., the space of bi-directional unit vectors, due to the antipodal symmetry of diffusion. We write the stick components ν_{ij} in terms of the geodesic distance on $\mathbb{RP}^2$, that is, $\cos d(\mathbf{g}_i, \mathbf{u}_j) = \mathbf{g}_i^T \mathbf{u}_j$. This leads to

$$\frac{d\nu_{ij}(\Theta)}{d\mathbf{u}_j} = -w_j S_0 \exp(-b\kappa_j(\cos d(\mathbf{g}_i, \mathbf{u}_j))^2) \frac{b\kappa_j \sin 2d(\mathbf{g}_i, \mathbf{u}_j)}{d(\mathbf{g}_i, \mathbf{u}_j)} \mathrm{Log}_{\mathbf{u}_j}(\mathbf{g}_i)$$

The derivatives $d\nu_{ij}/dw_j$ and $d\nu_{ij}/d\kappa_j$ are straightforward to compute and are not included here. These derivatives, combined with the expression in (8), define the update step in the gradient ascent in the M-step.

3   Sparsity Prior on Compartment Fractions

When fitting to a noisy DW signal with unknown number of fiber compartments, an increase in the number of sticks will generally improve the model fit. However, increasing the number of sticks beyond the true number of fiber compartments will overfit to the imaging noise. In real applications, we favor representation of a diffusion profile with as few compartments as possible. In terms of the parameters, this means we favor weighting fractions that concentrate on a minimal number of necessary compartments, rather than distribute equally upon all compartments. Therefore, we introduce a sparsity prior for the compartment fractions.

The l_p-norm with $p \leq 1$ is universally used as a sparsity (or concentration) measure, where the most common choice being the l_1-norm. However, the l_1-norm of the volume fractions $\|(w_0, \ldots, w_M)\|_1 = \sum_{j=0}^M w_j$ is constrained to be 1 in our case and cannot reflect sparsity level. Alternatively, we use the $l_{0.5}$-norm as the sparsity measure. That is,

$$C(w_0, w_1, \ldots, w_M) = \left(\sum_{j=0}^M w_j^{0.5}\right)^2, \tag{9}$$

where C gets its maximal value when all the fractions are equal, and its minimal value when one fraction equals to 1 and the rest equal to zero.

This term penalizes the number of compartments such that when a volume fraction, w_j, tends to zero during the optimization process, the derivative dC/dw_j tends to negative infinity, which results in pushing w_j faster toward zero. In that case, the value of w_j cannot increase anymore, the associated stick compartment will no longer correspond to a white matter fiber, and will be eliminated from the optimization process. We treat the sparsity penalty defined by (9) as a negative log prior on volume fractions, which results in an amended Q function

$$\hat{Q}(\Theta|\Theta^{(k)}) = Q(\Theta|\Theta^{(k)}) - \lambda_C \cdot C(w_0, \ldots, w_M), \tag{10}$$

where λ_C is a tunable coupling factor for the sparsity constraint. Thus, in the maximization step in the EM algorithm, the derivative of C is included in the gradient ascent update of the volume fractions.

4   Implementation Details

4.1   Initialization and Model Selection

In the proposed algorithm, the number of stick compartments is automatically selected using the sparsity constraint.

At the beginning of the estimation, the number of stick compartments is set to 3. A 2nd-order tensor is fit to the DW signal and its eigenvectors and eigenvalues are used to initialize the stick directions and diffusivity, respectively. Initial volume fractions are set to 0.25 equally for all stick and ball compartments.

During estimation, compartments with fractions driven to zero by the sparsity constraint are instantly removed from the model. In cases where small fractions of redundant compartments remain in the estimation results when the EM algorithm converges, a set of predefined fraction thresholds, W_1, W_2, and W_3, are applied to remove them. Given K stick compartments, those with fractions $w_j < W_K$ would be removed from the estimated model. If one or more compartments are removed by thresholding, the EM is continued with the reduced model until convergence again. Otherwise, the compartment number is determined. We then set $\lambda_C = 0$ and let the EM converge again, in order to eliminate the bias introduced by the sparsity constraint.

In our experiments, a universal set of fraction thresholds, $W_1 = 0.15$, $W_2 = 0.1$, and $W_3 = 0.05$, are used in all scenarios. These values are empirically selected from repetitive experiments and found to provide plausible results in synthetic data with various settings. The coupling factor, λ_C, can be set with respect to different b-value and SNR scenarios. In particular, we tune the value of λ_C to perform optimally on simulated training data (independent from the testing data in the results section) with the given b-value and SNR.

4.2   Assumptions on Diffusivity

It is known that indeterminacy prevents simultaneous estimation of diffusivities and volume fractions when the DW measurements are available for a single b-value only [13]. As we use the volume fractions for automatic model selection, constraining assumptions are made on diffusivity values to resolve parameter indeterminacy.

We first assume that the ball diffusivity is known and constant in a dataset, and let the algorithm determine the optimal fraction of the ball compartment for a given diffusivity. In practice, even though the ball diffusivity and volume fraction are in-determinant for a single voxel, we can estimate a common ball diffusivity from a *collection* of voxels. We discuss this process in the next section.

Secondly, we assume that all stick compartments in one voxel have the same diffusivity. This assumption helps to distinguish stick compartments from the ball. A stick compartment degenerates into a ball compartment when its diffusivity approaches zero. With this constraint, when a stick compartment is redundant, the EM algorithm inclines to decrease its fraction instead of its diffusivity, so it prevents the emergence of an additional isotropic compartment.

4.3   Estimating Ball Diffusivity

As the ball diffusivity is assumed to be known in the proposed estimation algorithm, its value needs to be determined from the given data. Yet, when the ball diffusivity and fraction are both unknown, indeterminacy between the two parameters prevents reliable estimation of either of them. To solve this problem, based on the assumption that the true ball diffusivity is constant in the dataset, we propose the following procedure to estimate its value. We first select a number of voxels with a single-fiber configuration. Then, we fit a ball-and-one-stick model to these voxels by alternating between estimating the diffusivities and the volume fractions, with the other fixed. After each iteration, the median of the diffusivities / fractions among all selected voxels are used to initiate the next round of estimation. After a few iterations, the median values would converge and the median ball diffusivity at convergence is taken as the ball diffusivity for the given dataset.

5   Results

5.1   Simulated Data

First, we tested the performance of the proposed method on simulated data. The clean DW measurements were synthesized using the ball-and-stick model with 64 gradient directions. In the simulation, all ball and stick compartments had the same volume fraction, $1/(M + 1)$, where M was the number of stick compartments simulated. The stick and ball diffusivities were derived to closely simulate real white matter and were set as 1.54×10^{-3} and 8.83×10^{-4}, respectively. The simulated DW signal was corrupted by Rician noise using a standard procedure where a complex Gaussian noise was added to the signal, and we took the modulus of the noisy signal in the complex domain.

The proposed method was evaluated at b-values of 2000 and 3000, and baseline SNRs of 15 and 20. For each scenario 100 noisy signal instances were generated to gather statistical evaluation of the estimation performance.

For each pair of b-value and SNR, we randomly picked 50 samples from the single-fiber signals and applied the method described in Section 4.3 to recover the ball diffusivity.

Parameter Estimation Accuracy. We assessed the accuracy of our algorithm in various cases that differed by the separation angle and the number of simulated compartments. We compared our results with the ball-and-stick estimation scheme proposed by Schultz et al. [11]. Also, to compare the reconstruction behavior between Rician and Gaussian noise models, we implemented a variant of our method where the Rician likelihood was replaced with the *Gaussian* likelihood. In this experiment, we fixed the number of stick compartments in both the algorithm of [11] and our algorithm (and, thus, turned off the sparsity prior by setting $\lambda_C = 0$).

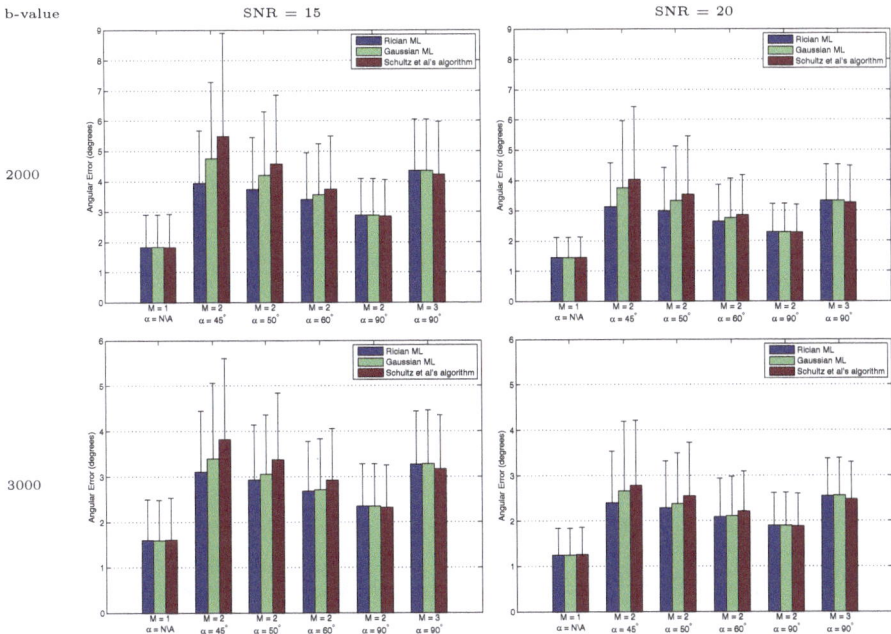

Fig. 1. Angular error of estimated stick directions (mean and standard deviation)

Figs. 1 and 2 show the errors in estimated stick directions and diffusivities, where M and α stand for the number of simulated compartments and the (minimum) separation angle between stick directions, respectively. When the separation angle is low, our method shows less bias in fiber orientations compared to the other two approaches. As the separation angle increases, or when there is only one stick component, the three methods perform similarly. As for diffusivity estimation, the proposed Rician ML algorithm consistently outperforms its opponents. Schultz et al.'s algorithm uses the same diffusivity for both ball and stick compartments, which would not adapt to the simulated situation, and therefore presents large diffusivity errors. Although the Gaussian and Rician ML methods perform similarly in terms of angular deviation in high-separation-angle scenarios, the Gaussian ML is less accurate in diffusivity estimation, due to the bias inherent to using a Gaussian approximation to the Rice distribution.

Model Selection. Now, we assume that the number of compartments is not known, and determine its value using the sparsity constraint on the volume fractions, as described in Section 4.1. The performance of the sparsity constraint was tested with both Rician and Gaussian noise models. The coupling factor, λ_C, ranged between 20 to 40, was chosen according to the b-value and SNR, using independent synthetic training data. The success rate of compartment number estimation is shown in Table 1. In most cases, the Rician model outperforms the

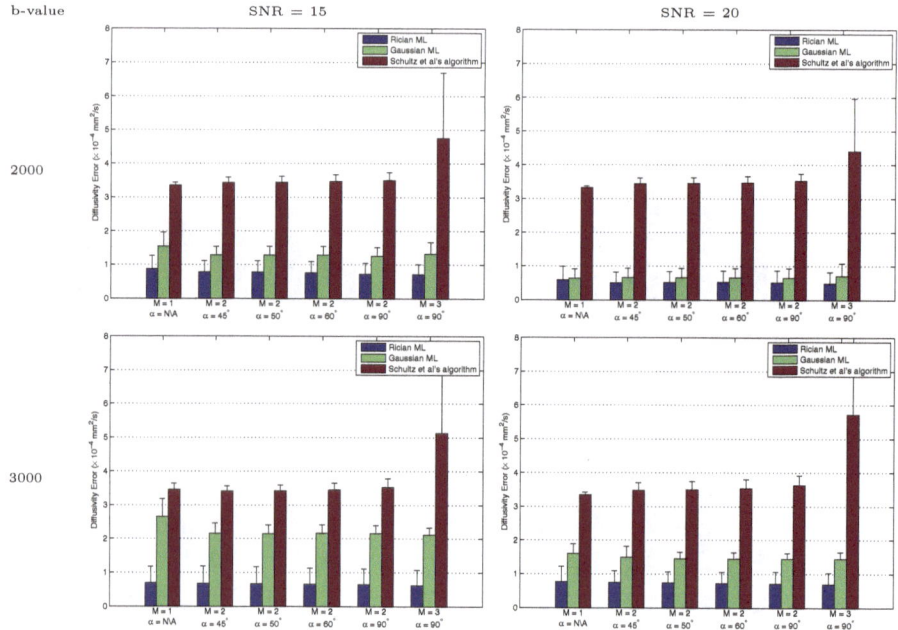

Fig. 2. Root mean square error of the estimated diffusivities

Gaussian one, especially at low SNRs. The only cases where the Gaussian ML performs better are at SNR=20 and a separation angle of 45°.

In addition, we compared the proposed model selection method with the Akaike Information Criteria (AIC). As shown in Table 1, AIC produces plausible results only for isotropic, or single fiber configurations. It is found that AIC is very conservative in choosing the optimal number of parameters, such that it always underestimates the number of compartments for complex diffusion structures. We have also found that the similar Bayesian Information Criteria (BIC) is even more conservative than the AIC.

5.2 In Vivo Brain Data

The human brain data was acquired on a 3T Siemens Allegra Tim Trio scanner using a b-value of 2000 s/mm². The scan was composed of 10 B0 volumes and 60 diffusion weighted volumes of matrix size $128 \times 128 \times 70$, and voxel size of $2 \times 2 \times 2$ mm³. The volumes were registered to a T_1 template with a voxel size of 1 mm³, and corrected for motion, eddy current, and EPI distortions. The Rician noise parameter σ was estimated from background voxels as $\hat{\sigma} = \sqrt{\mathrm{var}(S)/2}$. To determine the ball diffusivity in the brain data, 50 voxels were selected in the corpus callosum region, where the number of sticks was known to be 1. Following the procedure in Section 4.3, the ball diffusivity was estimated as 8.8294×10^{-4}.

We selected a $41 \times 41 \times 41$ region of the brain data for experimental evaluation. In the selected region, the SNR was estimated to be approximately 25. We chose

Table 1. Accuracy of number of compartments determination (in percentage)

	Compartment no.	0	1	2				3
	Separation angle	-	-	45°	50°	60°	90°	90°
Rician ML w/ Sparsity Prior	b-value = 2000 SNR=15	98	100	75	95	100	100	100
	SNR=20	100	100	83	99	100	100	100
	b-value = 3000 SNR=15	100	100	72	96	98	100	100
	SNR=20	100	100	71	98	100	100	100
Gaussian ML w/ Sparsity Prior	b-value = 2000 SNR=15	100	84	73	74	73	69	100
	SNR=20	100	96	90	91	90	86	100
	b-value = 3000 SNR=15	100	85	71	77	77	74	100
	SNR=20	100	96	89	91	93	93	100
Rician ML w/ AIC	b-value = 2000 SNR=15	100	100	0	0	0	29	0
	SNR=20	100	100	0	0	0	99	0
	b-value = 3000 SNR=15	100	100	0	0	0	83	0
	SNR=20	100	100	0	0	8	100	15

the sparsity prior coupling factor $\lambda_C = 75$ using a few synthesized training samples of the same b-value and SNR.

Figure 3(a) and (b) show the parameter estimation and automatic model selection results with the proposed method. It is easy to identify the corpus callosum where the one-stick model was selected, with a clear boundary against the isotropic background. Meanwhile, the 3-stick model was selected in the crossing region of the corpus callosum, cortical spinal and SLF. The pattern of the number of sticks is highly consistent with known anatomy of the white matter in the brain. Some erroneous model selection results can be spotted in the CSF, and at the boundary between the CSF and the white matter tracts, where 3 sticks are attributed. This is likely to result from an underestimated ball diffusivity.

As a comparison, we used the voxel classification method in Camino [14] to select the optimal order of spherical harmonics for the diffusion data, which applied Alexander et al.'s algorithm using an F-test [15]. In this method, three classes are detected with corresponding spherical harmonics orders 0, 2, and 4, which stand for isotropic diffusion, single directional diffusion tensor, and complex diffusion structures consisting of two or more fiber orientations, respectively. We set the background signal threshold as 100 and the thresholds for separating the three classes as 1×10^{-20}, 1×10^{-6} and 1×10^{-6}. As shown in Figure 3(d), the output of the F-test is noisy and does not match the anatomy well, especially in the crossing region of the three tracts.

We used the deterministic tractography tool in Camino to perform fiber tracking from our reconstruction results. The fibers were seeded in every voxel where our method detected one or more stick compartments. Following the tractography process, ROIs were used separately to select fiber bundles in the corpus callosum, cortical spinal and SLF, respectively, as shown in Figure 3(e) - (g). For the corpus callosum, tractography from the reconstructed ball-and-stick model reproduced the U-shaped callosal radiation and also the lateral transcallosal

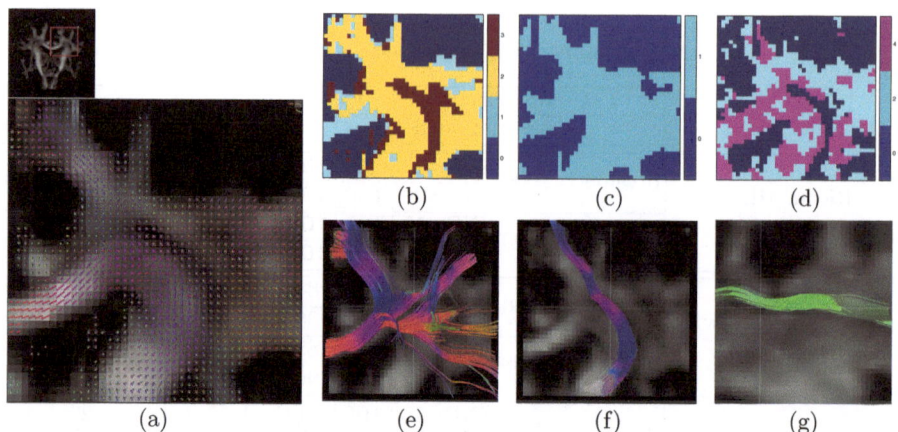

Fig. 3. Automatic model selection and reconstruction results on in vivo brain data. (a) Location of the selected section and the stick orientations (weighted by associated fractions) reconstructed with the proposed method; (b) stick compartment numbers estimated with the proposed method; (c) stick compartment numbers estimated with AIC; (d) the order of spherical harmonics selected by F-test; (e) - (g) tractography results from the reconstructed ball-and-stick models for (e) corpus callosum, (f) cortical spinal, and (g) SLF (sagittal slice).

fibers. In addition, the tractography yielded the cortical spinal going from bottom to top, as well as the SLF bundle in the front-back direction. All the three tracts crossed at the center region of the depicted section.

6   Conclusions

In this paper, we proposed a novel scheme for estimating parameters in a multi-compartment model that is composed of an isotropic "ball" compartment, and multiple perfectly linear "stick" compartments, under Rician noise assumption. Our scheme combines a robust Rician EM algorithm, and a sparsity prior on the volume mixing fractions to automatically select the number of compartments. Using simulated data, we showed that our formulation reduces bias in the estimation of fiber orientations, diffusivities, and number of compartments, compared to alternative schemes that rely on a Gaussian noise assumption. Furthermore, we applied the proposed algorithm to in vivo brain data and show that our method provides a clear distinction between different fiber populations, and is able to reconstruct fiber pathways that match known white matter structures such as the transcallosal fibers.

Acknowledgements. This project was supported in part by grants R01 MH084795, 5P41RR012553-14, and 8P41GM103545-14 from the National Institutes of Health.

References

1. Tournier, Calamante, F., Gadian, D.G., Connelly, A.: Direct estimation of the fiber orientation density function from diffusion-weighted MRI data using spherical deconvolution. NeuroImage 23(3), 1176–1185 (2004)
2. Descoteaux, M., Angelino, E., Fitzgibbons, S., Deriche, R.: Regularized, fast, and robust analytical Q-ball imaging. Magn. Res. Med. 58(3), 497–510 (2007)
3. Tuch, D.S., Reese, T.G., Wiegell, M.R., Wedeen, V.J.: Diffusion MRI of Complex Neural Architecture. Neuron 40(5), 885–895 (2003)
4. Behrens, T.E., Berg, H.J., Jbabdi, S., Rushworth, M.F., Woolrich, M.W.: Probabilistic diffusion tractography with multiple fibre orientations: What can we gain? NeuroImage 34(1), 144–155 (2007)
5. Liu, C., Bammer, R., Acar, B., Moseley, M.E.: Characterizing non-gaussian diffusion by using generalized diffusion tensors. Magn. Reson. Med. 51(5), 924–937 (2004)
6. Weldeselassie, Y.T., Barmpoutis, A., Atkins, M.S.: Symmetric positive-definite cartesian tensor orientation distribution functions (CT-ODF). In: Jiang, T., Navab, N., Pluim, J.P.W., Viergever, M.A. (eds.) MICCAI 2010, Part I. LNCS, vol. 6361, pp. 582–589. Springer, Heidelberg (2010)
7. Jiao, F., Gur, Y., Johnson, C.R., Joshi, S.: Detection of crossing white matter fibers with high-order tensors and rank-k decompositions. In: Székely, G., Hahn, H.K. (eds.) IPMI 2011. LNCS, vol. 6801, pp. 538–549. Springer, Heidelberg (2011)
8. Behrens, T.E.J., Woolrich, M.W., Jenkinson, M., Johansen-Berg, H., Nunes, R.G., Clare, S., Matthews, P.M., Brady, J.M., Smith, S.M.: Characterization and propagation of uncertainty in diffusion-weighted MR imaging. Magn. Reson. Med. 50(5), 1077–1088 (2003)
9. Hosey, T., Williams, G., Ansorge, R.: Inference of multiple fiber orientations in high angular resolution diffusion imaging. Magn. Reson. Med. 54(6), 1480–1489 (2005)
10. Caan, M., Khedoe, H., Poot, D., den Dekker, A., Olabarriaga, S., Grimbergen, K., van Vliet, L., Vos, F.: Estimation of diffusion properties in crossing fiber bundles. IEEE Transactions on Medical Imaging 29(8), 1504–1515 (2010)
11. Schultz, T., Westin, C.-F., Kindlmann, G.: Multi-diffusion-tensor fitting via spherical deconvolution: A unifying framework. In: Jiang, T., Navab, N., Pluim, J.P.W., Viergever, M.A. (eds.) MICCAI 2010, Part I. LNCS, vol. 6361, pp. 674–681. Springer, Heidelberg (2010)
12. Marzetta, T.L.: EM algorithm for estimating the parameters of a multivariate complex Rician density for polarimetric SAR. In: 1995 International Conference on Acoustics, Speech, and Signal Processing, vol. 5, pp. 3651–3654. IEEE (1995)
13. Scherrer, B., Warfield, S.K.: Why multiple b-values are required for multi-tensor models. Evaluation with a constrained log-Euclidean model. In: Proc. of the 7th IEEE International Symposium on Biomedical Imaging (ISBI), pp. 1389–1392 (2010)
14. Cook, P., Bai, Y., Nedjati-Gilani, S., Seunarine, K., Hall, M., Parker, G., Alexander, D.: Camino: Open-source diffusion-mri reconstruction and processing. In: 14th Scientific Meeting of the International Society for Magnetic Resonance in Medicine, vol. 2759 (2006)
15. Alexander, D., Barker, G., Arridge, S.: Detection and modeling of non-gaussian apparent diffusion coefficient profiles in human brain data. Magnetic Resonance in Medicine 48(2), 331–340 (2002)

Bayesian Segmentation of Atrium Wall Using Globally-Optimal Graph Cuts on 3D Meshes

Gopalkrishna Veni, Zhisong Fu, Suyash P. Awate, and Ross T. Whitaker*

Scientific Computing and Imaging (SCI) Institute, University of Utah

Abstract. Efficient segmentation of the left atrium (LA) wall from delayed enhancement MRI is challenging due to inconsistent contrast, combined with noise, and high variation in atrial shape and size. We present a surface-detection method that is capable of extracting the atrial wall by computing an optimal a-posteriori estimate. This estimation is done on a set of nested meshes, constructed from an ensemble of segmented training images, and graph cuts on an associated multi-column, proper-ordered graph. The graph/mesh is a part of a template/model that has an associated set of learned intensity features. When this mesh is overlaid onto a test image, it produces a set of costs which lead to an optimal segmentation. The 3D mesh has an associated weighted, directed multi-column graph with edges that encode smoothness and inter-surface penalties. Unlike previous graph-cut methods that impose hard constraints on the surface properties, the proposed method follows from a Bayesian formulation resulting in soft penalties on spatial variation of the cuts through the mesh. The novelty of this method also lies in the construction of proper-ordered graphs on complex shapes for choosing among distinct classes of base shapes for automatic LA segmentation. We evaluate the proposed segmentation framework on simulated and clinical cardiac MRI.

Keywords: Atrial Fibrillation, Bayesian segmentation, Minimum s-t cut, Mesh Generation, Geometric Graph.

1   Introduction

Segmentation of the heart's left atrium (LA) is a highly relevant problem in the clinical domain. In the context of medical imaging, delayed enhancement MRI (DE-MRI) has been shown to produce contrast in myocardium (heart wall) and in regions subjected to fibrosis and scarring [1]. So, these regions are associated with risk factors and treatment of atrial fibrillation (AF). Imaging with DE-MRI is therefore useful for the evaluation of potential effectiveness of radio-ablation therapy and for studying recovery. This AF recovery includes analysis of scarring as well as atrial shape and structural remodeling (SRM) after treatment.

---

* The authors would like to acknowledge the Comprehensive Arrhythmia Research and Management (CARMA) Center, and the Center for Integrative Biomedical Computing (CIBC) by NIH Grant P41 GM103545-14, and National Alliance for Medical Image Computing (NAMIC) through NIH Grant U54 EB005149, for providing Utah fibrosis data, and CIBAVision.

J.C. Gee et al. (Eds.): IPMI 2013, LNCS 7917, pp. 656–667, 2013.
© Springer-Verlag Berlin Heidelberg 2013

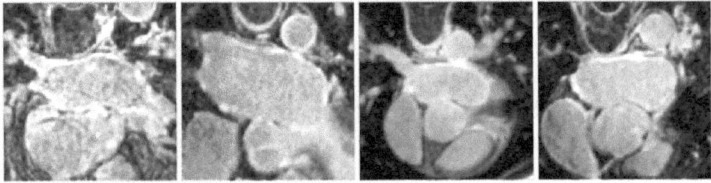

Fig. 1. Slices of left atrium DE-MRI images showing the challenges in segmentation

Automatic segmentation of the heart wall in this context is quite important; in a single clinic, hundreds of man hours are spent per month in manual segmentation. In DE-MRI images, this becomes a challenging task, because of relatively low and inconsistent contrast, high level of unwanted texture and noise, and high variability of atrial shape. Moreover, this problem gets aggravated by inaccuracies in cardiac gating and the SRM in chronic AF. Thus, this is a difficult image analysis problem, which also represents an ubiquitous challenge in a 3D medical segmentation: segmenting in the presence of relatively poor signal, high noise, and large variations in shape.

Several papers address the problem of segmenting the blood pool in MRI angiography (MRI-A) images [2, 3]. These methods make use of the relatively homogeneous brightness of the blood pool in MRI-A, which is well suited for deformable models or registration-based approaches. However, high-quality properly-aligned blood-pool images are often *not* readily available from DE-MRI protocols. Furthermore, due to thinness of the atrium wall, algorithms based on template registration fail as they often rely on coarse anatomical features. Figure 1 shows examples of DE-MRI images of the LA that depict its varying, low-contrast boundaries, high level of correlated noise, and high shape variability.

A variety of conventional segmentation methods have proven to be ineffective. One strategy to address these challenges is to introduce a prior on the segmentation problem, either in the form of probability on specific kinds of shapes or more generally on shape properties, such as smoothness. These priors are combined with image matching terms or simply feature detection to find some ideal compromise between the prior and the data. Level-set methods [4] rely on gradient-descent optimizations, which are sensitive to initializations and local minima. We have found such local optimizations to be particularly ill suited to this problem. Statistical models, such as active shape models [5] have been proven to be effective, but are also limited in their ability to deal with the small and large-scale shape variability. Generally, coarse-to-fine optimization strategies can help avoid local minima, but have proven inadequate for this segmentation problem, mostly because the features of interest (thin, brighter regions and small dark gaps between the atrium and nearby tissues) do not hold up under blurring. While recent developments addressing this problem [6] are promising, they rely on deformable models and/or image registration approaches that tend to also get caught in local minima.

The difficulty of segmentation in this context suggests that this problem would benefit from a global optimization strategy. Recently, Wu and Chen [7] described a scheme by which the problem of finding an optimal function value on a discrete grid (a *surface net* problem) is represented as a minimum *s-t* cut on a proper-ordered graph. Optimal solutions to the *s-t* cut are given by relatively efficient, polynomial-time algorithms. Li *et al.* [8] applied a version of this surface-net formulation to simultaneously segment multiple coupled surfaces in noisy images by including image-based costs and geometric constraints of the underlying graph. That approach has demonstrated some success in several challenging image segmentation problems [8–10]. This surface-net relies on the construction of a properly-ordered graph, which also defines the topology of the resulting segmentation. The construction of such graphs is challenging for complex and irregular anatomical structures, such as LA. Using naive offsets from a base mesh results in "tangling" between columns, and resulting cuts are not guaranteed to be valid surfaces or regions. Thus, these proper ordered graph-cut methods require a careful construction of the underlying graph.

The contributions of this paper are as follows. We show that a Bayesian formulation with a Markov random field prior can give rise to a certain type of surface-net problem, namely, a *VCE-Net*, which is solvable by the algorithm of Wu and Chen [7]. This formulation gives rise to soft penalties on surface smoothing and surface coupling, which, as we will show, is superior to the hard constraints described by Li *et al.*. The Bayesian formulation also gives rise to a set of *learned* feature detectors, so that the method does not rely on user-defined methods for characterizing edges or regions. We also propose a new method for the graph construction on irregular surfaces that avoids tangling. To address the variability in shapes, we process training examples into clusters to form multiple shape templates, that *compete* in our optimization scheme for the best segmentation. We evaluate the method on a set of synthetic examples and LA DE-MRI images with hand segmentations as the ground truth.

2   Methods

2.1   A Bayesian Formulation of Graph-Cut Segmentation

We treat the problem of segmentation as a maximum a-posteriori estimation. The proposed work differs from many previous Bayesian methods in two important aspects. First, we formulate the segmentation as estimation problem on a graph structure, rather than the image directly. Secondly, we obtain a global optimum to this problem by means of a graph-cut algorithm. The data for this formulation is the image data sampled at locations that are associated with the model. The prior is expressed as a Markov random field (MRF) on the location of the cut in the graph which is related to the formulation introduced by Ishikawa [11]. The graph, which forms a 3D mesh, must approximately adhere the shape to be segmented. It introduces a topological structure on the problem over which the Markov property is introduced.

We begin with a description of the graph structure and associated notation. The graph G is a proper-ordered graph with a set of columns, a neighborhood structure on those columns, and a consistent topological structure as one moves up and down the columns. We define the *base graph* $G^0 = (V^0, E^0)$, as a set of vertices $\{v_i^0 \in V^0\}$, and edges, $\{e_{i,j}^0 = (v_i^0, v_j^0) \in E^0\}$. For a proper-ordered graph, the vertices are arranged logically as a collection of (conceptually) parallel columns that have the same number of vertices. The entire graph G consists of an ordered set of copies of the base graph, and each vertex can be referenced by its column i and the position within that column l, e.g. v_i^l. The collection $G^l = (V^l, E^l)$ of vertices and edges at the same position l across all columns is called a *layer*. For ease of notation, an edge or vertex without a superscript, v_i or e_{ij}, is considered with respect to the base layer, which defines the topology of all columns. We let N be the number of columns and L be the number of vertices in each column (number of layers). The neighboring columns of the ith column are denoted as the set $\mathcal{N}_i$.

Above is the topological structure of the graph; here we describe its geometry. Each node in the graph has an associated position in the 3D volume/image, which we denote as $x_i^l = x(v_i^l) \in \mathbb{R}^3$. Associated with each x_i^l, there is a *set* of image coordinates, which form an image patch for that vertex, which we call $\mathcal{P}_i^l$. Associated with each patch is a probabilistic model of the intensity patterns one would find in the image at those locations, which is like the formulation of [5].

We now model a set of image measurements associated with a segmentation on the graph. We introduce a probabilistic model with respect to a single segmentation and extend that to coupled surfaces subsequently. We define the surface segmentation as a subset of nodes in the graph $\mathcal{S} \subset V$. Because we restrict the optimal cut to have only one vertex per column, we can parametrize the cut with respect to the base mesh, thus $\mathcal{S}$ can be represented as the function $S : V^0 \mapsto [0, \dots L - 1]$. Furthermore, $S(i)$, combined with the topology introduced by the base mesh and the 3D coordinates of the vertices describes a surface in 3D. Thus, we are describing a *surface estimation* problem.

For any given vertex in the graph, v_i^l, we can sample the image I as prescribed by the patch $\mathcal{P}_i^l$. We call the set of image patches for all vertices in the graph as I^V and the set of patches associated with segmentation to be I^S. For a particular segmentation, there is an associated patch I_i^S for each column i.

Now we introduce the probabilistic model, the posterior probability of a segmentation conditioned on image data as follows. Using Bayes rule and considering only terms in the optimization we have:

$$P(\mathcal{S}|I^V) \propto P(I^V|\mathcal{S})P(\mathcal{S}) \tag{1}$$

Next we introduce specific models. For the image intensity model we assume independence of image patches and use an isotropic Gaussian, with a mean for each column that is learned from a set of training examples. That is,

$$P(I^V|\mathcal{S}) \propto \Pi_{i=1}^N P(I_i^S) = \Pi_{i=1}^N \exp\left(-\frac{1}{2\sigma^2} \| I_i^S - \mu_i \|^2\right) \tag{2}$$

where μ_i is an average patch template learned for surface with physical locations of column i in training examples, and σ is a standard-deviation parameter associated with this data.

For the surface prior, we use a MRF on the function $S(i)$. Let $\mathcal{C} \subset V^0 \times V^0$ be the set of cliques in the base graph, defined by the neighborhood structure, and $C(S(j), S(k))$ is the pairwise clique potential. We use a Gibbs potential on these cliques for the MRF prior, which gives:

$$P(\mathcal{S}) = \exp\left(- \sum_{(v_j, v_k) \in \mathcal{C}} C(S(j), S(k)) \right),$$

(3)

where the clique potential $C(\cdot)$ typically takes the form $f(|S(j) - S(k)|)$. Here f is monotonic and convex (for optimization to be feasible). In this paper, we use $f(d) = \alpha d^{1+\gamma}; \gamma > 0$.

We minimize the negative log posterior to get the optimal segmentation as:

$$\text{argmin}_S \left[\lambda \sum_{i=1}^{N} \| I_i^S - \mu_i \|^2 + \sum_{(v_j, v_k) \in \mathcal{C}} C(S(j), S(k)) \right], \text{ where } \lambda = 1/(2\sigma^2).$$

(4)

Segmentation of LA wall requires extraction of epicardial and endocardial surfaces. So, we extend the model to two surfaces/segmentations, $\mathcal{S}^1, \mathcal{S}^2$:

$$P(\mathcal{S}^1, \mathcal{S}^2 | I^V) \propto P(I^V | \mathcal{S}^1, \mathcal{S}^2) P(\mathcal{S}^1, \mathcal{S}^2)$$

(5)

We use the same independence assumption with different mean patches for the different surfaces. As we use the MRF for intra-surface smoothness, we propose an inter-surface probability to model interactions between surfaces.

$$P(\mathcal{S}^1, \mathcal{S}^2) = \exp\left(- \sum_{(v_j, v_k) \in \mathcal{C}} C(S_j^1, S_k^1) \right) \exp\left(- \sum_{(v_j, v_k) \in \mathcal{C}} C(S_j^2, S_k^2) \right)$$

$$\exp\left(- \sum_{j=1}^{N} g(S_j^1 - S_j^2 - \Delta_j) \right),$$

(6)

where Δ_j is the ideal inter-surface distance, which may vary with column and learned from training examples, and $g(S_j^1 - S_j^2 - \Delta_j)$ must meet the same conditions of $f()$ in the clique penalty, but must also enforce $S_j^1 < S_j^2$. For this work we use

$$g(d) = \begin{cases} \alpha' d^{1+\gamma'} & d > -\Delta_j \\ \infty & d \leq -\Delta_j \end{cases}$$

(7)

The optimization problem for coupled surfaces is therefore:

$$\text{argmin}_{\mathcal{S}^1, \mathcal{S}^2} \left[\lambda \sum_{i=1}^{N} \left(\| I_i^{S^1} - \mu_i^1 \|^2 + \| I_i^{S^2} - \mu_i^2 \|^2 \right) \right.$$

$$\left. + \sum_{(v_j, v_k) \in \mathcal{C}} \left(C(S^1(j), S^1(k)) + C(S^2(j), S^2(k)) \right) + \sum_{j=1}^{N} g(S_j^1 - S_j^2 - \Delta_j) \right]$$

(8)

2.2   Graph Cut Formulation

From the objective functions in the previous section, we now construct a revised graph and define an optimal graph cut that is equivalent to the above optimization. The construction of the derived graph follows, generally, the method proposed by [7] for converting this optimization into an s-t cut. Wu et $al.$ [7] detail general strategies for solving $surface$-net problems of the type described by Eq. 8. They describe both the Vnet problem, which imposes hard constraints on inter-column behavior and the VCEnet problem, which allows for soft penalties. Previous work including [9, 10] shows the use of the Vnet solution for image segmentation. The Bayesian formulation in the previous section leads to a VCEnet problem, which we also extend to coupled surfaces.

We now briefly review the conversion to the graph-cut problem. The weights on vertices and edges on the extended graph are denoted by $w(v)$ and $c(e)$, respectively. Every vertex in the base layer is connected by a directed edge with a cost $+\infty$ to every other base vertex in its adjacent (neighboring) columns. This makes the base layer strongly connected. For each vertex in layer $l \in [1, L-1]$, a weight of $w_i^l = c_i^l - c_i^{l-1}$ is assigned. A directed edge $e_{i,j}^{l,l-1}$ with a cost $+\infty$ is let from that vertex to the one below it.

The MRF property is incorporated as follows. For every pair of adjacent columns in G, a sequence of directed edges, $e_i^{l,l-d}, d = \{l, ..., 0\}$ go from a vertex v_i^l in i-column to vertices v_j^{l-d} for all $j \in \mathcal{N}_i$, as shown in Figure 2(a). For notational convenience we first define an intermediate function to edge weights

$$q(e_{i,j}^{l,l-d}) = f(d), \quad d = 0, \ldots, l, \tag{9}$$

where $f(d)$ is the penalty, which derives from the clique potential, on the difference in the "height" of adjacent cuts. The weights on these edges are defined through a finite-difference scheme for second derivatives (along columns) of q:

$$w(e_{ij}^{l,0}) = q(e_{ij}^{l,1}) - q(e_{ij}^{l,0}) \tag{10}$$

$$w(e_{ij}^{l,m}) = q(e_{ij}^{l,m+1}) + q(e_{ij}^{l,m+1}) - 2q(e_{ij}^{l,m}), \quad m = 1, \ldots l-1. \tag{11}$$

For the penalty on $inter$-$surface$ distance, we extend the method of [8] to the VCEnet construction We construct two identical disjoint subgraphs, using the procedure above, one for each surface. In addition, a set of directed arcs are added between a pair of subgraphs such that the consistency is maintained between a pair of mutually interacting surfaces. To achieve this interaction, we include a set of arcs between corresponding columns of two subgraphs which are penalized by soft constraints. The formulation resembles the one above; however, all edges are between corresponding columns in the two subgraphs. For ease of notation, all references to vertices associated with the second/inner surface will have a hat (i.e., $\hat{\cdot}$). So, v_i^l and $\hat{v}_i^l$ are corresponding vertices on the two subgraphs. We denote edges between the two surface graphs with a $\tilde{\cdot}$.

Part of our design for this segmentation problem is that one surface should always lie inside the other surface (or "below", if we imagine all columns standing

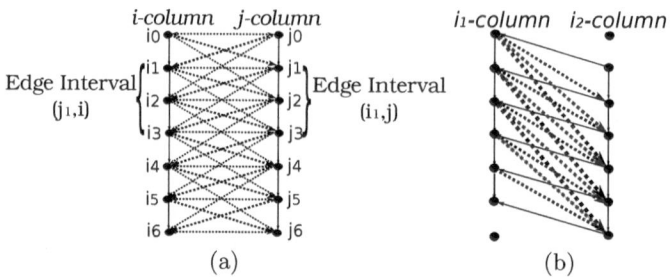

i-column j-column   *i₁-column i₂-column*

Edge Interval
(j₁,i)

Edge Interval
(i₁,j)

(a)   (b)

Fig. 2. (a) Inter-column arcs. (b) Inter-surface arcs. Blue arrows from column i_1 to i_2 represent arcs subjected to ideal inter-surface distance, Δ_i.

vertically). To achieve this, we include a directed edge between graphs, $\tilde{e}_{i,i}^{l,l+1} = (\hat{v}_i^l, v_i^{l+1})$ with weight $w(e_{i,i}^{l,l+1}) = +\infty$. Similarly, we construct a set of weighted edges that capture the second derivative of the inter-surface penalty when the inner/outer constraint is met as shown in Figure 2b.

$$\tilde{e}_{i,i}^{l,l+\Delta_i+d} = (v_i^l, \hat{v}_i^{l+\Delta_i+d}), \quad d = -\Delta_i + 1, \ldots \tag{12}$$

$$\text{and } w(\tilde{e}_{i,i}^{l,l+\Delta_i+d}) = g(d+1) - 2g(d) + g(d-1). \tag{13}$$

Subsequently, we obtain optimal segmentation of coupled surfaces by finding a minimum s-excess set in the derived graph, as described in Wu et al. [7]. This minimum s-excess set is computed by applying a minimum s-t cut in the transformed graph, G_{st}.

2.3   Building a Valid 3D Mesh

In the previous section, we described topology of the underlying graph based on a triangle structure per each layer. Here we describe the assignment of 3D positions to mesh vertices and triangulation of each layer so that these layers form a nested set of watertight meshes in 3D. This complete collection including a set of vertices, their 3D positions, and the prismatic topology of the nested meshes form a proper-ordered (PO) mesh.

For constructing the PO-mesh, we use an extension of the dynamic-particle-system method proposed by Meyer et al. [12]. This method computes thin-layers of triangular prisms that conform to shapes. A mesh is built using a template shape (described in the next section), which approximates the LA that we intend to segment. This template shape is represented as the zero level-set of a signed distance transform in the volume. So the following paragraph describes how to generate layers of high-quality meshes on top of this template.

The meshing strategy uses a cluster of points called particles. These particles are distributed on an implicit surface by interactively minimizing a potential function. The potential function based on pairwise distances defines a repulsive interaction between particles as, $U_{i,j}^{l,l} = \Phi(|x_i^l - x_j^l|)$. We denote the sum of this collection of repulsive potentials within each layer as $\mathcal{R}$. These particle systems have been shown to form consistent, nearly regular packings on complex surface [12]. Once points have been distributed on an implicit surface (with sufficient density), a Delaunay tetrahedralization scheme can be used to build a water-tight triangle mesh of the surface [13].

To build a nested set of surface meshes, we require a collection of offset surfaces, both inside and out, that not only inherit the topology of the base surface, but also represent valid, watertight 3D triangle meshes. This is crucial, because the cuts, which pass through vertices from different layers, must also form watertight triangle meshes. Thus, it results to bend the columns in order to avoid tangling of columns/triangles as the layers extend outward from the mean shape. For this, we introduce a collection of particle systems, one for each layer in the graph/mesh, and we couple these particles by an attractive force (Hooks law) between layers. Thus, there is an additional set of potentials of the form $U_{i,i}^{l,l+1} = |\boldsymbol{x}_i^l - \boldsymbol{x}_i^{l+1}|^2$, and we denote the sum of the attractive forces of neighboring particles between layers as $\mathcal{A}$.

To optimize an ensemble of particle systems for L layers, we perform gradient descent, using asynchronous updates, as in [12], on the total potential $\mathcal{R} + \beta \mathcal{A}$. Figure 3a illustrates a nested 3-layered mesh for one of the LA templates. The parameter β controls the relationship between attraction across layers and repulsion within layers and is tuned to prevent tangling. For this paper, we have used $\beta = 10$. The optimization requires an initial collection of particles. So, we place a particle at each point where the adjacent voxels have values on either side of the level set. This gives an average density of approximately one particle per unit surface area (in voxel units). The physical distance between layers must be inversely proportional to the particle density within layers. This is a compromise between the tangling that results from large offsets and the extra computation associated with many thin layers. Since a good mesh constraints the topology and the set of possible segmentations, we try different meshes based on the assumption that all good segmentations can be represented as spatially varying offsets of a mean. This corresponds to around 14,000 particles per each mesh layer for heart images and 2000 particles for simulated images. We have used a total of 30 layers, spaced at 0.5 pixels each, which gives each template a capture range of approximately 15 pixels.

2.4 Learning Template Meshes and Feature Detectors

Here we describe the construction of template shapes and the mechanism for computing costs on nodes from input images. The shapes of LA in the context of AF are highly variable. To address this, we rely on a *training set* of presegmented images. For this paper, the training set consisted of 32 segmented DE-MRI images of the LA. The work in this paper represents a prototype, and we anticipate a production-scale system that relies on hundreds of training images. These training images enable two things. First, training images give us a way of constructing a collection of PO-graphs, so that new images can be segmented as cuts through one of these graphs. Second, training images give us examples of

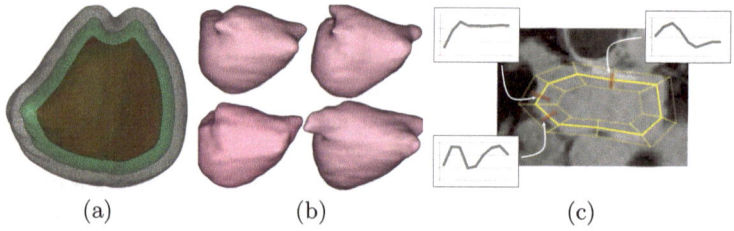

Fig. 3. (a) An example of several layers of PO-meshes for the LA.(b) Examples of average shapes, derived from k-means clustering on distance transforms of training images, around which the PO-meshes are constructed. (c) A mock up of a simplified PO-mesh in 2D with examples of feature detectors learned from the training data— actually P0-meshes for the LA have over 400,000 vertices.

patch profiles for the features that define epi- and endocardial surfaces, which leads to the costs at each node in the PO-graph.

We begin by clustering the examples based on their shapes. For this, we compute distance transforms of each endocardial surface. Training images are aligned via translation to ensure common center of mass for the blood pool (region bounded by the endocardium). This demands careful manual initialization of a template which will be handled in our future work by inducing other transformations. We then compute clusters using k-means using mean-squared distance metric between volumes. Based on the cluster residual curve, 5 clusters are chosen. However, one of the clusters has been removed from the test, because it contained only two (high distorted) examples. Surface meshes associated with the distance-transform means of these four clusters are shown in Figure 3b.

The cost associated with each vertex reflects the degree to which that vertex is a good candidate for a boundary, which will be found via a graph cut. At each vertex, the training data is used to derive a patch profile along a line segment, or *stick* perpendicular to the surface. We sample the stick at a spacing of one voxel. In our case, a patch size of 11 is considered along the normal direction of the surface. The intensity along each stick on each vertex of each template is computed by a weighted average of intensities of sticks for each feature point in each training image. Thus, for a particular vertex in a particular cluster, the intensities along a stick would correspond to an average of several hundreds of neighboring sticks from different images (that share the same blood-pool center). Thus the average stick at a vertex would be an isotropic Gaussian weighted average of all the nearby sticks (within the cluster) with standard deviation of 2 pixels. Figure 3c shows a diagram of the stick configuration and several stick intensity profiles for parts of a particular template.

3   Experiments and Results

For validation, we apply Bayesian framework based graph cut method on 100 simulated images of size $64 \times 64 \times 96$ voxels, and 30 DE-MRI images of the left atrium of size $400 \times 400 \times 107$ voxels. In all of our experiments, 30 mesh layers were generated, spaced at 0.5 voxels each, which gives each template a capture range

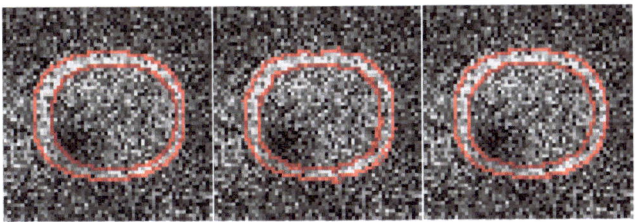

Fig. 4. Segmentation boundaries for outer and inner surfaces on synthetic data corresponding to ground truth, graph cuts with hard constraints and the proposed algorithm

of approximately 15 voxels. The scaling and exponential parameters, α and γ, for the convex function f of the graph's smoothness penalties are fixed as 300 and 2, respectively. The corresponding values for the function g of the graph's inter-surface penalties are set to 2 and 2, respectively. The values of these parameters reflect the complexity of surfaces and the inter-surface coupling between them.

To segment a given test image, we depend on the user input to position the template. The algorithm is robust to this position, as long as the nested mesh, corresponding to the template, does not lie outside or inside the desired surface (e.g. ± 5 voxels). We sample the input image along all of the sticks at all nodes. Then, we compute a posterior probability on each test stick with the corresponding template stick. This results in the assignment of costs, weights, edge capacities, and then an optimal cut. Likewise, we employ all of the learned templates to the input image, choosing the segmentation that produces the best average probability with the local intensity models for the optimal cut. A pair of optimal mesh surfaces are then recovered from the computed minimum s-t cut. Based on the extracted topological mesh structure, defined by the cut, it is scan converted to reproduce segmented volume(s).

In case of the simulated data, 30 training datasets and 100 test sets were considered for analysis. All these images include two oblong non-crossing surfaces with the inner surface translated randomly (Gaussian distribution) in 3D to mimic variations in heart-wall thickness; each image was corrupted with Rician noise ($\sigma = 30$ for the underlying Gaussian model) and a smoothly-varying bias field. Figure 4 illustrates the effectiveness of the proposed method in extracting smoother boundaries for outer and inner surfaces as compared to hard penalties.

We evaluated the segmentation accuracy for LA based on leave-one out strategy for a test dataset, against templates from the training data. We compared the segmented boundaries of epicardial and endocardial surfaces using our method to that of hard constraints. Since the geometric constraints and soft penalties in the proposed graph cut formulation are analogous to the energy based formulation in deformable models [4], we compared our results with level set based methods. Figure 5a presents segmentation boundaries for epicardial and endocardial surfaces obtained by the proposed algorithm along with others. The cost function image, derived from a-posterior probability, creates a platform on which graph cuts work. Figure 5b illustrates our segmentation result on cost function

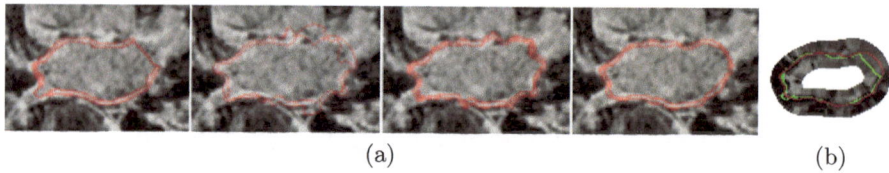

(a)   (b)

Fig. 5. (a) Surface boundaries of epi and endocardial surfaces corresponding to ground truth, level sets, graph cuts with hard constraints and proposed method. (b) Segmentation result of epicardial surface using the proposed algorithm (red) and ground truth boundary (green) overlaid on corresponding cost function image.

image corresponding to the epicardial surface. The rationale behind presenting this result is to show how the algorithm is able to extract smoother and accurate boundaries in some areas of the image where even the costs, which are derived from the sophisticated feature detector, could not be defined properly.

The qualitative comparison between the proposed method with others clearly indicates that our method surmounts other techniques in not only extracting correct surfaces, but also in maintaining smoothness along the surfaces and consistency in between them. The irregularity in the surfaces that we notice due to the hard constraints were greatly eliminated.

To evaluate the segmentation accuracy quantitatively, we used distance metric. The distance metric is based on the aggregate of pairwise distances between corresponding points on the ground truth and our segmentation. For each point on our segmented surface, we measure the distance to the nearest point on the ground truth; and vice-versa. For a perfect delineation of the boundary, all these distances would be zero. In the case of simulated examples, this distance metric which was computed over all the images came out to be 0.1879 voxels for the outer surface and 0.2639 voxels for the inner surface. For LA data, we obtained this metric value of 2.5068 voxels for epicardium and 2.6321 voxels for the endocardium. This indicates that the segmentations acquired by the proposed method lie very close to the ground truth.

For quantitative comparison, we studied Dice measures on heart wall using soft against hard constraints. The Dice metric provides the percent overlap between the ground truth and segmented regions. Figure 6 shows the histogram of Dice measures. In both simulated as well as LA cases, the metric values by inducing soft penalties on geometric constraints overpowered hard penalties. For synthetic data, the Dice values indicate excellent matches. However, in the case of myocardium, the dice values are little lower due to its varying thinness (2-6 mm) and undefined ground truth. The ground truth is a single hand segmentation from an expert. Therefore, much of the observed error is near the veins, which are subject to inter-rater variability, as the cutoff between atrium and vessel is not well defined. Also the ground truths for the wall do not form a complete boundary around the blood pool (even ignoring the vessels). Furthermore, we expect the improvement in results by increasing the number of training images so that more templates are formed in order to better match a given input image.

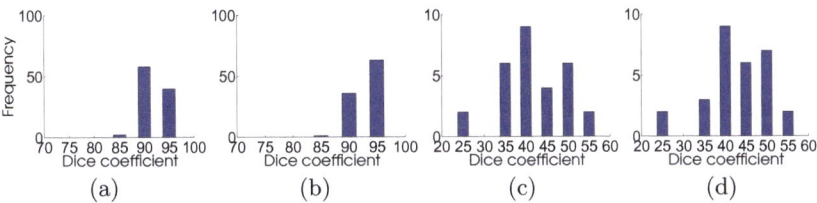

Fig. 6. Histogram of dice coefficients for the (a) middle region, graph cuts with hard constraints, (b) middle region, soft constraints, (c) heart wall, graph cuts with hard constraints, (d) heart wall, soft constraints

References

1. McGann, C.J., Kholmovski, E.G., Oakes, R.S., Blauer, J.J., Daccarett, M., Segerson, N., Airey, K.J., Akoum, N., Fish, E., Badger, T.J., DiBella, E.V., Parker, D., MacLeod, R.S., Marrouche, N.F.: New magnetic resonance imaging-based method for defining the extent of left atrial wall injury after the ablation of atrial fibrillation. J. American College of Cardiology 52(15), 1263–1271 (2008)
2. John, M., Rahn, N.: Automatic left atrium segmentation by cutting the blood pool at narrowings. In: Duncan, J.S., Gerig, G. (eds.) MICCAI 2005. LNCS, vol. 3750, pp. 798–805. Springer, Heidelberg (2005)
3. Karim, R., Mohiaddin, R., Rueckert, D.: Left atrium segmentation for atrial fibrillation ablation. In: SPIE Conference Series, vol. 6918 (2008)
4. Malladi, R., Sethian, J., Vemuri, B.: Shape modeling with front propagation: a level set approach. IEEE Transactions on PAMI 17(2), 158–175 (1995)
5. Cootes, T., Taylor, C., Cooper, D., Graham, J.: Active shape models-their training and application. Computer Vision and Image Understanding 61(1), 38–59 (1995)
6. Gao, Y., Gholami, B., MacLeod, R., Blauer, J., Haddad, W., Tannenbaum, A.: Segmentation of the endocardial wall of the left atrium using local region-based active contours and statistical shape learning. In: SPIE, vol. 7623 (2010)
7. Wu, X., Chen, D.Z.: Optimal net surface problems with applications. In: Widmayer, P., Triguero, F., Morales, R., Hennessy, M., Eidenbenz, S., Conejo, R. (eds.) ICALP 2002. LNCS, vol. 2380, pp. 1029–1042. Springer, Heidelberg (2002)
8. Li, K., Wu, X., Chen, D., Sonka, M.: Optimal surface segmentation in volumetric images-a graph-theoretic approach. PAMI 28(1), 119–134 (2006)
9. Dou, X., Wu, X., Wahle, A., Sonka, M.: Globally optimal surface segmentation using regional properties of segmented objects. In: CVPR, pp. 1–8. IEEE (2008)
10. Song, Q., Wu, X., Liu, Y., Smith, M., Buatti, J., Sonka, M.: Optimal graph search segmentation using arc-weighted graph for simultaneous surface detection of bladder and prostate. In: Yang, G.-Z., Hawkes, D., Rueckert, D., Noble, A., Taylor, C. (eds.) MICCAI 2009, Part II. LNCS, vol. 5762, pp. 827–835. Springer, Heidelberg (2009)
11. Ishikawa, H.: Exact optimization for markov random fields with convex priors. PAMI 25(10), 1333–1336 (2003)
12. Meyer, M., Kirby, R., Whitaker, R.: Topology, accuracy, and quality of isosurface meshes using dynamic particles. IEEE TVCG 12(5), 1704–1711 (2007)
13. Amenta, N., Bern, M., Eppstein, D.: The crust and the beta-skeleton: Combinatorial curve reconstruction. Graphic Models Image Proc. 60(2), 125–135 (1998)

Using Region Trajectories to Construct an Accurate and Efficient Polyaffine Transform Model

Gang Song, Yang Liu, Baohua Wu, Brian Avants, and James C. Gee

Penn Image Computing and Science Lab,
University of Pennsylvania, Philadelphia, PA, USA
songgang@seas,liuyang@sas,baohua@seas,
avants@grasp,gee@mail.med.upenn.edu
http://picsl.upenn.edu

Abstract. In this paper we propose a novel way to construct a diffeo-morphic polyaffine model. Each affine transform is defined on a local region and the resulting diffeomorphism encapsulates all the local transforms by a smooth and invertible displacement field. Compared with traditional weighting schemes used in combining local transforms, our new scheme guarantees that the resulting transform precisely preserves the value of each local affine transform. By introducing the trajectory of local regions instead of using regions themselves, the new approach encodes precisely each local affine transform using a diffeomorphism with one or more stationary velocity fields. Experiments show that our new polyaffine model is both accurate and efficient.

Keywords: Polyaffine, Transform, Diffeomorphism.

1 Introduction

The transform models applied in image registration have a wide span of degrees of freedom. The transform can be as simple as an affine transform [1], which is a linear function defined on the whole image domain and only requires 12 scalar parameters for an image of three dimensions. In contrast, one can also use a deformation field as the transform in a non-rigid image registration [2, 3], which has an arbitrary number of degrees of freedom at the cost of expensive computation and difficult optimization. Between these extremes of parameterization, many other transforms have been studied, such as B-Splines used in free-form deformation [4], Geodesic Interpolating Splines [5] and finite element method [6]. These transforms are capable of describing a wide range of non-rigid transforms while using fewer parameters than a dense displacement field.

The polyaffine transform is a parameterization for deformable maps that fills the gap between a global affine transform and a deformation field transform. It exploits the prior knowledge that for many applications of medical image registration, the underlying anatomical structure is comprised of multiple local

J.C. Gee et al. (Eds.): IPMI 2013, LNCS 7917, pp. 668–679, 2013.
© Springer-Verlag Berlin Heidelberg 2013

regions. An example of two lobes moving in different directions is illustrated in Fig. 1. Each local region is roughly rigid and can be approximated by a different local affine transform. The Polyaffine transform is a mathematical framework that fuses the local affine transforms through one non-rigid transform. Among different approaches like the piecewise affine transform [7, 8], a Log-Educlidean framework was first proposed in [9] especially to construct a smooth and invertible diffeomorphism, which can also be computed efficiently. This framework has been adopted in multiple image registration applications [9–13].

The key concept in [9] is to construct a stationary velocity field by fusing multiple regions with different affine velocity. The stationary velocity field is further integrated over time to generate an invertible transform. The construction method used in [9], however, as discussed in Section 2, cannot guarantee that the resulting final transform gives the exact same value of the input transforms in each local region 2. Our work reformulates the polyaffine transform as finding a feasible solution to a constrained problem. This new approach guarantees the local affine transformations are preserved. To achieve this, we demonstrate that the weight function used to fuse affine velocities has to be defined using a time-varying function in the framework of diffeomorphisms. The trajectory of each local affine region is proposed for computing the weight function in modeling a time-varying diffeomorphism with a series of stationary diffeomorphic transforms. With this new concept of region trajectory, our approach preserves each local transform and remains efficient in its implementation.

2   Methods

Consider a set of K affine transforms, $T_i(x) = A_i x + b_i$, each defined on a local region M_i. We want to integrate these local transforms into one transform $\phi(x)$ defined on the whole image domain Ω. For simplicity, these K local regions are subregions of Ω and do not overlap with each other. The polyaffine problem can be formulated as finding a feasible solution $\phi(x) : \Omega \to \Omega$ satisfying the constraints

$$\phi(x) = A_i x + b_i \text{ , when } x \in M_i \tag{1}$$

A direct way to construct such a ϕ is by simply averaging each local affine transform using a weight function w_i as in [14]: $\phi(x) = \sum_{i=1}^{K} w_i(x) T_i(x)$. A popular choice of weighting function is defined by the distance from the point x to each mask M_i: $w_i(x) \propto \exp(-\frac{\text{dist}(x, M_i)}{\sigma^2})$. Then the K weights $w_i(x)$ computed on the location x are further normalized such that $\sum_i w_i(x) = 1$.

This transform is smooth in the sense of its deformation gradient. However, one significant drawback is that it is not invertible in general [9]. To obtain the invertibility, i.e. making ϕ a diffeomorphism, the velocity field $v(x, t)$ was introduced in constructing ϕ in [9].

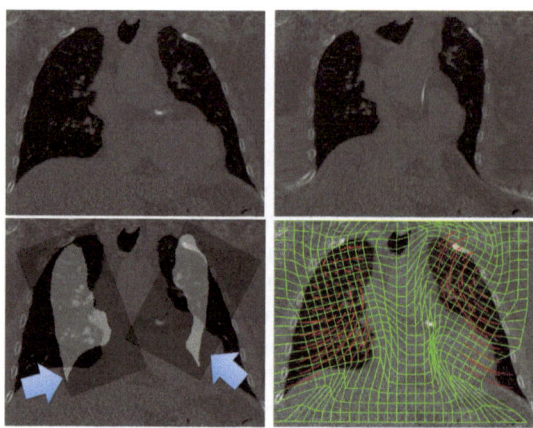

Fig. 1. Computed tomography images of two lung lobes moving in different directions. Top row: images before/after applying the transform. Bottom row: the two local affine transforms and the computed polyaffine transform using the proposed approach.

2.1   Diffeomorphism in Polyaffine Model

A diffeomorphism ϕ can be obtained by solving the ordinary differential equation over a time variable t:

$$\frac{\mathrm{d}\phi(x,t)}{\mathrm{d}t} = v(\phi(x,t),t) \tag{2}$$

At time $t = 1$, the diffeomorphism $\phi(x,1)$ can be obtained by integrating the velocity field $v(x,t)$ over time from $t = 0$ to 1. The affine transform $T(x) = Ax+b$ is an example of such a diffeomorphism. Using homogenous coordinates, an affine transform can be generated by a velocity field v [9]:

$$v(x,t) = Lx + u \text{ , with } \begin{bmatrix} L & u \\ 0 & 0 \end{bmatrix} = \log\left(\begin{bmatrix} A & b \\ 0 & 1 \end{bmatrix}\right) \tag{3}$$

Arsigny et al. proposed in [9] to first construct a velocity field v by fusing the K local affine velocity fields:

$$v(x) = \sum_i w_i(x)v_i(x), \text{ with } v_i(x) = L_ix + u_i, w_i(x) \propto \exp\left(-\frac{\mathrm{dist}(x,M_i)}{\sigma^2}\right) \tag{4}$$

It should be noted that here $v(x)$ is independent of t, i.e. $v(x) = v(x,t)$. Thus it is a stationary velocity field. To integrate ϕ from the velocity field v, a general approach is to discretize time from $t = 0$ to 1 into N time points. In the special case when v is stationary, an efficient recursive scaling-and-squaring method was proposed in [9] to compute the total field in only $\log N$ steps.

2.2   Polyaffine Transform Preserving Trajectories

Introducing the velocity field v as the generator for the transform guarantees the invertibility of the final transform. This, however, adds a new constraint in

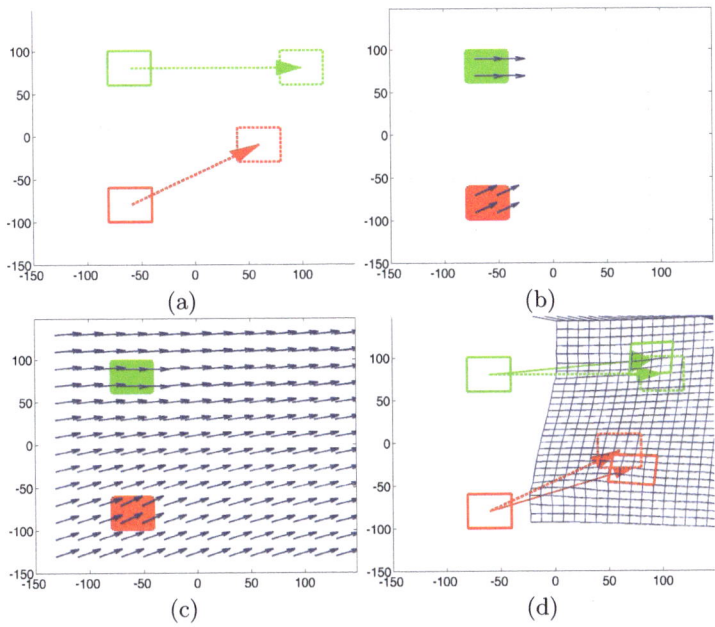

Fig. 2. Polyaffine transform using the previous approach [9]. (a) Two input affine transforms are shown in red and green. The starting and ending locations are indicated by the boxes in solid and dashed lines respectively. (b) The input local regions (shown as red and green areas) for each transform with their velocity plotted inside. (c) Computed velocity field using Eqn. 4, interpolated from the input local regions. (d) The resulting transform. The ending locations of each local region are plotted as boxes in solid lines at the arrow heads. The solid arrows (the result) deviate from the dashed arrows (the input), showing that local transforms are not preserved precisely.

finding a feasible solution to Eqn. 1. Instead of requiring the resulting transform $\phi(x)$ to match each local affine transform $T_i(x)$ within M_i at $t = 1$, it requires the velocity $v(x)$ to match each transform at all times from $t = 0$ to 1. Thus we can specialize the problem of Eqn. 1 into a more restricted one:

$$v(\phi(x,t),t) = v_i(\phi(x,t),t) \text{ for } x \in M_i \tag{5}$$

The solution of the new problem Eqn. 5 ensures that the whole temporal trajectory (from $t = 0$ to 1) for all x in M_i matches T_i. Indeed, given the uniqueness of the solution to the O.D.E of Eqn. 2, we have $\phi(x,t) = T_i(x,t)$ for $x \in M_i$ since $T_i(x) = A_i x + b_i$ is the solution when $v(\phi(x,t),t) = v_i(\phi(x,t),t)$. A natural solution of $\phi(x,t)$ in Eqn. 5 is to use a time-varying weight function to define the time-varying velocity field at any time t:

$$v(y,t) = \sum w_i(y,t)v_i(y) \text{ , with } y = \phi(x,t) \text{ and}$$
$$w_i(y,t) \propto \exp\left(-\frac{\text{dist}(y,\phi(M_i,t))}{\sigma^2}\right) \tag{6}$$

The weight $w_i(y,t)$ needs to be defined over t by tracking each M_i at time t, $\phi(M_i, t) = \{\phi(x,t), x \in M_i\}$. If a point $y = \phi(x,t)$ belongs to the i-th transform, the weight w_i should have:

$$w_i(y,t) = 1 \text{ and } w_{j \neq i}(y,t) = 0 \text{ for } x \in M_i . \tag{7}$$

This new definition of velocity field is different from the one used in [9], i.e. Eqn. 4, where it only matches v_i at time $t = 0$. The new definition of the weight w_i depends on t and needs to track the trajectory of the local mask M_i.

The definition in Eqn. 4 [9] could not guarantee that the velocity $v(\phi(x,t),t)$ is still dominated by T_i when a point $x \in M_i$ at $t = 0$ moves to a new location $\phi(x,t)$ at time t. Thus it could not preserve the trajectory of each local affine region. This makes it an inviable solution to Eqn. 5 (illustrated in Fig. 2).

2.3   Extend Local Region to Trajectory of Local Region

Although Eqn. 6 gives a feasible solution to Eqn. 5, it also eliminates the nice property of stationary velocity and is inefficient in computation. We propose a novel way to define a stationary velocity field v which still satisfies Eqn. 5. Define the trajectory of the region M_i from time t_1 to t_2 as notation $M_i^*|_{t_1}^{t_2} = \cup_{\tau=t_1}^{t_2} \phi(M_i, \tau)$.

Without loss of generality, we first assume that these region trajectories do not overlap in the spatial domain Ω. Define a new stationary weighting function $w(x)$ independent of t:

$$v(y) = \sum w_i(y)v_i(y) \tag{8}$$
$$\text{with } w_i(y) \propto \text{dist}(y, M_i^*|_0^1)$$

Since for $i \neq j$, $M_i^*|_0^1 \cap M_j^*|_0^1 = \varnothing$, for $x \in M_i$ we have $\text{dist}(\phi(x,t), M_i^*|_0^1) = 0$ and $\text{dist}(\phi(x,t), M_{j \neq i}^*|_0^1) \gg 0$. Thus the new stationary $w(x)$ still satisfies the same property of the time-varying version of $w_i(x,t)$ in Eqn. 7: $w_i(T_i(x,t)) = 1$ and $w_{i \neq j}(T_i(x,t)) = 0$ for $x \in M_i$. By introducing the region trajectory $M_i^*|_0^1$, the proposed stationary weight w_i gives the same ϕ as the time-varying version in Eqn. 6. The only difference between the two resulting ϕ is in the intermediate areas outside of $\cup_{i=1}^K M_i$.

When comparing the proposed stationary weight in Eqn. 8 and its generalized time-varying version in Eqn. 6, one should notice that $w(y,t)$ in Eqn. 6 is defined on the spatial-temporal domain $\Omega \times [0,1]$, while $w(y)$ in Eqn. 8 is a "squeezed version" that collapses the region trajectory M_i^* along the temporal axis into the spatial domain. The result using the proposed weight for the case in Fig. 2 is shown in Fig. 3, where our solution clearly preserves the input affine transform.

2.4   Series of Stationary Velocity Field for Trajectory Collision

One critical assumption in eliminating t from Eqn. 6 is that all trajectories $M_i^*|_0^1$ do not overlap in the spatial domain, $M_i^*|_0^1 \cap M_j^*|_0^1 = \varnothing$. Otherwise it will be

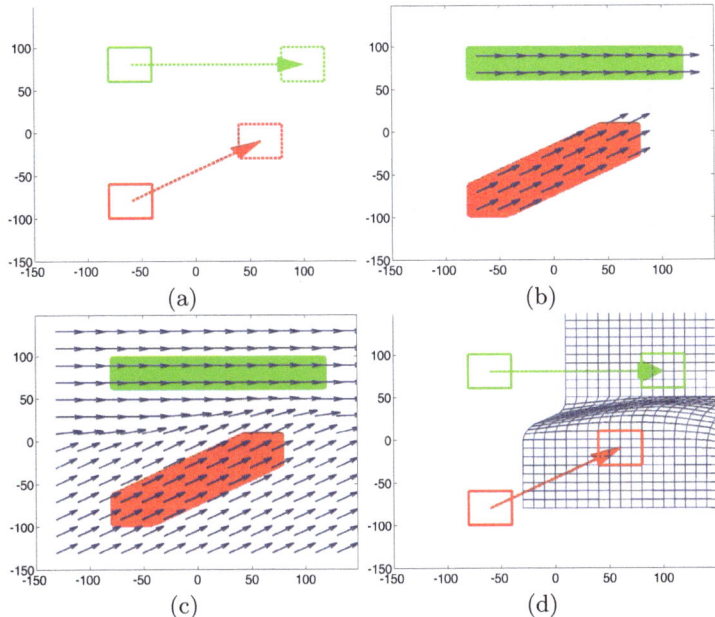

Fig. 3. Polyaffine transform using our proposed method. (a) Two input affine trans-forms (same as in Fig.2(a)) are shown in red and green. The starting and ending locations are indicated by the boxes in solid and dashed lines respectively. (b) The tra-jectories of the input local regions (shown as red and green areas) for each transform with their velocity plotted inside. (c) Computed velocity field using Eqn. 8, interpolated from the input region trajectories. (d) The resulting transform. The ending locations of each local region are plotted as boxes in solid lines at the arrow heads. The solid arrows (the result) are overlapped with the dashed arrows (the input), showing that local transforms are preserved precisely.

ambiguous to determine which local affine transform should be used when a point y belongs to multiple trajectories.

This non-collision assumption is nevertheless not true in general. Consider two local affine transforms T_1 and T_2 in Fig. 4, defined on region M_1 and M_2 respectively. The end of trajectory of M_1, $T_1(M_1)$, is overlapped with the starting position of M_2. In this case, for point y inside $T_1(M_1) \cup M_2$, it is ambiguous to define its weight $w_i(y)$ using Eqn. 8.

Our solution to this dilemma is to find a period from time t_1 to t_2 so that the trajectories within this period are not overlapped. By the time $t = 1$ when M_1 moves to $T_1(M_1)$, M_2 also moves to $T_2(M_2)$ and $T_1(M_1) \cap T_2(M_2) = \varnothing$. In general we need at any time $\tau_1, \tau_2 \in [t_1, t_2]$, no local regions are overlapped, $\phi(M_i, \tau_1) \cap \phi(M_j, \tau_2) = \varnothing$. When these trajectories are disjoint in the spatial-temporal domain, such $[t_1, t_2]$ is feasible. Thus it is possible to break the time from 0 to 1 into a sequence of $C + 1$ time points $[t_0, \ldots, t_C]$, such that

$$t_0 = 0 \text{ and } t_{k+1} = \max_{\tau} \{\tau | M_i^*|_{t_k}^\tau \cap M_j^*|_{t_k}^\tau = \varnothing, \forall i \neq j\} \qquad (9)$$

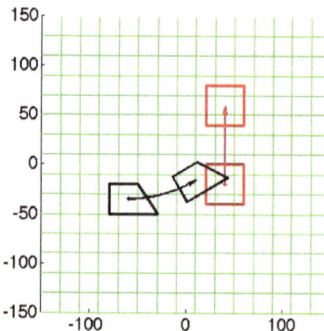

Fig. 4. The trajectories of two local regions overlap. Each arrow represents an input local transform, plotted in black and red. The boxes at the arrow tails are the starting locations of each input transform; the boxes at the heads are the ending locations.

For each non-collision period $[t_{k-1}, t_k]$, a stationary velocity v^k and its associated weight function are defined in the same way as in Eqn. 8. For each stationary velocity v^k, its transform ϕ^k is computed using the efficient scaling-and-squaring method in [9]. The final transform ϕ is the concatenation of these C diffeomorphism transforms and is also a diffeomorphism: $\phi = \phi^C \circ \cdots \circ \phi^2 \circ \phi^1$.

3   Implementation

We have proposed the notion of region trajectory to construct the polyaffine model. Unlike previous models, our polyaffine transform guarantees that the final transform is the exact value of $T_i(x)$ in each individual local region M_i. Before we discuss some of our implementation details, here is the summary of the construction steps:

1. Compute the collision time points $\{t_0 = 0, t_1, \ldots, t_C = 1\}$ using Eqn. 9.
2. Construct the stationary velocity v^k for each collision period $t = t_{k-1}$ to t_k.
3. Compute the corresponding diffeomorphism ϕ^k from v^k.
4. Concatenate all ϕ^k to get the final diffeomorphism ϕ.

3.1   Choice of Weight Function

A common practice to define the weight function $w_i(x)$ is to use the distance between the point x to the region M_i [9], or its trajectory M_i^* in our case. The weight is computed using a Gaussian function [9], or other decreasing functions [10]. The weights are further normalized by scale so that $\sum_i w_i(x) = 1$.

There are two drawbacks of using directly $\text{dist}(x, M_i^*)$. The first is a practical issue. For x in M_i^*, its distance to the j-th transform region trajectory cannot be infinite, and $w_{j \neq i}(x)$ is in general a small, nonzero scalar after

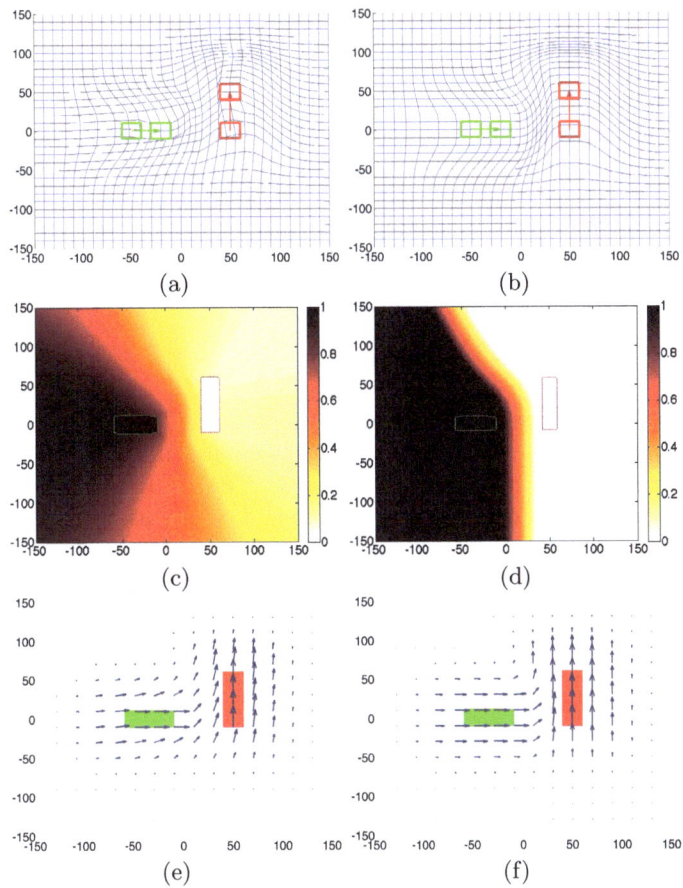

Fig. 5. Comparison of the transforms computed using (a,c,e) dist(x, M_i^*), and (b,d,f) dist$(x, \partial \overline{M}_i^*)$. (a,b) The transforms are constructed from the same input, one horizontal translation (green arrow) and one vertical translation (red arrow). (b) is visually more smooth than (a). (c,d) The weights $w(x)$ for the local vertical translation, range in $[0,1]$. (d) is more polarized except along boundary $\partial \overline{M}_i^*$. (e,f) The resulting velocity below the green trajectory has an upward vertical component in (e) but not in (f). Similar effects are seen on the right of the red trajectory. M_i^* are shown as green and red dotted boundaries in (c,d) and solid areas in (e,f).

normalization. Some arbitrary thresholding needs to be performed to approximate $w_{j \neq i}(x) = 0$. Finding a suitable σ in the Gaussian function for different regions is also arbitrary.

The second drawback is that such a distance does not consider the relative spatial configuration of different region trajectories. For example, in Fig. 5(b), there are two local transforms. One is a horizontal translation (on left), and the other is a vertical translation (on right). By examining the vertical component of the velocity field below the horizontal trajectory, it can be seen that there is some upward vertical velocity component, which comes from the small weights on the right vertical translation. Ideally, there should be no such vertical velocity around this region since the vertical velocity should be *blocked* by the horizontal trajectory on its left.

To eliminate this drawback, we propose a new weighting scheme by dividing the image into subdomains. The subdomains $\{\overline{M_i^*}\}$ are a partition of the whole image domain Ω. The subdomain $\overline{M_i^*}$ can be viewed as the region of influence of the trajectory M_i^* in the center. Based on this intuition, we use the distance to each trajectory to define the subdomain $\overline{M_i^*}$ as the the area containing all the points closer to M_i^* than other trajectories:

$$\overline{M_i^*} = \{x \in \Omega | \text{dist}(x, M_i^*) = \min_{j=1...K} \text{dist}(x, M_j^*)\} \tag{10}$$

Such a definition partitions the whole image domain Ω into K disjoint subdomains. The proposed weight is correspondingly defined by the distance from the point x to the boundary of the subdomain $\overline{M_i^*}$. If x is close to the boundary, the weights should be nonzero for all adjacent local transforms. If x is in the center and far away from the boundary, its weight should be polarized. Note that $\text{d}(x) = \text{dist}(x, \partial \overline{M_i^*})$, and σ is a constant. We can define w_i before normalization using a simple piecewise linear function.

$$w_i(x) \propto \begin{cases} 1 & \text{if } x \in \overline{M_i^*} \text{ and } \text{d}(x) > \sigma \\ 0.5 + \text{d}(x)/2\sigma & \text{if } x \in \overline{M_i^*} \text{ and } 0 \le \text{d}(x) < \sigma \\ 0.5 - \text{d}(x)/2\sigma & \text{if } x \notin \overline{M_i^*} \text{ and } 0 \le \text{d}(x) < \sigma \\ 0 & \text{if } x \notin \overline{M_i^*} \text{ and } \text{d}(x) > \sigma \end{cases} \tag{11}$$

An example of the computed weight function and the resulting transforms on two local affine transforms is illustrated in Fig. 5. Such a weighting scheme takes consideration of the relative position of each trajectory mask. Along the boundaries of the subdomains are the locations where the weighting matters most, while inside each subdomain it is dominated by one local transform. This can be viewed as an efficient approximate solution to the following equation:

$$w_i^* = \min \int \|\nabla w_i\|^2 dx, \text{where } w_i(x) = 1 \text{ for } x \in M_i \text{ and } w_i(x) = 0 \text{ for } x \in M_{j \ne i} \tag{12}$$

In one extreme case when each local region is one point and uniformly distributed, such a partition becomes the Voronoi diagram on the image domain if time $t = 0$ is only considered.

3.2 Computing Mask Trajectories and Their Collision

Another important implementation detail is how to efficiently compute each region trajectory M_i^* given its predefined velocity $v_i(x) = L_i x + u_i$. This is trivial when M_i is just a single point. However, when M_i is a region, there could be multiple trajectories. When a region can be efficiently parameterized as a polyhedron, one can track the trajectory of each vertex and compute the collision of any two polyhedra. Here we instead choose a simpler approximation by using a random point set to represent an arbitrary region.

For a region M, a point set $\{p_a\}$ is uniformly sampled inside using a sampling diameter d. The region can be then approximated by the union of dilations from the point set $\{p_a\}$ with distance d. The region M transformed at time t, $T(M, t)$, is also approximated by the dilation of the point set $\{T(p_a, t)\}$. The condition of collision detection in Eqn. 9 is implemented using:

$$M_i^*|_{t_1}^{t_2} \cap M_j^*|_{t_1}^{t_2} = \varnothing \Leftrightarrow \min_{\tau_i = t_1}^{t_2} \min_{\tau_j = t_1}^{t_2} \min_{a,b} \text{dist}(T_i(p_{i,a}, \tau_i), T_j(p_{j,b}, \tau_j)) < d \quad (13)$$

One interesting fact about the distance between the two point trajectories of a local affine region is that it is well bounded by a convex function of time variable t when the region deforms over time. For simplicity without using extra notations in the homogenous coordinates, suppose L is the logarithm of the affine matrix A (see Eqn. 3), we have $T(x, t) = \exp(tL)x$. We have the following theorem.

Theorem 1. $f(t) = \| \exp(tL)(p - q) \|$ *is bounded by a convex function for a given matrix L and any two points p and q.*

Proof 1

$$\| \exp(tL)(p-q) \| \leq \| \sum_{n=0}^{} \frac{(tL)^n}{n!} \| \|p-q\| \leq \sum_{n=0}^{} \frac{(t\|L\|)^n}{n!} \|p-q\| = \exp(t\|L\|)\|p-q\|$$

This bound ensures that if a sampling diameter d is small enough, the dilation of the point set $\{T(p, t)\}$ at time t should cover the mask $T(M, t)$ and thus is a good approximation.

4   Results

We evaluated the accuracy of our proposed approach using synthetic experiments. Two translation transforms were defined on two rectangular regions, similar to the inputs in Fig. 5. A scalar $r \in [0, 1]$ was used to control the relative range of the translation offset, $t_1 = r \times [100, 0]$ and $t_2 = r \times [0, 50]$. When $r = 0$, they were identity transforms; when r increased, the two affine trajectories overlap. The accuracy was evaluated by the difference between the resulting transform and the corresponding affine transform for each pixel in all regions, $e(x) = \|\phi(x) - (A_i x + t_i)\|$. The mean and variance of all $e(x)$ for $x \in M_1 \cup M_2$ were computed versus r.

We compared our proposed polyaffine construction using the region trajectory with the approach in [9] as the baseline, where the weight was computed based on the region only. When the translation was relatively small ($r < 0.3$), both methods had a good accuracy. However, when the translation increased, the error in the baseline method also increased quickly since the region trajectories became significantly different from the regions. In contrast, our approach still maintained a high accuracy with near-zero error. Similar results could be observed when comparing the case of two rotation transforms by changing the rotation angles (Fig. 4(b)).

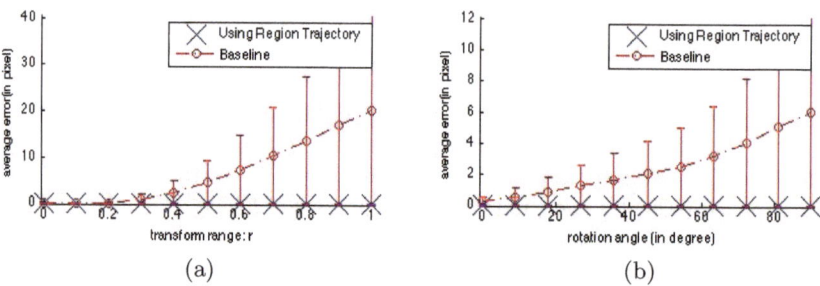

Fig. 6. Comparison of our proposed method and the baseline method [9], using (a) two local translation transforms and (b) two local rotation transforms. The x-axis corresponds to (a) the translation offset, or (b) the rotation angle. The y-axis corresponds to the average error of the resulting transforms in the local affine regions, with standard deviations plotted as error bars.

5   Discussion

In this work we presented a novel approach to constructing a polyaffine transform which can precisely preserve each affine transform using one diffeomorphism. The polyaffine problem is formulated as finding a feasible solution with a new constraint that preserves the affine trajectories of each local region. The natural solution uses a time-varying weight function, which is time and memory consuming in implementation. Our approach instead uses a composition of one or more diffeomorphisms of stationary velocities and is thus both efficient in computation and accurate in preserving the new constraints.

The key in constructing our weight function is to use the trajectory of each local region, instead of the region itself, to define the fusion weight for each local transform. In the case [9] when only the region is used in defining the weight, the affine velocity is only preserved at time $t = 0$. This may lead to inaccuracy in meeting the constraints. In contrast, our new approach preserves the affine velocity for any time t, and therefore preserves the affine transform.

Depending on the values of input affine transform and their regions, our approach requires one or more stationary velocity fields to preserve different affine velocities in each region over time. The number of stationary velocity fields are determined by the collision detection of region trajectories when collapsing them along the temporal direction. One real-life analogy to such a scheme is the traffic lights in an intersection. When two trajectories are overlapped at the intersection, a traffic light will indicate when the points along one direction should stop to allow the points along the other to pass the intersection, which solves the ambiguity in defining the velocity function at the intersection. Note that depending on the input affine transforms, there might be no collision and just one stationary velocity is enough.

References

1. Jenkinson, M., Smith, S.: A global optimisation method for robust affine registration of brain images. Medical Image Analysis 5(2), 143–156 (2001)
2. Thirion, J.P.: Image matching as a diffusion process: an analogy with maxwell's demons. Medical Image Analysis 2(3), 243–260 (1998)
3. Beg, M.F., Miller, M.I., Trouv, A., Younes, L.: Computing large deformation metric mappings via geodesic flows of diffeomorphisms. International Journal of Computer Vision 61(2), 139–157 (2005)
4. Rueckert, D., Sonoda, L., Hayes, C., Hill, D., Leach, M., Hawkes, D.: Nonrigid registration using free-form deformations: application to breast MR images. IEEE Transactions on Medical Imaging 18(8), 712–721 (1999)
5. Camion, V., Younes, L.: Geodesic interpolating splines. In: Figueiredo, M., Zerubia, J., Jain, A.K. (eds.) EMMCVPR 2001. LNCS, vol. 2134, pp. 513–527. Springer, Heidelberg (2001)
6. Ferrant, M., Warfield, S.K., Guttmann, C.R.G., Mulkern, R.V., Jolesz, F.A., Kikinis, R.: 3D image matching using a finite element based elastic deformation model. In: Taylor, C., Colchester, A. (eds.) MICCAI 1999. LNCS, vol. 1679, pp. 202–209. Springer, Heidelberg (1999)
7. Little, J., Hill, D., Hawkes, D.: Deformations incorporating rigid structures. Computer Vision and Image Understanding 66(2), 223–232 (1997)
8. Pitiot, A., Bardinet, E., Thompson, P.M., Malandain, G.: Piecewise affine registration of biological images for volume reconstruction. Medical Image Analysis 10(3), 465–483 (2006)
9. Arsigny, V., Commowick, O., Ayache, N., Pennec, X.: A fast and log-euclidean polyaffine framework for locally linear registration. Journal of Mathematical Imaging and Vision 33(2), 222–238 (2009)
10. Commowick, O., Arsigny, V., Isambert, A., Costa, J., Dhermain, F., Bidault, F., Bondiau, P.Y., Ayache, N., Malandain, G.: An efficient locally affine framework for the smooth registration of anatomical structures. Medical Image Analysis 12(4), 427–441 (2008)
11. Taquet, M., Macq, B., Warfield, S.K.: Spatially adaptive log-euclidean polyaffine registration based on sparse matches. In: Fichtinger, G., Martel, A., Peters, T. (eds.) MICCAI 2011, Part II. LNCS, vol. 6892, pp. 590–597. Springer, Heidelberg (2011)
12. Seiler, C., Pennec, X., Reyes, M.: Geometry-aware multiscale image registration via OBBTree-based polyaffine log-demons. In: Fichtinger, G., Martel, A., Peters, T. (eds.) MICCAI 2011, Part II. LNCS, vol. 6892, pp. 631–638. Springer, Heidelberg (2011)
13. Seiler, C., Pennec, X., Reyes, M.: Simultaneous multiscale polyaffine registration by incorporating deformation statistics. In: Ayache, N., Delingette, H., Golland, P., Mori, K. (eds.) MICCAI 2012, Part II. LNCS, vol. 7511, pp. 130–137. Springer, Heidelberg (2012)
14. Shepard, D.: A two-dimensional interpolation function for irregularly-spaced data. In: Proceedings of the 1968 23rd ACM National Conference, ACM 1968, pp. 517–524. ACM, New York (1968)

Extracting Evolving Pathologies via Spectral Clustering

Elena Bernardis, Kilian M. Pohl, and Christos Davatzikos

Section of Biomedical Image Analysis, Department of Radiology,
University of Pennsylvania, Philadelphia, PA 19104

Abstract. A bottleneck in the analysis of longitudinal MR scans with white matter brain lesions is the temporally consistent segmentation of the pathology. We identify pathologies in 3D+t(ime) within a spectral graph clustering framework. Our clustering approach simultaneously segments and tracks the evolving lesions by identifying characteristic image patterns at each time-point and voxel correspondences across time-points. For each 3D image, our method constructs a graph where weights between nodes capture the likeliness of two voxels belonging to the same region. Based on these weights, we then establish rough correspondences between graph nodes at different time-points along estimated pathology *evolution directions*. We combine the graphs by aligning the weights to a reference time-point, thus integrating temporal information across the 3D images, and formulate the 3D+t segmentation problem as a binary partitioning of this graph. The resulting segmentation is very robust to local intensity fluctuations and yields better results than segmentations generated for each time-point.

Keywords: 4D segmentation, longitudinal tracking, MRI white matter lesion.

1 Introduction

The diagnosis of white matter brain lesions often involves the analysis of longitudinal MR brain scans. This type of analysis can greatly benefit from accurately segmenting the lesions across the scans. However, the task is difficult to perform when done for each time-point individually as lesions are often hard to detect. They might appear very faint and white matter might be erroneously identified as lesions due to intensity fluctuations. These issues can be minimized by considering all time-points during segmentation, as lesions show up more clearly at later time-points and intensity fluctuations of white matter are not consistent across time-points. We propose an algorithm to extract 3D+t lesions by simultaneously capturing structural and temporal consistency in a spectral-graph framework.

While several 3D+t methods for temporally consistent healthy tissue segmentation [7,13,5,8,15] and for 3D lesion extraction [12,6,11,1] have been proposed in the literature, few approaches have been explored to study longitudinal lesion changes [14,9]. An atlas of a healthy population is often relied upon both for the temporally consistent segmentation of healthy tissues of adult brains [8], as well as for 3D lesion segmentation, which generally flag lesions as outliers. These outliers are detected by first estimating intensity distributions for the pathology and then incorporating contextual information in the classification [12], computing spatial posterior probabilities of each tissue in a

J.C. Gee et al. (Eds.): IPMI 2013, LNCS 7917, pp. 680–691, 2013.

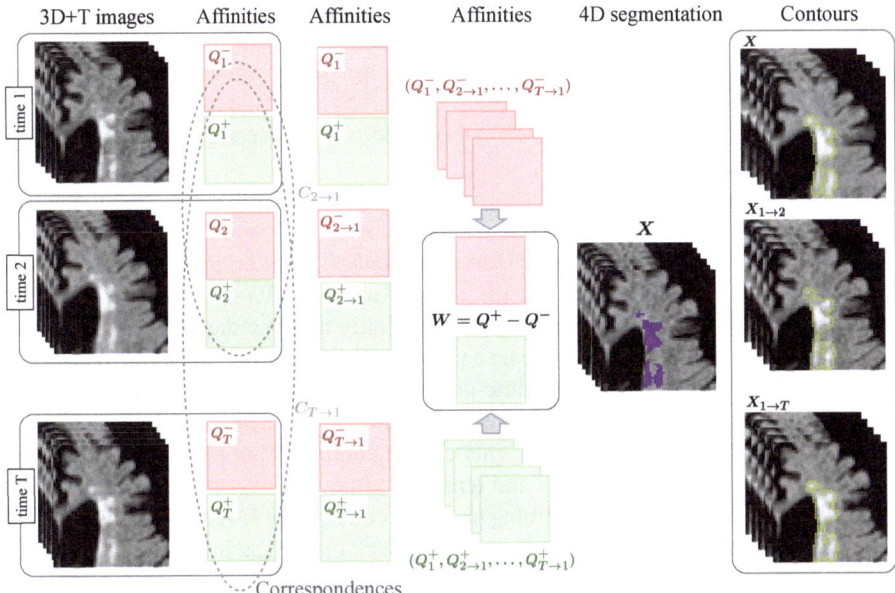

Fig. 1. Method Overview. First, we construct pairwise affinities Q_t^+ and Q_t^- for each 3D image I_t to capture the characteristic patterns of lesions vs. background. Second, we compute rough correspondences C between time-points by finding best affinities' matches. Affinities are then aligned to the first-time point and combined into one affinity matrix W, which now carries both structural and temporal information. Finally, we use spectral clustering to find the final 3D+t partition X, which is then back-projected to each I_t.

Bayesian framework [6], or adding topological constraints in addition to the statistical atlases [11]. Alternatively, [1] uses k-nearest neighbors classification to generate a label map outlining lesions. Adapting these lesion segmentation methods to the temporal domain is not straightforward as not only the lesions have to be interpreted as abnormal tissue not captured by the atlas, but their appearance across time-points has also to be taken into account. Alternatively, extensions to integrate spatial and temporal information in 3D+t lesion models include characterizing lesions by building a spatio-temporal lesion evolution model [14], or capturing implicit lesion information at each voxel by first computing displacement fields between time-points and then clustering the evolving lesions based on vector field operators [9].

We propose a method that does not rely on comparisons to healthy tissue, and that seamlessly integrates the lesion segmentation and tracking steps into one principled approach. We base our approach on spectral clustering [10,16], which has the ability to grasp the structural organization of an image from the global integration of local cues. Spectral clustering has been successfully used for the automatic segmentation of small, round structures (*e.g.* epithelial cells or lymphocytes) in 2D microscopic images [3], and extended to extract tubular structures in 3D microscopic images [4]. Images are represented by a graph, where nodes in the graph correspond to voxels in the image.

Weights associated to edges between graph nodes capture pair-wise affinities between voxels. Positive affinities indicate the likelihood of two voxels belonging to the same region while the opposite is true for negative affinities. By computing the top eigenvectors of this weight matrix, each voxel is represented by a point in the embedding space. The desired segmentation is obtained by straight-forward clustering of the voxels in this embedding space.

Our spectral graph method extracts lesions from longitudinal MR scans by defining grouping cues that distinguish lesions from healthy tissue. Specifically, we first construct pairwise affinities from each 3D image to characterize brighter regions of varying shapes and sizes. We then reduce the complexity of the 3D+t segmentation task by transforming it into a 3D one. We do so by explicitly tracking the graph nodes across time-points. For each node, we estimate a possible *evolution direction* of the pathology. Correspondences between adjacent time-points are then found by best affinities matching of the nodes along this direction. We use these correspondences to align each graph to a reference time-point, so that weights can be combined into one graph. This new graph now captures both structural and temporal affinities between nodes. To the best of our knowledge, this way of enforcing temporal consistency is very different in nature from any temporal consistent segmentation approach in medical imaging.

Our method is fully automatic and depends only on a few parameters. Additional time-points can be easily added to the graph as the method only requires computing the additional grouping cues at the new time-point as well as the projections to the previous one. Finally, our method is purely intensity-based and does not use any prior knowledge about the lesions other than that they are brighter than their background. While we test the approach only on longitudinal MR scans showing brain lesions, our method should be applicable to many other pathologies that full-fill these requirements.

2   Segmenting 3D+t Pathologies by Spectral Graph Partitioning

We segment lesions from 3D+t MR via a spectral graph theoretic framework. We assume the scans of each time are pose-corrected, so that across time-points healthy tissue remains constant and only the evolving pathology is changing.

An overview of our method is given in Fig. 1. For each time-point, we compute pairwise voxel affinities, called attraction Q_t^+ and repulsion Q_t^-, that capture differences between high and low intensity regions and whether two voxels might belong to a lesion region (Sec. 2.1). We then determine correspondences C_t between voxels at different time-points (Sec. 2.2) by tracking graph nodes. Given the correspondences, we map the affinities at each time-point to a reference to generate a new graph where weights now also carry temporal information (Sec. 2.3). The final 3D+t segmentation is found by partitioning this graph via spectral clustering (Sec. 2.4).

2.1   Creating a Graph for Each Time-Point: Computing Affinities in 3D

We start by constructing the graph $G_t(N, E, W_t)$ at each time point $t = 1, \ldots T$. Let I_t be the 3D scan associated with time-point t. Voxels of I_t are represented as nodes N in the graph and the $N \times N$ weight matrix W_t captures the affinity of the edges E

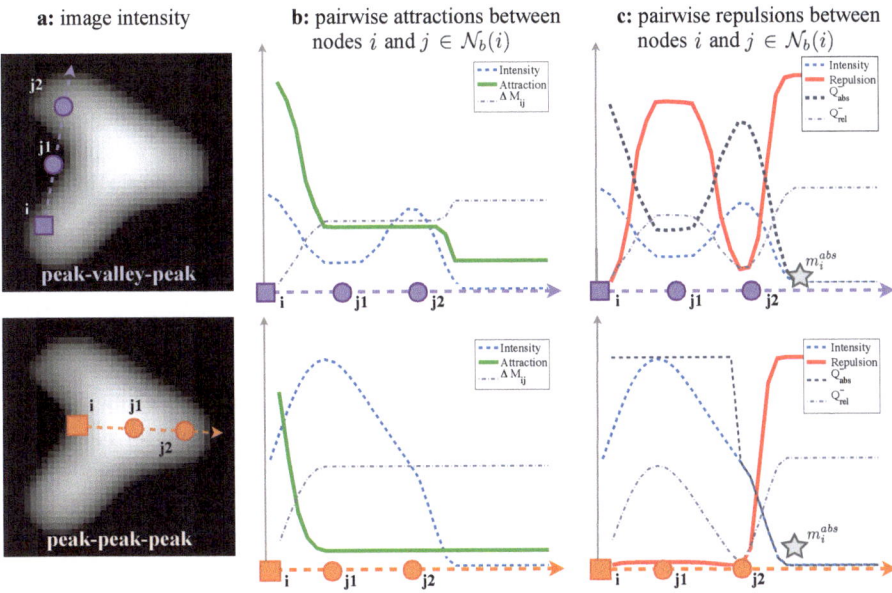

Fig. 2. Pairwise affinities. **a:** Image I_t with two neighboring nodes scenarios highlighted. In each case we plot, for $j \in \mathcal{N}_b(i)$, nodes at increasing radii of i along one direction b; **b:** intensities $I_t(j)$ (blue), maximum intensity differences ΔM_{ij} (gray) and final pairwise attractions $Q^+(i,j)$ (green). **c:** intensities I_j (blue) and final pairwise repulsions $Q^-(i,j)$ (red), computed as a function of relative and absolute repulsion terms $Q^-_{rel}(i,j)$ and $Q^-_{abs}(i,j)$ (both in gray). The absolute minimum m_i^{abs} (gray star) is only direction dependent so it remains constant for all $j \in \mathcal{N}_b(i)$.

between voxels. Affinities are composed of an attraction and a repulsion term, which we now define in further detail.

Attraction Q^+_t. Since lesions appear bright in Flair MR scans, attraction should be large between neighboring voxels with high and similar intensities. We measure this type of attraction between voxels (i, j) as a function of the maximum intensity difference $\Delta M_{ij} := \max_{s \in \text{line}(i,j)} |I_t(i) - I_t(s)|$ attained along the 3D line(i,j) connecting them, where $I_t(i)$ is the intensity at node i, and j is a node in i's neighborhood $\mathcal{N}(i) = \{j \in \mathcal{N}(i) | d(i,j) \leq r_a\}$ with attraction radius r_a. We then define the pairwise attraction $Q^+(i,j)$ between (i,j) as [2]:

$$Q^+_t(i,j) := \exp\left(-\frac{1}{\sigma_a^2}\left(\frac{\Delta M_{ij}}{\delta_i}\right)^2\right) \qquad (1)$$

where $\delta_i := |\max_{j \in \mathcal{N}(i)} I_j - \min_{j \in \mathcal{N}(i)} I_j|$ is the intensity range of the entire neighborhood $\mathcal{N}(i)$ and σ_a is a fixed parameter. Figure 2b visualizes $Q^+_t(i,j)$ and ΔM_{ij} along one sample line as j moves away from i. ΔM_{ij} enforces a decreasing affinity once j has passed the node with maximum intensity difference from i. Furthermore, scaling ΔM_{ij} by the neighborhood intensity range δ_i at each node effectively normalizes the affinities within each neighborhood. This scaling has also the effect of enhancing weaker intensity regions, thus allowing to capture faint regions near a salient one, which can be easily missed.

Repulsion Q_t^-. To extract brighter regions from the darker background, we add a repulsion term between background voxels and possible lesion ones. We denote high intensity regions by 'peaks' and low intensity regions by 'valleys'. Let the neighborhood of i be $\mathcal{N}(i) = \{j \in \mathcal{N}(i) | d(i, j) \leq r_r\}$ with repulsion radius r_r. A simple definition of repulsion between nodes i, j could be defined by their intensity difference:

$$Q_{rel}^-(i, j) := |I_t(j) - I_t(i)|. \tag{2}$$

Setting repulsion solely on Q_{rel}^- would ignore the relative location of i and j with respect to the peaks and valleys. We thus need to estimate whether i, j lie both on the same peak, both on peaks but are separated by a valley, or one on a peak and the other in a valley (illustrated in Fig. 2a). We achieve this by determining the minimum intensity $m_{ij}^{rel} := \min_{s \in \text{line}(i,j)} I_t(s)$ attained between i and j. We then measure for i and j the intensity difference to this minimum: $\Delta m_i := |I_t(i) - m_{ij}^{rel}|$ and $\Delta m_j := |I_t(j) - m_{ij}^{rel}|$ respectively. When the intensity of i is closer to the minimum compared to that of j, i.e. $\Delta m_i = \min(\Delta m_i, \Delta m_j)$, then the node i is adjacent to a region of higher intensity (since all nodes j are at higher intensity - as in the case of node i in the second row of Fig. 2), so we do not want i to repel its neighbors j. On the other hand, if j's intensity is closer, we then have the two possible scenarios illustrated in first row of Fig. 2 : peak(i)-valley(j_1) or peak(i)-valley-peak(j_2). In both cases, we want the repulsion term between i and j to capture the presence of the valley, *i.e.* a measure of the intensity drop attained between them. How much repulsion is added between these two nodes should depend on how much the intensity of node j differs from the absolute minimum intensity $m_i^{abs} := \min_{j \in \text{line}(i,k)} m_{ij}^{rel}$ (gray star in Fig. 2c) attained along the entire line (*i.e.* k is the farthest node along that direction line). We thus define:

$$Q_{abs}^-(i, j) := \begin{cases} |m_i^{abs} - I_t(j)| & \text{if } \Delta m_j = \min(\Delta m_i, \Delta m_j) \\ 1 & \text{otherwise.} \end{cases} \tag{3}$$

We can finally define the repulsion between nodes i, j as a function of Q_{rel}^-, weighted by a function of Q_{abs}^-:

$$Q_t^-(i, j) := \left[\exp\left(-\frac{1}{\sigma_{abs}^2} \left(\frac{Q_{abs}^-(i, j)}{\delta(i)} \right)^2 \right) \right] \left[1 - \exp\left(-\left(\frac{Q_{rel}^-(i, j)}{\sigma_{rel}} \right)^2 \right) \right] \tag{4}$$

where σ_{abs} and σ_{rel} are fixed parameters and δ_i is again the intensity range of the neighborhood $\mathcal{N}(i)$. Figure 2c illustrates how both $Q_{abs}^-(i, j)$ and $Q_t^-(i, j)$ vary for nodes lying on the same line with two different intensity scenarios. In the top row, we have the configuration peak(i)-valley(j_1) and peak(i)-valley-peak(j_2). In the bottom row, all three nodes i, j_1, j_2 belong to the same peak. The final repulsion $Q_t^-(i, j)$ is highlighted in a red.

The weights W_t at time-point t are then given by subtracting the repulsion Q_t^- from the attraction Q_t^+:

$$W_t = Q_t^+ - Q_t^-. \tag{5}$$

When repulsion is higher than the attraction between two nodes, the weights will have negative entries. This completes our definition of the graph G_t at time point t.

2.2 Establishing Correspondences between Time-Points

To combine the affinities computed at each time-point, we need to track the changes across the graphs $G_1, \ldots, G_T$. This is achieved in two steps. First, we compute the nodes' correspondences $C_{t \to t-1}$ from each time-point to the previous one. Then, we iteratively find the correspondences at each node to a reference time-point. We choose the first time-point as our reference for convenience since lesions only expand in time.

We start by finding the correspondences $C_{t \to t-1}$ to the previous time-point. Namely, for each for node i at time t, we find within the r_c radius neighborhood of i the node j at time $t-1$ whose affinities at $t-1$ best match the affinities of i at time t. To achieve this, we reformat the weights $W_t(i,:)$ of Eqn. 5 so that the affinities $W_t(i,:)$ at i can be written as a $1 \times J$ vector $W'_t(i,:)$, where J is the number of neighbors of i and entries in this vector correspond to the same neighborhood (relative) coordinates with respect to the center node i. Weights at each node are normalized by their outgoing connections, i.e. $\tilde{W}_t(i,:) = W'_t(i,:)[\sum_j W'_t(i,j)]^{-1}$. The correspondence of i to the previous time-point is then defined by the voxel which minimizes the dot product d between the corresponding normalized weights $\tilde{W}_t$:

$$C_{t \to t-1}(i) = \operatorname{argmin}_{j \in \mathcal{N}_e(i)} d(\tilde{W}_t(i,:), \tilde{W}_{t-1}(j,:)), \tag{6}$$

where we define the *eligible neighbors* $\mathcal{N}_e(i) \subset \mathcal{N}(i)$ based on the evolving direction of the lesion. Given that the contour of the lesion are closed, we can think of the contours always evolving along the normal of the contour. We therefore compute this direction based on the affinities W_t at each time-point.

Specifically, letting i_x, i_y, i_z be the 3D spatial coordinates of voxel i corresponding to node i, we define at each node the *evolution vector* $v_t(i) \in \mathbb{R}^3$:

$$v_t(i) = \sum_{j \in N(i)} W_t(i,j) \begin{pmatrix} j_x - i_x \\ j_y - i_y \\ j_z - i_z \end{pmatrix}. \tag{7}$$

For nodes near lesions, v_t will always point towards the center of the nearest highest intensity area, i.e. towards the interior of the lesion at that time-point. $\mathcal{N}_e(i)$ could be defined by nodes along $v_t(i)$ (for regions expanding from $t-1$ to t) or in the opposite direction $-v_t(i)$ (for regions contracting from $t-1$ to t). Since lesions only expand in time, we restrict $\mathcal{N}_e(i)$ to nodes in direction $v_t(i)$. Fig. 3a, shows sample vectors v_t.

Finally, we determine the correspondences at each node to the first time-point, setting $C_1(i) = i$, by iterating the following recursion:

$$C_{t \to 1}(i) = C_{t-1 \to 1}(C_{t \to t-1}(i)). \tag{8}$$

2.3 Graph Setup across Time-Points: Aligning Affinities

Once the correspondences $C_{t \to 1}$ have been computed, we can align the attraction and repulsion cues $Q_t^+(i,j)$ and $Q_t^-(i,j)$ computed in Sec. 2.1 to obtain the aligned graphs $G_{t \to 1}(N, E, W_{t \to 1})$. We compute the aligned attraction and repulsion, denoted by $Q_{t \to 1}^+$ and $Q_{t \to 1}^-$, separately to keep track of each cue's influence. For simplicity, we let $C_t(i) = C_{t \to 1}(i)$ in the remainder of this section.

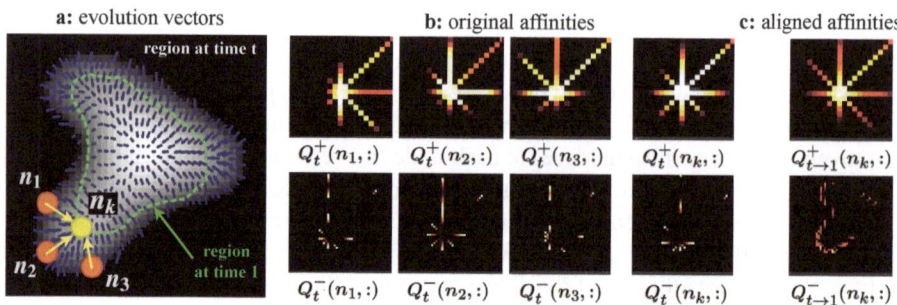

Fig. 3. Tracking temporal changes. **a:** Image I_t and *evolution vector* v_t at each node. Vectors for nodes n_1, n_2, n_3 are highlighted in yellow. For these nodes, we also illustrate on I_t, the corresponding node n_k at $t = 1$ (region boundary at $I_{t=1}$ traced in green); **b:** attraction Q_t^+ and repulsion Q_t^- for n_1, n_2, n_3, n_k; **c:** aligned attraction $Q_{t \to t-1}^+$ and repulsion $Q_{t \to t-1}^-$ at n_k.

One outstanding issue is what happens if multiple nodes at time t point to the same point at time 1, as well as those points at time 1 that have no correspondence at time t. We solve this issue by averaging as well as interpolating. For each node i that shifts to a new position k, i.e. $C_t(i) = k$ and $k = i$, we find all other nodes S that also shift to that location, i.e. $S = \{s \in S | C(s) = k\}$. A sample scenario is depicted in Fig. 3a. For each one, we obtain the aligned cues at the new node k by averaging the ones from the originating nodes (see Fig. 3b-c):

$$Q_{t \to 1}^{\pm}(C_t(i), :) = \frac{1}{|i \cup S|} \sum_{s \in \{i \cup S\}} Q_t^{\pm}(s, :).$$ (9)

For the remaining nodes, i.e. fixed nodes with $C_t(i) = i$ such that no other node maps to i (i.e. there are no other nodes s such that $C_t(s) = i$), we simply leave the affinities unchanged: $Q_{t \to 1}^{\pm}(i, :) = Q_t^{\pm}(i, :)$.

The cues can then be collapsed into one graph by normalizing attraction and repulsion separately and then combining them to obtain the final cues:

$$Q^{\pm} = \sum_{t=1}^{T} Q_{t \to 1}^{\pm} D_{Q_{t \to 1}^+}^{-1} + D_{Q_{t \to 1}^+}^{-1} Q_{t \to 1}^{\pm}$$ (10)

where D_Q is a diagonal matrix with entries $D(i, i) = \sum_j Q(i, j)$. We normalize each cue separately, to keep track of how they factor in at each node. The final weight matrix $W = Q^+ - Q^-$ contains pairwise affinities between nodes that capture both structural and temporal information between them.

2.4   Graph Segmentation via Spectral Clustering

We will now find the 3D+t segmentation X of our images by applying spectral partitioning on the constructed graph $G(N, E, W)$.

Spectral clustering is based on the following grouping criterion [16]:

$$\max \varepsilon = \frac{\text{within-group attraction}}{\text{total degree of attraction}} + \frac{\text{between-group repulsion}}{\text{total degree of repulsion}} \qquad (11)$$

Let the partition X of graph G be represented as a $N \times k$ binary matrix, so that $X(i, g)$ equals 1 if node i belongs to group g. The criterion can be then formulated in the following matrix form:

$$\text{maximize} \qquad \varepsilon(X) = \sum_{g=1}^{k} \frac{X_g^T W X_g}{X_g^T D X_g} \qquad (12)$$

$$\text{subject to} \qquad X \in \{0, 1\}^{N \times k}, \ X 1_k = 1_N \qquad (13)$$

where 1_N denotes the $N \times 1$ vector of 1's , and the weights are normalized by D, the diagonal matrix containing the *degrees* of $W = Q^+ - Q^-$, thus $D(i,i) = \sum_j Q^+(i,j) - Q^-(i,j)$. As was shown in the original framework [10], normalizing each node by its outgoing connections adds a sense of group balance. A near-global optimal solution can be computed by solving for the top k eigenvectors of the normalized matrix W [16]. Since we are seeking only a binary segmentation, the final voxel labeling can be obtained by simply thresholding the top second eigenvector (thus needing only $k = 2$).

The 3D+t segmentation mask can finally be displayed on each individual 3D image I_t by back-tracking the nodes to obtain the segmentations $X_{1 \to t}$ at each I_t.

3   Experiments

We apply our method to extract white matter lesions from longitudinal MR brain scans. We start by describing our data and provide implementation details for our method. We then illustrate results on 4D images and compare them to individual 3D segmentations.

Baseline and follow-up scans were acquired on 1.5-Tesla scanners, with a 36 months interval for the follow-ups. All modalities have been rigidly registered to T1 using **FSLs** Flirt tool. For the first group, images belong to subjects with diabetes-2 and $T = 2$ timepoints. The T1 images are skull-stripped using an automated tool and the brain masks are then manually corrected. For the second group, images belong to healthy subjects and lesions are due to normal aging, $T = 3$ and skull-stripping is not applied a priori. For all our experiments, we only use Flair image modalities so lesions always appear as higher intensity regions embedded within the brain's white matter.

By definition, white matter lesions lie solely within the white matter of the brain and, in Flair images, always have higher intensity than the average intensity of the brain. We observe that the darker regions, such as cerebrospinal fluid (CSF) and ventricles, on the other hand always have intensities lower than the average. To create stronger attraction and repulsion cues between regions, we 'invert' the darker regions by taking $I_t = |I_t - \text{mean}(I_t)|$ at each time-point. We therefore seek to extract lesions, CSF and

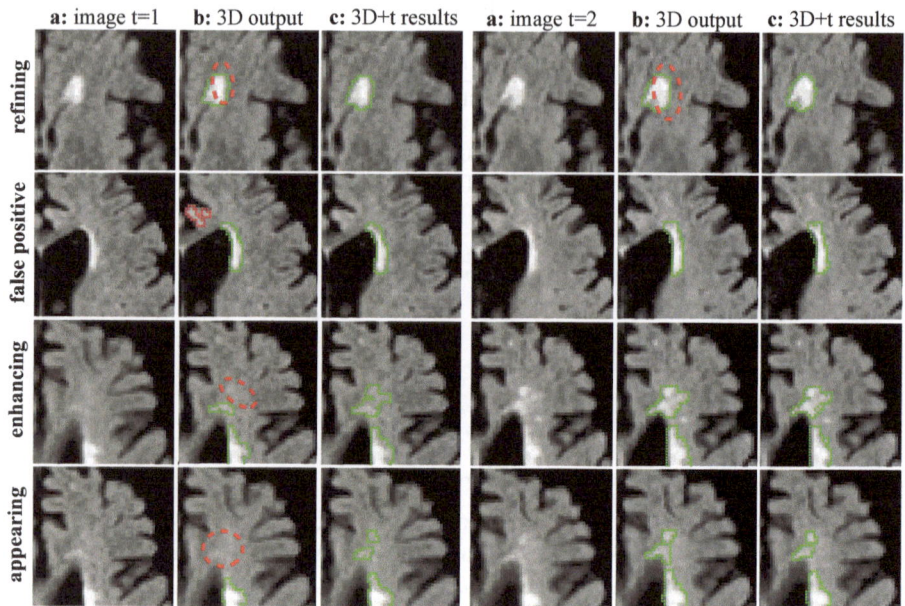

Fig. 4. 3D+t versus 3D segmentation. **a:** input I_t for 2 time-points; **b:** contours extracted from 3D segmentation X_t; **c:** contours extracted from our final 3D+t segmentation $X_{1 \to t}$. Both time-points benefit from each other. In each row, we illustrate different scenarios in which 3D+t improves over 3D by: (i) refining contours; ii) eliminating false-positives (*i.e.* lesions that disappear in time); (iii) enhancing fainter regions and segmenting regions that would otherwise not be detected, which includes (iv) enhancing at earlier time-points lesions that will appear at later times.

ventricles from their common white matter background. Once a segmentation is found for this new image, we simply threshold out regions below the original intensity average to obtain the final lesions.

We then apply our new graph construction to the I_t images. To compute affinities and correspondences, we adopt 3D neighborhoods $\mathcal{N}(i) = \{j \in \mathcal{N}(i) | d(i, j) \le r$ and directions $b = (\theta, \phi)\}$ with radii $r_r = 30$ and $r_a = r_c = 10$ for repulsion, attraction and correspondences respectively. Neighbors are computed along spherical coordinate directions $[\theta = 0, \phi = \{0, \pm\pi/4, \pm\pi/2, \pm3\pi/4, \pi\}], [\theta = \pm\pi/2, \phi = \pm\pi/4],$ $[\theta = 0, \phi = \{\pm\pi/4, \pm\pi/2, \pm3\pi/4\}]$. We set $\sigma_a = \sigma_{rel} = 0.3$ and $\sigma_{abs} = 0.5$. Parameters are fixed for all images. We apply spectral clustering as described in Sec. 2.4, on the combined weight matrix $W = Q^+ - Q^-$ and use the online code provided by [16] to solve for the final segmentation X. Running time for clustering the final graph G with $W = Q^+ - Q^-$ is approximately 150 seconds for initial image sizes $[128, 128, 30]$. Figures 5 and 6 show 4D segmentation results for two different subjects, with $T = 2$ and $T = 3$ time-points respectively. For each $X_{1 \to t}$, we visualize the contours extracted from the final 4D segmentation binary masks.

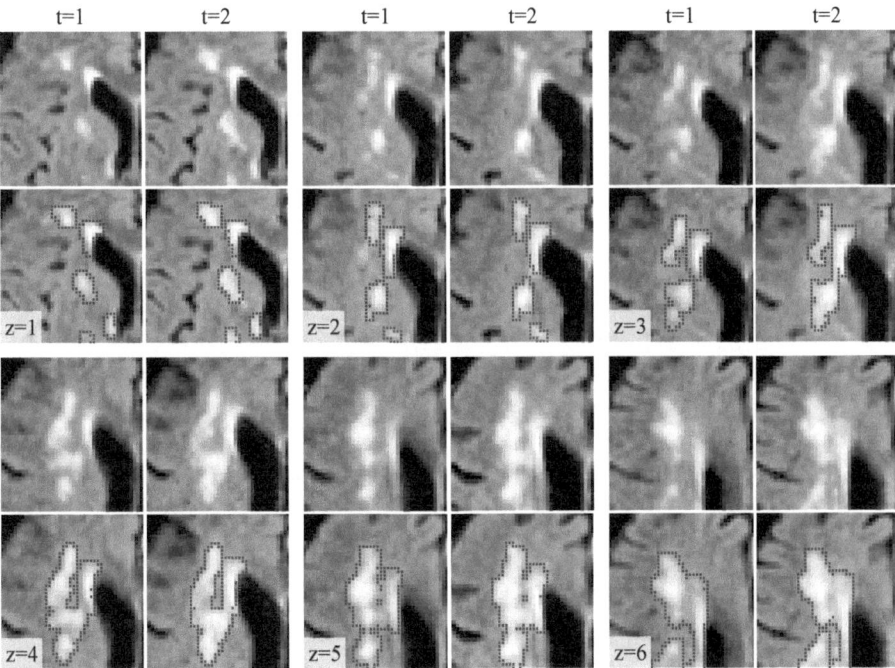

Fig. 5. Our 3D+t segmentation results for $T = 2$ time-points. Input images I_t together with final lesion contours extracted from $X_{1 \to t}$ at each time-point are shown for increasing z's. For better visualization, disconnected lesions in 3D are illustrated with different colors.

We compare our results with the individual 3D segmentations by applying spectral clustering directly on the individual weights $W_t = Q_t^+ - Q_t^-$ at each time-point t given by Eqn. 5. As illustrated for one subject in Fig. 4, advantages of 3D+t include: i) enhancing and/or detecting fainter regions at one time-point that appear more salient an another time; ii) refining boundaries; iii) eliminating false-positives, *i.e.* brighter regions due only to local intensity fluctuations at an earlier time-point that do not appear at later time-points. Clearly, if there is a consistent noisy region throughout all the time-points, the method would not be able to tell the difference. Note that appearing lesions are a special case of scenario (i): if a lesion appears at time t for the first time, all points on the contour of this new lesion will end up being matched to a single point at $t - 1$, corresponding to the center of the lesion at time t, thus defining an artificial 'seed' at $t - 1$. The appearing lesion will be properly detected at t and later time-points even if not present at the earlier ones. Alternatively, the lesion might be additionally enhanced if some faint region is already present but not sufficiently salient for a 3D segmentation to pick it up. As shown in Fig. 4, enforcing temporal consistency allows both earlier and later time-points to benefit from each other.

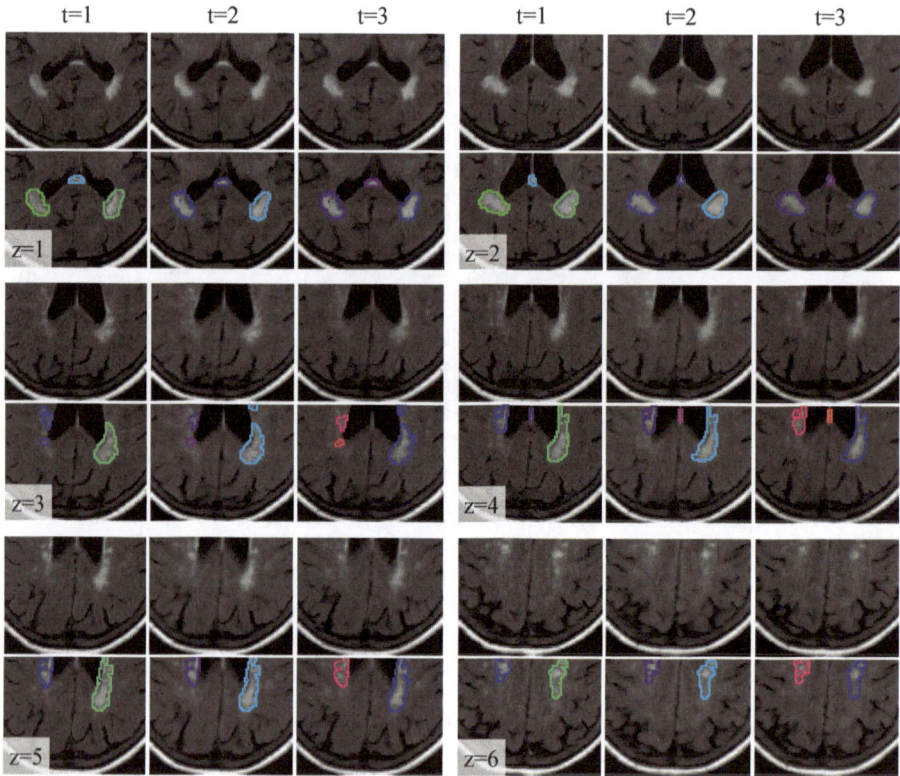

Fig. 6. Our 3D+t segmentation results for $T = 2$ time-points. Input images I_t together with final lesion contours extracted from $X_{1 \to t}$ at each time-point are shown for increasing z's. For better visualization, disconnected lesions in 3D are illustrated with different colors.

4   Conclusions

We segment evolving pathologies via spectral graph clustering. At each time-point, we construct affinities that properly capture structural agreement and yield good segmentations, even when used in isolation for 3D segmentation. Across time-points, we track nodes that lie within an estimated pathology evolution direction by finding best matches of node affinities. The computed correspondences are used to align and combine affinities across time-points. Our method relies on two assumptions: regions of interest have higher intensities than their common background (for affinities computations), and 3D images are linearly registered (for node tracking). While we applied the method only to expanding lesions, expansion of the regions of interest is not required.

Thanks to our graph construction, our final 3D+t segmentation has the same complexity as the 3D segmentations at each time-point. The method is scalable in time, as adding an additional time-point only requires computing the affinities and correspondences for the new image, and adding the aligned information to the already existing aligned graph from the other images for the final clustering step. As shown in our experiments, adding temporal information to segment the lesion allows all time-points to benefit from each other. Finally, while we used the correspondences only to enforce temporal consistency in the segmentation, they could also be used in future work to explicitly analyze the temporal shape changes of the extracted pathologies.

Acknowledgments. This project was supported in part by the Institute for Translational Medicine and Therapeutics' (ITMAT) and in part by NIH Grants UL1RR024134 and 5R01EB009234.

References

1. Anbeek, P., Vincken, K., Viergever, M.: Automated ms-lesion segmentation by k-nearest neighbor classification. In: Med. Image Comput. Comput. Assist. Interv. (July 2008)
2. Bernardis, E., Yu, S.X.: Robust segmentation by cutting across a stack of gamma transformed images. In: Cremers, D., Boykov, Y., Blake, A., Schmidt, F.R. (eds.) EMMCVPR 2009. LNCS, vol. 5681, pp. 249–260. Springer, Heidelberg (2009)
3. Bernardis, E., Yu, S.X.: Pop out many small structures from a very large microscopic image. Medical Image Analysis 15(5), 690–707 (2011)
4. Fragkiadaki, K., Zhang, W., Shi, J., Bernardis, E.: Structural-flow trajectories for unravelling 3D tubular bundles. In: Ayache, N., Delingette, H., Golland, P., Mori, K. (eds.) MICCAI 2012, Part III. LNCS, vol. 7512, pp. 631–638. Springer, Heidelberg (2012)
5. Habas, P., Kim, K., Corbett-Detig, J., Rousseau, F., Glenn, O., Barkovich, A., Studholme, C.: A spatiotemporal atlas of MR intensity, tissue probability and shape of the fetal brain with application to segmentation. NeuroImage 53(2), 460–470 (2010)
6. Prastawa, M., Gerig, G.: Automatic ms lesion segmentation by outlier detection and information theoretic region partitioning. In: Med. Image Comput. Comput. Assist. Interv. (September 2008)
7. Prastawa, M., Gilmore, J., Lin, W., Gerig, G.: Automatic segmentation of MR images of the developing newborn brain. Medical Image Analysis 9(5), 457–466 (2005)
8. Reuter, M., Fischl, B.: Avoiding asymmetry-induced bias in longitudinal image processing. NeuroImage 57(1), 19–21 (2011)
9. Rey, D., Subsol, G., Delingette, H., Ayache, N.: Automatic detection and segmentation of evolving processes in 3D medical images: Application to multiple sclerosis. Medical Image Analysis 6(2), 163–179 (2002)
10. Shi, J., Malik, J.: Normalized cuts and image segmentation. IEEE Trans. Pattern Analysis Machine Intelligence 22(8), 888–905 (2000)
11. Shiee, N., Bazin, P., Pham, D.: Multiple sclerosis lesion segmentation using statistical and topological atlases. In: Med. Image Comput. Comput. Assist. Interv. (October 2008)
12. Van Leemput, K., Maes, F., Vandermeulen, D., Colchester, A., Suetens, P.: Automated segmentation of multiple sclerosis lesions by model outlier detection. IEEE Transactions on Medical Imaging 20(8), 677–688 (2001)
13. Weisenfeld, N., Warfield, S.: Automatic segmentation of newborn brain MRI. NeuroImage 47(2), 564–572 (2009)
14. Welti, D., Gerig, G., Radü, E.-W., Kappos, L., Székely, G.: Spatio-temporal segmentation of active multiple sclerosis lesions in serial MRI data. In: Insana, M.F., Leahy, R.M. (eds.) IPMI 2001. LNCS, vol. 2082, pp. 438–445. Springer, Heidelberg (2001)
15. Xue, Z., Shen, D., Davatzikos, C.: CLASSIC: Consistent longitudinal alignment and segmentation for serial image computing. NeuroImage 30(2), 388–399 (2006)
16. Yu, S.X., Shi, J.: Understanding popout through repulsion. In: IEEE Proc. Computer Vision and Pattern Recognition, pp. 752–757 (2001)

Construction of Multi-scale Common Brain Networks Based on DICCCOL

Bao Ge[1], Lei Guo[2], Dajiang Zhu[3], Tuo Zhang[2,3], Xintao Hu[2],
Junwei Han[2], and Tianming Liu[3]

[1] College of Physics & Information Technology, Shaanxi Normal University, Xi'an, China
[2] School of Automation, Northwestern Polytechnical University, Xi'an, China
[3] Cortical Architecture Imaging and Discovery Lab, Department of Computer Science,
University of Georgia, Athens, GA, USA

Abstract. Modeling the human brain as a network has been widely considered as a powerful approach to investigating the brain's structural and functional systems. However, many previous approaches focused on a single scale of brain network and the multi-scale nature of brain networks has been rarely explored yet. This paper put forward a novel framework to construct multi-scale common networks of brains via multi-scale spectral clustering of fiber connections among DICCCOLs. Specifically, the recently developed and publicly released DICCCOLs provide the nodal structural and functional correspondence across individuals, and thus the employed multi-scale spectral clustering algorithm divided the DICCCOL landmarks and their connections into sub-networks with correspondences on multiple scales. Experimental results showed the promise of the constructed multi-scale networks in applications of structural and functional connectivity mapping. As an application example, these multi-scale networks are used to guide the identification of multi-scale common fiber bundles across individuals and to facilitate the bundle's functional role analysis, which could enable other tract-based and network-based analyses in the future.

Keywords: DTI, multi-scale common brain networks, fiber clustering, DICCCOL.

1   Introduction

Whole-brain anatomical and functional connectivity in living humans can be modeled as networks via diffusion MRI and fMRI data. Typically, network nodes are associated with distinct grey-matter regions of interest (ROIs), and edges are defined as fiber pathways or functional correlations between cortical ROIs. Then, graph theory based network analysis can be applied to reveal the brain's network properties in a variety of applications [1, 14, 15]. However, despite the growing importance of studying networks in the human brain mapping community, construction of brain network still faces two general challenges. The first is the lack of accurate nodal correspondence across individuals and populations. In general, there has been no gold standard for regional parcellation in the brain, which makes the definition of network nodes uncertain. For instance, network nodes can be defined by employing either template-based warping or based on certain parcellation criteria [5]. In fact, the

J.C. Gee et al. (Eds.): IPMI 2013, LNCS 7917, pp. 692–704, 2013.

template registration method has difficulty in dealing with the remarkable variation of cortical folding patterns in individual brains. Without the nodal correspondences between brain networks, many meaningful and comparative statistical measurements of network properties cannot be accurately performed. Second, many previous studies defined network nodes at a single spatial scale without consideration of the intrinsic multi-scale nature of brain networks. Essentially, recent research has demonstrated that the structural and functional connectivity occurs at multiple spatial levels [10, 14-15], and thus how to find the optimal scales and determine the number/size of nodes is vitally important to construct brain networks.

Recently, we developed and publicly released the DICCCOL (Dense Individualized and Common Connectivity-based Cortical Landmarks) system [1]. These identified and validated 358 group-wise consistent DICCCOL landmarks possess intrinsically-established structural and functional correspondences across individuals [1]. Importantly, they have been well reproduced in over 240 individual brains [1]. Thus, these 358 landmarks offer a universal and individuated brain reference system. In particular, these 358 landmarks can be accurately predicted in each individual brain with DTI data [1]. Thus, these DICCCOL landmarks can be used as the corresponding nodes for brain network construction to deal with the abovementioned first challenge. The DICCCOL software toolkit has been released on NITRC [11], and Figure 1(a) shows an example of these 358 DICCCOL landmarks.

In this paper, by treating the DICCCOL landmarks as the basic network nodes, we constructed the corresponding brain networks in multiple scales by an effective multi-scale spectral clustering algorithm [2]. Specifically, the DTI-derived fiber connection strength between DICCCOL landmarks is used as the feature of clustering based on the principle of functional segregation and integration [12]. Importantly, the correspondences are kept among the network nodes in multiple scales by group-wise averaging of the connectivity matrices across different subjects. Since the basic correspondences have been established by DICCCOLs, the optimal scales and the sizes/numbers of node are determined by the multi-scale spectral clustering. We have applied this novel methodology on a DTI dataset, and promising and meaningful results have been achieved. In particular, as an application example, the multi-scale networks are used to guide the multi-scale fiber clustering and reasonable results were obtained. Finally, we analyzed the functional roles for each sub-network and fiber bundle via meta-analysis [3] of the BrainMap fMRI activation database [7]. In general, the major methodological contributions of this paper are the introduction, evaluation and application of a general framework for multi-scale common network construction based on structural connectivity patterns and for multi-scale common fiber clustering, which can potentially enable other structural and functional modeling and mapping of brain networks in the future.

2   Methods

2.1   Overview

The flowchart of our multi-scale brain network construction includes the following steps. First, we pre-processed the raw DTI data, and tracked the whole-brain fibers via the streamline method. Then, we predicted the 358 corresponding and consistent

DICCCOL landmarks for each brain via the methods in [1]. By treating these DICCCOL landmarks as the primitive nodes, on which we computed the connectivity matrix based on the streamline fiber connections, then an effective multi-scale spectral algorithm was applied to determine the multiple scales and to cluster nodes into clusters with the optimal size/number.

2.2   Data Acquisition and Preprocessing

Nine healthy young adults recruited at The University of Georgia (UGA) under UGA IRB approval were scanned in a GE 3T Signa MRI system (GE Healthcare, Milwaukee, WI) using an 8-channel head coil at the UGA Bioimaging Research Center (BIRC), Athens, GA. Diffusion tensor imaging (DTI) data were acquired using the isotropic spatial resolution 2mm×2mm×2mm; parameters were TR 15.5s and TE min-full, b-value = 1000 with 30 DWI gradient directions and 3 B0 volumes acquired. Pre-processing of the DTI data included brain skull removal, motion correction, and eddy current correction. After the pre-processing, the whole-brain streamline tractography was performed using the MEDINRIA toolkit (FA threshold: 0.2; minimum fiber length: 20). Then, we predicted the DICCCOL landmarks using the open-source toolkit in [11].

2.3   The Dissimilarity Measure of Landmarks

The theory of functional segregation and integration considers that human brains might have been competitively selected to maximize the cost efficiency of parallel information processing in large-scale networks [12]. That is, brain evolution tends to increase its efficiency (favoring the selection of a few long-range axonal fiber connections mediating efficient information transfer between spatially distributed regions) while decrease the cost (favoring a high density of short-range local connections), like an economical small-world network. According to this principle, we can divide the brain network by its local connection or its DTI-derived streamline fiber connections. However, since current DTI and tractography techniques cannot track the local connection in gray matter, we can only seek alternative methods. In our previous paper [13], the local affinity was measured by using geodesic distance to construct multi-scale brain networks, in that those cortical regions with small distances are likely to connect each other by short-range intra-column connections. In this paper, instead, we adopt the DTI-derived fiber connection (long-range connection) as feature to divide the multi-scale networks.

Specifically, the connectivity strength between DICCCOL landmarks is defined as follows:

$$C^n(L_i, L_j) = \text{Fdensity} * \text{averFA}$$

where C^n measures the connectivity strength between landmark L_i to L_j of subject n, and L_i is the ith landmark and $averFA$ is the averaged FA (fractional anisotropy) value along those fibers. Therefore, the bigger the number of fibers passing two landmarks is, the stronger the fibers' orientation consistency is, and thus the higher is the connectivity strength of the two landmarks. That is, $C(L_i, L_j)$ means how likely the landmarks L_i and L_j belong to one sub-network. As an example, Fig.1(b) illustrates that those landmarks which have higher connectivity tend to be clustered into the same group. Here, it is assumed that the original spectral clustering algorithm [4] is adopted. For the convenience of visual evaluation, only two landmark groups are shown in Fig.1(b), that is, the red and green groups, respectively, which are likely to construct two sub-networks in the next section. This simple comparison experiment illustrates that the measurement can potentially reasonably group the DICCCOL landmarks. In order to keep the correspondences in other multiple scales, we averaged the connectivity strength between subjects, that is:

$$C = \sum_{n=1}^{N} C^n / N$$

Here, N is the number of subjects, and C^n is the connectivity matrix between the 358 DICCCOL landmarks of the nth subject. This averaged connectivity matrix aimed to eliminate inter-individual differences.

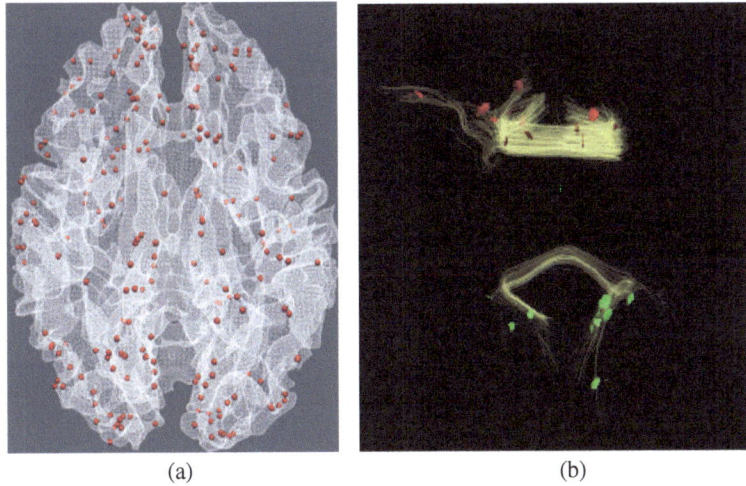

(a)   (b)

Fig. 1. (a) An example of DICCCOL landmarks (red spheres). (b) Two sub-networks which have strong connectivity within each network. Spheres in two colors represent two clusters here.

2.4   Multi-scale Clustering

By taking each DICCCOL landmark as the node of an undirected weighted graph and connecting each pair of landmarks by an edge, the input of a spectral clustering algorithm is thus a Gaussian similarity matrix associated with the graph, which can be expressed as $W_{ij}(\delta) = \exp\left(-\frac{D(L_i, L_j)}{\delta^2}\right)$, where D is the landmark distance function, which measures the dissimilarity between landmark L_i to L_j. Naturally, D is defined as 1/C. Here, δ is the length scale of the Gaussian similarity function. The smaller it is, the smaller is the 'neighborhood' of a DICCCOL landmark.

Traditional spectral clustering methods need to specify different sets of parameters. As a consequence, the partition results may be subject to variations and uncertainty. In contrast, the multi-scale spectral clustering algorithm [2] can automatically explore the data structures (that is, learn the optimal δ) and infers different plausible values for the number of clusters from a random walk perspective. It tries to seek a reasonable partition of the graph such that the random walk stays within the same cluster and seldom jumps between different clusters. The algorithm offers the tree structure partition of data points, starting by separation in a large scale, and then recursively partitioning each of the resulting sub-trees. Fig.2 illustrates how the basic random walk spectral clustering determines the optimal number of clusters using the following functions:

$$\Delta(M, \delta) = \max_{k} \left(\lambda_k^M(\delta) - \lambda_{k+1}^M(\delta) \right)$$
$$K(M, \delta) = \arg \max_{k} \left(\lambda_k^M(\delta) - \lambda_{k+1}^M(\delta) \right)$$

Here, λ_k is the kth eigenvalue, and λ_k^M is λ_k to the Mth power. The bigger $\Delta(M, \delta)$ is, the more distinguished is the structure revealed by it after a random walk of M steps. Here, δ for Fig.2 is fixed. However, we can learn δ and K simultaneously by changing δ. Thus each δ generates the curves of each Δ and K. For each δ, we identified the most distinguished structure with the highest Δ. Among all δ, we selected the most stable structure (staying the longest steps within the same cluster) with the highest stability measure. We recursively call the algorithm until the DICCCOL landmarks cannot be clustered furthermore, which finally resulted in a tree structure partition of data points. This procedure starts by separation in a large scale, and then recursively partitions each of the resulting sub-trees. More details of the algorithm can be found in [2, 13].

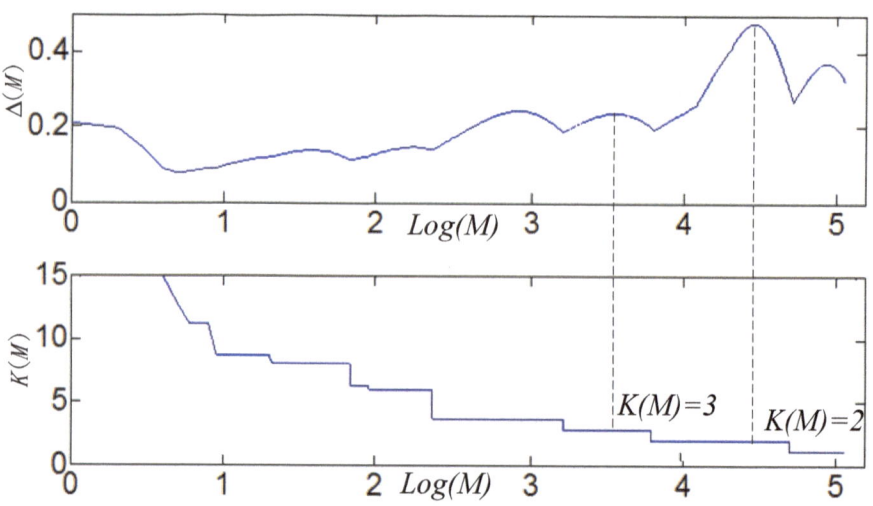

Fig. 2. The illustration for random walk spectral clustering

3   Experimental Results

3.1   Model of Multi-scale Brain Networks

The generated multi-scale brain networks via this proposed method are shown in Fig.3, each brain sub-network in one scale was divided again in the next scale, thus forming a tree structure from top-down. If we check from the left to the right, the most left column includes the clustered brain networks in each scale, and its sub-networks were shown in the right part. The clustered brain networks also include the leaf nodes from the upper layers. For the convenience of visual check, all the networks and sub-networks are represented as the overlay of all nine subjects at the same scale, and each brain sub-network was assigned with a different color. Altogether, the number of brain networks in scales 1~5 are 1, 5, 12, 17 and 20, respectively. We can see that the landmarks were reasonably clustered into groups across individuals.

Quantitatively, the consistencies within these sub-networks are stronger and stronger from scale 1 to 5. Figs. 4(a) and (b) show the connectivity strength matrices of every sub-network in scale 2 and 3, from which we can see that the consistency is higher for the higher scale. It is explained in (c), and the consistency curve also demonstrates this point. Here, the consistency is simply defined as the mean connectivity strength ("W" in section 2.4) within each network.

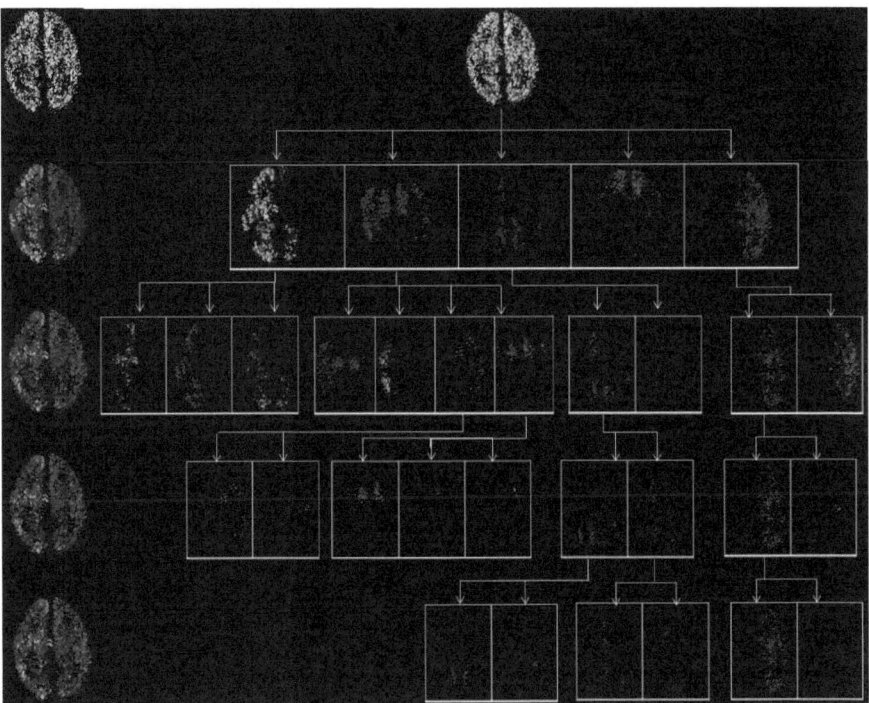

Fig. 3. Tree structure of the clustered multi-scale brain networks. Each sub-network in one scale was divided again in the next scale. All sub-networks are denoted by different colors, and each new sub-network in the next scale is designated a new color. The number of landmark clusters in scales 1~5 are 1, 5, 12, 17, 20 respectively.

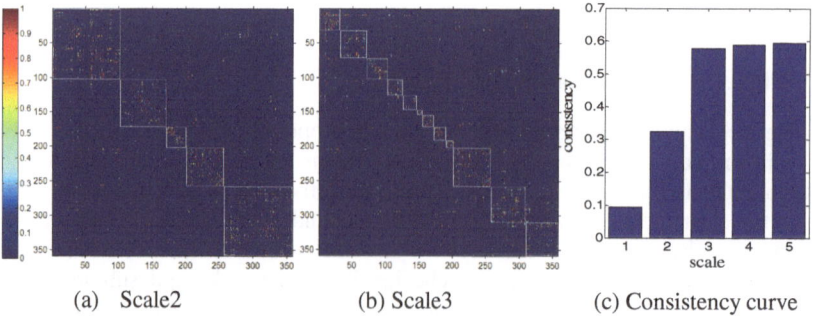

(a)   Scale2   (b) Scale3   (c) Consistency curve

Fig. 4. (a) and (b): The connectivity strength matrices of every sub-network in scale 2 and 3. (c) The consistency curve at all scales.

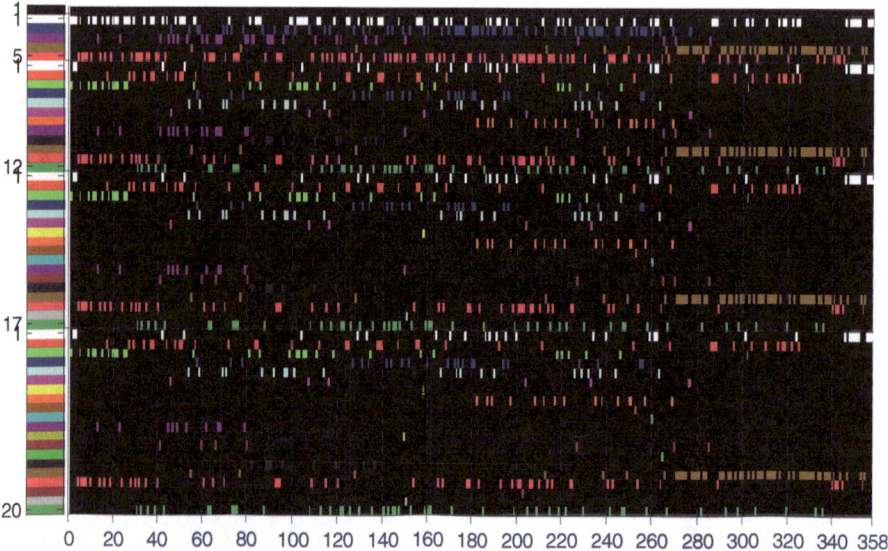

Fig. 5. The corresponding relationships between each sub-network and DICCCOL landmark ID included in each sub-network. The horizontal axis represents the 358 DICCCOL landmarks and the vertical axis represents every sub-network in scale 1~5. From top-down, the sub-network IDs are 1, 1~5, 1~12, 1~17 and 1~20 respectively. The color of each network and its corresponding landmarks are shown on the left and these colors are completely correspondent with those of all sub-networks in Fig.3. The colored rectangle in each row denotes the DICCCOL landmark ID included in this row sub-network.

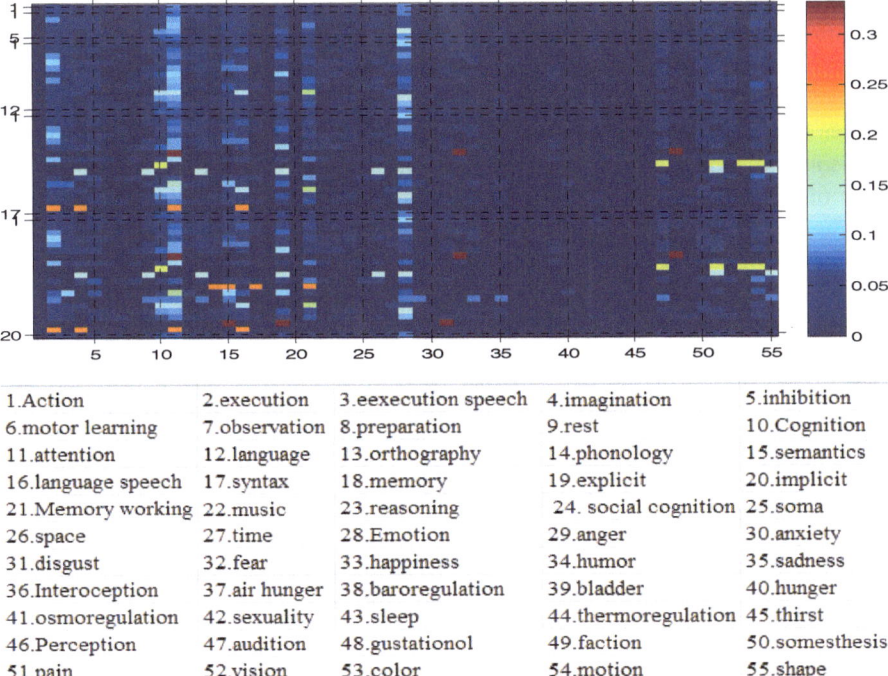

1.Action	2.execution	3.eexecution speech	4.imagination	5.inhibition
6.motor learning	7.observation	8.preparation	9.rest	10.Cognition
11.attention	12.language	13.orthography	14.phonology	15.semantics
16.language speech	17.syntax	18.memory	19.explicit	20.implicit
21.Memory working	22.music	23.reasoning	24. social cognition	25.soma
26.space	27.time	28.Emotion	29.anger	30.anxiety
31.disgust	32.fear	33.happiness	34.humor	35.sadness
36.Interoception	37.air hunger	38.baroregulation	39.bladder	40.hunger
41.osmoregulation	42.sexuality	43.sleep	44.thermoregulation	45.thirst
46.Perception	47.audition	48.gustationol	49.faction	50.somesthesis
51.pain	52.vision	53.color	54.motion	55.shape

Fig. 6. The percentage of functional roles of sub-networks. The horizontal axis represents the 55 functional behavioral domains used in the BrainMap database [7], which are listed in the bottom, and the vertical axis represents 55 sub-networks.

The significance of these sub-networks is that they can be cross-validated by the existing discovered functional or structural sub-networks [3]. Then, we provided a look-up table as shown in Fig.5, by which we can find how many sub-networks each network includes and which DICCCOL landmarks each sub-network includes. Furthermore, we can infer the functional roles of each sub-network by counting the functional roles of all landmarks within sub-network according to the recent meta-analysis results released in [3] based on the BrainMap database [7]. The percentage of each functional role of sub-network is shown in Fig.6. We can see that almost all the sub-network participate in some brain functional domains such as attention (11) and emotion (28), etc. We will provide a detailed functional analysis for sub-networks and fiber bundles in Section 3.3, because assigning fiber bundles with functional network roles is informative.

3.2   Prediction of Brain Networks in Individual Brains

We used another independent DTI dataset as a testing population to predict the multi-scale brain networks. The prediction procedure is straightforward under the guidance of the multi-scale network clustering results, since the Fig.5 already maps the multi-scale organization of the 358 DICCCOLs into the hierarchical brain networks. Because of the intrinsic correspondences established by the DICCCOLs, the group-wise clustered network in the previous section can be readily used as the models to predict the tree structure for the new individual brains, once the DICCCOL landmarks are predicted in the new subjects. Fig.7 shows that the predicted brain networks from the nine different subjects. In each scale, there are three networks. For comparison, all nine brain networks which are same as those in Fig.3 are put in the first column, and the second column shows the nine predicted brain networks. The color of each sub-network is the same as that of sub-network in Fig.3. It is evident that the predicted networks are very similar to those model networks. These results demonstrate the robustness of the multi-scale network construction framework, as well as the reproducibility of the DICCCOLs and the associated brain networks.

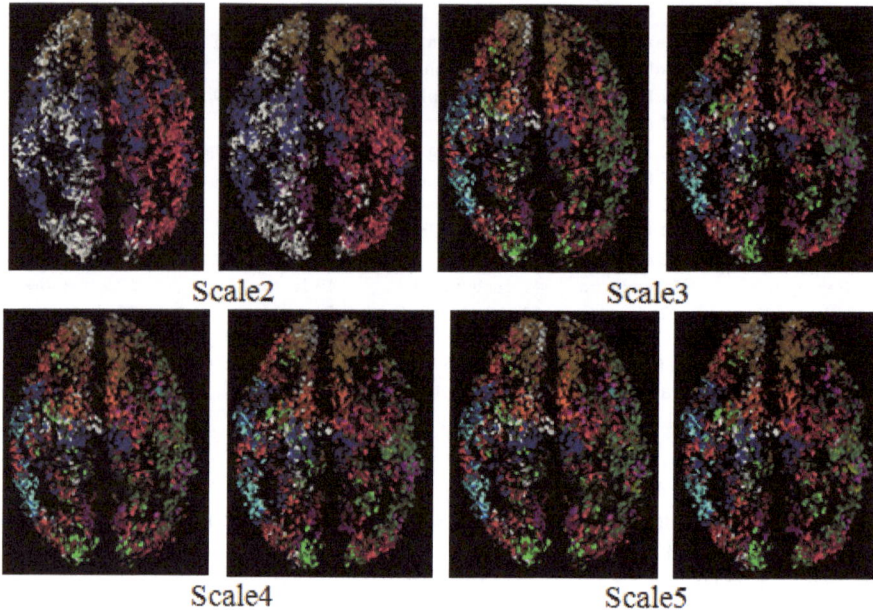

Scale2   Scale3

Scale4   Scale5

Fig. 7. The predicted multi-scale brain networks in nine different brains. Every brain network or sub-networks are overlaid by the nine different subjects. At each scale, for comparison, the left figure is the model network that corresponds to the left-most column in Fig.3, and the right is the predicted brain network.

3.3   Application in Identifying Common Fiber Bundles

Based on these multi-scale and corresponding brain networks obtained in section 3.1, we aim to identify common fiber bundles across individuals. First, we grouped all of the DTI-derived fibers connecting the pair of landmarks within each sub-network into the same fiber bundle, and then we selected those common fiber bundles across subjects at each scale. Fig.8 shows the common fiber bundles in scales 1-5. They have 1, 5, 11, 12 and 12 fiber bundles, respectively. The fiber bundles have the same colors as its corresponding sub-networks. It can be seen that there are stable and almost the same fiber bundles in scale 3~5. It is evident that the multi-scale networks are able to effectively guide the identification of consistent fiber bundle.

Furthermore, we computed the averaged Hausdorff distances of corresponding fiber bundles in different subjects for scales 2~5, similar to that in [6]. Each fiber bundle was represented by its exemplar of Hausdorff distance when computing the Hausdorff distances of corresponding fiber bundles. Then the averaged Hausdorff distances denote the degree of correspondence and consistency among these fiber bundles from different subjects, as shown in Table 1. We can see that the averaged Hausdorff distance is relatively small in scales 2~5, indicating the accurate correspondence of fiber bundles. Finally, we averaged all the Hausdorff distances in the same scale, as shown in the last row, demonstrating that the fiber bundles and sub-networks are more consistent in higher scales. Table 1 also gives the corresponding relationships between fiber bundles and sub-networks, because not all sub-networks have its corresponding fiber bundles across different subjects.

Finally, Fig.9 shows that the identified fiber bundles in scale 2 and 3, in which we can see that the fiber bundles in scale 3 have more consistent shape. This demonstrated that sub-networks and corresponding fiber bundles are more consistent in higher scale. Also, guided by the relationships between fiber bundles and sub-networks, we assigned each fiber bundle with the corresponding the functional roles according to Fig.6, and the top 3 major functional roles are marked in Fig.9. It will be of interest for tract-based analysis [8, 9] in the future.

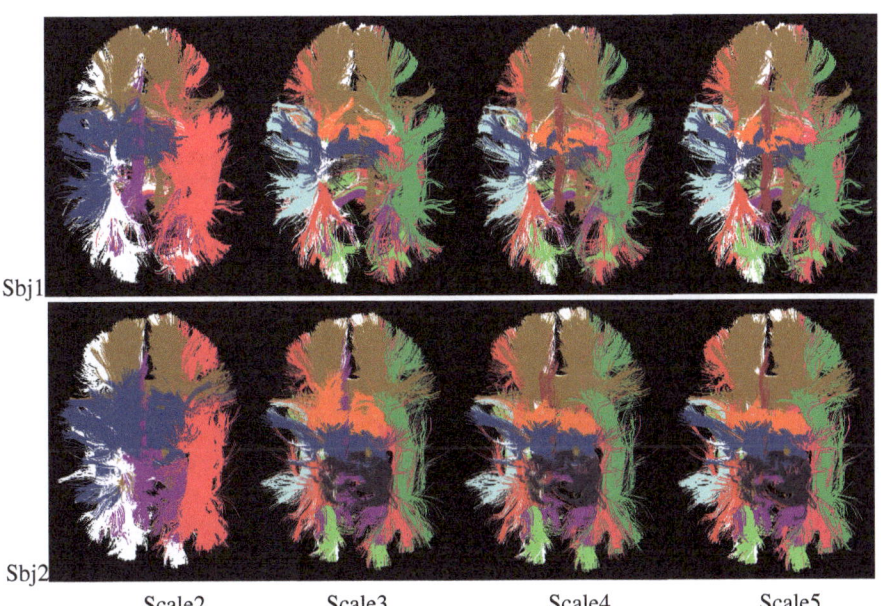

Sbj1

Sbj2

Scale2   Scale3   Scale4   Scale5

Fig. 8. The multi-scale common fiber bundles based on common brain networks from randomly selected two subjects. The fiber clusters were assigned with different colors, and the corresponding fiber bundles across different brains have the same color. Furthermore, these fiber bundles have the same colors as its corresponding sub-networks. The scales here correspond to the same set of scales in Fig. 3. The number of fiber bundles in scales 2~5 are 5, 11, 12, 12, respectively.

Table 1. The averaged Hausdorff distance (mm) of common fiber bundles between subjects in multi-scale and the corresponding relationships between fiber bundles and sub-networks. "null" represents that there are no common fiber bundles found in this sub-network.

		Scale2	Scale3	Scale4	Scale5
Sub-network ID	1: 13.84		1: 8.92	1: 8.92	1: 8.92
			2: 5.58	2: 5.58	2: 5.58
			3: 6.20	3: 6.20	3: 6.20
	2: 10.47		4: 6.49	4: 6.49	4: 6.49
			5: 4.02	5: 4.02	5: 4.02
		6: null		6: null	6: null
				7: null	7: null
		7: 3.81		8: 2.57	8: 2.57
				9: null	9: null
				10: null	10: null
	3: 8.49	8: 7.46		11: 2.87	11: 1.96
					12: null
				12: 3.58	13: 2.68
					14: null
		9: 2.95		13: 2.95	15: 2.95
	4: 9.56	10: 9.56		14: 9.56	16: 9.56
	5: 12.03	11: 8.73		15: 4.69	17: 3.59
					18: null
				16: null	19: null
		12: 6.94		17: 6.94	20: 6.94
average		10.88	6.42	5.36	5.12

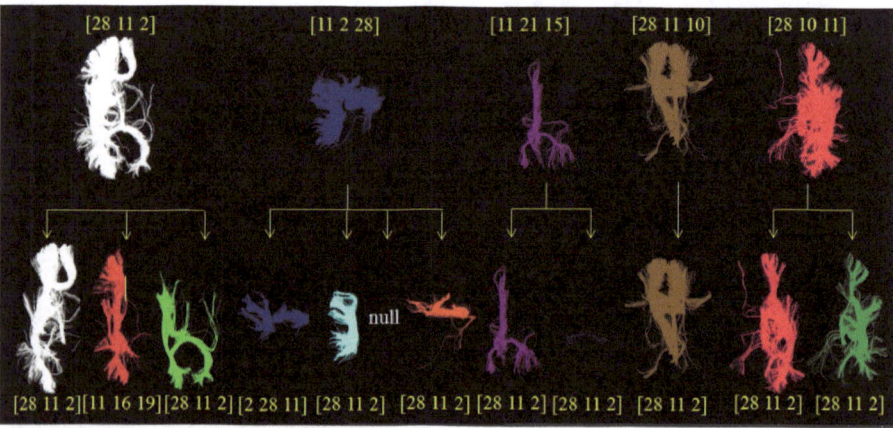

Fig. 9. The fiber bundles in scale 2 and 3. The first row shows the 5 fiber bundles identified via the 5 sub-networks at scale 2, and the second row shows the 11 fiber bundles identified via the 12 sub-networks at scale 3. The three major functional roles are marked by the indices of 55 networks in Fig.6 on each fiber bundle.

4   Conclusion

This paper proposed a novel method to construct the multi-scale common brain networks across individuals via an improved multi-scale spectral clustering of fiber connection strength. The obtained multi-scale common networks can be interpreted from the theory of functional integration of brain. The method has also been applied to identify common fiber bundles across subjects, and reasonable results were obtained. In general, our results on multi-scale brain networks and fiber bundles demonstrate the remarkable regularity of structural brain architecture, despite the noticeable variation across individuals as well. Experimental results have demonstrated that brain networks and fiber bundles are naturally organized in a multi-scale fashion, which can be reproduced and predicted across individuals and populations.

In the future, the work in this paper can be extended and enhanced in the following directions. First, the computational framework can be further extensively evaluated and validated by larger scale datasets. Second, these common multi-scale structural brain networks can be potentially widely used as the basis for many other brain network-level modeling and analyses such as functional interactions and dynamics. Also, the common multi-scale brain networks can be potentially used to examine the possible alterations in structural and functional connectivities in brain disorders. Finally, based on the multi-scale structural networks derived from DTI data, fMRI datasets can be used to model the multi-scale functional information flows on these structural networks for better understanding of the relationship between brain structure and function and for the elucidation of functioning mechanism of the brain.

References

1. Zhu, D., Li, K., Guo, L., et al.: DICCCOL: Dense Individualized and Common Connectivity-Based Cortical Landmarks. Cereb. Cortex 23(4), 786–800 (2012)
2. Azran, A., Ghahramani, Z.: Spectral methods for automatic multiscale data clustering. In: CVPR, pp. 190–197 (2006)
3. Yuan, Y., Jiang, X., Zhu, D., et al.: Meta-analysis of functional roles of DICCCOLs. Neuroinformatics (2012), http://www.ncbi.nlm.nih.gov/pubmed/23055045
4. von Luxburg, U.: A tutorial on spectral clustering. Statistics and Computing 17, 395–416 (2007)
5. Zalesky, A., Fornito, A., Harding, I.H., et al.: Whole-brain anatomical networks: does the choice of nodes matter? Neuroimage 50(3), 970–983 (2010)
6. Ge, B., et al.: Resting State fMRI-guided Fiber Clustering: Methods and Applications. Neuroinformatics (2012), http://www.ncbi.nlm.nih.gov/pubmed/23065648
7. Laird, A.R., Eickhoff, S.B., Kurth, F., Fox, P.M., Uecker, A.M., Turner, J.A., Robinson, J.L., Lancaster, J.L., Fox, P.T.: ALE meta-analysis workflows via the BrainMap database: Progress towards a probabilistic functional brain atlas. Frontiers in Neuroinformatics 3(23), 1–11 (2009)
8. Gerig, G., Gouttard, S., Corouge, I.: Analysis of Brain White Matter via Fiber Tract Modeling. In: IEEE EMBS, vol. 2, pp. 4421–4424 (2004)
9. Maddah, M., Grimson, W., Warfield, S.: Statistical Modeling and EM Clustering of White Matter Fiber Tracts. In: ISBI, vol. 1, pp. 53–56 (2006)

10. Zhang, D., Raichle, M.E.: Disease and the brain's dark energy. Nature Reviews Neurology 6(1), 15–28 (2010)
11. http://www.nitrc.org/projects/dicccol_0_1
12. Achard, S., Bullmore, E.: Efficiency and cost of economical brain functional networks. PLoS Comput. Biol. 3, e17 (2007)
13. Ge, B., Guo, L., Zhang, T., et al.: Construction of Multi-scale Brain Networks via DICCCOL Landmarks. In: ISBI (in press, 2013)
14. Kennedy, D.N.: Making Connections in the Connectome Era. Neuroinformatics 8(2), 61–62 (2010)
15. Hagmann, P., Cammoun, L., Gigandet, X., Gerhard, S., Grant, P.E., Wedeen, V., Meuli, R., Thiran, J.P., Honey, C.J., Sporns, O.: MR connectomics: Principles and challenges. Journal of Neuroscience Methods 194, 34–45 (2010)

Rotation Invariant Features for HARDI

Evan Schwab[1], H. Ertan Çetingül[3], Bijan Afsari[1],
Michael A. Yassa[2], and René Vidal[1]

[1] Center for Imaging Science, Johns Hopkins University
[2] Department of Psychological and Brain Sciences, Johns Hopkins University
[3] Imaging and Computer Vision, Siemens Corporation, Corporate Technology

Abstract. Reducing the amount of information stored in diffusion MRI (dMRI) data to a set of meaningful and representative scalar values is a goal of much interest in medical imaging. Such features can have far reaching applications in segmentation, registration, and statistical characterization of regions of interest in the brain, as in comparing features between control and diseased patients. Currently, however, the number of biologically relevant features in dMRI is very limited. Moreover, existing features discard much of the information inherent in dMRI and embody several theoretical shortcomings. This paper proposes a new family of rotation invariant scalar features for dMRI based on the spherical harmonic (SH) representation of high angular resolution diffusion images (HARDI). These features describe the shape of the orientation distribution function extracted from HARDI data and are applicable to any reconstruction method that represents HARDI signals in terms of an SH basis. We further illustrate their significance in white matter characterization of synthetic, phantom and real HARDI brain datasets.

Keywords: rotation invariance, spherical functions, feature extraction, diffusion magnetic resonance imaging, orientation distribution functions.

1 Introduction

Diffusion magnetic resonance imaging (dMRI) is a non-invasive imaging technique that can be used to characterize the white matter (WM) architecture of the brain in normal and diseased patients [1]. In particular, extracting scalar features (or biomarkers) from dMRI data has become an integral part of group/ longitudinal studies of WM changes in brain connectivity related to development, neurodegeneration, or disease [2]. Since diffusion tensor imaging (DTI) is currently the de facto standard in clinical neuroimaging, the vast majority of the studies assessing WM connectivity and its impairment employ features derived from DTI, e.g., mean diffusivity (MD), fractional anisotropy (FA), relative anisotropy (RA), linear/planar/spherical anisotropies (LA/PA/SA) [3, 4]. However, DTI is limited by its inability to resolve intra-voxel complexities like fiber crossings. This causes DTI-based features to severely lack specificity [5]. Hence, there is a strong need for deriving new scalar measures for characterizing

J.C. Gee et al. (Eds.): IPMI 2013, LNCS 7917, pp. 705–717, 2013.

the WM integrity, especially from more generic and versatile diffusion representations such as higher-order tensors [6, 7] and orientation distribution functions
(ODFs) [8–10], which describe the tissue microstructure with greater accuracy
and detail.

Few scalar features have been derived from the aforementioned representations
[11], with the most popular ones being the fractional multifiber index (FMI) [12],
generalized anisotropy (GA) [13] and generalized fractional anisotropy (GFA) [8].
Recently, [14] used a polynomial approach to extract geometric characteristics
from spherical functions (e.g., ODFs) and proposed new scalar measures such as
peak fractional anisotropy (PFA) and Total-PFA. Furthermore, [5] presented the
concept of the integrity basis for 2nd and 4th order tensors, as well as two standard bases called the basic and principal invariants, expanding the works of [15]
and [16] on the principal invariants of the 4th order tensor.

In this paper we propose a new framework for extracting a large set of rotation
invariant features from the spherical harmonic (SH) representation of HARDI signals and ODFs. The advantage of this framework is its generality. In fact, we derive
a family of rotation invariant features that can be extracted from any spherical
function written in an SH basis. Numerous HARDI reconstruction methods [11]
such as Spherical Deconvolution (SD), Diffusion Orientation Transform (DOT),
Spherical Polar Fourier Imaging (SPFI), Bessel Fourier Orientation Reconstruction (BFOR) model spherical functions like the Ensemble Average Propagator
(EAP), Fiber Orientation Distribution (FOD), and Apparent Diffusion Coefficient (ADC) using an SH basis. Our framework can be applied to any of these
spherical functions to extract a new set of scalar values. In addition, any continuous function of these scalar values can be used to generate additional features
that can be significant for a specific experiment or application.

The remainder of the paper is organized as follows. Section 2 lays the theoretical
groundwork for spherical functions and provides the derivation of a new set of
rotation invariant features. Section 3 applies our theory to HARDI signals and
ODFs and Section 4 evaluates our features on synthetic, phantom and real data.

2   Rotation Invariant Features for Spherical Functions

2.1   Spherical Harmonic Representation of Spherical Functions

Our framework for extracting features from HARDI signals is based on a theorem
first proved for functions represented by a Fourier basis [17]. This theorem was
recently extended to continuous spherical functions represented in an SH basis
[18, 19]. The (standard) SH basis are complex-valued functions defined as

$$Y_l^m(\theta, \phi) = \sqrt{\frac{2l+1}{4\pi} \frac{(l-m)!}{(l+m)!}} P_l^m(\cos\theta)e^{im\phi} , \quad l = 0, 1, 2, \ldots, \quad -l \leq m \leq l, \quad (1)$$

where P_l^m is the associated Legendre polynomial of degree l and order m, $\theta \in$
$[0, \pi]$, and $\phi \in [0, 2\pi)$. For a real continuous spherical function $f : \mathbb{S}^2 \to \mathbb{R}$,

we can write $f = \sum_{l=0}^{\infty} \sum_{m=-l}^{l} \hat{f}_{l,m} Y_l^m$, where $\hat{f}_{l,m}$ are the SH coefficients that parametrize f.

We can approximate f using a finite SH basis representation of degree up to L, giving us $(L+1)^2$ basis elements. Given the vector of SH coefficients $\hat{\boldsymbol{f}} = [\hat{f}_{l,m}]$, [19] constructed an $(L+1)^2 \times (L+1)^2$ matrix T_L, which is an analogue to the Toeplitz matrix of the Fourier representation. The matrix T_L is constructed as follows. Let $g(u) = \sum_{l=0}^{L} \sum_{m=-l}^{m=l} \hat{g}_{lm} Y_{lm}(u)$ be a spherical function and let $\hat{\boldsymbol{g}}$ be its vector of SH coefficients of length $(L+1)^2$. Then [19] shows that the coefficients $\widehat{\boldsymbol{fg}}$ of the product of two spherical functions, $f(u)g(u)$, can be obtained as

$$T_L(f)\hat{\boldsymbol{g}} = \widehat{\boldsymbol{fg}}. \tag{2}$$

Here, $T_L(f)$ is a matrix whose rows and columns are indexed by the pair $(l_1 m_1, l_2 m_2) = (l_1(l_1+1) + m_1, l_2(l_2+1) + m_2)$, where $l_i = 0, 1, 2, \ldots, L$ and $-l_i \le m_i \le l_i$, for $i = 1, 2$. The entry of $T_L(f)$ at index $(l_1 m_1, l_2 m_2)$ is defined as

$$T_L(f)_{l_1 m_1; l_2 m_2} = \sum_{l=|l_1-l_2|}^{l_1+l_2} \hat{f}_{l, m_1 - m_2} G(l, l_2, l_1; m_1 - m_2, m_2, m_1), \tag{3}$$

where $G(l_1, l_2, l_3; m_1, m_2, m_3)$ is a real constant Gaunt Coefficient (See [19] Appendix A). As an important note, $T_L(f)$ is not Toeplitz. However its structure embodies many of the same properties of the Toeplitz form for the Fourier case.

We can rewrite T_L as a linear combination of matrices of Gaunt Coefficients

$$T_L(f) = \sum_{l=0}^{L} \sum_{m=-l}^{m=l} \hat{f}_{lm} G_{lm}, \tag{4}$$

where $G_{lm}(l_1(l_1+1) + m_1, l_2(l_2+1) + m_2) = G(ll_2l_1; mm_2m_1)$. Note that the Gaunt coefficient matrices G_{lm} are sparse since $G(ll_2l_1; mm_2m_1)$ is zero unless $m = m_1 - m_2$, so this formulation is more computationally efficient and intuitive.

With the above notation, we have the following extension of the Eigenvalue Distribution Theorem to continuous spherical functions [17, 18], which asserts that the eigenvalues of $T_L(f)$ are distributed as the function f itself.

Theorem 1. (Eigenvalue Distribution Theorem on $\mathbb{S}^2$) *Let $f(u)$ be a continuous spherical function and let $T_L(f)$ be the Toeplitz-like matrix defined in (4). Furthermore let F be any continuous function defined on the range of f. Then*

$$\lim_{L \to \infty} \frac{F(\lambda_1^{(L)}) + \cdots + F(\lambda_{(L+1)^2}^{(L)})}{(L+1)^2} = \frac{1}{4\pi} \int_{\mathbb{S}^2} F(f(u)) d\sigma(u), \tag{5}$$

where $\{\lambda_k^{(L)}\}_{k=1}^{(L+1)^2}$ are the real eigenvalues of T_L with $\lambda_1^{(L)} \le \lambda_2^{(L)} \le \cdots \le \lambda_{(L+1)^2}^{(L)}$ and $d\sigma(u)$ is the area element in $\mathbb{S}^2$.

2.2 Spherical Harmonic Coefficients of Rotated Spherical Functions

Let $\mathbf{R} = \mathbf{R}(\alpha, \beta, \gamma) = \mathbf{R}_z(\gamma)\mathbf{R}_y(\beta)\mathbf{R}_z(\alpha)$ be an element of the rotation group SO(3), parameterized by the Euler angles $\alpha, \gamma \in [0, 2\pi), \beta \in [0, \pi]$, where $\mathbf{R}_z$ and $\mathbf{R}_y$ represent rotations about the z and y axes respectively. To understand the effect of $\mathbf{R}$ on the SH coefficients $\hat{f}_{lk}$ of a spherical function f, let us define

$$A_{km}^l(\mathbf{R}(\alpha, \beta, \gamma)) = e^{-ik\gamma}P_{km}^l(\cos(\beta))e^{-im\alpha}, \tag{6}$$

where P_{km}^l are the generalizations of the associated Legrendre polynomials, computed by a recurrence relation of Jacobi polynomials. As shown in [20], the SH coefficient $\hat{f}_{lm}^{\mathbf{R}}$ of the rotated function $f_{\mathbf{R}}(u) = f(\mathbf{R}u)$ is a linear combination of the SH coefficients $\hat{f}_{lk}$, for $k = -l, \ldots, l$, of the function f, which is given by

$$\hat{f}_{lm}^{\mathbf{R}} = \sum_{k=-l}^{l} \hat{f}_{lk} A_{km}^l(\mathbf{R}). \tag{7}$$

We can see that the rotation of $\hat{f}$ is localized to each set of coefficients of degree l. Therefore we can write the $(L+1)^2 \times (L+1)^2$ matrix $\mathbf{A}(\mathbf{R})$ as a block diagonal matrix where each block is of the form $[\mathbf{A}^l]_{km} = A_{w(k,l)w(m,l)}^l(\mathbf{R})$ with $w(k, l) = k+l+1, l = 0, 2, \ldots L$ and $|k| \leq l$. Furthermore, it is shown in [21] that each block $\mathbf{A}^l$ is unitary, i.e., $(\mathbf{A}^l)^\top \mathbf{A}^l = \mathbf{I}_{(2l+1)\times(2l+1)}$, hence the entire block matrix $\mathbf{A}(\mathbf{R})$ is also unitary. Rewriting equation (7) in matrix form leads to

$$\hat{f}_{\mathbf{R}} = \mathbf{A}^\top(\mathbf{R})\hat{f}. \tag{8}$$

In other words, a 3D rotation of the domain of the spherical function f by $\mathbf{R}$ induces an $(L+1)^2$-dimensional rotation of its SH coefficients by $\mathbf{A}^\top(\mathbf{R})$.

2.3 Invariance of the Eigenvalues of T_L under a Rotation on $\mathbb{S}^2$

Let $f(u) = \sum_{l=0}^{L}\sum_{m=-l}^{m=l} \hat{f}_{lm}Y_{lm}(u)$ and $g(u) = \sum_{l=0}^{L}\sum_{m=-l}^{m=l} \hat{g}_{lm}Y_{lm}(u)$ be two continuous spherical functions with vectors of SH coefficients $\hat{f} = [\hat{f}_{lm}]$ and $\hat{g} = [\hat{g}_{lm}]$, respectively. Using the definition of T_L in (2), [19] shows that

$$\hat{g}^* T_L(f)\hat{g} = \int_{\mathbb{S}^2} f(u)|g(u)|^2 d\sigma(u). \tag{9}$$

Let $\hat{g}_{\mathbf{R}^\top} = \mathbf{A}^\top(\mathbf{R}^\top)\hat{g}$ be the SH coefficient vector of $g_{\mathbf{R}^\top}(u) = g(\mathbf{R}^\top u)$ and let $\hat{g}_{\mathbf{R}}^* = \hat{g}^*\mathbf{A}(\mathbf{R}^\top)$ be the SH coefficient vector of $g_{\mathbf{R}}(u) = g(\mathbf{R}u)$. We have that

$$\hat{g}_{\mathbf{R}}^* T_L(f)\hat{g}_{\mathbf{R}^\top} = \int_{\mathbb{S}^2} f(u)|g_{\mathbf{R}^\top}(u)|^2 d\sigma(u) = \int_{\mathbb{S}^2} f(u)|g(\mathbf{R}^\top u)|^2 d\sigma(u) \tag{10}$$

$$= \int_{\mathbb{S}^2} f(\mathbf{R}u')|g(u')|^2 d\sigma(u') = \int_{\mathbb{S}^2} f_{\mathbf{R}}(u')|g(u')|^2 d\sigma(u') = \hat{g}^* T_L(f_{\mathbf{R}})\hat{g},$$

where $u' \doteq R^\top u \implies d\sigma(u') = |R^\top| d\sigma(u)$ and $|R^\top| = 1$. Since in addition $\hat{g}^* A T_L(f) A^\top \hat{g} = \hat{g}_R^* T_L(f) \hat{g}_{R^\top}$, we have proved the following important relation:

$$A T_L(f) A^\top = T_L(f_R). \tag{11}$$

This implies that the eigenvalues of $T_L(f)$ are equal to the eigenvalues of $T_L(f_R)$. Furthermore, using the spectral decomposition of $T_L(f) = U \Lambda U^* = A^\top V \Lambda V^* A$ we have $U^* = V^* A$, hence $A = VU^*$, where U and V are the sorted matrices of eigenvectors for $T_L(f)$ and $T_L(f_R)$, respectively, and Λ is the diagonal matrix of sorted eigenvalues. This result is equivalent to the following statement:

For a continuous spherical function f of degree L, the eigenvalues of $T_L(f)$ are invariant under rotation of the domain of f on $\mathbb{S}^2$.

Notice that this result holds only for spherical functions of degree L. In the case HARDI reconstruction, where the signals are approximated by a spherical function of degree L, the eigenvalues of T_L will be approximately equal to the eigenvalues of T_L after rotation. We will discuss this in more detail in Section 3.2.

3   Invariant Features for HARDI Signals and ODFs

In Section 2 we developed a framework for extracting a large set of rotation invariant scalar features from any continuous spherical function. In this section, we apply this framework to the case of HARDI signals and ODFs.

3.1 Spherical Harmonic Representation of HARDI Signals and ODFs

Let S_0 be the baseline MRI signal and let $S(\theta, \phi)$ be the continuous HARDI signal along (θ, ϕ). Following [10], we define the continuous ODF, p, as:

$$p(\vartheta, \varphi) = \frac{1}{4\pi} + \frac{1}{16\pi^2} FRT\{\nabla_b^2 \ln(-\ln(\frac{S(\theta, \phi)}{S_0}))\}, \tag{12}$$

where FRT is the Funk-Radon transform, ∇_b^2 is the Laplace-Beltrami operator on $\mathbb{S}^2$, $\vartheta \in [0, \pi]$ and $\varphi \in [0, 2\pi)$. Since the HARDI signals are real and symmetric, we will use the modified SH basis to represent ODFs. This basis is defined as:

$$Y_j = \begin{cases} \sqrt{2} Re(Y_l^{|m|}) & \text{if } -l \le m < 0, \\ Y_l^0 & \text{if } m = 0, \\ \sqrt{2}(-1)^{m+1} Im(Y_l^m) & \text{if } 0 < m \le l, \end{cases} \tag{13}$$

where $Re(\cdot)$ and $Im(\cdot)$ are the real and imaginary parts, respectively, and $j \doteq j(l, m) = \frac{l^2+l+2}{2} + m$ for $l = 0, 2, 4, \ldots$ and $-l \le m \le l$. For degree up to L, there are $R = \frac{(L+1)(L+2)}{2}$ basis elements. It is important to note that when constructing our T_L matrices we must first convert to the equivalent complex standard basis. To express p in terms of the modified SH basis, let

$$s(\theta, \phi) \doteq \ln(-\ln(\frac{S(\theta, \phi)}{S_0})) = \sum_{j=1}^{\infty} c_j Y_j(\theta, \phi). \tag{14}$$

Since $\nabla_b^2(Y_j(\theta, \phi)) = -l_j(l_j + 1)Y_j(\theta, \phi)$, and $FRT(Y_j(\theta, \phi)) = 2\pi P_{l_j}(0)Y_j(\vartheta, \varphi)$, where $P_{l_j}(0)$ is the Legendre polynomial of degree l_j at 0, we have

$$p(\vartheta, \varphi) = \frac{1}{4\pi} + \frac{1}{16\pi^2} \sum_{j=1}^{\infty} (-2\pi P_{l_j}(0))l_j(l_j + 1)c_j Y_j(\vartheta, \varphi) = \sum_{j=1}^{\infty} \tilde{c}_j Y_j(\vartheta, \varphi), \quad (15)$$

where $\tilde{c}_1 = \frac{1}{2\sqrt{\pi}}$ and $\tilde{c}_j = -\frac{1}{8\pi} P_{l_j}(0)l_j(l_j + 1)c_j$ for $j > 1$.

We can see that HARDI data gives us two particular spherical functions that encode biological information of dMRI: the HARDI signal, s, and the ODF, p. In the above formulation, both of these functions are continuous. In practice, the HARDI signals are measured at a finite number, G, of fixed gradient directions $(\theta_i, \phi_i)_{i=1}^G$, usually in the range of 30 to 200 points, and p is estimated from s using another set of M discrete points on the sphere, $(\vartheta_i, \varphi_i)_{i=1}^M$. Using discrete approximations of s and p, with an R-dimensional SH basis of degree L, we have

$$s = \mathbf{B}c, \quad (16)$$

where $s \doteq [\ln(-\ln(\frac{S(\theta_1, \phi_1)}{S_0})), \ldots, \ln(-\ln(\frac{S(\theta_G, \phi_G)}{S_0}))]^\top$, $\mathbf{B} \in \mathbb{R}^{G \times R}$ is a matrix whose i-th row is $\mathbf{B}_i = [Y_1(\theta_i, \phi_i), \ldots, Y_R(\theta_i, \phi_i)]$, and $c = [c_1, c_2, \ldots, c_R]^\top \in \mathbb{R}^R$. Then

$$p = \frac{1}{4\pi}\mathbf{1} + \frac{1}{16\pi^2}\mathbf{CLP}c = \mathbf{C}\tilde{c}, \quad (17)$$

where $\mathbf{1}$ is the $M \times 1$ vector of ones, $\mathbf{C}$ is the $M \times R$ SH basis matrix whose i-th row is $\mathbf{C}_i = [Y_1(\vartheta_i, \varphi_i), \ldots, Y_R(\vartheta_i, \varphi_i)]$, $\mathbf{L}$ is the $R \times R$ diagonal matrix of Laplace-Beltrami eigenvalues with $\mathbf{L}_{jj} = -l_j(l_j + 1)$, $\mathbf{P}$ is the $R \times R$ diagonal Funk-Radon transform matrix with $\mathbf{P}_{jj} = 2\pi P_{l_j}(0)$ and $\tilde{c}$ is defined as in (15).

3.2 Approximate Rotation Invariance Using a Finite SH Basis

In Section 2.3 we showed that, for a continuous spherical function f of degree L, the eigenvalues of the matrix $T_L(f)$ are invariant with respect to a rotation of the domain of f. In Section 3.1 we showed how to approximate HARDI signals and their ODFs, s and p, respectively, by continuous spherical functions of degree L. Notice, however, that the eigenvalues of $T_L(s)$ and $T_L(p)$ need not be invariant with respect to rotations of the raw HARDI signals. This is because the raw HARDI signals may not admit an expansion of degree L in terms of the SH basis.

In practice, however, we expect the HARDI signals to be well approximated by low-degree models, hence the eigenvalues of $T_L(s)$ and $T_L(p)$ should be approximately invariant with respect to rotations for large enough L. To verify this, we used the multi-tensor model in [22] to generate three noiseless HARDI signals of 1-, 2-, and 3-fiber ODFs. We applied two different rotations to each one of these HARDI signals and approximated the resulting nine HARDI signals by an SH expansion of degree $L = 4$. The two plots in column 1 of Fig. 1 show the 25 eigenvalues of $T_L(s)$ and $T_L(p)$, respectively, in increasing order. Notice

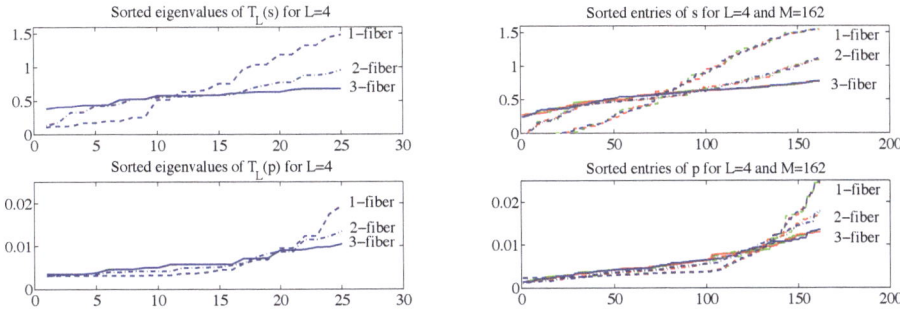

Fig. 1. Comparing the rotational invariance of the eigenvalues (first column) to that of the spherical function values (second column) using a discretization of the continuous function. The first row is the HARDI signal and the second row is the ODF. The plots show the sorted eigenvalues and sorted function values for nine different signals and ODFs, obtained by rotating three different signals with 1, 2, and 3 fibers, respectively. Observe the almost perfect overlap of the curves corresponding to 1-, 2-, or 3-fiber ODFs in the first column and the misalignment of the curves in the second column.

that the three curves of eigenvalues corresponding to 1-, 2-, or 3-fibers align almost perfectly, showing that the eigenvalues of T_L are approximately invariant to rotations in spite of the finite approximation by an SH basis of degree $L = 4$.

Now, since the eigenvalues of T_L give only approximately invariant features due to the use of a finite degree L, we might wonder why not using other approximately invariant features instead. For example, the maximum and minimum values of s are invariant to rotations. More generally, if we look at the entries of s, which correspond to samples of s at different directions on a fixed grid on $\mathbb{S}^2$, then the sorted entries of s should be approximately invariant to rotations. To verify this, we plot in column 2 of Fig. 1 the sorted entries of s and p (in increasing order) for the same nine HARDI signals described before. Notice that the three curves of 1-, 2-, or 3-fibers do not align as well as the corresponding curves in column 1. This shows that the sorted discrete values of s and p are not as invariant to rotations as are the eigenvalues of $T_L(s)$ and $T_L(p)$, respectively.

Given the (approximate) invariance of the eigenvalues of $T_L(s)$ and $T_L(p)$, we can use Theorem 1 to generate a large number of rotation invariant features for describing HARDI signals. For example, we can use the minimum and maximum eigenvalues, $\lambda_{\min}$ and $\lambda_{\max}$, respectively, which approximate the minimum and maximum of the spherical function. We can also use the range of the eigenvalues, $\lambda_{\max} - \lambda_{\min}$, as another feature. In addition, the variance of the eigenvalues will be closely related to the variance of the spherical function values and can be used as another feature. We also considered features such as the mean, median and mode of the eigenvalues as well as the determinant, trace, 2-norm and Frobenius norm of T_L. But the beauty of this framework is that one can use any continuous function of the eigenvalues, which provides a very rich set of features for a particular application. Furthermore, the choice of which spherical function to use (s, p or another) is also up to the user and can be determined

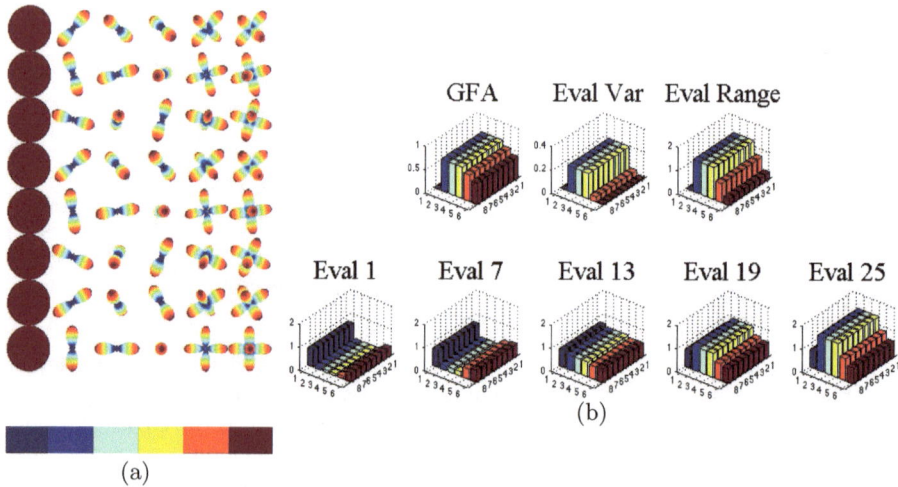

Fig. 2. Synthetic ODF field of 0-, 1-, 2-, and 3-fiber ODFs with various rotations and no noise. The graphs in 2(b) are colorcoded by the color bar in 2(a) to indicate each column of the ODF field while each row is a different rotation of each ODF. The constant height of each color in the bar graphs indicate the invariance of the eigenvalues under rotation and the relative differences in values for ODFs with varying number of crossing fibers.

based on the application or experiment. For different experiments (Section 4) we use the eigenvalues associated to both the HARDI signal, s and the ODF p. Furthermore, we can even extend L by zeropadding the coefficient vector of our spherical function using the method in [23] to extract a larger number of features, of which the values such as minimum, maximum, range and variance of eigenvalues will better approximate the distribution of the function values.

4   Validation

Synthetic Data. We first test the proposed HARDI features on synthetic data of isotropic, 1-, 2-, and 3-fiber ODFs generated using the multi-tensor model in [22]. For the synthetic ODF field in Fig. 2(a) we plot the variance and range of the eigenvalues of $T_L(s)$ in Fig. 2(b). Observe from the constant height of the bars in each color of the bar graph that these values are rotation invariant, as predicted. Observe also from the distribution of the bar graphs in Fig. 2(b) that these features give information about the shape of each ODF. In particular, notice that the maximum eigenvalue of the 1-fiber ODFs is greater than that for the 2- and 3-fiber ODFs. This is also apparent from Fig. 1. We can also see that the minimum eigenvalue of the 3-fiber ODFs is greater than that of the 2-fiber and 1-fiber ODFs, also as seen in Fig. 1. When interpreting the results for ODFs, we can additionally use the fact that p is a probability distribution. Thus, if the variances of each peak in our ODF are the same, as was the case in our synthetic

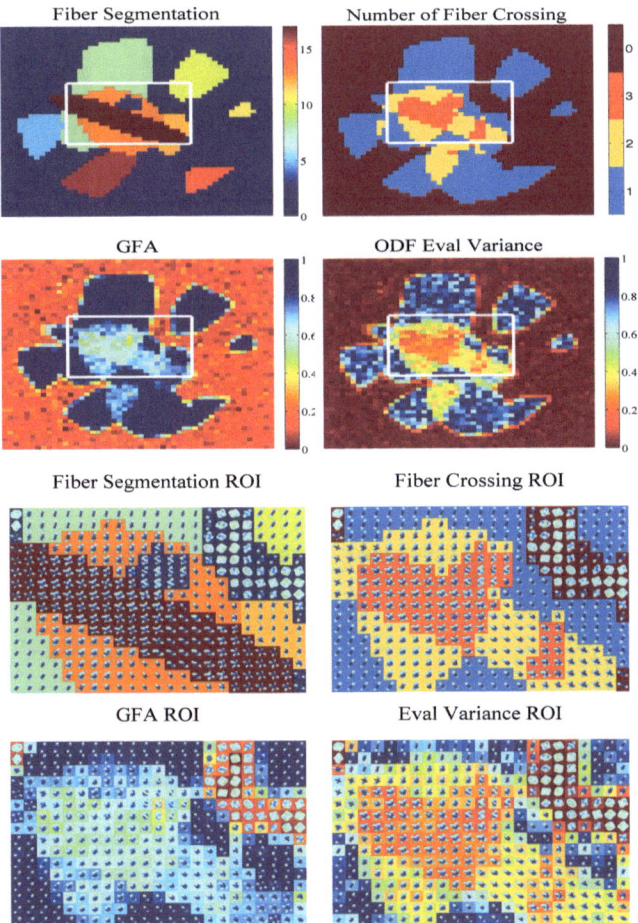

Fig. 3. ISBI 2013 HARDI Phantom. First Row: The left image is the ground truth fiber segmentation of a slice of the phantom dataset, where we've identified an intricate region of crossing fibers. The right image is a count of the number of fibers that cross in a given voxel, ranging from 0 to 3. Second Row: GFA and eigenvalue variance of the phantom slice. We notice here the stricking similarity between the plot of crossing fibers and the eigenvalue variance whereas the GFA is unable to reveal this information. Third/Fourth Row: Close up of the ROI with ODFs.

experiments, we know that the maximum of a 1-fiber ODF will be greater than that for the 2- and 3-fiber ODFs since the area under the curve must sum to 1. This information is also encoded in the range of the eigenvalues. Furthermore, the variance of the eigenvalues indicate how the values are spread out, revealing information about the relative roundedness of the ODF, where a lower variance indicates a rounder shape and a higher variance indicates a thinner shape.

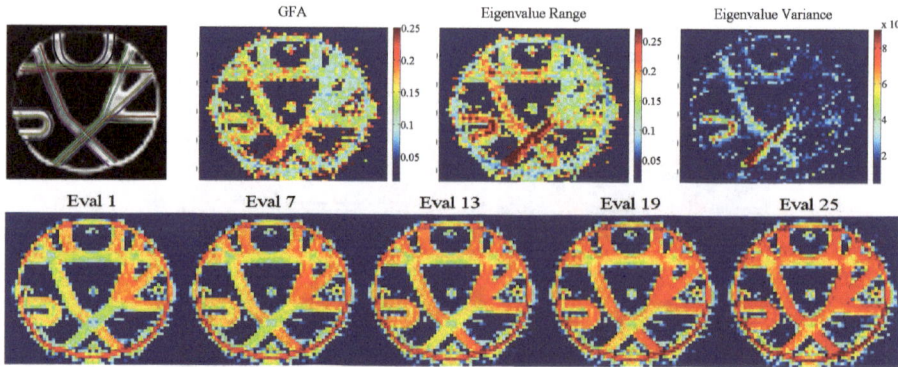

Fig. 4. Fiber Cup Phantom. We show the ground truth and GFA compared to the eigenvalue variance and range scalar maps and several eigenvalues of $T_4(s)$ where Eval 1 is the smallest eigenvalue and Eval 25 is the largest (Red: high, greenish blue: low).

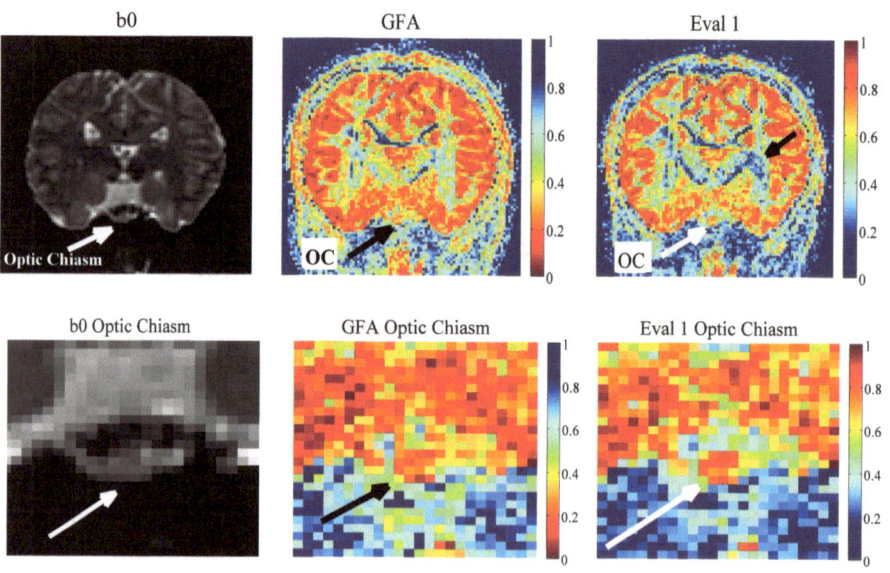

Fig. 5. Real HARDI scalar maps of the optic chiasm fiber crossing. The bottom arrows identify the location of the optic chiasm. We can distinguish the chiasm in the Eval 1 map while the GFA is noisier. The top arrow in the whole brain Eval 1 map indicates a region where there is more detail to highly anisotropic fiber tracts than the GFA.

Phantom Data. We also evaluate our method on two different phantom datasets. The first one is taken from the ISBI 2013 HARDI Reconstruction Challenge, which consists of 20 fiber bundles crossing at various angles within a $50 \times 50 \times 50$ spherical volume.[1] We used a subset of the dataset imaged at 64

---

[1] http://hardi.epfl.ch/static/events/2013_ISBI/download.html

gradient directions with $b = 3000s/mm^2$ and SNR of 30. We selected z slice 38 to demonstrate our method on the intricate crossing region shown in Fig. 3. In the top left we present an approximate ground truth segmentation of the fibers by using the given center and radius information for each fiber in the dataset. The image in the top right is a count of the number of fibers that cross in a single voxel based on the ground truth segmentation. The two figures in the second row compare the GFA to the variance of the eigenvalues of $T_L(p)$. Notice that the GFA mostly distinguishes isotropic regions from anisotropic ones, while the variance is able to discern regions with 0, 1, 2, or 3 crossing fibers, approximately matching the ground truth. The remaining two rows show a more detailed view of the central region, with the ODF estimates at each voxel.

Secondly, in Fig. 4, we experimented on the Neurospin MR phantom dataset provided for the MICCAI 2009 Fiber Cup [24, 25]. Analyzing our new scalar maps of eigenvalue range and variance of the Fiber Cup dataset we notice a higher degree of detail. We see more variety of values along the fiber travelling from top right to bottom left. Also very importantly, each new map reveals more details about the shape of the topmost U-shaped kissing fiber, over and above the GFA maps. Furthermore we show each individual eigenvalue and display a progression of values. In particular, the minimum and maximum eigenvalues, Eval 1 and Eval 25, respectively, reveal more detail in the crossing fiber regions. In Eval 1 the crossing regions show up greenish-blue, on the lower end of the spectrum. The same regions in Eval 25 also show lower values with color yellow. As noticed in the synthetic experiments, crossing fibers exhibit a lower range of eigenvalues when compared to single fiber ODFs.

Real HARDI Data. The optic chiasm is the location where two fibers leading from the right and left hemispheres intersect as they travel from the optic tract to the optic nerve. It has been identified as a unique region of two fiber crossing as well as kissing on either side using DTI tractography [26]. In Fig. 5 we analyze the fiber crossing of the optic chiasm and calculate the GFA and minimum eigenvalue feature for this ROI in a $112 \times 112 \times 64$ real human brain HARDI dataset acquired with 127 gradient directions and $b = 1000s/mm^2$. The minimum eigenvalue map is able to more concretely distinguish the crossing center red region from the yellow region of the optic tract extending from left and right.

5   Conclusion

We have developed a general framework for extracting rotation invariant features from any spherical function using an SH basis. In particular, we extracted features from ODFs of HARDI signals, but any other spherical function used in the numerous methods of HARDI reconstruction and fiber orientation estimation can be substituted here to obtain features valuable for a particular application. These features reduce the complexity of dMRI data to measurable and comparable scalar values that could be used as biomarkers in the detection of neurological diseases.

Acknowledgements. This work was supported by NIH grants 5T32EB010021-03, R01 EB008432 and P50 AG05146.

References

1. Jones, D.K.: Diffusion MRI: Theory, Methods, and Application. Oxford University Press (2010)
2. Smith, S.M., Jenkinson, M., Johansen-Berg, H., Rueckert, D., Nichols, T.E., Mackay, C.E., Watkins, K.E., Ciccarelli, O., Cader, M.Z., Matthews, P.M., Behrens, T.E.: Tract-based spatial statistics: Voxelwise analysis of multi-subject diffusion data. NeuroImage 31(4), 1487–1505 (2006)
3. Basser, P.: Inferring microstructural features and the physiological state of tissues from diffusion weighted images. NMR in Biomedicine (1995)
4. Westin, C.F., Maier, S.E., Mamata, H., Nabavi, A., Jolesz, F.A., Kikinis, R.: Processing and visualization for diffusion tensor MRI. Medical Image Analysis 6(2), 93–108 (2002)
5. Ghosh, A., Papadopoulo, T., Deriche, R.: Biomarkers for HARDI: 2nd & 4th order tensor invariants. In: IEEE International Symposium on Biomedical Imaging, pp. 26–29 (2012)
6. Barmpoutis, A., Hwang, M.S., Howland, D., Forder, J.R., Vemuri, B.C.: Regularized positive-definite fourth order tensor field estimation from DW-MRI. NeuroImage 45(1), S153–S162 (2009)
7. Barmpoutis, A., Vemuri, B.C.: A unified framework for estimating diffusion tensors of any order with symmetric positive-definite constraints. In: IEEE International Symposium on Biomedical Imaging, pp. 1385–1388 (2010)
8. Tuch, D.: Q-ball imaging. Magnetic Resonance in Medicine 52(6), 1358–1372 (2004)
9. Tristan-Vega, A., Westin, C.F., Aja-Fernandez, S.: Estimation of fiber orientation probability density functions in high angular resolution diffusion imaging. NeuroImage 47(2), 638–650 (2009)
10. Aganj, I., Lenglet, C., Sapiro, G., Yacoub, E., Ugurbil, K., Harel, N.: Reconstruction of the orientation distribution function in single- and multiple-shell q-ball imaging within constant solid angle. Magnetic Resonance in Medicine 64(2), 554–566 (2010)
11. Assemlal, H.E., Tschumperlé, D., Brun, L., Siddiqi, K.: Recent advances in diffusion mri modeling: Angular and radial reconstruction. Medical Image Analysis 15(4), 369–396 (2011)
12. Frank, L.R.: Characterization of anisotropy in high angular resolution diffusion-weighted mri. Magnetic Resonance in Medicine 47(6), 1083–1099 (2002)
13. Ozarslan, E., Vemuri, B.C., Mareci, T.H.: Generalized scalar measures for diffusion mri using trace, variance, and entropy. Magnetic Resonance in Medicine 53(4), 866–876 (2005)
14. Ghosh, A., Deriche, R.: Extracting geometrical features & peak fractional anisotropy from the odf for white matter characterization. In: IEEE International Symposium on Biomedical Imaging, pp. 266–271 (2011)
15. Fuster, A., van de Sande, J., Astola, L., Poupon, C., ter Haar Romeny, B.: Fourth-order tensor invariants in high angular resolution diffusion imaging. In: MICCAI 2011 Workshop on Computational Diffusion MRI (2011)
16. Basser, P.J., Pajevic, S.: Spectral decomposition of a 4th-order covariance tensor: Applications to diffusion tensor MRI. Signal Processing 87(2), 220–236 (2007)

17. Grenander, U., Szego, G.: Toeplitz Forms and their Applications. University of California Press (1958)
18. Okikiolu, K.: The analogue of the strong Szego limit theorem on the 2 and 3-dimensional spheres. Journal of the American Mathematical Society 9, 345–372 (1996)
19. Shirdhonkar, S., Jacobs, D.: Non-negative lighting and specular object recognition. In: IEEE Conference on Computer Vision and Pattern Recognition (2005)
20. Cetingul, H.E., Afsari, B., Vidal, R.: An algebraic solution to rotation recovery in hardi from correspondences of orientation distribution functions. In: IEEE International Symposium on Biomedical Imaging (2012)
21. Chirikjian, G., Kyatkin, A.: Engineering Applications of Noncommutative Harmonic Analysis: With Emphasis on Rotation and Motion Groups. CRC Press (2000)
22. Descoteaux, M., Angelino, E., Fitzgibbons, S., Deriche, R.: Regularized, fast and robust analytical Q-ball imaging. Magnetic Resonance in Medicine 58(3), 497–510 (2007)
23. Schwab, E., Afsari, B., Vidal, R.: Estimation of non-negative ODFs using the eigenvalue distribution of spherical functions. In: Ayache, N., Delingette, H., Golland, P., Mori, K. (eds.) MICCAI 2012, Part II. LNCS, vol. 7511, pp. 322–330. Springer, Heidelberg (2012)
24. Fillard, P., Descoteaux, M., Goh, A., Gouttard, S., Jeurissen, B., Malcolm, J., Ramirez-Manzanares, A., Reisert, M., Sakaie, K., Tensaouti, F., Yo, T., Mangin, J.F., Poupon, C.: Quantitative evaluation of 10 tractography algorithms on a realistic diffusion mr phantom. NeuroImage 56(1), 220–234 (2011)
25. Poupon, C., Rieul, B., Kezele, I., Perrin, M., Poupon, F., Mangin, J.F.: New diffusion phantoms dedicated to the study and validation of high-angular-resolution diffusion imaging (HARDI) models. Magnetic Resonance in Medicine 60(6), 1276–1283 (2008)
26. Hofer, S., Karaus, A., Frahm, J.: Reconstruction and dissection of the entire human visual pathway using diffusion tensor MRI. Frontiers in Neuroanatomy 4(15) (2010)

Geodesic Shape Regression
in the Framework of Currents

James Fishbaugh[1], Marcel Prastawa[1], Guido Gerig[1], and Stanley Durrleman[2]

[1] Scientific Computing and Imaging Institute, University of Utah
[2] INRIA/ICM, Pitié Salpêtrière Hospital, Paris, France

Abstract. Shape regression is emerging as an important tool for the statistical analysis of time dependent shapes. In this paper, we develop a new generative model which describes shape change over time, by extending simple linear regression to the space of shapes represented as currents in the large deformation diffeomorphic metric mapping (LDDMM) framework. By analogy with linear regression, we estimate a baseline shape (intercept) and initial momenta (slope) which fully parameterize the geodesic shape evolution. This is in contrast to previous shape regression methods which assume the baseline shape is fixed. We further leverage a control point formulation, which provides a discrete and low dimensional parameterization of large diffeomorphic transformations. This flexible system decouples the parameterization of deformations from the specific shape representation, allowing the user to define the dimensionality of the deformation parameters. We present an optimization scheme that estimates the baseline shape, location of the control points, and initial momenta simultaneously via a single gradient descent algorithm. Finally, we demonstrate our proposed method on synthetic data as well as real anatomical shape complexes.

1 Introduction

Shape regression is of crucial importance for statistical shape analysis. It is useful to find correlations between shape configuration and a continuous scalar parameter such as age, disease progression, drug delivery, or cognitive scores. When only few follow-up observations are available, regression is also a necessary tool to interpolate between data points and provide a scenario of continuous shape evolution over the parameter range [5,13]. Longitudinal studies also require to compare such regressions across different subjects [5,8,10,11].

Extending traditional scalar regression for shape is not straightforward as shape intrinsically live on a Riemannian manifold. Therefore, methods differ according to the choice of metric on the shape space and the corresponding regression function. In [5], a piecewise geodesic method has been proposed, which extends piecewise linear regression for shape time-series. In [7,16] second-order models have been proposed which are controlled by the acceleration of shape changes or the deviation from geodesic paths. Non-parametric regression has been proposed in [3], extending kernel regression to Riemannian manifolds. In [9]

J.C. Gee et al. (Eds.): IPMI 2013, LNCS 7917, pp. 718–729, 2013.

geodesic regression is proposed as a straightforward extension of linear regression on Riemannian manifolds. Geodesic regression is fully characterized by the baseline shape (the intercept) and the tangent vector defining the geodesic at the baseline shape (the slope). Therefore, it seems well adapted for longitudinal studies, since different regressions could be compared by transporting baseline and tangent vectors from subject to subject, using parallel transport for instance [12].

Methods in [5,7,14] are based on the large deformation diffeomorphic metric mapping (LDDMM) paradigm, which is well suited for regression purposes since it is built on a continuous flow of diffeomorphisms that model continuous shape changes over a time period. In [14], geodesic regression is proposed in the LD-DMM framework for image data. Extending it for geometric data such as curves and surfaces is challenging for at least two reasons.

First, images seen as measures on $\mathbb{R}^3$ inherit from a linear structure which eases the estimation of the baseline image (images could be averaged by averaging grey levels for instance). Curves or surfaces could be also embedded into a vector space if we assume point correspondences between shapes [2]. Alternatively, we can avoid explicit correspondence by embedding shapes into the space of currents, which defines a generic metric which can handle both surfaces and curves or any mix of them. However, the average of surfaces in the space of currents is usually not a surface anymore [5]. To overcome this limitation, we will use here the new formulation initiated in [6], which allows to optimize a given template in the space of currents, while preserving its topology.

Second, the parameterization of the deformations in the LDDMM setting is given by a scalar momenta map (which plays the role of the tangent vector defining the geodesic path), which has the same dimension as the images. For point data, the parameterization is given by one momentum vector at every point of the baseline shape. The dimension of this parameterization explodes when shape complexes are analyzed. To overcome this limitation, we will use the control point formulation in the LDDMM setting that has been introduced in [4]. Consequently, our geodesic model characterizes complex evolution with a small number of parameters (defined by the user), compared to [5,7] which require vectors at every shape point and every time point in the discretization.

2 Methods

2.1 Shape Regression

In shape regression, the goal is to estimate a continuous shape evolution from a discrete set of observed shapes $\mathbf{O}_{t_i}$ at time t_i within the time interval $[t_0,\ T]$. Here we consider shape to be generic geometric objects that can be represented as curves, landmark points, or surfaces in $2D$ or $3D$. Shape evolution is modeled as the geodesic flow of diffeomorphisms acting on a baseline shape $\mathbf{X}_0$, defined as $\mathbf{X}(t) = \phi_t(\mathbf{X}_0)$ with t varying continuously within the time interval determined by the observed data. The baseline shape $\mathbf{X}_0$ is continuously deformed over time to match the observation data $(\mathbf{X}(t_i) \sim \mathbf{O}_{t_i})$ with the rigidity of the evolution controlled by a regularity term. This setting is naturally expressed as a variational problem, described by the regression criterion

$$E(\mathbf{X}_0, \phi_t)) = \sum_{i=1}^{N_{obs}} ||(\phi_{t_i}(\mathbf{X}_0) - \mathbf{O}_{t_i})||_{W^*}^2 + \text{Reg}(\phi_t)$$

$$= \sum_{i=1}^{N_{obs}} D(\mathbf{X}(t_i), \mathbf{O}_{t_i}) + L(\phi_t) \tag{1}$$

where D represents the squared distance on currents ($||\cdot||_{W^*}^2$) and L is a measure of the regularity of the time-varying deformation ϕ_t.

2.2   Control Point Parameterization of Deformations

We adopt a discrete parameterization of deformations, where dense diffeomorphisms of the underlying space are built by interpolating momenta located at control points [4]. Let $\mathbf{c}_0 = \{c_1, ..., c_{N_c}\}$ be a finite set of control points which carry initial momenta vectors $\alpha_0 = \{\alpha_1, ...\alpha_{N_c}\}$, together referred to as the initial state of the system $\mathbf{S}_0 = \{\mathbf{c}_0, \alpha_0\}$.

The set of control point positions $\mathbf{c}_0$ and initial momenta α_0 serve as initial conditions for the geodesic equations, which define the time evolution of the system of control points and momenta, given by

$$\begin{cases} \dot{c}_i(t) = \sum_{p=1}^{N_c} K(c_i(t), c_p(t))\alpha_p(t) \\ \dot{\alpha}_i(t) = -\sum_{p=1}^{N_c} \alpha_i(t)^t \alpha_p(t) \nabla_1 K(c_i(t), c_p(t)) \end{cases} \tag{2}$$

where K is the interpolating kernel assumed (without loss of generality) to be Gaussian: $K(x, y) = \exp(-|x - y|^2)/\sigma^2)$. These equations describe the evolution of the state of the system $\mathbf{S}(t) = \{c_i(t), \alpha_i(t)\}$ and can be written in short as $\dot{\mathbf{S}}(t) = F\mathbf{S}(t)$

Thanks to the geodesic equations, the trajectories of control points $c_i(t)$ and $\alpha_i(t)$ now parameterize the *time-varying* velocity field $v(x, t)$ defined at any point in space x and time t as

$$\dot{x}(t) = v(x, t) = \sum_{p=1}^{N_c} K(x, c_p(t))\alpha_p(t). \tag{3}$$

which can be written in short as $\dot{x}(t) = G(x(t), \mathbf{S}(t))$.

The time-varying velocity field $v(x, t)$ can then be used to build the flow of deformations $\phi_t(x)$ in the spirit of the LDDMM framework by integrating the ODE: $\dot{\phi}_t(x) = v(\phi_t(x), t)$. Using the coordinates of the baseline shape $\mathbf{X}_0$ as initial conditions, integrating this ODE computes the deformation of the baseline shape from time t_0 to T. Therefore the flow of diffeomorphisms is fully determined by the initial state of the system $\mathbf{S}_0$: the set of initial control points $\mathbf{c}_0$ and initial momenta vectors α_0.

2.3 Minimization of Regression Criterion

The geodesic flow of diffeomorphisms ϕ_t in the criterion (1) is parameterized by N_c control points and momenta vectors $\mathbf{S}_0 = \{\mathbf{c}_0, \boldsymbol{\alpha}_0\}$, which act as initial conditions for the flow equations (2). The baseline shape $\mathbf{X}_0$ can then be deformed according to this flow by applying equation (3). Therefore we seek to estimate the position of the control points, initial momenta, and position of the points on the baseline shape such that the resulting geodesic flow of the baseline shape best matches the observed data. An overview of our control point formulation of geodesic shape regression is shown in Fig. 1. With all elements of our framework defined, geodesic shape regression can now be described by the specific regression criterion

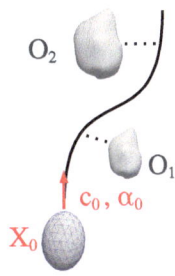

Fig. 1. Overview of geodesic regression with estimated parameters in red

$$E(\mathbf{X}_0, \mathbf{S}_0) = \sum_{i=1}^{N_{obs}} \frac{1}{2\lambda^2} D(\mathbf{X}(t_i), \mathbf{O}_{t_i}) + L(\mathbf{S}_0) \tag{4}$$

subject to

$$\begin{cases} \dot{\mathbf{S}}(t) = F(\mathbf{S}(t)) & \text{with } \mathbf{S}(0) = \{\mathbf{c}_0, \boldsymbol{\alpha}_0\} \\ \dot{\mathbf{X}}(t) = G(\mathbf{X}(t), \mathbf{S}(t)) & \text{with } \mathbf{X}(0) = \mathbf{X}_0 \end{cases} \tag{5}$$

where λ^2 is used to balance the importance of the data term and regularity, $L(\mathbf{S}_0) = \sum_{p,q} \alpha_{0,p}^t K(c_{0,p}, c_{0,q}) \alpha_{0,q}$ is the regularity term defined by the kinetic energy of the control points. The first part of (5) describes the trajectory of the control points and momenta as in (2). The second equation of (5) represents flowing the baseline shape along the deformation defined by $\mathbf{S}(t)$ as in (3).

As shown in the appendix, the gradients of the criterion (4) are

$$\nabla_{\mathbf{S}_0} E = \xi(0) + \nabla_{\mathbf{S}_0} L \qquad\qquad \nabla_{\mathbf{X}_0} E = \theta(0) \tag{6}$$

where the auxiliary variables $\theta(t)$ and $\xi(t) = \{\xi^c, \xi^\alpha\}$ satisfy the ODEs:

$$\begin{aligned} \dot{\theta}(t) &= -\partial_1 G(t)^t \theta(t) + \sum_{i=1}^{N_{Obs}} \nabla_{\mathbf{X}(t_i)} D(t_i) \delta(t - t_i) & \theta(T) &= 0 \\ \dot{\xi}(t) &= -(\partial_2 G(t)^t \theta(t) + d_{\mathbf{S}(t)} F(t)^t \xi(t)) & \xi(T) &= 0 \end{aligned} \tag{7}$$

The gradient is computed by first integrating equations (2) forward in time to construct the flow of diffeomorphisms. The deformations are then applied to the baseline shape by integrating forward in time equation (3). With the full trajectory of the deformed baseline shape, one can compute the gradient of the data term $\nabla_{\mathbf{X}(t_i)} D(t_i)$, corresponding to each observation. The ODEs (7) are then integrated backwards in time, with the gradients of the data term acting as jump conditions at observation time points, which pull the geodesic towards target data. The final values of the auxiliary variables $\theta(0)$ and $\xi(0)$ are then used to update the location of the control points, the initial momenta, and the location of the points on the baseline shape.

The method, summarized in Algorithm 1, is implemented via a gradient descent scheme. The parameters of the algorithm are the tradeoff between data matching and regularity λ, the standard deviation of the deformation kernel σ_V, and the standard deviation of the metric on currents σ_W. The value of σ_V controls the scale at which points in space move in a correlated manner, while the value of σ_W controls the scale at which shape differences are considered noise. The algorithm also requires an initial baseline shape. For surfaces, initialization consists of an ellipsoid for each connected component of the shapes, which defines the number of shape points as well as the connectivity, which is preserved during optimization.

Algorithm 1. Geodesic shape regression

Input: $\mathbf{X}_0$ (initial baseline shape), O_{t_i} (observed shapes), t_0 (start time), T (end time), σ (tradeoff), σ_V (std. dev. of deformation kernel), σ_W (std. dev. of currents metric)

Output: $\mathbf{X}_0, \mathbf{c}_0, \boldsymbol{\alpha}_0$

1   $\boldsymbol{\alpha}_0 \leftarrow 0$
2   Initialize control points $\mathbf{c}_0$ on regular grid with spacing σ_V
3   **repeat**
4   {Compute path of control points and momentum (forward integration)}
5       $c_i(t) = c_i(0) + \int_{t_0}^{T} \sum_{p=1}^{N_c} K(c_i(s), c_p(s))\alpha_p(s)ds$
6       $\alpha_i(t) = \alpha_i(0) - \int_{t_0}^{T} \sum_{p=1}^{N_c} \alpha_i(s)^t \alpha_p(s)\nabla_1 K(c_i(s), c_p(s))ds$
7   {Compute trajectory of deformed baseline shape (forward integration)}
8       $x_k(t) = x_k(0) + \int_{t_0}^{T} \sum_{p=1}^{N_c} K(x_k(s), c_j(s))\alpha_j(s)ds$
9   {Compute the gradient of the data term for each observation}
10      $\nabla_{\mathbf{X}(t_i)} D(t_i)$
11   {Compute auxiliary variable $\theta(t)$ (backward integration)}
12      $\theta_k(t) = \theta_k(T) + \int_{T}^{t} \sum_{p=1}^{N_c} \alpha_p(s)^t \theta_k(s)\nabla_1 K(x_k(s), c_p(s))$ $-$
13          $\sum_{i=1}^{N_{obs}} \nabla_{x_k(t_i)} D\delta(s - t_i)ds$
14   {Compute auxiliary variable $\xi^c(t)$ (backward integration)}
15      $\xi_k^c(t) = \xi_k^c(T) - \int_{T}^{t} \sum_{p=1}^{N_x} \alpha_k(s)^t \theta_p(s)\nabla_1 K(c_k(s), x_p(s)) +$
16          $(\partial_c F^c)\xi_k^c(s) + (\partial_c F^\alpha)\xi_k^\alpha(s)ds$
17   {Compute auxiliary variable $\xi^\alpha(t)$ (backward integration)}
18      $\xi_k^\alpha(t) = \xi_k^\alpha(T) - \int_{T}^{t} \sum_{p=1}^{N_x} K(c_k(s), x_p(s))\theta_p(s) +$
19          $(\partial_\alpha F^c)\xi_k^c(s) + (\partial_\alpha F^\alpha)\xi_k^c(s)ds$
20   {Compute gradients}
21      $\nabla_{\mathbf{c}_0} E = \xi^c(0) + \nabla_{\mathbf{c}_0} L$
22      $\nabla_{\boldsymbol{\alpha}_0} E = \xi^\alpha(0) + \nabla_{\boldsymbol{\alpha}_0} L$
23      $\nabla_{\mathbf{X}_0} E = \theta(0)$
24   {Update control points, momenta, and baseline shape}
25      $c_i(0) \leftarrow c_i(0) - \varepsilon \nabla_{c_i} E$ $\alpha_i(0) \leftarrow \alpha_i(0) - \varepsilon \nabla_{\alpha_i} E$ $x_i(0) \leftarrow x_i(0) - \varepsilon \nabla_{x_i} E$
26 **until** *Convergence*
27 **return** $\mathbf{X}_0, \mathbf{c}_0, \boldsymbol{\alpha}_0$

---

3 Results

Synthetic Transformations. We explore the ability of the geodesic regression model to capture simple synthetic transformations applied to a real anatomical surface. We consider the amygdala surface extracted from a 4 year old child and investigate translation and scaling. For both experiments, we initialize the baseline shape to be an ellipse, as shown in Fig. 2, which defines the topology of the baseline shape, which will remain unchanged during optimization. We define 12 control points on a

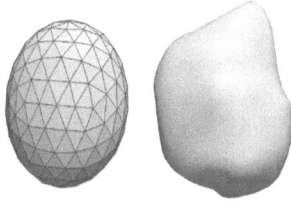

Fig. 2. Initial baseline shape and observed amygdala

regular grid and parameters $\sigma_V = 12$ mm, $\sigma_W = 5$ mm, and $\lambda = 0.1$. Both experiments contain three shape observations spaced one time unit apart.

For both experiments, the baseline shape estimated by our method closely matches the amygdala surface at the earliest time point and the dynamics of shape evolution are well captured by the geodesic model (Fig. 3). However, very accurate matching of the target shapes is not the goal with a geodesic model (and is generally not possible). The power of the model lies in the low dimensional parameterization of shape evolution, which facilitates statistical analysis. These experiments demonstrate the compactness of the geodesic model – continuous shape evolution is described by the baseline shape and 12 momentum vectors.

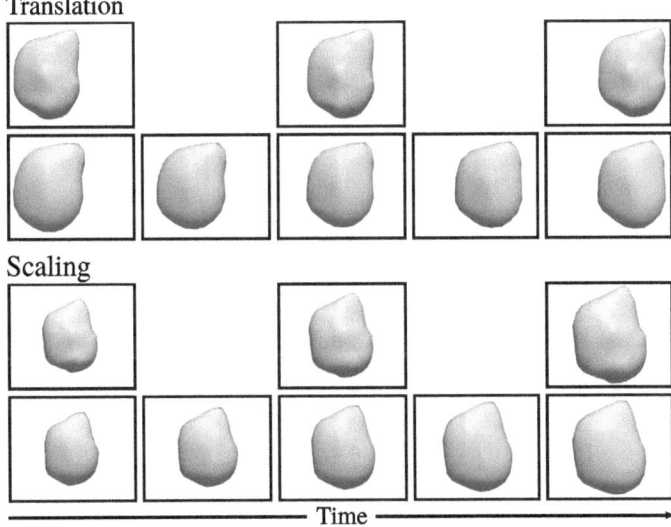

Fig. 3. For both translation and scaling panels, the top row shows discrete shape observations of the amygdala surface, while the bottom row shows shapes estimated during geodesic regression at observation times as well as intermediate stages. Our method estimates a baseline shape and momenta vectors that capture shape evolution.

Synthetic Tumor Evolution. Next, we apply our geodesic model to study tumor evolution over time. Using `TumorSim` [15], we simulate three differing tumor scenarios : a slowly deforming tumor, a rapidly deforming tumor, and a tumor which infiltrates rather than deforming surrounding tissue. We obtain four observations in the time span of one year, obtained at the same baseline time 0, 5 ± 1, 8 ± 1, and 12 months. This mimics the acquisition of real medical images, which are not necessarily acquired at the same time for every patient. The simulated images and tumor segmentations are shown in Fig. 4.

In order to compare the differing tumor evolutions, we leverage the control point formulation. We establish a common reference space which is shared among each geodesic model by placing 125 control points on a regular grid with 12 mm spacing and freeze these locations during optimization. We estimate a geodesic model for each tumor scenario, using parameters $\sigma_V = 12$ mm, $\sigma_W = 5$ mm, $\lambda = 1.0$, and initialize the baseline shape with an ellipse.

The estimated baseline tumor and initial momenta are displayed in Fig. 5 for each of the three tumor scenarios. The magnitude of the momenta describing the rapidly deforming tumor are the largest among the three tumor scenarios, which is also evident in the speed of growth overlaid on the baseline tumor. The orientation of the momenta vectors encode the direction of tumor growth, which highlight the differences in the way each tumor evolves. We note that the initial momenta vectors do not differentiate well between deforming and infiltrating tumors, as the infiltration process cannot be described by tumor shape alone. However, the estimated baseline shape and dynamics of shape change are well captured by the geodesic model for all three tumor scenarios.

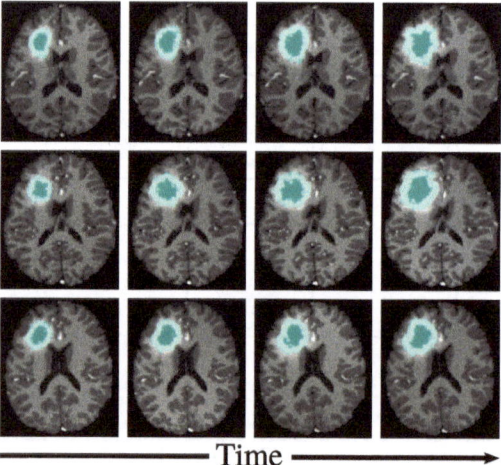

Fig. 4. Four observations of synthetic tumor evolution. **Top)** Slowly deforming tumor. **Middle)** Rapidly deforming tumor. **Bottom)** Tumor which infiltrates surrounding tissue. The first two cases show different degrees of deformation in surrounding tissue and ventricles, while the third has little deformation.

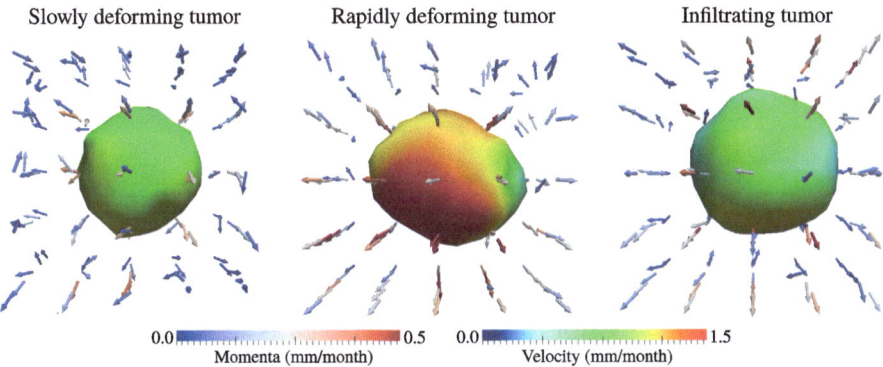

Fig. 5. Baseline shape and initial momenta for geodesic models of tumor evolution. Our regression framework captures the different tumor growth characteristics, with momenta vectors constrained to be in the same coordinates for comparison purposes.

Pediatric Subcortical Development. We next investigate the application of geodesic shape regression to model pediatric subcortical development. Three subcortical shapes are considered as a multi-object shape complex: putamen, amygdala, and hippocampus. The structures were obtained from MRI of a healthy child scanned at approximately 9, 13, and 24 months of age. Geodesic regression was conducted using 126 control points and parameters $\sigma_V = 8$ mm, $\sigma_W = 6$ mm, and $\lambda = 1.0$. To improve speed of convergence, we initialize the baseline shapes for each subcortical structure with an ellipse that has been coarsely registered to its corresponding subcortical shape. Regression was conducted on all shapes simultaneously, resulting in one deformation of the ambient space.

Several snapshots of the evolution of subcortical structures is shown in Fig. 6, with estimated baseline shape shown at 6 months. From 6 to 26 months, all subcortical structures increase in size, with the putamen demonstrating the most dramatic growth. The evolution of the putamen is characterized by accelerated growth at the superior anterior and inferior posterior regions, while the hippocampus grows mostly at the extreme posterior region, expanding and bending at the tip. The geodesic model is able to capture interesting non-linear growth patterns with few parameters; the full time evolution is modeled by three baseline shapes and 126 momenta vectors.

This experiment demonstrates the applicability of the geodesic model in characterizing pediatric subcortical development. Our regression framework simultaneously handles multiple shapes, including those with complex geometry. Multi-object regression allows for a more complete analysis, compared to an independent treatment of each subcortical structure, which ignores potentially important spatial relationships between structures. This single subject experiment can also be extended to a population analysis thanks to the control point formulation of deformations. As with the previous tumor experiment, one can fix the control point locations for all subjects. The differences between and within populations can be quantified by exploring the variability between

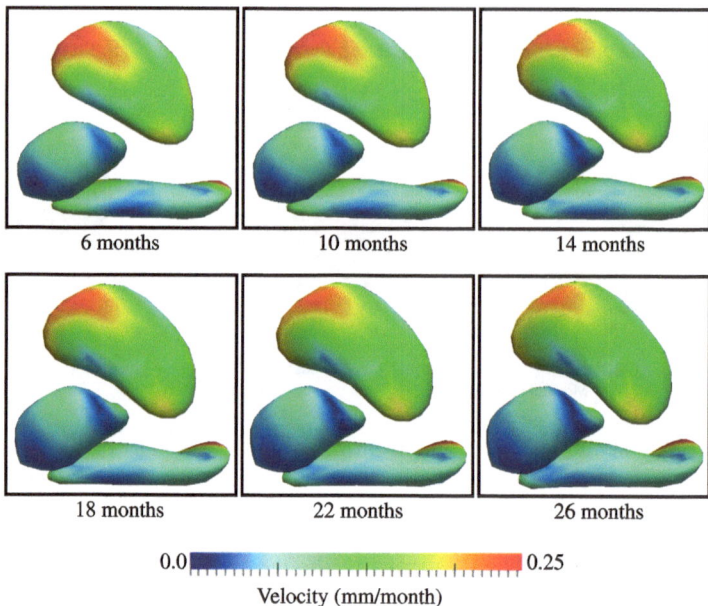

6 months   10 months   14 months

18 months   22 months   26 months

0.0 ▮▬▬▬▬▬▬▬▬▬▬▬▬ 0.25

Velocity (mm/month)

Fig. 6. Snapshots of subcortical shape evolution after geodesic regression on a multi-object complex: putamen, amygdala, and hippocampus

estimated baseline shapes, and between initial momenta at identical locations for all subjects.

White Matter Fibers in Early Brain Development. Finally, we study early brain development by considering the evolution of white matter connections from birth to 2 years of age. For this experiment, we have diffusion tensor imaging (DTI) data from 17 subjects with scans obtained at clustered time points of 2 ± 2, 12 ± 2 months, and 24 ± 2 months. We extract the genu fiber tract from each DTI using the framework of [1]. In our experiment, we use 26 genu fiber tracts which are represented as a collection of $3D$ curves. By considering fiber geometry obtained from multiple subjects, the estimated geodesic model can be considered as the development of the genu tract for an average child. We initialize the baseline shape with the genu fiber bundle from the atlas space, define 75 control points on a regular grid, and set parameter values as $\sigma_V = 5$ mm, $\sigma_W = 8$ mm, and $\lambda = 0.1$.

The average development of the genu tract estimated by our geodesic model is summarized in Fig. 7, which shows several snapshots on the genu fibers over time. The elongation of the fibers reflects the myelination process that occur during early development, where myelin sheaths grows to cover white matter regions outward to the cortex. Our geodesic regression framework handles the multiple fiber structure that form the genu fiber bundle, using the currents framework to match the curvilinear fiber structures.

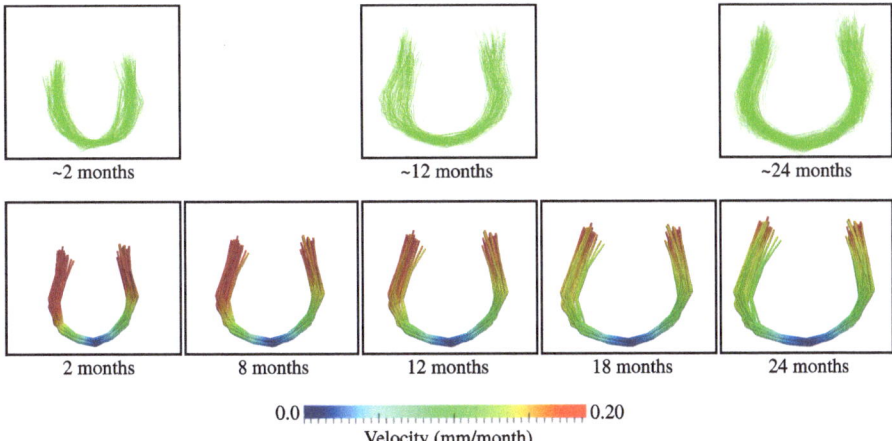

Fig. 7. Average development of genu fiber tract from 2 to 24 months. Top row shows observed data for all subjects, which is clustered around 2, 12, and 24 months. Bottom row shows genu fiber tracts estimated from geodesic regression at several time points with velocity of fiber development displayed on the surface of the estimated fibers.

4   Conclusions

We have presented a geodesic regression model for shapes represented as currents in the large deformation diffeomorphic metric mapping (LDDMM) framework where dense diffeomorphisms are built using a control point formulation. This provides a discrete and low dimensional parameterization of large diffeomorphic transformations, decoupling the parameterization of deformations from the specific shape representation. By representing shapes as currents, our regression model can seamlessly handle both surfaces and curves, or any combination of them represented as multi-object complexes. This is a powerful representation that incorporates potentially important spatial relationships between anatomical shapes into the regression framework.

By analogy with linear regression, our generative geodesic model is fully characterized by a baseline shape (intercept) and initial momenta vectors (slope). We have introduced an optimization scheme which estimates the baseline shape, location of the control points, and initial momenta simultaneously via a single gradient descent algorithm. Finally, we presented results from experiments carried out on a diverse collection of shape data, demonstrating the widespread applicability of our geodesic shape regression framework. Future work will focus on incorporating the geodesic model into a framework for the statistical analysis of longitudinal data. We will explore approaches which simultaneously estimate a population baseline as well as momenta for individual subjects in homologous locations. We will also explore methods for transporting baseline shapes and momenta vectors between subjects and between population groups to enable hypothesis testing on 4D growth models.

Acknowledgments. This work was supported by NIH grant RO1 HD055741 (ACE, project IBIS) and by NIH grant U54 EB005149 (NA-MIC).

References

1. Basser, P., Pajevic, S., Pierpaoli, C., Duda, J., Aldroubi, A.: In vivo fiber tractography using DT-MRI data. Magnetic Resonance in Medicine 44(4), 625–632 (2000)
2. Datar, M., Cates, J., Fletcher, P., Gouttard, S., Gerig, G., Whitaker, R.: Particle based shape regression of open surfaces with applications to developmental neuroimaging. In: Yang, G.-Z., Hawkes, D., Rueckert, D., Noble, A., Taylor, C. (eds.) MICCAI 2009, Part II. LNCS, vol. 5762, pp. 167–174. Springer, Heidelberg (2009)
3. Davis, B., Fletcher, P., Bullitt, E., Joshi, S.: Population shape regression from random design data. In: ICCV, pp. 1–7. IEEE (2007)
4. Durrleman, S., Allassonnière, S., Joshi, S.: Sparse adaptive parameterization of variability in image ensembles. IJCV, 1–23 (2012)
5. Durrleman, S., Pennec, X., Trouvé, A., Braga, J., Gerig, G., Ayache, N.: Toward a comprehensive framework for the spatiotemporal statistical analysis of longitudinal shape data. IJCV, 1–38 (2012)
6. Durrleman, S., Prastawa, M., Korenberg, J.R., Joshi, S.C., Trouvé, A., Gerig, G.: Topology preserving atlas construction from shape data without correspondence using sparse parameters. In: Ayache, N., Delingette, H., Golland, P., Mori, K. (eds.) MICCAI 2012, Part III. LNCS, vol. 7512, pp. 223–230. Springer, Heidelberg (2012)
7. Fishbaugh, J., Durrleman, S., Gerig, G.: Estimation of smooth growth trajectories with controlled acceleration from time series shape data. In: Fichtinger, G., Martel, A., Peters, T. (eds.) MICCAI 2011, Part II. LNCS, vol. 6892, pp. 401–408. Springer, Heidelberg (2011)
8. Fishbaugh, J., Prastawa, M., Durrleman, S., Piven, J., Gerig, G.: Analysis of longitudinal shape variability via subject specific growth modeling. In: Ayache, N., Delingette, H., Golland, P., Mori, K. (eds.) MICCAI 2012, Part I. LNCS, vol. 7510, pp. 731–738. Springer, Heidelberg (2012)
9. Fletcher, P.: Geodesic Regression on Riemannian Manifolds. In: Pennec, X., Joshi, S., Nielsen, M. (eds.) MICCAI MFCA, pp. 75–86 (2011)
10. Hart, G., Shi, Y., Zhu, H., Sanchez, M., Styner, M., Niethammer, M.: DTI longitudinal atlas construction as an average of growth models. In: Gerig, G., Fletcher, P., Pennec, X. (eds.) MICCAI STIA (2010)
11. Liao, S., Jia, H., Wu, G., Shen, D.: A novel longitudinal atlas construction framework by groupwise registration of subject image sequences. NeuroImage 59(2), 1275–1289 (2012)
12. Lorenzi, M., Ayache, N., Pennec, X.: Schild's ladder for the parallel transport of deformations in time series of images. In: Székely, G., Hahn, H.K. (eds.) IPMI 2011. LNCS, vol. 6801, pp. 463–474. Springer, Heidelberg (2011)
13. Mansi, T., Voigt, I., Leonardi, B., Pennec, X., Durrleman, S., Sermesant, M., Delingette, H., Taylor, A.M., Boudjemline, Y., Pongiglione, G., Ayache, N.: A statistical model for quantification and prediction of cardiac remodelling: Application to tetralogy of fallot. IEEE Trans. on Medical Imaging 9(30), 1605–1616 (2011)
14. Niethammer, M., Huang, Y., Vialard, F.-X.: Geodesic regression for image timeseries. In: Fichtinger, G., Martel, A., Peters, T. (eds.) MICCAI 2011, Part II. LNCS, vol. 6892, pp. 655–662. Springer, Heidelberg (2011)

15. Prastawa, M., Bullitt, E., Gerig, G.: Simulation of brain tumors in mr images for evaluation of segmentation efficacy. Medical Image Analysis 13(2), 297–311 (2009)
16. Vialard, F., Trouvé, A.: Shape splines and stochastic shape evolutions: A second-order point of view. Quarterly of Applied Mathematics 70, 219–251 (2012)

A   Differentiation of the Regression Criterion

Consider a perturbation $\delta\mathbf{S}_0$ to the initial state of the system $(\mathbf{c}_0, \boldsymbol{\alpha}_0)$, which leads to a perturbation of the motion of the control points $\delta\mathbf{S}(t)$, a perturbation of the template shape trajectory $\delta\mathbf{X}(t)$, and a perturbation of the criterion δE

$$\delta E = \sum_{i=1}^{N_{obs}} \left((\nabla_{\mathbf{X}(t_i)} D(t_i))^t \delta\mathbf{X}(t_i) \right) + (\nabla_{\mathbf{S}_0} L)^t \delta\mathbf{S}_0. \tag{8}$$

The perturbations $\delta\mathbf{S}(t)$ and $\delta\mathbf{X}(t)$ satisfy the ODEs:

$$\begin{aligned} \delta\dot{\mathbf{S}}(t) &= d_{\mathbf{S}(t)} F(t)\delta\mathbf{S}(t) & \delta\mathbf{S}(0) &= \delta\mathbf{S}_0 \\ \delta\dot{\mathbf{X}}(t) &= \partial_1 G(t)\delta\mathbf{X}(t) + \partial_2 G(t)\delta\mathbf{S}(t) & \delta\mathbf{X}(0) &= \delta\mathbf{X}_0 \end{aligned} \tag{9}$$

Let $R_{st} = \exp\left(\int_s^t d_{\mathbf{S}(u)}F(u)du\right)$ and $V_{st} = \exp\left(\int_s^t \partial_1 G(u)du\right)$. The first ODE is a linear homogeneous ODE with well known solution

$$\delta\mathbf{S}(t) = R_{0t}\delta\mathbf{S}_0 \tag{10}$$

The second ODE is a linear inhomogeneous ODE with solution

$$\delta\mathbf{X}(t_i) = \left(\int_0^{t_i} V_{ut_i}\partial_2 G(u)R_{0u}du\right)\delta\mathbf{S}_0 + V_{0t_i}\delta\mathbf{X}_0 \tag{11}$$

which can now be plugged into (8). After arranging terms we have

$$\begin{aligned} \delta E = \sum_{i=1}^{N_{obs}} &\left[\int_0^{t_i} R_{0u}{}^t\partial_2 G(u)^t V_{ut_i}{}^t \nabla_{\mathbf{X}(t_i)}D(t_i)du \right]^t \delta\mathbf{S}_0 + [\nabla_{\mathbf{S}_0} L]^t \delta\mathbf{S}_0 \\ &+ \sum_{i=1}^{N_{obs}} \left[V_{0t_i}{}^t \nabla_{\mathbf{X}(t_i)}D(t_i) \right]^t \delta\mathbf{X}_0 \end{aligned} \tag{12}$$

Letting $\theta(t) = \sum_{i=1}^{N_{obs}} V_{tt_i}{}^t \nabla_{\mathbf{X}(t_i)}D(t_i)\mathbf{1}_{\{t \leq t_i\}}$, $g(t) = \partial_2 G(t)\theta(t)$, and $\xi(t) = \int_t^{t_i} R_{tu}{}^t g(u)du$ leads to the gradient of the criterion written as

$$\begin{cases} \nabla_{\mathbf{S}_0} E = \displaystyle\int_0^{t_i} R_{0u}{}^t g(u)du + \nabla_{\mathbf{S}_0} L = \xi(0) + \nabla_{\mathbf{S}_0} L \\ \nabla_{\mathbf{X}_0} E = \theta(0) \end{cases} \tag{13}$$

where auxiliary variables $\theta(t)$ and $\xi(t)$ satisfy the ODEs

$$\begin{aligned} \dot{\theta}(t) &= -\partial_1 G(t)^t\theta(t) + \sum_{i=1}^{N_{Obs}} \nabla_{\mathbf{X}(t_i)}D(t_i)\delta(t - t_i) & \theta(T) &= 0 \\ \dot{\xi}(t) &= -(\partial_2 G(t)^t\theta(t) + d_{\mathbf{S}(t)}F(t)^t\xi(t)) & \xi(T) &= 0. \end{aligned} \tag{14}$$

Multinomial Probabilistic Fiber Representation for Connectivity Driven Clustering

Birkan Tunç[1], Alex R. Smith[1], Demian Wasserman[2], Xavier Pennec[3], William M. Wells[2], Ragini Verma[1], and Kilian M. Pohl[1]

[1] Section of Biomedical Image Analysis, University of Pennsylvania
[2] Brigham and Women's Hospital, Harvard Medical School
[3] INRIA - Sophia Antipolis

Abstract. The clustering of fibers into bundles is an important task in studying the structure and function of white matter. Existing technology mostly relies on geometrical features, such as the shape of fibers, and thus only provides very limited information about the neuroanatomical function of the brain. We advance this issue by proposing a multinomial representation of fibers decoding their connectivity to gray matter regions. We then simplify the clustering task by first deriving a compact encoding of our representation via the logit transformation. Furthermore, we define a distance between fibers that is in theory invariant to parcellation biases and is equivalent to a family of Riemannian metrics on the simplex of multinomial probabilities. We apply our method to longitudinal scans of two healthy subjects showing high reproducibility of the resulting fiber bundles without needing to register the corresponding scans to a common coordinate system. We confirm these qualitative findings via a simple statistical analyse of the fiber bundles.

Keywords: Tractography, connectivity, fiber clustering, log odds.

1 Introduction

Research in the area of fiber clustering has resulted in subject- as well as population-specific characterization of the white matter brain structures[1,2]. Clustering algorithm group fibers into feature-based bundles. The resulting fiber bundles delineate different characteristics of white matter regions depending on which features are described by the underlying fiber representation. Existing fiber representations and clustering techniques mostly rely on geometrical features, such as their shape and placement in the 3D space [3]. Groupings based on these features give a brief picture of the structure of the white matter but largely fail to provide information for the further analyses of their neuroanatomical functions, i.e connectivity between brain regions [4]. In this work, we address this issue by proposing a multinomial representation of fibers based on brain connectivity.

We first introduce multinomial feature vectors, called *connectivity vectors*, which capture the posterior probabilities of a voxel being connected to a set of ROIs. A fiber is encoded by the voxels it passes through as well as the corresponding connectivity vectors at those voxels. We then create a compact multinomial

J.C. Gee et al. (Eds.): IPMI 2013, LNCS 7917, pp. 730–741, 2013.

representation for the whole fiber by fusing the corresponding connectivity vectors via the *logit* transformation. The *logit* transform enables us to map the connectivity vectors, which are members of the M dimensional simplex $\mathbb{S}^M$, to the Euclidean space $\mathbb{R}^M$, where norm and inner product are defined naturally. In other words, we can perform all calculations in $\mathbb{R}^M$ without needing to pay attention to the geometric properties of the manifold spanned by connectivity vectors in $\mathbb{S}^M$.

We complete our representation with the definition of a distance measure, which is essential for clustering. The Hausdorff distance is one of the most popular distances for fibers represented by their geometrical features [5]. However, such a distance does not account for the neuroanatomical functions of fibers neither allow any statistical inference. In [6], authors use kernel density estimation to transform such distances into probabilities and apply it to statistical decision modelling. An alternative was recently proposed by [7], who measure the possible diffusion pathways between predefined ROIs and fibers via the Mahalanobis distance. We also propose the use of the Mahalanobis distance for fibers represented by the connectivity vectors in $\mathbb{R}^M$. We show that the distance is invariant to the parcellation biases over ROIs by proving that this metric is a specific instance of the family of prior invariant distances on $\mathbb{S}^M$. This property is important for clustering as it allows us to ignore implementations issues related to the calculation of the probabilities, e.g. representing fibers by likelihoods or posteriors.

One of the most important characteristic of the proposed representation is the fact that individual fibers and fiber bundles are treated as statistical objects invariant to the image coordinate system. Although it is possible to perform longitudinal or population based studies by analyzing fibers via 3D coordinates [6], an important novelty of the proposed work is the use of informative posteriors related to the connection of fibers to ROIs. In addition, our representation enables the analysis for these type of studies without needing to register the fibers to a common coordinate system. Finally, it allows hypothesis driven statistical analysis over fiber bundles, and can be thought as a first step in creating a probabilistic fiber atlases. This type of analysis requires the bundles to be comparable across the scans to be studied. We evaluate the reproducibility over our approach by applying our representation to the base line and follow up scans of two different subjects. The results are consistent allowing us to visually pinpoint the same fiber bundle across scans as well as perform statistical analyses on the bundles for quantitatively comparison.

2   Fiber Representation

We now describe our representation whose encoding of fibers is based on their connections to ROIs. These connections are captured at each voxel of the fiber by multinomial vectors, called *connectivity vectors*. We derive a compact representation of fibers, called *connectivity signature*, by fusing these connectivity vectors via the logit function. We complete the description of our representation by deriving a metric naturally inferred from the space spanned by the connectivity signatures.

2.1   Multinomial Fiber Representation

We view fibers as a collection of voxels and their corresponding probabilistic connectivity vectors. Specifically, let $\mathbb{R}^M$ denote M-dimensional real space and

$$\mathbb{S}^M \equiv \{\mathbf{u} = (u_0, \ldots, u_M) \in \mathbb{R}^M : u_0 + \ldots + u_M = 1;\ u_i > 0 \text{ for } i \in \{0, \ldots, M\}\},$$

is the M-dimensional simplex. u_0 is usually defined as $u_0 = 1 - \sum_{i=1}^{M} u_i$ so that the vector $\mathbf{u} \equiv (u_0, u_1, \ldots, u_M) \in \mathbb{S}^M$ has M degrees of freedom. In the remainder, we therefore represent $\mathbf{u}$ only by its independent components, i.e. $\mathbf{u} \equiv (u_1, \ldots, u_M)$, and mention u_0 where necessary. With respect to our representation, the multinomial vector $\mathbf{u}(x) \in \mathbb{S}^M$ captures the posterior probability of a given voxel x being connected to the ROIs (for instance gray matter regions) $\{G_1, \ldots, G_M\}$ in the image I. We compute the posteriors based on the outcome of probabilistic tractography (see Section 3 for further details). We call $\mathbf{u}(x)$ the *connectivity vector* and formally define it as

$$\mathbf{u}(x) \equiv \Big(p(G_1|I, x), \ldots, p(G_M|I, x) \Big). \tag{1}$$

We note that the probability $p(G_0|I, x) = 1 - \sum_{i=1}^{M} p(G_i|I, x)$ is the posterior probability that a given voxel x is not connect to any ROI. Furthermore, we could have $\mathbf{u}(x)$ represent likelihoods instead of posteriors. The reason we prefer using posterior probabilities is their superiority in terms of connectivity interpretations. The multinomial vector itself simply explains all possible connections of a voxel. We also assume that the connectivity vectors $\mathbf{u}(x)$ are independently drawn from a logistic normal distributions [8] for each voxel x. A popular alternative would have been the Dirichlet distribution [9,10]. However, any Dirichlet distribution can be approximated with a suitable logistic normal distribution [11]. In addition, the logistic normal distribution better fits into the modelling performed in the remainder of this article.

The main intuition behind this probabilistic representation is to enhance the results of deterministic tractography with the notion of uncertainty. This uncertainty is especially helpful in fiber clustering as it provides additional information for separating fibers with respect to just the two regions marking the fiber's ends. This observation leads us to the following definition: A *fiber* $\mathbf{f}$ in the image I is a collection of voxels x and corresponding *connectivity vectors* $\mathbf{u}(x) \in \mathbb{S}^M$. For sake of clarity, connectivity vectors, $\mathbf{u}(x)$, will from now on be denoted as $\mathbf{u}$.

One way to represent a fiber is now as a matrix composed of the connectivity vectors $\mathbf{u}$. Figure 1(a) shows a red fiber inside a bundle of the Corpus Callosum together with its matrix representation in Figure 1(b). As expected, the matrix clearly favours two regions, which are the ones touched by the ends of the fiber. Furthermore, the matrix also implicitly encodes geometric properties of the fiber by the changes in the multinomial distribution when moving along the path.

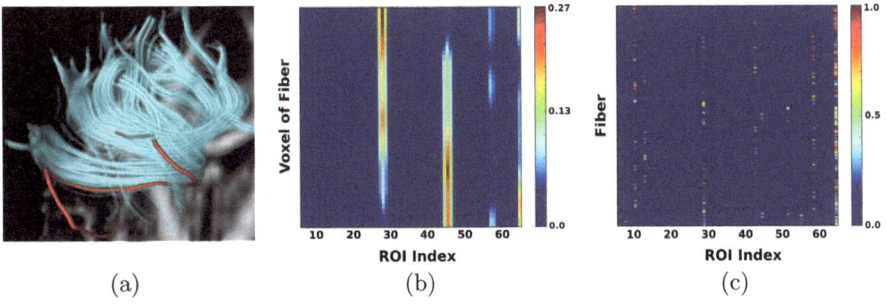

Fig. 1. (a) A fiber bundle from Corpus Callosum together with the (b) set of connectivity vectors **u** of the fiber in red and (c) connectivity signatures $\mathcal{F}$ of all individual fibers in the bundle. The x-axis of both matrices represents the ROI index. Blue indicates low and red high probabilities being connected to a specific ROIs. Note, how the connectivity vectors implicitly represent the geometry of the fiber in red. The connectivity signature on the other side summarizes the favoured regions by the whole bundle, which seem to be six.

2.2 Log Odds Representation of Fibers

Representing fibers as collections of multinomial vectors enables in-depth analyses over individual fibers. However one may want a more compact representation that can be used for immediate reasoning such as "which regions does the fiber connect with the highest probabilities ?". To derive such a compact representation, we now map the multinomial random vectors **u** from the simplex $\mathbb{S}^M$ to the Euclidean space $\mathbb{R}^M$. By doing so, we can compress the set of connectivity vectors representing a fiber without the constraints of the simplex.

Given that **u** is drawn from a logistic normal distribution, the most suitable homeomorphism between $\mathbb{S}^M$ and $\mathbb{R}^M$ is the *logit* transform [8]. The *log odds vector* $\mathbf{v}(x) \in \mathbb{R}^M$ is then defined as the logit transform of the *connectivity vector* $\mathbf{u}(x)$:

$$\mathbf{v}(x) \equiv logit(\mathbf{u}(x)) = \ln(\mathbf{u}(x)/u_0). \tag{2}$$

The inverse is called the *logistic* function $\sigma(\cdot)$ mapping $\mathbf{v} \in \mathbb{R}^M$ to $\mathbf{u} \in \mathbb{S}^M$

$$\mathbf{u} \equiv \sigma(\mathbf{v}) = \frac{e^{\mathbf{v}}}{1 + \sum_{j=1}^{M} e^{v_j}}. \tag{3}$$

Similar to the definition of a *fiber* **f**, a *log odds fiber* **l** is then defined as a collection of voxels x and corresponding *log odds vectors* $\mathbf{v}(x)$.

To define a compact representation of the *log odds fiber* **l**, we parametrize it with respect to the discrete arc length $s \in [0, 1]$, where $\mathbf{l}(s) \equiv \mathbf{v}(x)$. Furthermore, we introduce the weight function $w(s) \in [0, 1]$ enabling us to emphasize specific parts of the fiber. Our compact representation is motivated by the assumption that the connectivity vectors $\mathbf{u}(x)$ are independently drawn for each voxel x as well as the fact that the normalized multiplication between $\mathbf{u}(x)$ translates to the sum of $\mathbf{v}(x)$ [12]. A natural definition for a *compact log odds fiber representation*, $\mathbf{F} \in \mathbb{R}^M$, is thus by the weighted sum of the log odds vectors across the fiber

$$\mathbf{F} \equiv \sum_s w(s) \cdot \mathbf{l}(s) \,. \tag{4}$$

Now, the compact multinomial representation for a fiber is the sigmoid function applied to $\mathbf{F}$:

$$\mathcal{F} \equiv \sigma(\mathbf{F}) \,, \tag{5}$$

We call $\mathcal{F}$, the *connectivity signature* of fiber $\mathbf{f}$ as this multinomial vector summarizes the connectivity of $\mathbf{f}$ to the ROIs. One of the most useful properties of the logit transformation is that $\mathbf{v} \in \mathbb{R}^M$ is drawn from a multivariate Gaussian defined by $\mathcal{N}(\boldsymbol{\mu}, \boldsymbol{\Sigma})$ as $\mathbf{u} \in \mathbb{S}^M$ is drawn from a logistic normal distribution [8] (see Section 2.1). Thus, the *log odds representation* $\mathbf{F}$ of a fiber is again drawn from a Gaussian distribution since the summation of independent normally distributed random variables is also another normally distributed random variable. Furthermore, the *connectivity signature* $\mathcal{F}$ must then also be drawn from the logistic normal distribution.

An important property of the proposed log odds fiber representation is the fact that the mean and covariance have real statistical meanings unlike in other representations, such as in [7]. For instance, if we apply the inverse logit function to $\boldsymbol{\mu}$, we get a multinomial vector in $\mathbb{S}^M$ which summarizes the average connection probabilities of fiber bundles. Similarly, $\boldsymbol{\Sigma}$ gives the covariances among connection probabilities of different ROIs.

We end this discussion by pointing out that all the fibers extracted from an image I can be represented by a matrix composed of their *connectivity signatures*. Figure 1(c) shows an example of such a matrix representing fibers seeded from Corpus Callosum. Note, that the matrix represents all fibers independent of the image orientation. Assuming the generation of fibers is stable across scans, this matrix thus provides a mechanism for performing statistics on fibers among a set of scans without needing to register them beforehand. These assumptions will be justified by the experiments of Section 3.

2.3   Metrics in $\mathbb{S}^M$ and $\mathbb{R}^M$

Applications such as fiber clustering rely on metrics that properly measure the distance between fibers. We now define such a metric for our proposed fiber representation. Specifically, let $\mathbf{F}_1$ and $\mathbf{F}_2$ be the compact log odds representations of two fibers with $\mathcal{F}_1$ and $\mathcal{F}_2$ being their corresponding multivariate counterparts. As in our model log odds fibers $\mathbf{F}$ are normally distributed, a natural metric is the Mahalanobis distance

$$d(\mathbf{F}_1, \mathbf{F}_2) = \sqrt{(\mathbf{F}_1 - \mathbf{F}_2)^T \boldsymbol{\Sigma}^{-1} (\mathbf{F}_1 - \mathbf{F}_2)} \,, \tag{6}$$

where $\boldsymbol{\Sigma}$ is the covariance matrix of their distribution. An alternative motivation behind the Mahalanobis distance is its independence to the prior. In the remainder of this section, we will derive this property by first constructing Riemanian manifolds of the commutative Abelian group $\mathbb{S}^M$ as defined in [12], whose metrics are independent of the prior. We then show the equivalence of the Mahalanobis distances to a specific subset of these metrics. Finally, we discuss the importance of the prior invariance for the implementation of our representation.

In [12], the addition operation, $\oplus$, between connection signatures $\mathcal{F}_1$ and $\mathcal{F}_2 \in \mathbb{S}^M$ is defined as $\mathcal{F}_1 \oplus \mathcal{F}_2 \equiv \sigma(logit(\mathcal{F}_1) + logit(\mathcal{F}_2)) = \sigma(\mathbf{F}_1 + \mathbf{F}_2)$ while the inverse is $\mathcal{F}^{-1} \equiv \sigma(-logit(\mathcal{F}))$. Now, let $\mathbf{1}^T \equiv (1, \dots, 1)$ then the corresponding tangent space is $\mathcal{T}\mathbb{S}^M \equiv \{w \in \mathbb{R}^{M+1} \mid \mathbf{1}^T w = 0\}$ as the inner product of $\mathbf{1}$ with any curve on the Simplex $u^\epsilon = u + \epsilon \cdot w + O(\epsilon^2) \in \mathbb{S}^M$ has to be one, i.e. $\mathbf{1}^T u^\epsilon = 1$. Thus, the logarithm function, $LOG : \mathbb{S}^M \to \mathcal{T}\mathbb{S}^M$, projecting the simplex to the tangent space, is

$$LOG(\mathcal{F}) = \frac{1}{M^2}(M\mathbf{I} - \mathbf{1}\mathbf{1}^T)\ln(\mathcal{F}),$$

where $\mathbf{I}$ is the identity matrix. Finally, the family of prior invariant metrics on the commutative Abelian group $\mathbb{S}^M$ is defined by

$$d_R(\mathcal{F}_1, \mathcal{F}_2) = \sqrt{LOG(\mathcal{F}_1^{-1} \oplus \mathcal{F}_2)^T G_R LOG(\mathcal{F}_1^{-1} \oplus \mathcal{F}_2)}, \qquad (7)$$

where the concentration matrix G_R is positive definite. We show the prior invariance of $d_R(\cdot, \cdot)$ by denoting the posterior as $\mathbf{u}^{pst} \equiv \left(p(G_1|I, x), \dots, p(G_M|I, x)\right)$, the normalized likelihood as $\mathbf{u}^{lkh} \equiv \left(p(x|I, G_1), \dots, p(x|I, G_M)\right)$ and the prior as $\mathbf{u}^{pri} \equiv \left(p(G_1), \dots, p(G_M)\right)$. According to [12], adding the prior to the likelihood via $\oplus$ is equivalent to Bayes' rule as $\mathbf{u}^{pst} = \mathbf{u}^{lkh} \oplus \mathbf{u}^{pri}$ and the identity $(\mathbf{u}_1 \oplus \mathbf{p})^{-1} \oplus (\mathbf{u}_2 \oplus \mathbf{p}) = \mathbf{u}_1^{-1} \oplus \mathbf{u}_2$ holds for any $\mathbf{u}_1, \mathbf{u}_2, \mathbf{p} \in \mathbb{S}^M$. Then, the distance $d_R(\mathbf{u}_1^{lkh}, \mathbf{u}_2^{lkh})$ defined on $\mathbb{S}^M$ is invariant to priors as

$$d_R^2(\mathbf{u}_1 \oplus \mathbf{p}, \mathbf{u}_2 \oplus \mathbf{p})$$
$$= LOG\left((\mathbf{u}_1 \oplus \mathbf{p})^{-1} \oplus (\mathbf{u}_2 \oplus \mathbf{p})\right)^T G_R\, LOG\left((\mathbf{u}_1 \oplus \mathbf{p})^{-1} \oplus (\mathbf{u}_2 \oplus \mathbf{p})\right)$$
$$= LOG(\mathbf{u}_1^{-1} \oplus \mathbf{u}_2)^T G_R LOG(\mathbf{u}_1^{-1} \oplus \mathbf{u}_2) = d_R^2(\mathbf{u}_1, \mathbf{u}_2)$$

so that

$$d_R(\mathbf{u}_1^{lkh}, \mathbf{u}_2^{lkh}) = d_R(\mathbf{u}_1^{lkh} \oplus \mathbf{u}^{pri}, \mathbf{u}_2^{lkh} \oplus \mathbf{u}^{pri}) = d_R(\mathbf{u}_1^{pst}, \mathbf{u}_2^{pst}). \qquad (8)$$

If we now define $\boldsymbol{\alpha} \equiv (1, 0, \dots, 0)$ and specify the concentration matrix as $G_R \equiv M^2(\mathbf{I} - \boldsymbol{\alpha}\mathbf{1}^T)\boldsymbol{\Sigma}^{-1}(\mathbf{I} - \mathbf{1}\boldsymbol{\alpha}^T)$ then the resulting Riemannian metric is equivalent to the Mahalanobis distance of Equation (6): $d^2(\mathbf{F}_1, \mathbf{F}_2) = d_R^2(\mathcal{F}_1, \mathcal{F}_2)$. Thus, the Mahalanobis distance is invariant to any prior, i.e. bias shared among fibers. One of these factors are the priors of ROIs corresponding to their size and shapes. The probabilities in connectivity vectors $\mathbf{u}$ (and therefore in $\mathcal{F}$) are highly correlated with the partitioning of ROIs since shapes and size of these regions will change the fraction of fibers reaching them. Another important conclusion from the prior invariance is that distances between fibers are not impacted by ones choice of calculating posterior probabilities or normalized likelihoods for the definition

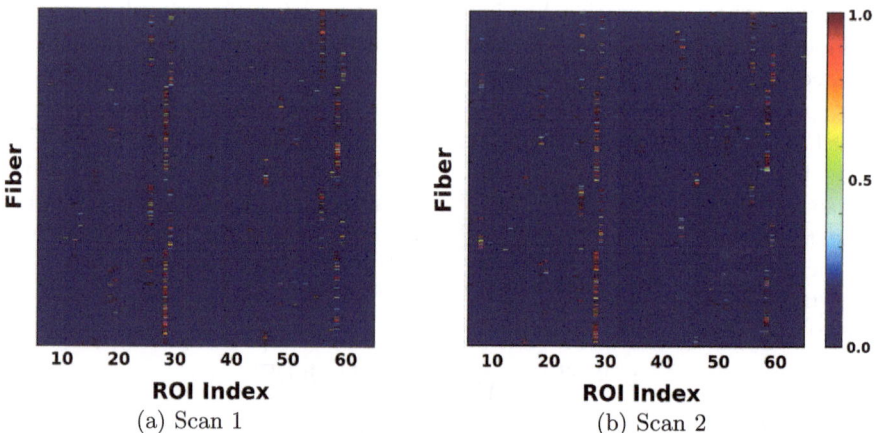

Fig. 2. Connectivity signatures of Corpus Callosum corresponding to different scans of a subject. The x-axis represents ROI index. Each row corresponds to connectivity signature $\mathcal{F}$ of a fiber. Colors indicate the connection probabilities to ROIs. Note, the common patterns of connections even though the scans are not registered or fibers are not ordered.

of the multinomial vectors $\mathbf{u}$. In summary, choosing the Mahalanobis distance as a metric for fibers greatly simplifies the implementation of our representation due to its invariance to priors.

We end this section by revisiting one more time the multivariate logistic-normal (MLN) distribution that is assumed as a prior over vector $\mathbf{u} \in \mathbb{S}^M$. One important property is that MLN distribution has more flexibility than the popular Dirichlet distribution, which is the conjugate of the multinomial. The Dirichlet distribution has a single concentration parameter, while MLN has a covariance matrix. This relation corresponds to the distinction between Mahalanobis distance, which is parameterized by a covariance matrix, and KL divergence or the Fisher metric, which have no such parameter. The invariance properties that we have described above may be of some interest to the community that uses MLN for modeling and analysis.

3   Fiber Clustering

We now apply the proposed representation for the clustering of fibers. Our goal is to test the consistency of the corresponding fiber bundles on longitudinal scans as well as across subjects. Consistency across scans is important for the reliability of studies analyzing the changes in the bundles.

3.1   Clustering Algorithm

Our experiment is based on T1 and DTI images of 2 female subjects. Each subject was scanned twice two weeks apart. The scans were acquired on a

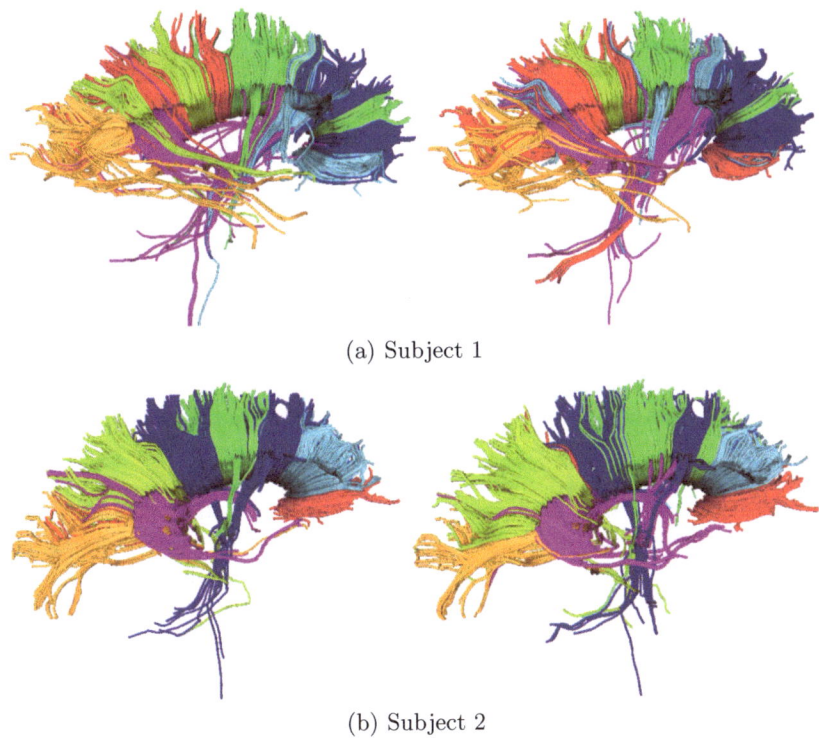

(a) Subject 1

(b) Subject 2

Fig. 3. Results showing reproducibility of fiber bundles with the proposed representation. Images show clustering of Corpus Callosum with 7 clusters for two subjects. Left and right images correspond to different scans of a subject. Note, the intra-subject consistency for both subjects.

Siemens 3T VerioTM scanner using a single-shot, spin-echo, echo-planar sequence (TR/TE=11400/78ms, b-value 1000 s/mm2, and 64 gradient directions). We separately created a gray matter parcellation for each DTI scan by applying FreeSurfer to the corresponding T1 image, which was affinely aligned to the DTI [13]. Note, the deformation map created by FreeSurfer is only defined for the gray matter. Inverting the map thus does not accurately register the DTI scan to the atlas of FreeSurfer. Analyses based on our fiber representation has no use for such registrations as our statistical model is invariant to the image coordinate system.

The log odds representations of fibers are created by first extracting the fibers using a streamline tractography [14] and then computing the corresponding connectivity vectors via probabilistic tractography [15]. Specifically, we perform the following steps: (1) create fibers via streamline tractography seeded from the Corpus Collosum, (2) for each fiber, run the probabilistic tractography seeded at each voxel defining the fiber, (3) for each voxel x of the fiber, compute the multinomial vector $\mathbf{u}(x)$ of Equation 1 by defining the posterior probability

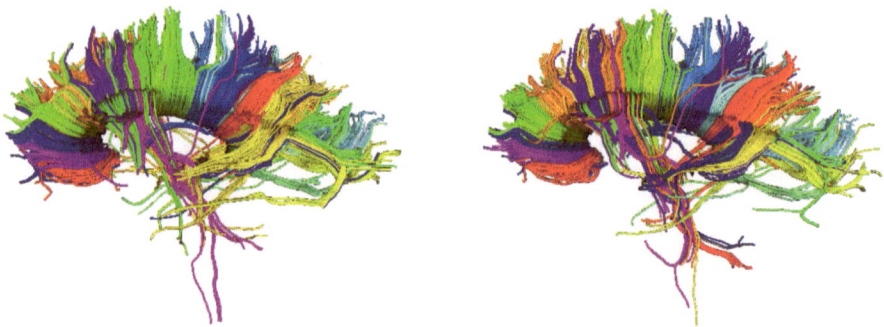

Fig. 4. Results showing reproducibility of fiber bundles with the proposed representation. Images show clustering of Corpus Callosum of Subject 1, with 25 clusters. Left and right images correspond two different time point scans of the subject. Intra-person consistency is excellent even with a fine grain clustering.

$p(G_i|I, x)$ as the fraction of fibers seeded at this voxel and reaching ROI G_i, (5) calculate the log odds vector $\mathbf{v}(x)$ by Equation 2, (6) generate the final log odds representation, $\mathbf{F}$, via Equation 4. Finally, we compute the connectivity signatures, $\mathcal{F}$, of Equation 5 for visualization and interpretation purposes.

Based on this protocol, we expect our clustering approach to produce very similar fiber bundles for the two time points of each subject.

To cluster the fibers, one could make the simplifying assumption that all fibers are drawn from a common Gaussian distribution.While this model is simple to implement, the resulting fiber bundles of our data set were very inconsistent as the assumption of all fibers being drawn from a single Gaussian distribution is not realistic. We discovered that the multinomial representations of fibers seeded at different white matter (WM) regions greatly vary due to the drastic differences in the connectivity of different WM regions.

We thus instead assume that the fibers are drawn from a mixture of logistic normal distributions in $\mathbb{S}^M$, which is a mixture of Gaussians in $\mathbb{R}^M$. We estimate the mixture of Gaussians via the Expectation-Maximization (EM) procedure [16]. By doing so, we implicitly make use of the Mahalanobis distance between fibers and mixture components' mean vectors for assigning fibers to mixture components. Hence, the mixture assignment is driven by the Mahalanobis distance thus still inheriting the proposed invariance to the common priors.

The clustering was solely performed on the connectivity signatures, such as the one shown in Figure 2. While the numbers of fibers and their orderings are different across the matrices, the matrices themselves are independent of the image coordinate system. They thus do not need to be registered for evaluating the reproducibility of our method.

3.2 Clustering Results

Finally, we review the fiber bundles extracted by our approach for the two subjects with two time points. Figure 3 shows the outcome of our approach for

Table 1. The average symmetric KL divergence between the mean signature values of matching bundles of two subjects (S1, S2) and two time points (T1, T2). The intra-person distances are always lower than that of inter-person.

	S1-T1	S1-T2	S2-T1	S2-T2
S1-T1	0	1.68	1.92	3.01
S1-T2	1.68	0	3.05	3.63
S2-T1	1.92	3.05	0	1.24
S2-T2	3.01	3.63	1.24	0

assigning the tracts to 7 fiber bundles. The consistency between the results of baseline and follow up is evident for both subjects. Similarly, there is a high consistency between subjects. We further challenge the repeatability of the algorithm by increasing the number of clusters. Figure 4 shows the outcome with 25 fiber bundles for a single subject. Even with such a fine grain clustering, intra-person consistency is excellent making it possible to pinpoint corresponding fiber bundles across these scans. This qualitative assessment seem to indicate that the proposed clustering algorithm exhibits a strong repeatability in terms of fiber groupings. The results in Figure 3,4 were generated without registering the DTI images. Thus, the consistency in clustering justifies the invariance of our proposed metric to priors over ROIs since individual registrations tend to have minor changes in shapes and sizes of ROIs.

We complement this qualitative interpretations with a quantitative assessment, which also provides an example on doing statistical analysis based on our representation. Fiber bundles generated by the clustering can be treated as statistical objects as each fiber is represented by a multinomial vector. One may assume each bundle as a distribution of such multinomial vectors and then can compare these distributions across scans. We do by representing each fiber bundle via its mean connectivity signature and then comparing signatures across scans via the symmetric KullbackLeibler (KL) divergence which is defined by

$$KL(\bar{\mathcal{F}}_1, \bar{\mathcal{F}}_2) = \frac{1}{2} \sum_{i=1}^{M} \left(\ln \left(\frac{\bar{\mathcal{F}}_1(i)}{\bar{\mathcal{F}}_2(i)} \right) \bar{\mathcal{F}}_1(i) + \ln \left(\frac{\bar{\mathcal{F}}_2(i)}{\bar{\mathcal{F}}_1(i)} \right) \bar{\mathcal{F}}_2(i) \right) \qquad (9)$$

where $\bar{\mathcal{F}}_j(i)$ is the ith element of the mean connectivity signature $\bar{\mathcal{F}}$ of a fiber bundle in scan j.

Our comparison of bundles across scans specifically focus on those pairs that match, i.e. have the lowest divergence score. Figure 5 shows the matched fiber bundle from four different scans and their corresponding symmetric KL-Divergence scores with respect to the first scan. First, we note that the score seems to reflect the geometrical properties of the bundle. The more similar the bundles look, the lower the score. Second, as expected, the bundle of the follow up scan of the same subject received the lowest score.

Table 1 lists the average symmetric KL divergence of the four different scans clustered into 7 bundles (see Figure 3). The average symmetric KL divergence was computed across the 7 bundles that best matched between scans. Note,

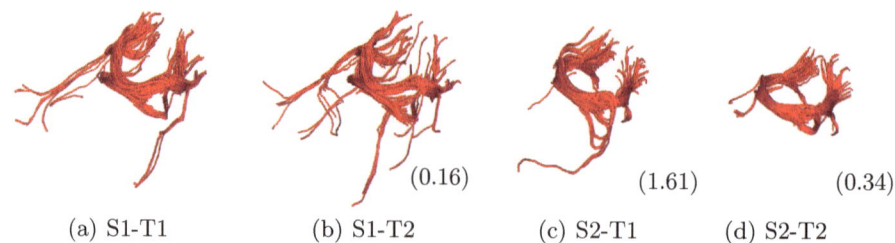

| | (0.16) | (1.61) | (0.34) |
| (a) S1-T1 | (b) S1-T2 | (c) S2-T1 | (d) S2-T2 |

Fig. 5. Same fiber bundle in four different scans of two subjects (S1, S2) and two time points (T1, T2). Matching of bundles is performed by KL divergence measure. The values in parentheses are the distances from the first bundle. Thank to our multinomial representation, corresponding fiber bundles across scans can be matched by using probabilistic measures like KL divergence.

the values of intra-subject pairs are always lower than values of inter-subject pairs. These quantitative results seem to echo the qualitative assessment that the bundles generated via our representation are highly consistent.

4   Conclusion

We developed a multinomial representation of fibers decoding their connectivity to gray matter regions. We simplified clustering these fibers into bundles by deriving a compact encoding of that representation via the logit transformation. Furthermore, we created a distance measure that is invariant to parcellation biases by deriving the family of prior invariant metrics on the simplex of multinomial probabilities. We applied our method on longitudinal scans of two healthy subjects showing high reproducibility of the resulting fiber bundles without needing to register the corresponding scans to a common coordinate system. We confirmed these qualitative findings by measuring the symmetric KL-Divergence of bundles across scans.

Acknowledgements. This work was supported by Institute for Translational Medicine and Therapeutics (ITMAT), NIH (UL1RR024134, R01MH092862, R01MH074794, P41RR013218, P41EB015898, P41RR019703, P41EB015902, P41RR013218), and French ANR-blanc Karametria.

References

1. Zhang, Y., Zhang, J., Oishi, K., Faria, A., Jiang, H., Li, X., Akhter, K., Rosa-Neto, P., Pike, G.B., Evans, A.C., Toga, A.W., Woods, R.P., Mazziotta, J.C., Miller, M.I., van Zijl, P.C.M., Mori, S.: Atlas-guided tract reconstruction for automated and comprehensive examination of the white matter anatomy. NeuroImage 52(4), 1289–1301 (2010)

2. Hagmann, P., Kurant, M., Gigandet, X., Thiran, P., Wedeen, V.J., Meuli, R., Thiran, J.P.: Mapping human whole-brain structural networks with diffusion MRI. PloS One 2(7), 597 (2007)
3. Guevara, P., Poupon, C., Rivire, D., Cointepas, Y., Descoteaux, M., Thirion, B., Mangin, J.F.: Robust clustering of massive tractography datasets. NeuroImage 54(3), 1975–1993 (2011)
4. Lenglet, C., Campbell, J.S.W., Descoteaux, M., Haro, G., Savadjiev, P., Wassermann, D., Anwander, A., Deriche, R., Pike, G.B., Sapiro, G.: Mathematical methods for diffusion MRI processing. NeuroImage 45(1), 111–122 (2009)
5. Gerig, G., Gouttard, S., Corouge, I.: Analysis of brain white matter via fiber tract modeling. In: International Conference on Biomedical and Health Informatics, p. 426 (2004)
6. O'Donnell, L.J., Wells III, W.M., Golby, A.J., Westin, C.-F.: Unbiased groupwise registration of white matter tractography. In: Ayache, N., Delingette, H., Golland, P., Mori, K. (eds.) MICCAI 2012, Part III. LNCS, vol. 7512, pp. 123–130. Springer, Heidelberg (2012)
7. Wang, Q., Yap, P.-T., Jia, H., Wu, G., Shen, D.: Hierarchical fiber clustering based on multi-scale neuroanatomical features. In: Liao, H., Edwards, P.J., Pan, X., Fan, Y., Yang, G.-Z. (eds.) MIAR 2010. LNCS, vol. 6326, pp. 448–456. Springer, Heidelberg (2010)
8. Aitchison, J., Shen, S.: Logistic Normal Distributions: Some Properties and Uses. Biometrika 67(2), 261–272 (1980)
9. Bouguila, N., Ziou, D., Vaillancourt, J.: Unsupervised learning of a finite mixture model based on the dirichlet distribution and its application. IEEE Transactions on Image Processing 13(11), 1533–1543 (2004)
10. Neal, R.M.: Markov chain sampling methods for dirichlet process mixture models. Journal of Computational and Graphical Statistics 9(2), 249–265 (2000)
11. Aitchison, J., Begg, C.B.: Statistical diagnosis when basic cases are not classified with certainty. Biometrika 63(1), 1–12 (1976)
12. Pohl, K.M., Fisher, J.W., Bouix, S., Shenton, M.E., McCarley, R.W., Grimson, W.E.L., Kikinis, R., Wells, W.M.: Using the logarithm of odds to define a vector space on probabilistic atlases. Medical Image Analysis 11(5), 465–477 (2007)
13. Desikan, R., Segonne, F., Fischl, B., Quinn, B., Dickerson, B., Blacker, D., Buckner, R., Dale, A., Maguire, R., Hyman, B., Albert, M., Killiany, R.: An automated labeling system for subdividing the human cerebral cortex on mri scans into gyral based regions of interest. NeuroImage 31(2) (2006)
14. Cook, P.A., Bai, Y., Gilani, N.S., Seunarine, K.K., Hall, M.G., Parker, G.J., Alexander, D.C.: Camino: Open-Source Diffusion-MRI Reconstruction and Processing. In: Scientific Meeting of the International Society for Magnetic Resonance in Medicine, p. 2759 (2006)
15. Friman, O., Farneback, G., Westin, C.F.: A bayesian approach for stochastic white matter tractography. IEEE Transactions on Medical Imaging 25(8), 965–978 (2006)
16. Dempster, A.P., Laird, N.M., Rubin, D.B.: Maximum likelihood from incomplete data via the em algorithm. Journal of the Royal Statistical Society B 39(1), 1–38 (1977)

Reliable Selection of the Number of Fascicles in Diffusion Images by Estimation of the Generalization Error*

Benoit Scherrer**, Maxime Taquet**, and Simon K. Warfield

Computational Radiology Laboratory, Department of Radiology
Boston Children's Hospital, 300 Longwood Avenue, Boston, MA, 02115, USA

Abstract. A number of diffusion models have been proposed to overcome the limitations of diffusion tensor imaging (DTI) which cannot represent multiple fascicles with heterogeneous orientations at each voxel. Among them, generative models such as multi-tensor models, CHARMED or NODDI represent each fascicle with a parametric model and are of great interest to characterize and compare white matter properties. However, the identification of the appropriate model, and particularly the estimation of the number of fascicles, has proven challenging. In this context, different model selection approaches have been proposed to identify the number of fascicles at each voxel. Most approaches attempt to maximize the quality of fit while penalizing complex models to avoid overfitting. However, the choice of a penalization strategy and the trade-off between penalization and quality of fit are rather arbitrary and produce highly variable results. In this paper, we propose for the first time to determine the number of fascicles at each voxel by assessing the generalization error. This criterion naturally prevents overfitting by comparing how the models predict new data not included in the model estimation. Since the generalization error cannot be directly computed, we propose to estimate it by the 632 bootstrap technique which has low bias and low variance. Results on synthetic phantoms and in vivo data show that our approach performs better than existing techniques, and is robust to the choice of decision threshold. Together with generative models of the diffusion signal, this technique will enable accurate identification of the model complexity at each voxel and accurate assessment of the white matter characteristics.

1 Introduction

Diffusion tensor imaging (DTI) is well known to be unable to represent the diffusion signal arising from multiple fascicles crossing in one voxel. Various approaches have been proposed to overcome this limitation. Among them, generative models such as multi-tensor models [12,9], CHARMED [2] or NODDI

---

* This work was supported in part by NIH grants R01 RR021885, R01 EB008015, R03 EB008680, R01 LM010033, UL1 RR025758-03 and 1U01NS082320. MT is supported by F.R.S-FNRS.
** These authors contributed equally.

J.C. Gee et al. (Eds.): IPMI 2013, LNCS 7917, pp. 742–753, 2013.

[13] seek to represent the signal contribution from different populations of water molecules such as the signal contribution from unrestricted diffusion and from each individual fascicle. These models are based on underlying biological assumptions and are of great interest to characterize and compare white-matter properties. For example, assessment of the free water diffusion arising from the extracellular space may be useful for the characterization of edema or inflammation [8]. Modeling of each individual fascicle may be useful to characterize properties such as the fascicle density, the axonal diameter distribution or the myelin integrity. This is not feasible with the tensor representation of the signal in DTI which conflates the signal contribution from multiple sources. However, accurate estimation of a generative model requires identification of the number of fascicles present in each voxel, which corresponds to identifying the appropriate model complexity. This remains a challenging and open problem.

Assessing the number of fascicles at each voxel is a model selection problem. To date, most approaches select between diffusion models of different complexity by minimizing the fitting error. Because both the model estimation and assessment is achieved on the same dataset, this favors complex models and may overfit the data. For this reason, the criterion usually integrates a component penalizing complex models.

The most common criterion for the selection of generative diffusion models is the F-test. Alexander *et al.* [1] compare the spherical harmonic expansion of the ADC truncated at different orders by means of a series of ANOVA F-Tests. In this strategy, complex models are penalized by their necessity to significantly decrease the fitting error when compared to simpler models. Kreher *et al.* [5] use F-tests to select the appropriate number of fascicles by observing the variance of the ADC. Scherrer and Warfield [9] use a similar F-test strategy applied to the signal residuals rather than the ADC. Besides the F-test, other approaches based on the quality of fit have been proposed. Behrens *et al.* [3] used a Bayesian Automatic Relevance Determination (ARD) approach which starts with the most complex model and gradually prune the unnecessary variables. However, this was shown inefficient in tractography and required to manually force the number of fascicles [6]. The Bayesian Information Criterion (BIC), a weighted sum of the fitting error and a penalizing term, has been suggested as well but was shown to yield suboptimal results, even on synthetic data [10].

A more reliable paradigm to avoid overfitting when selecting between models is to compare how each model performs for *new data* not included in the model estimation. This relates to the *generalization error* (GE). Typically, a model not complex enough to represent a dataset will have a large GE, and so will a too complex model which overfits the data. To the best of our knowledge, minimization of the GE has never been used to determine the number of fascicles at each voxel. Leave-one-out cross validation follows this paradigm. However, it does not lead to a consistent estimate of the model [11] and its results are highly variable. Other cross-validation methods, such as K-fold cross validation, reduce this variance at the cost of a higher bias. By contrast, the 632 bootstrap method proposed by Efron [4] reduces this variability while remaining almost unbiased.

In this paper we use for the first time the 632 bootstrap (B632) method to determine the number of fascicles present in each voxel from diffusion-weighted images. Section 2 introduces the methods used, from the definition of the generalization error (Section 2.1) to the use of its estimate in the selection of the number of fascicles (Section 2.5). Section 3 presents results on both synthetic phantoms and in vivo data. Finally, Section 4 discusses the results and concludes.

2   Material and Methods

In this section, we present the generalization error minimization framework and how it can be utilized to perform model selection and determine the number of fascicles in each voxel. We start by explaining the fundamental difference between generalization error and fitting error. We then introduce different methods to estimate the generalization error, and explain why the 632 bootstrap should be used in this context. We subsequently provide an expression to estimate the variance of generalization error. Finally, we detail how these methods are applied to the problem of selecting the number of fascicles at each voxel.

2.1   Generalization Error and Fitting Error

Let $z = \{z_1, ..., z_n\}$ with $z_i = (x_i, y_i)$ be the set of n observed data points, in which x_i are inputs to the model (e.g., the b-values and gradient directions in diffusion images, see Section 2.5) and y_i are outputs (e.g., the signal attenuation in diffusion images). These data are used to build a generative model $r_z(x)$ that tries to predict the output y from an input x. Ideally, the optimal model would minimize the *generalization error*, that is the error made on a new hypothetical data point $z_0 = (x_0, y_0)$. The generalization error conditional on the observed data is :

$$E_g|z = E_{z_0 \sim F}\left[|y_0 - r_z(x_0)|^2 \big| z\right],\tag{1}$$

where $E[.]$ is the statistical expectation and $z_0 \sim F$ indicates that the expectation is taken over the new data point that follows the distribution F. To account for the variability of the observed data points, the unconditional generalization error can be defined as the expectation of (1) over all z :

$$E_{g,n} = E_{z_i \overset{\text{iid}}{\sim} F}\left\{E_g|z\right\} = E_{z_i \overset{\text{iid}}{\sim} F}\left\{E_{z_0 \sim F}\left[|y_0 - r_z(x_0)|^2 \big| z\right]\right\},\tag{2}$$

where the index n indicates that n samples were used to optimize the model r_z. The generalization errors (1) and (2) cannot be directly computed because the distribution F is unknown. One simple solution would be to estimate $F(z)$ by the empirical distribution $\hat{F}(z) = \frac{1}{n} \forall z \in z$. For the conditional generalization error (1), this yields the following estimate:

$$\begin{aligned}\hat{E}_g^{\text{fit}} &= E_{z_0 \sim \hat{F}}\left[|y_0 - r_z(x_0)|^2 \big| z\right] \\ &= \frac{1}{n}\sum_{i=1}^{n}|y_i - r_z(x_i)|^2,\end{aligned}\tag{3}$$

that is the common *fitting error*. This estimate is a biased estimate of E_g since the data z are used both to optimize the parameters of the model r_z and to estimate its error. In particular, in many modeling problem (including multi-fascicle modeling), it is always possible to find a model that yields $\hat{E}_g^{fit} = 0$ provided that it is complex enough. In the following sections, we will therefore explore other estimates of E_g and investigate their bias and variance.

2.2   Cross-Validation Estimates

To circumvent the overfitting problem of $\hat{E}_g^{fit}$, one could estimate the model by omitting one data point in the training sample z and evaluate the model prediction for this data point. This is the idea behind the leave-one-out cross-validation (LOOCV) method. Let $z_{(-i)}$ be the training samples without z_i. The resulting estimate of the generalization error reads:

$$\hat{E}_g^{CV} = \frac{1}{n} \sum_{i=1}^{n} |y_i - r_{z_{(-i)}}(x_i)|^2. \tag{4}$$

This is an unbiased estimator of the generalization error $E_{g,n-1}$. For large n, the bias of $\hat{E}_g^{CV}$ as an estimator of $E_{g,n}$ is positive but low. Its variance, however, is large, leading to high root mean squared errors, despite the low bias [4].

The variance of the LOOCV can be decreased by keeping more than one element out of the dataset at each iteration of model training and testing. This defines K-fold cross-validation methods. They result in unbiased estimates of $E_{g,n-\frac{n}{K}}$ which, however, present an increased bias for the estimation of E_g.

2.3   632 Bootstrap

The bootstrap smoothing method can be used to lower the variance of the cross-validation estimate [4]. This technique estimates E_g in (2) by providing two different estimates for the distribution F. The distribution F of z_0 is estimated by the empirical distribution $\hat{F}$ and the distribution F of z is estimated from bootstrap samples $z_{(-i)}^*$ of the empirical distribution $\hat{F}_{(-i)}$ which excludes the sample z_i used for testing. Formally, an expression of the estimator comes by inverting the order of the expectations in (2) and by subsequently replacing the distributions F by their estimates:

$$\hat{E}_g^{BS} = \frac{1}{n} \sum_{i=1}^{n} E_{\hat{F}_{(-i)}} \left[|y_i - r_{z_{(-i)}^*}(x_i)|^2 \right].$$

An equivalent expression of $\hat{E}_g^{BS}$ that is closer to its implementation is:

$$\hat{E}_g^{BS} = \sum_{i=1}^{n} \left[\sum_{b=1}^{B} \delta(N_i^b) \left| y_i - r_{z_{(-i)}^*}(x_i) \right|^2 \middle/ \sum_{b=1}^{B} \delta(N_i^b) \right], \tag{5}$$

where N_i^b is the number of times sample i is used in the training set of the bth bootstrap replicate and $\delta(x)$ is the Dirac function. The factor $\delta(N_i^b)$ guarantees that sample i can be used as a testing sample in bootstrap replicate b.

Much like cross-validation, the bootstrap estimate is biased because it relies on fewer point than the number n of available samples. LOOCV uses $(n-1)$ points and its bias is therefore limited. By contrast, $\hat{E}_g^{\text{BS}}$ uses, on average, $[1-(1-\frac{1}{n})^n]n$ points which is approximately equal to $0.632n$ for large n. This makes the bias of $\hat{E}_g^{\text{BS}}$ more critical. Efron [4] proposed to counterbalance the positive bias of $\hat{E}_g^{\text{BS}}$ by the negative bias of $\hat{E}_g^{\text{fit}}$, introducing the 632 bootstrap estimator:

$$\hat{E}_g^{632} = 0.368\,\hat{E}_g^{\text{fit}} + 0.632\,\hat{E}_g^{\text{BS}}. \tag{6}$$

The coefficients are defined so that the testing samples used to estimate $\hat{E}_g^{632}$ are at the same average distance from the training sample as would be a random point drawn directly from F [4]. This estimator has outperformed others in many applications, mostly when the signal-to-noise ratio is moderate to low [7].

2.4   Standard Error of the Difference Estimator

In many model selection problems including the estimation of the number of fascicles from DWI, model classes are nested: simpler models are particular cases of complex models. A more complex model can be arbitrarily close to a simpler one and its improvement of the generalization error may be due to chance alone. To reliably select between the two models, we need to assess whether this improvement is statistically significant.

Assessing the statistical significance of the difference in generalization error estimates between a model A and a model B, $\hat{\Delta}_{AB}^{632} = \hat{E}_{g,A}^{632} - \hat{E}_{g,B}^{632}$, requires the standard error of this difference to be estimated. After rearranging the terms of $\hat{\Delta}_{AB}^{632}$, taking advantage of the linearity of the expectation, we have:

$$\hat{\Delta}_{AB}^{632} = \frac{0.368}{n}\sum_{i=1}^{n} E_{z_i \overset{\text{iid}}{\sim} \hat{F}}\left[\left|y_i - r_{\mathbf{z}}^A(x_i)\right|^2 - \left|y_i - r_{\mathbf{z}}^B(x_i)\right|^2\right]$$

$$+ \frac{0.632}{n}\sum_{i=1}^{n} E_{z_i \overset{\text{iid}}{\sim} \hat{F}_{(-i)}}\left[\left|y_i - r_{\mathbf{z}_{(-i)}^*}^A(x_i)\right|^2 - \left|y_i - r_{\mathbf{z}_{(-i)}^*}^B(x_i)\right|^2\right]$$

$$\triangleq \frac{0.368}{n}\sum_{i=1}^{n}\hat{\Delta}_{AB,i}^{\text{fit}} + \frac{0.632}{n}\sum_{i=1}^{n}\hat{\Delta}_{AB,i}^{\text{BS}} \triangleq 0.368\,\hat{\Delta}_{AB}^{\text{fit}} + 0.632\,\hat{\Delta}_{AB}^{\text{BS}} \tag{7}$$

One could estimate the standard error of $\hat{\Delta}_{AB}^{\text{BS}}$ as $[\sum_i(\hat{\Delta}_{AB,i}^{\text{BS}} - \hat{\Delta}_{AB}^{\text{BS}})^2/n^2]^{1/2}$. This would assume that the $\hat{\Delta}_{AB,i}^{\text{BS}}$ are independent, which is not the case. A better estimate can be obtained by the *delta-method-after-bootstrap* approach [4]. This method is nonparametric and allows the computation of the standard error for any statistics that (1) is smooth in the observed data z, (2) is invariant under permutations of the points z_i and, (3) only depends on the empirical distribution $\hat{F}$. With this method, one can show that the standard error of $\hat{\Delta}_{AB}^{\mathrm{BS}}$ can be estimated by:

$$\hat{SE}^{\mathrm{BS}} = \left[\sum_{i=1}^{n} \hat{D}_i^2 \right]^{1/2} \text{ with } \hat{D}_i = \left(2 + \frac{1}{n-1} \right) \frac{\hat{\Delta}_{AB,i}^{\mathrm{BS}} - \hat{\Delta}_{AB}^{\mathrm{BS}}}{n} + \frac{\sum_{b=1}^{B} (N_i^b - \bar{N}_i) \bar{q}^b}{\sum_{b=1}^{B} \delta(N_i^b)}$$

$$\text{and } \bar{q}^b = \sum_{i=1}^{n} \delta(N_i^b) \left[\left| y_i - r_{\mathbf{z}_{(-i)}^*}^{A}(x_i) \right|^2 - \left| y_i - r_{\mathbf{z}_{(-i)}^*}^{B}(x_i) \right|^2 \right],$$

where $\bar{N}_i$ is the average N_i^b over all B bootstrap replicates. The same approach cannot be used for the standard error of $\hat{\Delta}_{AB}^{\mathrm{fit}}$ because it is a non-smooth function of the samples $\mathbf{z}$. Efron [4] proposes to estimate the standard error of $\hat{\Delta}_{AB}^{632}$ as:

$$\hat{SE}^{632} \approx \frac{\hat{\Delta}_{AB}^{632}}{\hat{\Delta}_{AB}^{\mathrm{BS}}} \hat{SE}^{\mathrm{BS}}. \tag{8}$$

To infer whether a model A is better than a model B, the estimate of the difference between their generalization errors (7) can be compared to the estimate of the standard error of this difference (8). This is the cornerstone of the selection of the number of fascicles problem.

2.5   Selection of the Number of Fascicles

The main idea to identify the number of fascicles at each voxel is to progressively increase the complexity of the model as long as a substantial decrease in the generalization error can be achieved and to stop when the decrease is no more significant or when the generalization error starts to increase. More specifically, the steps for the selection of the number of fascicles are:

1. For each pair of consecutive models (model with $m - 1$ fascicles and m fascicles), compute the difference of generalization error estimates using (7). Let $\Delta_m = \hat{\Delta}_{m-1,m}^{632}$ be this difference. To use expression (5) for this estimate, the bootstrap replicates must be identical for all models.
2. Compute the standard error s_m of the estimate Δ_m using (8).
3. Select the model with m_{opt} fascicles such that:

$$m_{\mathrm{opt}} = \inf \left\{ m \big| \Delta_m - \theta^{\mathrm{B632}} s_m \geq 0, \Delta_{m+1} - \theta^{\mathrm{B632}} s_{m+1} < 0 \right\}, \tag{9}$$

where θ^{B632} is the number of standard error above which the difference should be to be deemed significant. For this expression to hold, we set $s_0 = \Delta_0 = \Delta_M = 0$ and $s_M = 1$, where M is the maximum number of fascicles.

We could compare every model to every other one and extend the selection rule (9) to express the need for a model to be significantly better than all the simpler ones and not significantly worse than the more complex ones. In our experiment, we did not observe a difference between the two rules. Rule (9) has the advantage that it can be applied as the model complexity is progressively increased, avoiding the need to optimize further complex models at voxels where a simple model has already been selected.

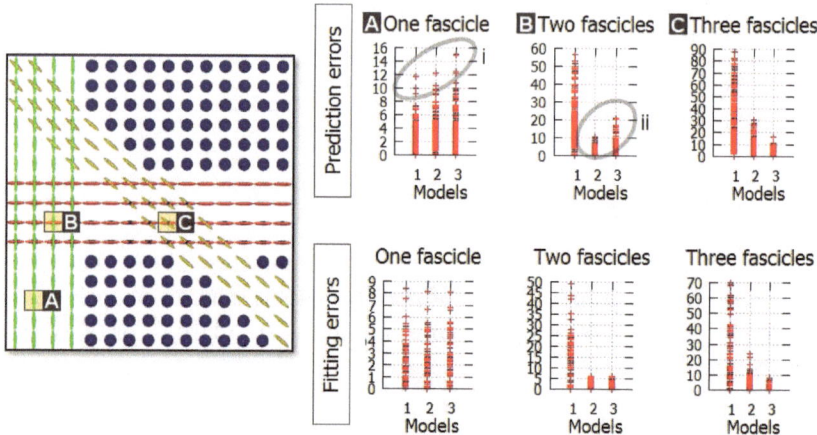

Fig. 1. (Left) Synthetic phantom used in our experiment, containing isotropic areas (blue balls), 1-fascicle areas [A], 2-fascicle areas [B] and three fascicle areas [C]. (Right) The repartition of the prediction errors, as used in the 632 bootstrap estimator, discriminates the three models, since more complex models may have higher prediction errors. On the contrary, the fitting error, as used in the F-test model selection, always decreases when the model complexity increases, due to overfitting.

2.6   Experimental Setup

Our proposed approach for the selection of the number of fascicles could be used with any generative model of the diffusion signal. In this work, we considered a multi-fascicle model in which each fascicle is represented by a tensor and the diffusion of free water is represented by an isotropic tensor. This amounts to considering the following generative model for the formation of the diffusion signal S for a b-value b and a gradient direction $\boldsymbol{g}$:

$$S = S_0 \left(f_0 e^{-bD_{\mathrm{iso}}} + \sum_{i=1}^{m} f_i e^{-b\boldsymbol{g}^T \boldsymbol{D}_i \boldsymbol{g}} \right),$$

where S_0 is the signal with no diffusion sensitization applied, $D_{\mathrm{iso}} = 3.0 \times 10^{-3} \mathrm{mm}^2/s$ is the diffusion of free water in the brain at 37°C, f_i are the volumetric fractions of occupancy associated with each compartment ($\sum_{i=0}^{m} f_i = 1$), m is the number of fascicles of the model and $\boldsymbol{D}_i$ is the tensor representing the fascicle $i \in [1, m]$. Such model requires a DWI acquisition that images multiple non-zero b-values [9]. We employed the CUSP gradient encoding scheme [9] which achieves short echo time and high SNR. This acquisition was composed of five $b = 0$, 30 DW images at $b = 1000$ and 30 DW images between $b = 1000$ and $b = 3000$. The parameters of each model were estimated using a maximum a posteriori approach. We focused on model complexity ranging from $m = 0$ (isotropic diffusion) to $m = 3$ fascicles. We investigated the performance of our B632 model selection approach with both synthetic phantoms and in vivo data.

We compared it to the F-test on the signal residuals [9], for which the null hypothesis is that the fitting error of models with $m - 1$ and m fascicles are equivalent by assessing the F-score:

$$F_{m-1,m} = \frac{n - 1 - |\mathcal{M}_m|}{|\mathcal{M}_m| - |\mathcal{M}_{m-1}|} \frac{\text{SSE}_{m-1} - \text{SSE}_m}{\text{SSE}_{m-1}} > \theta^{\text{F}-\text{test}}, \qquad (10)$$

where n is the number of data, $\theta^{\text{F}-\text{test}}$ is the F-score threshold above which the null hypothesis is rejected, and $|\mathcal{M}_m|$ and SSE_m are respectively the number of parameters and the sum of squared errors (fitting error) for a model with m fascicles. Various synthetic phantoms of size 15×15 were generated. The tensor profile $\boldsymbol{D}_i$ representing an individual fascicle was chosen to match typical in vivo data (trace of $2.1 \times 10^{-3} \text{mm}^2/s$ and FA of 0.8). We considered regions with 0, 1, 2 and 3 fascicles (Fig. 1). The simulated DWI were corrupted by various Rician-noise levels. In vivo imaging was achieved on a healthy volunteer using a Siemens 3T Trio scanner with a 32-channel head coil and the following parameters : FOV=220mm, 68 slices, matrix=128×128, resolution=$1.72 \times 1.7 \times 2mm^3$.

3   Results

3.1   Synthetic Phantom Experiments

Synthetic phantoms offer a ground truth against which results of the model selection can be compared. We investigated the performance of the B632 and F-test approaches under four different SNR : 10dB, 20dB, 30dB and 50dB. Both the B632 and the F-test approaches require determination of a threshold (see (9) and (10)). We investigated the influence of $\theta^{\text{F}-\text{test}}$ by evaluating the F-test model selection with $3 < \theta^{\text{F}-\text{test}} < 150$. Similarly, we evaluated the influence of θ^{B632} by computing the B632 model selection with $0 < \theta^{\text{B632}} < 13$. Note that $\theta^{\text{F}-\text{test}}$ is a threshold on the F-score while θ^{B632} is the number of standard error above which a model m is considered better than a model $m - 1$ (see (9)). The maximum number of bootstrap replicates for B632 was set to 150. We counted the number of errors between the ground truth and the automatic model selection results and reported the error rate.

The overall minimum error obtained by choosing the optimal thresholds is consistently higher with the F-test (Fig. 2a) than with B632 (Fig. 2b). The table in Fig. 2c summarizes those errors. In practice, the SNR is unknown and so the choice of threshold cannot depend on it. The overall minimum error rate are therefore lower bounds for what can actually be achieved in practice. The increase in error rate compared to this lower bound, due to the choice of a single threshold, is more dramatical with the F-test than with B632 (Fig. 2c, bottom rows). In particular, at 10dB, the error rate almost doubles compared to its lower bound with the F-test, while it increases only by a few percents with B632.

Finally, the evolution of the error rate with the number of bootstrap replicates assesses the stability of the estimate and allows the definition of a minimum number of bootstrap replicates required to achieve good performances. Fig. 2d shows that the error rate becomes stable after approximately 50 replicates.

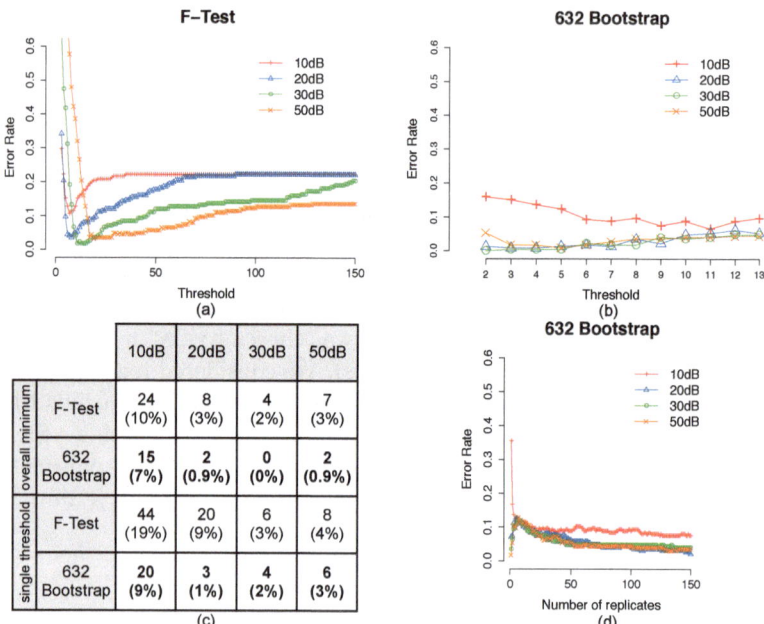

Fig. 2. Evaluation on simulated data for various noise levels. (a) For the F-test, the dependence of the error rate with the threshold $\theta^{F-\text{test}}$ shows that no single threshold can be used to achieve good performance at all noise levels. (b) The error rate is less sensitive to the threshold θ^{B632} set on the generalization error estimate. (c) Number of errors out of the 225 voxels and error rate for optimal thresholds chosen independently for each SNR (top rows) and jointly for all SNR (bottom rows). B632 leads to fewer error than the F-test, in both scenarios. The difference is more striking when a single threshold is used for all SNR. (d) The 632 bootstrap estimate reaches a close to optimal value after about 50 replicates.

3.2   In-Vivo Data: Robustness to Pre-processing

The results on the synthetic phantom suggest that the F-test model selection is not robust to changes in the characteristics of the image. In particular, if a threshold is optimized for some SNR, it will yield suboptimal results at another SNR. The acquisition of DWI is usually followed by several steps of preprocessing before the diffusion model is estimated. Some of these steps aim at improving the SNR. We may wonder whether the model selection is robust to these pre-processing step.

As an illustration, we applied the model selection methods on an in-vivo acquisition before and after automatic motion correction based on coregistration of all the DW images. The acquisition was not corrupted by any significant subject motion, and therefore this step mostly introduces a smoothing due to the interpolation when coregistering the images. Results in Fig. 3 show that the F-test model selection is strongly affected by this preprocessing step. With a threshold

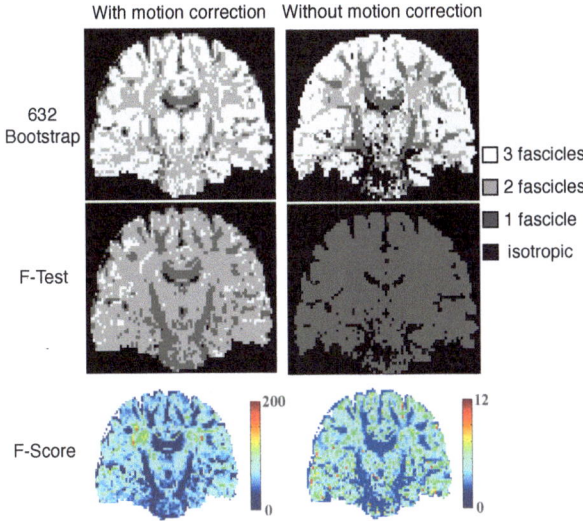

Fig. 3. Maps of the number of fascicles as detected with B632 and F-test for DWI with and without motion correction. Motion correction mostly introduced interpolation since no significant motion was present in this scan. B632 yields similar results in both cases, while the F-test selection fails to detect areas of more than one fascicle. This is due to the reduced perceived signal to noise ratio after motion correction, which affects the result of the F-test, as shown by the map of the F-score for the comparison between one and two-fascicle models.

of $\theta^{\mathrm{F-test}} = 15$, the map of the number of fascicles after motion correction does not resemble that before motion correction. In the latter, only one-tensor models and isotropic diffusion models were selected, while two- and three-tensor models are detected at many locations after motion correction. To observe two- or three-tensor models in the second map, one would need to decrease $\theta^{\mathrm{F-test}}$ since the SNR is lower, which is consistent with the synthetic results of Fig. 2(a). By contrast, for a constant $\theta^{\mathrm{B632}} = 8$, the maps of the number of fascicles detected with B632 are consistent across both images and follow the traits of the anatomy.

3.3   In Vivo Data: Cross-Testing Validation

Experiments based on in vivo data cannot rely on any ground truth to assess the error rates of the methods. To objectively compare the performance of the F-test and the B632 model selection approaches, we performed a cross-testing analysis. This procedure consists in repeatedly splitting the dataset into an *estimation set* and a *testing set*. In our experiments, we considered 70% of the data for estimation and the remaining 30% for testing. Both the model selection and estimation of the MFM parameters were carried out with the estimation set while the testing set was used to assess the performance of the two approaches. The threshold parameters were set to respectively $\theta^{\mathrm{F-test}} = 15$ and

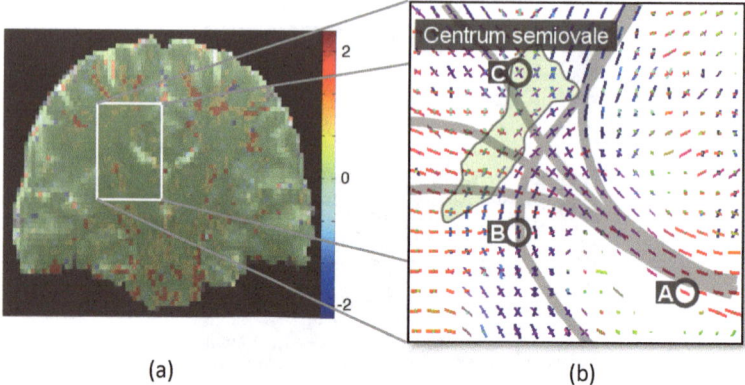

(a)   (b)

Fig. 4. (a) Comparison of the F-test and B632 model selection approaches using cross-testing. Difference between the testing error when using F-test model selection and B632 model selection. It shows that the testing error is significantly lower (positive values) when using B632. (b) Illustration that B632 and MFM estimation enables reliable detection of the number of fascicles that matches the known anatomy. (a) body of the corpus callosum, (b) crossing of the corpus callosum and the cortico-spinal tracts and (c) centrum semiovale which contains three fascicle orientations.

$\theta^{B632} = 8$. The performance of the approaches was assessed by computing the mean-square prediction error on the testing set. We repeated the estimation-testing process 30 times and computed the average testing error. Fig 4 shows that the testing error with B632 is lower than with F-test. More precisely, a paired t-test on the differences between the testing errors at each voxel shows that B632 is significantly better than F-test ($p < 10^{-12}$) with an mean improvement of 0.56.

4   Discussion and Conclusion

The estimation of the generalization error allows a reliable selection of the optimal model. Results on both synthetic and in vivo data show the improved performance over model selection based on the F-test.

Validating the models by means of an external dataset, as done in Section 3.3, seems the most objective validation method. Arguably, the generalization error is therefore what all model selection approaches attempt to minimize. However, unlike the fitting error, the generalization error cannot be computed and model selection criteria can be viewed as bypasses to this conceptual limitation. In this interpretation, the fitting error is, itself, an estimate of the generalization error. Complexity penalization could then be seen as heuristic methods to correct for the high bias of this estimate. The 632 bootstrap estimate, on the other hand, directly estimates the generalization error paying attention to remove as much bias and unnecessary variance as possible.

Computing the fitting error is a lot faster than computing the 632 bootstrap which requires several estimations of the model (one for each of the B bootstrap replicates). For this reason, model selection and estimation using B632 is about

B times slower. Different approximations could be used to decrease the computational time, such as estimating sticks instead of tensors during the model selection step and defining a stopping criterion on the number of bootstrap replicates based on the current estimate of the generalization error.

In a future work, we will apply the proposed approach to select between a broader class of generative diffusion models of the diffusion signal. This will enable appropriate identification of the model complexity at each voxel and accurate assessment of the white matter characteristics.

References

1. Alexander, D.C., Barker, G.J., Arridge, S.R.: Detection and modeling of non-gaussian apparent diffusion coefficient profiles in human brain data. Magn. Reson. Med. 48(2), 331–340 (2002)
2. Assaf, Y., Basser, P.J.: Composite hindered and restricted model of diffusion (CHARMED) MR imaging of the human brain. NeuroImage 27(1), 48–58 (2005)
3. Behrens, T.E.J., Berg, H.J., Jbabdi, S., Rushworth, M.F.S., Woolrich, M.W.: Probabilistic diffusion tractography with multiple fibre orientations: What can we gain? NeuroImage 34(1), 144–155 (2007)
4. Efron, B., Tibshirani, R.: Improvements on cross-validation: The .632 + bootstrap method. Journal of the American Statistical Association 92(438), 548–560 (1997)
5. Kreher, B., Schneider, J., Mader, I., Martin, E., Hennig, J., Il'yasov, K.: Multitensor approach for analysis and tracking of complex fiber configurations. Magnetic Resonance in Medicine 54(5), 1216–1225 (2005)
6. Miller, K.L., et al.: Diffusion imaging of whole, post-mortem human brains on a clinical MRI scanner. Neuroimage 57(1), 167–181 (2011)
7. Molinaro, A., Simon, R., Pfeiffer, R.: Prediction error estimation: a comparison of resampling methods. Bioinformatics 21(15), 3301–3307 (2005)
8. Pasternak, O., Westin, C., Bouix, S., Seidman, L., Goldstein, J., Woo, T., Petryshen, T., Mesholam-Gately, R., McCarley, R., Kikinis, R., et al.: Excessive extracellular volume reveals a neurodegenerative pattern in schizophrenia onset. The Journal of Neuroscience 32(48), 17365–17372 (2012)
9. Scherrer, B., Warfield, S.K.: Parametric Representation of Multiple White Matter Fascicles from Cube and Sphere Diffusion MRI. PLoS ONE 7(11) (2012)
10. Schultz, T., Westin, C.-F., Kindlmann, G.: Multi-diffusion-tensor fitting via spherical deconvolution: A unifying framework. In: Jiang, T., Navab, N., Pluim, J.P.W., Viergever, M.A. (eds.) MICCAI 2010, Part I. LNCS, vol. 6361, pp. 674–681. Springer, Heidelberg (2010)
11. Shao, J.: Linear Model Selection by Cross-Validation. Journal of the American Statistical Association 88(442), 486–494 (1993)
12. Tuch, D.S., Reese, T.G., Wiegell, M.R., Makris, N., Belliveau, J.W., Wedeen, V.J.: High angular resolution diffusion imaging reveals intravoxel white matter fiber heterogeneity. MRM 48(4), 577–582 (2002)
13. Zhang, H., Schneider, T., Wheeler-Kingshott, C.A., Alexander, D.C.: Noddi: practical in vivo neurite orientation dispersion and density imaging of the human brain. Neuroimage 61(4), 1000–1016 (2012)

IDiff: Irrotational Diffeomorphisms
for Computational Anatomy

Jacob Hinkle and Sarang Joshi

Scientific Computing and Imaging Institute,
Department of Bioengineering, University of Utah, Salt Lake City, UT

Abstract. The study of diffeomorphism groups is fundamental to computational anatomy, and in particular to image registration. One of the most developed frameworks employs a Riemannian-geometric approach using right-invariant Sobolev metrics. To date, the computation of the Riemannian log and exponential maps on the diffeomorphism group have been defined implicitly via an infinite-dimensional optimization problem. In this paper we the employ Brenier's (1991) polar factorization to decompose a diffeomorphism h as $h(x) = S \circ \psi(x)$, where $\psi = \nabla \rho$ is the gradient of a convex function ρ and $S \in \mathrm{SDiff}(\mathbb{R}^d)$ is a volume-preserving diffeomorphism. We show that all such mappings ψ form a submanifold, which we term $\mathrm{IDiff}(\mathbb{R}^d)$, generated by irrotational flows from the identity. Using the natural metric, the manifold $\mathrm{IDiff}(\mathbb{R}^d)$ is flat. This allows us to calculate the Riemannian log map on this submanifold of diffeomorphisms in closed form, and develop extremely efficient metric-based image registration algorithms. This result has far-reaching implications in terms of the statistical analysis of anatomical variability within the framework of computational anatomy.

Keywords: image registration, computational anatomy, Helmholtz-Hodge decomposition, irrotational, polar factorization.

1 Introduction

Over the last decade, the field of computational anatomy has substantially matured and several approaches have been developed for the study of anatomical variations that are evident within medical images. The most theoretically developed and principled approaches are based on the Riemannian geometry of groups of diffeomorphisms of three-dimensional Euclidian space, $\mathbb{R}^3$, and its submanifolds (points, curves and surfaces) on which these groups act. Fundamental to this approach is the computation of geodesics which provide *normal coordinates* via the Riemannian log and exponential maps allowing for statistical analysis of anatomical variability. Despite the elegance of the theory, universal adoption has been limited by the computational complexity of the resulting optimization problems, especially the need for infinite dimensional optimization to compute the geodesic and the log map. To mitigate the computational complexity, recently some [7] have suggested abandoning the intrinsic Riemannian geometric

J.C. Gee et al. (Eds.): IPMI 2013, LNCS 7917, pp. 754–765, 2013.

approach and taking an extrinsic Eulerian view of deformation based on stationary vector fields.

One of the major contributions of this paper is the use of the remarkable result by Brenier [3] concerning the polar factorization of diffeomorphisms (analogous to the polar factorization of matrices) to define a submanifold of irrotational diffeomorphisms which we call IDiff($\mathbb{R}^d$). In this paper we show that this
infinite-dimensional submanifold is generated by irrotational velocity fields and
that furthermore using the natural metric this submanifold is flat, meaning that
sectional curvature in every direction is 0. This theoretical result has far reaching consequences: for example, within this space the intrinsic or Fréchet mean
is guaranteed to be unique. Another consequence of this remarkable result is
that we are able to derive in closed form the Riemannian log map and compute
the distance between any two diffeomorphisms within IDiff in closed form. In
this paper we begin to explore the applications of this by developing extremely
computationally efficient and numerically stable image registration algorithms.

2   Mathematical Background and Notation

Although diffeomorphisms in the context of image registration have been extensively studied for completeness we review the basic set up. A compactly sup-
ported diffeomorphism φ is a bijective map from $\mathbb{R}^d$ to $\mathbb{R}^d$ such that both φ
and its inverse φ^{-1} are smooth and have compact support. The identity transformation id is a diffeomorphism as well as the composition of any two. As the
inverse of a diffeomorphism is also a diffeomorphism, it implies that the set of all
diffeomorphisms forms a group. The Lie algebra $\mathfrak{g}$ of the compactly supported
diffeomorphism group of Diff($\mathbb{R}^d$) consists of all compactly supported smooth
vector fields on $\mathbb{R}^d$, equipped with the Lie bracket of vector fields.

Given a time dependent vector field $v(x,t)$ one defines a path in Diff($\mathbb{R}^d$) via
the O.D.E:

$$\frac{d\varphi(x,t)}{dt} = v(\varphi(x,t),t), \text{ with initial condition: } \varphi(x,0) = x.$$

One induces a right invariant metric by choosing a differential operator L which
acts on velocity fields. This operator determines the norm of a velocity field,
$\|v\|^2 = \int (Lv(x), v(x))dx$. The dual space of the Lie algebra, $\mathfrak{g}^*$ consists of vector-
valued distributions. The velocity, $v \in \mathfrak{g}$, maps to its dual deformation momenta,
$m \in \mathfrak{g}^*$, via the operator L such that $m = Lv$. Using this norm geodesics
are defined as energy minimizing paths between their endpoints. The distance
between id and diffeomorphism ϕ is defined via the optimization problem:

$$d(id, \phi)^2 = \inf \left\{ \int_0^1 \|v(\cdot, t)\|^2 dt, \text{ subject to: } \varphi(\cdot, 1) = \phi \right\}.$$

EPDiff for Geodesic Evolution: Given the initial velocity, $v_0 \in \mathfrak{g}$, or equivalently, the initial momentum, $m(0) = m_0 \in \mathfrak{g}^*$, the geodesic path $\varphi(t)$ satisfies
the EPDiff equation [1,8]:

$$\frac{d}{dt}m = -\operatorname{ad}_v^* m = -(Dv)^T m - Dmv - (\operatorname{div} v)m \tag{1}$$

where D denotes the Jacobian matrix, and the operator ad^* is the dual of the negative Jacobi-Lie bracket of vector fields [8,1,12]: $\operatorname{ad}_v w = -[v, w] = (Dv)w - (Dw)v$.

3 Polar Factorization of Diffeomorphisms and IDiff: The Space of Irrotational Diffeomorphisms

Brenier's [3] polar factorization of diffeomorphisms states that any diffeomorphism φ of $\mathbb{R}^d$ can be uniquely written as a composition

$$\varphi = S \circ \psi, \quad \text{where } \psi = \nabla\rho \tag{2}$$

for some convex function $\rho : \mathbb{R}^d \to \mathbb{R}$ and where $S \in \operatorname{SDiff}(\mathbb{R}^d)$ is a measure-preserving diffeomorphism. This decomposition is analogous to the classical polar factorization of matrices. Just as an invertible matrix can be written as product of a positive definite matrix and a unitary matrix, the Jacobian of the deformation ψ, $D\psi = H\rho$ is the Hessian of the convex function ρ, and as such is a symmetric positive-definite matrix, and as S is volume-preserving its Jacobian DS has determinant 1 every where and is unitary. Brenier's polar factorization of $\operatorname{Diff}(\mathbb{R}^d)$ is intimately connected to the Helmholtz-Hodge decomposition of vector fields, which has proven useful for modeling incompressible deformation in computational anatomy [6]. The Helmholtz-Hodge decomposition states that any compactly supported square-integrable C^2 vector field $v \in \mathfrak{g}$ can be written as $v = \nabla f + \operatorname{curl} A$ where $f \in H^1(\mathbb{R}^d)$ and $A \in H^{\operatorname{curl}}(\mathbb{R}^d)$. This constitutes a decomposition of $\mathfrak{g}$ into two linear subspaces: one containing irrotational vector fields represented as gradients of scalar Sobolev functions and one containing incompressible (divergence-free) vector fields represented as curls of Sobolev vector fields. We will denote by $\mathfrak{g}_P$ the subspace of irrotational vector fields and by $\mathfrak{g}_S$ the subspace of divergence-free vector fields, so that $\mathfrak{g} = \mathfrak{g}_P \oplus \mathfrak{g}_S$. Further more assuming compact support, f is uniquely determined by the divergence of v and f satisfies Poisson's equation:

$$\operatorname{div}(v) = g, \quad \Delta f = g, \tag{3}$$

where Δ is the Laplacian operator and $g \in L^2(\mathbb{R}^d)$. Define the space $\operatorname{IDiff}(\mathbb{R}^d)$ to be the space of diffeomorphisms $\psi(1)$ for which there exists a smooth path $\psi(t)$ of diffeomorphisms satisfying

$$\psi(0) = id \quad \text{and} \quad \frac{d}{dt}\psi(t) = v(t) \circ \psi(t) \qquad \forall t \in [0,1] \tag{4}$$

for some time-varying collection of $v(t) \in \mathfrak{g}_P$. This implies that every $\phi(1) \in \operatorname{IDiff}(\mathbb{R}^d)$ is determined by a time-varying H^1 scalar field $f(t)$:

$$\frac{d}{dt}\psi(t) = (\nabla f(t)) \circ \psi(t). \tag{5}$$

By Liouville's theorem, all such ψ have symmetric positive-definite Jacobian matrices and can be written as the gradient of a convex function. This definition mimics that of $\mathrm{SDiff}(\mathbb{R}^d)$, the space of compactly-supported incompressible diffeomorphisms of $\mathbb{R}^d$. It is to be noted that although $\mathrm{SDiff}(\mathbb{R}^d)$ is a subgroup of diffeomorphisms of $\mathbb{R}^d$, $\mathrm{IDiff}(\mathbb{R}^d)$ is a not a subgroup as $\mathfrak{g}_P$ is not closed with respect to Lie bracket. Just as the with symmetric positive definite matrices, composition of two irrotational diffeomorphisms is not necessarily an irrotational diffeomorphism.

4   Metric and Geodesics on $\mathrm{IDiff}(\mathbb{R}^d)$

The Helmholtz-Hodge decomposition assumes that the divergence of v is square-integrable, so the most natural inner product to induce on irrotational vector fields is the one induced via the L^2 inner product on it divergence, the natural inner product on $\mathfrak{g}_P$ becomes:

$$\langle v, w \rangle_{\mathfrak{g}_P} = \langle \mathrm{div}\, v, \mathrm{div}\, w \rangle_{L^2} = \langle \mathrm{div}\, \nabla f, \mathrm{div}\, \nabla h \rangle_{L^2} = \int_\Omega \Delta f(x) \Delta h(x) dx \quad (6)$$

where Δ is the Laplacian operator. Notice that with the above inner product if g is the divergence of v, the norm of v is simply the L^2 norm of g:

$$\|v\|_{\mathfrak{g}_P}^2 = \|\mathrm{div}\, v\|_{L^2(\mathbb{R}^d)}^2 = -\int (\nabla \mathrm{div}\, v(x))^T v(x) dx = \|g\|_{L^2(\mathbb{R}^d)}^2. \quad (7)$$

This is the $\dot{H}^1$ metric, $\langle -\Delta v, w \rangle$, restricted to $\mathfrak{g}_P$, which follows from the fact that $\mathrm{curl}\, v = 0$ in $\mathfrak{g}_P$ and the identity $\Delta v = \nabla \mathrm{div}\, v - \mathrm{curl}\, \mathrm{curl}\, v$.

Letting $\psi_1, \psi_2 \in \mathrm{IDiff}(\Omega)$ be two diffeomorphisms, a geodesic between ψ_1 and ψ_2 is a path $\alpha(t) \in \mathrm{IDiff}(\mathbb{R}^d)$ connecting ψ_1, ψ_2 that minimizes

$$S(\alpha) = \frac{1}{2} \int_0^1 \|\dot{\alpha}(t)\|^2 dt = \frac{1}{2} \int_0^1 \int |(\Delta f(t))(x)|^2 dx dt. \quad (8)$$

Geodesics on $\mathrm{IDiff}(\mathbb{R}^d)$ are actually minimizing curves in all of $\mathrm{Diff}(\mathbb{R}^d)$ with the constraint that the right-trivialized velocity lie in $\mathfrak{g}_P$ at all times, and are sub-Riemannian geodesics on the Lie group $\mathrm{Diff}(\mathbb{R}^d)$. The theory of sub-Riemannian geodesics in Lie groups has been studied previously [5]. We define the momentum associated with the velocity v as $m = -\nabla \mathrm{div}\, v = -\nabla g$. Geodesics in $\mathrm{IDiff}(\mathbb{R}^d)$ satisfy the constrained Euler-Poincaré equation 1 with the constraint that v is curl free. Substituting $m = -\nabla g, v = \nabla f$ and $\mathrm{div}\, v = g$ the constrained Euler-Poincaré equation simply becomes:

$$\frac{d}{dt} \nabla g = -Hg \nabla f - (Hf)^T \nabla g - g \nabla g. \quad (9)$$

The Hessian matrix is always symmetric and notice that $\nabla(g^2) = 2g \nabla g$, so we can rewrite this using the product rule as

$$\nabla \frac{d}{dt} g = -\nabla \left(\nabla g^T \nabla f + \frac{1}{2} g^2 \right). \quad (10)$$

Along with our boundary conditions on g this implies that

$$\dot{g} + \nabla g^T v = -\frac{1}{2}g^2. \tag{11}$$

The left-hand side has the form of a material derivative, suggesting a change to Lagrangian coordinates. Introducing $\gamma(t) = g \circ \psi(t)$, implying $\dot{\gamma} = \dot{g} \circ \psi + ((\nabla g)^T v) \circ \psi$ we see that

$$\dot{\gamma}(t) = -\frac{1}{2}\gamma(t)^2, \quad \text{or} \quad \gamma(t) = \frac{\gamma(0)}{\frac{1}{2}t\gamma(0) + 1}. \tag{12}$$

Using the shorthand $g_0 = g(0)$ and the assumption $\psi(0) = id$, we arrive at

$$g(t) \circ \psi(t) = \frac{g_0}{\frac{1}{2}tg_0 + 1}. \tag{13}$$

The quantity $g(t)$ is, by definition, the divergence of the velocity at time t. Using the well-known Liouville's formula we relate this directly to the determinant of the Jacobian matrix of the diffeomorphism ψ as follows:

$$|D\psi(t)| = \exp\int_0^t (\text{div } v) \circ \psi ds = \exp\int_0^t \frac{g_0}{\frac{1}{2}sg_0 + 1}ds = \left(\frac{1}{2}tg_0 + 1\right)^2. \tag{14}$$

Using the solution of the EPDiff equation we can explicitly write the expression for the distance in $\text{IDiff}(\mathbb{R}^d)$ between the identity and any irrotational diffeomorphism ψ. As the metric is simply the L^2 norm of g, by conservation of momenta along a geodesic we have

$$d(id, \psi)^2 = \|g_0\|_{L^2(\mathbb{R}^d)}^2 = 4\int_{\mathbb{R}^d} (\sqrt{|D\psi|} - 1)^2 dx. \tag{15}$$

The simplicity of the above formula comes from the fact that by solving the EPDiff equation, g_0 is essentially the log map on $\text{IDiff}(\mathbb{R}^d)$ with the $\dot{H}^1$ metric.

5   Curvature of $\text{IDiff}(\mathbb{R}^d)$

We now use the relationship between g_0 and $|D\psi|$ to show that the curvature of $\text{IDiff}(\mathbb{R}^d)$ with the $\dot{H}^1$ metric is 0. Define the following mapping from ψ to the divergence of its initial velocity field:

$$P : \text{IDiff}(\mathbb{R}^d) \to L^2(\mathbb{R}^d) \tag{16}$$
$$P(\psi) = 2(\sqrt{|D\psi|} - 1) = g_0. \tag{17}$$

We first need the following Lemma:

Lemma 1. *The pushforward of a vector field $u \circ \psi \in T_\psi \text{IDiff}(\mathbb{R}^d)$ under the mapping P is given by the formula*

$$TP(u \circ \psi) = \sqrt{|D\psi|}(\text{div } u) \circ \psi. \tag{18}$$

Proof. Let ψ_s be a family of irrotational diffeomorphisms indexed by the real variable s and satisfying

$$\psi_0 = \psi, \quad \frac{d}{ds}|_{s=0}\psi_s = u \circ \psi. \tag{19}$$

Then the pushforward of the vector field u is defined as

$$TP(u \circ \psi) = \frac{d}{ds}|_{s=0}P\psi_s. \tag{20}$$

A straightforward computation then yields

$$TP(u \circ \psi) = 2\frac{d}{ds}|_{s=0}\sqrt{|D\psi_s|} = \sqrt{|D\psi|}(\operatorname{div} u) \circ \psi. \tag{21}$$

Theorem 1. *The mapping P is an isometry from* $\mathrm{IDiff}(\mathbb{R}^d)$ *into an open subset of* $L^2(\mathbb{R}^d)$.

Proof. As the pushfoward is only zero for divergence-free vector fields, Lemma 1 directly implies that P is injective on $\mathrm{IDiff}(\mathbb{R}^d)$. To prove that P is furthermore an isometry, we compute the pullback of the L^2 metric for any two vector fields $u \circ \psi, w \circ \psi \in T_\psi \, \mathrm{IDiff}(\mathbb{R}^d)$:

$$\langle u, w \rangle_{P*} = \langle TP(u \circ \psi), TP(w \circ \psi) \rangle_{L^2(\mathbb{R}^d)}. \tag{22}$$

Plugging in and performing a change of variables, we have

$$\langle u, w \rangle_{P*} = \int \sqrt{|D\psi(x)|}(\operatorname{div} u) \circ \psi(x)\sqrt{|D\psi(x)|}(\operatorname{div} w) \circ \psi(x)dx \tag{23}$$

$$= \int |D\psi(x)|(\operatorname{div} u) \circ \psi(x)(\operatorname{div} w) \circ \psi(x)dx \tag{24}$$

$$= \langle \operatorname{div} u, \operatorname{div} v \rangle_{L^2(\mathbb{R}^d)}, \tag{25}$$

which is our right-invariant metric on $\mathrm{IDiff}(\mathbb{R}^d)$, proving that P is a local isometry. By the uniqueness of Brenier's polar factorization, the mapping P is injective, completing the proof. □

The property that P is an isometry is remarkable in that it implies (since $L^2(\mathbb{R}^d)$ is a flat vector space) that with the $\dot{H}^1$ metric, $\mathrm{IDiff}(\mathbb{R}^d)$ has zero Riemannian curvature[1]. Another important consequence is that under P, geodesics in $\mathrm{IDiff}(\mathbb{R}^d)$ map to straight lines in $L^2(\mathbb{R}^d)$. The image of P consists of all L^2 functions with values strictly greater than -2, implying that geodesics can leave this open subset in finite time. Given an initial velocity field, this blow-up time is determined by the minimum value of its divergence g_0 and Eq. 14.

---

[1] This has been observed very recently in [2] for the special case of $d = 1$ where $\mathrm{IDiff}(\mathbb{R}^1) = \mathrm{Diff}(\mathbb{R}^1)$ as the only compactly-supported measure-preserving diffeomorphism of the real line is the identity mapping.

The P map is injective, so given $g_0 \in L^2(\mathbb{R}^d)$, there is a unique irrotational diffeomorphism $\psi \in \mathrm{IDiff}(\mathbb{R}^d)$ in the inverse image $P^{-1}(g_0)$. Computation of ψ is equivalent to computing the exponential map in $\mathrm{IDiff}(\mathbb{R}^d)$. We are unaware of a closed-form method for computing ψ, but it may be computed numerically using Eq. 13 to compute $g(t) = \operatorname{div} v(t)$ at each time, then solving for the velocity field $v(t)$ and integrating the flow.

6   Irrotational Image Registration

Consider a registration problem in which two images $I_0, I_1 \in L^2(\mathbb{R}^d)$ are given and one wishes to find an irrotational deformation $\psi \in \mathrm{IDiff}(\mathbb{R}^d)$ that best matches the two images. Analogous to the LDDMM approach, we introduce the energy functional

$$E(\psi) = \frac{1}{2\sigma^2}\|I_0 \circ \psi^{-1} - I_1\|^2_{L^2(\mathbb{R}^d)} + d(id, \psi)^2 \tag{26}$$

where d denotes the geodesic distance within $\mathrm{IDiff}(\mathbb{R}^d)$. However, unlike with general LDDMM, the distance term can now be evaluated in closed form only using ψ:

$$E(\psi) = \frac{1}{2\sigma^2}\|I_0 \circ \psi^{-1} - I_1\|^2_{L^2(\mathbb{R}^d)} + 4\|\sqrt{|D\psi|} - 1\|^2_{L^2(\mathbb{R}^d)}. \tag{27}$$

This allows us to take the Sobolev variation of E with respect to ψ directly by first taking the L^2 variation and then sharping it using the inverse of the metric. Let $\nabla c \in \mathfrak{g}_P$ be a perturbation of ψ, and let $\psi_s \in \mathrm{IDiff}(\mathbb{R}^d)$ be a family of irrotational diffeomorphisms parametrized by the real variable s, satisfying

$$\psi_0 = \psi \quad \text{and} \quad \frac{d}{ds}|_{s=0}\psi_s = (\nabla c) \circ \psi. \tag{28}$$

Then the variation of E with respect to ψ in the direction of ∇c is computed via

$$(\delta E, \nabla c) = \frac{d}{ds}|_{s=0}E(\psi_s) \tag{29}$$

$$= \frac{d}{ds}|_{s=0}\frac{1}{2\sigma^2}\int_\Omega (I_0 \circ \psi_s^{-1}(y) - I_1(y))^2 dy + 4\int_\Omega (\sqrt{|D\psi_s(x)|} - 1)^2 dx \tag{30}$$

$$= \frac{1}{\sigma^2}\int_\Omega (I_0 \circ \psi^{-1}(y) - I_1(y))\nabla(I_0 \circ \psi^{-1}(y))^T \nabla c(y) dy \tag{31}$$

$$+ 4\int_\Omega (\sqrt{|D\psi(x)|} - 1)\frac{1}{\sqrt{|D\psi(x)|}}\frac{d}{ds}|_{s=0}|D\psi_s(x)|dx. \tag{32}$$

Using $\frac{d}{ds}|_{s=0}|D\psi_s(x)| = (\operatorname{div}\nabla c) \circ \psi(x)|D\psi(x)|$ and the fact that, for compactly supported vector fields, the adjoint of the divergence is the negative gradient, we have

$$(\delta E, \nabla c) = -\frac{1}{\sigma^2} \int_\Omega \text{div} \left((I_0 \circ \psi^{-1}(y) - I_1(y)) \nabla (I \circ \psi^{-1}(y)) \right) c(y) dy \tag{33}$$

$$+ 4 \int_\Omega (\sqrt{|D\psi|} \circ \psi^{-1}(y) - 1) \sqrt{|D\psi|} \circ \psi^{-1}(y) \Delta c(y) |D\psi^{-1}(y)| dy. \tag{34}$$

Now we use the identity $(D\psi^{-1}) \circ \psi(x) = (D\psi)^{-1}(x)$ and self-adjointness of the Laplacian to simplify this to

$$(\delta E, \nabla c) = -\frac{1}{\sigma^2} \int_\Omega \text{div} \left((I_0 \circ \psi^{-1}(y) - I_1(y)) \nabla (I_0 \circ \psi^{-1}(y)) \right) c(y) dy \tag{35}$$

$$+ 4 \int_\Omega c(y) \Delta \left(1 - \sqrt{|D\psi^{-1}(y)|} \right) dy. \tag{36}$$

By adjointing the gradient in the left-hand side we see that since this must hold for all c, we have

$$\text{div} \, \delta E = \frac{1}{\sigma^2} \text{div} \left((I_0 \circ \psi^{-1} - I_1) \nabla (I_0 \circ \psi^{-1}) \right) + 4\Delta (\sqrt{|D\psi^{-1}|} - 1). \tag{37}$$

In order to convert δE to the Sobolev variation of E, we solve the following for the scalar function b:

$$\Delta^2 b = \frac{1}{\sigma^2} \text{div} \left((I_0 \circ \psi^{-1} - I_1) \nabla (I_0 \circ \psi^{-1}) \right) + 4\Delta (\sqrt{|D\psi^{-1}|} - 1) \tag{38}$$

then update ψ via $\psi(x) \mapsto \psi(x) - \epsilon(\nabla b) \circ \psi(x)$ for some step-size ϵ. In practice, as ψ is never needed we directly update only ψ^{-1} via $\psi^{-1}(y) \mapsto \psi^{-1}(y + \epsilon \nabla b(y))$.

Notice that this allows ψ^{-1} to be optimized directly in a gradient-based scheme without the need for numeric integration of geodesic equations or adjoint equations.

7   Symmetric Image Registration

In this section, we present an image registration approach that is symmetric with respect to swapping of the input images. Consider re-weighting the image match term by the square root of the Jacobian determinant.

$$E(\psi) = \frac{1}{2\sigma^2} \int |I_0 \circ \psi^{-1}(y) - I_1(y)|^2 \sqrt{|D\psi^{-1}(y)|} dy + d(id, \psi)^2. \tag{39}$$

Now using the change of variables $x = \psi^{-1}(y)$

$$E(\psi) = \frac{1}{2\sigma^2} \int \|I_0(x) - I_1 \circ \psi(x)\|^2 \sqrt{|(D\psi^{-1}) \circ \psi(x)|} |D\psi(x)| dx + d(\psi^{-1}, id)^2. \tag{40}$$

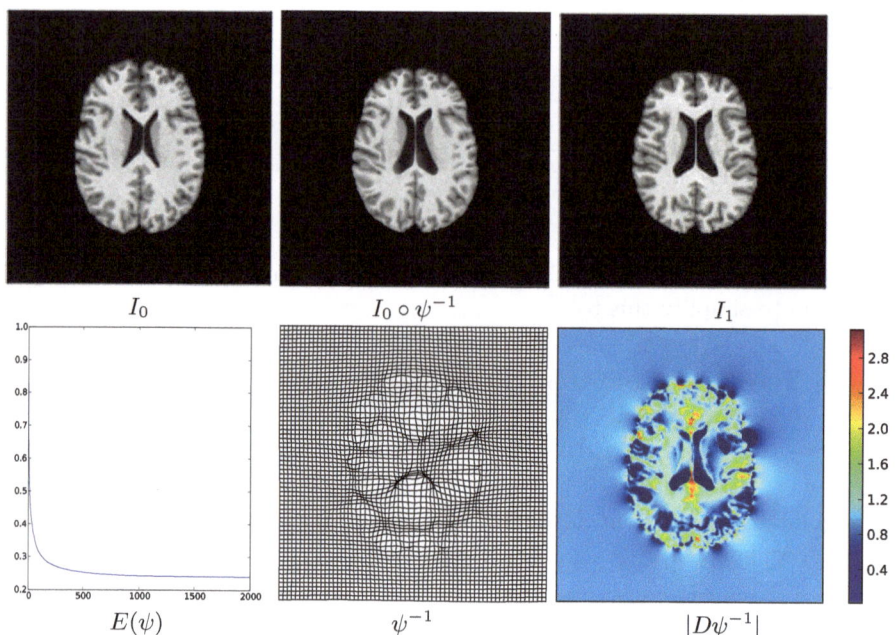

$$I_0 \qquad I_0 \circ \psi^{-1} \qquad I_1$$

$$E(\psi) \qquad \psi^{-1} \qquad |D\psi^{-1}|$$

Fig. 1. Neuroimaging study, symmetric irrotational registration results. The algorithm was run with inputs I_0, I_1 to generate the irrotational diffeomorphism ψ. The plot of energy $E(\psi)$ at each iteration is shown on the left in the lower column showing good convergence, along with the estimated deformation ψ and its Jacobian determinant.

Using the inversion-invariance of our metric we rewrite the cost functional as

$$E(\psi) = \frac{1}{2\sigma^2} \int |I_0(x) - I_1 \circ \psi(x)|^2 \sqrt{|D\psi(x)|}\,dx + d(id, \psi)^2. \qquad (41)$$

This has the same form as the original function in which the first image I_0 was deformed to match I_1, but instead we match I_1 to I_0. So the introduction of the square-root Jacobian determinant into the image match term has the effect of making the image registration problem invariant under relabeling of the input images. This resembles the "square-root trick" used in one dimension to develop parametrization-invariant metrics on time-series data [9] and planar curves [11].

Computing the variation of this functional is very similar to the method in the previous section, and leads us to the following biharmonic equation:

$$\Delta^2 b = \frac{1}{\sigma^2} \operatorname{div}\left((I_0 \circ \psi^{-1} - I_1)\sqrt{|D\psi^{-1}|}\nabla(I_0 \circ \psi^{-1})\right) \qquad (42)$$

$$+ \Delta\left(\left(4(1 - \sqrt{|D\psi^{-1}|}) - \frac{1}{4\sigma^2}|I_0 \circ \psi^{-1} - I_1|^2\right)\sqrt{|D\psi^{-1}|}\right). \qquad (43)$$

After solving this equation for b, we take the gradient then update ψ just as we did in the asymmetric case.

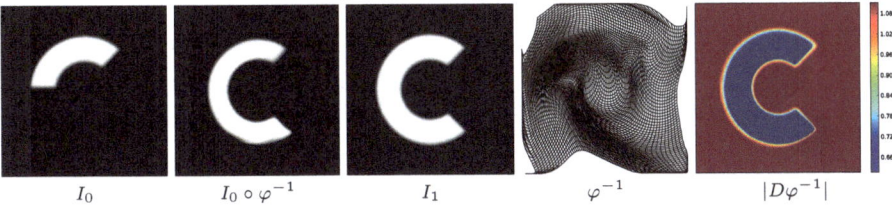

I_0 $I_0 \circ \varphi^{-1}$ I_1 φ^{-1} $|D\varphi^{-1}|$

Fig. 2. Synthetic study, symmetric hybrid image registration results. Shown here are the input image I_0, along with the deformed image $I_0 \circ \varphi^{-1}$, the target image I_1, the deformation φ^{-1}, and its Jacobian determinant $|D\varphi^{-1}|$.

Neuroimaging Study. We have implemented the symmetric irrotational image registration algorithm and applied it to two structural MRI images. Figure 1 shows the result of symmetric irrotational image registration. Notice that even without allowing any local rotation, the two images are matched quite well. In the bottom row is shown the energy at each iteration, indicating very stable convergence. Also notice that the Jacobian determinant clearly indicating regions of expansion and contraction. In our irrotational matching method, the Jacobian determinant entirely characterizes the diffeomorphism.

8   Pseudo-riemannian Hybrid Irrotational/Incompressible Registration

In this section we present an extension of the irrotational-only algorithms which allows an incompressible component to be estimated without any penalty. The right invariant metric on $\mathrm{IDiff}(\mathbb{R}^d)$ defined in Section 4 is also a right-invariant Riemannian pseudo-metric on all of $\mathrm{Diff}(\mathbb{R}^d)$. The null space of this metric consists of precisely all divergence-free vector fields, which is the Lie algebra $\mathfrak{g}_S$ associated with the group of volume-preserving diffeomorphisms $\mathrm{SDiff}(\mathbb{R}^d)$. Consider registration using a general diffeomorphism $\varphi = S \circ \psi$, where $S \in \mathrm{SDiff}(\mathbb{R}^d)$. Using the polar factorization of $\mathrm{Diff}(\mathbb{R}^d)$, we replace $E(\psi)$ with the functional

$$E(\psi, S) = \frac{1}{2\sigma^2} \int |I_0 \circ \psi^{-1} \circ S^{-1} - I_1|^2 \sqrt{|D\psi^{-1} \circ S^{-1}|} dy + d(id, \psi)^2. \quad (44)$$

Equation 44 is rewritten in terms of φ^{-1} only, using the fact that $|DS| = 1$:

$$E(\varphi) = \frac{1}{2\sigma^2} \int |I_0 \circ \varphi^{-1} - I_1|^2 \sqrt{|D\varphi^{-1}|} dy + 4 \int (\sqrt{|D\varphi^{-1}|} - 1)^2 dy. \quad (45)$$

This is optimized by decomposing the Sobolev variation of $E(\varphi)$ using the Helmholtz-Hodge decomposition into irrotational and incompressible components, then performing gradient descent steps in either component. The irrotational updates are performed exactly as described in the previous section, and since the incompressible updates do not effect the Jacobian determinant, the incompressible update direction $w \in \mathfrak{g}_S$ is found by simply solving

$$\Delta w = -\frac{1}{\sigma^2} \left(I_0 \circ \varphi^{-1} - I_1 \right) \sqrt{|D\varphi^{-1}|} \nabla(I_0 \circ \varphi^{-1}) \qquad (46)$$

and projecting onto the space of divergence-free vector fields $\mathfrak{g}_S$. This projection has been discussed previously in the literature and is performed efficiently in the Fourier domain while simultaneously solving the above Poisson's equation [6].

Synthetic Example. In order to test the performance of our algorithms in the presence of large deformation, a simulated experiment was also performed. Two synthetic two-dimensional datasets were generated, simulating a completed "C" and a half C. In Fig. 2 are shown the results of the hybrid image registration algorithm. Notice that the deformed half C image, $I_0 \circ \varphi^{-1}$, agrees very well with the full C image, I_1 and that this is achieved while maintaining a diffeomorphic transformation. Since we penalize the L^2 norm of the root Jacobian, the Jacobian determinant of the overall deformation is distributed very evenly across the entire deforming region, instead of being concentrated at a single advancing edge.

9   Multi-scale and Scale Independence of the Metric

Along the way, we have noted that the Helmholtz-Hodge decomposition leads us naturally to the $\dot{H}^1$ metric we use, which is essentially the Laplacian metric restricted to IDiff($\mathbb{R}^d$). This metric is also quite natural in the sense that it is spatial scale-independent. The Green's function of the Laplacian is given by $K(x, y) = \frac{1}{|x-y|}$. Clearly then, any scaling of the domain has the simple effect of multiplying this kernel by a constant factor, or equivalently changing the speed of the geodesics. By contrast, the commonly used Sobolev metric $s - \Delta$ has as its Green's function $K(x, y) = e^{-s|x-y|}$. Changing of the spatial scale in this case has the effect of changing the bandwidth and in fact changes the curvature of the space. The Laplacian metric allows phenomena at all scales to influence the image registration. This follows from the recently-developed theory of multiscale image registration [4,10] along with the fact that the Laplacian kernel can be written as an integral of $s - \Delta$ kernels as follows: $\frac{1}{|x-y|} = \int_0^\infty e^{-s|x-y|} ds$.

10   Discussion

We have shown that Brenier's polar decomposition of compactly-supported diffeomorphisms, along with the divergence metric on the irrotational component leads to novel new image registration algorithms. Furthermore, Theorem 1 shows that with this metric, the IDiff($\mathbb{R}^d$) component can be isometrically embedded in the flat vector space $L^2(\mathbb{R}^d)$, a fact that underlies the efficiency of our new algorithms. Even more importantly, it has far reach statistical implications, allowing statistics to be performed in IDiff($\mathbb{R}^d$) without the difficulties that often accompany statistics on curved manifolds. In particular, parallel transport of a vector field $w \in \mathfrak{g}_P$ along a curve in $\psi(t) \in \mathrm{IDiff}(\mathbb{R}^d)$ is path-independent and can be conveniently computed in closed form using only the divergence $h(t) = \mathrm{div}\, w(t)$ and the diffeomorphism at times 0 and 1:[2] $h(1) = h(0)\sqrt{|D\psi^{-1}(1)|/|D\psi^{-1}(0)|}$. Flatness also enables simplification of other intrinsic methods involving the covariant derivative and curvature tensor such as geodesic regression and Jacobi fields, principal geodesic analysis, as well as Riemannian polynomials and splines.

Acknowledgements. The authors thank Xavier Pennec and Marco Lorenzi for discussions about irrotational diffeomorphisms, as well as Peter Michor and Martin Bauer for invaluable discussions on the flatness of diffeomorphism spaces on $\mathbb{R}^1$, all of which occurred primarily at the Workshop on Geometry and Statistics 2012 organized by University of Copenhagen and Aarhus University. This work was supported by NIH grants 5R01EB007688, P41 RR023953 and 5R21HL110059-02.

References

1. Arnol'd, V.I.: Sur la géométrie différentielle des groupes de Lie de dimension infinie et ses applications à l'hydrodynamique des fluides parfaits. Ann. Inst. Fourier 16, 319–361 (1966)
2. Bauer, M., Bruveris, M., Michor, P.W.: The homogeneous Sobolev metric of order one on diffeomorphism groups on the real line. arXiv preprint math-ap/1209.2836 (2012)
3. Brenier, Y.: Polar factorization and monotone rearrangement of vector-valued functions. Communications on Pure and Applied Mathematics 44(4), 375–417 (1991)
4. Bruveris, M., Risser, L., Vialard, F.X.: Mixture of kernels and iterated semi-direct product of diffeomorphism groups. arXiv preprint arXiv:1108.2472 (2011)
5. Fedorov, Y., Jovanović, B.: Integrable nonholonomic geodesic flows on compact Lie groups. arXiv preprint math-ph/0408037, 115–152 (2006)
6. Hinkle, J., Szegedi, M., Wang, B., Salter, B., Joshi, S.: 4D CT image reconstruction with diffeomorphic motion model. Medical Image Analysis 16(6) (2012)
7. Lorenzi, M., Ayache, N., Pennec, X.: Regional flux analysis of longitudinal atrophy in Alzheimer's disease. In: Ayache, N., Delingette, H., Golland, P., Mori, K. (eds.) MICCAI 2012, Part I. LNCS, vol. 7510, pp. 739–746. Springer, Heidelberg (2012)
8. Miller, M.I., Trouvé, A., Younes, L.: Geodesic shooting for computational anatomy. Journal of Mathematical Imaging and Vision 24(2), 209–228 (2006)
9. Piccioni, M., Scarlatti, S., Trouvé, A.: A variational problem arising from speech recognition. SIAM J. Appl. Math. 58(3), 753–771 (1998)
10. Sommer, S., Lauze, F., Nielsen, M., Pennec, X.: Kernel bundle EPDiff: Evolution equations for multi-scale diffeomorphic image registration. In: Bruckstein, A.M., ter Haar Romeny, B.M., Bronstein, A.M., Bronstein, M.M. (eds.) SSVM 2011. LNCS, vol. 6667, pp. 677–688. Springer, Heidelberg (2012)
11. Srivastava, A., Klassen, E., Joshi, S.H., Jermyn, I.H.: Shape analysis of elastic curves in euclidean shapes. IEEE Trans. Pattern Anal. and Machine Intel. 33(7), 1415–1428 (2011)
12. Younes, L., Arrate, F., Miller, M.I.: Evolutions equations in computational anatomy. NeuroImage 45(1), S40–S50 (2009)

---

[2] Due to space limitations, we omit the derivation, which follows from Lemma 1.

Joint Modeling of Imaging and Genetics

Nematollah K. Batmanghelich[1], Adrian V. Dalca[1],
Mert R. Sabuncu[2], and Polina Golland[1] for the ADNI

[1] Computer Science and Artificial Intelligence Laboratory, MIT, Cambridge, MA
[2] Martinos Center for Biomedical Imaging, Charlestown, MA
{kayhan,adalca,msabuncu,polina}@csail.mit.edu

Abstract. We propose a unified Bayesian framework for detecting genetic variants associated with a disease while exploiting image-based features as an intermediate phenotype. Traditionally, imaging genetics methods comprise two separate steps. First, image features are selected based on their relevance to the disease phenotype. Second, a set of genetic variants are identified to explain the selected features. In contrast, our method performs these tasks simultaneously to ultimately assign probabilistic measures of relevance to both genetic and imaging markers. We derive an efficient approximate inference algorithm that handles high dimensionality of imaging genetic data. We evaluate the algorithm on synthetic data and show that it outperforms traditional models. We also illustrate the application of the method on ADNI data.

Keywords: Imaging Genetics, Bayesian Models, Variational Inference, Probabilistic Graphical Model.

1 Introduction

In this paper, we propose a generative probabilistic model for genetic variants associated with a disease using imaging data as an intermediate phenotype. The search for genetic variants that increase the risk of a particular disorder is one of the central challenges in medical research, and has been traditionally performed via genome-wide association studies (GWAS). Such studies examine each genetic marker and its correlation with the incidence of the disease independently of all other genetic markers in the study. However, some variants may have a weak but cumulative effect that cannot be identified by traditional GWAS analysis [12]. Imaging genetics introduces imaging-based biomarkers as a promising intermediate phenotype (i.e., endo-phenotype) between genetic variants and diagnosis. Imaging provides a rich quantitative characterization of disease and promises to aid in identifying genetic variations that are correlated with the clinical variables [1, 17]. Furthermore, multivariate analysis using imaging endo-phenotypes promises to stratify the population in more informative ways than the binary diagnosis. A commonly used approach in imaging genetics is to isolate image-based features affected by the disease, and then identify the relevant genetic markers that explain the observed image variations. In this work, we jointly model image-based phenotypes and clinical indicators to identify genetic variants associated with the disorder.

Imaging genetics presents numerous challenges in clinical studies due to the relatively small number of subjects and extremely high dimensionality of images (hundreds

J.C. Gee et al. (Eds.): IPMI 2013, LNCS 7917, pp. 766–777, 2013.

of thousands of voxels) and genetic data (millions of single nucleotide polymorphisms (SNPs)). To address the problem of high dimensionality and small sample size, earlier algorithms considered only a few imaging candidates (voxels, regions, or other biomarkers) or only a few genetic markers in the analysis [5, 15]. The reduced joint dataset is then analyzed in a univariate testing framework, where each pair of a candidate genetic variant and an imaging biomarker is tested for association via a standard statistical test. Examples include using activation maps of the prefrontal cortex to find SNPs associated with schizophrenia [15], and searching for changes of gray matter volume correlated with the Alzheimer's Disease risk factor APOE gene [5].

More recently, genome-wide voxel-wise analysis has been demonstrated using univariate methods [18]. Unfortunately, massive univariate analysis has several limitations. Due to multiple comparisons, a corrected conservative significance level is selected to limit the false positive rate, but this also dramatically reduces the power of the test. Moreover, the univariate methods are unlikely to identify weaker variants that jointly create an additive effect.

Multivariate techniques aim to overcome shortcomings of univariate analysis [9,20]. A common approach is to use multivariate regression combined with regularization to extract a sparse set of coefficients for correlated genetic variants and image features. For example, low rank representations can be approximated via sparse reduced rank regression (sRRR) [19, 20], Partial Least Squares (PLS) [9] or Canonical Correlation Analysis (CCA) [9]. Unfortunately, these unsupervised methods do not use the subject class label (e.g., diagnosis) directly, and thus the detected genetic markers and image features are not immediately related to the disease of interest. The image features relevant to the disease are identified separately from modeling the relationship between the genetic and imaging data. For example, sRRR has been demonstrated using brain regions pre-selected for Alzheimer's disease (AD) via Linear Discriminant Analysis [19]. In contrast, we model and estimate relevant genetic variants in the context of a particular disease. Our method is applicable to any set of image biomarkers, such as anatomical regions, tissue appearance, or functional measures. We are motivated by applications to the AD and use local measures of atrophy as image features.

Our model includes a common assumption of genetic studies that only a small set of SNPs is associated with any particular disease. This subset of genetic markers induces variation in certain image-based features, and a subset of these measures exhibits changes that are discriminative with respect to the disease phenotype. Therefore, if a brain region is irrelevant to the target disease, it is ignored even if its measures are highly correlated with some genetic variants.

In the remainder of the paper, we define a generative model for the relationship among genetic, imaging and disease measures, derive an efficient inference algorithm to identify relevant brain regions and genetic loci, and demonstrate the method on synthetic data and the ADNI study [13]. We show that our algorithm outperforms standard univariate and regression analysis for genetic variant detection on synthetic data and yields promising results on real data.

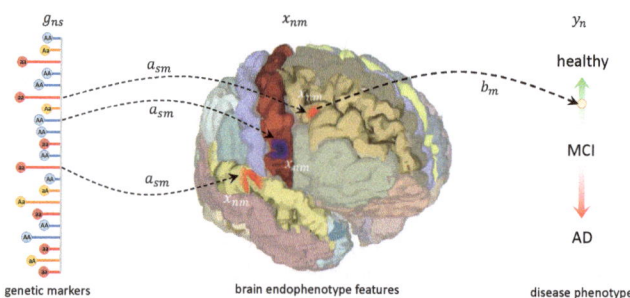

Fig. 1. A schematic illustration of the relationship between genetic, imaging and clinical measures in our model

2   Model

Our model structure is illustrated schematically in Fig.1. We are motivated by anatomical brain studies, but the model is general.

Let y_n be the disease phenotype (0 or 1) for subject n in the study ($1 \leq n \leq N$). Let $\mathbf{x}_n$ and $\mathbf{g}_n$ be vectors of M imaging biomarkers (features) and S genetic markers (SNPs) for subject n, respectively. We capture the overall process via two coupled regression models: a logistic regression predicts class label y_n from image features $\mathbf{x}_n$; a ridge regression associates genetic variants $\mathbf{g}_n$ with image features $\mathbf{x}_n$. The graphical model in Fig.2 presents the relationships among variables of the model. All variables are summarized in Table 1. Below, we first define the relationship between imaging features and the disease phenotype and then specify the generative model for the relationship between SNPs and image features. Note that we do not model a direct link between genetic variants and disease label, but it is captured indirectly through image features.

2.1   From Imaging Features to Disease Phenotype

We adopt a Bayesian model based on logistic regression for predicting binary class label y_n from image features $\mathbf{x}_n$ [2]:

$$p(y_n|\boldsymbol{\eta}, \mathbf{x}_n) = \left[\psi(\boldsymbol{\eta}^T\mathbf{x}_n)\right]^{y_n} \left[1 - \psi(\boldsymbol{\eta}^T\mathbf{x}_n)\right]^{1-y_n}, \qquad (1)$$

where $\psi(a) = \frac{1}{1+e^{-a}}$ is the logistic function and $\boldsymbol{\eta} \in \mathbb{R}^M$ are the regression coefficients that we treat as latent random variables. Similar to prior work [3], we propose to use a *spike-and-slab* prior to promote sparse solutions for the regression coefficients $\boldsymbol{\eta}$ [7,14]:

$$p(\boldsymbol{\eta}; \beta, \sigma_\eta^2) = \prod_{m=1}^{M} \left[(1 - \beta)\delta(\eta_m) + \beta\mathcal{N}(\eta_m; 0, \sigma_\eta^2)\right],$$

where $\delta(\cdot)$ is the Delta Dirac distribution concentrated at 0, parameter β controls sparsity ($0 \leq \beta \leq 1$), and $\mathcal{N}(\cdot; \mu, \sigma^2)$ is a Gaussian distribution with mean μ and variance σ^2. In a deterministic regression context, one can view the spike-and-slab prior

Table 1. Notation and variables used throughout the paper

Model Variables

x_{nm}	Image feature m in subject n.
g_{ns}	Genetic variant s in subject n.
y_n	Disease phenotype (class label) of subject n: 0 - healthy, 1 - diseased.
η_m	Regression coefficient for image feature m in the imaging part of the model.
$b_m \in \{0,1\}$	Indicator variable that selects image feature m.
$a_{sm} \in \{0,1\}$	Indicator variable that selects SNP s for modeling image feature m.
v_{sm}	Regression coefficient for SNP s for modeling feature m.
β	Prior probability for selecting image features.
α	Prior probability for selecting genetic variants.
σ_η^2	Variance of η_m.
σ_0^2	Variance of noise in the genetic to image regression.

Variational Variables

ρ_m	Probability of selecting feature m.
τ_s	Probability of selecting SNP s.
ξ_n	Tightness of lower bound for the logistic function.
ν_m, ς_m	Imaging parameters for feature m.
$\vartheta = \{\mathbf{V}, \boldsymbol{\tau}, \boldsymbol{\rho}, \boldsymbol{\xi}, \boldsymbol{\nu}, \boldsymbol{\varsigma}\}$	Set of variational parameters that we optimize when fitting the model.

as a combination of ℓ_0 and ℓ_2 norms for regularization. We find it convenient to introduce a latent Bernoulli random variable b_m that selects the regime for the regression coefficient η_m:

$$p(b_m) = \beta^{b_m}(1-\beta)^{1-b_m}, \qquad p(\eta_m|b_m; \sigma_\eta^2) = \begin{cases} \delta(\eta_m), & \text{if } b_m = 0, \\ \mathcal{N}(\eta_m; 0, \sigma_\eta), & \text{if } b_m = 1. \end{cases} \quad (2)$$

2.2 From Genetics Variants to Imaging Features

In modeling the relationship between genetics and imaging, we treat image features relevant for disease prediction differently from all other image features. If feature m is relevant for disease prediction (i.e., $b_m = 1$), variations in the values of this feature are explained by a sparse subset of the genetic variants $\mathbf{g}_n \in \mathbb{R}^S$. We define $\mathbf{a}_m \in \{0,1\}^S$ to be a vector of latent Bernoulli random variables that specify a subset, or *mask*, of relevant genetic markers that affect feature m, and arrive at the second regression component of our model:

$$x_{nm} = \sum_{s=1}^{S} (a_{sm} v_{sm}) g_{ns} + \epsilon_{nm} = \langle \mathbf{a}_m \odot \mathbf{v}_m, \mathbf{g}_n \rangle + \epsilon_{nm}, \quad (3)$$

where $\mathbf{v}_m$ is the vector of regression coefficients, $\epsilon_{nm} \sim \mathcal{N}(\cdot; 0, \sigma_0^2)$ is the noise in the image feature m in subject n, and $\langle \cdot, \cdot \rangle$ and $\odot$ denote the inner and element-wise products, respectively. While an obvious modeling choice for regression coefficients $\{v_{sm}\}$ would be to treat them as latent random variables with a spike-and-slab prior, the large number of such variables ($S \times M$) makes it computationally intractable. We therefore model regression coefficients $\{v_{sm}\}$ as unknown but deterministic variables.

If image feature m is irrelevant for predicting disease (i.e., $b_m = 0$), we do not model genetic contributions, and assign the probability mass uniformly between the observed feature values, i.e., $p(x) = \frac{1}{N}\delta(x - x_{nm})$. Furthermore, we set $a_{sm} = 0$ with probability 1 for all s.

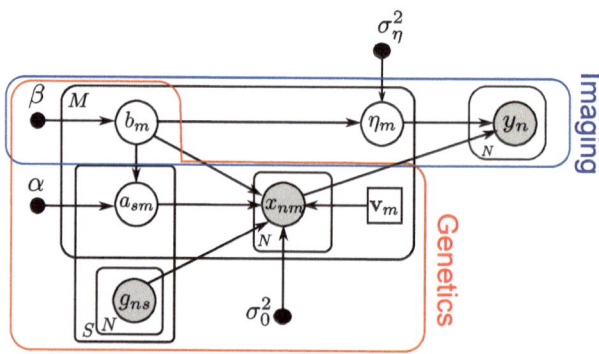

Fig. 2. Graphical representation of the generative model. Hollow circles denote random variables, solid circles represent hyper-parameters, and shaded circles represent observed variables. The rectangle containing $\mathbf{v}_m$ represents deterministic variables to be estimated. The plates indicate conditionally independent instantiations.

Combining the two regimes, we obtain the genetic selection prior:

$$p(a_{sm}|b_m;\alpha) = \begin{cases} \delta(a_{sm}), & \text{if } b_m = 0, \\ \alpha^{a_{sm}}(1-\alpha)^{1-a_{sm}}, & \text{if } b_m = 1, \end{cases} \qquad (4)$$

and the image feature likelihood:

$$p(x_{nm}|b_m,\mathbf{a}_m,\mathbf{g}_n;\mathbf{v}_m,\sigma_0^2) = \begin{cases} 1/N, & \text{if } b_m = 0, \\ \mathcal{N}(x_{nm};\langle \mathbf{a}_m \odot \mathbf{v}_m,\mathbf{g}_n\rangle,\sigma_0^2), & \text{if } b_m = 1. \end{cases} \qquad (5)$$

2.3 Complete Model

We define $\mathcal{Z} = \{\boldsymbol{\eta},\mathbf{b},\mathbf{A}\}$ to be the set of latent variables, $\mathcal{D} = \{\mathbf{X},\mathbf{y}\}$ to be the set of data variables that we model, and $\pi = \{\sigma_\eta^2,\sigma_0^2,\alpha,\beta\}$ to be the set of hyper-parameters. Here $\mathbf{y} = [y_1;...;y_N]$, and $\mathbf{X} = [\mathbf{x}_1;...;\mathbf{x}_N]$. Combining the elements of the model in Eqs. (1)-(5), we construct the joint distribution of the hidden variables $\mathcal{Z}$ and modeled variables $\mathcal{D}$ given genetic markers $\mathbf{G} = [\mathbf{g}_1;...;\mathbf{g}_N]$:

$$p(\mathcal{D},\mathcal{Z}|\mathbf{G};\mathbf{V},\pi) = \prod_{n=1}^{N} p(y_n|\boldsymbol{\eta},\mathbf{x}_n) \prod_{m=1}^{M} p(b_m)p(\eta_m|b_m)p(x_{nm}|b_m,\mathbf{a}_m,\mathbf{g}_n;\mathbf{v}_m) \prod_{s=1}^{S} p(a_{sm}|b_m).$$

3   Inference

Our goal is to compute the posterior probability $p(\mathcal{Z}|\mathcal{D};\mathbf{G},\mathbf{V},\pi)$ of the latent variables that summarizes genetic and imaging influences in our model. Because of coupling of variables in the joint model, computing the posterior distribution is intractable, necessitating approximation via sampling or variational methods. Due to the amount of data and its dimensionality, sampling is computationally impractical. We therefore derive a Variational Bayes approximation [2] that estimates the lower bound for the log-likelihood $p(\mathcal{D}; \mathbf{G}, \pi)$ and seeks distribution q that minimizes the cost functional:

$$F(q) = \int q(\mathcal{Z}) \ln \frac{p(\mathcal{D}, \mathcal{Z}|\mathbf{G}; \mathbf{V}, \pi)}{q(\mathcal{Z})} d\mathcal{Z}. \tag{6}$$

The optimal distribution q provides an approximation to the posterior distribution $p(\mathcal{Z}|\mathcal{D}; \mathbf{G}, \pi)$ [2]. We choose a factorization for the distribution q that captures most model assumptions and yet is computationally tractable:

$$q(\boldsymbol{\eta}, \mathbf{b}, \mathbf{A}) = \prod_{m=1}^{M} q(b_m) q(\eta_m|b_m) \prod_{s=1}^{S} q(a_{ms}|b_m), \tag{7}$$

where:

$$q(b_m) = \rho_m^{b_m} (1 - \rho_m)^{1-b_m}, \qquad q(\eta_m|b_m) = \begin{cases} \delta(\eta_m), & \text{if } b_m = 0, \\ \mathcal{N}(\eta_m; \nu_m, \varsigma_m), & \text{if } b_m = 1, \end{cases}$$

$$q(a_{sm}|b_m) = \begin{cases} \delta(a_{sm}), & \text{if } b_m = 0, \\ \tau_s^{a_{sm}} (1 - \tau_s)^{1-a_{sm}}, & \text{if } b_m = 1. \end{cases} \tag{8}$$

Variational parameters $\rho_m, \nu_m, \varsigma_m$ and τ_s of the approximating distribution q define the optimization space. In this formulation, the estimate of τ_s is interpreted as relevance of the genetic variant s. The estimate of ρ_m provides a measure of relevance for image feature m. We define $\{\boldsymbol{\tau}, \boldsymbol{\rho}, \boldsymbol{\nu}, \boldsymbol{\varsigma}\}$ to be the set of all parameters $\tau_s, \rho_m, \nu_m, \varsigma_m$.

Given the parametrization above, all terms in the cost function $F(q)$ can be optimized analytically, except for the logistic regression term $p(y_n|\boldsymbol{\eta}, \mathbf{x}_n)$. For this term, we employ the variational treatment [8] that leads to improved accuracy over Laplace approximation [2] and has been successfully used in prior work [3]. Specifically, we replace the logistic function with its lower bound:

$$\psi(x_n) \geq \psi(\xi_n) \exp\left\{ \frac{1}{2}(x_n - \xi_n) + \frac{1}{2\xi_n}(\psi(\xi_n) - \frac{1}{2})(x_n^2 - \xi_n^2) \right\}, \tag{9}$$

where ξ_n controls the tightness of the lower bound for subject n and should be optimized.

We define $\vartheta = \{\mathbf{V}, \boldsymbol{\tau}, \boldsymbol{\rho}, \boldsymbol{\nu}, \boldsymbol{\varsigma}, \boldsymbol{\xi}\}$ to be the full set of parameters of distribution q, where $\mathbf{V}$ and $\boldsymbol{\xi}$ are deterministic parameters of the model, and the rest are parameters of q. Using Eqs. (7)-(9), we can maximize $F(q) = F(\vartheta)$ by updating elements of the variational parameter vector ϑ. We omit the derivations due to space constraints, but summarize the resulting updates in Appendix A.

Every update iteration reduces the cost function $F(\vartheta)$, which in turn brings q closer to the posterior distribution $p(\mathcal{Z}|\mathcal{D}, \mathbf{G}; \mathbf{V}, \pi)$.

Our imaging genetics regression bears resemblance to previously demonstrated sRRR regression [20] that considers $\mathbf{X} = \mathbf{GV}$. Our update for $\mathbf{V}$ can be viewed as a solution of a system of linear equations:

$$\mathbf{X} = \left(\mathbf{G} + (\mathbf{G}^{\mathbf{T}})^{\dagger} diag\left(\frac{1 - \boldsymbol{\tau}}{\boldsymbol{\tau}} \right) \right) \mathbf{V},$$

where † indicates a pseudo-inverse, and the second term $diag(\frac{1-\tau}{\tau})$ weighs the SNPs based on their importance. We do not impose rank or sparsity constraints on the regression coefficients matrix $\mathbf{V}$, although they can be added in a fashion similar to [20].

4   Results

We evaluate our model on synthetic data using univariate tests and the sRRR method [20] as baseline algorithms. We also illustrate our method on the ADNI dataset, where we recover several top SNPs associated with the risk of AD.

4.1   Synthetic Data

We generate synthetic data to match a realistic scenario as much as possible. In this section, minor allele frequency (MAF) refers to the frequency of the less common allele in the population at a particular genetic location. A genetic marker (or SNP) g_{ns} is represented by the count of minor alleles at location s in subject n, i.e., $g_{ns} \in \{0, 1, 2\}$. We employ the widely used population genetics software package PLINK [16] to simulate 1,020 SNPs with a minor allele frequency uniformly sampled from an interval [0.05, 0.95], for 400 healthy subjects and 400 patients. For SNPs relevant to the disease, the heterozygote odds ratio is defined as the ratio of patients to controls with $g_{ns} = 1$, normalized by the same ratio for $g_{ns} = 0$. Similarly, one can define the homozygote odds ratio. These ratios control the disease risk in the patient population. The simulated SNPs are split into three sets:

- Set $\mathcal{G}_1$ includes 20 disease causative SNPs that affect selected areas of simulated images. The odds ratio is set to 1.125 for heterozygote SNPs, with a multiplicative homozygote risk. Other odds ratios yield similar results (we tested 1.0625 to 1.5, not shown due to space constraints).
- Set $\mathcal{G}_2$ includes 20 SNPs that are *irrelevant* to the disease (i.e., odds ratio is 1) but affect other areas in simulated images.
- Set $\mathcal{G}_3$ includes 980 *null* SNPs that are independent of both label and images.

Based on the class labels and the genetic variants, we generate image voxels, organized in several sets:

- Voxels in set $\mathcal{I}_1$ are affected by causative SNPs ($\mathcal{G}_1$), and thus are indirectly associated with the disease. These voxels are separated into three regions. Voxel intensity in this set is correlated with genetics:

$$c_{nk}^r = \mathbf{w}_r^T \mathbf{g}_n^{\mathcal{G}_1} + \epsilon_{nk}^r, \qquad 1 \le r \le 3, \tag{10}$$

where c_{nk}^r is the intensity value of voxel k in region r for subject n. The region weights $\mathbf{w}_r$ are drawn from a normal distribution $\mathcal{N}(\cdot; 0, 1)$, and ϵ_{kn}^r is Gaussian noise. Our experiments explore a range of values for the noise variance σ_{noise}^2.
- Voxels in set $\mathcal{I}_2$ are determined by non-causative SNPs $\mathcal{G}_2$, and thus are irrelevant to disease. We dedicate one region to this category:

$$c_{nk}^4 = \mathbf{w}_4^T \mathbf{g}_n^{\mathcal{G}_2} + \epsilon_{nk}^4. \tag{11}$$

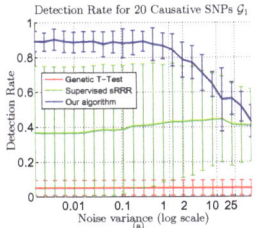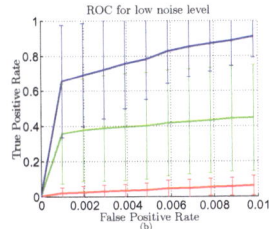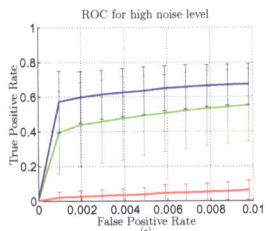

Fig. 3. Summary of results. (a) Detection rates for our algorithm (blue), the supervised sRRR pipeline (green), and the genetic t-test (red) as a function of image noise for causative SNPs in $\mathcal{G}_1$ at a false positive rate of 1%. (b,c) ROC curves for low ($\sigma^2_{noise} = 1.2$) and high ($\sigma^2_{noise} = 21.4$) noise levels are shown up to the selected false positive threshold of 1%.

- Voxels in set $\mathcal{I}_3$ are related to the disease but are not related to genetic markers, and are therefore not helpful in causative SNP detection. In fact, such features confuse the detector as they get selected as relevant to disease at the cost of features in $\mathcal{I}_1$. We generate these voxels as follows:

$$c^5_{kn} \sim \begin{cases} \mathcal{N}(0.5, 1), & \text{if } y_n = 1, \\ \mathcal{N}(-0.5, 1), & \text{if } y_n = 0. \end{cases}$$

- Voxels in set $\mathcal{I}_4$ are not relevant to either label or genetic markers. These voxels are sampled from $\mathcal{N}(0, \sigma^2_{noise})$.

We use the synthetic data to evaluate detection of disease causative SNPs with our method. We observe that our algorithm is not sensitive to the hyper-parameters, which we set as follows: $\log \frac{\beta}{1-\beta} = -1$, $\log \frac{\alpha}{1-\alpha} = -3$, $\sigma^2_\eta = 1$, and σ^2_0 to the variance of image features. As a first baseline, we perform univariate Bonferroni corrected t-tests directly between SNPs and class labels, omitting imaging. As a second baseline, which we refer to as *supervised sRRR*, we perform univariate voxel filtering using class labels, followed by sRRR multivariate regression between surviving voxels and genetic variants to recover relevant SNPs [20]. We compare the methods in different image noise regimes by varying the variance σ^2_{noise} in Eqs (10)- (11), and run 50 different independent simulations for each noise regime.

Fig.3(a) reports detection rates (TP) of disease causative SNPs in $\mathcal{G}_1$. To set the detection thresholds we fix the false positive rate to 1%. We observed similar behavior for a broad range of low false positive rates (not shown). We focus our experiments on low false positive rates because at higher rates false detections become comparable with, and ultimately overwhelm true detections. We find that for a given false positive rate, our algorithm detects significantly more disease causative SNPs in $\mathcal{G}_1$ than the baseline algorithms, and has lower standard deviation than the supervised sRRR pipeline. The direct univariate t-tests only detect SNPs that have a very strong independent association with disease label. To illustrate the behavior of the methods at different false positive rates, we report the receiver operating characteristic at two different noise levels in Fig.3(b,c). Our approach achieves a better detection than the baseline methods.

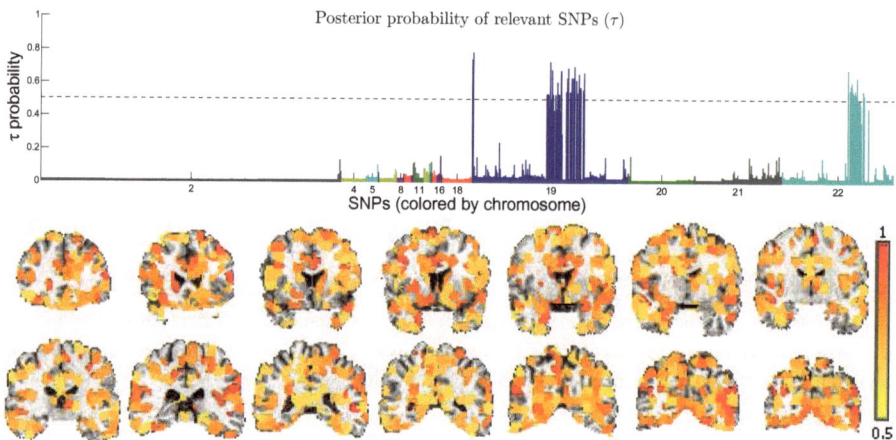

Fig. 4. Results on ADNI dataset. Top: Posterior probability τ_s (colored by chromosome), with 41 SNPs passing a $\tau = 0.5$ threshold. Bottom: Image features ($\rho_m > 0.6$) overlayed on a template MR image, with color intensities proportional to values of ρ.

4.2 ADNI Dataset

We apply our method on a subset of the Alzheimers Disease Neuroimaging Initiative (ADNI) dataset that includes T1-weighted MR images and 620,000 genetic variants for 228 AD patients and 187 normal controls (NC). All images were pre-processed and non-rigidly aligned to a common [4]. We compute the tissue density map, indicating expansion or contraction of gray matter using the determinant of the Jacobian of the deformation field. The map values in the template space are proportional to the volume of structures in the original brain scan. To reduce image dimensionality, we aggregate voxels into *supervoxels* using spatial $k-$means clustering [11] and obtain about 1700 supervoxels. We define our image features x_{nm} as the average value of the tissue density map in a supervoxel. We use a SVM classifier to asses the discriminative power of the resultant features and obtain 86% classification rate of AD versus NC, close to the state-of-the-art results [4]. We used the ENIGMA protocol to pre-process the genotype data[1]. Briefly, PLINK was used to eliminate SNPs on the basis of standard quality control criteria, e.g., low MAF (< 0.01), poor genotype calling (call rate $< 95\%$) and deviations from Hardy–Weinberg equilibrium ($P < 1 \times 10^6$). We then performed imputation using the Mach software[2]. Finally, we pre-selected 960 SNPs that have the strongest association with AD overlapped with SNPs reported in a prior AD-GWAS study involving over 16,000 individuals [6].

We ran our algorithm with 10 initializations, and selected the run that achieved the lowest value of the cost function. As before, we set: $\log \frac{\beta}{1-\beta} = -1$, $\log \frac{\alpha}{1-\alpha} = -3$ and $\sigma_\eta^2 = 1$. We set $\sigma_0^2 = \omega \cdot \sigma_x^2$, where we sweep $\omega \in [0.1, 0.9]$ and σ_x^2 is the variance of image features. Fig.4 illustrates the posterior probabilities of SNP relevance τ, averaged

---

[1] http://enigma.loni.ucla.edu/protocols/genetics-protocols/
[2] http://www.sph.umich.edu/csg/abecasis/MaCH/index.html

Table 2. Summary of selected SNPs with the highest posterior probability τ_s

rank	τ_s	SNP (Gene)	chr	rank	τ_s	SNP (Gene)	chr
1	0.78	APOE-ϵ4	19	6	0.68	rs6857 (PVRL2)	19
2	0.74	APOE-ϵ3	19	7	0.68	rs75843224	22
3	0.73	rs283812 (PVRL2)	19	8	0.67	rs59007384 (TOMM40)	19
4	0.70	rs5117 (APOC1)	19	9	0.66	rs66626994 (APOC1P1)	19
5	0.69	rs75627662	19	10	0.65	rs12721051 (APOC1)	19

over the swept parameters. We list the top SNPs in Table 2. The top variants are APOE-ϵ4 and APOE-ϵ3, which are strongly correlated with AD [6]. We also detect variants on APOC1, TOMM40 and PVRL among our top hits, all of which are on chromosome 19 and have been frequently reported [6]. Similarly, several chromosome 22 variants are identified [10]. Fig.4 illustrates the average posterior probability of feature relevance ρ. Among high probability regions are hippocampus and temporal lobe, which have been frequently reported to undergo significant shrinkage in AD [4], and are associated with memory.

5   Conclusion

We proposed and demonstrated a unified framework for identifying genetic variants and image-based features associated with the disease. We capture the associations between imaging and disease phenotype simultaneously with the correlation from genetic variants and image features in a probabilistic model. We derive an algorithm that iteratively refines the relevant variants using disease phenotype and imaging features. It also isolates representative features that are discriminative with respect to the disease and are modulated by the genetic variants. We demonstrated the benefit of simultaneously performing these two tasks in simulations and in a context of a real clinical study.

Acknowledgements. This work was supported by NIH NIBIB NAMIC U54-EB005149, NIH NCRR NAC P41-RR13218 and NIH NIBIB NAC P41-EB-015902, NIH K25 NIBIB 1K25EB013649-01, AHAF pilot research grant in Alzheimer's disease A2012333, NSERC CGS-D and Barbara J. Weedon Fellowship.

References

1. Batmanghelich, N.K., Taskar, B., Davatzikos, C.: Generative-discriminative basis learning for medical imaging. IEEE Trans. Med. Imaging 31(1), 51–69 (2012)
2. Bishop, C.M.: Pattern recognition and machine learning. Springer, New York (2006)
3. Carbonetto, P., Stephens, M.: Scalable Variational Inference for Bayesian Variable Selection in Regression, and its Accuracy in Genetic Association Studies. Bayesian Analysis 7, 73–108 (2012)
4. Fan, Y., Batmanghelich, N., Clark, C.M., Davatzikos, C., ADNI: Spatial patterns of brain atrophy in MCI patients, identified via high-dimensional pattern classification, predict subsequent cognitive decline. Neuroimage 39(4), 1731–1743 (2008)

5. Filippini, N., Rao, A., Wetten, S., Gibson, R.A., et al.: Anatomically-distinct genetic associations of APOE epsilon4 allele load with regional cortical atrophy in Alzheimer's disease. Neuroimage 44(3), 724–728 (2009)
6. Harold, D., Abraham, R., Hollingworth, P., Sims, R., et al.: Genome-wide association study identifies variants at clu and picalm associated with Alzheimer's disease. Nat. Genet. 41(10), 1088–1093 (2009)
7. Hernandez-Laborto, J.M., Hernandezi-Lobato, D.: Convergent Expectation Propagation in Linear Models with Spike-and-Slab Priors (December 2011)
8. Jaakkola, T.S., Jordan, M.I.: Bayesian Paramater Estimation via Variational Methods. Statistics and Computing (10), 25–37 (2000)
9. Le Floch, E., Guillemot, V., Frouin, V., Pinel, P., et al.: Significant correlation between a set of genetic polymorphisms and a functional brain network revealed by feature selection and sparse Partial Least Squares. Neuroimage 63(1), 11–24 (2012)
10. Lee, J.H., Cheng, R., Graff-Radford, N., Foroud, T., et al.: Analyses of the national institute on aging late-onset Alzheimer's disease family study: implication of additional loci. Archives of Neurology 65(11), 1518 (2008)
11. Lucchi, A., Smith, K., Achanta, R., Knott, G., Fua, P.: Supervoxel-based segmentation of mitochondria in em image stacks with learned shape features. IEEE Trans. Med. Imaging 31(2), 474–486 (2012)
12. Lvovs, D., Favorova, O.O., Favorov, A.V.: A polygenic approach to the study of polygenic diseases. Acta Naturae 4(3), 59 (2012)
13. Mueller, S.G., Weiner, M.W., Thal, L.J., Petersen, R.C., et al.: The Alzheimer's disease neuroimaging initiative. Neuroimaging Clinics of North America 15(4), 869 (2005)
14. O'Hara, R.B., Sillanpää, M.J.: A Review of Bayesian Variable Selection Methods: What, How and Which. Bayesian Analisis 4(1), 85–118 (2009)
15. Potkin, S.G., Turner, J.A., Guffanti, G., Lakatos, A., et al.: A genome-wide association study of schizophrenia using brain activation as a quantitative phenotype. Schizophr. Bull. 35(1), 96–108 (2009)
16. Purcell, S., Neale, B., Todd-Brown, K., Thomas, L., et al.: PLINK: a tool set for whole-genome association and population-based linkage analyses. Am. J. Hum. Genet. 81(3), 559–575 (2007)
17. Sabuncu, M.R., Van Leemput, K.: The Relevance Voxel Machine (RVoxM): A Bayesian Method for Image-Based Prediction. In: Fichtinger, G., Martel, A., Peters, T. (eds.) MICCAI 2011, Part III. LNCS, vol. 6893, pp. 99–106. Springer, Heidelberg (2011)
18. Stein, J.L., Hua, X., Lee, S., Ho, A.J., et al.: Voxelwise genome-wide association study (vGWAS). Neuroimage 53(3), 1160–1174 (2010)
19. Vounou, M., Janousova, E., Wolz, R., Stein, J.L., et al.: Sparse reduced-rank regression detects genetic associations with voxel-wise longitudinal phenotypes in Alzheimer's disease. Neuroimage 60(1), 700–716 (2012)
20. Vounou, M., Nichols, T.E., Montana, G., ADNI: Discovering genetic associations with high-dimensional neuroimaging phenotypes: A sparse reduced-rank regression approach. Neuroimage 53(3), 1147–1159 (2010)

Appendix A

We define $\mathbf{X} \in \mathbb{R}^{N \times M}$ to be a matrix of all image features (each row is a subject), $\mathcal{J}(x,y) := (1-x)\log(\frac{1-x}{1-y}) + x\log(\frac{x}{y})$, and use $diag(\cdot)$ to transforms a vector into a diagonal square matrix or the diagonal of a square matrix into a vector. $\mathcal{E}_m = \langle \cdot \rangle_{q|b_m=1}$

denotes expectation with respect to q conditioned on $b_m = 1$ of the genetics-to-image regression. We define $\mathbf{Q} = \mathbf{G}^T\mathbf{G}$, and $\mathbf{D} = diag(diag(\mathbf{Q}) \odot \frac{1-\tau}{\tau})$.

Parameters of the genetic part of the model are updated as follows:

$$\mathcal{E}_m := \sum_n \langle x_{nm} - \mathbf{g}_n^T(\mathbf{v}_m \odot \mathbf{a}_m)\rangle_{q|b_m=1} = \qquad (12a)$$

$$(\mathbf{x}^m)^T\mathbf{x}^m + \mathbf{v}_m^T(\mathbf{Q} \odot (\boldsymbol{\tau}\boldsymbol{\tau}^T - diag(\boldsymbol{\tau}^2 - \boldsymbol{\tau})))\mathbf{v}_m - 2(\mathbf{x}^m)^T\mathbf{G}diag(\boldsymbol{\tau})\mathbf{v}_m,$$

$$\mathbf{v}_m = diag(\boldsymbol{\tau})\mathbf{D}^{-1}\mathbf{G}^T[\mathbf{U}_O((I + \Sigma_O)^{-1})\mathbf{U}_O^T]\mathbf{x}^m, \qquad (12b)$$

$$\log\frac{1-\tau_s}{\tau_s} = \log\frac{1-\beta_s}{\beta_s} + \frac{2}{\sum_m \rho_m}\sum_{m=1}^M \frac{\rho_m}{2\sigma_0}\frac{\partial\mathcal{E}_m}{\partial\tau_s}. \qquad (12c)$$

$\mathbf{U}_O\Sigma_O\mathbf{U}_O^T$ is the Singular Value Decomposition of $\mathbf{GD}^{-1}\mathbf{G}^T$, whose complexity $\mathcal{O}(N^3)$ is not expensive for a modest number of subjects N. $\mathbf{x}^m$ denotes column m of matrix $\mathbf{X}$. In Eq.(12c), the posterior log-odds ratio is updated by adding the prior log-odd ratio and a weighted sum of the derivatives of the regression error terms for all m with respect to τ_s. Moreover, we obtain

$$\xi_n^2 = \mathbf{x}_n^T(diag(\boldsymbol{\nu}^2 + \boldsymbol{\varsigma}^2))\mathbf{x}_n, \qquad (13a)$$

$$1/(\varsigma_m)^2 = (\mathbf{X}^T\mathbf{X})_{mm} + 1/\sigma_\mu^2, \qquad (13b)$$

$$\nu_m = (\varsigma_m)^2((\mathbf{X}^T\hat{y})_m - \sum_{j\neq m}(\mathbf{X}^T\mathbf{X})_{jm}\rho_j\nu_j), \qquad (13c)$$

$$\log\frac{1-\rho_m}{\rho_m} = \log\frac{1-\alpha}{\alpha} + \log\frac{\sigma_\mu}{\varsigma_m} + \sum_{s=1}^S \mathcal{J}(\tau_s,\beta_s) - \frac{1}{2}(\frac{\nu_m}{\varsigma_m})^2 + \frac{\mathcal{E}_m}{2\sigma_0^2} + \log\sigma_0. \quad (13d)$$

Eq.(13b)-(13c) update the mean and standard deviations of the normal distributions in the approximate posterior. Eq.(13d) updates posterior probability of the relevance of region m.

Author Index